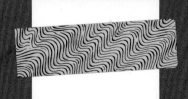

PATIENT TRANSPORT
PRINCIPLES & PRACTICE

FIFTH EDITION

PATIENT TRANSPORT

PRINCIPLES & PRACTICE

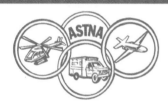

AIR & SURFACE TRANSPORT NURSES ASSOCIATION

Edited by

Reneé Semonin Holleran, FNP-BC, PhD, CEN, CCRN (emeritus),CFRN and CTRN (retired), FAEN
Former Chief Flight Nurse
University Air Care
Cincinatti, Ohio
Former Manager
Adult Transport Services
Intermountain Life Flight
Salt Lake City, Utah

Allen C. Wolfe, Jr., MSN, CNS, APRN, CFRN, CCRN, CTRN, CMTE
Director of Clinical Education/Critical Care Clinical Nurse Specialist
Air Methods Corporation
Denver, Colorado

Michael A. Frakes, MSc, APRN, CCNS, CFRN, CNPT, EMTP, FACHE
Director, Clinical Care
Director, Organizational Quality
Boston Med Flight
Boston, Massachusetts

ELSEVIER

ELSEVIER

3251 Riverport Lane
St. Louis, Missouri 63043

PATIENT TRANSPORT: PRINCIPLES & PRACTICE, FIFTH EDITION   ISBN: 978-0-323-40110-4

Copyright © 2018 by Elsevier, Inc. All rights reserved.

Notices

Knowledge and best practice in this field are constantly changing. As new research and experience broaden our understanding, changes in research methods, professional practices, or medical treatment may become necessary.

Practitioners and researchers must always rely on their own experience and knowledge in evaluating and using any information, methods, compounds, or experiments described herein. In using such information or methods they should be mindful of their own safety and the safety of others, including parties for whom they have a professional responsibility.

With respect to any drug or pharmaceutical products identified, readers are advised to check the most current information provided (i) on procedures featured or (ii) by the manufacturer of each product to be administered, to verify the recommended dose or formula, the method and duration of administration, and contraindications. It is the responsibility of practitioners, relying on their own experience and knowledge of their patients, to make diagnoses, to determine dosages and the best treatment for each individual patient, and to take all appropriate safety precautions.

To the fullest extent of the law, neither the Publisher nor the authors, contributors, or editors, assume any liability for any injury and/or damage to persons or property as a matter of products liability, negligence or otherwise, or from any use or operation of any methods, products, instructions, or ideas contained in the material herein.

Previous editions copyrighted 2010, 2003, 1996, and 1991.

Library of Congress Catalonging-in-Publication Data

Names: Holleran, Reneé Semonin, editor. | Wolfe, Allen C., Jr., editor. |
 Frakes, Michael A., editor. | Air & Surface Transport Nurses Association
 (U.S.)
Title: Patient transport : principles & practice / Air & Surface Transport
 Nurses Association ; edited by Reneé Semonin Holleran, Allen C. Wolfe,
 Jr., Michael A. Frakes.
Other titles: ASTNA patient transport.
Description: Fifth edition. | St. Louis, Missouri : Elsevier, [2018] |
 Preceded by ASTNA patient transport / Air and Surface Transport Nurses
 Association ; edited by Reneé Semonin Holleran. 4th ed. c2010. | Includes
 bibliographical references and index.
Identifiers: LCCN 2017027351 | ISBN 9780323401104 (paperback : alk. paper)
Subjects: | MESH: Emergency Nursing | Air Ambulances | Transportation of
 Patients | Emergency Medical Services
Classification: LCC RC1097 | NLM WY 154.2 | DDC 362.18/8--dc23 LC record available at
 https://lccn.loc.gov/2017027351

Senior Content Strategist: Sandy Clark
Senior Content Development Manager: Laurie Gower
Associate Content Development Specialist: Elizabeth Kilgore
Publishing Services Manager: Jeffrey Patterson
Book Production Specialist: Carol O'Connell
Design Direction: Patrick Ferguson

Last digit is the print number: 9   8   7   6   5   4   3   2   1

 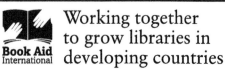

Working together
to grow libraries in
developing countries

www.elsevier.com • www.bookaid.org

Contributors

Anthony Baca, MBA, MSN, APRN, ACNP, LP, CCRN, CFRN
Clinical Manager
PHI Air Medical, Texas/California Division
Acute Care Nurse Practitioner
Medical Center of Plano
Emergency & Critical Care
Plano, Texas

Eric Bauer, MBA, FP-C, CCP-C, C-NPT
Clinical Education Manager
Air Methods Corporation
Clinical Services
Aurora, Colorado
CEO–Founder
FlightBridgeED, LLC
Scottsville, Kentucky

Stefan Becker
Head of Corporate Development
Member of Management
Swiss Air-Ambulance Ltd
Rega-Center
Zurich, Switzerland

Tammy Bleak, BSN, MBA, RN, C-NPT
Manager/Flight Nurse
Intermountain Life Flight, Children's Services
Salt Lake City, Utah

Molly Bondurant, RN, BSN, CFRN, CMTE
Chief Flight Nurse
Dartmouth Hitchcock Medical Center, DHART
Lebanon, New Hampshire

Jason Cohen, DO, FACEP, FCCM
Chief Medical Officer
Boston MedFlight
Bedford, Massachusetts
Faculty
Brigham and Women's Hospital, Departments
    of Emergency Medicine and Surgery
Boston, Massachusetts

Patricia Corbett, RN, BSN, CPHRM, CMTE
Director of Clinical Risk Management and Compliance
Air Methods Corporation, Clinical Services
Englewood, Colorado

Kelly Edwards, NRP, FP-C, MPA
Flight Paramedic, Air Methods
Valdosta, Georgia
Past President, International Association of Flight and
    Critical Care Paramedics
Snellville, Georgia

Jan L. Eichel, RN, BA, CFRN, EMT-P
Director of Clinical and Communications Operations
West Michigan AirCare
Kalamazoo, Michigan
Associate Executive Director, CAMTS
Anderson, South Carolina

Tonya Elliott, MSN, RN, CCTC, CHFN
Program Development Specialist
MedStar Heart and Vascular Institute
Washington, DC

Vahé Ender, NRP, FP-C, C-NPT
Critical Care Transport Paramedic
Boston MedFlight
Bedford, Massachusetts

Cheryl Erler, DNP, CNE, RN
Director, Doctor of Nursing Practice Program
School of Nursing
Purdue University
West Lafayette, Indiana

Kathleen Flarity, DNP, PhD, CEN, CFRN, FAEN
Research Nurse Scientist
UCHealth, Aurora, Colorado
Colonel, United States Air Force
Assistant Clinical Professional
School of Medicine, Department of Emergency Medicine
University of Colorado
Aurora, Colorado

Eileen Frazer, RN, CMTE
Executive Director, CAMTS
Anderson, South Carolina

Luke Gasowski, BS, BSRT, RRT-ACCS-NPS, FP-C, CCP-C, NRP
Critical Care Flight Paramedic Respiratory Therapist–Clinical Base Supervisor
Air Methods, LifeNet of New York
Syracuse, New York

Clyde Gentry, RN, CFRN, EMT-A
Flight Nurse Specialist
Metro Life Flight
Metro Health Medical Center
Cleveland, Ohio

Michael D. Gooch, DNP, ACNP-BC, FNP-BC, ENP-C, CFRN, CTRN, CEN, TCRN, NREMT-P
Flight Nurse
Vanderbilt University Medical Center–Life Flight
Instructor in Nursing
Vanderbilt University School of Nursing
Nashville, Tennessee
Emergency Nurse Practitioner
TeamHealth
Columbia, Tennessee
Faculty
Middle Tennessee School of Anesthesia
Madison, Tennessee

Cindy Goodrich, RN, MS, CCRN
Clinical Educator and Flight Nurse
Airlift Northwest
Seattle, Washington

Robert L. Grabowski, MSN, RN, CNP, AGACNP-BC, CPNP-AC, CEN, CCRN, CFRN, EMT-P
Acute Care Nurse Practitioner
Metro Life Flight
MetroHealth Medical Center
Cleveland, Ohio

Teresa Greenwood, RN, CEN, CFRN
Flight Nurse
AirMethods
San Tan Valley, Arizona

Jonathan D. Gryniuk, FP-C, CCP-C, NRP, RRT, CMTE
CAMTS Representative/Past President
International Association of Flight and Critical Care Paramedics
Snellville, Georgia
Regional Safety Director
Air Methods Corporation
Corporate Safety
Englewood, Colorado

Michel Hall, BA, RN, BSN, CFRN, MHRD/OD
Flight Nurse/Education Coordinator
LifeFlight Eagle
Kansas City, Missouri

Krista Haugen, RN (BSN), MN, CEN
Director, Patient Safety & Medical Risk Management
Med-Trans Corporation
Lewisville, Texas

Timothy L. Hudson, PhD, RN, FACHE
U.S. Army

Fred Jeffries, FP-C, MTSP-C
Clinical Team Educator/Flight Paramedic
Boston MedFlight
Boston, Massachusetts

Jonathan Johnson, BSN, RN, NRP, CFRN, CMTE
Trauma Clinician
Trauma Services Department
Children's Healthcare of Atlanta
Atlanta, Georgia

Tina Johnson, BSN, CFRN, CPEN, CEN, CMTE
Assistant Manager
Children's Healthcare of Atlanta, Critical Care Transport
Atlanta, Georgia

Mark Larson, MBA, BSN, BA, EMPT-P
Flight Paramedic
LifeStar of Kansas
Topeka, Kansas
Emergency Room Nurse
Olathe Medical Center, ECC
Olathe, Kansas

Leslie S. Lewis, DNP, APRN, CPNP-AC, CCRN, C-NPT, CPEN, CPN, EMT-LP, FP-C, CCP-C
Acute Care Nurse Practitioner/Neonatal Pediatric Transport
Medical City Children's Hospital
CHSU, PICU, Transport
Dallas, Texas

Kyle Madigan, MSN, CMTE, CFRN, CTRN, CEN, CCRN
Director
Dartmouth Hitchcock Advanced Response Team (DHART)
Dartmouth Hitchcock Medical Center
Lebanon, New Hampshire

Heather McLellan, MEd, BN, RN, CFRN, CEN
Associate Professor
Mount Royal University
School of Nursing and Midwifery
Registered Nurse
Foothills Medical Centre
Emergency Department
Calgary, Alberta
Canada

David J. Olvera, NRP, FP-C, CMTE
Clinical Education Manager
Air Methods Corporation, Aurora
Clinical Services
Aurora, Colorado

Christopher T. Paige, FNP-BC, CFRN, CEN, NREMT-P
United States Air Force Nurse Corps

Chad Poggemeyer, RRT, NPS, NRP, F-PC
Flight Paramedic
Star Care
Crete, Nebraska
Respiratory Therapist
Nebraska Heart Hospital, Respiratory Care
Lincoln, Nebraska

Carol Rhoades, RN, MSN
Nurse Director
Intermountain Medical Center, Intermountain Life Flight
Salt Lake City, Utah

James Rutherford, MSN, RN, ACNP-BC, CFRN, EMT-B
Flight/Acute Care Nurse Practitioner
MetroHealth, Cleveland Metro Life Flight
Cleveland, Ohio

Kevin Schitoskey, RN, MSN, CFRN, TCRN, CMTE
Regional Director of Strategic Operations
Med-Trans Corporation
Bend, Oregon

Clayton Smith, CFC
Supervisor CQI, Training
PHI Air Medical, Communications
Phoenix, Arizona

Charles Swearingen, BS
Clinical Education Manager
Air Methods Corporation, Clinicial Services
President
Meducation Specialists, LLC
Denver, Colorado

Leslie C. Sweet, RN, BSN
Manager, Medical Communication and Education
Medical Affairs
HeartWare International, Inc
Framingham, Massachusetts

Denise Treadwell, CRNP, MSN, CFRN, CEN, CMTE
President
AirMed International, LLC
Birmingham, Alabama

Cathleen Vandenbraak, BSN, MBA/MHA, CEN, CCRN, CFRN
Nurse Clinical Education Coordinator
Thomas Jefferson University Hospital, JeffSTAT
Philadelphia, Pennsylvania
Nursing Supervisor
Paoli Hospital, Nursing Administration
Paoli, Pennsylvania

Kathryn Wade, RN, MSN, CFRN, CEN, CLNC
Flight Nurse
Air Methods Corporation
Sahuarita, Arizona

Reviewers

David Alexander, MD, MC, CFC, FAAEP
Flight Surgeon
Operational Flight Medicine
NASA
Houston, Texas

Aaron E. Bell, MSN, ACNP-BC, CFRN, RN, EMT-B
Critical Care Transport RN
Boston MedFlight
Bedford, Massachusetts

Laura M. Criddle, PhD, ACNS-BC, CEN, CPEN, CFRN, TCRN, NR-P, FP-C, CCP-C, FAEN
Clinical Nurse Specialist, Trauma Care After Resuscitation Programs
Scappoose, Oregon

Jan L. Eichel, RN, BA, CFRN, EMT-P
Director of Clinical and Communications Operations
West Michigan AirCare
Kalamazoo, Michigan
Associate Executive Director, CAMTS
Anderson, South Carolina

Arnold W Facklam III, MSN, FNP-BC, FHM
Nurse Practitioner
Lee Physician's Group, Critical Care
Lee Memorial Hospital
Fort Myers, Florida
Nurse Practitioner
Cape Coral Hospital, Critical Care
Cape Coral, Florida

Malisa C. Frakes, BSN, RNC-NIC
Neonatal Intensive Care Unit
University of Massachusetts Memorial Medical Center
Worcester, Massachusetts

Steven D. Glow, MSN, FNP, RN, Paramedic
Associate Clinical Professor
Montana State University
College of Nursing
Missoula, Montana

Jennifer Griffin, RRT, RCP, EMT-B
Wake Forest Baptist Medical Center
Department of Respiratory Care
Winston-Salem, North Carolina

Michel Hall, BA, RN, BSN, CFRN, MHRD/OD
Flight Nurse/Education Coordinator
LifeFlight Eagle
Kansas City, Missouri

Kevin High, RN, MPH, MHPE, CEN, CFRN, EMT
Trauma Resuscitation Manager
Senior Associate in Emergency Medicine
Department of Emergency Medicine/Emergency Services
Clinical Associate/Vanderbilt LifeFlight
Vanderbilt Medical Center
Nashville, Tennessee

Ray Hummel, MSN, RN, ACNP, CEN, CFRN
Flight Nurse
Mercy Air–California

Jill Johnson, DNP, APRN, FNP-BC, CCRN, CEN, CFRN, APRN
Chamberlain College of Nursing
Department of Emergency Education
Lexington, Kentucky

Kent Johnson, ATP, BS
Chief Pilot
Intermountain Healthcare
Life Flight
Salt Lake City, Utah

Dawn Johnston, RN, BSN, MBA, CFRN, NREMT-P
Flight Nurse
Marketing Coordinator
West Michigan AirCare
Kalamazoo, Michigan

Scott Jordan, BSN, RN, CCRN
Clinical Nurse Manager
Formerly MedSTAR Transport
Washington Hospital Center
Washington, DC

James Pace
Lead Pilot
University Air Care and Mobile Care
Cincinnati, Ohio

Kenneth J. Panciocco, Jr., EMT, CFC, CMTE
Director of Communications
Boston MedFlight
Bedford, Massachusetts

Tamara (Tammy) Rush, MSN, RN, C-NPT, EMT
Registered Nurse, Pediatric Trauma
Brenner Children's Hospital
Winston-Salem, North Carolina

Joseph Peter Santiago, RN, BSN, MBA, CEN, CFRN, EMT-P, CMTE
Registered Professional Nurse, Practice Operations
Albany Medical Center
Albany, New York

Sam Schaab, RN, BSN, CFRN, EMT
Director of Clinical Operations
LifeFlight of Maine
Central Maine Medical Center
Lewiston, Maine

Dennis S. Schmidt, RN, BSN, NRAEMT, MTSP-C
Flight Nurse, Safety Officer
University of Cincinnati Medical Center, Air Care
 & Mobile Care
Cincinnati, Ohio

Wade Scoles, RRT-NPS, EMT
Clinical Simulation Lab Coordinator
Providence Sacred Heart Medical Center
Spokane, Washington

Stephanie Steiner, MSN, ACNP-C, CPNP-AC, CFRN
Acute Care Nurse Practitioner
Cleveland Clinic, Critical Care Transport Services
Case Western Reserve University, School of Nursing
Cleveland, Ohio

Jacqueline C. Stocking, RN, PhD(c), MSN, MBA, NEA-BC, CMTE, CEN, CFRN, FP-C, CCP-C, NREMT-P
University of California Davis Health System
Internal Medicine
Sacramento, California

Capt. Andrew S. Warburton, RN, BSN, CCRN, NREMT
Flight Nurse
Cleveland Clinic, Critical Care Transport Services
Cleveland, Ohio
Nurse Corps Staff Development Officer
190th Fighter Wing, Ohio Air National Guard
Swanton, Ohio

Will White, LTC, BSN, MS
Director, Army Trauma Training Department
US Army, Ryder Trauma Center, Army Trauma
Miami, Florida

Gordon H. Worley, MSN, FNP-C, EMT-P, CFRN, CEN, CPEN, FAWM
Nurse Practitioner
Department of Emergency Medicine
Woodland Healthcare
Woodland, California
Sutter Amador Hospital
Jackson, California

Cheryl Wraa, MSN, RN, FAEN, TCRN
Director, Trauma Care After Resuscitation Programs
Laurelwood Education
Scappoose, Oregon

Preface

The Air & Surface Transport Nurses Association (ASTNA) recognized the need for a comprehensive textbook that provided a foundation for the art and science of transport nursing more than 20 years ago. The first edition of this book was edited by Genell Lee (the "Brown Book"), and the second, third, and fourth editions were edited by Reneé Semonin Holleran. The fourth edition won the American Journal of Nursing *Book of the Year Award in* 2011.

This is the fifth edition of *Patient Transport: Principles & Practice* and the final one Reneé will be editing. Two new editors, Michael A. Frakes and Allen C. Wolfe, Jr., joined this project in 2015. As it has been said by many, "time marches on."

This edition contains updates to previous chapters as well as some new chapters. The book follows as closely as possible the newest edition of the *Critical Care Transport Core Curriculum.* Content has been updated and reviewed. We have also included additional international input since the transport of patients continues to be a worldwide challenge. To help prepare transport nurses for the Certified Flight Registered Nurse (CFRN) and the Certified Transport Registered Nurse (CTRN), a new

Evolve site accompanies this edition with 350 questions. This text is also recommended for preparing for the Certified Flight Paramedic (FP-C) and the Certified Critical Care Paramedic (CCP-C).

Patient transport is a unique, multidisciplinary process. This text has been used for the past 20 years as one of the resources for patient transport all over the world. This edition again demonstrates why.

"You must be the change you want to see in the world" (Mahatma Gandhi). This will continue to be one of the major challenges we all face in today's world. Please use the wisdom of the authors in this book, and we always invite you to share your unique insights with us.

Reneé Semonin Holleran, FNP-BC, PhD, CEN, CCRN (emeritus), CFRN and CTRN (retired), FAEN

Allen C. Wolfe, Jr., MSN, CNS, APRN, CFRN, CCRN, CTRN, CMTE

Michael A. Frakes, MSc, APRN, CCNS, CFRN, CNPT, EMTP, FACHE

Foreword

This marks the fifth edition of a textbook originally intended to serve the needs of the National Flight Nurses Association (NFNA). Just as the transport industry has grown and changed, so have we. Now as the Air & Surface Transport Nurses Association, we have made changes to this textbook to include a variety of different transport modalities. This was done in an effort to address the various challenges nurses face when caring for patients during transport.

We have gone to great lengths to expand on the themes of the original text and update content. As the abilities of critical care transport providers evolve, so must we by offering valuable information to assist in these situations.

The appreciation that ASTNA has for the editors, authors, and reviewers is unmeasurable. Without their commitment to improving patient care and their love of transport medicine, this text would not have become a reality. We offer a heartfelt thank you for their dedication and expertise.

It is what each of you do every day to ensure excellence in patient care and safe returns of our teammates and patients that makes all the difference. Thank you for your dedication!

Brian Solada, RN, CFRN, CMTE
President
Air & Surface Transport Nurses Association (ASTNA)

Acknowledgments

It has been stated that patient transport cannot be done in a vacuum. It requires a dedicated team of professionals to provide competent care focused on a safe transport environment. We all depend on our team members (whether pilots, nurses, paramedics, physicians, respiratory therapists, communication specialists, mechanics, or other personnel) to deliver care to the critically ill or injured patients of all ages, some even before birth. We need the support of each member of our teams to accomplish a safe and successful transport. The information in this book has been expanded to include the roles of all these individuals.

We wish to recognize the hard work of Elizabeth Kilgore and Carol O'Connell in preparing this fifth edition. We also would like to recognize the dedication of Lynne Shindoll, who did not give up on the creation of a fifth edition of this book.

Contents

Section VII   Professional Issues

1

History of Patient Transport

STEFAN BECKER, RENEÉ SEMONIN HOLLERAN, AND KELLY EDWARDS

Introduction

The history of patient transport started when the first injured or sick persons were carried, dragged, or otherwise moved to care providers. During the Middle Ages the first systems began to be established for moving war casualties to care providers. These early methods saw little change until the late 18th century and beyond, when it was recognized that the rapid transport of injured soldiers reduced morbidity and mortality.

After the world wars there had been dramatic changes in patient transport in both military and civilian settings. The usefulness of airplanes, and later helicopters, for patient transport was realized in the 20th century and quickly spread. As these changes in the modality and the proliferation of transport took place, the training of care providers during transport was gaining attention. Patients were increasingly being transported in specialized vehicles with care providers trained beyond the basic requirements of ambulance crews.

Critical care transport is the term used to describe this new level of patient transport service. Critical care patients have an acute, life-threatening medical condition that requires intervention and care typically beyond the scope and capability of advanced life-support care providers. As critical care transport has grown, so have the requirements in education, training, and certification for the care providers.

This chapter will detail the pertinent history of critical care transport and its origins in patient transport. The second part of the chapter will examine the history of the main professions involved and the professional associations that are part of the critical care transport industry.

Origins of Patient Transport

The first documented record of moving injured patients to care providers was in the 11th century during the Crusades. The Knights of St. John treated and transported injured soldiers after learning first-aid techniques from Arab and Greek physicians. The impetus for providing care was likely both altruistic and monetary—any soldier who carried an injured comrade to medical treatment often received a small payment. Regardless, this may be the genesis of the first emergency medical transport and treatment providers. By the 1400s, rudimentary ambulance systems using carts were common for transporting injured soldiers after battle.[1-4]

Serious interest in resuscitation and care began in the 18th century. One of the first organized efforts to establish resuscitation systems started in 1767 in Amsterdam by a group of wealthy men called the Society for the Recovery of Drowned Persons. This group recommended the use of rapid transport of patients to hospitals capable of providing resuscitation care. These early groups were the first to conceive of a civilian patient transport, but little progress was made other than rudimentary stretchers and they were dependent on volunteers.[1-11]

In 1792 French surgeon Dominique Jean Larrey was dismayed by how long injured soldiers would lay on the battlefield before being evacuated for care. Dr. Larrey was convinced that many deaths could be prevented with timely evacuation from the battlefield, including evacuation during the battle. He designed different tow and four-wheeled carts that were more maneuverable for carrying injured soldiers. He called these carts the *ambulance volante* (the flying ambulance).

Larrey's design proved to be very successful for both transporting medical personnel to the battlefield to provide care and transporting injured soldiers from the battlefield to field hospitals. This was the first recorded use of a patient evacuation system to reduce the mortality and morbidity of injured soldiers. Dr. Larrey is credited with creating the first official military medical corps and a system for moving injured soldiers.[1-16]

Although some hospitals in Europe and England had a rudimentary stretcher service, something similar to a civilian ambulance service did not appear in London until 1832. A special carriage for cholera patients was used to transport them to the hospital for care. The *London Times* reported that the use of these carriages allowed the patient to receive definitive care quicker and could even allow for fewer hospitals that were further apart. Despite this initial innovation, patient transport via ambulance did not spread in the United Kingdom until the 1880s with the St. John Ambulance Association and a number of towns adopting ambulance carriages.[1-16]

In the United States American surgeon Jonathan Letterman developed a plan for a medical treatment and evacuation system. This system became the US Ambulance Corps, and it used its own personnel, vehicles, and facilities. Instituted in 1862 at the Battle of Antietam, it was a resounding success and became enshrined in military doctrine. By 1917 the Ambulance Corps had evolved into the US Army Ambulance Service and had grown to include the utilization of trains, automobiles, and steamboats.[1-16]

In 1865 Cincinnati Commercial Hospital started the first hospital-based ambulance service in the United States (Fig. 1.1). By 1869, Bellevue hospital in New York City had established its own ambulance service staffed by hospital physicians. The rapidly increasing call volume for the Bellevue ambulance forced the hospital to begin staffing the ambulances with orderlies or staff with no medical training. As a result, mortality rates increased, and the focus shifted to the rapid transport of the patient to the hospital.[1-16]

By 1899, The Michael Reese Hospital in Chicago received the first motorized ambulance. This new ambulance was capable of an astounding top speed of 25 kilometers per hour (16 miles per hour) and promised a smoother and quicker transport to the hospital. The motorized ambulance was quickly adopted by other hospital ambulance services.[1-16]

In 1905, the first motorized ambulance designed for military use was the Palliser Ambulance, which was named for Captain John Palliser of the Canadian Militia. This unique design featured three wheels (one at the front and two at the rear) and was essentially a modified heavy tractor encased in bulletproof steel sheets. The British followed quickly behind the Canadians in introducing a limited number of automobile ambulances and commissioned several motorized ambulance vans based on a double-decker bus design.[1-16]

By 1909 the first mass-produced automobile-based ambulance designs began to appear. James Cunningham, Son & Company in Rochester, New York, designed the Model 774 automobile ambulance. Their design featured a 32-horsepower engine, electric headlights, pneumatic

tires, room for an attendant, a suspended cot system, and even a large external gong as a warning device. This design was the culmination of the changing ideas of ambulance use for civilians, because ambulance crews had increasingly become centered on a driver and a patient care attendant.[1-16]

Following the world wars (and the Korean War; Fig. 1.2) physicians had become increasingly interested in the quality of care provided to patients during transport. In 1946 the British National Health Services Act required local authorities to provide ambulances "where necessary," and ambulances were gradually adopted throughout the United Kingdom. Initially staffed by volunteers, professionals were introduced gradually. In 1964 British ambulances were restructured to provide care to patients and not just affect transport. This was a result of an earlier horrific rail crash resulting in the death of 112 people with 340 injured, most of whom waited a considerable amount of time to receive care.[12]

Physicians in the rest of the world were similarly concerned with ambulances being able to provide care as well as transport patients. By the 1960s the work of Safar and Elam had demonstrated the benefit of resuscitation techniques (which would become cardiopulmonary resuscitation) outside of the hospital setting. In Ireland in 1966, a mobile coronary care ambulance was introduced that successfully used new pharmaceuticals and devices (such as the defibrillator). Similar advanced ambulances went into service throughout Europe and the United States soon afterward.[1-3]

The publication of the paper "Accidental Death and Disability: The Neglected Disease of Modern Society" by the National Institutes of Health in 1966 had a profound effect on emergency medical services in the United States.[14] This paper pushed for the Department of Transportation to set national standards for ambulances and emergency medical technicians, which was still largely unregulated. In 1969 President Lyndon Johnson's Committee on Highway Traffic Safety recommended the creation of a national certification agency to establish uniform standards for training and examination of personnel active in the delivery of emergency ambulance service. The first paramedic programs started in Miami in 1969, and other cities in the United States quickly followed. By the 1970s the Emergency Medical Service (EMS) started to resemble what it is today.

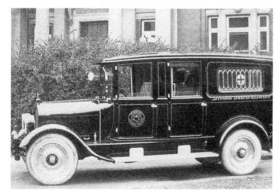

• **Fig. 1.1** Early ambulance dispatched from Cincinnati Hospital to transport patients. (Courtesy University Hospital, Cincinnati, Ohio.)

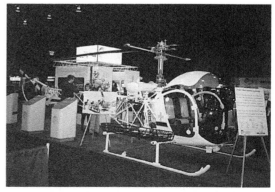

• **Fig. 1.2** Helicopter used to transport patients during the Korean War.

As the requirements and use of ambulances changed, there was the need for a new design. By the 1970s a standard car chassis was unable to carry the weight and meet the performance demands for ambulance use. Ambulance designers and manufacturers turned to van and light truck chassis to solve this problem. The result was the first van-based ambulances followed by truck chassis box-mounted style ambulances. As ambulance use has changed and matured, ambulance design has also evolved to meet the technical, performance, safety, and human ergonomic requirements for emergency medical services.[1-16]

Origins of Air Medical Transport

There is a persistent myth that air transport of patients originated with the Prussian siege of Paris in 1870. This myth likely has its roots in Jules Verne's story *Robur le Conquerant,* published in 1866, which described rescuing shipwrecked sailors by balloon. There is no conclusive primary evidence that any patients were ever evacuated by balloon at the Siege of Paris; it was likely only a proposed plan that never came to fruition. Balloons were used during that battle to carry mail in and out of the city during the siege as well as some important military personnel and civilians, but not significantly injured personnel.[17-19]

In 1890 M. de Mooy, chief of the Dutch Medical Service, began to seriously pursue the concept of transporting injured patients by balloon. He proposed a method of suspending stretchers from balloons that could move patients out of the front line and to field hospitals further away. During this time, it was a radical departure from the traditional means of patient transport and met with resistance from critics. These first experiments in changing the traditional means of patient transport would not become reality until aviation became more established.[17-19]

Fixed-Wing Transport

In December of 1903 the Wright brothers made their famous successful flight in Kill Devil Hills, North Carolina. This event marked the beginning of the new era of machine-powered aircraft flight. More important was the Wright brothers, continued success in developing better planes and showcasing them to the rest of the world at demonstrations in Europe and the United States.[17-21]

Soon medical personnel realized the potential of the airplane. In 1909 Captain George Grosman from the US Army Medical Corps and Lieutenant Albert Rhoades of the Coast Auxiliary Corps designed and constructed a plane to transport patients. The plane design required a physician to be the pilot and to sit next to the patient during the flight. Unfortunately they were unsuccessful, and the plane crashed during the initial test flight. The US government put a halt on the project, but 3 years later it would change its position.[17-21]

This change in position may be attributable to European experiments with airplanes and wounded soldier evacuation. In 1912 Emilie Raymond, a medical doctor and French senator, proposed using airplanes as ambulances for the military. By 1913 the French were pushing for the Geneva Convention to be extended to provide protection for air ambulances (although their efforts were met with scorn at first). French medical officer Gautier famously said that airplanes would "revolutionize war surgery if [it] could be adapted as a means of transport for the wounded."[19-22]

It was in 1915, during World War I, that the first successful aeromedical evacuation occurred. During the Serbian retreat from the Albanian mountains, French Captain Dangelzer and Lieutenant Paulhan evacuated wounded men from Mitrovica to Valona by airplane. Although this spurred more interest in airplane use for patient transport, it was 1917 by the time modifications were made to a Dorand AR II aircraft to make space in the fuselage specifically for patient stretchers. In 1918 two of these modified planes were used to evacuate patients from the Battle of Flanders. These initial successes demonstrated the viability of air medical evacuation.[19-22]

During the International Conference of the Red Cross in 1923, attendees debated the role and use of air ambulances. The result of these debates led to a supplement to the Geneva Convention that provided protection of air medical units from belligerent action. Medical aircraft were prohibited from carrying any armament or photographic equipment, they could not fly over (or even approach) the battle lines, and all air medical units had to have the Red Cross insignia prominently displayed.[19-22]

The French continued to expand on the use of air medical evacuation following World War I. During the smaller conflicts in Morocco and Syria after World War I, they used airplanes to evacuate the wounded. By 1925 the French had established the Medical Air Transport Service. This service not only introduced the concept of flying the wounded, but it also introduced flying surgeons and doctors to the patients. This concept was not as successful because of safety and logistical concerns, and the focus of the Medical Air Transport Service remained on evacuating the wounded back to the medical facilities. By 1929 the French had 43 aircraft assigned to the Medical Air Transport Service.[19-22]

Other countries were far behind the French efforts, and mostly relied on an informal system of volunteers. The British used a system of volunteer aviators operating under the British Red Cross Society. The US Army was modifying de Havilland airplanes to accommodate two patients and a physician. In 1926 the United States made its first successful air medical evacuations in Nicaragua. Other European countries were cautiously following the French and/or British examples in a limited fashion.[23-26]

In 1928 the first civilian air medical airplane service was established in Australia. The Australian Inland Mission sought to provide medical services to people in remote areas of the Australian Outback. Initially they provided clinics or hospitals in remote communities. As they struggled to provide medical personnel for these locations, Lieutenant Clifford Peel suggested using airplanes to fly physicians out to these isolated locations. From that suggestion, the Australian Inland Mission Air Medical Service was finally created in 1928 when enough funds were raised—10 years after Lieutenant Peel's suggestion.[23-26]

The Australian Inland Air Medical Service completed 50 flights in its first year, relying on fund raising and donations for financial support. By 1932 their service had become so successful and popular that there was a push for a network of "flying doctors" across Australia. In 1934 the Australian Aerial Medical Service was formed and created sections across the continent with coverage areas. In 1942 the service was renamed the Flying Doctor Service, and in 1955 the appellation Royal was added.[23-26]

Today the Royal Flying Doctor Service of Australia operates 66 aircraft at 23 locations. They provide transport of health care personnel to remote locations, transport of patients from remote locations, telehealth services, education, and consultation for remote health care providers. The service is still run as a not-for-profit organization and relies on community support for funding.[23-26]

The first civilian air ambulances in the United Kingdom started in 1933 with the evacuation of a patient from the Isle of Islay in Scotland. Eventually the U.K. Department of Health for Scotland sponsored the development of air ambulances for Scotland (which continues to this day as the Scottish Ambulance Service Air Wing). In 1934 the first civilian air ambulance service was established in Africa by French nurse and pilot Marie Marvingt, and by 1957 a group of surgeons would establish the Flying Doctors in Africa. Austin Airways started operating in Canada in 1934, becoming the first North American private air ambulance. Swiss Air-Rescue (REGA) was established in 1952, and not only flies patients in Switzerland but also retrieves Swiss citizens from anywhere in the world.[25]

From its beginnings in wartime, the airplane has played a significant role in patient transport. It has continued to be an important part of the health care system, especially in rural or underserved areas of the world. It has also become a valuable asset in transporting patients to specialty care facilities or repatriating injured or sick citizens back to their home country.

Patient Transport by Helicopter

Leonardo da Vinci was likely the first person to conceive an idea for what could be considered a helicopter. His "aerial screw" design dates back to 1493 and consisted of a platform with a helical screw driven by a rudimentary turning system powered by humans. Although his design was never created, and likely would not have flown as designed, it illustrates that the rotor wing/vertical flight concept has existed for a long time.[17-26]

Contrary to popular misconception, it was French engineer Paul Cornu that designed and built the first rotary wing (helicopter) aircraft to achieve flight. Like the Wright brothers, he was primarily a bicycle manufacturer that tinkered with aviation designs. In 1907 he successfully flew his

twin rotor helicopter for 30 seconds. Although his early work had limited success, it proved the concept of rotor wing flight.[17-26]

In 1909 Russian Engineer Igor Sikorsky returned from Paris (then the center of the aviation world) and began designing rotor wing aircraft. By 1910 Sikorsky had designed a helicopter capable of flight that also overcame the technical problems of controlling the aircraft in flight. By 1912 Sikorsky had designed helicopters able to carry passengers and even developed plans for airplanes with multiple engines. Sikorsky and his significant early contributions have cemented his place as the "father" of the helicopter.[17-26]

German engineer Henrich Focke built on Sikorsky's successful work. In 1936 he created the dual rotor FA-61, which is generally considered to be the first practical and functional helicopter because it could fly at a speed of about 90 kilometers per hour (56 miles per hour) with a 230-km (143-mile) range and ceiling limit of 3427 m (11,243 feet). The conflict in Europe (which would grow to become World War II) spurred Focke to iterate improvements. By 1940 the dual rotor FA 223 Drache ("dragon") became the first helicopter to enter into mass production as World War II threw most of the world into conflict. Although few of the Drache were made, it could reach speeds and altitudes twice that of the FA-61 and carry a significant amount of ordinances.[17-26]

Although Sikorsky was successful in Russia, he immigrated to the United States in 1919 where there was more opportunity and a chance to escape the economic turmoil of Europe. Sikorsky formed the Sikorsky Manufacturing Corporation in 1923. In 1929 he developed the first twin-engine airplane in America, the S-29. The financial success of the S-29 allowed Sikorsky to work on new helicopter designs, leading to the VS-300 design in 1940. The VS-300 used a single main rotor with an antitorque tail rotor, which is the most common configuration of helicopters today.[17-26]

Because of the helicopter's ability to get into smaller areas than airplanes, the US Army quickly realized the potential of Sikorsky's work. It commissioned Sikorsky to develop helicopters for military use, and they were initially used to position special military units in remote areas. In April 1944 the helicopter was first used to evacuate a patient; a US Army Sikorsky YR-4B transported a wounded British soldier from more than 100 miles behind Japanese lines in Burma.[4,11,17-26]

The military focus on helicopters until now was on their role either as combat aircraft or as troop transports. When the United States entered into the Korean War, the helicopter gained a new focus, casualty evacuation. Two weeks after the start of the conflict, Marine Corps pilots used their HMR-161 helicopters to evacuate patients. A special helicopter unit was soon formed with the express purpose of patient evacuation from the front lines to the Mobile Army Surgical Hospitals.[4,11,17-26]

This new unit used the smaller, and unarmed, Bell 47 helicopter that could transport two patients on external patient litters. During the course of the Korean War, over

20,000 medical evacuations by helicopter took place. The combination of rapid transport by helicopter and nearby surgical hospitals greatly reduced the casualty rate, cementing the helicopter as a tool for rapid patient transport (see Fig. 1.2).[4,11,17-26]

In 1958 a California businessman named Bill Mathews decided to organize a civilian air medical service based on the successes of helicopters in Korea. Mathews lived in the small northern city of Etna, California, and partnered with the town physician, Granville Ashcroft, to transport patients. The helicopter was even used to transport medications for the town pharmacist during emergencies. This short-lived service was the first civilian helicopter medical operation in the United States. Meanwhile, REGA had conducted its first use of helicopter rescue in 1952 and fully embraced its use by 1959.[4,11,17-26]

During the Vietnam War, the care and transport of injured personnel continued to expand. During the conflict, over 200,000 injured were evacuated by helicopter to field hospitals and even further. A significant change in this conflict was the use of a much larger helicopter, the Bell UH-1 (often referred to as a Huey). The UH-1 could carry more patients and personnel inside the aircraft, allowing army medics to provide care during the transport. A more comprehensive system had developed, which allowed the injured to be evacuated to field hospitals while receiving care and then often transported to specialty care later by airplane or helicopter.[4,11,17-26]

During the 1960s Europeans as well as Americans had begun to embrace the use of helicopters for civilian medical transport. REGA was setting an example for helicopter use in Europe. They presented their rescue tools (the rescue line and horizontal net) and techniques for helicopters to attendees at their first helicopter symposium in 1966. REGA is believed to be the first civilian helicopter service to routinely use a hoist for rescue operations. When REGA began to exhaust its financial resources in the late 1960s, the Swiss government declined to fund it further. Instead, REGA offered a patronage system to the public: in exchange for a minimum donation, Swiss citizens received free emergency air transport. This system has fundamentally remained unchanged to this day and has been copied or modified by many other air medical services (Fig. 1.3).[4,11,17-26]

The publication of "Accidental Death and Disability: The Neglected Disease of Modern Society" by the National Institutes of Health in 1966 had a profound effect on emergency medical services in the United States. This paper pushed for the Department of Transportation to set the national standards for ambulances and emergency medical technicians, which before this were largely unregulated. In addition to setting the standards for modern emergency medical services, this paper provided an impetus for the growth of civilian air medical services based on the military model.[4,11,14,17-26]

In 1969 the US government implemented two programs to study the effect of medical helicopters on mortality and morbidity rates: Coordinated Accident Rescue Endeavor,

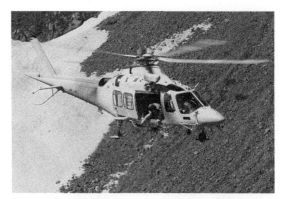

• **Fig. 1.3** Swiss Air-Rescue (Courtesy REGA).

State of Mississippi (Project CARESOM) and the Military Assistance to Safety and Traffic (MAST) in Texas. CARESOM used purchased helicopters located and staffed at three geographically different hospitals, whereas MAST used military helicopters and personnel to augment civilian emergency medical services. Both programs were successful at demonstrating the need for civilian air medical services.[4,11,14,17-26]

Meanwhile, the state of Maryland received a grant to purchase Bell Jet Ranger model helicopters. Maryland purchased four of them and strategically placed them throughout the state for quick response to emergency calls. The helicopters were staffed with a paramedic that was also trained as a law enforcement agent. When the helicopter was not being used for patient transport, it could be (and often was) used for law enforcement activity. The Maryland State Police Aviation Command still functions in this manner today, albeit with much larger aircraft than the Bell Jet Ranger.[4,11,14,17-26]

In Europe, Germany began operating its first civilian medical helicopter in 1970. Christoph 1, named after St. Christopher, was a resounding success. By 2015 Germany had over 75 medical helicopters with a combination of government and nonprofit programs. England was slower to develop its air medical services, outside of the Scottish Ambulance Service Air Wing, and that air medical services funded by charities did not take root until 1980.[4,11,14,17-26]

In 1972 the first hospital-based helicopter medical program was established at Loma Linda Medical Center in California, but financial difficulties ended the program after 6 months. In that same year, St. Anthony's Hospital in Denver started its Flight for Life program with an Alouette III helicopter. Flight for Life is still in operation today, making it the longest-running hospital-based flight program in the United States (Fig. 1.4).[4,6,11,27-30]

The National Highway and Transportation Safety Administration (NHTSA) released a study in 1972 on helicopter use in emergency medical services and transport. NHTSA stated that the use of helicopters was of limited use in urban settings, and a follow-up study in 1981 suggested that air ambulances were not equipped to handle critically ill or injured patients. The criticism led the Federal Aviation Administration to demand better equipment and specially

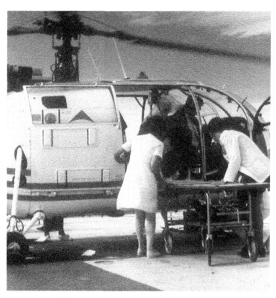

• **Fig. 1.4** Nurses unloading helicopter.

trained crews for air ambulances, and many individual states started to set requirements for air ambulances.[4,6,11,27-30]

In the 1980s hospital-based helicopter air medical programs opened at a rapid pace in the United States. By the late 1980s over 150 programs were in operation, and that number continued to rise. By 2003 the number of air medical helicopters had increased to 540, and by 2015 the number had nearly doubled from 2003. Europe and the rest of the world have seen similar growth in air medical programs, but not at the same pace as the United States.[4,6,11,27-30]

In the Gulf War of 1990 the US military underwent a significant shift in its medical response system. Before the collapse of the Soviet Union, the military focus on casualty evacuation had centered on conflict as part of smaller isolated incidents or a larger conflict in the European continent. By 1991 US personnel were stationed in the Middle East, and the Air Force Medical Service was the only substantial medical presence.[4,6,11,27-30] In 45 days the Air Force had deployed 15 hospitals, and before the offensive operation Desert Storm the Air Force and Army were prepared to evacuate 3600 patients per day from the front line to hospitals by helicopter and 1000 to 2000 per day from these hospitals back to military hospitals in Europe or America. Although the casualty rate never came close to these estimates, it showed the preparation and commitment to air medical evacuation by the military.[4,6,11,27-30,32]

In 1994 there was a marked change in battlefield trauma care standards. The US special operations forces community began to develop and embrace the doctrine that would become tactical combat casualty care. This doctrine and approach focused on preventing battlefield deaths by focusing on the quick stabilization of immediate life-threatening injuries and delaying treatment for injures that were not immediately life-threatening. The doctrine also emphasized the use of "damage control" treatment by using tourniquets

and hemostatic agents instead of more complicated or time-consuming treatments.[4,6,11,27-30,32]

The combined US military operations in the Middle East precipitated by the events of 9/11 built on lessons learned regarding medical evacuation in previous conflicts. The military medical doctrine continued to focus on rapid and aggressive care and transport to definitive surgical care. Helicopters were still used for rapid evacuation of injured personnel to nearby surgical care, followed by later evacuation via airplane to hospitals in Europe or America for long-term treatment. This system, along with new practices and treatments, significantly reduced mortality among injured personnel. Lessons learned by medical personnel have slowly disseminated into civilian medicine, including air medical programs.[4,6,11,27-30,32]

Air Medical Program Models

Although air ambulance programs outside the United States have mostly remained nonprofit/charity or governmental programs, the United States has several different models of operation. Today there are four basic models of air medical programs in the United States. The oldest is the so-called "traditional model," in which hospitals or another health care agency contracts a third-party operator to provide aircraft, pilots, and maintenance, while providing medical personnel and management themselves. These programs have declined recently as other air medical program models have emerged and hospitals look to cut costs (Fig. 1.5).[4,6,11,27-30,32,33]

Next is a "community-based model," in which a company manages the helicopters, personnel, and support separate from a specific local hospital/health care agency. This model can be organized as a for-profit agency or as a nonprofit agency, but the key to the model is that the company running the program is not a governmental agency. Generally this model is very similar to a private ambulance service in which the company bears all of the costs and seeks reimbursement for services from insurance, Medicaid/Medicare, or private payment.[4,6,11,14,27-30,32,33]

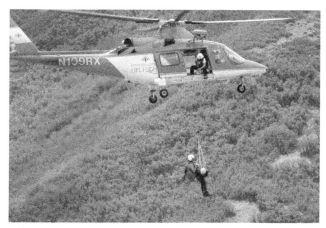

• **Fig. 1.5** Intermountain Life Flight Hoist Rescue Operation. (Photo courtesy Intermountain Life Flight.)

One of the newest models is the so-called "alternative delivery model" or "hybrid model," which is a mix of the traditional and community-based model. In this model, a partnership exists between a health care agency and a private company. The specifics can vary, but the partnership allows both the private company and the health care agency to contribute something to the program. Sometimes this partnership can also be between a private company and a governmental agency to provide air medical services to a specific region or underserved area.[4,6,11,14,27-30,32,33]

The third model of the helicopter EMS (HEMS) is the "government-operated" version, in which governments take direct responsibility for providing air ambulance operations in specific regions. This is the least common of the models in the United States; most of these programs operate as part of a law enforcement agency such as the Maryland State Police Aviation Command.[4,6,11,27-30]

Nursing in Critical Care Transport

Florence Nightingale is generally considered the founder of modern nursing practice. She was one of the first nurses to practice outside the confines of a hospital and was in charge of the Female Nursing Establishment of the English General Hospitals during the Crimean War. Her leadership helped reduce the mortality rate from 47% to less than 3%.[4,6,11,27-30]

In the United States Clara Barton became the symbol of nursing practice. She was committed to providing aid to all patients needing care, regardless of race, creed, or belief. She was an advocate of providing care to patients on the battlefield during the American Civil War, and in 1882 she founded the American Red Cross. Since Nightingale and Barton, nurses have been actively involved in the care of patients at the front lines of conflict and involved in their care during transport.[4,6,11,27-30]

The first flight nurse, and founder of flight nursing, was Marie Marvingt (1875–1963). She was a trained surgical nurse, licensed pilot, and even designed an airplane that was capable of carrying a stretcher. Following World War I, she devoted herself to advocating for air medical evacuation. She gave thousands of seminars and conferences on the subject, and established the first civilian air medical service in Africa in 1934. She also appeared in two documentaries on air ambulances, and in World War II she served as a surgical nurse. In 1955 at age 80, she earned a helicopter pilot license and even flew a supersonic fighter jet. Marie Marvingt remains the most decorated woman in the history of France, and her contribution to air medical transport and flight nursing cannot be overstated (Fig. 1.6).[4,6,11,22,27-30]

American Flight Nursing starts with the Emergency Flight Corps, formed in 1933 by Lauretta M. Schimmoler, who pressured the US military to open a flight nurse training program in 1942 at the 349th Air Evacuation Group. This training program was a 6-week course that included flight physiology and transport considerations for patients. To enter the program, a nurse had to apply and work for 6 months at an Army Air Force Hospital. Once a candidate

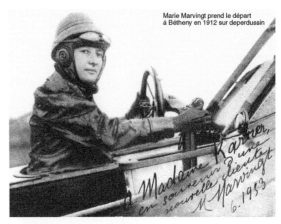

Marie Marvingt prend le départ á Bétheny en 1912 sur deperdussin

• **Fig. 1.6** Marie Marvingt, Reims, 1912. (From Hargrave L. The pioneers: aviation and aeromodeling–interdependent evolutions and histories. www.ctie.monash.edu.au/hargrave/marvingt.html; Accessed June 1, 2008.)

was approved and completed the training program at the 349th Air Evacuation group, a nurse could request the designation "Flight Nurse" from the Commanding General of the Army Air Force. This designation was highly prized because it represented the elite of the nursing corps (Fig. 1.7 and Boxes 1.1 and 1.2).[4,6,11,22,27-30]

During World War II 1.5 million patients had been flown with flight nurses in attendance. By the end of the war 217 nurses had died (or were missing) in the line of duty. Following World War II flight nurse training was conducted by the US Air Force (which had separated from the US Army). Flight nurses were used during the Vietnam and Korean wars,

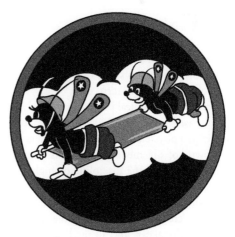

• **Fig. 1.7** Bees insignia. Insignia of the US Army Air Force's School of Air Evacuation was a dark blue disk with two honeybees, whose bodies were or (gold) and sable (black) with argent (white) wings bearing stars, carrying a brown litter, all in front of an argent cloud. Blue and gold are the Air Corps colors. The honeybees, helmeted and wearing Red Cross armbands, are indicative of the industry displayed by the personnel of the organization. The litter is symbolic of evacuation of the sick and wounded, and the cloud is indicative of the area in which the mission is performed. The insignia was designed by Mrs. Don Rider of Buechel, Kentucky, who was greatly impressed by the work of the air evacuation personnel during the flood in Louisville in 1942.

• BOX 1.2   Flight Nurses' Creed

I will summon every resource to prevent the triumph of death over life.

    I will stand guard over the medicines and equipment entrusted to my care and ensure their proper use.

    I will be untiring in the performance of my duties, and I will remember that upon my disposition and spirit will in large measure depend the morale of my patients.

    I will be faithful to my training and to the wisdom handed down to me by those who have gone before me.

    I have taken a nurse's oath reverent in man's mind because of the spirit and work of its creator, Florence Nightingale. She, I remember, was called the "lady with the lamp."

    It is now my privilege to lift this lamp of hope and faith and courage in my profession to heights not known by her in her time, Together with the help of the flight surgeons and surgical technicians, I can set the very skies ablaze with life and promise for the sick, injured and wounded who are my sacred charges.

    ...This I will do, I will not falter, in war or in peace.

David N.W. Grant
Major General, USA
Air Surgeon

---

although their role remained as care providers inside field hospitals or during the transport of a patient from a field hospital to definitive or long-term care.[4,6,11,22,27-30]

The first civilian air medical programs in the United States were hospital-based programs. As a result, they often used a nurse along with a physician as the care providers. The expansion and growth of air medical programs throughout the United States has led to the discipline of flight nursing becoming a specialty type of nursing outside the military. By 1991 the Certified Flight Registered Nurse (CFRN) examination had been created to reflect the role specialization. A large number of critical care and air medical programs worldwide use nurses as part of the care team, and some programs use nurses exclusively (Fig. 1.8).[4,6,11,22,27-30]

Paramedics in Critical Care Transport

The history of the paramedic can be traced back to early ambulance squads that provided aid during World War I. Although these squads provided little more than transportation of the injured, they did possess some basic first-aid

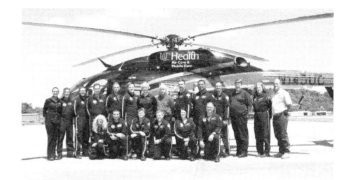

• Fig. 1.8 University Air Care air medical transport crew. (Photo courtesy University Hospital, Cincinnati, Ohio.)

training. In World War II, the military corpsman was a soldier trained to provide battlefield care to a wounded soldier. The corpsman evolved into the field medic, who was capable of providing more advanced care and preparing a patient for helicopter evacuation. During the Vietnam War, the field medics were responsible for providing initial care and care for the injured soldier during the helicopter evacuation to a field hospital.[1-13]

As civilian ambulance services took root and spread, the focus began to shift to the training of the attendants and the care given during transport. By the 1960s ambulance attendants were generally trained and certified to some degree, but there was a noted disparity in the training requirements from country to country, and even within regions of the same country. In the United States the 1966 paper "Accidental Death and Disability: The Neglected Disease of Modern Society" along with President Lyndon Johnson's Committee on Highway Traffic Safety resulted in the standardization of emergency medical technicians and paramedic training programs by the Department of Transportation. The paramedic standards developed by the United States were the framework for paramedic programs throughout the world.[1-14]

In 1975 the paramedic profession gained official recognition as a health care occupation by the American Medical Association. As air medical programs began to emerge worldwide, many countries saw them as an extension of ambulance service and placed paramedics in them. In the United States paramedics were used as part of an air medical program as the number of programs grew and air medical helicopters began providing prehospital care and response.[31-35]

The paramedic profession has grown and evolved as health care needs and the medical transport system has changed. The educational requirements and training for paramedics often includes associate-level or bachelor-level degrees, and specialty disciplines and certifications for paramedics, such as the Certified Flight Paramedic (FP-C) and Critical Care Paramedic (CCP-C), are available. Today most air and critical care transport medical programs worldwide use paramedics as part of the care team, and some countries and programs exclusively use paramedics.[31-35]

Recent Patient Transport History in the 20th and 21st Centuries

As the transport industry continues to grow and expand from its roots, several attempts have been made to describe what patient transport is, what impact it has, and how it might evolve.[36-43]

Several summits and surveys have been conducted and published within the transport environment that especially focus on air medical transport. The primary focus of these has been to identify where the field of patient transport is now and where it should be in the future. Table 1.1 provides a summary of a number of these events and publications including their focus and potential direction for transport safety, patient care, and research.

These issues continue to be important components related to patient transport, whether by air or ground. Associations have developed that address specific parts of the transport industry. The following section contains information about the primary associations involved in patient transport.

Associations

The critical care and air medical industry is home to a multitude of member organizations that advocate for their members, profession, and the industry as a whole. Although this is not an exhaustive list, it covers some of the more significant associations that play a part in critical care or air medical transport.

Association of Air Medical Services

The American Society of Hospital-Based Emergency Air Medical Services, now known as the Association of Air Medical Services (AAMS), was established in 1980 as a nonprofit trade association.[37] Members of AAMS are the companies, associations, and related organizations that have a stake in critical care and medical transport. AAMS seeks to represent and advocate on behalf of their membership to enhance their ability to deliver quality, safe, and effective medical care and medical transportation for every patient in need. An example of AAMS advocacy includes Vision Zero, which focuses on safety in the transport environment, and publication of position papers that support the roles of transport programs in patient care.

Air and Surface Transport Nurses Association

The National Flight Nurses Association (NFNA), now known as the Air and Surface Transport Nurses Association (ASTNA), is a membership association that advocates for nurses involved in patient transport.[38] The NFNA was founded in 1981 by a group of dedicated flight nurses. These nurses *developed* standards of practice including a

TABLE 1.1 Industry Summits and Publications 20th and 21st Centuries

Summit	Focus
1985 Safety Summit	Concern about escalating HEMS accidents focused on pilot fatigue Recommended 12-hour shifts for pilots
2000 Safety Summit	Increase in number of HEMS accidents from 1988 to 2000 Development of AMSAC
1991 AAMS Air Medical Reimbursement Congress	Focused on coverage, reimbursement, billing, and cost-effectiveness
1996 AAMS Air Medical Transport Summit	What objective information existed that described patient transport and what needed to be identified and in what specific areas of transport including: transport of specific patient populations such as neonatal and pediatric patients, economic advantage of helicopter transport, and airway management
2003 Air Medical Leadership Congress: Setting the Health Care Agenda for the Air Medical Community	Focused on safety, medical care, cost/benefit, and regulatory/compliance
A Blueprint for Critical Care Transport Research (2013)	"Go Zone" research ideas Safety Human factors Outcomes Utilization Financial Clinical care issues Education/training
AIRMED World Congress	Has been organized for over 30 years to address international issues related to defining the future of professional aeromedical services

AAMS, Association of Air Medical Services; *AMSAC,* Air Medical Safety Advisory Council; *HEMS,* Helicopter emergency medical services.

safety committee that started the CONCERN Network, which is a communications system developed to relay critical incidents and processes from one program to another.

In addition, the Flight Nurse Advanced Trauma Course was an appointed committee that revised a course focused on advanced trauma care by flight nurses. This course originally was a part of the Advanced Trauma Course from the American College of Surgeons. It is now known as the Transport Nurse Advanced Trauma Course. This course provides knowledge, competencies, and skills for all who provide care in the transport environment.

In 1991 ASTNA partnered with the Board for Certified Emergency Nurses to develop both the CFRN and the Certified Transport Nurse certification examinations.

ASTNA is also responsible for the *Air and Surface Transport: Principles and Practice* text. This is a multidisciplinary, comprehensive text that addresses the principles and practice of patient transport. This text was the dream of a flight nurse named Carol Wickman and brought to fruition by Genell Lee as the text *Flight Nursing Principles and Practice* published in 1991. The fourth edition of the text *Air and Surface Transport Nursing: Principles and Practice* was awarded the *American Journal of Nursing* Book of the Year in 2011.

ASTNA is recognized worldwide as the professional organization for nurses practicing in the critical care transport industry.

International Association of Flight and Critical Care Paramedics

The National Flight Paramedic Association, now known as the International Association of Flight and Critical Care Paramedics (IAFCCP), was founded in 1984 and formally incorporated in 1986.[34,35] Although originally founded as a nonprofit association to represent the interests of flight paramedics, the association has expanded its depth and representation into critical care transport both in the air and on the ground. The IAFCCP is committed to providing education, representation, and advocating for the critical care and flight paramedic profession. Transport safety has remained a paramount concern for the association, and they have partnered with various other industry and governmental organizations in support of transport safety initiatives.

In 1998 founding association board member and past president Tim Hynes was killed in a tragic air medical crash in Utah. Tim's loss reaffirmed the association's commitment to averting future industry tragedies. In 2000 the association's Flight Paramedic of the Year Award was renamed the Tim Hynes Award and annually recognizes an association member for their outstanding contributions in leadership, education, and safety. In 2013 the IAFCCP facilitated the creation of a separate charity named the Tim Hynes Foundation. The foundation's goal is to create opportunities through career development, access to education, and programs to improve leadership abilities that will reinforce and advance medical transport safety. Currently, the foundation provides an annual scholarship to the Safety Management Training Academy.

The IAFCCP has furthered its dedication to transport safety by its continued support and membership with the industry's principal accrediting organization, the Commission on Accreditation of Medical Transport Systems (CAMTS). The IAFCCP was present at the first inaugural meeting of CAMTS in 1990 and has maintained steady representation on their board of directors to maintain a voice in developing and implementing industry standards that impact the role of critical care and flight paramedics. In 2016 the IAFCCP furthered its position as an international advocate for paramedic practice by serving as a founding member organization to the Commission on Accreditation of Medical Transport Systems–Europe (CAMTS-EU), which is based in Zurich, Switzerland.

In 2000 the IAFCCP undertook its most visible step in standardizing the practice of flight paramedicine with the introduction of the FP-C. To maintain the highest level of currency and applicability of the examination, the IAFCCP assisted in the creation of the Board for Critical Care Transport Paramedic Certification (BCCTPC) and turned over control of the examination process to this organization while maintaining representation on their Board of Directors. The BCCTPC subsequently expanded their examination offerings to include the CCP-C examination, which has become the first nationally accepted certification for critical care paramedics. Both the FP-C and CCP-C are currently recognized by CAMTS and have been embraced by the international transport community as well, with the first European offering of the FP-C examination occurring in Germany in 2009. The IAFCCP continues to directly support its membership through the examination process by providing a variety of examination preparatory courses, review texts, and discounts.

The IAFCCP continues to foster positive working relationships with other air medical and EMS industry organizations and has continued its pledge of advocacy by participating in several governmental meetings and lobbying activities. In 2010 the IAFCCP participated in the Federal Interagency Committee of EMS meeting; the 2011 EMS stakeholder's meeting in Washington, DC; and in the 2012 National Association of Emergency Medical Technicians, "EMS on the Hill Day." The association continues as a supporting organization of both the annual Air Medical Transport Conference and the Critical Care Transport Medicine Conference.

Commission on Accreditation of Medical Transport Systems

CAMTS is an independent, nonprofit agency established in 1990 (as Commission for the Accreditation of Air Medical Service [CAAMS]) that audits and accredits fixed-wing and rotary wing air medical transport services as well as ground interfacility transport services in the United States based on a set of industry-established criteria.[39]

The idea of CAMTS came from individuals in the transport environment who were concerned about the number of accidents and lack of standards in the air transport industry. Lead by a flight nurse, Eileen Frazer, who is now the CAMTS Executive Director, representatives from all who are involved in patient transport established standards that encompass the education and training of personnel, the function and safety of transport vehicles, and medical care of ill and injured patients.

CAMTS first enacted its Accreditation Standards in 1991, which were developed by its member organizations as well as with extensive public comment and input. The criterion includes patient care standards, safety standards, and logistical and financial standards. The 10th edition of these standards was published in 2015.

International Association of Medical Transport Communications Specialists

The International Association of Medical Transport Communications Specialists (IAMTCS), formerly known as the National Association of Air Communication Specialists (NAACS), was founded in 1989.[40] IAMTCS is a not-for-profit professional organization whose mission is to provide advocacy in medical patient logistics for operational control air and ground communications specialists. IAMTCS has helped create standards and training tools for communication specialists in critical care and air medical transport with the Certified Flight Communicator certification.

Air Medical Physician Association

The Air Medical Physician Association (AMPA) is an international organization committed to patient-focused, quality critical care transport medicine by promoting excellence in medical direction, research, education, safety, leadership, and collaboration.[41] AMPA published the *Principles and Direction of Air Medical Transport,* which is a comprehensive text that lays the foundation for transport medicine. The second edition of this text, published in 2015, provides additional information and tools to assist medical directors and transport team members in providing safe and competent care in the transport environment. AMPA is the largest worldwide professional organization of physicians dedicated to air medical and critical care ground transport.

National Emergency Medicine Service Pilots Association

The National EMS Pilots Association (NEMPSA) was founded in 1984.[42] NEMSPA is a professional organization dedicated to serving pilots involved in the air medical transport industry and to improving the quality and safety of those services. It has published position papers such as "Night Vision Goggles in Helicopter Emergency Medical Services, Sleep and Fatigue Management," and created online tools for Risk Assessment and Helipad Safety. NESMPA

is recognized worldwide as the professional organization for pilots operating specifically in air medical transport.

Summary

Patient transport has existed since patients required movement for definitive care, originating with the transport of patients from the battlefield to areas of safety.

Transport nursing originated through the work of nursing pioneers, such as Florence Nightingale, Clara Barton, Marie Marvingt, and Lauretta M. Schimmoler, whose theories and work became integral to patient care before and during transport. As the principles of flight and transport care were incorporated into civilian care, hospital-based transport programs were started and staffed by nurses.

Paramedics have been involved in patient transport since the beginning of the 20th century from their origins as battlefield care providers. Their role in critical care transport has continued to expand to critical care paramedics and flight paramedics.

In 1988 the US Department of Transportation published the Air Medical Crew National Standard Curriculum. This publication encompasses basic and advanced curriculum for the education and training of air medical transport teams. In 1990 the CAAMS, now known as CAMTS, began evaluating both helicopter and fixed-wing air medical transport services.

We must be familiar with and take pride in our origins as we forge into the future. Combining the expertise of many professions provides optimum patient care during all modes and phases of the transport process.[43]

Bibliography

1. Air ambulance history. http://www.100yearsofnursing.ca/english/content/SK_19.html; 2016 Accessed 09.07.16.
2. Barkley K. *The Ambulance.* New York, NY: Exposition Press; 1990.
3. Bell R. *The Ambulance: A History.* Jefferson, NC: McFarland & Company; 2009.
4. Blumen I. (Editor in Chief). *Principles and Direction in Air Medical Transport.* 2nd ed. Salt Lake City, UT: Air Medical Physicians Association; 2015.
5. Dick W. Anglo-American vs. Franco-German emergency medical services system. *Prehosp Disaster Med.* 2003;18(1):29-35.
6. Donahue P. *Nursing: The Finest Art.* 2nd ed. St. Louis: Mosby; 1996.
7. Eisenberg M, Pantridge J, Cobb L, et al. The revolution and evolution of cardiac care. *Arch Intern Med.* 1996;12(26):1-15.
8. Browne B, Jacobs L, Pollack C. *Emergency Care and Transportation of the Sick and Injured.* 7th ed. Sudbury, MA: Jones & Bartlett; 1999.
9. Gonsalves D. Historical background of emergency medical services in the United States. *Emerg Care Q.* 1988;4(3):77.
10. Haller J. *Battlefield Medicine: A History of the Military Ambulance from the Napoleonic Wars through World War I.* Carbondale, IL: Southern Illinois University Press; 1992.
11. Holleran RS. *Prehospital Nursing: A Collaborative Approach.* St. Louis, MO: Mosby; 1994.

12. Link MM, Coleman HA. *Medical Support of the Army Air Forces in World War II*. Washington, DC: Society for Military History; 1955.

13. McCall W. *The American Ambulance: 1900-2002*. Hudson, WI: Enthusiast Books; 2002.

14. Division of Medical Sciences, Committee on Trauma and Committee on Shock. *Accidental Death and Disability: The Neglected Disease of Modern Society*. Washington, DC: National Academy of Sciences-National Research Council; 1966.

15. Porter R. *The Greatest Benefit to Mankind: A Medical History of Humanity*. New York: Knopf; 1999.

16. Skandalakis P, et al. To afford the wounded speedy assistance: Dominique Jean Larrey and Napoleon. *World J Surg*. 2006; 30(8):1392-1399.

17. Carter G. The evolution of air transport systems: a pictorial review. *J Emerg Med*. 1986;6(6):499-504.

18. *Helicopter EMS: Part I: A Brief History*. http://www.emsworld. com/article/10319182/helicopter-ems; 2016 Accessed 10.07.16.

19. McNab A. Air medical transport: "hot air" and a French lesson. *J Air Med Trans*. 1992;11(8):15-16.

20. Ortiz J. The Revolutionary Flying Ambulance of Napoleon's Surgeon. *U.S. Army Med Dep J*. 1998;8:17-25.

21. WWII helicopter evacuation. http://olive-drab.com/od_medical_ evac_helio_korea.php; 2016 Accessed 09.07.16.

22. Lam DM. Marie Marvingt and the development of aeromedical evacuation. *Aviat Space Environ Med*. 2003;74(8):863-868.

23. Royal Flying Doctor Service. Our history. https://www. flyingdoctor.org.au/about-the-rfds/history/; 2016 Accessed 09.07.16.

24. History of Queensland Ambulance Service. http://www.ambulance. qld.gov.au/about/; 2016 Accessed 10.07.16.

25. Rega History. https://en.wikipedia.org/wiki/Rega_(air_rescue); 2016 Accessed 09.07.16.

26. State of Mississippi. *Extension of Project CARESOM: Final Report*. Jackson, MI: State Press; 1971.

27. Bader GB, Terhorst M, Heilman P, et al. Characteristics of flight nursing practice. *Air Med J*. 1995;14(4):214-218.

28. Grimes M, Mason J. Evolution of flight nursing and the National Flight Nurses Association. *Air Med J*. 1991;10(11):19-22.

29. Thomas F. The early years of flight nursing. *Hospital Aviation*. 1986;5(10):6-8.

30. Lee G. History of flight nursing. *J Emerg Nurs*. 1987;13(4):212.

31. Wheeler D, Poss W. Pediatric Transport Medicine. In: Wheeler D, Wong H, Shanley T, eds. *Resuscitation and Stabilization of the Critically Ill Child*. London: Springer-Verlag; 2009:125-136.

32. Kuehl A, ed. *Prehospital Systems and Medical Oversight*. 3rd ed. Overland Park, KS: National Association of EMS Physicians; 2000.

33. Jaynes C, Werman H, White L. A blueprint for critical care transport research. *Air Med J*. 2013;32(1):30-35.

34. International Association of Flight and Critical Care Paramedics. http://www.iafccp.org/; 2016 Accessed 09.07.16.

35. International Board of Specialty Certification. http://www. ibscertifications.org/about/about-us; 2016 Accessed 06.08.16.

36. Thomas F, Robinson K, Judge T, et al. The 2003 Air Medical Leadership Congress: findings and recommendations. *Air Med J*. 2004;23(3):20-36.

37. Association of Air Medical Services. http://aams.org/; 2016 Accessed 09.07.16.

38. Air and Surface Transport Association. http://aams.org/; 2016 Accessed 09.07.16.

39. Commission on Accreditation of Medical Transport Systems (CAMTS). http://www.camts.org/; 2016 Accessed 09.07.16.

40. International Association of Medical Transport Communication Specialists. Available at http://www.iamtcs.org; 2017. Accessed 18.01.17.

41. Air Medical Physicians Association. http://www.ampa.org/; 2016 Accessed 09.07.16.

42. National Association of EMS Pilots. http://www.nemspa.org/ index.php; 2016 Accessed 09.07.16.

43. Mattera C, Hutton K, Allenstein T. No box of chocolates. *Air Med J*. 2001;20(5):4-5.

2

Members of the Transport Team

RENEÉ SEMONIN HOLLERAN, DENISE TREADWELL, AND JONATHAN D. GRYNIUK

Patient transport has become a widespread theme in the provision of care for many ill and injured patients, as cited by the National Highway Traffic Safety Administration in the *2006 Guide for Interfacility Patient Transfer*. Interfacility and emergent patient transports have continued to increase in recent years.[1] Transport may be required for a patient to receive emergent lifesaving care from the prehospital setting or a technological advancement not available at a referring facility. Critical care transport is a collaborative practice and process. The scope and mission of the transport program, types of patients transported, and regulations of state nursing boards and emergency medical services (EMS) authorities contribute to transport team configurations. In the United States transport teams are composed of a registered nurse (RN) and a paramedic.[2] In other parts of the world the team may be composed of a physician or a "rescue man." It is most important that the members of the transport team reflect the level of care needed by the patient. The transport program must be able to safely and competently provide the level of care described in their mission statement and scope of care.

A team approach to patient transport is paramount. The goals of a transport team are to maintain or enhance the level of care from the referring facility or agency and render interventions as appropriate. This chapter provides an overview of some of the members of the transport team.

Transport Team Members (Air and Surface)

With advances in medical care came the need to maintain the care for increasingly complex cases that required a critical care–like setting during transport. The role of the transport professional has evolved over time to include individuals from all disciplines. Crew pairing may involve professionals with similar training and experience or differing skill sets and education. Both configurations have demonstrated benefits in consideration of the patient demographic, scope of practice, mode of transport, and accepted or recognized clinician practice.

The flight paramedic has played a pivotal role in the development of air medical transport. Transport professionals require education, training, experience, and continuous evaluation of competence. Transport providers must be physically and emotionally ready to meet the demands of patient care during transport. Although some general characteristics do exist among these professionals, the specific responsibilities and practice protocols depend on the type of service provided, the crew matrix, the type of vehicles used for transport, and state regulations.[3]

In 1970, the Maryland State Police instituted the first statewide EMS helicopter service. This multifaceted air transport, air rescue, and police program was staffed by emergency medical technician-paramedics/police officers (trooper paramedic) and has remained in continuous operation to this day.[4] In 1998, the Emergency Nurses Association and the National Flight Nurses Association (now known as the Air and Surface Transport Nurses Association [ASTNA]) released a joint position paper that described the role of nursing in the prehospital environment.[5] This document denotes that nurses who practice in the prehospital care environment need to be appropriately educated to function successfully in that role. It further recommends that nurses who practice must be regulated by the state boards of nursing in the state(s) in which the transport nurse practices in place of EMS agencies governing nursing practice. The different training and expertise of nurses, paramedics, respiratory therapists (RTs), and physicians compliments the transport team, providing focused care for patients requiring transport. The evolution to air rescue has required those professionals that routinely practice within the confines of the hospital to leave that setting and learn the nuances of providing care in the out-of-hospital arena. Simultaneously, specialized skills that were once reserved for the hospital setting have found their way into the paramedic scope of practice.[6,7]

ASTNA acknowledges that staffing with the most appropriate health care provider reduces the risk of poor patient outcomes. State boards of nursing, local EMS regulations, and even some national EMS and physicians' associations have provided input into the practice of transport professionals. Clinical staffing models configured based on the level of care required by the patient during the transport have been routinely accepted within the transport industry; however, no consistent nexuses recognized beyond state and local regulations exist today.

The Commission on Accreditation of Medical Transport Services (CAMTS) has defined the levels of care required based on the scope of care to include basic life support (BLS), advanced life support (ALS), emergency critical care, and specialty care. The expertise of the health care professional should include established tenure within the area of expertise and age-specific life-support and advance trauma training. The health care professional should also demonstrate a merit of knowledge specific to the scope of care with the successful completion of industry-specific advanced certifications.[8]

Both ASTNA and the International Association of Flight and Critical Care Paramedics Association have developed position papers that address some of the issues identified with the nurse practicing outside the hospital and paramedic providing critical care beyond the routine care provided by the field paramedic. The customary hospital-specific orientation or prehospital training does not include the knowledge and skills needed to deliver patient care in the transport setting.[5,9,13]

Although nurse paramedic team configurations are the predominant dynamic, respiratory care practitioners (RCPs) are also often valued members of the critical care transport teams. RCPs typically work in hospitals, in which they perform assessments, diagnostics, intensive critical care procedures, and patient interventions for all patient populations, from the neonate to the geriatric.[10]

Respiratory care requires education in physics (gas laws), biology, pharmacology, chemistry, and microbiology. An RT possesses specific skill sets to perform multiple clinical interventions valued in the out-of-hospital critical care setting. For example, RTs are often trained in arterial line and chest tube insertion; intubation; surgical airways; medication administration (inhalation and parenteral); and managing high-technology medical equipment such as mechanical ventilation, intraaortic balloon pump, and pulmonary artery catheter monitoring.[10]

The American Association of Respiratory Care has a section for surface and air transport members that provides specific information about the roles of a transport RT. Like the other members of the transport them, the qualifications, education, and training for transport RTs are based on the scope of practice of the transport program and the program for which they may work. This training should include safety, survival, and operating within individual transport vehicles.[10]

Invasive hemodynamic monitoring, administration of blood products, initiation and titration of vasoactive and sedative medications, and analysis of a variety of laboratory data through portable devices has become an integral part of medical transport. It is not uncommon to have varying patient populations including adult cardiac patients with an intraaortic balloon pump or a left ventricular assist device to the preterm infant undergoing extracorporeal membrane oxygenation requiring the expertise of the transport professional. The pairing of different disciplines or supplementing a standing team with a specialty care provider allows for team diversity to meet the needs of today's transport patients.[11]

Physicians

Physicians may contribute to the care provided by the team directly or indirectly: directly, as a member of the critical care transport team, and indirectly through the provision of medical direction or clinical oversight responsible for all aspects of care provided, or as a liaison with specialty care physicians. The level of expertise of transport physicians may range from that of resident physician to that of an experienced board-certified physician specialist.

In programs in which physicians are not used as transport team members, control of medical direction of the transport team is often provided by assigning a physician responsible for the actions of the transport team. This medical control physician has the responsibility of overseeing that the correct team (e.g., adult, pediatric, neonatal), appropriate team configuration (e.g., RN/paramedic, RN/RN, RN/RT, specialty care team), equipment (e.g., ALS, BLS, specialized), and mode of transport (e.g., helicopter, fixed-wing, ground) are selected to meet the patient's transport medical needs and that appropriate medical backup is available to the nonphysician transport team.

The Medical Director, as cited by Air Medical Physician Association (AMPA) "Medical Direction and Medical Control of Air Medical Services" position paper, must be authorized to practice; actively involved in the care of critically ill and injured patients specific to the program's defined mission set; and experienced and knowledgeable in transport medical service appropriate to the program's scope of care.[12,13] The medical director must possess qualifications appropriate to ensure the quality of medical care provided.

Physician Medical Director

The primary responsibility of the physician medical director is to provide administrative medical oversight and medical quality management and improvement over the transport program. Specifically, the physician medical director's role includes but is not limited to (1) helping develop, review, and approve medical protocols or guidelines; (2) provide oversight of medical crew member training; (3) provide oversight of medical control physicians; (4) provide quality improvement oversight for the medical care rendered by the transport service; (5) provide support for medical team members; and (6) assist in the clarification and resolution of transport issues that may arise during the transport or from the referring or receiving agency.

The educational and experiential qualifications of an individual medical director are dictated by the mission profile of the relevant service. For patients who need specialty transports, medical direction may remain with the program medical director. Specialty trained physicians (i.e., neonatologist, pediatric, adult critical care–trained) may be consulted or the responsibility to provide medical control or oversight for specific cases may be delegated to that individual.[12,13]

The CAMTS standards provide educational and clinical recommendations for physicians involved in critical care transport. Moreover, AMPA offers robust resources for medical directors in their course, Medical Director Core Curriculum and in the textbook *Principles and Direction of Air Medical Transport.*[5,10-12,14,15]

Identify Medical Protocols For the transport service that does not routinely use physicians as transport team members, the medical director is responsible for identifying, reviewing, and approving medical protocols or guidelines that enable the transport team to initiate care treatments and procedures considered outside the routine practice of their individual disciplines. Although the transport medical physician director may not directly write these protocols, the transport medical physician is ultimately responsible for the content and accuracy of these protocols. Team members, in conjunction with the medical director, develop and revise policies, protocols, or guidelines that guide medical care.

Ensure Adequate Training The medical director is actively involved in the development of training that ensures that the transport team members can meet the expected level of medical care related to the transport environment. Prospective training occurs through introduction courses to emergency and critical care transport. Such training includes altitude physiology, transport medical care, and advanced procedures (i.e., difficult airway management, chest tube insertion, arterial line insertion, central line insertion, management, etc.). In addition to the initial training, the medical director is actively involved in continuous training and updating of the transport team members regarding new innovations in patient care. The use of items identified in quality improvement retrospective reviews of transport care via run/chart review provides feedback for reinforcing or modifying care delivered by the transport team members.

Oversight of Medical Control Physicians One role of the medical director is to ensure that physicians who provide medical control are educated to the mission and capabilities of the transport service. Clinical discrepancy between medical control and medical flight team members can arise. Under these circumstances, the medical director clarifies the recommended standard of practice for the transport service to both parties. Likewise, control physicians can determine whether additional training may be necessary for selected team members. Contacting the medical director regarding these training issues ensures that proper steps can be taken by the medical director to reduce medical mishaps.

During the transport, the control physician serves as the sounding board and provides medical support to the transport team members. This support may be done before transport so the physician can provide the transport team members with information regarding the patient's status and with possible diagnostic or therapeutic suggestions. This support can also be provided during the transport, when the transport team recognizes that additional medical input may be beneficial in diagnosing or providing care to the patient.

After the transport, the transport team may discuss the possible diagnostic and therapeutic options related to the patient's condition. Such interactions are beneficial because the transport team members gain additional insight and the medical director recognizes any need for additional transport team training.

Continuous Quality Improvement One of the most important roles of the medical director is to provide quality improvement of the medical care provided by the medical team. Carrubba noted[12] that the medical director is specifically responsible for the following:

- Empowerment of flight crew members to identify quality improvement issues and to develop appropriate strategies to study these issues
- Recognition of pertinent quality assurance/continuous quality improvement (CQI) expertise both within and outside the program
- Internal collaboration with institutional quality management coordinators to link the air medical quality management plan to the organizational quality management program
- Contribution of time, knowledge, and action to all aspects of quality management in the program
- Vigorous support for the acquisition of necessary resources and executive-level commitment for all quality management activities.

Resolving Conflict That Arises during the Transport Conflict can arise among transport team members, particularly when a nurse, paramedic, or RT and a physician disagree about patient treatment, but also may occur with the referring or receiving physician. Most often such conflict is a result of a difference in perspectives. When such conflicts occur, the team member and the physician should work together to resolve the issue. Physicians must attempt to understand transport team members' concerns related to the delivery of patient care. Likewise, the transport team member must recognize that the physician may have a different perspective of the issue related to patient treatment. The best patient care results from a collaborative effort between the team member and the physician. Medical directors can serve as a go-between to resolve these conflicts.

Communication Specialists

Communication is the first step in the transport process. The National Association of Air Medical Communication Specialists has developed a description of the role of the communication specialist in the transport process. In addition operational control is an integral component of communications and the transport process, which ensures that the operator who holds the aircraft-operating certificate issued by the Federal Aviation Administration (FAA) is fully aware and involved in each movement of the aircraft throughout the transport. More components of the role of the communication specialist, particularly specific functions, are discussed in Chapter 6.

The communication specialist is responsible for obtaining patient information; initiating the operational control process for the transport; the tracking of the transport (air or ground); and notification of appropriate personnel before, during, and after the transport process. The transport team must always remember that the communication specialist is the "voice" of the transport team and should be treated as a team member and included in decision making and stress management.

Pilots

Clinical team and pilot interactions play a critical role in the performance of air medical teams. Team-level and organizational factors may enhance or impede the ability of well-trained individuals to work together effectively and efficiently. Each team member's position must be clearly stated and defined, which establishes structure and determines the flow of communication.

The National EMS Pilots Association is dedicated to pilots involved in patient transport and focused on improving the quality and safety of air medical transport.

Pilot-in-Command Qualifications

The FAA mandates that the pilot-in-command (PIC) is responsible for the safety of the aircraft, crew, and passengers as stated in the Federal Aviation Regulations, Part 91. The pilot is accountable for nonmedical aspects of the flight and has final authority in all flight-related issues. CAMTS outlines the PIC qualifications for both rotorcraft-helicopter and fixed-wing aircraft.[16,17]

The PIC must help maintain a balanced predictable environment while responding to changing situations. This responsibility implies that shifts of balance occur and that each crew member should understand that they have the responsibility to participate fully and professionally in every flight.

The PIC must establish clear leadership and command authority and appropriately apply the use of authority based on the current situation. He or she will ensure the safety of the flight through strict adherence to the Federal Aviation Regulations as well as the general operations manual of their employer, which may be an air operator company rather than the transport program itself. The pilot must command respect but at the same time create an atmosphere conducive to crew participation.

Transport team members assist in flight-related duties as outlined by the individual program or vendor's policies or general operations manual and as reinforced by the PIC. Flight team members offer assistance in a variety of flight duties. Some of their contributions include air or ground traffic sightings, hazard and obstacle sightings, obstacle avoidance procedures (landing zones), cargo (medical equipment) securing, passenger briefing, radio monitoring, and minor participation in the computation of weight and balance requirements.

When time and safety permit, the pilot may also assist the flight team by helping load and unload patients. In addition, the pilot can transport needed medical equipment to the flight team and relay medical information to the receiving hospital.

To optimize program safety, an expectation of safety must override all other considerations. The adage "all to go, one for no" reflects the expectation that any member of the transport team can turn down a flight for safety concerns, and a program's safety environment must support such decision making. Although an administrative request for justification is reasonable, unjust consequences toward pilots or other transport team members should not exist for turn-downs/flight aborts. Team members should feel safe to prioritize decision making on the basis of established safety practices, program minimums, and previous flight experience.

The bond between established team members and the air medical staff could become quite strong. The eight goals for a successful relationship between the pilot and transport team members (personal communication, Dry Michelle North, June 2002) are as follows:
1. Communicate positively.
2. Direct assistance as needed.
3. Announce decisions clearly.
4. Offer assistance.
5. Acknowledge the actions of others.
6. Be specific.
7. Know and understand the team's aviation roles and responsibilities.
8. Be vigilant in understanding the interaction between the team members, the machine, and the environment.

Emergency Vehicle Operators

Drivers of the ground units or mobile intensive care units are often referred to as emergency vehicle operators (EVOs). The EVO is an active team member, but is primarily responsible for the safe operations of the vehicle at all times. The individual must be trained, licensed, and qualified to practice safely and professionally within the unit. He or she must demonstrate proficiency in the mechanical operations of the vehicle, routine vehicle maintenance, emergency vehicle operation as regulated by state and local authorities, proper use of the communication equipment, operation of the patient care equipment and knowledge of the supplies, driving adeptness in varying weather, and familiarity with the service area. The EVO may participate in the loading and unloading of the patient and be an active transport team member when the vehicle is not in motion.

Program Manager

In most critical care transport programs, the program manager or director is responsible for coordinating the administrative activities of the transport service. The program director may be an RN, physician, pilot, paramedic, or administrator.

CAMTS provides some recommendations for the role of a program manager.

The major responsibilities of the program director include formulating administrative policies, directing CQI activities, managing vehicle contracts, negotiating medical equipment purchases or leases, navigating vendor's relationships, maintaining the communications system, preparing and monitoring components of the budget, participating in strategic planning and marketing, serving as a resource for problem solving, and serving as community liaison.

The Association of Air Medical Services offers a Medical Transport Leadership Institute that has a mission to enhance the management of medical transportation services. This 2-year program offers courses in human resource management, leadership and administration, financial operations, program development, and asset management.[18] Program directors, medical crew supervisors, operators, lead pilots, and other leadership personnel in critical care transport are provided with a framework to strengthen or develop their leadership and administrative skills. A graduate-level program is also offered, which expands on foundational concepts, providing further opportunity for interactive dialog and problem solving. Networking with proven transport industry leaders is a daily occurrence at all levels and provides excellent opportunity for participants to realistically hone their acquired skills.

Each critical care transport program dictates the role of the program director. The transport team must know and understand the director's role in the program and the program's organizational chart and how the transport team functions in the program.

Other Members of the Transport Program

Depending on the structure of the transport program, there may be many different types of leadership positions. Theses may include Chief Flight Nurse, Safety Officer, Business Manager, and Medical Manager. Each of these positions should come with defined job descriptions and recommended qualifications. The addition of transport team members will depend on the size of the program operations or the type of model that a particular program uses.

Summary

For effective patient transport, multiple resources are necessary. The mission of the transport service designs the transport team and defines the roles of all disciplines involved. The patient and the patient's needs determine the members of the team. Patient transport depends on organized professional components cohesively working together to ensure both safe and competent patient care.

References

1. Glenn. Guide for interfacility patient transfer. http://m.paems.org/forms/system-protocol-manual/interfacility-cct-protocols.pdf; 2006.
2. Coons J, Zalar C. 2015 Air Medical Safety Survey. *Air Med J.* 2016;35(3):120-125.
3. Kupas F, Wang H. Critical Care Paramedics—A Missing Component for Safe Interfacility Transport in the United States. *Ann Emerg Med.* 2014;64(1):17-18.
4. Critical Care Transport Program (CCEMTP). *University of Maryland Baltimore Campus.* Available at http://ehspace.umbc.edu/ccemtp; August 2008.
5. Air & Surface Transport Nurses Association (ASTNA). *Role of the Registered Nurse in the Out-of-Hospital Environment.* Denver, CO: ASTNA; 2015.
6. Sjolin H, Lindstrom V, Rinsted C, Kurland L. What an ambulance nurse needs to know: A content analysis of curricula in the specialist nursing programme in prehospital emergency care. *Int Emerg Nurs.* 2015;23:127-132.
7. Treadwell D, Arndt K, Werth R. *Standards for Critical Care and Specialty Transport.* Aurora, CO: Air and Surface Transport Association; 2015.
8. Commission on Accreditation of Medical Transport Systems. *Accreditation Standards.* 10th ed. Anderson, SC: CAMTS; 2015.
9. International Association of Flight & Critical Care Paramedics (IAFCCP). *Critical Care Paramedic Position Statement.* Snellville, GA: IAFCCP; 2009.
10. American Association for Respiratory Care. http://www.aarc.org/?s=Air+Transport+Section; 2016.
11. Blumen I, et al. *Principles and Direction of Air Medical Transport.* Salt Lake City, UT: Air Medical Physicians Association; 2015.
12. Carrubba C. Role of the medical director in air medical transport. In: Blumen I, ed. *Principles and Direction of Air Medical Transport.* Salt Lake City, UT: Air Medical Physicians Association; 2015:90.
13. Carrubba C. Role of the medical director in air medical transport. In: Blumen I, ed. *Principles and Direction of Air Medical Transport.* Salt Lake City, UT: Air Medical Physicians Association; 2015:89-96.
14. Air Medical Physician Association (AMPA). *Medical Direction & Medical Control of Air Medical Services.* Salt Lake City, UT: AMPA; 2012.
15. Air Medical Transport Leadership Institute. http://aams.org/events/mtli/; 2016 Accessed 06.07.16.
16. Federal Aviation Administration. Pilot in command. http://www.faa.gov/about/initiatives/cabin_safety/regs/legal/media/pic_responsibility_fa_duty_rest.pdf; 1997 Accessed 23.09.16.
17. U.S. Department of Transportation. Rules and regulations. In: *Federal Aviation Regulations.* Part 91. Washington, DC: Federal Aviation Administration.
18. Raynovich W, Hums J, Stuhlmiller D, Bramble J, Kasha T, Galt, K. Critical care transportation by paramedics: a cross-sectional survey. *Air Med J.* 2013;32:280-282.

3

Preparation for Practice

DENISE TREADWELL, JONATHAN D. GRYNIUK, AND RENEÉ SEMONIN HOLLERAN

Critical care patient transport requires skilled and experienced personnel to meet the needs of complex cases in a challenging environment. It also necessitates clinical competency, critical thinking skills, and flexibility. The education, clinical proficiency, and knowledge needed to provide this care before, during, and after the transport must be diverse and comprehensive. Transport teams vary and may be composed of registered nurses (RNs), paramedics, physicians, respiratory therapists, or others, as dictated by patient needs. Although no central reporting agency can identify who makes up a transport team, most teams within the United States continue to be staffed by RNs and paramedics.[1-8] However, all team members must possess some basic information; for example, aircraft or ground vehicle safety, use of radios or communication devices, and survival training. Transport team staffing and education should be commensurate with the mission statement and scope of care of the medical transport service. The transport vehicle, by virtue of how it is staffed and medically equipped, becomes a patient care unit specific to the needs of the patient. The team that transports that patient must be appropriately educated and trained in patient management before, during, and after the transport process.[1-8]

The makeup of a transport team varies across the world. The Commission on Accreditation of Medical Transport Systems (CAMTS)[6] defines team members on the basis of the mission of the transport. Table 3.1 describes the different types of missions and teams that may be involved in transport with use of the CAMTS definitions.

Qualifications for Transport Practice

Transport Nurse

The RN has had a role in patient transport and the prehospital environment for numerous years. Discussion continues about what qualifications a nurse should have to practice. State and local emergency medical services (EMS) regulations and even some national EMS and physicians' associations have provided input into transport nursing practice. The Air & Surface Transport Nurses Association (ASTNA)[1] developed a position paper that addresses some of these issues. The preparation for patient care required to practice nursing, along with the appropriate experience and education, provides a sound foundation for practice in the prehospital and transport environments. However, that preparation rarely includes the skills needed to deliver patient care in the prehospital environment. ASTNA supports State Boards of Nursing, or in other countries, the equivalent regulatory bodies for the profession of nursing. It believes that services providing critical care transport are functional extensions of hospital emergency departments and critical care or specialty units and that staffing for these services minimally consists of at least one professional, an RN. ASTNA pursues recognition by state EMS agencies or their equivalent for the unique role of an RN to practice in the prehospital environment. The RN who practices in the out-of-hospital and transport environment must be properly prepared to deliver patient care safely and competently in this exceptional and challenging environment.[1]

In 2015, ASTNA published a specific position paper that recommends the qualifications a transport nurse should have before being hired as a member of a transport team. These qualifications are summarized in Box 3.1.[2]

The advanced practice nurse (APRN) has been a part of many transport teams for years, especially neonatal nurse practitioners. As the role of the APRN has developed and grown, some services have included them, especially the acute care nurse practitioner who has been specifically educated to manage the critically ill or injured patient. However, as previously noted, transport teams need to be composed of the appropriate members based on their mission and scope of service.[7]

Transport Paramedic

The International Association of Flight and Critical Care Paramedics (IAFCCP; formerly the International Association of Flight Paramedics) supports the utilization of the paramedic in air medical and critical care transport environments.[8] However, there have been several definitions of paramedic practice in the transport environment leading to confusion in role identity. Most definitions are determined by the area of the country (and even the world) in which the paramedic practices. The certified flight paramedic (FP-C)

TABLE 3.1	Transport Team Definitions
Mission	**Definition**
Critical care	Critical care is defined as transport from a scene or clinical setting of a patient whose condition warrants care commensurate with the scope of practice of a physician or registered nurse
Advanced life support	Advanced life support mission is defined as transport from an emergency department, critical care unit, or scene of a patient who needs care commensurate with the scope of practice of an EMT-P
Basic life support	A basic life support is defined as the transport of a patient from an emergency department or scene who requires care commensurate with the scope of practice of an EMT-B
Specialty care	These team members have a specific specialty and are added to the regularly scheduled transport team (e.g., neonatal, pediatric, perinatal, IABP transports).

EMT-B, Emergency medical technician-basic; *EMT-P,* emergency medical technician-paramedic; *IABP,* intra-aortic balloon pump.

• BOX 3.1   Qualifications for Transport Nurses

- Registered nurse (with appropriate state/provincial licensure)
- Minimum 3 years' critical care or emergency department experience
- Specialty certification commensurate with previous experience (CEN, CCRN, CFRN, or CTRN within 2 years of hire)
- Basic cardiac life support or equivalent
- Age-specific ACLS and/or PALS, NRP, PEPP, and ENPC or equivalent
- TPATC, ATLS, or equivalent
- Objective assessment of the transport nurse applicant's qualifications for transport based on, but not limited to, the following characteristics:
  - Educational and experiential background
  - Technical and clinical competence
  - Leadership Skills
  - Critical thinking skills
  - Proficient communication and interpersonal skills
  - Appreciation of public and community relations

ACLS, Advanced cardiac life support; *ATLS,* advanced trauma life support; *CCRN,* critical care registered nurse; *CEN,* certified emergency nurse; *CFRN,* certified flight registered nurse; *CTRN,* certified transport registered nurse; *ENPC,* Emergency Nursing Pediatric Course; *NRP,* Neonatal Resuscitation Program; *PALS,* pediatric advanced life support; *PEPP,* Pediatric Education for Prehospital Professionals; *TPATC,* Transport Professional Advanced Trauma Course.

---

examination and the certified critical care paramedic (CCP-C) certifications were developed to help clarify what preparation is necessary for an advanced role as a paramedic performing air medical and critical care ground transport, respectively. Box 3.2 provides a summary of the IAFCCP's recommendations for the qualifications for flight and critical care transport paramedics.[8-10]

Respiratory Therapist

Many transport teams include a respiratory therapist as either a primary member of the team or as an additional team member when the needs of the patient require respiratory management. Ventilatory management has become an integral part of the management of critically ill and injured patients. In many cases, this care includes the use of ventilatory equipment and assessment parameters that many transport teams have not been trained on or may not consistently use.

When the respiratory therapist is a primary member of the team, he or she must complete the same education and training as other team members. The therapist's role on the team must be well defined and again within the scope of practice in the geographic area in which he or she practices.[7]

Physicians

Transport teams continue to be composed of two team members. The most common is the RN/paramedic team. However, physicians have been members of transport teams in some areas of the United States and the world since the inception of hospital-based helicopter programs.[11] Reasons cited for the use of a physician as a part of a transport team include medical/clinical judgment, technical skills, clinical experience, and the marketing value of having a physician on board.[11,12]

The transport environment can provide physicians with valuable training experience. The physician can bring medical expertise, possibly reduce medical legal issues, and provide important public relations in the prehospital environment.[7]

Preparation for Practice

The CAMTS standards provide an outline for the initial training program requirements for each of the mission types (air or surface/ground) for transport programs.[6] These requirements provide a strong framework on which a program's initial orientation and continuing education are built. A summary of these requirements is found in Box 3.3.[6,9]

A comprehensive orientation can be provided in numerous ways. With the use of adult learning principles, an educational program can be designed that uses self-directed learning packets, traditional lecture with discussion, or case scenario teaching.[3-5]

In addition to the didactic information, a practical component of skills training is needed. This training should

---

• BOX 3.2 | **Qualifications for a Transport Paramedic**

- Minimum of 3 years' experience or full-time employment as a paramedic in a busy advanced life support EMS system
- Education
  - Primary: Successful completion of the paramedic National Standard Curriculum or equivalent
  - Secondary: Successful completion of a critical care education program that meets or exceeds the educational objectives of this position statement, including didactic sessions, practical sessions, skill proficiency demonstration, and clinical rotations
  - Tertiary: Continuing mentored didactic education, skill maintenance, and clinical opportunities that maintain the educational objectives of this position statement
- Certifications
  - Advanced Cardiac Life Support
  - Adult and Pediatric International Trauma Life Support/ Prehospital Trauma Life Support/Advanced Trauma Life Support
  - Pediatric Advanced Life Support/Advanced Pediatric Life Support
  - Neonatal Resuscitation Program
  - Or an equivalent education in each of the previously mentioned areas
- Knowledge
  - Assessment of the critically ill or injured patient
  - Advanced adult and pediatric airway management including, but not limited to, the following:
    - RSI intubation
    - Alternative and rescue airways
    - Surgical cricothyroidotomy
    - Continuous waveform capnography to monitor $ETCO_2$
  - Mechanical and noninvasive ventilation theory, troubleshooting, and competence
  - Chest tube thoracostomy management and insertion (if applicable)
  - Obtain and maintain peripheral venous, central venous (if applicable), and/or intraosseous access
  - Administration of blood and blood products
  - ECG monitoring and 12-lead ECG interpretation
  - Defibrillation; cardioversion; and transcutaneous and transvenous pacing monitoring, maintenance, and treatment
  - Circulatory management and support including invasive hemodynamic monitoring and IABP management (theory, transport considerations, troubleshooting, and operations, if applicable)
  - Intracranial pressure monitoring and management
  - Pharmacology included in the National Standard Curriculum augmented by knowledge of analgesics, antibiotics, antidysrhythmics, antiepileptics, paralytics, sedatives, and vasoactive medications

- Laboratory value interpretation including arterial blood gas analysis
- Targeted radiology study interpretation
- Patient management:
  - Acute respiratory emergencies
  - Cardiovascular emergencies
  - Hypertensive emergencies
  - Shock and multiorgan system failure
  - Infectious diseases
  - Neurologic emergencies including stroke and intracranial hemorrhage
  - Trauma
  - Spinal cord injury
  - Burn
  - Trauma in pregnancy
  - Pediatric trauma
  - Critical pediatric emergencies
  - Obstetric emergencies
  - Neonatal emergencies (if applicable)
  - Environmental emergencies
  - Poisoning/toxic exposure/hazardous material awareness
  - Bioterrorism
- Transport medicine:
  - Safety
    - Vehicle operations and emergency procedures
    - Critical care transport equipment
    - Patient/family factors
    - Human factors (including but not limited to AMRM or equivalent)
    - Evaluation of appropriateness for transport based on required level of care
  - Transport logistics
  - Critical care transport equipment (ventilator, IABP, neonatal isolette, etc.)
  - Patient packaging for safety and accessibility
  - Radio and communication technology
  - Transport physiology
  - Interaction and communication with medical oversight
  - Medical provider communication/transfer of care
  - Documentation
- Quality management: understanding principles and best practice.
- Certification examination: successful completion of a critical care paramedic certification examination. Along with the FP-C, the IAFCCP recognizes the CCP-C as a valid certification examination for the critical care paramedic.

AMRM, Air medical resource management; *CCP-C,* Critical Care Paramedic Certification Examination; *ECG,* electrocardiogram; *EMS,* Emergency Medical Service; *ETCO₂,* end tidal carbon dioxide; *FP-C,* certified flight paramedic, *IABP,* intraaortic balloon pump; *IAFCCP,* International Association of Flight and Critical Care Paramedics; *RSI,* rapid sequence induction.

---

include various inpatient and prehospital care clinical experiences and an invasive skills laboratory.[4-6]

After the initial education and training is complete, the new transport team member needs to complete an internship or preceptorship, which provides further role definition, recognition of the need for additional education or training, and an opportunity to "put into practice" all the previous learning. Although evaluation is an ongoing process, a final evaluation during the orientation process assists new transport team members in assessing their experience and the need for any further education.

Adult Learning Principles

Incorporation of adult learning principles and the use of various teaching methods should be included in a comprehensive orientation program. Adult learning today is influenced by generational differences, technology advancements,

• BOX 3.3   Commission on Accreditation of Medical Transport Systems Initial Training Program Requirements

Didactic Component

- Advanced airway management
- Altitude physiology/stressors of flight
- Anatomy, physiology, and assessment for adult, pediatric, and neonatal patients (specific to the program's scope of care)
- Cardiac emergencies and advanced cardiac critical care
- Didactic education that is mission specific and specific to the scope of care and patient population
  - Burn emergencies (thermal, chemical, and electrical)
  - Compliance issues and regulations
  - Disaster and triage EMS radio communications
  - Environmental emergencies
  - Equipment education: airway, breathing, and circulation equipment; defibrillators; pacemakers; monitors; IABP, etc.
- Hemodynamic monitoring devices such as pacemakers, AICD, intraaortic balloon pump, central lines, pulmonary arterial and arterial catheters, ventricular assist devices, and ECMO
  - High-risk obstetric emergencies defined as "a transport that is directly related to pregnancy that may endanger the mother or fetus of a gestational age greater than 20 weeks"
  - Highway scene safety management
  - Human factors: crew resource management and air medical resource management
  - Infection control and prevention
  - Just culture or equivalent education
  - Mechanical ventilation and respiratory physiology for adult, pediatric, and neonatal patients specific to the program's scope of care and equipment
  - Metabolic endocrine emergencies
  - Multitrauma (chest, abdomen, and facial)
  - Neonatal emergencies (respiratory distress, surgical, and cardiac)
  - Oxygen quality controls include: hazard awareness, how to reach cylinder levels, basic understanding of CGA connections, how to safely transport liquid oxygen cylinders

(if used), and knowledge of cylinder durations as per local and national regulations
- Pediatric medical emergencies
- Pediatric trauma
- Pharmacology
- Quality management: didactic education that supports the medical transport service's mission statement and scope of care
- Respiratory emergencies
- Safety and risk management training
- Scene management/rescue/extrication
- Sleep deprivation, sleep inertia, circadian rhythms, and recognizing signs of fatigue
- State EMS rules and regulations: province or government rules reading surface and air transport
- Stress recognition and management
- Toxicology
- Transport vehicle orientation/safety and procedures as appropriate and in-transport procedures/general vehicle safety including all types of vehicles the team may be exposed to, including depressurization procedures for fixed-wing vehicles (as appropriate)

Clinical Component (on Basis of the Program's Scope of Care)

- Critical care (adult, pediatric, and neonatal)
- Emergency care (adult, pediatric, and neonatal)
- Invasive procedures on mannequin equivalent for practicing of invasive procedures
- Neonatal intensive care
- Obstetrics
- Pediatric critical care
- Prehospital care
- Tracheal intubations (and alternative airway management)

AICD, Automatic implantable cardiac defibrillator; *CGA,* Compressed Gas Association; *ECMO,* extracorporeal membrane oxygenation; *EMS,* Emergency Medical Service; *IABP,* intraaortic balloon pump.

---

and differing learning styles. These should be considered in the development of any orientation or educational program for new team members. Adult learning also requires various educational techniques including but not limited to traditional lecture with discussion, case presentation/scenario-based teaching, Internet-based learning, multimedia applications, simulation training, and self-directed learning packages.[13-15] In addition to the didactic component, transport nursing practice requires additional skills with a practical clinical component. These skills should include various prehospital care and inpatient clinical experiences in addition to simulation training with tools such as synthetic models and mannequins or computer simulations.[13-16]

Simulation training also has become a popular and common method of providing orientation, ongoing clinical skills, and exposure to uncommon clinical problems. Many transport programs are no longer part of a hospital system, so finding clinical environments for education and practice has become limited.[13] As noted by Alfes et al.,[16,17] there is minimal literature describing the ideal way to orient transport team members to the critical care transport

environment. Simulation training can be standardized based most appropriately on the scope and mission of the transport service.

After the initial education and training is complete, standard practice is for a new transport team member to participate in a period of preceptorship or internship. This period allows for further role clarification and definition, provides an opportunity to put into practice all the learning from the initial education, and allows for recognition of the need for additional education or training.

Because of the variety of adult learning styles in today's education world and the knowledge that adult learners progress at a different paces, emphasis and due consideration are needed in the evaluation of progress through the period of preceptorship. The duration of orientation and preceptorship for new team members varies according to the needs of the transport program and the individual member. Using a survey, Alfes et al.[16] identified that transport teams reported the most helpful resources that assisted them in the development of their role as a new transport member were case reviews, additional time in the mode of transportation they were to use with a preceptor, and experiences with task trainers and mannequins.

Competency-Based Education

Competency-based learning is a method of education that allows for flexibility and builds on previous knowledge. Competency-based instruction provides an opportunity for regular feedback and assessment of competency at the end of the various stages of the program, which provides positive response for progression through to the next stage and the ability to assess competency development as the transport nurse learns. An example is advanced airway management skills. The plan is an outline of requirements for competency in advanced airway skills. The orientation member then initiates the plan (Do, as shown in Fig. 3.1). An assessment of the member's ability to perform advanced airway management is done, and the plan is then modified.

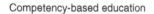
Competency-based education

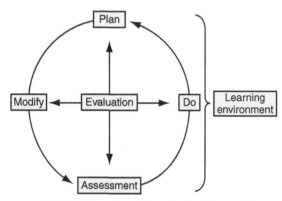

• **Fig. 3.1** Competency-based education model.

Evaluation is continuous. Fig. 3.1 illustrates the use of this model.

ASTNA[1,2,18] has developed a list of the minimal competencies that are recommended for nurses who practice in the transport environment. A summary of these competencies is found in Box 3.4.

In addition, Johnson[14] has also developed a competency-based manual that provides several references and outlines for the orientation of transport personnel.

Each transport program, on the basis of the program's mission and scope of practice, has a standard of technical competencies and skills necessary for clinical practice. During the orientation period, new staff members are required to demonstrate competence in the specified requisites for progression to independent practice. Once demonstrated, these skills are built on by the novice practitioner and provide a continuing checklist for the experienced provider for continuing professional development. Additional individual skill sets, or a blend of technical, interpersonal, and critical thinking as identified in a specific job description, need to be measurably shown by the end of the orientation program. These objectives may also form the basis for an annual performance development review or personal evaluations within the transport program. Feedback regarding performance from a variety of sources, including peer reviews, self-reflection, and posttransport debriefings, provides honest evaluation and is often powerful motivation for self-development.

ASTNA recommends that clinical competencies be evaluated with use of written examinations, simulated practice/skills laboratories, transport preceptor/mentor supervised skills practiced during actual transports, case presentations, and oral examinations conducted by peers and the medical director. Staff meetings offer excellent opportunities to teach both new and experienced transport personnel using case studies from actual transports.

• **BOX 3.4** **Air and Surface Transport Nurses Association–Recommended Competencies for Transport Nurses**

Advanced patient assessments skills to include anatomy, pathophysiology, assessment, and treatment for the age group and patients that are transported by the program (e.g., neonatal, pediatric, adult, geriatric):
• Acute and chronic respiratory disease
• Cardiovascular abnormalities
• Surgical problems
• Infectious diseases
• Musculoskeletal abnormalities
• Neurologic and spinal cord emergencies
• Gastrointestinal emergencies
• Genitourinary disorders
• Integumentary disruption
• Hematologic disorders
• Metabolic/endocrine disorders
• Genetic/disorders of dysmorphology
• Disorders of the head, eyes, ears, nose, and throat
• Trauma
• Environmental and toxicologic emergencies
• Adult and child maltreatment

• Airway management (basic and advanced)
• Vascular access
• Medication administration
• Intraaortic balloon pump management
• Ventricular assist device management
• Needle decompression
• Chest tube insertion
• Pericardiocentesis
• Pacing devices
• Immobilization skills
• Twelve-lead electrocardiographic interpretation
• Arrhythmia analysis and treatment
• Invasive monitoring
• Fetal heart monitoring
• Radiographic interpretation
• Interpretation and treatment of clinical laboratory data
• Thermoregulation
• Psychological/bereavement support and crisis intervention
• Transport equipment management

Coaching, mentoring, and clinical supervision programs should be available to new transport team members. Mentors fulfill a different role than that of the preceptor. They help new nurses in a role to deepen their knowledge and develop professionally, whereas clinical supervision allows the practitioner to share clinical, organizational, developmental, and emotional experiences with another professional to enhance knowledge and skills.

Continuing Professional Development

Continuing professional development has a fixed portion of training determined by standards, regulations, and the transport program, including skills/technical training, occupational health and safety, and local and state requirements. Additional sources of continuing education may include current textbooks related to transport, professional journals, online discussion forums, and continuing education courses.

Commission on Accreditation of Medical Transport Systems Recommendations

CAMTS outlines specific components of transport education and skills that should be reviewed annually (Box 3.5).[6]

In addition to these requirements, transport team members have a further responsibility to identify their own educational needs aside from any regulatory or accreditation standard requirements. As discussed previously, adult learners need a variety of experiences to learn and remain competent. Team members must maintain and continue to gain knowledge to meet patient needs and carry on the growth of the profession of transport nursing. This continuing education is an important part of the development and maintenance of expert practice in the field of transport nursing.

Clinical Decision Making

Clinical decision making or clinical judgment is a process in which the clinician identifies, prioritizes, establishes plans, and evaluates data, which leads to the formation of a judgment to provide patient care.[19,20] In transport nursing, complex clinical decisions are made on a daily basis, in collaboration (Fig. 3.2) with other health professionals and transport team members. In dealing with increasing patient complexity and technological advancement, transport nurses must rely on sound decision-making skills to deliver up-to-date evidenced-based care and help facilitate positive patient outcomes.

Reflective Practice

The use of reflective practice (application of learning experiences and current evidenced-based knowledge) in clinical decision making enhances patient care delivery. A higher level of learning is achieved by applying learned material to current situations. This application of reflective practice associated with learning from experience is an important strategy for health professionals who engage in continual learning.[21] The act of reflection is seen as a way of promoting the development of autonomous, qualified, and self-directed health professionals.

• BOX 3.5 Commission on Accreditation of Medical Transport Systems Continuing Education/Staff Development

Didactic

- Hazardous materials recognition and response
- Human factors: crew resource management
- Infection control
- State EMS rules and regulations in relation to ground and air transport
- Stress recognition and management
- Survival training

Clinical/Laboratory

- Critical care (adult, pediatric, and neonatal)
- Emergency/trauma care
- Invasive procedures laboratories
- Labor and delivery
- Prehospital experience
- Skills maintenance program documented to comply with the number of skills required in a set period according to the policy of the medical transport service (e.g., endotracheal intubations, chest drains)
- Clinical competency maintained by currency in the following or equivalent as appropriate for position description, mission statement, and scope of care:
  - BLS: documented evidence of current BLS certification according to the AHA

- ACLS: documented evidence of current ACLS according to the AHA
- ATLS: according to the American College of Surgeons, ATLS audit, ATLS for Nurse or TPATC
- PALS or APLS according to the AHA and ACEP, or equivalent education
- NRP: documented evidence of current NRP according to the AHA or American Academy of Pediatrics
- Nursing certifications (such as CEN, CCRN, CTRN, and especially CFRN) are strongly encouraged; if required in position descriptions, certifications must be current

ACEP, American College of Emergency Physicians; *ACLS,* advanced cardiac life support; *AHA,* American Heart Association; *APLS,* advanced pediatric life support; *ATLS,* advanced trauma life support; *BLS,* basic life support; *CCRN,* Critical Care Registered Nurse; *CEN,* Certified Emergency Nurse; *CFRN,* Certified Flight Registered Nurse; *CTRN,* Certified Transport Registered Nurse; *EMS,* Emergency Medical Service; *NRP,* Neonatal Resuscitation Program; *PALS,* pediatric advanced life support; *TPATC,* Transport Professional Advanced Trauma Course.

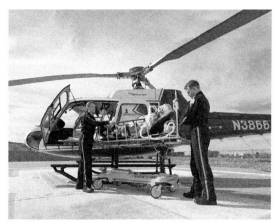

• **Fig. 3.2** Transport nurse and paramedic. (Courtesy Air Methods Corporation.)

Engagement in reflective practice is associated with improvement in the quality of care, stimulation of personal and professional growth, and closing of the gap between theory and practice. If nurses are not thinking autonomously on a regular basis, they risk losing competence in their decision-making abilities.[21]

Certification

Certification is defined by the American Board of Nursing Specialties as the formal recognition of specialized knowledge, skills, and experience demonstrated by achievement of standards identified by a nursing specialty to promote optimal health outcomes.[22,23] Certification in nursing first began in the 1940s. Since that time, the number of certifications offered in nursing and other health care–related professions has greatly increased.

Several studies have shown the value of certification.[24-27] The benefits of certification include increased job satisfaction, personal achievement, demonstration of knowledge of a specific body of nursing, commitment to the profession of nursing, increased credibility, indication of professional growth, enhancement in personal confidence in clinical abilities, and promotion of recognition from other health professionals.[24-27]

With the vast overlap of knowledge among nursing specialties, nurses sometimes are unsure about which certification they should obtain. Multiple certifications are available in nursing, including specialty and advanced practice certifications. A point to consider is what knowledge is needed by the specific specialty one practices. For example, the transport nurse may choose to take the Certified Emergency Nurse (CEN), Critical Care Registered Nurse (CCRN), Certified Flight Registered Nurse (CFRN), or Certified Transport Registered Nurse (CTRN) examination. Each examination reflects specific areas pertinent to transport nursing. For example, the CFRN addresses issues specific to flight nursing, such as landing zone and scene safety and aircraft operations.

Transport Nursing Certification

Transport nursing has two specialty certifications, CFRN and CTRN. In some states, additional certifications are required for nurses to practice. For example, in California, certifications are needed for the mobile intensive care nurse or the prehospital health professional.

The CFRN and the CTRN were created through the work of ASTNA (formally known as the National Flight Nurses Association) and the Board of Certification for Emergency Nursing. A member of ASTNA is appointed to the Board, and transport nurses are item writers for the examinations. More information about these examinations, as well the elements that are evaluated on the examinations, is available at http://www.bcencertifications.org/Home.aspx.

ASTNA publishes the *Flight and Ground Transport Nursing and Paramedic Core Curriculum*, which contains the knowledge needed for transport nursing practice. ASTNA also publishes review manuals and has other materials available for review for preparation for both the CFRN and the CTRN examinations. More information about these resources can be found at http://astna.org/.

Applicants must be sure that the certification organization is legitimate. Various certification programs offer examinations that are not psychometrically sound. To eliminate confusion, certifying organizations are now usually accredited.

Flight and Critical Care Paramedic Certification

Although most air medical programs have expanded the flight paramedic's role to that of a critical care provider, some programs continue to provide basic paramedic-level care in the flight environment. This diversity in flight paramedic practice has clouded the definition of the practice. There is a group of flight paramedics who define the practice as the ability to perform paramedic skills in the air medical environment; however, most flight paramedics define their practice as that of a critical care provider.

To combat this ambiguity and the lack of a nationally recognized flight paramedic examination, the National Flight Paramedics Association (now the IAFCCP) introduced the FP-C examination. This examination was created on the premise that most flight paramedics function as critical care providers. Therefore the certification process that defines the practice of the flight paramedic is not only based on an understanding of basic paramedic skills and flight physiology but also incorporates an understanding of critical care theory and practice. Specific recommendations for attaining and maintaining basic competencies are outlined in the IAFCCP position statement.[28]

Following the success of the FP-C examination, a separate board, the Board for Critical Care Transport Paramedic Certification (BCCTPC), was created to oversee the continued development of the FP-C examination. Many of the same issues causing confusion related to flight paramedic practice also plague ground critical care paramedic practice. As a result, the BCCTPC pioneered the creation and implementation of a critical care ground transport–specific paramedic certification, the CCP-C. Both the FP-C and CCP-C examinations are available via either paper and pencil or computer and currently consist of 125 questions. The focus of the examination is on the knowledge level of experienced paramedics who work with flight or critical care transport teams. The examination is not meant to test entry-level knowledge. In January 2016, the BCCTPC moved to expand its role within specialty certifications, thus forming the International Board of Specialty Certification (IBSC), which currently oversees the FP-C and CCP-C examinations as well as a variety of other specialized transport and paramedic certifications.[28-30] Box 3.6 contains a summary

of the types and numbers of questions that are now on the FP-C and CCP-C examinations.[28-30]

The title FP-C or CCP-C denotes a transport professional with a broad expanse of knowledge. The FP-C and CCP-C examinations are not regionally specific. Regional practice and state laws are understood to direct the flight or critical care paramedic's ability to perform certain procedures or administer specific medications. However, the IBSC and IAFCCP does not believe that this precludes the necessity of the transport paramedic to maintain a basic knowledge of these skills or medications.

The FP-C and CCP-C examinations demonstrate, through written or computer-based testing, the ability to provide care beyond what may be allowed within a specific locale. By adopting this philosophy, successful completion

---

• BOX 3.6 Examination Content

Examination Content for Certified Flight Paramedic[28-30]

There are 125 questions, and the candidate is provided 2.5 hours to complete the examination. The certification process is focused on the knowledge level of accomplished, experienced paramedics currently associated with a flight and/or critical care transport team(s). The questions on the examination are based in sound paramedicine. The candidate is expected to maintain a significant knowledge of current ACLS, PALS, NALS, and ITLS/PHTLS standards. This examination is not meant to test entry-level knowledge; rather it tests the experienced paramedic's skills and knowledge of critical care transport. As you prepare for the examination, please consider that there are a variety of mission profiles throughout the spectrum of transport medicine. Please remember this examination tests the candidate's overall knowledge of the transport environment and not the specifics of one individual program. Just because your program does not complete IABP transports, it does not mean you will not have questions related to these types of transports. Likewise, if your program does not perform SAR, you still need to understand this information for the examination.

Question Category	Number of Questions on Examination
Trauma management	12
Aircraft fundamentals, safety, and survival	14
Flight physiology	7
Advanced airway management techniques	11
Neurologic emergencies	7
Critical cardiac patient	18
Respiratory patient	8
Toxic exposures	3
Obstetric emergencies	4
Neonates	5
Pediatric	9
Burn patients	5
General medical patient	16
Environmental	6

Examination Content for Certified Critical Care Paramedic[28-30]

There are 125 questions, and the candidate is provided 2.5 hours to complete the examination. The certification process is focused on the knowledge level of accomplished, critical care paramedics providing patient care in the prehospital, interhospital, and hospital environment. The questions on the examination are based in sound paramedicine. The candidate is expected to maintain a significant knowledge of current ACLS, PALS, NALS, and ITLS/PHTLS standards. This examination is not meant to test entry-level knowledge; rather it tests the experienced paramedic's skills and knowledge. As you prepare for the examination, please consider that there are a variety of mission profiles throughout the spectrum of transport medicine. Please remember this examination tests the candidate's overall knowledge of the transport environment and not the specifics of one individual program. Just because your program does not complete IABP transports, it does not mean you will not have questions related to these types of transport. Likewise, if your program does not provide neonatal transport, you still need to understand this information for the examination.

Question Category	Number of Questions on Examination
Trauma patient management	12
Transport fundamentals, safety, and survival	9
Advanced airway management techniques	12
Neurologic patient	11
Cardiac patient	12
Respiratory patient	12
Toxic exposure and environmental patient	12
Obstetric patients	9
Neonatal and pediatric patient	15
Burn patients	9
General medical patient	9

ACLS, Advanced cardiac life support; *IABP,* intraaortic balloon pump; *ITLS,* international trauma life support; *NALS,* neonatal advanced life support; *PALS,* pediatric advanced life support; *PHTLS,* prehospital trauma life support; *SAR,* search and rescue.

of the FP-C and CCP-C examination should be viewed as the pinnacle achievement in transport paramedic practice. Successful completion of the FP-C and CCP-C examinations denotes the ability of the transport paramedic to practice with equal proficiency and without regional discrimination in both prehospital and interfacility transport.

Summary

Transport professionals require experience, advanced skills, and continuing education so that the transport team is able to function autonomously and in collaboration with all others who may be involved in the transport process. Patient care and management during transport occurs in diverse multidimensional situations. The development of a sound orientation and strong preceptorship training program, in conjunction with continuing values-based professional development, provides the transport nurse with the skills and ability to care for patients in diverse and sometimes difficult situations. All of these experiences contribute to retaining a highly skilled nursing staff in a diverse environment.

Certification holds value for health care and health care providers in many ways. Certified transport team members demonstrate to the consumer and the employer that nurses and paramedics have achieved a certain level of knowledge in a specific area of transport care. Certification also confirms pride in one's profession and in one's specialty.

References

1. Air & Surface Transport Nurses Association (ASTNA). *Role of the Registered Nurse in the Out-of-Hospital Environment.* Denver, CO: ASTNA; 2015.
2. Air & Surface Transport Nurses Association (ASTNA). *Qualifications, Orientation, Competencies, and Continuing Education for Transport Nurses.* Denver, CO: ASTNA; 2015.
3. Air & Surface Transport Nurses Association (ASTNA). *Staffing of Critical Care Transport Services.* Denver, CO: ASTNA; 2015.
4. Bader GB, Terhorts M, Heilman P, et al. Characteristics of flight nursing practice. *Air Med J.* 1995;14(4):214-218.
5. Blumen I, ed. *Principles and Direction of Air Medical Transport. Advancing Air & Ground Critical Care Transport Medicine.* 2nd ed. Salt Lake City, UT: Air Medical Physicians Association; 2015.
6. Commission on Accreditation of Medical Transport Systems. *Accreditation Standards.* 10th ed. Anderson, SC: Commission on Accreditation of Medical Transport Systems; 2015.
7. Stocking J. Crew configuration. In: Blumen I, ed. 2015. *Principles and Direction of Air Medical Transport. Advancing Air & Ground Critical Care Transport Medicine.* 2nd ed. Salt Lake City, UT: Air Medical Physicians Association; 2015:50-56.
8. International Association of Flight and Critical Care Paramedics. Preparatory Outline for FP-C and CCP-C Exams. Available at http://www.iafccp.org/?page=ExamPrep; 2016 Accessed 01.05.16.
9. International Association of Flight and Critical Care Paramedics. FAQs About Critical Care and Flight Paramedicine. Available at http://www.iafccp.org/?page=CareerFAQ; 2016 Accessed 01.05.16.
10. Gryniuk J. The role of the certified flight paramedic as a critical care provider and the required education. *Prehosp Emerg Care.* 2001;5(3):290-292.
11. Stone K. The air medical crew: Is a flight physician necessary. *J Air Med Transp.* 1991;10(11):7-10.
12. Taylor C, Jan S, Curtis K, et al. The cost-effectiveness of physician staffed Helicopter Emergency Medical Service (HEMS) transport to a major trauma centre in NSW, Australia. *Injury, Int. J. Care Injured.* 2012;43(11):1843-1849.
13. Grisham L, Vickers V, Biffar D, et al. Case study feasibility of air transport simulation training: a case series. *Air Medical Journal.* 2016;35(5):308-313.
14. Johnson J. *Competency Based Orientation and Continuing Education for Critical Care Transport.* Denver, CO: Air and Surface Transport Nurses Association; 2007.
15. Knapp B. Competency: an essential component of caring in nursing. *Nurs Admin Q.* 2004;28(4):285-287.
16. Alfes C, Steiner S, Rutherford-Hemming T. Challenges and resources for new critical care transport crewmembers: a descriptive exploratory study. *Air Med J.* 2016;35(4):212-215.
17. Alfes M, Steiner S, Manacci C. Critical care transport training: new strides in simulating the austere environment. *Air Med J.* 2015;34(4):186-187.
18. Treadwell D, et al. *Standards Critical Care Specialty Transport.* Aurora, CO: ASTNA; 2015.
19. Pugh D. A Phenomenologic study of flight nurses' clinical decision-making in emergency situations. *Air Med J.* 2012; 21(2):29-36.
20. Miller M, Babcock D. *Critical Thinking Applied to Nursing.* St. Louis, MO: Mosby; 1996.
21. Goudreau J, Pepin J, Larua C, et al. A competency-based approach to nurses' continuing education for clinical reasoning and leadership through reflective practice in a care situation. *Nurse Educ Pract.* 2015;15(6):572-578.
22. AACN American Association of Critical Care Nurses Board of Certification. Available at http://www.aacn.org. Accessed 06.07.16.
23. American Board of Nursing Specialties American nurses credentialing center. Available at www.nursingcertification.org. Accessed 06.07.16.
24. Wyand CA. Current factors contributing to professionalism in nursing. *J Prof Nurs.* 2003;19(5):251-261.
25. Straka KL, Ambrose HL, Burkett M, et al. The impact and perception of nursing certification in pediatric nursing. *J Pediatr Nurs.* 2014;29(3):205-211.
26. Boev C, Xue Y, Ingersoll GI. Nursing job satisfaction, certification, and healthcare-associated infections in critical care. *Intensive Crit Care Nurs.* 2015;31(5):276-284.
27. Frazer E, Holleran RS. Education and certification for patient transport. *Air Med J.* 2016;35(11):101-102.
28. International Board of Specialty Certification, About Us. Available at https://www.ibscertifications.org/about/about-us. Accessed 31.05.16.
29. International Board of Specialty Certification, Exam Preparation, FP-C. Available at https://www.ibscertifications.org/resource/pdf/FP-C%20EXAM%20OUTLINE.pdf. Accessed 31.05.16.
30. International Board of Specialty Certification, Exam Preparation, CCP-C. Available at https://www.ibscertifications.org/resource/pdf/CCP-C%20EXAM%20OUTLINE.pdf.

4

Transport Physiology

CHARLES SWEARINGEN

COMPETENCIES

1. Integrate pertinent gas laws and their effects in the transport environment.
2. Provide interventions to prevent the adverse effects of barometric pressure changes during patient transport.
3. Identify specific management of the stresses that may occur during transport.

Patient transport requires an understanding of the physiologic stresses that may occur in this environment. Understanding the concepts of transport physiology is crucial because they are the basis for the special skills used in transporting patients within the air medical environment via fixed-wing or rotor-wing (RW) aircraft.

This chapter includes a discussion on gas laws and their potential effect on patients and the transport team. It also includes information about the physiologic stresses of transport and effects on the patient and team during air medical transport.

Gas Laws

For optimal patient care in the air medical environment, transport personnel must possess in-depth knowledge of altitude physiology and the effects on the patient during transport. Altitude physiology exemplifies the concepts of the gas laws; the primary concern is the relationships among the interdependent variables of temperature, pressure, volume, and mass of gases. Before the gas laws are addressed, those factors that influence the behavior of gases need to be considered. The four basic variables that affect gas volumetric relationships are temperature, pressure, volume, and the relative mass of a gas or the number of molecules. These variables (*T, P, V,* and *n*) are defined as follows[1-11]:

1. *Temperature (T),* when expressed in degrees kelvin (K), indicates the level of energy of a gas sample and is referred to as absolute temperature, converted from temperature Celsius (°C) or Fahrenheit (°F).

2. *Pressure (P),* defined as absolute or total exerted pressure, is conventionally expressed in atmospheres (torr) or as a given column of mercury in millimeters (mm Hg) or of water balancing the pressure in centimeters (cm H_2O).

3. *Volume (V)* is expressed in cubic units, such as cubic meters (m^3), cubic centimeters (cm^3), or in liters (L).

4. *Relative mass* of a gas or number of molecules *(n)* or ions is expressed in gram molecules (the molecular weight of the substance in grams). Gas laws govern the body's physiologic response to barometric pressure changes by these four variables. When the transport team is caring for the air transport patient, these changes become particularly important on ascent and descent.

Boyle's Law

Boyle's law, which originated from experiments conducted by Robert Boyle in 1662, states that at a constant temperature, the volume of gas is inversely proportional to its pressure. This law applies to all gases and may be expressed as follows:

$$P_1 \times V_1 = P_2 \times V_2 \text{ or } P_1/P_2 = V_2/V_1$$

where V_1 is initial volume, V_2 is final volume, P_1 is initial pressure, and P_2 is final pressure.

Thus at a constant temperature, the volume of a gas is inversely proportional to the pressure. The gas in a balloon, for example, expands as the balloon ascends. This occurs because there is less pressure as the balloon ascends higher into the atmosphere, and the balloon expands because of decreased pressure.

The effects of this law can be seen in several clinical situations. As an unpressurized aircraft ascends, patients can exhibit pneumothorax expansion, rupture of air endotracheal tube cuffs, and gastric distention—all because of Boyle's law. If gas expansion within outpatients is ever a concern, consider requesting the pilot to fly at the lowest, safest altitude. It is important to always be aware of the effects of Boyle's law on the patients.[1-11]

Dalton's Law (Law of Partial Pressure)

Dalton was a chemist who observed in 1803 that the total pressure of a mixture of gasses is equal to the sum of the partial pressures of each gas in the mixture. Dalton's law is expressed in the following formula:

$$P = P_1 + P_2 + P_3 + \dots P_n$$

P is the total pressure of the gas mixture, and P_1, P_2, and P_3 are partial pressures of each gas in the mixture.

The partial pressure of each gas in the mixture is derived from the following equation[12]:

$$P_1 = F_1 \times P$$

where P_1 is the partial pressure of gas 1, F_1 is the fractional concentration of gas 1 in the mixture, and P is the total pressure of the gas mixture.[1-11]

In other words, the pressure a gas mixture exerts is due to the fraction of each individual gas multiplied by the barometric pressure. Thus each individual gas present in a mixture exerts a partial pressure that when summed equals the total pressure of the gas.[1-11]

A mathematic illustration of Dalton's law is shown in the following example, in which the partial pressure of oxygen (PO_2) at sea level is calculated:

$$PO_2 = 20.95 \ (21\%) \times 760 \ \text{mm Hg} = 159.6$$

Barometric pressure, or atmospheric pressure, is the pressure exerted against an object or a person by the atmosphere (Table 4.1). At sea level, this pressure is 15 psi, or alternatively measured as 760 mm Hg and 760 torr. Increased altitude results in decreased barometric pressure. Barometric pressure multiplied by the concentration of a gas is equal to the partial pressure of the gas[1-11]:

$$\text{barometric pressure} \times \text{gas concentration} = \text{gas partial pressure}$$
$$760 \ \text{mm Hg} \times 21\% \ O_2 = 159.6 \ \text{mm Hg} \ PO_2^{\text{a}}$$

Charles' Law

An additional development in the early formulation of the laws of ideal gases came from the French physicist Jacques Charles who concluded that, "When pressure is constant, the volume of a gas is very nearly proportional to its absolute temperature." This law is expressed as follows[1-11]:

$$V_1/V_2 = T_1/T_2 \ \text{or} \ V_1/T_1 = V_2/T_2$$

---

[a]Note: Oxygen concentration remains at 21%, regardless of altitude. However, oxygen availability decreases with altitude because the oxygen molecules are farther apart, which could potentially result in hypoxia.

TABLE 4.1			
Summary of the Stages of Hypoxia Gas Law	**Action**		**Practical Application**
Boyle's law	↑ Altitude = ↓ Pressure = ↑ Volume		With higher altitudes, gases expand: pneumothoraces get bigger, ETT cuffs can expand and rupture, free air in the stomach can expand and prevent adequate ventilation
Dalton's law	Total pressure = $P_1 + P_2 + P_3 \dots P_n$		As altitude increases, the partial pressure decreases, therefore, supplemental O_2 is needed at higher and higher altitudes
Charles' law	↑ Temperature = ↑ Volume		As the air heats up, it expands and therefore is less dense, colder air is therefore more dense; this allows a wing to create more lift, thus the aircraft can pick up heavier patients or cargo
Gay-Lussac's law	↓ Pressure = ↓ Temperature		At higher altitudes, pressure will decrease and thus will be cooler; clinicians and patients may need more warmth, and oxygen tank pressures may change between takeoff and at altitude (colder temperatures shrink gases)
Henry's law	↑ Pressure = ↑ Gas solubility		At depth, a diver is subjected to incredibly high pressures, which pushes nitrogen molecules very close together; this increases the solubility of nitrogen and should the diver comes up too fast, this nitrogen will quickly come out of solution and cause decompression illness
Graham's law	↑ Diffusion = ↓ Molecular weight		Lower molecular weight molecules have higher diffusion rates
Fick's law	↑ Partial pressure = ↑ Oxygenation ↑ Surface area ↓ Thickness		By adding FiO_2 and PEEP, partial pressure and surface area will be increased, and the thickness of the alveolar capillary membrane will decrease

ETT, Endotracheal tube; *PEEP,* positive end expiratory pressure.

where V_1 is initial volume, V_2 is final volume, T_1 is initial absolute temperature, and T_2 is final absolute temperature.

Thus the volume is directly proportional to the temperature when expressed on an absolute scale with all other factors constant (P and n are constant).[13] Consequently, if a mass of gas is kept under a constant pressure as the absolute temperature of the gas is increased or decreased, the volume increases or decreases accordingly.[1-11]

Charles' law describes how aircraft, especially RW aircraft, are affected by atmospheric temperatures. In colder months, the air is denser because gases contract as temperature decreases. The contracting of gases in cold temperatures illustrates a decreasing volume with higher density. An aircraft's wing can produce greater lift in cold temperatures; therefore the transport team may be able to transport a bariatric patient in an aircraft in the winter that it could not pick up in the summer. This law affects aircraft but has little effect on the human physiology because humans normally maintain a constant temperature, not to mention the heat needed to expand our physiologic gases would damage our tissue irreparably.[1-11]

Gay-Lussac's Law

Gay-Lussac's law relates pressure and temperature and is expressed as follows:

$P_1/T_1 = P_2/T_2$ where V and n are constant. Thus the pressure of a gas when volume is constant is directly proportional to the absolute temperature for a constant amount of gas.[1-11] As the transport team ascends into the atmosphere, it is subjected to less pressure; therefore, as altitude increases, pressure and temperature decrease. Ultimately, as passengers and equipment travel higher in an unpressurized aircraft, they will experience colder temperatures. This means the passengers may need warmer clothes at altitude and oxygen tanks may reflect lower pressures than what was measured before takeoff. Additionally, oxygen tanks stored outside of an aircraft will reflect lower pressures while at altitude because the cold air will cause the oxygen within the tank to contract, thus lowering the internal pressure.[1-11]

Henry's Law

Henry's law deals with the solubility of gases in liquids. The law states: "The quantity of gas dissolved in 1 cm^9 (1 mL) of a liquid is proportional to the partial pressure of the gas in contact with the liquid." The absolute amount of any gas dissolved in liquid under conditions of equilibrium is dependent on the solubility of the gas in the liquid, the temperature, and the partial pressure of the gas.[9] A simpler variation is the weight of a gas dissolved in a liquid is directly proportional to the weight of the gas above the liquid.[1-11]

Ultimately, gases can be forced to dissolve into a solution (like body fluids); as the pressure over a fluid rises, more gas is dissolved into the fluid. This means as high pressure is removed, the gas will want to come out of solution. This can be illustrated by a soda can being opened. Before opening, the contents of the can have been pressurized, allowing the CO_2 to be dissolved into the soda. Once the can is opened, the pressure in the can becomes the same as the atmospheric pressure (much less than when the can was pressurized), and the gas violently escapes. When a scuba diver ascends too rapidly from a deep dive, nitrogen bubbles can form in the blood and cause a form of decompression sickness that acts like CO_2 released from soda.

Graham's Law (Law of Gaseous Diffusion)

Graham's law states that the rate of diffusion of a gas through a liquid medium (such as the membranes throughout the body) is directly related to the solubility of the gas and inversely proportional to the square root of its density or gram molecular weight.[9] In other words, Graham's law simply states substances with lower molecular weights will dissolve faster through a membrane and that gases with higher solubility stay in liquids longer.[b] This does not have a direct impact on patient care or equipment management but is discussed to offer a thorough review of the gas laws that will be experienced.

Fick's Law

Fick's Law is another diffusion law that states that the diffusion rate of a gas is proportional to the difference in partial pressure and the surface area of the membrane, and is inversely proportional to the thickness of the membranes. This law directly relates to oxygenation with respect to ventilator management. By increasing the FiO_2, the partial pressure of oxygen delivered to a patient is increased, resulting in an increasing SpO_2. In a disease process like emphysema the alveolar walls are destroyed, which shrinks the surface area of the alveoli. This results in decreased oxygenation. In patients with congestive heart failure, pulmonary edema is present, which increases the thickness of the alveolar capillary membranes. This increased thickness reduces oxygenation. Therefore to increase oxygenation in patients on a mechanical ventilator, the FiO_2 (partial pressure) would be increased and positive end expiratory pressure added, which both increases surface area and thins the alveolar capillary membrane.[1-11]

Stresses of Transport

Multiple stresses that may be caused by air medical transport have been identified. According to the US Air Force,[3] which has done the most research about stresses related to flight, the eight classic stresses of flight are as follows:

- Hypoxia
- Hyperventilation
- Barometric pressure changes

---

[b]Note: Carbon dioxide is more soluble than oxygen.

- Gastrointestinal (GI) changes
- Thermal changes
- Decreased humidity
- Noise
- Vibration
- Fatigue
- Gravitational forces
- Aircraft motion
- Cabin Pressurization

Additional stresses related to transport include the following:

- Spatial disorientation
- Flicker vertigo
- Fuel vapors

Hypoxia

Within the air medical environment, different types of hypoxia are found. An understanding of the terms *hypoxia*, *hypoxemia*, and *hypercapnia* is essential to establish a foundation of knowledge about the effects of decreased partial pressure of oxygen.

Hypoxia is a general term that describes the state of oxygen deficiency in the tissues. It refers to a decrease in tissue oxygen or an oxygen supply inadequate to meet tissue needs.[1-5,10,11,13,14] Hypoxia disrupts the intracellular oxidative process and impairs cellular function.[10,11]

Many factors may interfere with a blood cell's ability to carry oxygen to the body. Anemia, altitude, alcohol, medications, carbon monoxide poisoning, and heavy smoking can all decrease the blood's ability to absorb and transport oxygen.

Hypoxemia refers to a decrease in arterial blood oxygen tension (PaO_2). A normal PaO_2 does not guarantee adequate tissue oxygenation; conversely, a low PaO_2 may not indicate tissue hypoxia and may be clinically acceptable.[1-5,10,11,13,14]

Hypercapnia refers to an increased amount of carbon dioxide in the blood.[10,15,16]

Four Stages of Hypoxia

Four stages of hypoxia need to be considered when examining its effects on human pathophysiology. These four stages are divided by altitude. The first stage is the *indifferent stage.* The physiologic zone for this stage starts at sea level and extends to 10,000 feet. In this stage the body reacts to the lessened availability of oxygen in the air with a slight increase in heart rate and ventilation. Night-vision deterioration occurs at 5000 feet. The second stage is the *compensatory stage,* which occurs from 10,000 to 15,000 feet. In this stage, the body attempts to protect itself against hypoxia. Increases in blood pressure, heart rate, and depth and rate of respiration occur. Efficiency and performance of tasks that require mental alertness become impaired in this stage. The third stage is the *disturbance stage,* which occurs between 15,000 and 20,000 feet. This stage is characterized by dizziness, sleepiness, tunnel vision, and cyanosis. Thinking becomes slowed, and muscle coordination decreases. The *critical stage* is the fourth stage of hypoxia. This stage occurs between 20,000 and 30,000 feet and features marked mental confusion and incapacitation followed by unconsciousness, usually within a few minutes.[11] Table 4.1 contains a summary of the stages of hypoxia and its effects on humans.

Types of Hypoxia

Based on the physiologic effects elicited on the body, hypoxia can be divided into four different types: hypoxic hypoxia, hypemic hypoxia, stagnant hypoxia, and histotoxic hypoxia.

Hypoxic hypoxia is a deficiency in alveolar oxygen exchange. A reduction in PO_2 in inspired air or the effective gas exchange area of the lung may cause oxygen deficiency. The result is an inadequate oxygen supply to the arterial blood, which in turn decreases the amount of oxygen available to the tissues.[10] Decreased barometric pressure at high altitudes causes a reduction in the alveolar partial pressure of oxygen (PaO_2). The blood oxygen saturation, which is 98% at sea level, is reduced to 87% at 10,000 feet and 60% at 22,000 feet. This reduction in the amount of oxygen in the blood decreases the availability of the oxygen to the tissues and causes an impairment of body functions.[10] Hypoxic hypoxia is also referred to as altitude hypoxia because its primary cause is exposure to low barometric pressure. Hypoxic hypoxia interferes with gas exchange in two phases of respiration: ventilation and diffusion. During the ventilation phase, a reduction in PaO_2 may occur. Specific causes include breathing air at reduced barometric pressure, strangulation/respiratory arrest/laryngospasm, severe asthma, breath holding, hypoventilation, breathing gas mixtures with insufficient PO_2, and malfunctioning oxygen equipment at altitude. Causes of reduction in the gas exchange area include pneumonia, drowning, atelectasis, emphysema (chronic obstructive pulmonary disease), pneumothorax, pulmonary embolism, congenital heart defects, and physiologic shunting. Some causes of diffusion barriers are pneumonia and drowning.[9,11]

Hypemic hypoxia is a reduction in the oxygen-carrying capacity of the blood. If the number of red blood cells per unit volume of blood is reduced, as from various types of anemia or from a loss of blood, the oxygen-carrying capacity and thus the oxygen content of the blood are reduced.[9] Even with normal ventilation and diffusion, cellular hypoxia can occur if the rate of delivery of oxygen does not satisfy metabolic requirements as from poor saturation of oxygen to the red blood cell.[1-5,10,13,14] Hypemic hypoxia interferes with the transportation phase of respiration and causes a reduction in oxygen-carrying capacity. Specific causes of hypemic hypoxia include anemia, hemorrhage, hemoglobin abnormalities, use of drugs (e.g., sulfanilamides, nitrites), and intake of chemicals (e.g., cyanide, carbon monoxide).[1-5,10,13,14] Carbon monoxide is significant to air medical crews because it is present in the exhaust fumes of both conventional and jet-engine aircraft. It is also present in cigarette smoke and any fire or smoke situations. Carbon monoxide binds with hemoglobin 200 times more readily than does oxygen and displaces oxygen to form carboxyhemoglobin.[1-5,9,13,14]

Stagnant hypoxia occurs when conditions result in reduced total cardiac output, pooling of the blood within certain regions of the body, a decreased blood flow to the tissues, or restriction of blood flow.[9] Stagnant hypoxia interferes with the transportation phase of respiration by reducing systemic blood flow. Specific causes include heart failure, shock, continuous positive-pressure breathing, acceleration (g forces), and pulmonary embolism. A reduction in regional or local blood flow may be caused by extremes of environmental temperatures, postural changes (prolonged sitting, bed rest, or weightlessness), tourniquets (restrictive clothing, straps), hyperventilation, embolism by clots or gas bubbles, and cerebral vascular accidents.[1-5,9,13,14]

Histotoxic hypoxia (tissue poisoning) occurs when metabolic disorders or poisoning of the cytochrome oxidase enzyme system results in a cell's inability to use molecular oxygen.[1-5,9,13,14] Histotoxic hypoxia interferes with the utilization phase of respiration because of metabolic poisoning or dysfunction. Since every cell of the body needs oxygen and sugar to engage in metabolism, without oxygen normal metabolism cannot occur. Poisons such as carbon monoxide, cyanide, and alcohol all prevent oxygen from cellularly uniting with sugar, and anaerobic metabolism is allowed to occur.[1-5,9,13,14] It is important to mention that carbon monoxide poisoning can cause both hypemic and histotoxic hypoxia, but it has a greater effect on histotoxic hypoxia.[1-11]

Effective Performance Time and Time of Useful Consciousness

These two terms are frequently used synonymously but are not without difference. *Effective performance time* (EPT) denotes the amount of time an individual can perform useful flying duties in an environment of inadequate oxygen.[7,11] *Time of useful consciousness* (TUC) refers to the elapsed time from the point of exposure to an oxygen-deficient environment to the point at which deliberate function is lost.[5,7,8,11] EPT more accurately refers to critical (functional) performance than does TUC. With the loss of effective performance in flight, an individual is no longer capable of taking the proper corrective or protective action.[5,7,8,11] Thus for air medical personnel the emphasis is on prevention.

In addition to altitude, factors that influence TUC are rate of ascent and an individual's physical fitness, physical activity, temperature, individual tolerance, and self-imposed stresses, such as smoking, intake of alcohol and medication, and fatigue.[10] Another factor that dramatically reduces both EPT and TUC is rapid decompression, which occurs when a quick loss of cabin pressure occurs in a pressurized aircraft at high altitudes. On decompression at altitudes above 10,058 m (33,000 feet), an immediate reversal of oxygen flow in the alveoli takes place, caused by a higher PO_2 within the pulmonary capillaries, which depletes the blood's oxygen

TABLE 4.2	Average Time of Useful Consciousness for Nonpressurized Aircraft	
Altitude (in feet)	**Time**
18,000 and lower	30 min
25,000	3–5 min
30,000	90 sec
35,000	30–60 sec
40,000 and higher	15 sec or less

reserve and reduces the EPT at rest by up to 50%. Exercise also reduces the EPT considerably.[5,7,8,11] Table 4.2 presents altitude and TUC.

Causes

Hypoxia has the three following causes: (1) high altitude, (2) hypoventilation, and (3) pathologic condition of the lung.

Characteristics

The onset of hypoxia may be gradual or insidious. Intellectual impairment occurs, demonstrated by slowed thinking, faulty memory of events, lessened immediate recall, delayed reaction time, and a tendency to fixate.

Early Signs and Symptoms

The individual symptoms of hypoxia can be identified in subjects under safe and controlled conditions in an altitude chamber. Once recognized, these symptoms do not vary dramatically in similar time exposures or among subjects. Hypoxia can be classified by objective signs (those perceived by an observer) or subjective symptoms (those perceived by the subject).[17] Signs and symptoms that appear on both lists in Table 4.3 may be seen by observers and recognized by the hypoxic subject when they occur.[10,15-17]

Cyanosis has been determined to be an unreliable sign of hypoxia because the oxygen saturation must be less than 75% in persons with normal hemoglobin levels before it is detectable.[10,15-17]

Treatment

The treatment for hypoxia is administration of 100% oxygen. The type of hypoxia needs to be determined so that treatment can be administered accordingly. The following are required steps for transport team members:

1. **Administer supplemental oxygen under pressure.** Provision of adequate supplemental oxygen is the prime consideration in the treatment of hypoxia. Consideration must be given to the altitude and the cause of the oxygen deficiency. Equipment malfunction or altitude exposure above 12,192 m (40,000 feet) cannot be corrected without the addition of positive pressure.[c]

---

[c]Positive-pressure breathing is the opposite of normal breathing.

TABLE 4.3	Signs and Symptoms of Hypoxia
Objective Signs	**Subjective Symptoms**
Confusion	Confusion
Tachycardia	Headache
Tachypnea	Stupor
Seizures	Insomnia
Dyspnea	Change in judgment or personality
Hypertension	
Bradycardia	Dizziness
Arrhythmias	Blurred vision
Restlessness	Tunnel vision
Slouching	Hot and cold flashes
Unconsciousness	Tingling
Hypotension (late)	Numbness
Cyanosis (late)	Nausea
Euphoria	Euphoria
Belligerence	Anger

The physiologic requirements for breathing are as follows:

Normal	**Positive Pressure**
Inspiration—active	Inspiration—passive
Expiration—passive	Expiration—active

The proper method of positive pressure breathing is as follows:

Inhale slowly → Pause → Exhale forcibly → Pause

2. **Monitor breathing.** After a hypoxic episode, the resulting hyperventilation must be controlled to achieve complete recovery. A breathing rate of 12 to 16 breaths per minute or slightly lower aids recovery.
3. **Monitor equipment.** The most frequently reported causes of hypoxia are lack of oxygen discipline and equipment malfunction. A conscientious preflight check of equipment and frequent in-flight monitoring reduce this hazard. Inspection of oxygen equipment when hypoxia is suspected may detect its cause. Ground-transport team members must also conduct the same careful inspection of their equipment before and after transport to prevent any problems with their oxygen-delivery system during transport. Correction of a malfunction should bring immediate relief of the hypoxic condition. If treatment for hypoxia does not remedy the situation, oxygen contamination should be suspected. Use of an alternative oxygen source, such as the emergency oxygen cylinder or portable assembly, should be considered. Descent should be initiated as soon as possible, and the contents of the oxygen system should be analyzed.
4. **Descend.** Increasing the ambient oxygen pressure by descending to lower altitudes, particularly below 3048 m (10,000 feet), is also beneficial. Descent to a lower altitude

compensates for malfunctioning oxygen equipment that may have caused the hypoxia.[10,15,16]

The primary treatment of hypoxia for any patient being transported is prevention. The transport team must remember that the patient's condition is already compromised and that stresses related to transport increase the risk of patient hypoxia unless the transport team continuously monitors the patient and accurately anticipates the oxygen needs of the patient during transport.

Hyperventilation

Hyperventilation at altitude is an important consideration for air medical personnel and for the air medical patient. Hyperventilation is of concern because it produces changes in cellular respiration. Although the causes are unrelated, the symptoms of hyperventilation and hypoxia are similar and often result in confusion and inappropriate corrective procedures. Despite increased knowledge, training, and improved life-support equipment, both hypoxia and hyperventilation are hazards in flying and diving operations.[10,17] *Hyperventilation* is an abnormal increase in the rate and depth of breathing that upsets the chemical balance of the blood[10,11,15,16]; it is commonly caused by psychological stress (e.g., fear, anxiety, apprehensiveness, anger) and environmental stress (e.g., hypoxia, pressure breathing, vibration, heat). Certain drugs such as salicylates and female sex hormones also cause or enhance hyperventilation, and any condition that creates metabolic acidosis results in hyperventilation at high altitudes.[10,11,15,16]

Treatment

At high altitudes, hyperventilation and hypoxia are treated in the same way because of similarities in the signs and symptoms. The following steps describe the treatment:
1. Administer 100% oxygen.
2. Begin positive-pressure breathing, which is the same as supplemental oxygen under pressure.
3. Regulate breathing and watch for hyperventilation.
4. Check equipment.
5. Descend.

The treatment for hyperventilation in the air medical patient is administration of oxygen. If treatment is successful, the amount of oxygen in the blood increases. Oxygen transfers from air to blood 20 times slower than carbon dioxide, and carbon dioxide transfers 20 times faster from blood to air than oxygen, which explains why the amount of carbon dioxide in the blood is directly associated with ventilation. When a patient is hyperventilating from anxiety, the act of putting a mask on the face to administer oxygen probably heightens the anxiety and increases tidal volume. Tidal volume must be reduced.[17] More favorable responses can be obtained by talking to patients to distract them, identifying causes of hyperventilation, and suggesting specific exercises to reduce respiratory rate. Several helpful exercises include the following:
1. The patient should count to 10 slowly while exhaling.
2. The patient should inhale and exhale only 10 times per minute.

3. Using a watch with a second hand, the patient should set a respiratory rate between 10 and 12 breaths per minute.
4. The air medical team member can provide counter-pressure by suggesting isometric or active-passive exercises[6] that cause the patient to hold the breath and reduce the respiratory rate.

Barometric Pressure Changes

Boyle's law states that at a constant temperature, the volume of a gas is inversely proportional to the pressure. On ascent, gases expand; on descent, gases contract. Therefore trapped or partially trapped gases within certain body cavities (e.g., the GI tract, lungs, skull, middle ear, sinuses, teeth) expand in direct proportion to the decrease in pressure.[2,5,8,10,11,15,17,18]

Middle Ear

The *middle ear cavity* is an air-filled space connected to the nasopharynx by the eustachian tube. The eustachian tube has a slit-like orifice at the throat end that allows air to vent outward more easily than inward. During ascent, air in the middle ear cavity expands but normally vents into the throat through the eustachian tube when a pressure differential of approximately 15 mm Hg has been reached. A mild fullness is usually detected but disappears as equalization occurs. This constitutes the *passive process.*[4,5] On descent, however, a different situation exists. The eustachian tube remains closed unless actively opened by muscle action or high positive pressure in the nasopharynx. If the eustachian tube opens, any existing pressure differential is immediately equalized. If the tube does not open regularly during descent, a pressure differential may develop. If this pressure differential reaches 80 to 90 mm Hg, the small muscles of the soft palate cannot overcome it, and either reascent or a maneuver that is not physiologic is necessary to open the tube.[10,11,15,16,19] On descent, equalization of pressure in the middle ear can be accomplished by performing the Valsalva's maneuver, yawning, swallowing, moving the lower jaw, topical administration of vasoconstrictors, or use of a bag-valve mask. These procedures are examples of the *active process.*

Gum chewing is not recommended as a method of pressure equalization because it causes swallowing of air, causing gastric distention and discomfort.

Barotitis Media *Barotitis media,* frequently referred to as an ear block, results from failure of the middle ear space to ventilate when going from low to high atmospheric pressure (i.e., on descent).[10,11,15,16] Pressure in the middle ear becomes increasingly negative, and a partial vacuum is created. As the pressure differential increases, the tympanic membrane is depressed inward and becomes inflamed, and petechial hemorrhages develop. Blood and tissue fluids are drawn into the middle ear cavity, and if equalization with ambient pressure does not take place, perforation of the tympanic membrane occurs. Severe pain, tinnitus, and possibly vertigo and nausea can accompany acute barotitis.[10,11,15,16] Priority is placed on patient briefing before flight and adequate instructions for air medical crews. The ears should be cleared on descent with the methods previously described. Patients who are sleeping should be awakened before descent so they can clear their ears in the normal manner.

Patients with colds or upper respiratory tract infections must be closely monitored during both ascent and descent for swollen eustachian tubes, which interferes with normal equalization procedures.[10,11,15,16] Air medical crew members with upper respiratory tract infections should not fly.

If an ear block occurs, mild vasoconstrictors should be administered early, and the plane should reascend to a higher altitude until symptoms lessen or the patient's ear block clears. If patients have ear pain during ascent, which rarely occurs, air medical personnel should not have them execute a Valsalva's maneuver because that would only aggravate the problem; instead, personnel should have them swallow or move their jaw muscles or administer a mild vasoconstrictor.[3] Either the Politzer bag or a source of compressed air may be used. A patient's nose should be sprayed with a decongestant solution to attain maximal shrinkage of the mucosa. For the Politzer bag method, the olive tip is placed in one nostril, the nose is compressed between the air medical crew member's fingers, and the patient is then instructed to say "kick, kick, kick" while the bag is squeezed, increasing the pressure in the nasopharyngeal cavity to the point at which the eustachian tube is opened and the middle ear space ventilated.[3]

In review, the treatment is as follows:
1. Patient performs Valsalva's maneuver.
2. Crew member administers vasoconstrictor spray.
3. Crew member administers Politzer bag or bag-valve mask.
4. Aircraft reascends.

Delayed Ear Block A *delayed ear block,* which occurs after the flight is terminated, results from breathing 100% oxygen during flight. As the ears clear during descent, 100% oxygen is forced into the middle ear cavity.[3,10] In addition, the absorption of oxygen by the middle ear and mastoid mucosa also contributes to the relatively negative pressure in those cavities. The patient may be symptom free immediately after flight, but if the oxygen in the middle ear is not replaced with air, the surrounding tissues absorb it, creating a negative pressure within the cavity. Delayed barotitis media occurs when oxygen absorption is the primary factor in the development of a pressure differential.[3,10,18] This condition causes a tightness or "stopped-up" sensation in the ears and slight to possibly severe pain. To prevent delayed ear problems, the patient should perform the Valsalva's maneuver periodically after the flight.[3] However, if a flight is completed in the late-evening hours or during the night and the individual retires a short time later, a significant pressure differential may develop during sleep because of the combined effects of oxygen absorption and infrequent swallowing.[19] Patients who are maintained on 100% oxygen during flight are especially susceptible to this problem.[10,11,15,16]

Flight crew members who continue to have ear pain after flight can treat it with decongestants and analgesics. If symptoms persist, flying at high altitudes should be avoided until the symptoms subside. If the team member has had a ruptured tympanic membrane, several days to weeks may be needed before it heals, and they should not fly until cleared.[1]

Barosinusitis (Sinus Block)

The sinuses usually present little problem when subjected to changes in barometric pressure. Because a free flow of air exists between the sinus cavities and the exterior, the sinuses automatically equalize with ambient pressure when the air in them expands or contracts.[1]

Barosinusitis is an acute or chronic inflammation of one or more of the paranasal sinuses produced by the development of a pressure difference, usually negative, between the air in the sinus cavity and that of the surrounding atmosphere.[2,19] Common causes of barosinusitis are colds and upper respiratory tract infections. Patients with such problems should be closely monitored during ascent and descent.[2,19] The symptoms of barosinusitis are usually proportional to its severity and may vary from a mild feeling of fullness in or around the involved sinus to excruciating pain. Pain can develop suddenly and be incapacitating.[2,19] Another symptom is possible persistent local tenderness. The immediate treatment for barosinusitis is to reascend until the pressure within the sinus equals the cabin pressure, administer vasoconstrictors to reduce swelling, and descend as gradually as possible to afford every opportunity for pressure equalization.[2,19]

Barodontalgia

Barodontalgia, or aerodontalgia, is a toothache that is caused by exposure to changing barometric pressures during actual or simulated flight.[2,19] The precise cause of barodontalgia has not been determined; however, exposure to reduced atmospheric pressure is obviously a significant factor. This exposure is evidently a precipitating factor, with disease of the pulp the primary cause. Pressure changes do not elicit pain in teeth with normal pulps, regardless of whether a tooth is intact, carious, or restored.[2,19]

Some pathologic conditions may cause no symptoms at ground level but be adversely affected by a change in barometric pressure. Barodontalgia commonly occurs during ascent, with descent bringing relief.[4] Moderate to severe pain that usually develops during ascent and is well localized generally indicates direct barodontalgia. The patient or crew member is frequently able to identify the involved tooth. This condition can usually be prevented by high-quality dental care with an emphasis on slow, careful treatment of cavities and the routine use of a cavity varnish. Indirect barodontalgia is a dull, poorly defined pain that involves the posterior maxillary teeth and develops during descent.[10] If patients have tooth pain during descent, especially involving the upper posterior teeth, they may have barosinusitis and should be treated accordingly.[2,19]

A crew member who undergoes dental treatment involving deep restorations should be restricted from flying for 48 to 72 hours after treatment to allow time for the dental pulp to stabilize.[2,19]

Gastrointestinal Changes

Gas contained within body cavities is saturated with water vapor, the partial pressure of which is related to body temperature. In determining the mechanical effect of gas expansion, one must account for the noncompressibility of water vapor, which causes wet gases to expand faster than dry gases.[2,19] The stomach and intestines normally contain a variable amount of gas at a pressure that is equivalent to the surrounding barometric pressure. On ascending to high altitudes, however, the gases in the GI tract expand. Unless the gases are expelled by belching or the passing of flatus, they may produce pain and discomfort, make breathing more difficult, and possibly lead to hyperventilation or syncope.[2,19] Severe pain may cause a vasovagal reaction that consists of hypotension, tachycardia, and fainting. Abdominal massage and physical activity may promote the passage of gas. If this treatment is unsuccessful, a descent should be initiated to an altitude at which comfort is achieved.[19] Because the possibility of decompression does exist, however, certain precautionary measures should be taken to reduce the chances of GI gas-expansion difficulties. Such measures include avoiding hasty and heavy meals before flight, such as gas-forming foods; carbonated beverages; and foods that are not easily digested.[2,11,19] Normally, the average GI tract has approximately 1 L of gas present at any one time. Wet gas expands its original volume at 9000 feet.

One useful example is a pediatric patient with abdominal distention. Gas expansion in the abdominal cavity, if untreated, can increase to such a volume that it raises the diaphragm. With diaphragmatic crowding, lung volume and expansion are decreased. If this distention is large enough, the great blood vessels in the area are compressed, which alters the blood supply to vital organs.[2,10,11]

Patients with ileus (bowel obstruction) or recent abdominal surgery should have a gastric tube placed before transport. The gastric tube should not be clamped but should be vented for ambient air or low intermittent suction during transport. After abdominal surgery, pockets of air may remain in the abdominal cavity. For this reason, general recommendations are that patients not be transported by air until 24 to 48 hours after the surgery. Patients who have undergone colostomy should be advised to carry extra bags because of more frequent bowel movements that result from gas expansion.[9-11,15,16] Colostomy bags should be empty and properly vented before air medical transport. Penetrating wounds allow ambient air to travel along the wound tract. According to Boyle's law, penetrating wounds to the eyes, neck, thorax, abdomen, and lower extremities can cause the introduction of emboli, in addition to irreparable damage to nerves and surrounding tissues.

Thermal Changes

An increase in altitude results in a decrease in ambient temperature. Consequently, cabin temperature fluctuates considerably depending on the temperature outside the aircraft.[3] The ratio of altitude to temperature is fairly constant from sea level to approximately 35,000 feet. Temperature decreases by 1°C for every 100-m (330-feet) increase in altitude. From flight level (FL) 350 to FL 990, the temperature fluctuates from ±3°C to 5°C. The temperature remains relatively isothermic at approximately −50°C from FL 350 to FL 990.[2,10] Vibration and thermal change, depending on whether the change is to greater heat or more cold, can have either an antagonistic or a synergistic effect. The body's primary response to heat exposure is vasodilation and activation of cooling mechanisms. Exposure to cold and vibration stimulate vasoconstriction and decreased perspiration.[2] Exposure to whole-body vibration appears to interfere with the normal human cooling responses in a hot environment by reducing blood flow and decreasing perspiration.[6] Turbulence can be produced by high and low temperature changes in the air. Turbulence increases stress during flight by promoting fatigue and increasing one's susceptibility to motion sickness and disorientation.

The transport team must also keep in mind that some medications can also interfere with the maintenance of a constant body temperature. Sedatives, analgesics, some psychoactive agents, and neuromuscular blocking agents are only a few examples of the medications that can place the patient at risk for problems with body temperature regulation.

Both hyperthermia and hypothermia increase the body's oxygen requirement. Hyperthermia increases the metabolic rate, and hypothermia increases energy needs because of shivering, increasing the body's oxygen consumption.[3] Air medical crews can facilitate maintenance of adequate body temperature with blankets, warm clothing, and warm liquids.[6] An additional way to facilitate thermoregulatory control is with a first-aid thermal blanket, which is sometimes called a space blanket.

Decreased Humidity

Humidity is the concentration of water vapor in the air; as air cools, it loses its ability to hold moisture. Because temperature is inversely proportional to altitude, an increase in altitude produces a decrease in temperature and, therefore, a decrease in the amount of humidity. The fresh-air supply is drawn into the aircraft cabin from a very dry atmosphere.[3] Before takeoff, small amounts of moisture are present in the cabin air from clothing and other items on board that retain moisture, in addition to expired air from crew members, patients, and other passengers. As the aircraft altitude increases, the air exhausted overboard carries

away trapped moisture. Eventually, all the original moisture is lost. The only moisture that remains is supplied by crew members, patients, other passengers on board, and the fresh-air system.[2,4,6] For example, on a typical flight of a military jet aircraft known as a C-141 Starlifter, which is a high-speed, high-altitude, long-range aircraft used for troops, cargo, and air medical transport, less than 5% relative humidity remains after 2 hours of flying time. Relative humidity decreases to less than 1% after 4 hours.[2,4,6,10] Propeller-type aircraft are not as dry inside because they do not fly as high; the lowest relative humidity levels reached on typical propeller aircraft flights range from 10% to 25%.[8] Patients and air crew members may become significantly dehydrated because of the decreased humidity at high altitudes. The ventilation systems on aircraft draw off what little moisture there is and contribute further to the decrease in the percentage of humidity. For a healthy person, low humidity results in nothing more than chapped lips, scratchy or slightly sore throat, and hoarseness. Steps that the medical crew member can take to minimize problems caused by decreased humidity include mouth care, use of lip balm, and adequate fluid intake. Patients who receive in-flight oxygen therapy are twice as susceptible to dehydration because oxygen itself is a drying agent. Humidified oxygen should be used on extended patient transports. The transport team must be certain that when humidifiers are used they are changed often to prevent contamination.

Patients who are unconscious or unable to close their eyelids must be provided with eye care. The administration of artificial tears and the taping shut of lids prevent corneal drying. Before transport, patients with compromised conditions predisposed by age, diet, or preexisting medical or surgical complications need special consideration with respect to decreased humidity.

Transport team members should also maintain adequate fluid intake to prevent dehydration. Water or other appropriate liquids need to be available during both air and ground transport.[20]

Noise

Sound is any undulatory motion in an elastic medium (gaseous, liquid, or solid) capable of producing the sensation of hearing. Normally, the medium is air.[12,20] *Sound waves* are variations in air pressure above and below the ambient pressure.[12,20] Sound is described in terms of its intensity, spectrum, and time history. The *intensity* of a sound wave is the magnitude by which the pressure varies above and below the ambient level. It is measured with a logarithmic scale that expresses the ratio of sound pressure to a reference pressure in decibels (dBs), which are the units used to describe levels of acoustic pressure, power, and intensity.[20] The *spectrum* of a sound represents the qualities present distributed across frequency. The frequency of periodic motion (e.g., sound and vibrations) is the number of complete cycles of motion taking place in a unit of time, usually 1 second. The international standard unit of frequency is the hertz (Hz), which is 1 cycle per second.[12] *Pressure–time histories* describe variations in the sound pressure of a signal as a function of time. The frequency content is not quantified in pressure–time histories of signals, so analytic techniques must be applied to the signal to obtain frequency or spectrum characteristics.[9,20]

Theoretically, sound waves in open air spread spherically in all directions from an ideal source. Because of this spherical dispersion, the sound pressure is reduced to half its original value as the distance is doubled, which is a 6-dB reduction in sound pressure level.[9,20] Hence, several factors are involved in the creation of sound. In relation to the definition of sound, it is usually easier to think of sound as comprising intensity, which is commonly thought of as merely loudness, in decibels; frequency, in cycles per second and pitch; and duration.

Thus noise, which is dependent on sound, can be more easily defined. *Noise* may be defined subjectively as a sound that is unpleasant, distracting, unwarranted, or in some other way undesirable.[9,20] The human hearing mechanism has a wide range and is fairly tolerant, but at times in an aircraft this tolerance is exceeded, with the following potential effects:

- Communications in the form of speech and other auditory signals inside the aircraft or air-to-air or air-to-ground may be degraded.
- The sense of hearing may be temporarily or permanently damaged.
- Noise, acting as a stress, may interfere with patient care and safe transport.
- Noise may induce varying levels of fatigue.[9,20]

The A-level of a decibel (dBA) is a unit of noise measurement that correlates most closely with the way a human ear accommodates sound or noise. The dBA is a single measurement that incorporates both amplitude and the selective frequency response features that most closely parallel those of the human ear. When ambient noise levels exceed 80 to 85 dBA, a person must usually shout to be heard.[9,20] Essentially, unprotected exposure to noise can produce one or more of the following three undesirable auditory effects: interference with effective communication, temporary threshold shifts (auditory fatigue), or permanent threshold shifts (sensorineural hearing loss).[9,20] Auditory fatigue incurred by noise is frequently accompanied by a feeling of "fullness," high-pitched ringing, buzzing, or a roaring sound in the ears (tinnitus). Tinnitus usually subsides within a few minutes after cessation of the noise exposure; however, for some individuals, the tinnitus may continue for several hours.[3] Most of the truly significant forms of undesirable response to acoustic noise, such as nausea, disorientation, and excessive general fatigue, are associated with only very intense noise, which air medical personnel rarely encounter during normal airlift operations.[9,20] Other hazards of exposure are loss of appetite and interest, diaphoresis, salivation, nausea or vomiting, headache, fatigue, and general discomfort.

Noise in the transport environment also impairs the ability of the transport team to perform patient assessment before and during transport. Aircraft noise, sirens, and traffic and crowd noise can interfere with the evaluation of breath sounds, auscultation of blood pressure, or even when obtaining patient information. Propeller aircraft noise is a loud tonal noise from piston or turbo propeller engines in the cabin. A beating noise may occur when the tonal noises from two propellers are at similar levels but differ slightly in frequency. Rotorcraft cabin noises can come from impulsive, periodic, and broadband noises from rotors and structures such as the gearbox. The noise from a helicopter contains both high-level and low-frequency noise. Jet aircraft also produce high frequency–level noise that increases with liftoff and climbing out.[9-12,15-17,20]

Transport team members need to rely on monitoring devices to measure patient blood pressure and monitor oxygen saturation, tube placement, and overall perfusion. Visible signs of distress or discomfort such as increased respiratory rate, changes in skin color, and grimacing may provide additional information about a patient's condition and comfort in a noisy transport environment.

Table 4.4 provides an example of the numbers of decibels that result from certain sources. Whenever the noise cannot be controlled at a desirable level, ear protection devices that attenuate the noise on its way from the surrounding air to the tympanic membrane must be worn, whether in an aircraft or ground transport vehicles. Such devices include helmets, earplugs, and earmuffs. Because effectiveness can vary considerably depending on a device's basic performance and personal fit, all transport team personnel should be carefully instructed regarding quality and size selection and techniques for use.[10] Earplugs are inert devices, and headsets and earmuffs are occluding devices. Earplugs must fit tightly to offer the maximum allowable attenuation; the only requirement for using airtight earplugs during flight operations is that the plugs be removed before descent. Pressure changes that result from decreased altitude tend to pull the plugs inward toward the tympanic membrane.[3] Transport team members should have their hearing evaluated on a yearly basis.

The Commission on Accreditation of Medical Transport Systems[13] requires that all RW personnel wear helmets during

TABLE 4.4　Decibels and Source

Decibels	Source
60	Normal conversation at 1 m
80	Garbage disposal
88	Propeller aircraft flyover at 1000 feet
90	Noisy factory Cockpit of light aircraft
103	Jet flyover at 1000 feet
117	Jet on runway in preparation for takeoff
110–130	Construction site during pile driving

patient transport operations. This requirement should help decrease the risk of hearing damage related to RW transport and will hopefully improve team member communications during transport.[13]

A patient's hearing, particularly that of an unconscious patient, needs to be protected during transport; therefore a headset or earmuffs should be placed on all patients.

Vibration

Vibration is the motion of objects relative to a reference position (usually the object at rest) and is described relative to its effect on humans in terms of frequency, intensity (amplitude), direction (regarding anatomic axes of the human body), and duration of exposure.[3,9-12,15-17,20] Most vehicles contain two principal sources of vibration: the first originates within the vehicle (specifically, the power source), and the second comes from the environment, which encompasses the terrain over which the land vehicle travels, the turbulence of the air through which the aircraft flies, or the status of the sea in which the ship sails.[2,9,10] Thus both air and ground vehicles cause vibration.

Helicopter vibration occurs with broadly similar intensity in all three axes of motion. Large differences in the amplitudes of specific harmonics in different modes of flight may exist, but the overall amplitude of vibration tends to increase with airspeed and with the loading of the aircraft. Vibration is usually worse during transition to the hover position.[3,9-12,15-17,20]

In fixed-wing aircraft, any vibration from the power source is usually at a higher frequency than in helicopters. The main source of vibration encountered in fixed-wing aircraft is the atmospheric turbulence through which the aircraft flies. Consequently, the most severe vibration usually occurs during storm-cloud penetration or during high-speed low-level flight. The response of the aircraft to atmospheric turbulence is determined by the aerodynamic loading on the wings. An aircraft with a large wing area relative to its weight undergoes greater amplitude low-frequency excursions from level flight because of turbulence.[2,9-12,15-17,20]

Resonance frequencies of body structures produce a more pronounced effect than do nonresonant frequencies.[9] Vibration between 1 and 12 Hz has been firmly established to cause performance decrement in the cockpit. For example, low-frequency vibration can induce motion sickness, fatigue, shortness of breath, and abdominal and chest pain.[9] Research has established that a human's sensitivity to external vibration is highest between 0.5 and 20 Hz because the human system absorbs most of the vibratory energy applied within this range, with maximal amplification between 5 and 11 Hz. The most physiologically harmful frequencies lay between 0.1 and 40 Hz.[9]

When the human body is in direct contact with a source of vibration, mechanical energy is transferred, some of which is degraded into heat within those tissues that have dampening properties. The response to whole-body vibration is an increase in muscle activity to maintain posture and possibly to reduce the resonant amplification of body structures. This response is reflected in an increase in metabolic rate under vibration and a redistribution of blood flow with peripheral vasoconstriction. The increase in metabolic rate during vibrations is comparable with that seen in gentle exercise. Respiration is increased to achieve the necessary increase in elimination of carbon dioxide (CO_2).[2-4,9,10,13] Disturbances in dynamic visual acuity, speech, and fine-muscle coordination result from vibration exposure.[2-4,9,10,13] The effects of vibration on the body can be reduced by attention to the source of vibration, modification of the transmission pathway, or alteration of the dynamic properties of the body.[2-4,9,10,13] Pain from injuries such as fractures or disease states can be increased, which causes the need for additional analgesia and sedation. Sensors, electrodes, leads, endotracheal tubes, and intravenous lines may become disconnected or dislodged. Vibrations then could make replacement of these during the transport difficult.[2-4,9,10,13]

Vibrations can also interfere with transport equipment such as cardiac and blood pressure monitors. The equipment should be secured in the transport vehicle in a manner least conducive to vibrations.

Aircraft manufacturers have eliminated severe vibrations by improving designs and materials; however, some vibrations still occur as a result of engine operation, flap and landing gear extension and retraction, and general aircraft movement. To minimize reactions to vibrations in either air or ground transport vehicles, transport crew members should properly secure patients, encourage and assist them with position changes, and provide adequate padding and skin care.[2-4,9,10,13]

Fatigue

All the many operational stresses of transport may induce fatigue to some degree. Fatigue is an inherent stress of transport duties. Erratic schedules, hypoxic environments, noise and vibration, and imperfect environmental systems eventually take their toll; therefore, in transport, fatigue is always a potential threat to safety.[9-12,15-17,20]

Fatigue is the end product of all the physiologic and psychological stresses of flight associated with exposure to altitude.[9-12,15-17,20] Fatigue can also result from self-imposed stressors regardless of the type of transport. Box 4.1 shows self-imposed stresses that can have disastrous results.

Gravitational Force

In terms of practical application for civilian air medical transports, the effects of g force are limited and, in most cases, negligible. For an examination of force as a stress of flight, an understanding of mass, speed, velocity, and acceleration is helpful to clarify the concepts of exerted forces.

Speed is the rate of movement of a body regardless of the direction of travel. *Velocity* is the rate (magnitude) of change of distance and direction of travel of an object and is, therefore, a vector quantity. The velocity of a body changes if its speed or direction of travel changes. It is expressed as the rate of change of distance in a specified direction. *Acceleration* is the rate of change of velocity of an object, and like velocity, it is a vector quantity.[5]

Weight is the force exerted by the mass of an accelerating body.[3,5] *Mass* is a measure of the inertia of an object (e.g., its resistance to acceleration).[3,5] Newton's three laws of motion define the relationship between motion and force[3,5]:

1. **Newton's First Law of Motion.** Unless it is acted on by a force, a body at rest will remain at rest and a body in motion will move at a constant speed in a straight line.
2. **Newton's Second Law of Motion.** When a force is applied to a body, the body accelerates, and the acceleration is directly proportional to the force applied and inversely proportional to the mass of the body.
3. **Newton's Third Law of Motion.** For every action, there is an equal and opposite reaction.

Two types of acceleration must be considered: linear and radial. *Linear acceleration* is produced by a change of speed without a change in direction. In conventional aviation, prolonged linear accelerations seldom reach a magnitude that could produce significant changes in human performance because most aircraft do not exert sufficient thrust to produce extended changes in linear velocity. However, significant linear accelerations that last 2 to 4 seconds are produced during catapult-assisted takeoffs and arrested landings and when reheat is engaged in certain high-performance aircraft. Large prolonged linear accelerations occur during the launching of spacecraft and during slowing on reentry into the Earth's atmosphere. *Radial acceleration* is produced by a change of direction without a change of speed. Such accelerations occur when the line of flight is changed. Aircraft maneuvers are, by far, the most common source of prolonged acceleration in flight. Accelerations on the order of 6 to 9*g* or more can be maintained for many seconds by circular flight in agile military aircraft.[3,5]

When the main interest is the effect of acceleration on humans, the direction in which an acceleration or inertial force acts is described with the use of a three-axis coordinate system (X, Y, and Z), in which the vertical (Z) axis is parallel to the long axis of the body. Considerable confusion can result if a clear distinction is not made between the applied acceleration and the resultant inertial force because these, by definition, always act in diametrically opposite directions.[3,5]

Aircraft Motion

Because space is three-dimensional, linear motions in space are described with reference to three linear axes, and angular motions with three angular axes. In aviation, customary terms are the longitudinal (fore-aft), lateral (right-left), and vertical (up-down) linear axes and the roll, pitch, and yaw angular axes.[3,5]

Linear Axes	Angular Axes
Longitudinal axis (fore-aft)	Axis of roll
Lateral axis (right-left)	Axis of pitch
Vertical axis (up-down)	Axis of yaw

The relationship of this three-axis system with its action on humans is illustrated in Table 4.5.

Long-Duration Positive Acceleration

The crews of agile aircraft are frequently exposed to sustained positive accelerations ($+g_z$) with changes in the direction of flight, either in turns or in recovery from dives. Exposure to positive acceleration usually causes deterioration of vision before any disturbance of consciousness. For example, exposure to $+4.5$ g_z typically produces complete loss of vision, or "blackout," but hearing and mental activity remain unaffected. Exposure to a positive acceleration stress somewhat greater than that required to produce blackout results in unconsciousness. At moderate levels of acceleration (5–6*g*), blackout precedes loss of consciousness, but at higher accelerations, unconsciousness occurs before any visual symptoms occur.[3,5]

Long-Duration Negative Acceleration

Flight conditions that cause negative accelerations ($-g_z$) are outside loops and spins and simple inverted flight and recovery from such maneuvers. Tolerance for negative acceleration is much lower than that for positive acceleration, and the symptoms produced by even -2 g_z are unpleasant and alarming. Furthermore, low levels of negative acceleration produce serious decrements in performance.[1,2,3,5,14,18]

Long-Duration Transverse Acceleration

Accelerations of long duration acting at right angles to the long axis of the body ($+g_x$) rarely occur in present-day conventional flight. They are usually confined to catapult launches, rocket-assisted and jet-assisted takeoffs, and carrier landings, although forces more than -2 g_x may build

TABLE 4.5 **Three-Axis Coordinate System for Describing Action on Humans regarding Direction of Acceleration and Inertial Forces**

Direction of Acceleration	Direction of Resultant Inertial Forces	Physiologic and Vernacular Descriptors	Standard Terminology
Headward	Head to foot	Positive g Eyeballs down	$+g_z$
Footward	Foot to head	Negative g Eyeballs up	$-g_z$
Forward	Chest to back	Transverse A-P-G Supine g Eyeballs in	$+g_x$
Backward	Back to chest	Transverse P-A-G Prone g Eyeballs out	$-g_x$
To the right	Right to left	Left lateral g Eyeballs left	$+g_y$
To the left	Left to right	Right lateral g Eyeballs right	$-g_y$

up during flat spins. However, the forces in these maneuvers are small relative to human tolerance and do not cause problems.[1,2,5,14,18]

The definitions of the effects of g forces given here are applicable to high-performance aircraft, mostly fighter type, and to emergency situations. The longitudinal axis is most important in air medical transports. However, the effects of g forces are usually encountered only with forces greater than 1.5g.

Cabin Pressurization

The pressure environment that surrounds the Earth can be divided into the four zones: physiologic, physiologically deficient, space-equivalent, and space. These zones are characterized according to their physiologic effects as follows:

Physiologic zone: From sea level to altitudes up to 10,000 feet.

Physiologically deficient zone: Altitudes from 10,000 to 50,000 feet.

Space-equivalent zone: Altitudes from 50,000 to 250,000 feet.

Space: Altitudes beyond 250,000 feet.

In the physiologic zone, humans are well adapted. Although middle ear or sinus problems may be experienced during ascent or descent in this zone, most physiologic problems occur outside this zone and when proper protective equipment is not used. In the physiologically deficient zone, protective oxygen equipment is mandatory because the decrease in barometric pressure results in oxygen deficiency and causes altitude hypoxia.[8-12,15-18,20] Additional problems may result from trapped and evolved gases. Travel in the space-equivalent and space zones requires either a sealed cabin or a full-pressure suit.

Generally, the most effective way to prevent physiologic problems is to provide an aircraft pressurization system so the occupants of the aircraft are never exposed to pressures outside the physiologic zone. In cases in which ascent above the physiologic zone is necessary, protective oxygen equipment must be provided.[8-12,15-18,20] Aircraft pressurization consists of increased barometric pressure within crew and passenger compartments, which reduces the cabin altitude, creating near-the-Earth atmospheric conditions within the aircraft.[18] Commercial passenger aircraft normally pressurize to the equivalent of 5000 to 8000 feet, with the aircraft ascending a bit over 40,000 feet (FL 400).[8,12,15,17] The conventional method, used in virtually all current aircraft, is to draw air from outside the aircraft, compress it, and deliver it into the cabin. The desired pressure is maintained within the cabin with control of the flow of compressed gas out of the cabin and to the atmosphere. The continuous flow of air ventilates the compartment; in most aircraft, this flow of air also controls the thermal environment within the cabin.[18]

The difference between the absolute pressure within an aircraft and that of the atmosphere immediately outside an aircraft is called the *cabin differential pressure.* Differential pressure is frequently controlled so that it varies with aircraft altitude. The two principal aircraft pressurization systems, isobaric and isobaric-differential, are described as follows[5]:

Isobaric system: Isobaric control maintains a constant cabin pressure while the ambient barometric pressure decreases. Many military and civilian aircraft are equipped with isobaric pressurization systems. This pressurization increases the comfort and mobility of the passengers, negates the necessity for the routine use of oxygen equipment, and minimizes fatigue.

Isobaric-differential system: Tactical military aircraft are not equipped with isobaric pressurization systems because the added weight severely limits the range of the aircraft and the large pressure differential increases the danger of rapid decompression during combat situations. Instead, these aircraft are equipped with an isobaric-differential cabin pressurization system. The isobaric function controls cabin pressure until a preset pressure differential is reached. With continued ascent, the preset differential is maintained. Thus the apparent cabin altitude progressively increases as the aircraft ascends.

In air medical transports, cabin pressurization is especially important. Not only does it protect the occupants from the physiologic hazards of altitude, but it also provides more effective control of cabin temperature and ventilation, promotes greater mobility and comfort, and reduces fatigue. Cabin pressurization does not eliminate all problems, however. Cabin pressure can be lost as a result of structural failure, such as a window or a door blowing out, or through a mechanical malfunction of pressurization equipment.[4]

Decompression

A loss of cabin pressure is referred to as *decompression*. Aircraft decompression can be slow and gradual, over a period of several minutes, or it can be sudden, within a matter of seconds.[4,10] The risk of injury from decompression increases in proportion to the ratio of the area of the defect to the volume of the cabin and to the ratio of cabin pressure before and immediately after the decompression.[6,9] The following factors control the rate of decompression[15,16]:

- Volume of the pressurized cabin: The larger the cabin, the slower the rate of decompression if all other factors are constant.
- Size of the opening: The larger the opening, the faster the rate of decompression. The most important factor is the ratio between the volume of the cabin and a cross-sectional area of the opening.
- Pressure differential: The initial pressure gradient between the initial cabin pressure and the initial ambient pressure directly influences the rate and severity of decompression. The greater the differential, the more severe the decompression.
- Pressure ratio: Time is directly related to the pressure ratio between the cabin and ambient pressures. The greater the ratio, the longer the decompression.
- Flight pressure altitude: The altitude at which decompression occurs relates directly to the physiologic problems that occur after the incident.

Box 4.2 illustrates the physical characteristics of decompression.

The physiologic effects of rapid decompression are hypothermia, gas expansion, hypoxia, and decompression sickness. Hypoxia is by far the most important hazard of cabin decompression of an aircraft flying at high altitudes.[15,16] The rapid reduction of ambient pressure produces a corresponding drop in the PO_2 and reduces the alveolar oxygen tension. A two- to threefold performance decrement occurs, regardless of altitude. The reduced tolerance for hypoxia after decompression is caused by (1) a reversal in the direction of oxygen flow in the lungs, (2) diminished respiratory activity

---

> **• BOX 4.2 Physical Characteristics of Decompression**
>
> **Slow Decompression**
>
> Onset is insidious and gradual and can occur without detection. Signs and symptoms are the same as for hypoxia. Decompression can be determined by checking the cabin altimeter.
>
> **Rapid Decompression**
>
> Onset is immediate, in 1 to 3 seconds, and is accompanied by noise, flying debris, and fog.
>
> **Noise**
>
> When two different air masses collide, a sound is heard that ranges from a swish to an explosion.
>
> **Flying Debris**
>
> On decompression, rapidly rushing air from a pressurized cabin causes the velocity of airflow through the cabin to increase rapidly as the air approaches the opening. Loose objects, such as maps, charts, and unsecured medical equipment, can be extracted through the orifice. Dust and dirt hamper vision for a short period of time.
>
> **Fog**
>
> During rapid decompression, both temperature and pressure suddenly decrease. This decrease reduces the capacity of air to contain water vapor and causes fog. The dissipation rate of fog is fairly rapid in fighter aircraft but considerably slower in larger multiplace aircraft.
>
> Modified from Chase NB, Kreutzman RJ: Army aviation medicine. In: DeHart RL, ed. *Fundamentals of Aerospace Medicine*. Philadelphia, PA: Lea & Febiger; 1985; Heimbach RD, Sheffield PJ: Decompression sickness and pulmonary overpressure accidents. In DeHart RL, ed. *Fundamentals of Aerospace Medicine*. Philadelphia, PA: Lea & Febiger; 1985.

at the time of decompression, and (3) decreased cardiac activity at the time of decompression.[15,16]

Crew members and passengers must protect themselves from the potential physiologic hazards caused by loss of cabin pressure. Because hypoxia is the most immediate hazard, all occupants must breathe 100% oxygen. Air medical personnel must first ensure that they are breathing 100% oxygen before attempting to assist their patients. Patients who already have oxygen deficiencies, such as patients with coronary disease, anemia, or pneumonia, must be closely monitored after decompression. After the prevention or correction of hypoxia, descent is made to an altitude below 10,000 feet, if possible.[3,9-12,15-17,20]

Decompression Sickness

The first human case of decompression sickness was reported in 1841 by M. Triger, a French mining engineer who noticed symptoms of pain and muscle cramps in coal miners who had been working in an air-pressurized mine shaft.[12,15-17] Because tunnel workers were first to have the syndrome now known as decompression sickness, early terminology describing this disorder was related to that occupation, hence, the names *caisson disease* and *compressed-air illness*.[2,5,15,16]

A distinct difference is found between compressed-air illness and *subatmospheric decompression sickness*, although they share the same colloquial nomenclature for the common manifestations. Classically, the main manifestations are limb pain (the bends), respiratory disturbances (the chokes), skin irritation (the creeps), various disturbances of the central nervous system (the staggers), and cardiovascular collapse (syncope). These symptoms of subatmospheric decompression sickness virtually always subside or disappear during descent to ground level. Rarely, however, does recovery occur after recompression to ground level, and in some cases, the severity of the symptoms may increase, accompanied by a generalized deterioration in the individual's condition, which is known as *postdescent collapse*.[2,5,15,16]

Although the finer points of the pathologic processes that underlie some of the manifestations of altitude decompression sickness remain unknown, the basic mechanism is supersaturation of the tissues with nitrogen.[9,12,15-17,20] Because the partial pressure of nitrogen in the inspired air falls with ascent to higher altitudes, nitrogen is carried by the blood from the tissues to the lungs, in which it exits the body in the expired gas. In addition, because the solubility of nitrogen in the blood is relatively low and some tissues contain large amounts of nitrogen, the rate of fall of the absolute pressure of the body tissues, which is associated with the ascent in altitude, is greater than the rate of fall of the partial pressure of nitrogen in the tissues. These tissues therefore become supersaturated with nitrogen. In certain circumstances, supersaturation gives rise to the formation of bubbles of gas, the main constituent of which is initially nitrogen, in specific tissues of the body. Gas exchange is the governing mechanism in the formation of the bubbles, and these bubbles subsequently grow in size through the diffusion of nitrogen and other gases such as oxygen and carbon dioxide from surrounding tissues.

The driving pressure for bubble formation in a fluid is the difference between the partial pressure of the gas dissolved in the fluid and the absolute hydrostatic pressure.[12] Henry's law can be applied as follows: the amount of a gas that dissolves in a solution and remains in that solution is directly proportional to the pressure of the gas over the solution. Nitrogen is metabolically inert. At sea level, the amount of nitrogen dissolved in the body tissues and fluid is in equilibrium with the ambient pressure. At higher altitudes, nitrogen evolves in a manner similar to the formation of bubbles in a carbonated beverage when the bottle cap is removed. Decompression sickness is not usually encountered below a pressure altitude of FL 250.[4] The clinical manifestations of decompression sickness are shown in Box 4.3.[15,16]

In a small number of cases, circulatory collapse or postdecompression collapse may occur. The clinical symptoms vary. Typically, the patient becomes anxious, develops a frontal headache, and feels sick. Facial pallor, coldness, and sweaty extremities may occur, and peripheral cyanosis almost always occurs. General or focal signs of neurologic involvement, such as weakness of the limbs, apraxia, scotomata, and convulsions, may occur. Arterial blood pressure is generally well maintained until late in the development of the illness. Finally, in the worst cases, coma supervenes. Recovery can

---

• BOX 4.3   Clinical Manifestations of Decompression Sickness

Skin

Paresthesia (numbness or tingling sensation)
Mottled or diffuse rash of short duration
Itching
Cold or warm sensations

Joints

"Bends" pain (mild to severe) in muscles and joints, caused by nitrogen bubbles in the joint space
Pain is mild at onset, becomes deep and penetrating, and eventually becomes severe
Pain usually affects (in order) knee, shoulder, elbow, wrist or hand, and ankle or foot
Pain increases with motion

Lungs

"Chokes" (rare in both diving and aviation)
Deep sharp pain under sternum
Dry cough
Inability to take a normal breath
Attempted deep breath causes coughing (frequently paroxysmal)
Condition progresses to collapse if exposure to altitude is maintained
"False chokes" (caused by breathing cold dry oxygen, which dries the throat and causes irritation and a nonproductive cough)

Brain

Visual disturbances
Headache
Spotty motor or sensory loss, or both
Unilateral paresthesia
Confusion
Paresis
Seizures

---

occur at any stage, but in the past, it has been rare once coma has developed.[2,5,15,16]

In addition to supersaturation of the tissues with nitrogen, other factors that influence susceptibility are the rate of ascent, altitude, time of exposure, reexposure to high altitude, body fat, age (if greater than 40 years), exercise before and after flight, presence of infection, and alcohol ingestion.[2,5,15,16]

The primary treatment of decompression sickness that arises at high altitudes is recompression to ground level as rapidly as possible. Breathing 100% oxygen also relieves the tissue hypoxia produced by the reduction of local blood flow. The actual management of a case of serious decompression sickness depends on geographic location and the availability of a suitable hyperbaric chamber. Therefore the order of preference of available treatment is as follows[8,15,16,18]:

1. Immediate hyperbaric compression with or without intermittent oxygen breathing should be administered.
2. Where no chamber facility exists, air medical personnel should treat circulatory collapse and arrange for early transfer to a hyperbaric chamber where this facility is available at a reasonable time or distance (less than 6 hours of travel time). Surface transport is preferable; flight to a suitable

chamber should be at an altitude below 1000 feet if possible and not higher than 3000 feet.

3. Air medical crew members should administer full supportive treatment for circulatory collapse if no possibility exists of transfer within a reasonable time to a hyperbaric chamber.

Transport team members should not fly for at least 12 hours after diving.

Additional Stresses of Transport

Spatial Disorientation

Spatial disorientation is described as an individual's inaccurate perception of position, attitude, and motion in relation to the center of the Earth.[1] When persons experience spatial disorientation, they cannot correctly interpret or process the information they are given by their senses. Spatial disorientation primarily occurs during air transport.

During flight, the following three systems are involved in maintenance of equilibrium: visual, vestibular, and proprioceptive. These systems combine to allow the appropriate interpretation of input. However, the visual system plays the most important role.

Spatial disorientation can cause the following visual illusions[1,5]:

- Cloud formations being confused with the horizon or ground.
- Water or desert appearing to be farther away than it is.
- During night flights, the perception is that another aircraft is moving away when it is actually getting closer.

These visual illusions can cause significant motion sickness, which may render pilots or transport team members incapable of performing their duties or providing patient care. Spatial disorientation can also lead to misinterpretation of a landing area and result in a crash.

To prevent spatial disorientation, transport team members should use proper scanning techniques, never stare at lights, get adequate rest and nutrition, and provide conscious patients with a tactile reference during transport.

Flicker Vertigo

Flicker vertigo can occur when transport team members and patients are exposed to lights that flicker at a rate of 4 to 20 cycles per second.[1,5,10] It can cause nausea and vomiting. In severe cases, it can cause seizures and unconsciousness. Flicker vertigo commonly occurs when sunlight flickers through the rotor blades of a helicopter or an airplane propeller. It has also been triggered by light from rotating beacons against an overcast sky.

Transport team members or patients with a history of seizures are at risk for flicker vertigo. Wearing a hat with a bill and sunglasses can prevent flicker vertigo. Adequate rest and stress management may also decrease the risk.

Fuel Vapors

Both ground and air transport can expose transport crew members and patients to fuel vapors. Jet fuel, diesel fuel, and gasoline are a few examples of what may be used in transport vehicles. Exposure to fuel vapors can cause altered mental status, nausea, and eye inflammation.[1,5,10]

Fuel vapors may be an indication of a problem in the transport vehicle and, when detected, should be immediately reported by the transport team. Adequate ventilation can help decrease the effects of exposure.[1,5,10]

Summary

To become an effective health care provider in the transport environment, each transport team member must be thoroughly familiar with the effects of the stresses of transport on the human body. Implementation of correct interventions is an essential responsibility of each team member to minimize the effects of the stresses of transport.

CASE STUDY

Transport Physiology 1

A 70-year-old man with a history of a nonembolic stroke is being transported via RW aircraft for treatment of sepsis. His vital signs are blood pressure 84/59 mm Hg, pulse rate 120 beats per minute (bpm; sinus tachycardia), respiratory rate (intubation on transport ventilator) 14 bpm, and rectal temperature 97°F.

He has been prepared for transport in a BK 117. When the pilot begins to turn the rotors, the flight nurse notices that the patient's eyes are blinking rapidly and he begins to have a generalized tonic-clonic seizure. The monitor shows ventricular fibrillation, but a pulse can be palpated.

The transport nurse asks the pilot to stop the engines so that the team may obtain resuscitation assistance from the referring hospital personnel. As the rotors slow down, the patient's seizure activity ceases. After a quick evaluation and administration of 2 mg of lorazepam, the transport team prepares to leave again. Once again, with the turning of the rotors, the patient has the same symptoms.

This time, the transport nurse covers the patient's eyes with a towel and the seizure activity ceases. The team keeps the patient's eyes covered throughout the transport without further seizure activity.

Discussion

Although flicker vertigo is not a common condition, sunlight flickering through rotor blades can trigger seizure activity in persons with seizure disorders or neurologic disorders that may place a patient at risk for seizures. This patient had had a recent stroke. Other clues that made the transport nurse consider flicker vertigo as the cause of this man's seizures are as follows:

- The patient care platform positioned the patient's face in front of a window.
- The day was sunny.
- The activity ceased when the rotor blades stopped and began again with start-up.

CASE STUDY

Transport Physiology 2

A 9-month-old infant was involved in a one-car MVC with frontal impact. Upon impact the infant was secured in a car seat. His vital signs are 82/58 mm Hg, pulse rate of 162 bpm (sinus tachycardia), respiratory rate 70 bpm, oxygen saturations 88%, and rectal temperature is 97°F. The patient appears very fatigued and is exhibiting see-saw respirations.

You and your partner decide to intubate the patient. The intubation is performed without incident. You package the patient for transport and prepare to transition the patient to the aircraft. An isolette is used to transport the infant. Just prior to departing the small county ER, the patient is on the mechanical ventilator and monitoring devices, and the patient seems to be stabilized. Upon departure, the patient's blood pressure is 91/61 mm Hg, pulse rate of 154 bpm, and the oxygen saturation is 96%.

The pilot launches the aircraft and it reaches cruise altitude. Within minutes, the patient's blood pressure drops to an undetectable value, the carotid pulse weakens, and the oxygen saturations drops to 76%. The tracheal tube is confirmed to be in the correct placement between the vocal cords. An isotonic crystalloid fluid bolus is administered. The FiO_2 is increased on the ventilator to 1.0. The patient's vitals do not correct with these treatments. Your partner makes a comment about how high up the aircraft is. You question the pilot as to your altitude and he replies 9500 feet.

You request the pilot descend to the lowest safest altitude and needle decompress the chest with an 18-gauge IV catheter into the 4th intercostal space at the anteaxillary line. This results in an immediate return of stable vital signs.

Discussion

The patient developed a tension pneumothorax. The initial impact of the MVC caused a very small, undetectable pneumothorax. When the pilot ascended to 9500 feet, the lower pressure at this altitude allowed the pneumothorax to develop into a tension pneumothorax, as predicted by Boyle's Law. A critical care transport team needs to be proactive in protecting their patients from the dangers of high flying.

References

1. Blumen I, Callejas S. Air Transport physiology: a reference for air medical personnel. In: Blumen I, Lemkin DL, eds. *Principles and Direction of Air Medical Transport*. Salt Lake City, UT: Medical Physicians Association; 2006.

2. Brashers V. Structure and function of the pulmonary system. In: McCance K, Huether S, eds. *Pathophysiology: The Biologic Basis for Disease in Adults and Children*. 7th ed. St. Louis, MO: Elsevier; 1225-1247.

3. Department of the Air Force. *Aeromedical Evacuation*. Washington, DC: US Air Force Pamphlet No 10-1403; 2011.

4. Egan F, Spearman CB, Sheldon RL. Gases, the atmosphere and the gas laws. In: Scanlon CL, Spearman CB, Sheldon RI, eds. *Egan's Fundamentals of Respiratory Therapy*. 4th ed. St. Louis, MO: Mosby; 1982.

5. Hawkins H. The aircraft cabin and its human payload. In: Orlady HW, ed. *Human Factors in Aviation*. 2nd ed. Aldershot, UK: Avebury Technical; 1993.

6. Kenefick W, Cheuvront SN, Castellani JW, et al. Thermal stress. In: Davis J, Johnson R, Stepanek J, eds. *Fundamentals of Aerospace Medicine*. 4th ed. Philadelphia, PA: Wolters Kluwer; 2008.

7. Martin TE. Clinical aspects of aeromedical transport. *Current aspects of aeromedical transport*. 2003;14(3):131-140.

8. Polikoff LE, Giuliano JS. Up, up and away: Aeromedical transport physiology. *Clin Pediatr Emerg Med*. 2013;14(3):222-230.

9. Thibeault S. *Transport Professional Advanced Trauma Course Manual*. 6th ed. Aurora, CO: Air and Surface Transport Nurses Association; 2015.

10. Woodward GA, ed. *Guidelines for Air and Ground Transport of Neonatal and Pediatric Patients*. Elk Grove Village, IL: American Academy of Pediatrics; 2007.

11. Clark Y, Stocking J, Johnson J. *Flight and Ground Transport Nursing Core Curriculum*. Denver, CO: Air and Surface Transport Nurses Association; 2007.

12. Rood GM. Noise and communication. In: Ernsting J, King P, eds. *Aviation Medicine*. 2nd ed. London: Butterworth; 1988.

13. Commission on Accreditation of Medical Transport Systems (CAMTS). *Accreditation Standards*. 10th ed. Anderson, SC: Author; 2015.

14. Banks RD, Brinkley JW, Allnutt R, et al. Human response to acceleration. In: Davis J, Johnson R, Stepanek J, eds. *Fundamentals of Aerospace Medicine*. 4th ed. Philadelphia, PA: Wolters Kluwer/Lippincott Williams & Wilkins; 2008.

15. Van Hoesen K, Bird N. Diving medicine. In: Auerbach P, ed. *Wilderness Medicine*. 6th ed. Philadelphia, PA: Elsevier Mosby; 2012:1520-1549.

16. Van Hoesen K, Bird N. Diving medicine. In: Auerbach P, ed. *Wilderness Medicine*. 6th ed. Philadelphia, PA: Elsevier Mosby; 2012:1549-1562.

17. Stepanek J, Webb JT. Physiology of decompressive stress. In: Davis JR, Johnson R, Stepanek J, eds. *Fundamentals of Aerospace Medicine*. 4th ed. Philadelphia, PA: Wolters Kluwer/Lippincott Williams & Wilkins; 2008.

18. Pickard JS, Gradwell DP. Respiratory physiology and protection against hypoxia. In: Davis JD, Johnson R, Stepanek J, eds. *Fundamentals of Aerospace Medicine*. 4th ed. Philadelphia, PA: Wolters Kluwer/Lippincott Williams & Wilkins; 2008.

19. Phelan JR. Otolaryngology in aerospace medicine. In: Davis J, Johnson R, Stepanek J, eds. *Fundamentals of Aerospace Medicine*. 4th ed. Philadelphia, PA: Wolters Kluwer/Lippincott Williams & Wilkins; 2008.

20. Smith D, Gooman JR, Grosveld FW. Vibration and acoustics. In: Davis JR, Johnson R, Stepanek J, eds. *Fundamentals of Aerospace Medicine*. 4th ed. Philadelphia, PA: Wolters Kluwer/Lippincott Williams & Wilkins; 2008.

5

Scene Operations and Safety

MARK LARSON

COMPETENCIES

1. Perform an initial scene evaluation to identify safety hazards.
2. Explain the purpose of the Incident Command System.
3. Identify potential hazardous materials and who to notify.
4. Verbalize general procedures for the decontamination process.
5. Understand general extrication principles/hazards as they apply to scene safety.
6. Define actions to take (e.g., THREAT) in an active shooter scenario.

Critical care transport personnel, particularly those working in rotor-wing aircraft, frequently participate in on-scene patient care. They are often preceded to the scene by other rescue personnel who have already managed scene hazards, freed trapped victims, and begun patient care. Nevertheless, extrication and scene management are important concepts for the transport team to understand thoroughly. Although familiarity with extrication, scene management, and hazardous material management exercises should be included in transport team initial and recurrent training, only transport team members with the appropriate training and appropriate personnel protective equipment (PPE) should participate in extrication or hazard management. More complex technical rescues, including hazardous materials response, trench collapse, confined space, and rope rescue situations, are "high-risk, low-frequency" events that require specially coordinated, equipped, trained, and competent rescue personnel.

Most often, the transport teams will operate in an environment in which other personnel manage the scene, extrication, and specialty rescues, while maintaining high situational awareness and attention to their personal safety. The failure of proper awareness and the failure to exercise personal and team restraint can result in direct injury, exposure, or contamination to both rescuers and victims and may delay patient care and transport. Even if a patient is safely removed from an incident, inattention to decontamination may result in a transport vehicle being taken out of service for an extended period of time

Scene Management

Prearrival/En Route Considerations

Scene evaluation begins when the communications center obtains information about possible problems and circumstances the rescuers may confront. The communication specialist should continue to seek information that could aid the rescuers throughout the incident, such as time of day, weather conditions, location, terrain, and number of victims, as well as information about fire, spilled fuel, toxic chemicals, overturned or entangled vehicles, and downed electrical lines. While approaching the scene, observe the terrain and attempt to understand the mechanism of injury, whether there was a head-on impact or rollover, the general speed of the vehicles, and other hazards that may present themselves as a result of the accident (i.e., downed lines, narrow bridges, or poor landscape access). For air operations, the opportunity to survey this information may be limited if one is being directed to a landing zone away from the accident. Information such as wind direction and speed is more easily gathered during daylight hours; vision at night can be limited, even with night vision goggles.

Before arrival, the communication center should relay contact information for on-scene providers. This information will be important for hazard communication, landing zone information for air operations, and postarrival deployment information.

At the scenes of roadway incidents there must be an adequate traffic control zone in which responders can operate (Fig. 5.1). This may directly abut an active traffic lane, so responders must be attentive to the boundaries of their safe work area. All responders, particularly all members of the transport team who will exit the vehicle, should wear traffic vests for visibility and safety. The traffic control zone, including roadways being used as landing zones or staging areas, should be blocked off with larger, well-lit emergency vehicles parked at an angle to deflect traffic away from the scene.[1] The team should discuss ingress and egress before approaching the scene, should be aware of hazards, and should understand vehicle loading options.

At the scene, the risk of a secondary incident involving property damage or personal injury to responding personnel

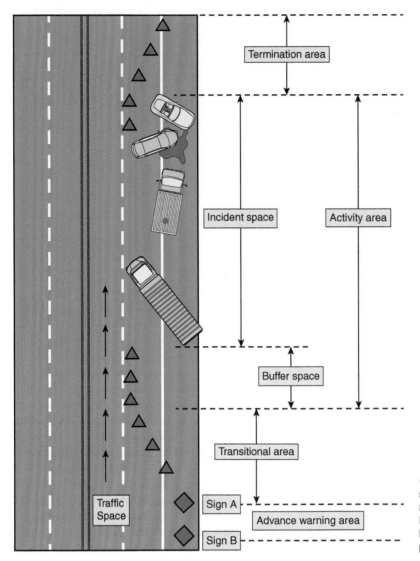

• **Fig. 5.1** Traffic control zone at roadway accident scene. (From *Federal Emergency Management Association publication*. United States Fire Administration–Traffic Incident Management Systems. Publication FA-330, Fig. 3.5. <https://www.usfa.fema.gov/downloads/pdf/publications/fa_330.pdf; 2012.)

is real. Factors associated with secondary incidents include the following:

- Lack of training
- Lack of situational awareness
- Failure to establish a sufficient traffic control zone for roadway incidents
- Improper positioning of apparatus
- Inappropriate use of scene lighting
- Failure to use safety equipment[1]

Proper placement of the helicopter is also essential in avoiding a second incident. Even with over four decades of civilian helicopter Emergency Medical Service (EMS) operations in the United States, landing zone incursions still occur. Landing zones should be secured by law enforcement or fire departments. The landing area may be of sufficient distance from the incident that it requires a second traffic control zone to be established, in which case the transport team should consider themselves as part of two separate incidents, with a need to operate safely in both and to plan the transit between scenes carefully.[1] If helicopters are left

running at the scene, a tail guard must be in place. Personnel leaving and approaching the aircraft should do so within sight of the pilot (Fig. 5.2). Landing zone requirements and operations are discussed elsewhere in this book.

Approach to the Incident

Once the vehicle has arrived safely, providers still must consider scene safety carefully in approaching the incident; never compromise the rescuers to aid the victims. The area should be appropriately secured by the referring agencies, and high situational awareness around the incident is imperative. Even with appropriate protective equipment, rescuers are at risk of injury. Defer to specialty expertise: the utility company should secure downed electrical lines, the fire department contains and controls hazardous materials, and scene security is usually provided by law enforcement personnel. Onlookers and the media should be kept well back from the operation (Box 5.1).

It is important not to lose sight of equipment being used at the scene. Fire hoses, extrication tools, stabilization

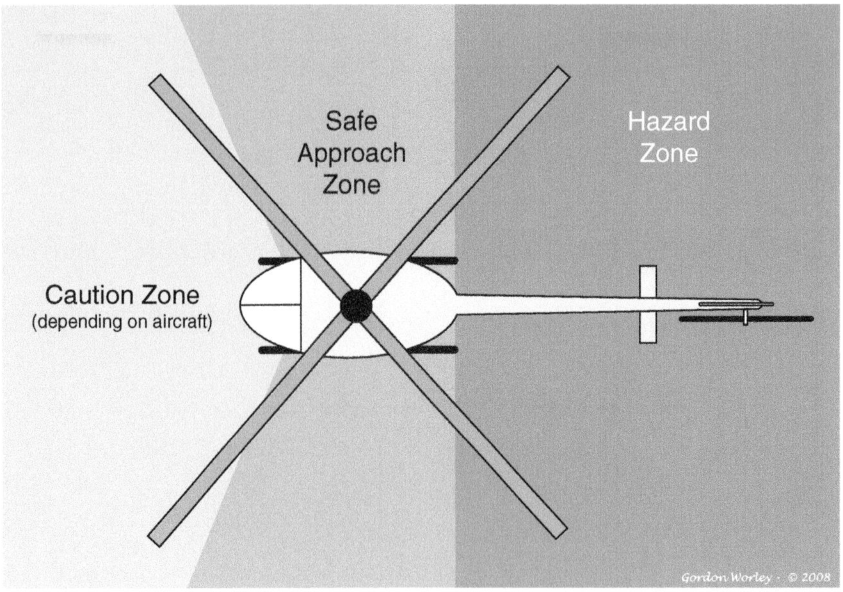

• **Fig. 5.2** Landing zone safety.

• BOX **5.1** **Scene Management Guidelines**

- Never compromise rescuers to aid victims.
- Evaluate the situation for potential safety hazards (e.g., traffic, utilities, gasoline, propane, fuel oil, water, sanitary systems, movement of vehicles, release of high-pressure systems).
- Report arrival to Incident Command and follow deployment instructions.
- Secure the accident scene and any traffic flow that may endanger rescuers.
- Wear personal protective equipment appropriate to the hazards on the scene (e.g., traffic vests, gloves, eye protection).
- Gain access to the patient only if trained and properly protected.
- Defer to specialty expertise for rescue and hazard management.

---

devices, and other equipment have a way of taking up much of the ground around an accident. Awareness of the ground around your feet can prevent an injury. Lighting around the scene is important for all personnel involved in the extrication for safety and ease of work.

Incident Command System

The Incident Command System (ICS) is a management method designed to clarify command relationships at incidents, to foster interagency cooperation, and to offer maximum flexibility for achieving strategic goals. The use of a common terminology facilitates communication and, during an incident, ICS allows transitions with only minimal adjustments—it is easily scalable in real time, both for expansion and contraction. Any incident that taxes the assets of the responding rescuers is considered a mass casualty incident (MCI), ranging from a three-patient motor vehicle crash in a resource-limited area to an event with overwhelming geographic scope or casualties. The ICS is designed to work effectively across the spectrum from minor incidents to complex MCIs or geographically disparate events.[1,2]

One or more individuals must always have authority over the incident, known as the command function. This can be a single person, the Incident Commander, or it may be a group of people who exert a unified command. Once command is established, usually by the most senior person in the initial response team, there are clear rules for the transfer of command and for the chain of command. Another key feature of ICS is a modular organization, allowing subgroups of the response team to be deployed to address needs. This modular function is what allows expansion and contraction, which is the feature that preserves the span of control (no individual is accountable for more than 3 to 7 people; Fig. 5.3).[1,2]

There are five functional areas for major incidents: command, operations, planning, logistics, and finance/administration. For most incidents, command and operations are in place and planning, logistics, and finance/administration often are not deployed, except on very large-scale, extended duration incidents. Field personnel will usually be involved under the Operations component, which consists of an Ops branch and may include a dedicated air operations branch. A staging area may also be assigned under Operations. Divisions and Groups are components that may be under the Branches, depending on the size of the incident, and may be responsible for search and rescue (SAR) or triage, for example.[1,2]

One essential feature of the ICS is that members report to their designated supervisor, who has a known location and assignment within the pyramid of the command structure. For the transport team, this requires identification of the appropriate supervisor, a clear report to that person, and following the given assignment. The transport team will generally report to the commander for operators, or some subpart of the Operations group. The team rarely reports directly to the Incident Commander.[1,2]

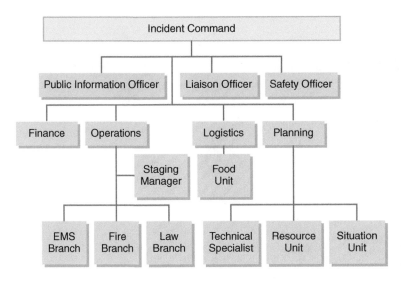

• **Fig. 5.3** Sample incident command structure. (Modified from Sanders MJ, Lewis LM, Quick G, et al. *Mosby's Paramedic Textbook*. 3rd ed. St Louis, MO: Elsevier/Mosby; 2007.)

Hazardous Materials Emergencies

The Department of Transportation (DOT) defines hazardous material as any substance or material that could adversely affect the safety of the public, handlers, or carriers during transportation. Emergencies that involve hazardous materials occur in all areas of the United States, and transport teams are likely to be involved in the care of those who have been injured. The key for the transport team, and all responders, is to remain a safe distance away until the hazard is identified, to avoid entering the scene and risking danger to themselves, and to avoid contaminating themselves and their vehicles by ensuring that patients are adequately decontaminated before entering the treatment area. When a hazardous material can be identified from a number or by name, emergency service personnel may obtain advice about the emergency from agencies that assist in the management of hazardous materials such as the Chemical Transportation Emergency Center (CHEMTREC) and the US DOT.[2-4]

Not every transport vehicle or locality containing hazardous materials is marked with a placard that identifies the specific materials on board. More often they have placards that identify only the category of material carried or a four-digit identification number (Fig. 5.4). The Emergency Response Guidebook (ERG), carried in all first response vehicles, provides the first responders with general information about hazardous materials. It focuses on protection of the responders and the general public and is meant to be used only during the initial response. The book is broken down into six color-coded sections, each dealing with different aspects of a hazmat response. The ERG has been around since 1973 and is still widely used throughout the world.[2-4]

The National Fire Protection Agency has developed a diamond sign to designate the different types and severity of hazards present on site. This diamond is made up of four different colored boxes, each representing a specific hazard class: blue for health hazard, red for flammability, yellow for reactivity, and white for special hazards. The special hazard box will also contain identification letters, such as AS (as-phyxiant), W (water reactive), or O (oxidizing agent). The three colored boxes will have a number between 0 and 4, representing increasing level of risk in the specific category.[2-4]

The shape of a transport vehicle or container can also provide some basic information. Rail and road transport units may have certain identifying characteristics. All pressure vessels will have rounded ends. High-pressure vessels will have fittings only at the top of the rounded vessel, whereas lower pressure containers may have fittings elsewhere. Flammable products will be in containers with an oval cross-sectional shape and fittings on the bottom of the tank. Compressed gas transport trailers have multiple smaller rounded tanks stacked together, whereas a trailer containing corrosives will usually have a large black ring around the center of the trailer.[2-4]

Transport teams responding to the scene of hazardous material emergencies follow these general guidelines[2-4]:
- Land the aircraft uphill, upwind, and far enough away from the scene to prevent rotor wash from spreading hazardous materials. Pilots should avoid flying over the top of hazardous materials areas.
- Keep out of low areas in which heavier-than-air vapors can accumulate.
- Hazardous Materials crews will establish "hot," "warm," and "cold" zones of operation. Transport teams should always stage in the Cold Zone to prevent risk of personal injury or contamination of the aircraft. Only hazardous materials responders trained to the technician or operations levels should operate in the Warm Zone, and only those trained to technician level should work in the Hot Zone (Fig. 5.5).[2]
- Rescuers should wear PPE that is appropriate for the situation, including respiratory and splash protection, as dictated by the nature of the hazardous material. Flight suits and flight uniforms are classified as Level D protection, the lowest level of protection possible.
- If there is a fire, some corrosive materials react violently with water. If attempting to extinguish a small fire, use dry chemical or carbon dioxide extinguishers.
- Stay away from the ends of tank vehicles.
- Cool down uninvolved containers exposed to heat.

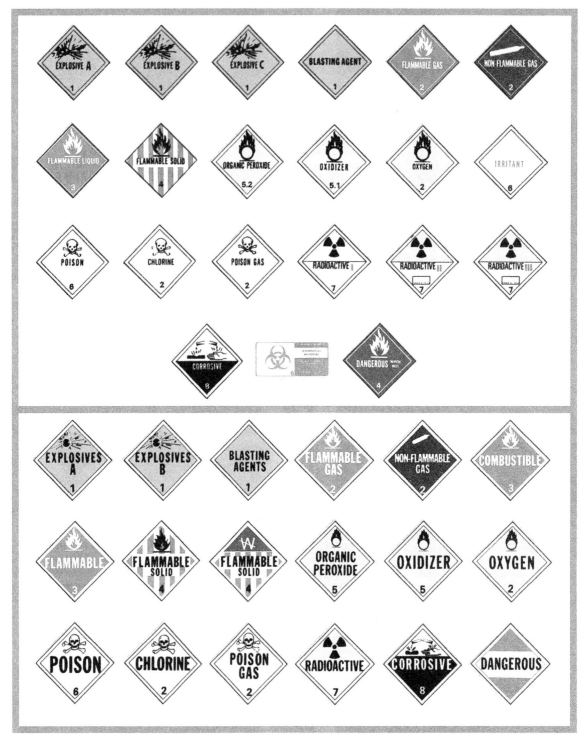

• **Fig. 5.4** Hazardous materials warning placards and labels. (From Sanders MJ, Lewis LM, Quick G, et al. *Mosby's Paramedic Textbook.* 3rd ed. St Louis, MO: Elsevier/Mosby; 2007.)

Decontamination

The following steps have been recommended for use when a person needs decontamination after exposure to a hazardous material. The decontamination corridor is called the Warm Zone and is located between the hot and cold zones. This zone should be the only point of entry and exit to the Hot Zone:

1. An entry point should be established for the "dirty" victims and rescuers to remove their clothing.

2. Surface decontamination should be performed with plenty of water unless the contaminant requires another decontaminant.
3. PPE should be removed and stored.
4. Other clothing may have to be removed, depending on the level of contamination.
5. Contaminated personnel and victims should be washed at least twice. Whenever possible, warm water with detergent should be used for decontamination.

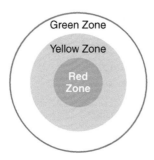

Red Zone—Hot (Contamination) Zone	Yellow Zone—Warm (Control) Zone	Green Zone—Cold (Safe) Zone
• Protective gear needed, highest potential for exposure • Number of personnel limited to those critical or necessary	• Surrounds contamination zone, decontamination takes place here • Prevents the spread of contamination • Protective gear needed • Emergency care and decontamination are performed	• Personnel sheds contaminated gear before entering, free from contamination • Normal care (triage, stabilization) and treatment here • Planning and staging area

• **Fig. 5.5** Safety zones for hazardous materials incident.

6. Victims and personnel should be medically evaluated.
7. Injured individuals should be transported for definitive care.
8. The decontamination site must be cleaned up and contaminated materials disposed.
9. All equipment that has been used should be decontaminated and cleaned.
10. Contaminated clothing should never be taken home and cleaned or transported with the patient. Remember that clothing may be evidence.
11. Decontamination procedures must meet Occupational Safety and Health Administration requirements 29 CFR 1910.120.

Radioactive Material Emergencies

Radioactive material emergencies are one variant of hazardous material emergencies. The degree of hazard varies greatly depending on the type and quantity of the radioactive material, and individual risk varies with time of exposure, distance from the source, and available shielding. Exposure can also come from inhalation, ingestion, or skin absorption. Although some radioactive materials may burn normally, they do not, as a class, ignite rapidly. Runoff from fire control or dilution activities can cause water pollution and thus spread the probability of contamination.[3,4]

Again, knowledge of the hazard is important. If only the yellow, black, and white "Radioactive Material" placards are visible and the material being carried cannot otherwise be identified, people nonessential to the firefighting or rescue operation should be kept at least 150 feet upwind of the area; greater distances may be advised by the radiation authority. Rescuers will only enter the spill area to save a life, will stay only the shortest possible time, and will have to wear full protective equipment and a positive-pressure breathing apparatus. Persons and equipment exposed to the radioactive material must then be detained until the radiation authority arrives or other instructions are received.[3,4]

Ensure that patients have undergone appropriate decontamination before being placed in any transport vehicle. Defer to expertise for determining appropriate decontamination. If the victim is not appropriately decontaminated, both the team and the transport vehicle can be contaminated if they are not protected. If the transport vehicle is contaminated, it needs to be taken out of service and decontaminated according to decontamination codes and guidelines.[3,4]

Transportation Emergency Scenes

Vehicle Extrication

Extrication teams at incidents will vary according to the location, resources, and emergency preparedness model. Rescue may be a function of a regularly responding team, or may be designated for a dedicated crew trained for most scenarios. These teams usually train on a regular basis with their equipment and are familiar with the needs required to free the entrapped patient. Transport teams should not participate in rescue or operate around rescue scenes without sufficient protective equipment (this is most easily described as the minimum equipment that the rescue team will wear for their evolutions).[5]

Any unanticipated vehicle movement is both unacceptable and unsafe for rescuers and occupants, so rescue crews should stabilize the vehicle before entry to prevent any unexpected movement. This is accomplished by some combination of placing cribbing blocks underneath the vehicle, flattening tires, and attaching stabilizing lines or struts. Before proceeding with patient extrication, rescue personnel should always ensure that the vehicle's tires are chocked, the key/engine is turned off, the transmission is placed in park, and, whenever possible, the vehicle's battery is disconnected.[5]

In approaching a patient who is presumed to be entrapped, always remember to "try before you pry." The simplest solution is usually the fastest and safest for the rescuer. Entry to the patient may be gained by simply unlocking an undamaged door, not necessarily the one nearest the patient, and opening it.[5]

The transport team may enter a vehicle after donning protective clothing, if trained or directed by a trained individual, and if the vehicle is stabilized and deemed safe. Flight suits and regular EMS uniforms are considered the lowest level of protective equipment. Entering a car in which a heavy rescue is about to take place requires that the medical personnel wear the same level of protective equipment as the other public safety personnel working on the rescue. Entry can be made through the car doors or by breaking out the glass and crawling through the windows. If the vehicle is lying on its side, access may be gained through the topside car door or rear window.[5]

The basic principle of extrication is that the rescuers should remove the vehicle from the victim rather than the other way around. If the vehicle is on its side, the extrication may be performed through the roof. If the vehicle is on its wheels or roof, extrication is conducted through the doors. If the vehicle is resting on its side and has been stabilized, extrication can be achieved by cutting an upside down U in the roof. The vehicle should be stabilized in the side position, the occupants should be warned of the very loud noise about to begin, and a heavy aluminized blanket should cover the occupants for their safety. After a three-sided U-shaped cut is made in the roof, the metal flap should be folded down to provide a smooth edge to move the victims across on their way out.[5]

Rescue personnel inside an upright vehicle should first unlock the doors and use interior handles while their partners use exterior handles to open the doors. Hydraulic "jaws" can be used to force a door open or remove the door for better access to the patient. They can also be used to force a seat backward on the tracks or make relief cuts in the vehicle floor for ease of moving the dash off victims' legs by a hydraulic ram or piston. High-volume, low-pressure air bags are used to lift a vehicle off a patient and can be rapidly deployed. Only trained individuals should operate this equipment for the safety of the patient and the rescuer.[5]

Occasionally, a victim's thorax becomes wedged between the forward-displaced seat and the rearward-displaced steering wheel/column, or a victim's feet and legs become trapped under the downward-displaced dashboard and the accelerator or brake pedal. A quick option to create more room between the victim, the seat, and the steering wheel is to manually slide the seat back, if it remains operational. Multiple rescuers should control the seat and the patient to avoid unnecessary movement and possible risk of further injury.[5]

Rescuers must also be aware of the hazard of air bags. Most recently built cars are equipped with these safety devices. Studies have documented the effectiveness of air bags in decreasing serious injuries to drivers and passengers. However, air bags can also cause injuries such as facial abrasions and lacerations and contusions to the chest and upper extremities. Undeployed air bags may be a potential hazard to the rescuer

---

• BOX 5.2 Considerations for Vehicles with Air Bags

- Disconnect or cut both battery cables. Always cut or disconnect the negative side first. Secure both cables so they do not spring back and touch each other or the battery.
- Avoid placing personnel or objects in front of the air bag deployment path.
- Do not mechanically displace or cut through the steering column until the system has been deactivated. Charts are available that indicate how long the air bag may take to deactivate. Some may take up to 30 minutes.
- Do not cut or drill into the air bag module.
- Do not apply heat in the area of the steering wheel hub.
- Be aware of other air bags within the vehicle (e.g., the side air bag).

---

and can cause injuries similar to those reported in accidents in which the air bag has deployed. Box 5.2 describes considerations for vehicles with air bags.[6,7]

Downed Aircraft

The crash of even a light aircraft requires the response of a variety of emergency service units, including fire, rescue, EMS, and law enforcement. It is helpful to have good prearrival information including the following:

1. Type of aircraft (e.g., small passenger plane, commuter aircraft, large commercial jet, military transport plane, military fighter aircraft, helicopter).
2. Whether the wreckage is on fire.
3. Identification numbers and markings of the aircraft. Military aircraft are marked "US Air Force," "US Navy," and so forth. Commercial aircraft show the name of the carrier. Private aircraft may have a combination of letters and numbers that constitute the identification number.
4. Status (e.g., on fire, damaged, collapsed) of any structures struck by the aircraft or its components.
5. Status of people in those structures, if known.
6. Vehicles that were struck by the aircraft or parts of it and the status of any persons inside the vehicles, if known.
7. Structures that appear to be endangered by encroaching fire, spilled fuel, military ordnance, and so on.

If the transport team arrives at the crash site before emergency service units, team members must proceed with caution. Survivors of the crash or persons who have been ejected from the aircraft may be lying anywhere about the site, including on the roadway leading to the crash site. There is a likelihood of a fuel spill and contamination of the occupants. If the aircraft is military, crew members must avoid both the front and rear ends of any externally mounted tanks or pods because these may be containers for missiles or rockets. The crew must be careful not to disturb any armament thrown clear of the aircraft, which may explode if improperly handled. No one should move body parts or components of the aircraft unless movement is necessary to care for injured persons.

Railroad Incidents

In the event of an accident involving a train, an essential prerequisite is to stop all other train activity in the area. The engineer of a train that is traveling at 60 mph has approximately 1 second to determine whether a collision is imminent and activate the emergency-braking system. The train will travel a distance of 7920 feet (1.5 miles). After the engineer applies the emergency brake, a train will continue for two-thirds of a mile before stopping, even when traveling at only 30 mph.

The universal railroad signal to stop a train before it reaches a grade crossing is to send a person to a point 1.5 to 2 miles from the grade crossing and swing a lighted flare slowly back and forth horizontally at right angles to the track. The locomotive engineer should acknowledge the signal with two whistle blasts and then stop the train. The engineer might either misinterpret or disregard other signs and not stop the train. A flare can be waved day or night. If a flare is not available, a flashlight, battery-powered hand light or lantern can be waved at night; a flag or other brightly colored object can be used during daylight.

Similarly, if the incident is a vehicle-train collision at an intersection, the actual accident scene may be a significant distance from the intersection or impact area. This can present several problems in locating patients. A wide area at the impact site narrowing to the front of the train would be appropriate for searching for patients. Any clues that may be present in the vehicle as to the number of patients would be helpful, such as car seats, purses, toys, and so forth.

For any railroad incident, locate the conductor promptly. The conductor is in charge of the train and has documents that show whether the train is carrying hazardous materials. If the conductor and other train members are incapacitated, the crew member can look in the documentation drawer for information about the train cargo. Car movement waybills and a consist should be available. *Waybills* are documents that describe the cargo and identify the shipper and receiver. The *consist* is a car-by-car listing of the contents of each rail car.

Do not imperil rescuers to aid victims. First, power to the train must be disrupted. Electric locomotives operate from an overhead electricity system that carries an 11,000-V alternating current. The overhead power must be disconnected by pressing the pantograph down button in the locomotive control cab. A derailed electric locomotive with a pantograph that remains in contact with overhead wires poses the same electrocution threat as power lines that rest on a vehicle if rescuers contact the locomotive and the ground at the same time. Steam generators are powered by diesel fuel. Fuel shutoff controls are located on each side of the car body under a cover plate marked Fuel Shutoff. The rescuer should lift the plate and pull the ring straight out 2 inches; the generator will stop running within 1 to 2 minutes.

When the power is secured, ultimately the train will need to be searched. Again, do not imperil rescuers: rescuers should not go under or near any unstabilized derailed cars that are piled high when passing close to the wreckage. A precariously perched car can come plunging down without warning. When searching for injured crew members in the locomotive, the crew will observe forward and rear cabin doors. If access cannot be achieved by opening these doors inward, a rescuer can come in through the sliding cabin windows. The entire cabin area, including nose section, boiler room, and electrical power transmission areas, should be searched for injured persons.

Searching the train for injured passengers requires sliding open the side or end car doors or entering through an emergency window. The crew should check the entire car, including the toilet and baggage areas. Side-entry doors on passenger cars may be locked and require tools to open. Side doors that slide in the car body panels have electric locks. The conductor and crew members have a skeleton key necessary to open this type of door latch. Access through dual-paned emergency exit windows is accomplished by shattering the outer tempered glass with a heavy, sharp, pointed tool, removing the inner window's rubber molding, and using a pry bar to remove the inner Lexan window.

Motor Coach Crashes

Vehicles, such as buses, equipped with diesel engines do not need continued electrical power to run the engine once it has been started. If possible, the rescuers should stop the engine by using the emergency stop button located on the driver's left-hand-side switch panel. If the engine does not stop with this button, most buses can be stopped by discharging a carbon dioxide fire extinguisher into the engine air intake located at the left rear corner of the coach. A dry chemical extinguisher will not be as effective, and the carbon dioxide should be aimed inward and toward the front of the coach.

Do not place anything under any portion of the coach until it is securely stabilized. The air suspension system bellows may deflate without warning, in which case the body of the coach may drop suddenly to within inches of the roadway.

The rescuers should enter the coach through the front door if possible, but only after the vehicle is stabilized. Again, ensure that anyone entering the vehicle is wearing proper safety equipment. Door unlocking and unlatching mechanisms can be found under the right-side wheel well, behind the front medallion, or to the left of the driver's seat, depending on the make and model of the bus. If the rescuers cannot enter through the front door, they can enter the bus through the windshield by removing the rubber locking strip from around the pane and then removing the pane. For a bus equipped with a restroom, access is possible by opening the small flap at the right rear window and lifting the latch bar to open the window. If the bus is lying on its side, entry may be possible through a roof access hatch or rear emergency window. Bus accidents are likely to overwhelm local rescue resources because of the high number of potential victims.

Electrical Emergencies

High-voltage lines are common on roadside utility poles. Wooden poles are sometimes used to support conductors of as much as 500,000 V. *Always* assume a downed line is charged ("hot") until a representative from the power company says otherwise. Energized downed lines may or may not arc and may or may not burn. Importantly, when an interruption of current flow is sensed in most power distribution systems, automatic devices may restore the flow two or three times over a period of minutes. No assurance can be given that a dead line at the scene of a vehicle accident will not become energized again unless it is disconnected from the system by a representative of the power company. Depending on the distances between poles, the danger zone may be as large as 600×1500 feet.

Any rescuer should stop the approach immediately if a tingling sensation is felt in the legs and lower torso. This sensation signals energized ground; current is entering through one foot, passing through the lower body, and leaving through the other foot. This current flow is possible because of the condition known as *ground gradient,* which means the voltage is greatest at the point of contact with the ground and then diminishes as the distance from the point of contact increases. If a tingling sensation is felt, the safest procedure is to bend one leg at the knee and grasp the foot of that leg with one hand, turn around, and hop to a safe place on one foot. This maneuver ensures that the body does not complete a circuit between sections of ground energized with different voltages.

Similarly, discourage ambulatory accident victims from leaving their vehicles until conductors that are either touching or surrounding the wreckage can be deenergized.

Rescues from Unique Locations

Wilderness Rescue

When considering rescue from wilderness locations, the mnemonic TOMAS will help with planning and safety[8]

T: Terrain (exposure, cliffs, water, forest, vegetation, hiking terrain, snow)
O: Obstacles (trees, loose rock, debris, wires, daylight, rotor wash, blade clearance)
M: Method (type of insertion and location, landing near or remote from patient, hover load)
A: Alternatives (wait for SAR, ferry SAR personnel, relocate patient, no go/abort mission)
S: Safety (first, last, always)

Confined Spaces

A worker may fall and be injured while working inside the confined space, including mines and caves. If any doubt exists about the quality of the air within the structure, rescuers should wear self-contained breathing units and a full set of protective clothing. Rescuers not certified in confined space rescue should attempt nonentry retrieval of victims via tag lines or other means without physically entering the confined space.[9,10]

The rescuer should consult with the plant safety engineer or manager at the confined space location. If a knowledgeable person is not present (as in a multiple-injury situation), the Confined Space Entry Permit, which should be displayed

near the entrance to the vessel, should be located and should provide helpful information about the following[9]:
• Requirements for special protective clothing
• The atmosphere in the confined space
• Presence of toxic, flammable, radioactive, or explosive materials
• Requirements for safety harnesses or equipment
• Requirements for respiratory protection
• The need for standby personnel before entry

The confined space can be further secured by having plant personnel close feed valves and charging chutes. A rescuer or other responsible person should be assigned to guard any valves or chutes to ensure that they are not inadvertently opened during the rescue operation. Additionally, plan personnel should deenergize any internal equipment by opening the main disconnect switch and installing a lockout device. The padlock key should be secured until the rescue operation is over.[9]

Construction Site Emergencies

If a transport team member is near a piece of construction equipment when aiding a sick or injured operator and the engine of the machine is still running, the team member should not touch any of the operating levers, pedals, or other controls but should ask another operator to shut down the engine. If the injured operator can communicate, the transport team member should ask how to shut down the machine. If another operator is not available and the sick or injured operator cannot provide instructions in the shutdown procedure and if the equipment is gasoline-powered, the medical team member should turn the key or master switch to the "off" position. If this does not work, the injured party should be moved away from the equipment and law enforcement should be charged with the safety of the machine.

Trench Collapse

Workers and emergency service personnel can be buried under tons of earth when unsupported trench walls collapse. Sheeting and shoring a trench is a labor-intensive task but absolutely necessary if a rescue operation is to be performed safely. The steps to be followed in case of a trench collapse are as follows[10]:
• Maintain a safe distance from the scene.
• Determine who is in charge.
• Assess the immediate injury problem. Determine whether the rescue team will operate in rescue mode or recovery mode; if the patient is obviously deceased, lives of rescuers should not be risked and all operations should proceed slowly and methodically to prevent unnecessary harm or injury to rescuers.
• Determine how many people are buried.
• Determine last known location of people who are buried. Look for tools, clothing, personal belongings, heavy equipment, machinery, or pipe locations. If an open pipe end is near the location of the trench collapse, victims may have dived into open pipe ends before being buried. If the pipe can be accessed safely through an access point,

rescuers should attempt communication inside the pipe to check whether victims may be inside the pipe.

- Control hazards by controlling traffic and spectator movement. All heavy equipment on scene must be parked, turned off, and locked out and tagged out. Heavy equipment should never be used during a rescue situation to dig out the patient.
- Make the trench and the trench lip safe.
- Ventilate the trench.
- Position a safety observer.
- Provide a second means of egress from the trench with ladders placed at opposite ends of the collapse site.
- If the trench cannot be made safe, dig to the angle of repose.

Once access to the trapped victims has been achieved, the rescuers can dig them out by hand and remove the mechanisms of entrapment. First, a rescuer should uncover each victim's head and chest and initiate emergency care measures. When all the victims have been assessed and the airway, breathing, and circulation have been treated, the rescuers can work to free them completely. Then, as the victim is freed, the victim should be secured to an extrication device and removed from the trench.[10]

Law Enforcement–Related Situations

Law enforcement officials expect the cooperation of other emergency personnel with a police emergency. A cooperative relationship must exist to successfully mitigate a situation.

Explosive Materials Emergencies

There are four types of injuries seen with explosions: fragmentation, overpressure, impact, and head. Fragmentation injuries occur from fragments exploding and traveling at a high rate of speed that penetrate the body and do immeasurable damage. Overpressure injuries happen when a shock wave travels through the air and damages gas-containing organs in the body. Lungs are the most susceptible and can show a delayed affect as the damage starts to build. These patients will need to be monitored for the potential of an injury to progress. Impact injuries are a result of the body being thrown by the force of the explosion and striking an object on landing or injuries by objects landing on the patient. Head injuries may consist of open wounds or a closed head injury. Violent movement from falls and pressures can cause significant damage to the brain and other structures. Spinal injuries can be associated with trauma to the head and should be suspected.[11]

Intentional explosions are meant to cause massive damage and loss of life. Rescuers must watch out for any secondary devices that are present and intended for the first responders. These devices may take the form of pipe bombs, backpacks, small packages, or a large vehicle or van. Larger communities have bomb disposal units that can clear an area. Structures around the blast must be watched for potential collapse issues.

It is common for rescuers to run into the scene to start to render care, but caution is warranted when entering a bomb scene. Full PPE is necessary because of the potential for widespread and large quantities of blood-borne pathogens.

Explosions may also be intentionally contaminated with biological or radioactive materials.

Active Shooter

Active shooter (AS) situations usually involve one or more suspects participating in a random or systematic shooting spree with the intent to harm or commit mass murder. These scenarios can easily fall into the category of an MCI. Law enforcement and EMS must focus on preparation to respond to these events with the intention of saving as many lives as possible.[12,13]

Recently a group, convened by the American College of Surgeons and the Federal Bureau of Investigation in Hartford, Connecticut, developed a concept aimed at increasing survivability in one of these incidents. Clinical evidence shows that the greatest cause of death in penetrating trauma is hemorrhage, and the Hartford Consensus identifies hemorrhage control as the most important requirement in response to an AS/MCI. The consensus also described necessary compression of the traditional hot, warm, and cold zones of safety in such incidents.[12,13]

The acronym THREAT outlines critical actions during an AS/MCI[12]:

T: Threat suppression
H: Hemorrhage control
R/E: Rapid extrication to safety
A: Assessment by medical providers
T: Transport to definitive care

Other on-scene precautions in these situations include the following[12]:
- Cautious approach to the scene, lights/sirens off early, distance approach.
- Look out for secondary devices.
- Be prepared to withdraw to safe area.
- Work in pairs.
- Responders must be easily identifiable.
- Advise hospitals early.
  See Figure 5.6.

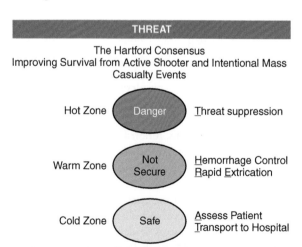

THREAT

The Hartford Consensus
Improving Survival from Active Shooter and Intentional Mass Casualty Events

Hot Zone — Danger — Threat suppression

Warm Zone — Not Secure — Hemorrhage Control Rapid Extrication

Cold Zone — Safe — Assess Patient Transport to Hospital

• **Fig. 5.6** Response to active shooter/intentional mass casualty incidents. (From Schneidman D, Jacobs LM, Burns KJ. Strategies to enhance survival in active shooter and intentional mass casualty events: a compendium. *Bull. Am. Coll. Surg.* 2015;100(1S):16-17.)

Firearms

A weapon found at the scene of an emergency must be left in the exact position in which it was discovered. Rescuers should assume the weapon is loaded and in operating order even if it appears otherwise. Law enforcement officers should be called.

If the weapon must be moved for any reason before police officers arrive, that task should be delegated to a trustworthy person. Only one person should handle the weapon until it can be turned over to the police officers. If a camera is available, a photograph can be taken of the weapon in place, with reference points, such as doors, windows, furniture, and so on, that will help investigators accurately place the weapon included in the picture. A photograph that shows only the weapon is useless. The number of live and expended rounds in a revolver, their position in the cylinder, and the status of the round under the hammer all may be important to investigators.[14]

A party handling the weapon should pick it up with the grips held between the fingers. Although this seems inconsistent with the policy of preserving fingerprints, it is the safe way to handle a handgun, and recognizable fingerprints cannot usually be recovered from checked grips. When carrying the weapon, the person should keep the barrel pointed in a safe direction, preferably skyward.[14]

Evidence Preservation

Many investigations have been seriously hindered because emergency service personnel inadvertently disturbed or destroyed articles of evidence at the scene of a crime. Investigators look at everything; something that seems of little importance may be a valuable piece of evidence to law enforcement personnel.

The transport team must keep unauthorized persons from the crime scene and not touch, kick, or otherwise move anything unless necessary during the rescue or during efforts to care for victims. Mental notes of possible clues can be extremely helpful later in the investigation, such as the position of a weapon, overturned furniture, or pooled blood. Clothing should be cut away from any deformities caused by trauma (e.g., bullet holes, stab wounds). Hands should be covered and sealed with paper bags to protect any evidence that may be present. As soon as rescue or emergency care activities are completed, observations can be shared with the investigating officers.[14]

At vehicle crash scenes, items of significance to accident investigators are tire marks, runoff from radiators and crankcases, blood, broken glass, vehicle trim, motor parts, and even clods of dirt turned up by a vehicle's wheels. To assist police investigators at the scene of a vehicle accident, the transport team should first rope off the crash site so physical evidence can be preserved in place and then keep spectators from picking up or moving pieces of debris. Photographs of the bottom of victim's shoes can help see if braking had been applied. Noting if seatbelts were present, cut, or unlatched can also indicate who was driving or assist in the investigation.[14]

Summary

Although the transport team may not be directly involved in extrication or rescue activities, crew members should be prepared to help the rescue effort and not endanger themselves so that they are unable to help the injured after they are rescued. Scene management of various incidences should be a component of all transport teams.

Air and ground transport teams can offer additional medical care and rapid transport to those injured in all types of incidents. Only transport teams that have had appropriate training, carry the correct equipment, and have experience performing rescues should be the rescuers. Without the proper equipment and training, the rescue crew may find themselves in need of rescue.

References

1. Federal Emergency Management Association publication. United States Fire Administration–Traffic Incident Management Systems. Publication FA-330, March 2012.
2. Sanders MJ. *Mosby's Paramedic Textbook.* 4th ed. St. Louis, MO: Mosby; 2014.
3. Occupational Safety and Health Administration. *Hazardous Materials,* 29 CFR 1910.120 (2013). Available online at http://www.ecfr.gov/cgi-bin/text-idx?SID=a0438214500657c983296 01f8fb58a02&mc=true&node=se29.5.1910_1120&rgn= div8. Accessed March 12, 2017.
4. Welles WL, Wilburn RE, Ehrlich JK, et al. New York hazardous substance emergency events surveillance: learning from hazardous substances releases to improve safety. *J Hazard Mater.* 2004;115:39-49.
5. Sweet D. *Vehicle Extrication Levels: I & II: Principles and Practices.* Burlington, MA: Jones & Bartlett Learning; 2011.
6. Poremba J. Airbag dangers firefighters face. FireRescue 1 News. Available at http://www.firerescue1.com/firefighter-safety/articles/1168850/; 2011. Accessed March 12, 2017.
7. National Highway Transportation and Safety Administration. *Emergency Rescue Guidelines for Air Bag Equipped Vehicles,* 1997. Available at http://link.houstonlibrary.org/portal/Emergency-rescue-guidelines-for-air-bag-equipped/iiafXVWPhog/. Accessed March 12, 2017.
8. Cooper DC, LaValla PH, Stoffel RC. Search and rescue. In: Auerbach P, ed. *Wilderness Medicine.* 6th ed. Philadelphia, PA: Mosby; 2011.
9. Hudson SE, McCurley LH, Mortimer RB. Caving and cave rescue. In: Auerbach P, ed. *Wilderness Medicine.* 6th ed. Philadelphia, PA: Mosby; 2011.
10. Martinette Jr CV, Zawlocki R. *Trench Rescue: Level I & II: Principles and Practices.* 3rd ed. Boston: Jones & Bartlett Learning; 2015.
11. Polk JD. Response to blast injuries. *JEMS,* June 2012. Available at http://www.jems.com/articles/2012/06/response-blast-injuries.html; 2012. Accessed March 12, 2017.
12. Schneidman D, Jacobs LM, Burns KJ. Strategies to enhance survival in active shooter and intentional mass casualty events: a compendium. *Bull Am Coll Surg.* 2015;100(1S):16-17.
13. US Department of Homeland Security: FEMA. 2013. Fire/Emergency Medical Services Department Operational Considerations and Guide for Active Shooter and Mass Casualty Incidents. September 2013.
14. Sharma BR. Clinical forensic medicine-management of crime victims from trauma to trial. *J Clin Forensic Med.* 2003;10:267-273.

6

Communications

CLAYTON SMITH

COMPETENCIES

1. Demonstrate knowledge about communications systems and their use in patient transport.
2. Apply appropriate communication skills before, during, and after transport.
3. Demonstrate the use of appropriate communication equipment to provide safe and competent patient transport.

*C*ommunication encompasses more than the use of a radio or telephone; it is a total system that ensures the smooth operation of routine daily patient transports while guaranteeing optimal patient care and transport team safety (Fig. 6.1). No one perfect communications system exists for all transport programs. The communications system must meet the present and future needs of the program it serves.

All transport team members must have good communication skills and know how to operate any equipment they may use for communication.[1] Communication equipment is influenced by the geographic location of the program and the education and training of those who use the equipment.

All communication needs to be compliant with the Health Insurance Portability and Accountability Act of 1996 (HIPAA). Team members must remember that radio and verbal communications can be easily overheard and cause a breach of patient confidentiality.[1,2]

Because working in communications is a multifaceted role and applies to the physical equipment as well as an intangible human action, this chapter will focus on the two aspects of communications: physical hardware and the human component of communicating.

Communication Centers

The communication center is the physical point at which the coordination for different types of transport takes place. An integral part of the transport program, the communication center is the hub for all electronic traffic, communication, and coordination efforts that the communication specialists (CSs) bring together to provide a safe, seamless, and effective transport for the crews and patients. There are many models

of communication centers currently in existence. Some are single service models such as police or fire only. Other models incorporate multiple programs such as fire dispatch and emergency medical services (EMS) into one integrated center. Flight dispatch centers often stand alone as an independent entity because of the intricacy and degree of commitment it sometimes takes to successfully coordinate just one air medical transport. The Commission on Accreditation of Medical Transport Systems (CAMTS) standards dictate that a CS must be assigned to receive and coordinate all requests for the medical transport service.[3] Federal Aviation Regulation 135.79 requires that the Part 135 certificate holder must have procedures established for locating each flight for which a Federal Aviation Administration (FAA) flight plan is not filed.[4] CAMTS[3] lists the components that a communication center must contain (Box 6.1).

Communications Specialist

The complexities of organizing a communications system are unique with respect to its operation. Beyond dealing with electronic hardware and computer software, the program is faced with one of the most challenging of tasks—dealing with people.

Humans are both the strongest and the weakest points in a system. People represent a broad spectrum of personalities and opinions, and no two individuals are quite the same. A communications center, a communications specialist, and communication skills are mandatory to ensure a safe transport operation.

Roles and Responsibilities

The *communications specialist* (CS) is designated to coordinate requests for aircraft and ground responses. The title assigned to the person with the CS function varies from program to program. The only limitation is that the FAA uses the term *dispatcher* to designate the person who decides whether or not an aircraft takes off. Unless this is the case in a program, another title should be used.

The CS is responsible for coordinating intraagency and interagency communications pertaining to any phase of a transport, from a request to hospital admission. The role of

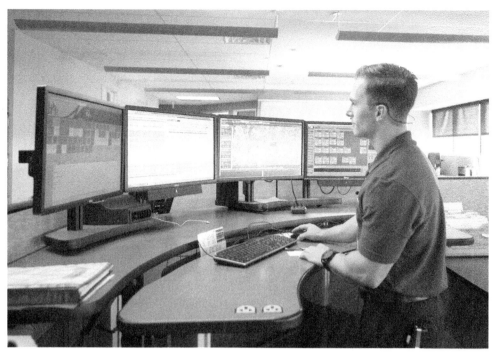

• **Fig. 6.1** Communications Center. (Courtesy Clayton Smith.)

• **BOX 6.1** **Components of a Communication Center**

At least one dedicated phone line.
A system for recording all incoming and outgoing telephone and radio transmissions, which should be stored for 90 days, with time-recording and playback capabilities.
Capability to notify the transport team and online medical direction for a request and during transport.
Back-up emergency power when power outages occur.
A status board to follow transport vehicles and show who is on the transport teams, weather status, and so on.
Local aircraft service area maps and navigation charts.
Road maps available for ground transport.
Communication policy and procedures manual.

From Commission on Accreditation of Medical Transport Systems. *Accreditation Standards*. 10th ed. Anderson, SC: The Commission on Accreditation of Medical Transport Systems; 2015.

---

the CS is to serve as a facilitator for the smooth integration of all the resources at the program's disposal, with the dual objectives of program safety and excellent patient care.

The CS must perform a variety of tasks including the following[5]:

- Listening intently
- Asking appropriate questions
- Accurately confirming what was said
- Reading maps (including using computer mapping software)
- Using spelling and professional grammar skills
- Using medical, aviation, and EMS terms
- Setting, evaluating, and resetting priorities
- Providing customer service and good public relations

Selection

Applicants for CS positions should be screened as thoroughly as applicants for transport team positions. Just as all persons who desire to be part of a transport team are not suited for the work, all persons who desire to be a CS may not be suited to the type of stress inherent in the job.[6,7]

The decision about whom to hire as a CS must be determined by each individual program. Certain minimal educational requirements must be met in any case, but some controversy has arisen about background requirements. Areas of controversy include the following:

1. Should the CS have medical field experience? If so, at what level and how much?
2. Should the CS have communications center experience? If so, what type of experience is acceptable, and how much experience is necessary?

Neither medical field experience nor communications center experience alone qualifies a person to be a CS, and neither does being a friend or relative of someone employed by the program.

CAMTS recommends that certifications, such as emergency medical technician, emergency medical dispatcher, and National Association of Air Medical Communication Specialists (NAACS) Certified Flight Communications Course, be encouraged and actually required by some transport programs.[3]

Training

Regardless of the background of the CS applicant, the person must be trained as a communications specialist. The

CAMTS standards that address communications state that the training of the designated communications specialist should be commensurate with the scope and responsibility of the Communications Center personnel. Box 6.2 contains a summary of the initial training. The NAACS has developed a specific course to train and educate the CS, and the components of this course are summarized in Box 6.3.

Training must be an ongoing process to ensure currency and proficiency. During training, the CS should be given a variety of situations, be allowed to make decisions, and discuss why decisions were made. Just as many transport teams use their "worst transports" to teach others, the "worst communication situations" presented and discussed with new CSs may assist them in future work.

The CS should undergo periodic testing on all elements of the position. This person must know everything about the program and be able to use that information at a moment's notice with a high degree of accuracy. In terms of communications procedures, the goal is 100% accuracy. For example, many programs periodically practice downed aircraft or communication loss exercises.

Communications Operations

Operations Control Centers

The FAA has determined that any helicopter air ambulance certificate holder that operates 10 or more helicopters must have an Operations Control Center (OCC).[8] Depending on the location of the communication center, many programs house the OCC in the same building because of the radio, Internet, and technological components that are required by both the OCC and the communications center.

Operational control (OC) requires the certificate holder to be responsible for all aspects of flight operations. The FAA recognized the challenge of maintaining a Part 135 OC with different companies joined together to provide separate services. The responsibility and authority of the OC should never be in question, and the FAA provides guidance with Order 8900.4. Flight operations consist of crew member training; currency and certification; aircraft maintenance and airworthiness; "weather minimums, proper aircraft loading, center of gravity limitations, icing conditions, and fuel requirements"; and flight-locating requirements.[9]

It is important that the roles and responsibilities of the OCC do not get confused with those of the CS or communication center. It is best practice to treat them as two separate entities, and communications with one department does not mean that the other will automatically relay that information, particularly involving weather issues.

Roles and Responsibilities

The FAA has compartmentalized OC duties into two tiers. The OC responsibilities for *Tier I* consist of the "assignment of crew and release of aircraft to revenue service."[4] Tier I also requires management to verify and maintain the level of quality of employees. *Tier II* represents the daily operations or how a specific flight is conducted. Generally, these duties are performed at a management level, but they may be delegated without removing responsibility from the certificate holder.

Alternative Sites/Backup Equipment

An alternative site and backup equipment should be identified and prepared by every transport program. A plan of action to deal with such a scenario, should it ever occur,

---

> **BOX 6.2** **Summary of the Commission on Accreditation of Medical Transport Systems Initial Training of Communication Specialists**

1. Medical terminology and how to obtain patient information
2. Knowledge of emergency medical system, including roles and responsibilities of various levels of training
3. State and local regulations that govern the EMS systems in which the transport service operates
4. Familiarization with equipment used in the prehospital environment
5. Knowledge of Federal Aviation regulations and Federal Communications Commission regulations pertinent to medical transport services
6. General safety rules and emergency procedures pertinent to medical transportation and flight following procedures
7. Navigation techniques/terminology and flight following and map skills
8. Weather interpretation
9. Radio frequencies used in medical and ground EMS
10. Assistance with hazardous material response
11. Stress recognition and management
12. Customer services
13. Quality management
14. Air medical crew resource management
15. Computer literacy and software training
16. Postaccident incident plan

EMS, Emergency Medical Services.

> **BOX 6.3** **Summary of the National Association of Air Medical Communication Specialists Training Course**

Postaccident incident plan
Flight following
Radio communications skills
Aviation weather
Aircraft emergencies
Medical terminology
Navigation and map usage
Customer service/public relations
Air medical crew resource management
Stress management
Federal Aviation Administration

should be annually reviewed. Each communications center must be able to continue operations at an alternative site with backup equipment if the primary communications center becomes inoperable.

Plans should also be in place for rapidly repairing or replacing any piece of essential equipment in the communications center.

Telephones

Each communications center must have at least one dedicated line for the medical transport service. Emergency telephone lines should not go through a switchboard; instead, they should be dedicated central office lines, so that if the switchboard fails, the communications center still has telephone communications. The number of incoming local and wide area telephone service lines should be based on the size of the service area and the projected volume of calls. Phone lines can be added relatively quickly when needed.

All calls made with emergency phone lines should be recorded as well as any outgoing call that pertains to requests for assistance or notifications.

Both wired and wireless communication systems are routinely used. Cellular phones are used by many transport services. However, their use should be guided by Federal Communications Commission (FCC) regulations on air medical transport vehicles. The FCC prohibits the use of cell phones in flight per FCC Code of Federal Regulations, Part 22, subpart H, Section 22.925. Cell phone use during ground transport should never interfere with patient care or safe driving.

Satellite phones may available as independent handheld devices or as part of the aircraft. The satellite tracking systems come with satellite phone communication. Both CS and transport team members need to be educated on how to use them.

Radios

The radio continues to be the key hardware element in medical transport communications systems. The crucial role of communication was especially recognized September 11, 2001, and during disasters such as Hurricane Katrina. The radio frequencies on which a program operates are assigned by the FCC on the basis of recommendations by the state chapter of Associated Public Safety Communications Officers, to which it has delegated responsibility for frequency coordination. The FCC issues licenses and assigns call letters. A program's assigned frequencies may be found in several radio bands (Box 6.4).

Included in the ultrahigh frequency (UHF) spectrum are the so-called *MED channels,* which are a set of 10 paired frequencies set aside by the FCC for the exclusive use of EMS units. The channels from MED 9 to MED 10 are frequency allocation channels used in metropolitan regions where UHF traffic is high. To use such a channel, an EMS unit calls the frequency allocation center, usually located in

---

> ### • BOX 6.4 Radio Bands
>
> VHF high-band FM (148–174 MHz): The radio signal in this band follows a straight line.
> VHF low-band FM (30–50 MHz): The radio signal in this band follows the curvature of the Earth and has the greatest range.
> VHF AM (118–136 MHz): This band is typically used for aviation-related communications.
> UHF (403–941 MHz): These ultrahigh frequencies have limited range and are most often used between ground units and base stations. They can be used for air-to-ground and ground-to-air communications for relatively short distances that fluctuate with the terrain.
> 800 MHz: Digital communication controlled by computers. They allow multiple agencies to communicate with each other and have higher frequency, less noise, and greater penetration outside of buildings.
>
> *AM,* Amplitude modulation; *FM,* frequency modulation; *MHz,* megahertz; *VHF,* very high frequency; *UHF,* ultrahigh frequency.

> ### • BOX 6.5 MED Channel Frequencies
>
> 463.000/468.000 MHz (MED-ONE)
> 463.025/468.025 MHz (MED-TWO)
> 463.050/468.050 MHz (MED-THREE)
> 463.075/486.075 MHz (MED-FOUR)
> 463.100/468.100 MHz (MED-SIX)
> 463.150/468.150 MHz (MED-SEVEN)
> 463.175/468.175 MHz (MED-EIGHT)
> 462.950/467.950 MHz (MED-NINE)
> 462.975/467.975 MHz (MED-TEN)

a fire department or ambulance service communications center, and requests assignment to a channel for the purpose of speaking with a specific hospital. The unit is then assigned an open channel or is told to stand by until one is available (Box 6.5).

The 800-MHz range has been assigned by the FCC because of overcrowding. These frequencies have a limited range because the signals are more line directed than the UHF and very high frequency (VHF) spectrums.

Some programs have their own private VHF. Others may choose to use one of the existing UHFs allocated for EMS use nationwide. Regardless, the same rules and principles apply when using any frequency spectrum.

Since September 11, 2001, and natural disasters such as Hurricane Katrina, a concerted effort has been made to make emergency and disaster management agencies interoperable. The advent of five mutual aid channels in the 800-MHz spectrum allows agencies from anywhere in the country to communicate to the incident command or units on the scene. One drawback has been that some agencies have given these frequencies different names, creating a myriad of names for the same channel (Box 6.6).

There are several basic types of radio systems[1,4,10,11]:

1. *Simplex system:* This system transmits in one direction at a time with a single frequency.

• BOX 6.6   New Mutual Aid Frequencies: Names and Renaming

Federal Standard

Mutual Aid 1: 866.0125
Mutual Aid 2: 866.5125
Mutual Aid 3: 867.0125
Mutual Aid 4: 867.5125
Mutual Aid 5: 868.0125

State of Ohio

Air Med 1: 867.0125
Air Med 2: 868.0125

Hamilton County, Ohio

I Call: 867.0125
I TAC 1: 866.5125
I TAC 2: 867.0125
I TAC 3: 867.5125
I TAC 4: 868.0125

---

2. *Full duplex system:* This system transmits and receives simultaneously with two frequencies (typically UHF).
3. *Half-duplex system:* This system transmits or receives in one direction at a time with two frequencies (typically UHF high band).
4. *Multiplex system:* This system transmits from two or more sources over the same frequency.

A repeater system is a type of half-duplex system that involves a base station repeater at an elevated site remote from the communications center. This system is particularly useful in regions with mountainous terrain. A repeater system receives a signal on one frequency and instantly retransmits it on a second frequency to the other radios in the system, extending the communications center's range. The process is reversed when the repeater receives signals coming into the base station.

Radio Use

All members of the transport team must know how radios work. Kane[1] noted that each team member must know how to properly use radios under normal circumstances; how to troubleshoot a radio under abnormal circumstances; and how improper use of a radio could make a straightforward call complex, stressful, and potentially unsafe.

Phone–Radio or Radio–Phone Patch

With a phone–radio or radio–phone patch, special circuits in the radio console permit a radio and telephone to be linked together, one direction at a time, so that the medical crew can speak to a person who is not in the communications center and vice versa. This capability is useful for programs that require voice contact with a medical control physician and for occasions when a member of the medical crew needs to speak with the receiving physician.

Programs that use a phone–radio or radio–phone patch have found that radio-like procedures must be used because transmissions are simpler. At times, this presents problems when patched through to persons who may not understand the system. Cellular telephones have supplanted this feature in many programs.

Squelch Control

Continuous Tone-Controlled Subaudible Squelch
A continuous tone-controlled subaudible squelch (CTCSS) circuit acts as a filter to others who use the radio's frequency. Only users of radios with the same tone-control frequency setting normally hear each other. This feature may be disabled when the tone of a transmitting radio is unknown or different or the radio operator wishes to monitor the entire frequency. *Private line* and *channel guard* are proprietary names for CTCSS.

Pagers

Two-way paging with use of **satellite communications** allows voiceless pages to be sent and an acknowledgment to be received with use of data terminals. The push-to-talk (PTT) method provides a nationwide service that combines instant communications with bases that use multiple transmitters across the country. These units offer global positioning system (GPS)–enabled tracking to locate aircraft or staff should a precautionary landing need to be made and the staff leave the aircraft for some reason. The units can be left on the aircraft; they are not transmitting in the air, and they are being pinged by the transmitters in the service area.

An extremely detailed needs assessment should be undertaken by qualified technical personnel before the implementation of any radio system. A program is ill advised to purchase a system identical to that of another program based solely on its recommendation.

Headsets and Foot Switches

The use of headsets rather than microphones should be considered in busy communications centers. When used in conjunction with a foot switch, a headset leaves the CS hands free, which is particularly desirable during operations in which only one CS is on duty. With more centers moving to a computer-based radio system, the PTT feature of traditional radios is being replaced by selecting a channel with a simple mouse click on the radio computer. In these systems the foot switch is replaced entirely, and the radio system is integrated into the daily use of the computers for transmissions.

The microphones used should be able to filter out background noises. A microphone placed on a bracket or gooseneck fixture attached to the console is preferable because it leaves the desktop space clear. When a headset microphone is used, it should be fairly close to the lips; proximity to the lips varies because of the varying speech characteristics of different people.

Communication Recorders

The CAMTS standards state that communication centers must have a system that records all incoming and outgoing telephone and radio transmissions with time-recording and playback capabilities. These recordings should be kept for a minimum of 90 days.

In most communication centers the recorders that use physical tapes have been upgraded to keep digital copies of all communications that enter and exit the center. Because of the availability and low cost of modern-day storage devices, this information can be kept for an indefinite amount of time. Because those recordings are usually only accessed by certain individuals, many centers use an immediate playback feature so the CS can review the last hour of transmissions in case he or she needs to double-check information or relisten to a report that was given over the radio.

Computers and Peripherals

Computers are an integral part of the well-equipped communications center. What a computer can do for a program is limited primarily by imagination and budget. Most communication centers operate multimonitor platforms on which a great deal of information can be displayed at a moment's notice. Depending on the individual program and the information technology infrastructure, most computer consoles are digitally backed up and can be accessed remotely, depending on the circumstances. Separate computers are generally used for different systems as a fail-safe; for example, if the computer-aided dispatch (CAD) system were to fail, then the Internet-based radios and communication systems would still be available because they were set up on a different computer system.

Computer-Aided Dispatch Systems

The **CAD** is the heart of the dispatch software that is used in modern-day dispatching (Fig. 6.2). In the past, multiple systems had to be used simultaneously by the CS to accomplish a string of tasks, but now they can all be completed within one integrated program. For dispatch centers that remain at the forefront of technological advancement, one would be hard-pressed to find loose paper, reference manuals, and large Rolodex references sitting around. Modern-day communication centers and transport team environments rely heavily on the CAD to ensure the transport is accomplished safely and effectively.

The CAD software often implements multiple systems into one functioning program; for example, it will usually have a built-in "library." This library can store information about agencies, locations, landing zones, hospitals, units, and any other data the CS may need to access. If a transport is entered into the CAD from Point A to Point B, the library is readily accessed to show phone numbers, addresses, important hazard information, and relevant notes

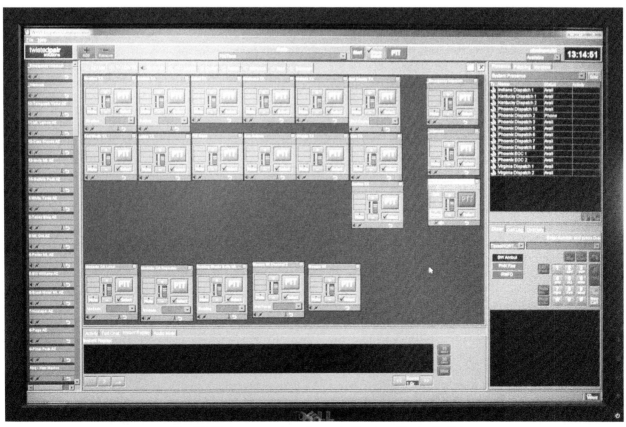

• **Fig. 6.2** Modern computer radio stack. (Courtesy Clayton Smith.)

pertaining to those points, and all information is immediately accessible to the CS. Because CADs are usually network based and share a common server, when one CS changes information (like a phone number within the CAD), all the other users on the network that access that library will be receiving the most up-to-date information. Communication centers routinely back up their CAD in the event of an outage or routine maintenance. Backups are quite easy to print and store for a permanent reference should a center experience a complete power or Internet outage.

In addition to the library feature, modern CAD software has the ability to page information to a crew-assigned cell phone in the form of a text, automatically alert the CS of critical updated information, and even incorporate mapping and distance features based on GPS points gathered from the units to determine which vehicle is the closest to a call. A modern flight CAD system can calculate the distance and heading that an aircraft must fly, where the closest airport is for fuel, and even estimate the time it will take the aircraft to fly to the scene or hospital based on its current location.

The main feature of the CAD, however, is the management of transport resources and crews. It is a vital tool for providing the multiple CSs who are working within the center access to the same up-to-date information regarding the location and status of the various transporting units. This server-based software, as well as technological communication advancements, allows the center to be remotely located from any particular unit or location if the need arises. Additionally, because of the increasing need for disaster preparedness and evacuation procedures, a server-based CAD system would allow the communication center to relocate to a different location and resume operations with nothing more than a bank of laptops and a high-speed Internet connection. Because of the vast degrees of complexity that a program may choose to implement with its CAD, it is important that transport team members understand the capabilities of their particular dispatch center and what they should expect as routine for the practices that have been implemented for their particular program.

Weather Radar

All pilots have access to FAA flight service weather information. Although the FAA generally does an excellent job, its reports may not be as current as desired at a given point in time. New weather tools are constantly being introduced. Great examples are available at http://weather.aero.

Weather radar display systems are available through several commercial services. These systems may be connected to the National Weather Service radar site in the region via telephone line or computer modem. All weather radar display systems provide displays and printouts of excellent quality. The display should be installed where the pilots have access to it. If the pilot needs an update while airborne, the CS may also have access to it. This situation may not be

a problem if the aircraft has its own weather radar. If a program has a computer-driven system, the CS can access the weather report from the communications center. An alternative to the phone-line system is to place a remote monitor in the communications center.[4] If the program does use an OCC, care must be taken so that the CS is taken out of the weather and risk analysis decision-making process; oftentimes those conversations are for the pilot, crew, and OCC specialist only. This is not to discourage the CS from voicing an opinion if he or she feels something is wrong; instead it is used to illustrate that weather decisions and discussions should be left to the trained OCC specialist if the program uses them.

Closed-Circuit Television/Web Cameras

The CS may need to have access to video scanning of the helipad or hangar ramp. Such scanning serves as a security system and enables the CS, who does not have direct visual contact with the program's parked aircraft, to see what is happening. Television monitors are available that may serve as a computer screen or as a video monitor by pressing a button, reducing the cost to the program. Web cameras also may be used to monitor aircraft and other areas of the transport service.

Maps

Technology has vastly improved "finding" EMS providers and referring hospitals. Mapping software is available that allows the CS to point and click on selected response sites, displaying coordinates for navigational purposes. GPS devices allow EMS to provide exact location information to both the communication center and the transport team. Many transport programs actually create websites with information about common destinations (hospitals and predesignated landing areas), which could save time and also affords an opportunity to review helipads and landing areas.

It is important to remember that technology is generally only as good as the operator, so CS, pilots, and transport team members must know how to use a map. An aviation sectional map or maps of the program's normal area of operations should be available in the communications center and on board transport vehicles. A compass radial overlay with a center string attached should be affixed to the map centered over the base of operations for backup if systems go down or are not functioning. A heavy dark line that radiates from base operations should be drawn on the map and marked off in 10-mile increments. This map enables the CS to rapidly obtain a heading and distance of a given point.

A street map should also be included of the metropolitan area around the base of rotary-wing operations. This map should be modified as previously mentioned. Topographic maps that show variations in terrain contour and various other maps that may be obtained from state or county highway departments prove useful in the communications center.

Policies and Procedures

A detailed policy and procedures manual is necessary for any organization that wishes to function in a systematically effective manner. The communications center manual must be a part of the program's overall policy and procedures manual. When the communications center manual is written, it should be carefully integrated with existing policies and procedures to minimize potential conflicting instructions to the CS.

The manual must cover all aspects of operation that have anything to do with communications. Each segment of the manual should be extremely detailed so that if a question arises about a specific item, it can be resolved by referring to the manual.

Communicating

Radios

Language

To effectively communicate within a program, standardized terminology should be used so that meanings are not lost or misinterpreted.

Generally, communication in plain language is preferable to using various codes; this precludes errors caused by the misunderstanding of a garbled coded transmission. Because of the broad area over which an air medical program operates, knowledge of codes for each of the many jurisdictions in the program's service area would be extremely difficult. Times should be communicated in the 24-hour clock format to ensure accuracy (Box 6.7).

Speaking

When initiating a radio transmission, a transport team member should begin with the name or call sign of the unit being called, followed by the member's own name or call sign. When older radio systems and poorly maintained new

• BOX 6.7	24-Hour Clock		
AM		**PM**	
1:00	0100	1:00	1300
2:00	0200	2:00	1400
3:00	0300	3:00	1500
4:00	0400	4:00	1600
5:00	0500	5:00	1700
6:00	0600	6:00	1800
7:00	0700	7:00	1900
8:00	0800	8:00	2000
9:00	0900	9:00	2100
10:00	1000	10:00	2200
11:00	1100	11:00	2300
Noon	1200	Midnight	2400 (0000)

systems are used, the speaker, when keying the microphone, should pause for a second before speaking to allow the radio to reach its maximal output level. This practice helps prevent the frequent problem of receiving incomplete messages. Another cause of this problem is speaking before keying the microphone.

The speaker should talk at a normal level; yelling into the microphone distorts the transmission. The speaker should know what to say before keying the microphone; speak clearly and concisely without irrelevant comments; attempt to control the voice level and intonation even when under stress; try to avoid transmissions that reflect disgust, irritation, or sarcasm; and avoid the use of profanity at all times. Radio transmissions are a measure of a program's professionalism, and both the media and a large population of citizens with scanners hear every word.

Transport team members must know how to properly operate the two-directional radio-intercom switch commonly found on headset cords in aircraft or ground vehicles. Many transport team members have been embarrassed when personal conversations or comments less than socially acceptable were broadcast over a wide area. This problem occurs less often in programs that operate pressurized aircraft, in which transport team members do not use a headset system.

Intracrew communications are also important. The pilot should keep the medical crew informed of any developments in a clear, complete message that leaves no doubt about what is happening. The following two anecdotes illustrate this point. Although the incidents are somewhat humorous now, the crews involved did not think so at the time. In the first incident, the crew received a badly scrawled note from the pilot, pushed through an opening behind his seat, just as the helicopter began an unexpected banking turn. The note read "I can't talk." The crew members looked at each other, each thinking that the pilot had had a cerebrovascular accident. They were about to get upset when the aircraft resumed straight and level flight. The pilot came on the intercom and explained that he could not talk on the medical radio, that he had spoken to approach control, and that he was returning to base for another aircraft. A more complete written message or advance warning on the intercom could have prevented a tense few moments for the crew.

In the second incident, the pilot of an outbound aircraft observed a transmission chip light blink on. In accordance with company policy, he immediately began a descent in preparation for landing. He told the crew "we're going down." The crew prepared themselves for a hard landing, and then began a vigorous discussion over the use of the one pillow on board. A normal landing was made, the mechanic arrived and corrected the problem, and the aircraft returned to its base. Once again, a more complete explanation would have prevented these tense moments.

During a flight, the pilot of an airport-based aircraft communicates with ground control, airport tower departure control, air route traffic control center, approach control, airport tower, and ground control again, in addition to the CS.

Hospital-based rotorcraft may or may not be near an airport but will be in communication with the appropriate segments of the air traffic control system and the program's own communications center. In either case, only the pilots should communicate with air traffic control. Aircraft on emergency scene flights also speak with units already on the scene.

Sterile cockpit (not speaking except in case of an emergency) must be practiced during takeoff and landing and any other critical phases of flight. Radio traffic should always be kept to a minimum to avoid unnecessary distractions, whether transporting via air or ground.

Transport teams in programs with multiple aircraft should also be aware that nonessential interaircraft conversations may make a telephone conversation or receipt of an essential transmission from another unit difficult for the CS.

If a team member asks the CS to make a telephone call, a minute or so should be allowed to pass before transmitting again to avoid interrupting the call.

If either party is having difficulty making a word understood, then that person should spell it using the phonetic alphabet (Box 6.8).

Portable Units

A program may elect to provide transport members with portable handheld radios for use on the ground outside the aircraft. These radios are particularly useful for programs that do emergency scene flights and during transfer flights for alerting the pilot to the imminent return of the crew with the patient.

• BOX 6.8 Phonetic Alphabet and Numbers

Phonetic Alphabet

A: Alpha
B: Bravo
C: Charlie
D: Delta
E: Echo
F: Foxtrot
G: Gulf
H: Hotel
I: India
J: Juliet
K: Kilo
L: Lima
M: Mike
N: November
O: Oscar
P: Papa
Q: Quebec
R: Romeo
S: Sierra
T: Tango
U: Uniform
V: Victor
W: Whiskey
X: X-ray
Y: Yankee
Z: Zulu

Phonetic Numbers

1: WUN
2: TOO
3: TREE
4: FOW-ER
5: FIFE
6: SIX
7: SEV-EN
8: AIT
9: NIN-ER
0: ZEE-RO

From *Federal Aviation Administration*. Available at https://www.faa.gov/regulations_policies/handbooks_manuals/aviation/media/remote_pilot_study_guide.pdf. Accessed March 28, 2017.

Cellular and satellite phones may also be used by transport team members for communication.

Aircraft Radios

Aircraft radios are usually integrated with the avionics package within the cockpit of the aircraft. These radios have more power and can transmit larger distances than most handheld radios. The antennae for these radios are often mounted on the belly of the aircraft so that during flight the radio transmission is broadcast down toward the earth where there is nothing obstructing the signal from the repeater tower to the aircraft. These radios are also used to talk with other air traffic, air traffic control, and the ground agency or security unit that is assisting in the crew's arrival to a particular destination.

Effective Communication

The effectiveness of the transport team as well as the communication team to provide and deliver exceptional service in a safe and efficient manner is directly related to the quality of communication delivered. High-quality communication is the responsibility of every individual involved with the transport to ensure that their message is being conveyed clearly and concisely. Because of the routineness of the messages that are relayed between the CS and the transport team, their importance can easily be lost within the sheer number of transmissions that can occur during a transport. This can result in a "desensitization" of the information that is being relayed, and the importance of delivering a clear message may be lost. If left unchecked, this will lead to unsuccessful attempts at getting the message through, incomplete transmissions born out of frustration, and a general dysfunction in the overall communication atmosphere between the teams. In posttransport reviews of situations with unfavorable outcomes, the root cause can frequently be traced back to an issue with communication. Remind yourself to
1. Never assume the intent, content, or meaning of the message if it is unclear.
2. Believe in positive intent for everyone involved.
3. Be clear and concise in transmissions, and ask for a repeat if the transmission is not clear.
4. Trust but verify the information received.

Sensitive Radio Traffic

When communicating information over the radio to the communications center, it is important to remember that these channels are oftentimes monitored by anyone who has access to a radio system and knows where the frequencies are published. Therefore patient identifiers and protected patient information should never be shared over the radio for any reason. It is sometimes necessary for the transport team to deliver patient information to the CS over the radio if they need to deliver a patient report to the receiving facility on behalf of the transport team. This is an acceptable and standard practice, but care must be used when delivering that information and it should never include any HIPAA-protected information including names, addresses, personal descriptions, or any other protected patient identifiers.

Additionally the communications team must use discretion when dispatching their units for a call. It is common for the media and news organizations to scan the radio frequencies and receive information for breaking news based on publicly available dispatch transmissions. One helicopter transport service was surprised to hear an actual recording of their CS dispatching an aircraft played over the nightly news for a high-profile call.

When dealing with the communication of patient information, it will always be best practice to censor out the patient identifiers and deliver the information in a sterile, factual, and straightforward way. A good habit is to always assume that someone unaffiliated with the transport is listening to your radio traffic.

Telephones

Often a requesting party's first impression of a program is created by the CS who answers the telephone. A courteous manner combined with comprehensive knowledge of the program helps give the caller the impression that the program is staffed by competent professional personnel.

Electronic Communication

Advances in communications technology in recent years has opened the door for new ways to communicate between the transport team and the CS. With the implementation of voice over Internet protocol (VoIP) radio communication, it is possible to integrate communications between a traditional radio frequency and the Internet. By transmitting the signal first via the Internet, the signal can then be broadcast locally to a unit or base once it is converted to a signal on a local frequency. With this technology the communication center can communicate with aircraft or ground units potentially thousands of miles away. The voice message travels via the Internet the majority of the distance, and then it is locally routed to a repeater that transmits the signal on a radio frequency that the unit is monitoring locally. When the unit responds back, the reverse process happens and the transmission is heard in the communication center with a negligible lag.

This advancement in Internet-based communication allows for the use of mobile phones and Internet-capable devices to transmit voice messages to a radio frequency even if they are out of the radio coverage area. With many different applications available for communicating on tablet and cell phone platforms, software companies are providing companion apps with their primary software packages that allow the users to utilize the features of the communication infrastructure that they have in place. Make sure you have

---

| • BOX 6.9 | Technology in Transport |

Companion applications used on smartphones and tablets can provide useful capabilities by using the cellular data network including:

- Textual-based communication
- Voice-based message transmissions
- The automatic sharing of information (like location or unit status) at the push of a button
- Charting, documentation, medical control, and sending information to receiving facilities
- Allowing transmissions to use a radio frequency by accessing the data network

---

a good understanding of the communication resources that your program provides (Box 6.9).

Medical Direction

Programs that operate with nurses or paramedics are included under medical direction regulations that vary from state to state. Whether communicating with their medical direction physician via radio, radiophone patch, satellite, or cellular phone, the medical crew should follow the medical reporting format used in the region. All reports should be to the point. Any treatment order received should be acknowledged by repeating the order verbatim. Medical direction that is delivered in the middle of a patient transport should be directly between the transport team and the physician. With the proliferation of applications used for smartphones and tablets, some charting and reporting platforms allow for face-to-face video conferencing or for sharing of pictures with the physicians. These communication outlets can provide a valuable tool for sharing information from the field with medical control. As with all patient-related activities, care should be taken in respecting the patient's rights when sharing medical information through this medium. Although this method is more secure than radio transmissions alone, the same precautions must be taken in protecting the patient's identity.

With the Media

Local news media usually have a high level of interest in the activities of any transport program. The CS must be able to politely but firmly deal with their calls when they interfere with operations. He or she must be aware of program policy with respect to giving out information and should refer the caller to the appropriate person if this is dictated by policy. Most programs have a designated individual that is responsible for handling media requests for information. Ask your program management who this person is and how they would like requests to be delivered.

In addition to the media, there are times when other agencies or businesses may call requesting information regarding a transport that was done by the transport team. Care must be taken when giving out information to other agencies that request it. It may be tempting or sound quite persuasive to deliver information to a detective or state agent looking for information regarding a patient that was recently transported, but you can still violate the patients' rights and HIPAA by sharing information with agencies and individuals who are not privileged to hear it. The CS must become familiar with his or her programs' specific media and information request policies regarding these types of requests.

Emergency Procedures

The operational procedures section of the policy and procedures manual should include a subsection that deals with procedures to be followed in the event of any unscheduled event that affects the use of the aircraft or directly involves the aircraft.

Postaccident Incident Plan

Every transport program must have a written plan in the event of an incident such as a vehicle accident. Each program should identify which incidents trigger this plan. The *postaccident incident plan* (PAIP) must be easily identified, readily available, and understood by all of the transport team members. CAMTS[3] recommends that at a minimum, the plan should include the following: a list of personnel to notify in order of priority; consecutive guidelines to follow in attempts to communicate with the aircraft or ambulance, initiate search and rescue or ground support, have a backup plan for transporting the patient or team, and have an aviation individual identified as the scene coordinator to coordinate activities at the crash site; a preplanned time frame to activate the PAIP for overdue vehicles; a method for ensuring accurate dissemination; coordination of transport of injured team members; a procedure to document all notifications, calls, and communications and to secure all documents and recordings related to the incident; a procedure to deal with releasing information to the press; resources available for critical incident stress management; and a process to determine whether the program will stay in service.

The program's specific utilization of the PAIP determines how frequent the CS and transport team will go through a PAIP situation. For some programs the PAIP is limited to accidents and injuries, loss of communications with the aircraft, and overdue aircraft incidents. Other programs use the PAIP as a notification system for a wider variety of situations including weather turnarounds, flight path deviations, forgetting medical equipment at the sending or receiving facility, unscheduled landings, flight plan diversions for fuel, or changes in patient condition. For programs that run the PAIP frequently, it becomes a well-rehearsed action with the notification and activation of the plan and is often used for both ground and air units. For other programs, the PAIP is reserved for critical accidents and incidents only. Be sure to be familiar with the program's PAIP policy and procedures.

Drills

The program's PAIP plan should also allow for scheduled drills. These drills are an excellent opportunity for the communication staff and the transport team to become familiar with the program's emergency procedures and operations. The ways in which program's implement drills can be as specific or creative as warranted. Some programs used their drills to host a "Safety and PR" event day for local agencies.

These drills begin with the CS getting the indication that something is wrong and the PAIP is activated. The unit participating in the drill initiates emergency procedures and involves the local responders in practicing for the emergency as well. Once the drill is complete, they can use that opportunity to go over loading zone safety and important public relations information with the responders. The drill is then reviewed and critiqued by a designated board and changes are recommended based on the information that was learned from the drill. Many programs find that the success of the drill is dependent on proper planning so that it happens in a safe and effective way. Additionally the review of the drill is critical in disseminating the information that was learned so everyone within the organization can benefit and be better prepared should a real emergency occur.

Critical Incident Stress Management

Each program should have a critical incident stress management plan in place in the event of an incident that causes the CS or the transport crew to have a strong reaction. The CS on duty at the time must be included in this plan. Depending on the situation, the CS may feel just as involved and affected as the transport crew. The CS may believe that he or she could have done something more or failed to do something, taking on unwarranted feelings of guilt. In adapting to the recognized stresses inherent in these types of situations, it is imperative that those involved reach out to their program's affiliated critical incident response team to seek further assistance in dealing with these complex situations.

Satellite Communication

As the name implies, satellite communication uses an infrastructure of complex communication satellites orbiting the Earth to provide two-way tracking and communication capabilities between individuals. Because the signal to transmit and receive via satellite travels in a more vertical pattern instead of laterally across the Earth, it is far less prone to interruptions or coverage area issues caused by obstructions in the terrain. Satellite communication and the upgrade in features that it provides has improved the ability to communicate in locations in which radio coverage or traditional cell phone service does not exist. The technology has become easier and more cost-effective to implement within the transport vehicles and mobile devices. Although conventional satellite tracking of transport vehicles has been around for many years, the ability to communicate and send messages through that same service is a newer advancement within the industry. Some units allow the transport team and the CS to communicate directly with either a text-based message or recorded voice transmission. This communication medium provides yet another outlet in expanding the service area and coverage for the transport vehicle. If the program incorporates such technology, it then must become familiar with the operation and transmission capabilities of the installed unit. There may come a time when that is the only possible way to communicate with the communications center.

Summary

Effective communication begins long before the first dispatch is delivered to the transport team. Communication encompasses both the understanding of the physical equipment as well as the components of communicating on an interpersonal level. The job of the transport team and the CS can be tense, leading to situations in which stress and an urgency to complete the tasks at hand overwrite the ability to communicate what is important in an effective and efficient way. Using the new technology to its maximum potential and setting a precedent of making effective communication a habit will provide an atmosphere in which the exchange of information contributes to the success of the various teams and the program overall.

References

1. Kane D. Communications. In: York-Clark D, Stocking J, Johnson J, eds. *Flight and Ground Transport Nursing Core Curriculum*. 2nd ed. Denver, CO: Air and Surface Transport Nurses Association; 2006.
2. American Academy of Pediatrics. *Air and Ground Transport of Neonatal and Pediatric Patients*. 3rd ed. Elk Grove, IL: American Academy of Pediatrics; 2007.
3. Commission on Accreditation of Medical Transport Systems. *Accreditation Standards*. 10th ed. Anderson, SC: CAMTS; 2015.
4. FAA. *Federal Aviation Administration*. available at http://www.faa.gov/regulations_policies; June 2008. Accessed March 28, 2017.
5. NAACS. *National Association of Air Medical Communications Specialists*. available at http://www.naacs.org; June 2008. Accessed March 28, 2017.
6. Rau W. 2000 Communications survey. *Air Med J*. 2000;6(2): 22–26.
7. Yocum K. A new look at hiring communication specialists. *Air Med J*. 1999;5(2):132–134.
8. *Federal Aviation Regulations and Aeronautical Information Manual*. Newcastle, WA: Aviation Supplies and Academics, Inc.; 2016 Edition.
9. Federal Aviation Administration. *FAA document N 8000.347, order 8400.10*. Vol 3. Washington, DC: FAA; 2006. chapter 6, section 5, dated 12/28/2006 appendix 1.
10. Illman P. *Pilot's Communication Handbook*. 5th ed. New York: McGraw-Hill; 1998.
11. Sholl S, Morse AM, Broome R, et al. Communications. In: Blumen IJ, ed. *Principles and Directions of Air Medical Transport*. Salt Lake City, UT: Air Medical Physicians Association; 2006.

7

Teamwork and Human Performance

FRED JEFFRIES

Introduction

Knowing the Enemy: The Problem of Human Error

To understand the role of teamwork and human performance in the transport medicine setting, it is useful to begin with an understanding of the challenges that we seek to overcome. The fact is, human beings make errors. Regardless of the degree of automation, or the extensiveness of the rules and procedures we put in place, medicine, aviation, and the movement of critically ill patients is a human endeavor. It is therefore imbued with all of the strengths and weaknesses that the human mind can bring to such challenges. These natural tendencies, rooted in our physiology, allow a consistent rate of error and mishap to continue despite our best attempts to engineer them out. As crew members and teammates, we are the source and the solution to many of these problems. The extent to which we understand how they occur, and how we can apply principles of teamwork and human performance to prevent, identify, and stop them, will determine our ability to function and thrive in an unforgiving practice environment. It should be noted that although it is often discussed in just such a context, the consequences of these errors are not limited to the safe or unsafe operation of the vehicles. The problem of human error reaches into all aspects of transport medicine, both operational and clinical. We become better, safer clinicians by learning to master how we function as a team and how we master ourselves to trap errors before they reach a level of consequence.

When mistakes and mishaps occur in medicine or the transport environment, they can be categorized in a variety of ways. Helmreich et al.[1] developed a modal classification scheme that classified error based on how the error occurred, resulting in five categories: procedural error, communication error, proficiency error, decision error, and intentional noncompliance. Other schemes have been contextually based and describe the timing or location of the error. The psychological approach, as described by Ferner and Aronson,[2] is used here because of its broad application and its ability to explain the causality of an event as opposed to merely describing one.

Slips and Lapses

A *slip* (sometimes referred to as a technical error) is an error caused by the failure of an individual to maintain the necessary attention on the task being performed. It results in performing a task incorrectly or in the wrong sequence. A *lapse* is caused by forgetting (and thereby omitting) a step in a planned sequence. Both slips and lapses are unintended and are skill-based mistakes. The error was not one of planning, but rather one of execution, because the person was correct in knowing what needed to be done but failed to perform that task correctly.[3]

Knowledge-Based Errors

Knowledge-based errors represent an ignorance of a required fact that was required to respond appropriately to a given circumstance. Unlike slips and lapses, this is an error of planning; the course of action was incorrect, even though the incorrect act may have been performed correctly. One type of knowledge-based error is the loss of situational awareness (SA). In dynamic environments the need to make timely and correct decisions requires that we not only observe our environment but correctly place our attention to understand what is happening around us and to our patient, and formulate an expectation regarding what will happen in the immediate future.[4] When we fail to perceive appropriate cues from our environment, or we cannot correctly interpret the cues we have, then we have a failure in our SA. Often this can manifest as task fixation, resulting in the failure to perceive everything else happening in the environment.

Rule-Based Errors

A rule in this context is simply a course of action prescribed by a given policy or procedure for a familiar or expected situation. They can often be expressed in IF/THEN propositions. For example, IF the patient is in congestive heart failure, THEN fluids should be avoided. The adoption of rules like this reduce cognitive burden, but the problem remains that there is a subset of congestive heart failure patients that would benefit from gentle fluid resuscitation. Add to this the natural tendency to force novel circumstances into the mold of previous events, and rule-based

The Tenerife Disaster (KLM Flight 4805 and Pan Am Flight 1736)

On March 27, 1977, two Boeing 747 aircraft sat on the tarmac of Los Rodeos Airport in Tenerife on the Canary Islands. Both had been bound for Las Palmas Airport but had been forced to divert to their current location because of an unexpected closure of the Las Palmas Airport after a terrorist bomb explosion. Now both aircraft were sitting just off the departure end of the runway waiting. Unlike the KLM flight, the Pan Am flight had not deplaned its passengers and was ready for departure 15 minutes later when Las Palmas Airport had been reopened. The Pan Am flight was parked behind the KLM flight, however, and was forced to wait for over 2 hours while the KLM flight reboarded and refueled.

With poor visibility and a fog bank laying across the airport dividing the runway in half, neither aircraft could see each other or the control tower once they began to taxi into position for takeoff; everyone was completely dependent on radio communication for coordination of their location on the airport and runways.[6] The control tower had instructed the KLM flight to back-taxi down the runway they intended to take off from, turn around at the end, and wait for takeoff clearance. The Pan Am flight was to follow behind the KLM flight on the same runway and turn off the active runway at about the halfway point. The Pan Am flight slowly back-taxied down the runway far behind and out of sight of the KLM flight. Meanwhile, the KLM aircraft had reached the other end of the runway and turned around.

On turning around, the KLM captain began to advance the throttles for takeoff, to which the KLM first officer said,

"wait a minute we don't have clearance yet." The KLM captain, rather than acknowledge the mistake, retarded the throttles and said, "No, I know that, go ahead and ask."[7] The KLM first officer then requested both the ATC clearance (which specifies the routing the plane will take after departure) and takeoff clearance (required to take off from the runway). As the first officer of the KLM flight received the ATC clearance (not clearance for takeoff), the captain of the KLM flight, mistakenly believing he was cleared for takeoff, released his brakes and began his takeoff roll. The first officer (for whom English was a second language) then communicated with the tower stating with surprise, "we are now at takeoff," which the control tower interpreted as meaning that they were in position for takeoff, not that they were beginning takeoff.[6] The tower responded by saying "okay" with a pause, and then told KLM to stand by for takeoff. The KLM first officer did not acknowledge the last message, and the control tower did not challenge him again.

At the same moment the tower was responding, the first officer of the Pan Am flight realized that the KLM flight may have interpreted the ATC clearance as takeoff clearance and quickly responded, "we are still on the runway." That transmission occurred simultaneously with the tower request to stand by for takeoff, resulting in both messages being barely audible and accompanied by a strong squeal heard in the KLM cockpit. The captain of the KLM flight commented on the quality of the radio transmission, and the collision killing 528 people in two fully loaded 747 aircraft occurred some 13 seconds later.

errors are born. Thus a distinction can be drawn between what is often described as good rules and bad rules. For a rule to be "good" it has to apply to the intended circumstance, and it must prescribe an appropriate course of action. A bad rule is one in which the situation at hand does not match the conditions the rule was intended to govern, or the action prescribed by the rule is unsuitable to the given situation.[5] When a rule-based error is committed, the individual fails either to apply or completely apply an appropriate good rule to the situation, or inappropriately applies a bad rule to the situation.

Combating Human Error

In the Tenerife disaster all of the aircraft functioned properly and the crews were experienced. A series of miscommunications and errors of judgment compounded to bring about a tremendous loss of life. To combat human error and its effects we must begin with the understanding that *error will occur.* Without acknowledging the possibility of error in our teammates and ourselves, we create an environment in which it becomes difficult to detect, confront, or learn from our mistakes. We may also create situations in which we create margins so close that small mistakes can have significant and lasting consequences. If, however, we understand the inevitability, it becomes less personal, and it

creates the mandate to be vigilant for its detection, requiring the formation of plans that do not require perfection. There are a host of measures used to accomplish this task, from how we engineer our technology and systems to how we build policy and procedures. For the ones out practicing in the transport environment, the team dynamic and the individual performances are the spheres in which we have the most impact and control. Teamwork and individual human performance are discussed together because in the transport medicine environment they are inseparable. The first prerequisite for effective team membership is individual development and competence, which is furthered and facilitated by effective coordination within a team. Without competent and effective individuals, teams are ineffective; without teams, the full potential of those individuals cannot be expressed.[7]

Teamwork

Value of Teamwork

The military theorist Charles Ardant D'Picq,[8] writing on unit cohesion and adversity, said:

> *Four brave men who do not know each other will not dare attack a lion. Four less brave men, but knowing each other*

United Flight 173

On December 28, 1978, United Flight 173 had been flying from New York to Portland, Oregon, and was on the approach to land when the flight crew experienced a landing gear malfunction.[9] Electing to abort the approach, the crew climbed and entered a holding pattern about 20 miles from the airport and orbited for about an hour while troubleshooting the gear malfunction and preparing the cabin and passengers for the possibility of an emergency landing.

At 1738 hours the captain reported that he had 7000 pounds of fuel remaining with the intention of orbiting for 10 to 15 more minutes before returning to land. That estimation proved to be erroneous, and 8 minutes later at 1746 hours the first officer asked the flight engineer, "how much fuel we got?" The flight engineer responded, "five thousand." The crew continued to discuss the landing gear until 2 minutes later the when the captain asked for the fuel weight if they landed in about 15 minutes, specifying he would like to have about 3400 pounds at landing. The flight engineer replied, "Not enough. Fifteen minutes is gonna really run us low on fuel here." At 1755 hours the flight engineer announced that the descent checklist was complete, at which time the first officer asked, "how much fuel you got now?" The flight engineer responded, "3000 pounds." At 1757 hours the captain sent the flight engineer to check on preparation in the cabin for a possible emergency landing, and he

returned at 1801 hours. The flight engineer then reported to the captain that, "we have about three on the fuel and that's it."

At that time the aircraft was only 5 nautical miles from the airport, turning away to continue holding. On hearing the flight engineer's report of the fuel, the captain said, "Okay, on touch down, if the gear folds…" never acknowledging the criticality of the fuel state. At 1803 hours the captain told Portland approach they had, "about 4000" pounds of fuel. At 1806 hours the captain announced his intention to turn back to the airport and begin the approach to land. He had just announced that intention to a flight attendant when the first officer announced, "I think you just lost number four…" followed by the flight engineer suggesting that they had better open the cross feeds. Ten seconds later the first officer told the captain "We're going to lose an engine," to which the captain replied, "Why?" The first officer repeated himself, and the captain again asked, "Why?" The first officer responded, "fuel."

The first engine flamed out from fuel starvation at 1807 hours. At that point the aircraft had traveled approximately 19 nautical miles from the airport. Six minutes later the remaining engines flamed out and Flight 173 crashed 6 nautical miles short of the airport. Only 10 of the 189 people on board were killed because of absence of a postcrash fire. One of those fatalities was the flight engineer.

well, sure of their reliability and consequently mutual aid, will attack resolutely. (p. 110)

This idea, that the familiarity and confidence in the abilities of teammates allows individuals to complete tasks that capable individuals cannot, hints at how the creation of an effective team improves our effectiveness in the delivery of care and the safe operation within the transport environment. Effective team members contribute to the collective pool of knowledge that allows the synthesis of ideas, creating new options for the team. Within highly effective teams, individual strengths offset other teammates' weaknesses, allowing for the team to be stronger and higher performing then the individuals that make it up. The result of this is an increase in the reliability of performance and a higher rate of successful completion of critical tasks. These benefits do not come without a cost, however, and the same quality that makes a team more effective can create traps that can weaken its performance. Interpersonal dynamics within the team, as well as personality and communication styles, can reduce performance or subject the team to the hazards of group think.

Foundation of Teamwork: Leadership and Followership

Teams are composed of leaders and followers, but within the dynamic context of transport medicine not only can that distinction shift quickly as circumstances change but the role of the follower should not be one of blind obedience. It is

possible within the span of a single call to have the roles of individuals shift. This may be because one crew member has more expertise in a given situation, and it may be because of the inclusion of different team members from outside the normal crew; for example, changes in the patient's condition may prompt the addition of an attending physician to the dynamic. These transitions of leadership do not absolve any of the team members from their responsibilities, but it does require a fluid and collaborative approach as the team encounters different spheres of authority in the course of a single call, moving between roles of leadership and followership. There are two types of teams in the operational transport team. First, there is the "crew," which is composed of clinicians and vehicle operators. This is what is typically described in the context of teamwork. There also is a second team composition at play. The "ad hoc team" is composed each time the crew goes out and interacts with the requesting agencies. One does not often receive patients in a vacuum, and often the transport team and the requesting agency work in cooperation or coordination for a period before the crew assumes full responsibility for the patient. Each time a new ad hoc team is formed, there is a critical point in the interaction in which the boundaries of the relationship, the norms of the group, and the scope of authority will be defined. Effective leaders typically address these three formative processes intentionally.[10]

Managing Boundaries

When a transport team arrives to receive a patient, they are almost always interacting with other services, clinicians, or institutions. Those entities will have their own rules, norms, values, and hierarchy. Entering and thriving in that realm requires respect for those systems, and the boundaries that separate outsiders from insiders should be softened quickly so effective communication and actions can be facilitated.

Establishing Group Norms

A norm is an unwritten set of informal rules that govern a group's behavior. Shortly after the formation of the ad hoc team, norms are communicated overtly or through example. Effective leaders communicate norms of safety, cooperation, and open communication. Modeling gratitude, acknowledging ideas, accepting feedback, or expressly stating risks and plans to mitigate them may help establish these norms. Kern[10] described the leader of a newly formed team establishing these norms in an early team briefing:

> The leader can simply state: "We need to all keep an eye on each other. Don't expect me to know everything, so speak up if you see something that is important to us. We need and expect everybody's input to get the job done safely and efficiently." (p. 131)

It is also clear how unconscious or unskillful actions could easily communicate the opposite of these norms when encountering our ad hoc teams.

Utilizing Appropriate Authority

When rapid action is required, an effective leader is capable of decisive unilateral action. That degree of decisive action is not frequently required, however, and an effective leader is capable of adjusting the tightness of control on the team depending on the capability of the members and the situation at hand.

As important as leadership is, equally important is the seldom-discussed role of followership. It is a commonly held fallacy that being a good follower is a temporary requirement on the way to a leadership position.[10] The truth is quite the opposite. Team membership in the transport medical environment means transitioning between leadership and followership roles quickly with adaptability and flexibility. The archetypal good follower is one with the ability to critically analyze the situation, who is not afraid to offer thoughts that contradict the prevailing opinions and can communicate those thoughts at the right time effectively.

Teamwork Barriers in the Tenerife Disaster

In the Tenerife case study above, in the KLM cockpit, the captain was also the head of the Flight Training Department for the airline. In analyzing the crew management style of the KLM captain, Rotisch et al.[7] concluded:

> The KLM cockpit crew behavioral profile centered on a captain who gave the appearance to the rest of the crew that all factors had been considered and a safe takeoff was ensured. Such a posture was undoubtedly enhanced by the captain's position in the company as Head of Flight Training Department. Whenever upper management captains fly line trips, there is a natural subtle tension in the cockpit atmosphere that is not found between regular line crewmembers. (p. 17)

This subtle tension may have been the reason the KLM first officer failed to further challenge the KLM captain once takeoff was initiated when it is apparent that the KLM first officer was not expecting the commencement of takeoff, nor did he believe that they had received clearance. After the takeoff roll had commenced, the KLM flight engineer asked if Pam Am was clear of the runway. It was asked in a tentative and unsure manner and was curtly dismissed by both pilots.

Formation of Group Norms in the Tenerife Disaster

Although the aircraft were parked waiting for takeoff, the cockpit voice recorder on the KLM aircraft captured several concerns expressed by the crew that may have contributed to them feeling pressure to depart the airport quickly. These discussions, led by the KLM captain, established the cockpit crew's priorities and shaped the norms that would contribute to the accident. First, there was a question of duty time, which is the maximum number of hours a pilot can be on duty in a row. KLM's governing body in Belgium had recently changed the rules, making duty time more difficult to calculate, and with no discretion on the part of the pilots. The KLM captain and first officer discussed their concern about further delays encroaching on duty time and risking violation. Second, there was concern over the weather. With visibility so limited, it was a real concern that the airport would close, and the aircraft would be delayed much longer. Although these types of delays are common for line personnel, it is possible that a captain in upper management may have felt more responsibility for maintaining the airline's schedule.[7]

Task Saturation and Barriers to Teamwork in Flight 173

The risk associated with the crew's preoccupation with the emergency exceeded the risk the emergency itself posed. Despite having the fuel quantity information available to them, and having the means to calculate their remaining flying time, the information was not correctly understood by the captain and was not effectively communicated. Only once did the flight engineer express his concern about the low-fuel state and provided no additional information or details to the captain who, even as engines began flaming out, still believed he had sufficient fuel on board.

Origins of Crew Resource Management

In the 1970s the airline industry had a problem. Several airline accidents had occurred with senior and experienced flight crews at the controls, and the accidents appeared to be caused by failures of interpersonal communications, decision making, and leadership.[11] Throughout the latter half of the 1970s, the National Aeronautics and Space Administration's Aerospace Human Factors Research Division had been tasked with studying the problems, and in 1979 it brought together the airline industry and key government agencies in a workshop to discuss their findings.[12] What was needed was improvement in teamwork, coordination, and an environment in which leadership encouraged subordinates' participation and critique. It was from here that the first generation of *cockpit* resource management (CRM) was born.

Early CRM training emphasized the communication and managerial styles of the individuals to correct the under assertiveness of junior crew members, while reducing the excessively authoritarian behavior of senior crew members.[11] These efforts were bolstered by the National Transportation Safety Board (NTSB) in 1979. They included in their findings and probable cause of Flight 173's crash after running out of fuel that neither "the first officer nor the flight engineer conveyed any concern about fuel exhaustion to the captain" and the "failure of the other two crew members to either fully comprehend the criticality of the fuel state or to successfully communicate their concern to the captain" contributed to the cause.[9] For the first time, the NTSB had listed the failure of the crew's communication as a contributor to the accident.

Throughout the 1980s CRM continued to evolve. The emphasis on modifying management style gave way to understanding cockpit group dynamics, emphasizing briefing strategies, SA, and breaking error chains. It was during this time that the name evolved as well. Recognizing that the concepts were really about the human interaction and not the equipment, the name changed to *crew resource management*. By the 1990s CRM was spreading beyond the cockpit into flight dispatchers, maintenance personnel, and cabin crew.

Operationalizing Teamwork: Crew Resource Management

Current concepts of CRM have at its center the understanding that error will occur, and that through the efficient use of all the resources available, in an appropriate and timely fashion, SA and improved decision making can be enhanced, making all aspects of operation safer. Its goal is primarily to recognize and voice that an error has occurred or is about to occur, or to mitigate that error once it has occurred. To accomplish this, CRM seeks to address core problems, such as workload management and delegation, maintenance of SA, use of authority and assertiveness, utilizing all available resources including other crew members, and improving interpersonal communication.[13]

Problems Crew Resource Management Had to Solve

Workload Management and Delegation

In a complex and technically advanced environment, how should workloads be managed and delegated to make the best use of the resources available to the crew? First, it must be understood that workload is not constant; rather, it is a constantly evolving state shifting during different phases of a transport. Within a team, workload may impact different crew members at different times. The clinical crew has a very low workload en route to a patient and has a very high workload during a resuscitation. Similarly the vehicle operator, be it an emergency medical technician (EMT) or

---

CASE STUDY

Elaine Bromiley

On March 29, 2005, Mrs. Elaine Bromiley, a 37-year-old mother, underwent elective surgery to her nose.[14] In her preoperative anesthesia note mouth opening was recorded as normal and neck movements as "slightly restricted" due to congenitally fused cervical vertebrae. No other note or particular concern was recorded, and the plan was for a general anesthetic with a laryngeal mask airway (LMA). At 0835 the anesthesia was induced with remifentanil and propofol, and an attempt was made to place the LMA. The muscular tone in the jaw proved to be too high and did not allow enough mouth opening. Believing that the patient was not deeply enough sedated, a repeat dose of propofol was given and a second attempt to place the LMA was made, as well as attempting placement with two smaller sizes of LMAs without success.

At 0837 Mrs. Bromiley's SpO_2 began to desaturate to 75%, and she became cyanotic and tachycardic. By 0839 her SpO_2 had fallen to 40% despite attempts to provide facemask ventilations with an oral airway. Shortly thereafter her heart rate began to fall precipitously. Having already fallen to 69 beats per minute (bpm), it was now in the 40s. Around 0841 the decision was made to transition to endotracheal intubation, and Mrs. Bromiley was given atropine and succinylcholine. It was about this time that the anesthesiologist was joined in the operating room (OR) by a second anesthesiologist from an adjoining OR. On the first

attempt at direct laryngoscopy (DL) a Connack-Lehane Grade IV (no laryngeal structure visible) was used. The SpO_2 remained less than 40%, although the heart rate had temporarily responded to the atropine and increased to the mid-60s.

Despite using a two-person technique, ventilation by facemask was described as extremely difficult and was ineffective at providing ventilations. The situation is now a can't-intubate-can't-ventilate emergency. Between 0847 and 0850 further attempts at DL intubation are made with a variety of instruments, without success. Fiberoptic attempts were made, but were unsuccessful because of blood in the airway.

At 0851 an additional anesthesiologist entered the OR and attempted DL intubations for an additional 4 minutes, and SpO_2 continued to remain less than 40%. At 0900 an LMA was placed successfully with a recovery of the SpO_2 to 90%. For the next 10 minutes, multiple additional attempts were made to intubate through the LMA with an occasional SpO_2 dipping as low as 49% but recovering to the 90s.

At 0910 it was decided to abandon the procedure and allow Mrs. Bromiley to awaken. At this point Elaine Bromiley had been profoundly hypoxic in excess of 20 minutes. She did not regain consciousness, and after being transferred to the intensive care unit (ICU) she died a few days later.

pilot, may have a very low workload during the stabilization but a very high workload during the transport phase. Understanding when the different team members have different workloads will help time communication and tasking during the transport.

Different crew members are tasked with different workloads at different times, but not all work has the same priority. *Critical tasks* are ones that must be performed correctly at the right time to prevent harm to the team or the patient. Vehicle operation often involves critical tasking. Addressing apnea is a critical tasking in the clinical management of a patient and must precede other lower-priority tasks. One of the challenges of a transport environment is when there are multiple critical tasks occurring within the vehicle. A helicopter departing an unimproved landing zone with a critical patient provides several critical tasks competing for attention. When presented with such situations, they are managed in the following priority—safety of the team first and safety of the patient second. *Important tasks* will evolve into critical tasks if they are not managed at the appropriate time. Replacing an intravenous vasopressor bag before it runs out is an important task because if it is not done, it will result in the patient's hemodynamic status declining, which prompts the critical task of resuscitating the blood pressure. A *routine task* is a procedural step that in and of itself is neither important nor critical, but may ensure a condition that allows such circumstances to be recognized or managed by its completion. The monitoring of blood pressure at a regular interval is a routine task that allows the identification of a situation that requires an important or critical task. Regardless of the timing of the workload, there are some consistencies in how individuals and teams react to different workloads.

Effects of High and Low Workloads Response to workloads has a curvilinear bell-shaped relationship in which an optimum workload is in the center and performance trails off in either direction as workloads are underloaded or overloaded. During *optimum workload* the individual or team is engaged and focused with enough reserve attention and energy to recognize and adapt to changes. This is in contrast to a team that is *underloaded.* In this state the team has very little to challenge them; as a result, they have an overall lower level of attention, boredom may set in, and they may miss important environmental or clinical cues that the situation is changing or a new hazard is present. In an *overloaded* state the team may begin to lose the larger picture as its attention begins to tunnel, SA begins to fail, and reasoning reverts to a pattern recognition mode in which team members begin reverting to old habits that have worked in the past. Additionally, overloaded teams may begin deviating from procedural standards and norms (Fig. 7.1).

Task Saturation When a team or team member begins to have difficulty maintaining routine tasks or upholding procedural standards and norms because of an increased workload, that team or individual is task saturated. Any additional workload requires the displacement of another task. Recognition of task saturation in yourself or teammates allows the team to adjust to make the most of its resources. The signs that a teammate or team is task saturated vary based on the situation. They may include erratic errors or inconsistent performance, deviation form from policy and procedure, indecision, fixation on a task or indication, distortion of time, or confused, halting speech. Scheduled tasks, medication doses, and record-keeping tasks may be missed. When task saturation is recognized, let the team know ("alright, we are task saturated right now"), and take steps to get caught up.

1. **Prioritize the critical tasks.** Ask the question: "What do we have to do now?" Then begin on those tasks. Set end points ("we need to get a vasopressor up") so that on its completion you can reassess the priorities.
2. **Delegate tasks as able.** In specialized teams there may be procedures or tasks that only particular members of the team can perform. Ensure that they are free to complete those tasks by delegating the other tasks to other team members.

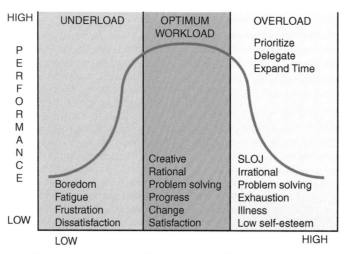

• **Fig. 7.1** Effects of high and low workloads. (Redrawn from Smith, D. (n.d.). CRM Resources, Workload Management, Briefings, Callouts, Checklist, Error Management, Darren Smith, Flight Instructor, CFI Homepage. Retrieved March 10, 2017, from http://www.cfidarren.com/crmworkload.htm.)

3. **Expand available time.** Routine or less important tasks can be put off to free resources to manage the crisis or high tasking for the moment.

4. **Manage distractions.** Distractions are tasks or attention drains that have no bearing on the safe performance of the tasks at hand. They may be dealt with using some of the previously mentioned techniques, or they may be ignored outright. In error-prone situations it may serve the team to develop a signal that the individual performing a task should not be interrupted for anything other than patient safety or crew safety. Similar to the use of a sterile cockpit during critical phases of flight, certain tasks have a high workload and high probability of error. Limiting communication to safety concerns prevents interruptions.

Task Saturation and Filtering Effects in the Tenerife Disaster One of the earliest points the KLM crew could have avoided the accident was when the control tower said, "Okay...standby for takeoff." That message, after the "okay," appears to never have been processed by the KLM crew. The reasons for their inability to process the message may have been task saturation at the time of takeoff and a filtering effect that prevented them from recognizing the transmission as coming from the control tower. Once the decision to take off had been made, and the throttles advanced, the crew became absorbed in the task of taking off. Little attention was left for lower-priority information once the KLM aircraft started takeoff. To be processed, the message would have to overcome the attention filter that screens out lower-priority information while individuals are engaged in activities requiring high degrees of concentration. The transmission that followed, "hold for takeoff," was distorted by the simultaneous transmission from the Pan Am crew, thus removing the familiar voice that had been controlling them, making it sound distant and unrelated. The transmission failed to make it past the two pilots' information filters.

It is interesting to note the respective workload of the pilots and the flight engineer at the time the KLM flight engineer questioned if Pan Am was clear of the runway. When the flight engineer was "curtly dismissed," the pilots were at a peak workload accelerating down the runway, their attention was saturated, and their filters closed to anything but the most critical pieces of information. The KLM flight engineer had just completed the largest portion of his work and was less tasked, with a more open filter. Although it is apparent that the KLM flight engineer did not hear the tower's instruction to "standby for takeoff," he may have heard the Pan Am first officer respond to the tower shortly after with "okay, we will report clear." Questioning what they will report clear of may have prompted the KLM flight engineer to question where Pan Am was clear of the runway.

Maintaining Situational Awareness

In essence, SA is knowing what is happening around you in such a way that you are able to anticipate near-future events. There are several processes that take place as we develop an SA of our environment moment by moment and a host of pitfalls that can be encountered as we do so. Individuals must perceive information from their environment, comprehend that information correctly, use that information to construct a model of what is about to happen in the near

---

CASE STUDY

Blood Pressure Control Error

A ground-based critical care team consisting of an experienced team member and new team member were dispatched to a community hospital for a 59-year-old male with a subdural hematoma. The patient was hemodynamically stable, awake and alert, and nonintubated. Transporting this patient by critical care was a precaution and presented no complexity or challenge to the crew.

On arrival at the bedside, the newest team member went to obtain report, while the experienced team member assessed the patient and packaged him for transport. Both tasks were completed at the same time, and when the new teammate returned to the bedside, the patient was ready to move to the ambulance as he asked, "did you get the story?" The experienced team member acknowledged his partner and said he had "gotten enough of it," but as they left the facility, both crew members had very different ideas about the cause of the head bleed. This was the first failure of CRM. They had an opportunity to share a mental model and make sure they were together in their thinking, but they did not take it. From report the new teammate had learned that the head bleed was caused by a fall yesterday and was traumatic in nature, whereas his partner believed the head bleed to be spontaneous in nature. This misalignment would come into play during the course of the transport when the patient's blood pressure began to climb to a point when their standing orders required them to control the mean arterial pressure as if it had been a spontaneous bleed. No such order existed for treating a traumatic head bleed.

After the blood pressure had cycled a couple of times and it was clear that the patient was in fact hypertensive, the more experienced crew member suggested starting nicardipine to lower the blood pressure. His teammate looked quizzical and suggested, "how about just some more fentanyl instead." It was clear to the experienced team member that his partner did not agree with the proposed treatment plan, but he did not question him about why. Instead he dismissed his partner's hesitation without acknowledging it, allowing himself to believe he knew the reason for his partner's hesitation (his newness to the program, lack of familiarity with standing orders, etc.), and proceeded with his proposed plan of care. This was the second and third failure of CRM. The experienced team member recognized the concern of his partner but failed to act on it, and his partner failed to assert himself enough to be heard and understood when he believed an error was about to occur. Although in this case no harm befell the patient, it is easy to see how it may have in a similar circumstance.

future, and base their actions off the results of that model. Each of those components—perception, comprehension, and projection—can have errors that render the individual's understanding of his or her situation incorrect and outdated, leading to impaired judgments and a potentially harmful outcome to the patient or team (see Fig. 7.1).

Feeding into a Common Situational Awareness *For SA to exist within a team, the members that constitute it must feed information forward to build a comprehensive understanding without overwhelming or disrupting the decision-making process.* When a team first encounters a challenge, whether clinical or operational, it begins a process of building its SA by observing and orienting to the environment and the challenges within which it is operating. This process, described by Colonel John Boyd as the "OODA Loop," describes how the individual cycles through a process of observing, orienting, deciding on an action, and then acting (Fig. 7.2).[15] The first task, observing, involves the team developing an awareness of those things around them that may impact the situation. When that team has a designated leader for either a portion of the task, or that is responsible for all of the operations, the leader must develop this understanding using information fed to him or her from technology and teammates. The problem is that each of these data points is obtained from a different, although similar, point of view. In a clinical interaction, this observation phase may involve understanding patient assessment, laboratory data, vital signs, the anxiety of the sending staff, and the wishes of the patient. In an operational context, this may include vehicle type and availability, weather conditions (present and forecast), patient stability, out-of-hospital time, crew resources, crew experience, patient risks, and so on. Each one of these points is delivered through the sender's point of view and is affected by past experience.

The team, or team leaders, then must place these data within a context and orient themselves and their team. The second phase of the loop focuses attention on one or more discrepancies or challenges presented in the situation and establishes their priorities within the greater context. For example, in a clinical setting, there is a low systolic blood pressure reading that has been observed by a teammate. This fact in isolation does not give the leader the information required to act. Is the patient a penetrating trauma patient? Should the lower blood pressure be accepted in the name of hypotensive resuscitation? Does the patient have a low blood pressure at baseline, so this is not a deviation at all? Without orientation to make sense of the observation, meaningful intervention becomes difficult. Thus the leader must assemble these pieces using his or her previous experience, analysis, and organizational guidelines, as well as his or her own observations and the information from teammates to decide on an appropriate action.

It is possible now to see how information delivered by a teammate with poorly calibrated urgency, or poor timing, can skew the orientation process and disrupt a decision-making process. This is particularly true when the situation presents itself as a crisis requiring immediate and decisive action. In the previous case study United Flight 173, the pilot-in-command (PIC) had prioritized the troubleshooting of his landing gear light. The flight engineer knew the diminishing fuel supply was becoming an increasing hazard to the safe completion of the flight, but pushed that information to the PIC in such a way that the urgency was not communicated and in language that allowed the PIC to misinterpret it as pounds of fuel instead of minutes remaining. In doing so the flight engineer's information was given a low priority in the PIC's orienting process and not considered as decisions were made about when to land.

Thus when information is forwarded to a leader, it is imperative that the crew member advancing that information ensures both that it is correctly timed and that the appropriate degree of urgency is appreciated by the leader receiving it. Poorly timed information delivered in a crisis

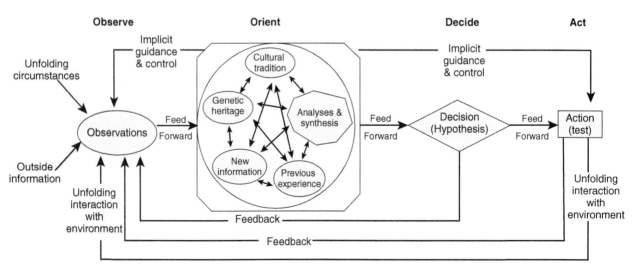

• **Fig. 7.2** The OODA loop. (Redrawn from Boyd J. The Essence of Winning and Losing. June 28, 1995. In Brehmer B. The Dynamic OODA loop: Amalgamating Boyd's OODA Loop and the Approach to Command and Control. 2006.)

situation results in the attention of the leader being temporarily placed on something that not only does not contribute to the solution but detracts from the resources available to meet the challenge.

Recognizing Lost Situational Awareness, and Recovering It

In the case study about Elaine Bromiley there was a fundamental loss of SA. There were sufficient staff and resources available, the procedure was elective, and the staff was experienced and well trained. The initial failure was not one of technique, but of awareness when the clinicians became fixated on completing the task and lost sight of the patient's safety. At no point did the two anesthesiologists or the ear, nose, and throat surgeon ever state out loud what was happening. Although the physicians seem to have been late in realizing that the patient was in trouble, the nursing staff present was experienced and was aware of the risk to the patient early on. They independently brought in the surgical airway tray, announced its presence, and called for an ICU bed for the patient. What the nursing staff detected was a state in which the team was no longer meeting the planned goals, had an increasing fixation and tunnel vision, and was experiencing unresolved discrepancies in the information they were receiving. These are key moments when the team may be able to recognize that they have lost SA in the moment. The clues, however, are extremely difficult to detect by the individuals involved in the crisis. This is why each team member must be allowed to express his or her concerns, and be heard by the team and its leader. Additionally, *the team must have a practiced response to loss of SA, either in the operational or clinical realms.* Those responses include the following:

1. **Announce the problem to the team.** State in clear terms what the problem or hazard is.
2. **Create time or space distance between the team and the hazard.** In a clinical setting this may involve slowing or stopping the decline of a particular vital sign and providing temporizing care while the specific solution to the condition is sought or readied. In an operational setting, like in an aircraft, this may be increasing altitude in response to an accidental encounter with instrument meteorologic conditions.
3. **Stabilize the condition.** In addition to reversing the impact of the problem condition, stabilizing the condition also involves avoiding unnecessary complications to the situation and creating an increasing degree of margin allowing for latitude of action.
4. **Give the team enough time to get caught up to the situation**. Once the team is out of immediate danger, or the patient has been stabilized, time should be taken to assess if the original plan is still the correct one, or if a new plan is required.

Although the nursing staff in the Elaine Bromiley case recognized the loss of SA, they did not feel they had a mechanism with which to raise their concerns to the physician team, nor did they feel they would be heard if they had. How to communicate within the team during a crisis is the next problem that the principles of CRM seek to solve.

Recognizing Lost Situational Awareness in the Blood Pressure Control Error One of the crew members recognized that there was a departure from the expected course of action and had unsettled disparities in the plan. Although he attempted to express these, his actions were ineffective and he took no additional action to assert his concern and reestablish the team's lost SA.

When and How to Communicate Within a Team

Each team member must have the skills and sensitivity to transmit information in an increasingly clear, bold, and concise manner as the team faces challenges and hazards. CRM seeks to improve safety of the team and the patient by emphasizing how to communicate effectively, recognize the barriers to effective communication, and overcome them. Communication within a team is a two-way process that begins with the sender encoding a message and transmitting it to the receiver. It is important when communicating within a team that both the content of the message and the tone with which it is delivered communicate the same meaning. Other considerations must be given to the volume that the situation requires and to the timing of the message. Sending information when the intended recipient is unable to receive it or process it is ineffective. Once the message is encoded, it is transmitted across the medium. That may be just a spoken word in a room, or it may be across a radio, a phone, or an aircraft's intercom system. One of the challenges in communicating in a transport environment is that often the nonverbal component of communication, responsible for expressing much of the message in routine face-to-face communications, is missing. This makes it even more important that the sender verifies that the message sent was the one received (Fig. 7.3).

At the center of CRM's focus on communication is the mandate that *it is the responsibility of the person sending the message to ensure that he or she is understood.* All too often what is said is not heard. Steps to ensure an effective message include the following:

1. Stating one idea at a time
2. Stating things simply
3. Encourage feedback
4. Repeat and explain as required

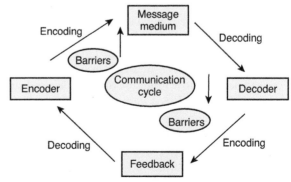

• **Fig. 7.3** Effective communication cycle. (Redrawn from Patil M, Patil S. Process of Communication, Two Way Process of Communication. July 26, 2013. Retrieved March 10, 2017. http://articles-junction. blogspot.com/2013/07/process-of-communication-two-way.html.)

In times of crisis when immediate action from the team is required, the order of communication also becomes important. For example, an air medical crew member sees an immediate hazard to the helicopter as it lands on a country road. There is a barbed wire fence obscured by high grass that poses a risk of striking the tail rotor if the aircraft continues to land in the direction it is currently moving. Time is short, and the first thing the crew member needs to express is the action that is required to avoid the accident; this is *directive communication.* "Abort!" or "Go around!" delivered with the appropriate degree of urgency and at an appropriate volume gives direction to the pilot to avoid the impact. Only then, after the aircraft is free of the hazard, does the crew member use *descriptive communication* to describe the reason for the direction given, "fence line, at 6 o'clock." There are times when certain hazards may be anticipated, either operationally or clinically. In those circumstances it can serve the team to brief specific language to be used if that hazard is encountered. If, for example, a team is moving a patient on an intraaortic balloon pump and the pump is being pulled behind the patient, it improves patient safety if before moving the patient the team states, "if at any point someone sees a problem during movement, say the word *stop,* and everyone immediately will stop movement." This seems intuitive, but often people will use more casual language, such as "hold on," "just a second," or even "ok" to indicate the need to stop. In a situation in which a snag or a stumble could result in displacement of the device sitting in the aorta, the delay while the team decodes the intent of the message could have dire results. Once the message is encoded by the sender and is transmitted across the medium, a variety of barriers may exist between the sender and the receiver. Understanding these barriers will aid the crew member in overcoming them.

Barriers to Communication

Nonassertive Behavior and Lack of Confidence

There are a variety of styles that individuals use to communicate ranging from passive on one side of the continuum to aggressive on the other side of the continuum. One of the challenges of working within a team is recognizing that different crewmates may be saying the same thing with very different styles, and we must be careful not to overlook or dismiss the message because it is delivered in a more passive style. Although one crew member may look at a situation and declare definitively, "No, this is not safe, I'm not doing it," another crew member may say, "I'm not sure if we should do this." These two messages may contain exactly the same concern, but it would be much easier to dismiss the latter. *Therefore we have a dual responsibility, both to acknowledge the concerns of our teammates even when they are expressed in a less assertive style, and to ensure that if we are the ones expressing concern, that appropriate assertiveness is used ensure our message is received and understood.*

Task Preoccupation

The relationship to workload and available attention for effective communication was discussed in the previous section.

This behavior may be evident in tasks requiring a high degree of concentration or ones that have high stakes attached to them. The act of intubating a critically ill patient serves as a good example. This is a high-stakes activity that has a great deal of social pressure on the person instrumenting the airway, because typically the majority of the team stops and waits while this task is completed. Task preoccupation may be avoided by empowering the team to intercede at a designated point if a team member goes beyond it; for example, the briefing at the beginning of the airway procedure states, "if the saturations fall below 95%, stop me, we will back out and bag the patient." Doing this makes it clear to the team that not only is it okay to stop you, but you are asking them to do it.

When a team member is task fixated and is not hearing you, using the person's proper name, title, or rank helps break through their focus and get your message heard. There may be times when a teammate's task fixation is severe enough to prompt more assertive behavior. The *two-challenge rule* is an agreement within a team. When an unsafe condition is present, the team will advise the team leader, or person performing the procedure, of that hazard or condition, e.g., "the saturations are falling." If that message is not acknowledged, then the team member repeats the message using the name or title of the individual, with an increased urgency and with a recommended action: "John, the sats are falling below 80%, we have to bag the patient." If the individual does not acknowledge the second message, then the teammate takes action to correct the problem. In this case he or she begins bagging the patient.

Rank and Experience Differences

When there is a significant difference in rank or experience between teammates, there can be a reluctance to challenge plans and question actions for fear of the consequences extending beyond the momentary situation. The experienced or ranking member expressly stating his or her openness to questions and his or her ability to make mistakes can overcome this barrier. The other pitfall of rank and experience can be *excessive professional courtesy,* which is a hesitancy of less senior or lower-ranking teammates to challenge or insult the more experienced or higher-ranking teammate's skills. Communication patterns in these situations tend to be passive and avoid direct confrontation.

Overcoming the Barriers: The Practice of Assertiveness Within a Team

Assertiveness is the ability of a teammate to state and maintain a position even if that position is contrary to the prevailing opinion of the group. Further, that individual maintains that opinion until he or she is persuaded by the facts, and is not swayed by the authority or personality of the other team members. Within the context of CRM, effective leaders expect and advocate for open and questioning communication from his or her crewmates. At the heart of assertiveness is the belief that each individual on the team has the right to express ideas and feelings, the right to be heard by the team, the right to be taken seriously, the right to ask for clarification, and the right to be treated with respect. *Teammates must speak up when they are unsure of instructions or a plan of action, when they believe they have a solution to the problem, or when they believe the crew or patient are in danger.* How we practice assertiveness in a high-stress environment, particularly with a high task loading, is as important as when we practice it. There are three key elements to communicating a concern in this setting:

1. Use the intended recipient's proper name or title.
2. State a specific concern.
3. State what you believe the consequence of that concern will be if it is not addressed.
4. Propose your solution.

In all of the case studies presented thus far, one member of the respective teams following this procedure may have prevented disaster. In the Tenerife disaster, had the flight engineer stated, "Captain (stating proper title) I am not sure we have been cleared for takeoff (stating specific concern) Pan Am may still be on the runway (perceived consequence), abort the takeoff (proposed solution)," the disaster may have been averted. In the case of Elaine Bromiley, had the nursing staff stated, "Doctor, the patients saturations are below 50%, we are in a can't-intubate can't-ventilate situation, we need to move to a surgical airway," her death may have been avoided.

Often, when time is less critical, a fifth step should be included: seeking feedback from the team. Conflicts within a team should be viewed as differences of opinion and approached open minded with a focus on finding the solution as opposed to defending positions.

CASE STUDY

Rob's Story

A flight crew departed a base in Northern California on a very dark night. The program at the time did not have night vision goggles, and the night was pitch black without a moon. The crew, consisting of two flight nurses and a pilot, had not worked together very much, and the pilot was a recent hire for the program. En route to the sending hospital, the aircraft had to fly over mountains and routinely maintained an altitude above 5500 feet. On this night, the crew member flying in the front seat noticed that the aircraft was flying several thousand feet lower than normal. The nurse raised his concern to the pilot, "Hey man, we are usually much higher than this." The pilot explained that he had set a GPS waypoint in a valley along his route, and if we flew to the waypoint they would be fine. The nurse considered this for a moment, knowing this was not the usual procedure and knowing that he could usually see the town's lights in the distance, replied, "Nope, either climb up to our usual altitude, or let's head back to base." The pilot, upset by the challenge, aggressively climbed, but soon the town lights appeared in the distance and the crew completed the transport. After the transport was complete the pilot and the flight nurse continued to argue, and it was decided that they would not fly any more that night. The next morning, with the chief pilot, base manager, and the flight nurse present, the pilot flew the route at the same altitude, to the same waypoint as the previous night. Had they continued their course the night before, they would have impacted terrain in the valley (R. LaCount, personal communication, 2009).

When we are called to act, and assertiveness is required, two factors often interfere with our decision to speak up and be heard. The first factor is our anticipation of the team's reaction, and the second is the perceived difference in rank or authority. Often in a team setting when something first appears to be going wrong, we look to the rest of the team and judge their reaction to it. If they do not appear to be concerned, then the individual with the concern is less likely to speak up. The second factor that may prevent speaking up is the belief that in doing so we would be questioning authority. *It is imperative that the senior crew empower the junior crew to speak up and question plans and actions.* Both of these factors are amplified in effect when an individual lacks confidence, believes a teammate is not approachable or is disinterested, fears reprisal, or is hesitant to invite conflict.

Sharing the Mental Model

A shared understanding of a task and the context of why it is being performed is the idea behind a shared mental model. This may take the form of recapping events, defining where the team is at in a problem, and deciding what the next steps are; this has been demonstrated to improve team performance.[16] This sharing of a mental model is often undertaken by the team leader but may be initiated by any member of the team as a means to bring some clarity to the situation. Additionally, mental model sharing provides the team leader the opportunity to invite alternate ideas and other observations from the team.

Lack of Shared Mental Model in the Blood Pressure Control Error In the case of Emily Bromiley both crew members recognized the change in the patient's status and the change in blood pressure. Because of a lack of a shared understanding of the patient's condition, the significance of that change held different meanings for the respective crew members, which promoted different and contradictory actions.

Recognizing Decision-Making Hazards

Strength of an Idea

When confronted with a time-sensitive emergency there is a tendency for an individual to grasp the first seemingly appropriate explanation or action without considering the alternatives. This is particularly true if the person offering up the solution is perceived to have expertise or authority. Once the group has grasped that one solution it can be extremely difficult to change directions, despite evidence to the contrary.

Groupthink

When a team has a high task loading, or during an emergency, raising an idea that is contrary to the prevailing thoughts of the team may be perceived by the individual as increasing the stress of the group and is thus avoided. Consequently, the single team member does not offer up information that conflicts with the group consensus, even if that information may be vital to the safe treatment or movement of the patient or the safety of the crew. As described by Janis,[17] the more cohesive the group is, the more individuals prioritize group harmony over the realistic exploration of options. This effect is intensified if the team leader is the person promoting the preferred solution.[17] Groupthink may be recognized as a rationalization of contrary evidence, peer pressure to conform, or self-censorship. When it is recognized begin by stating what you believe is happening: "We may be experiencing groupthink." Then state the immediate risks associated with the decision and ask for any other ideas.

Seeking the Perfect Solution

Seeking the perfect solution is a characteristic often found in newer team members. It is a tendency to seek the perfect solution or diagnosis at the exclusion of other appropriate and safe actions. This tendency may prevent any action from being taken and may allow the emergency to worsen. This tendency can be dealt with by first looking for safe, workable solutions and then improving on those solutions as time allows.[10]

Leadership

Most of what has been discussed in this chapter applies to the roles of leadership. The CRM principles of leadership seek to balance the authority of the team leader with the previously mentioned assertiveness of the team, thus allowing for decisive action when required and an environment open to input. As important as it is for the team to speak up when required, it is essential that the team leader does not hinder or withhold team input. He or she needs to encourage crew member input during planning and task completion, clearly stating the team's goals or intentions, and be flexible enough to change those plans if the team provides feedback that should be used. An additional role of leadership is the oversight of the team and to ensure that the team is operating within standard procedures. If situations require operation outside of the normal standard operating procedure, the team leader should discuss and announce such deviations.

Use of All Available Resources

Throughout all of this, the central theme has been that when confronting a challenge or a routine tasking, an effective team uses all available resources to ensure the safe care and movement of a patient. There are no separate CRM courses for EMTs, registered nurses, paramedics, pilots, or respiratory therapists. The principles applied here shape the interactions, regardless of the team makeup, to provide the safest possible means of moving a sick or injured patient.

Human Performance

Human performance at times of crisis is a matter of how well an individual or a team is prepared to meet the emergency, how well equipped that team is, and how well it manages acute stress. In the transport medicine environment we encounter environmental stressors, such as things that increase fatigue and weaken attention (e.g., workload, heat, noise, and sleep deprivation), but we also encounter acute stress. Acute stress is the result of situations that involve a novel situation, an unpredictable outcome, or a threat to the ego of an individual or team. The acute stress response is initiated by the sympathetic nervous system and is driven by the flight, fight, or freeze response, and it is mediated by the sympathetic nervous system. We must understand how these external stressors affect our ability as well as recognize the effects of acute stress and manage it accordingly to ensure maximum performance in this challenging environment.

Task Performance and External Stress

In 1908 Yerkes and Dodson developed a model that stated that different tasks require different degrees of arousal to complete, but at a certain point tasks requiring high-order thinking began to fail as arousal continued to climb, while simple tasks remain intact.[18] These findings have evolved over time to suggest an optimal stress performance zone, in which performance was enhanced at a moderate stress level and degraded as the individual became either understimulated (low stress) or overwhelmed (high stress). This theory became the ubiquitous "Inverted U" much propagated in discussions about stress and performance (Fig. 7.4).

This curvilinear representation of stress and performance suggests performance increases as stress levels increase, until it is impaired by excessive states of stress. Although this model is useful and explains aspects of individual performance at different stress levels, the problem with the model extrapolated from the work of Yerkes and Dodson is that different stressors affect performance differently, suggesting that there is no universal stress response.[19] For example, Broadbent described how loss of sleep affected speed but not accuracy of simple tasks, whereas heat stress affected accuracy but not speed and only typically at the beginning of a task. In his latter works Broadbent[20] demonstrated that increasing stress narrowed attention and limited the range

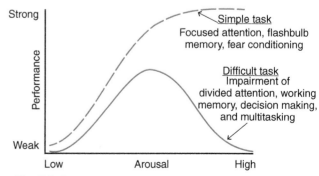

• **Fig. 7.4** Stress and performance. (Redrawn from Diamond DM, Campbell AM, Park CR, et al. "The Temporal Dynamics Model of Emotional Memory Processing," Neural Plasticity. 2007. doi:10.1155/2007/60803.)

of information that was being perceived and processed. What we are left with is a nonlinear understanding of the effect of stress on performance. It is not as easy as believing higher arousal states lead to improved performance until they do not; instead, the stress response will be dependent on the type of stressor.

Responses to External Stressors

Effects of Workload *Workload* can be understood as the relationship among the amount of work needing to be done (often referred to as task loading), the time available, and the amount of cognitive resource committed to the task (work capacity). It represents the cost to an individual's team as they attempt to adapt to that work with limited attention and concentration. The cost of high workloads can be exacted in the form fatigue, stress, and errors[21] as the required resources exceed those available. Common errors during high workloads include slower reaction times as well as errors in communication. When multiple concurrent demands are placed on a crew member, those tasks may interact in one of several ways. Tasks may interfere with each other by either confusing or competing with the other task, e.g., placing a central line competes and interferes with the task of maintaining SA of the patient's condition. The greater the requirement of attention (in this case to place a central line), the more likely the clinician is to lose sight of the patient's condition. When the clinician attempts to simultaneously perform both tasks, the limited resource of attention will result in a degradation of one or both of the tasks.[22] If the clinician elects to switch between tasks—first attending to the procedure, stopping, then attending to the understanding the patient's condition—before returning to the procedure, he or she may be more effective. The ability to effectively *task switch* is dependent on the degree of similarity among the tasks. The more *dis*similar a task is, the more effectively an individual can switch between them without seeing degradation in one of the tasks. Thus in the previously mentioned case, the more motor-based skill of placing a central line is significantly different from the primarily cognitive task of briefly assessing the patient's condition. Furthermore, the more practiced a task is, or the more expertise present in the individual, the less negative the effect when switching behaviors or simultaneously performing both tasks.[23]

Thermal Stress The effect of thermal stress, both heat and cold, on crew performance is related to the severity of those conditions, with the majority of cognitive impairment occurring in extremes of cold.[18] If a breakdown in thermal regulation is excluded from consideration, the predominant source of cognitive impairment involving information processing is a result of the distraction caused by the extremes of temperature. In terms of heat, initial exposure produced little effect on strength, but with exposure time, increases in fatigue,[24] decreases in vigilance,[25] and decreases in accuracy[26] all occurred. The effects seemed more likely to occur as temperatures increased above 85°F.

Effects of Noise Understanding the effect of noise on performance requires that first we describe the temporal characteristics of that stimulus (i.e., is the noise continuous or intermittent). Continuous noise seems to have little effect on simple task performance[27] at even relatively high decibel (dB) levels. As tasks become increasingly complex; however, continuous noise, especially above 95 dB, induces increasing numbers of errors, occasional slow responses, and some impairment of memory often occurring after approximately 30 minutes of exposure.[28]

In contrast to the continuous noise, intermittent noise appears to be significantly more disruptive than continuous noise, specifically if the intermittent noise comes at unpredictable intervals. When a new noise is present in the environment there is a notable decline in performance of an individual because the individual is more heavily loaded, thus performing additional tasks with more difficulty.[28] This effect will be minimized as the individual adapts to the noise and the task. As long as the tasks being performed are well practiced and the novel noises familiar, there should be little effect of performance. The performance of a new task, paired with the introduction of a novel noise, could result in a marked, although temporary, reduction in performance.

Effects of Fatigue It will come as little surprise that sleep deprivation results in performance degradation, including difficulty in monitoring data, increased distraction, focusing on the primary task while neglecting peripheral information, and delays in response and consistency.[29] Some of those fatigue effects may be moderated by failures of motivation during sleep-deprived states. Matthews and Desmond[30] demonstrated, while studying drivers, that when task demands are low, individuals had a harder time mobilizing sufficient effort to perform well, but when motivated to compete the task, many of the effects of fatigue can be mediated and performance preserved. The authors went on to suggest that interventions geared toward enhancing motivation would be more effective in mitigating fatigue in the short term than efforts geared at minimizing attention demands.

The degree of sleep deprivation has a linear relationship to the degree of impact on performance. In an experiment performed by Van Dongen et al.[31] the authors investigated the extent to which sleep can be restricted before the development of cognitive deficits. Two groups were assigned either 4 hours or 6 hours of sleep for a period lasting 3 days. Both groups demonstrated a linear reduction of cognitive performance but differed greatly in their ability to recognize their own impairment. After 3 days the group limited to 6 hours of sleep per night functioned at an equivalent level to an individual deprived of all sleep for 2 days, but they tended not to be aware of their inability to perform at normal levels. The effects of fatigue seem to be less evident when the tasks being performed are self-paced, but more apparent when the tasks are externally paced.[26]

Responses to Acute Stress

Acute stress is driven by fear, which is the recognition by an individual that something in the environment poses a danger to either the ego or the body (i.e., to their emotional well-being), or to the physical self. Imagine an experienced clinician responding to a cardiac arrest caused by an intentional overdose. It is likely that there is very little acute stress in that circumstance. It is not a novel situation for the experienced clinician, and he or she expects to perform well. Now imagine the same circumstance but the cardiac arrest immediately followed the administration of an overdose of a medication given by this same clinician. The patient's condition is no different, his physiology has not changed, but the stress level of the clinician has increased monumentally. What is different in the circumstance? The clinician in the second scenario is attached to the outcome and consequences of the resuscitation, resulting in an acute stress reaction to the event.

When acute stress presents itself the sympathetic nervous system adapts the body for a physical response; adrenal glands release adrenalin, muscles tense, blood pressure rises, and heart rate increases. This increase in heart rate has a correlation with performance and is a marker for the degree of stress the individual is under.

Stress and Heart Rate　As stress levels increase, the sympathetic surge drives heart rates higher with effects on our mentation and motor skills that are significantly different from high heart rates obtained during exercise. There are predictable points in this escalation when our performance begins to alter. Grossman and Christensen[32] described that when we first identify a threat, or are faced with a potential threat, our heart rates increase to between 90 and 115 bpm as our bodies begin to respond by increasing awareness, but we have not begun to prepare ourselves for the full flight or flight response yet. When faced with greater stress, or a more immediate danger, the authors described how our heart rates climb between 115 and 145 bpm, preparing us to make the most of our gross motor skills, and enhance our rapid visual and cognitive reaction time. The cost of this preparation is degradation in our fine motor skills, which is observed above heart rate of 115 bpm. Beyond 145 bpm our performance begins to drop off, with loss of peripheral vision, depth perception, and near vision, as well as auditory exclusion (Fig. 7.5).

After the Adrenaline　It is common after an acute stress reaction and a resolution of the emergency for there to be a period of almost giddiness. For example, after a particularly difficult or dicey intubation there is a collective release of the tension in the resuscitation bay or ambulance. Staff may start joking or talking about weekend plans. This is the result of the parasympathetic surge

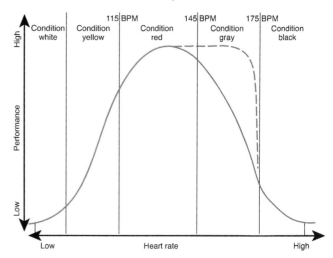

• **Fig. 7.5**　Stress and heart rate. (Redrawn from Grossman D, Christensen LW. *On Combat: The Psychology and Physiology of Deadly Conflict in War and Peace.* Millstadt, IL., 2008, Warrier Science Publication.)

that follows the high-stress encounter. It is also a time of danger for the patient and crew, because their guard is lowered.

Improving Performance Under Stress

Emotional Awareness

The ability of an individual's emotional awareness to mitigate stressor states is summarized by Staal[18]:

> There is some evidence to suggest that individuals with greater awareness of their emotional states—the ability to label their current feelings—perform better under stress than those unable to do so. Worchel and Yohai (1979) found that individuals who were able to label or identify the novel physiologic reactions they experienced under stress were less distressed by them and they performed better. Similarly, Gohm, Baumann, and Shiezak (2001) noted that individuals who are able to label or identify their emotional reactions to stressful events appear to have more attentional resources (perhaps due to engaging in fewer ruminations) to devote to tasks. The result is improved performance compared with those who are not able to label their emotional experience. It seems reasonable to conclude from these findings that cognitive appraisal is at least one explanatory mechanism. Those who can introspect and cognitively frame their experience are likely to feel better and improve their sense of control and predictability over their reactions than those unable to do so. These factors have previously been shown to be of value in reducing the negative effects of stress exposure. (p. 98)

Stress Inoculation

In an effort to fortify an individual or a team against some of the effects of stress, training can be developed to simulate those conditions before the team encounters them. What makes stress inoculation different from rehearsal and other psychomotor training is the increasingly realistic nature of the simulated encounters. Staal[18] explained that stress inoculation, through the successive approximation, "builds a sense of expectancy and outcome that is integrated into positive cognitive appraisal, a greater sense of mastery and confidence" (p. 98). Furthermore, it builds into routine what might have otherwise been an anxiety-producing situation.

Training Fine Motor Tasks With Stress in Mind When training for tasks or new procedures, repetition under increasing stress will develop a motor pattern that will remain intact despite higher levels of stress. Additionally the motor patterns can be learned in such a way that the effects of stress are minimized. How you anchor a hand while holding an instrument should not be designed for calm environments; instead, rehearse the skill assuming your fine motor skills will be impaired. How will you steady your hand? How will you support the instrument?

Tactical Breathing

Designed by the military, tactical breathing allows for a targeted reduction in heart rate and stress level during times of acute stress. Also referred to as box breathing, it involves breathing in 4 seconds, holding your breath for 4 seconds, exhaling 4 seconds, and holding the exhale for 4 seconds. Doing this several times before or during a stressful situation will help regulate your sympathetic surge and keep you in a heart rate range appropriate for the situation in which you find yourself (Fig. 7.6).

Focusing through the Parasympathetic Surge During the parasympathetic surge, after the adrenaline dump, it is important to maintain SA and focus on the next priorities. Reassess the patient and immediately establish the next series of actions and brief the team to keep them focused as well.

Conclusion

In transport medicine mistakes will be made; the environment is too dynamic, and the target is moving too fast to be perfect. The key to operating in this environment in a safe and effective way is to develop a team of people that are

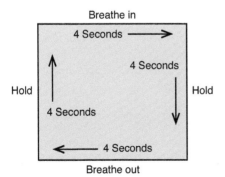

• **Fig. 7.6** Tactical breathing.

able to see clearly, maintain SA, and communicate to safeguard each other and the patients. This requires that we understand how we communicate in a team, what barriers may get in the way, how to overcome them, and how we as individuals respond and manage our external and acute stress reactions.

References

1. Helmreich RL, Klinect JR, Wilhelm JA. System safety and threat and error management: the line operations safety audit. *Proceedings of the Eleventh International Symposium on Aviation Psychology*. Columbus: The Ohio State University; 2001.
2. Ferner RE, Aronson JK. Clarification of terminology in medication errors: definitions and classification. *Drug Saf.* 2006;29(11): 1011-1022.
3. Aronson JK. Medication errors: definitions and classification. *Br J Clin Pharmacol.* 2009;67(6):599-604.
4. Endsley MR. Toward a theory of situational awareness in dynamic systems. *Human Factors.* 1995;37(1):32-64.
5. Reason J. *Human Error.* New York: Cambridge University Press; 1990.
6. McCreary J, Pollard M, Stevenson K, Wilson M. Human Factors: Tenerife revisited. *J Air Transp World Wide.* 1998;3(1): 23-32. Retrieved from http://ntl.bts.gov/lib/7000/7500/7585/jatww3-1wilson.pdf.
7. Rotisch PA, Babcock GL, Edmunds WW. *Human Factors Report on the Tenerife Accident.* Retrieved from www.project-tenerife.com; http://www.project-tenerife.com/engels/PDF/alpa.pdf; 1977.
8. Ardant D'Picq C. *Battle Studies: Ancient and Modern.* Harrisburg, PA: Military Service Publishing; 1947.
9. National Transportation Safety Board. *Aircraft Accident Report: United Airlines Inc.*, Douglas DC-8-54, N8082U, Portland, Oregon, December 28, 1978 (NTSB-AAR-79-7). Washington, DC: Government Printing Office; 1979.
10. Kern T. *Redefining Airmanship.* New York: McGraw-Hill; 1997.
11. Helmreich RL, Merritt AC, Wilhelm JA. The evolution of crew resource management training in commercial aviation. *Int J Aviat Psychol.* 1999;9(1):19-32.
12. Cooper GE, White MD, Lauber JK, eds. *Resource Management on the Flight Deck: Proceedings of a NASA/Industry Workshop* (NASA Conference Publication 2120). Washington, DC: Government Printing Office; 1979.
13. Kanki BG, Helmreich RL, Anca J. *Crew Resource Management.* New York: Academic Press; 2010.
14. Michael H. The case of Elaine Bromiley: independent review on the care given to Mrs. Elaine Bromiley on March 29, 2005. Retrieved from http://testing.chfg.org/resources/07_qrt04/Anonymous_Report_Verdict_and_Corrected_Timeline_Oct_07.pdf; 2005.
15. Brehmer B. 10th International Command and Control Research and Technology Symposium. In *The Dynamic OODA Loop: Amalgamating Boyd's OODA Loop and the Approach to Command and Control.* Symposium conducted at the Department of War Studies, Stockholm, Sweden. Retrieved from http://www.dodccrp.org/events/10th_ICCRTS/CD/papers/365.pdf; 2006.
16. Westli HK, Johnsen BH, Eid J, et al. Teamwork skills, shared mental models, and performance in simulated trauma teams: An independent group design. *Scand J Trauma Resusc Emerg Med.* 2010;18:47.

17. Janis IL. *Groupthink*. Boston: Houghton Muffin Company; 1982.
18. Staal MA. Stress, cognition, and human performance: A literature review and conceptual framework. Retrieved from Ames Research Center, Moffett Field: http://human-factors.arc.nasa.gov/flightcognition/Publications/IH_054_Staal.pdf; 2004.
19. Broadbent DE. Differences and interactions between stresses. *Q J Exp Psychol*. 1963;15:205-211.
20. Broadbent DE. *Decision and stress*. London: Academic Press; 1971.
21. Hart SG. *Task Loading Index*. Retrieved from Human Factors and Ergonomics Society: http://www.stavelandhfe.com/images/TLX_20_years_later_2006_Paper.pdf; 2006.
22. Hitch GJ, Baddeley AD. Verbal reasoning and working memory. *Q J Exp Psychol*. 1976;28:603-621.
23. Spelke E, Hirst W, Neisser U. Skills of divided attention. *Cognition*. 1976;4(3):215-230.
24. Enander AE. Effects if thermal stress on human performance. *Scand J Work Environ Health*. 1989;15:27-33.
25. Grether WF. Human performance at elevated environmental temperature. *Aerosp Med*. 1973;44(7):747-755.
26. Driskell JE, Johnson B, Hughes S, Batchelor C. *Development of Quantitative Specifications for Simulating the Stress Environments* [Report No. AL-TR-1991-0109]. 1992.
27. Stevens SS. Stability of human performance under intense noise. *J of Sound Vib*. 1972;21(1):35-56.
28. Broadbent DE. Human performance and noise. In: Harris CM, ed. *Handbook of Noise Control*. (2nd ed.). New York: McGraw-Hill; 1979.
29. Bartlett FC. Psychological criteria for fatigue. In: Floyd WF, Welford AT, eds. *Symposium on Fatigue*. London: H.K. Lewis; 1953.
30. Matthews G, Desmond PA. Task-induced fatigue states and simulated driving performance. *Q J Exp Psychol*. 2002;55(2):659-686.
31. Van Dongen HP, Maislin G, Mullington JM, Dinges DF. The cumulative cost of additional wakefulness: dose-response effects on neurobehavioral functions and sleep physiology from chronic sleep restriction and total sleep deprivation. *Sleep*. 2003;26(2):117-126.
32. Grossman D, Christensen LW. *On Combat: The Psychology and Physiology of Deadly Conflict in War and Peace*. Millstadt, IL: Warrier Science Publications; 2008.

8

Patient Safety

MICHEL HALL, KRISTA HAUGEN, TINA JOHNSON, JONATHAN JOHNSON, JAMES RUTHERFORD, KEVIN SCHITOSKEY, AND MICHAEL A. FRAKES

The first known statement addressing patient safety in health care was when Hippocrates declared, "I will never do harm to anyone," which has become the basis for the Hippocratic Oath. Other health care leaders, including Ignaz Semmelweiss (1857), Florence Nightingale (1863), Ernest Codman (1911), Robert Moser (1959), and Elihu Schimmel (1964), have put forth various patient safety concepts for centuries. It is interesting that Semmelweiss was derided and ignored by his contemporaries, died in an asylum, and the prescience of his work was not recognized until long after his death. In addition to his scientific contributions, perhaps his story should encourage persistence in today's patient safety advocates.

In the modern era, however, the Institute of Medicine (IOM), using information from the Harvard Medical Practice study, estimated that at least 98,000 Americans die each year from medical errors and compared that total to a "jumbo jet" crashing every day.[1] More recent research has suggested these numbers are much higher: up to 400,000 deaths and costs of at least $17.1 billion for measurable medical errors.[2]

These initiatives, and high-profile medical errors such as Josie King and the Quaid twins, have changed the way health care approaches patient safety and medical errors.[3,4] Incident-reporting systems continue to evolve and are changing how events, from near-misses through high-acuity errors impacting patients, are reported, tracked, and disclosed. Several organizations have been instrumental in the improvements in patient safety, including the Agency for Healthcare Quality and Research, the Institute for Healthcare Improvement, and the National Patient Safety Foundation. The 2005 Patient Safety Act was instrumental in promoting the creation of the Patient Safety Organizations, with the ultimate goal of encouraging voluntary and confidential adverse event reporting. The National Patient Safety Foundation has published a white paper follow up to the IOM report, titled "Free From Harm: Accelerating Patient Safety Improvement Fifteen Years After To Err Is Human."[5]

Errors can occur in all medical specialties and with all levels of experience. A paradigm shift in addressing risk and errors is the increased focus on system designs and ergonomic stressors, and also on human factors, including stress and fatigue. Another element of efforts to improve patient safety is a focus on the medical provider involved in the error. Universally, clinicians are hardworking and committed to caring. No one comes to work planning to commit an error or harm a patient. Dr. Albert Wu was the first to use the phrase "second victim" when discussing medical errors involving a patient, referring to the clinician involved in the error.[6] Affected clinicians can exhibit signs of anxiety, depression, and begin to doubt themselves in the clinical arena.

Organizational Characteristics Associated With Patient Safety

Health care organizations accept the inevitability of failure in both routine and sentinel events: hand hygiene compliance rates are reported at under 50% and wrong site/patient/procedure surgeries occur in 1 per 112,000 procedures.[7-9] At least 70%, and perhaps well over 90%, of surgical and critical care alarms are not relevant.[10,11] Imagine such performance in the operation of a nuclear reactor.

Health care, and particularly critical care transport, calls for extremely high performance because the milieu is characterized by the following:

- Hypercomplexity: This is the need for coordinating multiple systems and the variability of caring for patients, rather than machine-based systems.
- Tight coupling: Individual members depend on the successful performance of tasks by other individuals on the team.
- Complex communication networks: This uses multiple decision makers and the need for frequent, immediate feedback.
- Compressed operating times.
- High consequences of errors.

Highly reliable organizations maintain exemplary safety levels over a long time horizon. Rather than accepting failure as inevitable or acceptable, they maintain extremely safe operations with a collective mindfulness in which everyone values error identification and analysis of close calls for the lessons that can be learned. A commitment to reporting small problems and unsafe conditions allows them to be remedied before a substantial risk develops or error occurs.[7,12] The classic examples of such organizations are the United States nuclear navy and the United States nuclear power industry. Health care organizations and providers can benefit from such mindfulness, which is characterized by five elements:

1. Preoccupation with failure
2. Reluctance to simplify
3. Sensitivity to operations
4. Deference to expertise
5. Resilience

Preoccupation with failure describes a continued belief (even suspicion) that potential harms lurk constantly in the environment, rather than a paralyzing fear of error. This continuous alert for small signals creates a focus on predicting and preventing, rather than on reacting to, adverse events. The highly aware environment also counters the complacency that can come with relatively scarce events. For a health care organization, no news is not good news, but rather means that team members either are not recognizing or are not reporting unsafe conditions that will ultimately lead to harm. This shows that the foundation of high reliability is the reporting of near misses, trapped errors, unsafe conditions, and unsafe behaviors. The organization must encourage vigorous reporting and remove barriers to reporting. Moreover, it must view reports not by complacently congratulating the success of safety mechanisms, but with the knowledge that they identify calls for continued improvement.

Highly reliable organizations also understand that systems can fail in novel ways and do not assume that failure is the result of a single, simple cause. When a risk is identified, oversimplification of the explanation can miss a subtlety that, if addressed, could prevent a future failure. A failure unaddressed because of an overly simplified explanation allows risk to persist.

Sensitivity to operations is situational awareness at both the individual and organizational levels. Members are not only free to speak up about anomalies, potential errors, and actual errors, but they understand their obligation to do so. Individually, everyone involved in operations understands expected performance and always reports deviations from that expected performance. Desensitization to unsafe performance and practices creates a "culture of low expectations" that is a key cause of adverse events.[13] The organization understands that manuals and policies must constantly change because of the complexity and evolution of the workplace and work quickly to update training and resources.

Reliability requires both a clear organizational structure and a deference to expertise. Although these ideas may intuitively seem conflicting, they are not. In times of high operational tempo and when evaluating responses to detected risks or errors, experience and hierarchy are often inversely related to availability and do not necessarily equate with expertise. Health care is a classic example: senior leaders and clinicians are much less likely to be available for a complex nighttime case. At the time of an operation (a transport or patient care encounter), expertise lies with those at the operational level. Once the operational tempo has normalized (an individual event is over or crisis managed), participants report their outcomes and lessons learned and the organization marshals the expertise to understand and address identified future risks and deploys learnings across the organization.

At the same time, a clear organizational structure is required to ensure integration: the disparate parts of the organization benefit from evolving wisdom, and the focus on high-quality outcomes is ingrained in every part of the operation. Hierarchy also allows for accountability and resource allocation. Quality is a top-priority strategic goal in a highly reliable organization, with the board actively engaged in the quality plan, committed to the goal, and with the Chief Executive Officer leading the development of a proactive quality agenda. Cascading down the organization, proficiency with improvement tools and strategies is required for career advancement, and reward systems at all levels are linked with quality accomplishment. Performance improvement tools are accepted throughout the organization, and key quality measures are routinely reported internally and externally. Individual providers have performance improvement training relevant to their roles, and providers outside the leadership structure routinely lead performance initiatives.

Closely related to deference to expertise is resilience: the organization is not disabled by errors, but recognizes them quickly and responds quickly to them. The assumption is that, in spite of safeguards, systems may fail. In anticipation of that, teams are well trained to perform quick assessments; to work effectively in ad hoc teams that may include outsiders; have the necessary knowledge, tools, and resources; and have practiced responding to failures.

These traits of individuals and organizations must be so pervasive that they define the culture of the organization. Five intertwined concepts describe a culture best positioned for optimal patient safety: an informed culture supports a learning culture and relies on a reporting culture. The reporting culture cannot exist without a just culture and a culture of respect.[14-16]

An organization and the leaders of an organization must be fully informed about factors affecting whole-system safety and must act responsibly on those reports. The organization must learn from both reactive and proactive safety assessments and have the willingness to adapt and improve. To achieve this, leadership fosters a learning culture. Team members understand risks associated with their operational area and are encouraged not only to identify and report safety threats but actively to seek changes needed to resolve those threats. Leadership has accountabilities to provide the teams with the necessary knowledge, skills, and real or simulated experience to work safely. When presented with safety information, it must have the ability to use it to reach correct conclusions and an inherent willingness to make improvements.

As discussed, learning and informed cultures rely on a strong reporting culture, in which everyone is not only prepared to report errors and near-misses but understands their obligation to do so. It is not whether a reporting system exists, but whether errors, near-misses, and hazards are regularly reported. As leaders and operational personnel must freely share critical safety information without fear or punitive action, a reporting culture depends on how the organization handles blame and punishment.

James Reason famously posits that a so-called just culture is required to support a reporting culture and, subsequently, informed and learning cultures.[14,15] In many applications, the just culture has been carved out from the other necessary elements of a safety culture and is sometimes perverted into a no-blame approach to individual actions. A true just culture is one in which participants are encouraged to, and even rewarded for, providing important safety-related information. The organization's obligation not to "shoot the messenger" is met by an individual's duty to produce an outcome, follow a procedure, or avoid undue risk. Just as it is unacceptable to punish any error without consideration of the causal factors, it is equally unacceptable to give blanket immunity. There is culpability for repetitive at-risk behaviors and for behaviors involving recklessness or malice.

Leape and colleagues have suggested that disrespectful behavior is the root cause of the health care culture that threatens both patient safety and organizational culture by impairing communication, preventing compliance with guidelines and safe practices, undermining teamwork, and alienating patients.[17,18] To counter this, health care organizations must work actively to encourage a culture of respect.

Disrespectful behavior takes many forms. The most common behaviors are not obviously flagrant and disruptive practices, but rather are demeaning or condescending treatment of any other team member, passive-aggressive behaviors, and passive disrespect. Passive-aggressive behaviors are defined by negativism and intent to cause psychological harm, including refusing to do tasks, or doing them in a way intended to annoy others. They can include failing to follow through on agreements and deliberate delays or omissions in returning needed communications. Passive disrespect, on the other hand, is the spectrum of uncooperative behaviors not rooted in malice, yet still disrespectful to others and to the organization. These are the colleagues who are often accepted but labeled as "difficult." These providers may be apathetic, burned out, or frustrated, and they display behaviors such as chronic tardiness to appointments and in returning communications, poor collaboration, impatience with questions, and failure to follow safe practices.

An extremely safe organization requires staff at every level to be comfortable sharing information and concerns with others, and to be commended when they do so. Disrespectful behavior is a barrier to this information sharing, and the presence of disrespectful behavior in the environment is associated with increased risk for error.[19] Highly reliable organizations do not tolerate intimidating or disrespectful behavior from any member, with no exceptions made for even the most senior or most skilled members.

Provider Readiness

Each day, transport providers manage critically ill patients during one of the most vulnerable periods of the health care experience. Impaired providers present a risk to the patient, their partners, their employers, and to themselves. Impairment caused by chemical dependency is most commonly considered; it is important also to consider the risks caused by other impairments. For over 40 years, the American Medical Association has described providers who are "unable to practice medicine with reasonable skill and safety to patients because of physical or mental illness, including deterioration through the ageing process or loss of motor skill, or excessive use or misuse of drugs including alcohol."[20] Professional difficulties, such as stress from errors, malpractice, or litigation, and simple poor incompetent clinical performance also interfere with the ability to provide care within appropriate safety margins.[6]

Teams make fewer errors than individual providers, and the Agency for Healthcare Quality and Research and Department of Defense Patient Safety Program in 2006 released Team Strategies and Tools to Enhance Performance and Patient Safety (TeamSTEPPS) in an effort to reduce medical errors and bring a team approach to the multidisciplinary health care delivery.[21] Much like crew resource management, TeamSTEPPS incorporates concepts that help break down the hierarchical barriers in communication, increase situational awareness, and acknowledge that to err is human.[1] The concepts of effective teamwork are reviewed extensively in Chapter 7 of this book.

In addition to improved communication, provider readiness should also focus on initial education and ongoing clinical and technical proficiency. Current evidence links the lack of board certifications to poor outcomes in the in-patient setting.[22] Along with education and certification requirements, medical simulation can create realistic situations, which aids in the promotion of patient safety–centered care. Robert Wachter points out that "the adage of see one, do one, teach one is not much of an exaggeration."[22] Providers are challenged to make critical clinical decision and provide technical, high-risk procedures in unique environments. Advancements in simulation training have proven to be successful in providing an environment in which providers are able to navigate their learning curves without causing patient harm. It can also be an opportunity to provide challenging ongoing education that can be rooted in the organization's actual case experience or performance improvement processes. Simulation is also one of the few opportunities to exercise human factors skills.

However, simulation-based training comes with a price. High-fidelity human patient simulators can cost over $100,000, in addition to other considerations such as supplies, staff time, and travel. Nevertheless, compared with the cost of operational and teamwork errors and given the unique nature of the transport medical environment, the return on investment for quality simulation-based training seems favorable.

There is increasing interest across the health care community in evaluating the ongoing physical, technical, and mental function of providers, both in relation to physical fitness for duty and the ability to provide safe and effective patient care.[23]

In the continuous demand areas of health care and public safety, fatigue is a significant concern. Surprisingly, while the transportation industries have linked fatigue with poor outcomes, fatigue alone has not been clearly tied with poor health care outcomes. An oft-cited study showed that after 17 to 19 hours of sleeplessness, performance was equal to or worse than a blood alcohol content of 0.05%, and performance after longer sleepless periods reached or exceeded that of levels of legal intoxication.[24] Common sense would suggest that a sleep-deprived health care provider is more susceptible to making a medical error. Much of the medical fatigue research has been focused on residency programs. There is suggestion that confounders to a decisive link between fatigue and outcomes include variability in environments, the support of teams and team variability, and that the benefits from fatigue reduction may be balanced by the risks from increased provider-to-provider handoffs. Reductions in duty hours in medical residency programs do seem to improve quality of life.[25]

Although patient needs do not change regarding the time of day or day of week, medical errors are more common, and outcomes often worse, during nights and weekends.[26,27] It may be that there is greater access to support and supervision on weekdays, so there is more accountability during the times in which errors may be more visible, making providers more astute in their clinical decisions. In spite of the lack of absolute certainty, critical care transport providers and organizations must be attentive to the potential for safety risks associated with fatigue, night work, and weekend work.

Every industry, including medical transport, must be prepared to deal with strain between safety and productivity. Research suggests that health care providers experience different types of pressure, such as time pressure (having to perform tasks in a short period of time) and production pressure (having to "produce" at the expense of safety). An unnamed oil executive has been quoted as saying: "Safety is not our top priority. Our top priority is getting oil out of the ground. However, when safety and productivity conflict, then safety takes priority."[22] This statement can be echoed in many industries, including health care. Our top priority is patient care, which requires that safe care is provided to patients. On that point, conflicts must always be resolved in favor of the patient. When patient care and operational safety conflict, operational safety must take priority, which necessarily furthers patient safety.

Substance abuse rates and dependence are similar for health care professionals and the general public, estimated at up to 15%. Although abuse rates are similar, use rate not meeting the criteria for abuse or dependence may be up to five times that of the general public.[28,29]

It can be difficult to identify impaired providers. Often, the first indication is domestic discord. Physical, emotional, and behavioral alterations often precede detectable changes in work performance. Changes in work habits such as attendance, tardiness, decreased productivity, decreased charting skill, and conflicts with colleagues may indicate substance abuse. An actual clinical performance decline is usually one of the last signs of a substance use disorder.[28] Many of these signs and symptoms seem fairly obvious but are often overlooked and excused by colleagues, family, and friends. The American Medical Association clearly describes an ethical obligation to make objective reports about impaired, incompetent, and unethical colleagues, including those who behave inappropriately, and to ensure that identified deficiencies are either remedied or further reported.[20,29]

Impaired health care providers are usually intelligent and achievement oriented, giving them good potential for rehabilitation if they have the emotional intelligence to accept the need for recovery and to participate in the process. Reported recovery rates vary between 27% and 92% for physicians, which are likely better with at least 2 weeks of intensive therapy, and the percentage of nurses who reenter clinical practice ranges between 70.2% and 97.4%. In a conundrum for critical care transport providers, the recommendation is often that impaired providers return to work in areas of less stress and with less access to potential drugs of abuse. When providers return to work, self-vigilance and formal monitoring procedures are needed to maintain abstinence. Random alcohol- and drug-screening programs are essential: recovery and continued abstinence correlate with posttreatment monitoring and surveillance techniques.[28]

Error prevention takes preparation. Health care providers must be in a constant state of readiness to prevent medical errors and provide patient safety–centered care. Each must remain consciously aware of their actions to reduce error. Attention to communication, provider skill, fatigue, production pressure, and substance abuse are key elements in planning for reducing medical errors and improving patient safety.

Communication Tools: Checklists and Handoffs

Human recall is complicated by emotions, stress, fatigue, and haste. Providers may forget or may take a shortcut or "calculated risk." Any of those can end with disastrous consequences. The amount of information critical care transport providers are required to process during every transport can overwhelm the provider's ability to properly use it or convey it to others in a consistent, correct, and safe manner.

Human factors account for the majority of adverse events in aviation as well as in clinical medicine. The current safety paradigm is based on limiting human variability in otherwise safe systems, which requires strict procedural guidelines. Strict procedures lend themselves well to checklists as memory aids.[30] The aviation community has used checklists for some time; they are one factor associated with an improved safety profile. Box 8.1 describes what is

BOX 8.1 Origin of the Checklist

On October 30, 1935, the Boeing Model 299 crashed during a US Army Air Corps flight competition held to select the next-generation long-range bomber. After a normal taxi and takeoff, the 299 began a smooth climb and then suddenly stalled, falling to the ground and bursting into flames, killing two of five persons on board. The investigation revealed nothing mechanical had gone wrong and found "pilot error" as the cause of the crash.

The pilot was Major Ployer P. Hill, the US Army Air Corps Chief of Flight Testing. Major Hill had years of experience and expertise under his belt. The new Boeing Model 299 had four engines with multiple new features requiring adjustment and regulation. Hill had forgotten to release a new locking mechanism on the elevator and rudder controls. After the crash, the 299 was reported by newspapers as "too much plane for one man to fly." Boeing nearly went bankrupt.

A group of test pilots remained convinced that the Model 299 was flyable. Aeronautics had advanced so significantly that the Model 299 was not too much plane for one man to fly. It was too complicated to be left to the memory of the pilot—no matter how much experience and training. What was needed was a way of making sure that nothing was forgotten or overlooked. The answer was a checklist. Using the checklist, 12 Model 299s ended up flying over 1.8 million miles without a serious accident. The Army ended up accepting Model 299 and ordered almost 13,000 of them. We know it as the B-17 today.

From Schamel J. How the pilot's checklist came about. *Officer Rev Mag.* 2010;50(5):16.

believed to be the development of the first modern checklist.[31] Errors of ineptitude are mistakes made because providers do not make proper use of the knowledge they possess. Experts are human and all humans are subject to making mistakes. A simple checklist is essential to protect caregivers from these errors of ineptitude. Gawande developed a surgical checklist and applied it around the world with amazing success, as did Dr. Peter Pronovost, with a checklist intervention to reduce central line–associated bloodstream infections.[32,33] Well-designed checklists can improve outcomes.

Checklists are not a foolproof barrier to error, however.[34] A checklist can be used effectively, incompletely, or disregarded, thus negating the purpose for which it was created. The most common reasons for not using a checklist are staff resistance, function perceived as inappropriate or illogical, complacency with process or content, and the perception of it wasting time.[35]

Numerous checklists have been developed to prevent error such as the "challenge and response" performed by most critical care transport teams before departure, and procedural checklists are increasingly used (Tables 8.1 and 8.2). Most transport checklists have been studied in the context of interfacility transport.[36] Although prehospital and interfacility transport studies are limited, it makes sense that a well-designed checklist could prevent adverse events in the transport environment.

The question is: What constitutes a good checklist for transport? It is important to note that a checklist is not a teaching tool or algorithm, but a performance aid. Traits of a well-written checklist are described in Box 8.2, and

TABLE 8.1 Challenge and Response

EMS Service Provider Challenge	Flight Crew Response
Drugs, blood, radio, cell phone, chargers	Present
Equipment onboard, hard equipment secured with strap	Secured
Oxygen bottles secured	Secured
Lap belt for each flight crew member and passenger	Present
Adequate onboard oxygen with 50-psi source	Adequate >1000 if vent
Working inverter	Present
Working onboard suction	Present
STATCOM notified of ambulance/flight crew contact information and planned travel route	Notified
Flight Crew Challenge	**EMS Provider Response**
Patient condition/information is not presented to ambulance operator	Check
STAT personnel will advise the operator when out of lap belts	Done
One crew member will remain awake and in front with driver between 21:00 and 07:00	Check
Expected passengers, i.e., family members, additional medical help, and so forth	Done
Mode of Transport Briefing	
No emergency lights/siren unless directed by flight crew	Done
If emergency response is indicated, vehicle will stop at all traffic lights/stop signs	Done
Concerns regarding ride quality, road conditions discussed as needed	Done

EMS, Emergency medical services.
Courtesy Stat Medevac.

TABLE 8.2	Checklist

Intubation Preparation
Nasal cannula
Second oxygen source
BVM and O_2 on
Suction on and functioning
Functional IV line
Pulse oximeter and ECG monitor
10-mL syringe
Tube(s)
Stylette
Blade(s)
Handle
Light
Confirmation device
Commercial tube holder
Backup plan

BVM, Bag-valve-mask; *ECG,* electrocardiogram; *IV,* intravenous.
Courtesy Stat Medvac.

• BOX 8.2   Checklist Development

Laying the Groundwork

Are objectives straightforward and succinct?
For each item, ask the following questions:
- Is this step critical to safety? Is there a hazard or danger if it is missed?
- Is it already covered by other items?
- Is it actionable; is a specific response needed?
- Is it written to be read aloud for a verbal check?

Consider:
- Including items that will build communication among team members
- Involving team members in the checklist development process

Writing the Checklist

Use:
- Natural pauses in sentence structure to make verbal use easier
- Basic language and structure
- Minimal colors, use basic colors, if any
- Title that reflects objectives/purpose
- Length one page or shorter, with readable font
- Fewer than 10 items per pause point
- Date of creation/revision visible

Proofing

- Trial with team members in real or simulated situation, then revise based on response
- Evaluate adequacy of length, tone, effect
- Confirm that errors are intercepted before producing an adverse effect
- Is the checklist's length brief enough and easy to read?
- Does the checklist fit the usual workflow?
- Plan for future revisions and review of checklist

---

include clear, concise objectives, a design that is easy to read aloud, fits on one page, has been trialed with front-line users, and is continually reviewed and/or updated. One important item in checklists is the use of "pause points," which are natural breaks in workflow, and a limit to fewer than 10 items per pause point.[37]

Another approach that may help improve both handoff and checklist processes is incorporating a pause or a "safety check" with each transfer made by the team.[38] A safety check after giving a handoff can provide an opportunity to double-check that the appropriate information has been given as well as received. A pause can also be used on nonpatient legs of a transport: a safety check before leaving base or after delivering a patient can help ensure all equipment has been retrieved, which can directly impact patient safety if, for example, a medication bag or ventilator would have otherwise been left behind.

The complex and multivariate nature of critical care transport, combined with time pressures, the stress of critical situations, fatigue, and other human factors, can create ample opportunities for miscommunication of critical information. Communication failures result in 60% to 70% of sentinel events in the inpatient setting.[39] In a study of 60 surgical malpractice claims associated with poor communication, 43% involved poor handoffs.[40]

Transitions of care—the movement of patients between health care practitioners, settings, and home as their condition and care needs change—account for a significant number of medical errors, perhaps up to 80%.[41] Standardization of handoffs is one way to improve communication and continuity of care. One of the Joint Commission's National Patient Safety Goals requires a "standardized approach to handoff communications, including an opportunity to ask and respond to questions."

Mnemonics are examples of simple checklists that can ensure completeness and consistency during the patient handoff process. A large, multisite trial, the IPASS study, demonstrated a nearly 25% reduction in medical errors in a teaching hospital setting after implementation of a standardized handoff bundle including mnemonics.[42] Examples of using IPASS are seen in Tables 8.3 and 8.4. The SBAR

TABLE 8.3	IPASS Mnemonic	
I	Illness/severity	Stable, guarded, critical
P	Patient summary	Brief summary of patient condition and treatment plan
A	Action list	To-do items to be completed by the receiving clinical team
S	Situational awareness/ contingency plans	Directions in case of changes in patient status
S	Synthesis by receiver	Opportunity for "read back" to confirm understanding; receiver asks questions

TABLE 8.4	"IPASS the Baton" Mnemonic	
I	Introduction	Introduce yourself and your role; include the patient
P	Patient	Name, identifiers, sex, location
A	Assessment	Chief complaint, vital signs, symptoms, diagnosis
S	Situation	Current status/circumstances, code status, recent changes, response to treatments
S	Safety concerns	Critical laboratory values or reports, socioeconomic factors, allergies, alerts, i.e., fall, isolation precautions
The		
B	Background	Comorbidities, previous episodes, current medications, family history
A	Actions	Describe what actions were taken and what are still required along with rationale
T	Timing	Level of urgency and explicit timing and prioritization of actions
O	Ownership	Who is responsible, individual or team, including patient/family
N	Next	Identify anticipated changes, plans, contingencies

Copyright © 2012 by the American Academy of Pediatrics.

TABLE 8.5	SBAR Mnemonic	
S	Situation	What is going on with the patient: a problem statement?
B	Background	What is the background on this patient/situation?
A	Assessment	Observations/evaluation of patient's current status
R	Recommendations	Suggestions for continued care of the patient

• **BOX 8.3   MIVT Mnemonic**

M: Mechanism of injury
I: Injuries
V: Vital signs
T: Treatment

• **BOX 8.4   CHEATED Mnemonic**

C: Chief complaint
H: History
E: Examination
A: Assessment
T: Treatment
E: Evaluation
D: Disposition

• **BOX 8.5   CHATT or CHART Mnemonic**

C: Chief complaint
H: History
A: Assessment
T or Rx: Treatment
T: Transport/changes en route

• **BOX 8.6   DMIST Mnemonic**

D: Demographics
M: Mechanism of injury
I: Injuries
S: Vital signs
T: Treatment

method (Table 8.5) is more commonly used in the hospital setting because it may permit more effective modification to meet the needs of the transport professional's environment. Additional detailed components can be added under each category to capture the elements necessary for accurate and thorough communication. Other examples of mnemonics used in the prehospital setting to give report are MIVT, CHATT/CHART, CHEATED, and DMIST, which are seen in Boxes 8.3 to 8.6.

Another important consideration when using standard handoff methods or checklists is the process surrounding utilization. Effective communication goes far beyond simply using a standard handoff or checklist. Although standardization of handoffs and utilization of checklists can help decrease errors, simultaneously addressing other aspects that impact communication, such as distractions, situational awareness, training, and environmental factors, also helps to enhance the effectiveness of communication during patient handoffs [38] Standardized handoff training for critical care transport teams should include the desired rubric and training in effective communication and the impact of human factors on communication. Organizations should measure the effectiveness of the handoff tool in preventing or decreasing adverse events related to miscommunication during handoffs.

Some authors suggest a "pit stop" approach, which takes into consideration the comprehensive aspects of a handoff. This includes considerations regarding the environment, teamwork, equipment, and other human factors that may impact the ability to communicate critical information.[38] Regardless of the tool, specific factors associated with handoff effectiveness are culture, introductions, environment, time, standardization, direct communication with the team leader, and interdisciplinary feedback.[43,44] It is interesting that perceptions of professionalism improve the quality of handoffs, and rude behavior by any team member increases the risk for medical error.[19,45]

Teams can harness awareness of these factors to improve both giving and receiving handoff. The transport organization must enculturate the importance of a quality handoff in team members who will model that to requesting and receiving team providers on every transport. At the bedside, the team can set the tone for a handoff with introductions and a stated expectation that there will be a conscious pause in the action and attention to the handoff. When the environment is stabilized, a brief, organized handoff using the desired format can be delivered, followed with a specific request for feedback and questions from both the provider and nursing teams at the bedside.

Using simulation training as an opportunity to practice handoffs can also enhance effective communication as well as training with referring and receiving providers. Templates of handoff methods can be shared during outreach education to demonstrate what information is considered to be necessary for safe patient care and transport.

At the Bedside

They keys to patient and operational safety lie primarily in team performance and communication, which are described both in this chapter and, in excellent detail, in Chapter 7. Certain fundamental approaches specific to the care of patients are also important to review and to incorporate into routine clinical practice: medication safety is fundamental to all health care settings, and alarm management is a key to all critical care patient areas.

Providers are well versed in the "five rights" of medication administration, yet it is flaws in those basic steps that contribute to a significant number of medication errors. Box 8.7 restates the five rights. Other important considerations have extended this classic list, perhaps to nine steps. Various experts suggest including the following:

- Right documentation: This is entered *after* giving the medication.
- Right reason: This confirms the rationale for the ordered medication.
- Right assessment: This is used for contraindications before administration and for effects (and adverse effects) after administration.
- Right response.

Environmental and system factors can contribute to the failure to verify the rights, in spite of a provider's best efforts, including poorly designed medical devices, unclear handwritten orders, ambiguous drug labels, and uncertainty related to trailing zeroes and decimal points. In transport, in particular, systemic challenges to medication safety include poor lighting, distractions and interruptions, and limited or missed opportunities for effective independent cross-checks.[46]

> **• BOX 8.7** **Five Rights of Medication Administration**

1. Right patient
   a. Confirm the patient's identification.
      i. Use two identifiers.
      ii. Ask patient to identify himself/herself, if possible.
   b. Confirm the order.
   c. Use technology, such as a bar code system, if possible.
2. Right medication
   a. Check the medication label.
   b. Cross-check the medication with the order.
3. Right dose
   a. Check the order.
   b. Is this an appropriate drug and dose?
   c. If necessary, calculate the dose and cross-check with a partner.
4. Right route
   a. Check the order and appropriateness.
5. Right time
   a. Check the ordered frequency.
   b. Confirm when the last dose was given.

The transport environment is also fairly unique in the health care system because it has a continued absence of readily accessible pharmacist expertise, transfer of medications between institutions, lack of computer-controlled dispensing systems at the point of care, and continued provider compounding of infusions. Current targeted improvements for medication safety include using only kilogram weights, segregating neuromuscular blocking agents from other medications, delivering high-risk medications by programmable infusion pumps with error-reduction software, and ensuring that appropriate antidotes and reversal agents are readily available. When compounding medications, there should be an independent cross-check of the volume and material for both the medications and diluents.[47,48] To the greatest extent possible, transport teams should adopt hospital-designed medication safety best practices.

Clinical device alarms provide warnings of immediate or potential adverse patient conditions. A successful alarm system requires technical and human factor inputs: the device must provide accurate and appropriate alarms, and the provider needs to interpret and act on the data provided. The health care universe struggles with problems across this spectrum.[10,11,49] In the critical care transport environment, vehicle movement and ambient noise additionally increase the risk for failures of both alarm accuracy and detection.

The transport team initially optimizes patient safety simply by ensuring that all available monitors are used and available alarms are turned on. For transport teams, the combination of visual and auditory notification of alarm conditions is particularly important. In addition to basic vital sign monitoring of heart rate, respiratory rate, blood pressure, and oxygen saturation, this includes the alarms on specialty equipment such as ventilators and ventricular assist devices. Activating the alarms also requires that the alarm limits are set in ranges that identify key threats, minimize nuisance alarms, and provide enough time to manage the clinical situation identified by the alarm.

For transport, some alarms and monitors provide both important clinical information and immediate feedback for device-related problems. This includes transducing arterial lines both for the clinical data and for rapid detection of a disconnect and capnography in patients receiving sedatives or with airway appliances.

One use of proper monitoring and alarms is to detect device complications. Transport teams have a particular role in preventing inadvertent device removals during their care. The rates of in-transport adverse events are not well reported. For traditional Emergency Medical Service providers, older data suggest undetected endotracheal tube misplacement rates of up to 16%.[50,51] For interfacility transport, clinically significant events are conceivably at least as high as the 8% rate seen in intrahospital transport.[52] The use of specialty teams, both in and out of the hospital, makes patient transport significantly safer.[52-57]

Best practices to prevent inadvertent removal of vascular access devices, indwelling monitors, endotracheal tubes, gastric tubes, and other devices begin with clear identification of all *in situ* devices and communication of their presence to the team. Before the first patient movement, usually to the transport stretcher, ensure that all devices are well secured. Uncover the patient before moving to improve visibility and prevent sources of entanglement as well as to create a conscious pause and briefing before moving, which seems helpful.

Conclusion

Many of the principles associated with operational safety for critical care transport teams are the same as the principles associated with patient safety in health care. Teams and organizations will see a double benefit from attention to those common principles, and have a duty to their providers and patients to focus equal attention on all the factors associated with patient safety, operational safety, and the journey to the standard of high reliability.

References

1. Committee on Quality of Health Care in America, Kohn LT, Corrigan JM, Donaldson MS, eds. *To Err Is Human: Building a Safer Health System.* Washington, DC: National Academies Press; 2000.
2. Van Den Bos J, Rustagi K, Gray T, et al. The $17.1 billion problem: the annual cost of measurable medical errors. *Health affairs (Project Hope).* 2011;30(4):596-603.
3. Ornstein C. Dennis Quaid files suit over drug mishap. *Los Angeles Times.* December 5, 2007.
4. Niedowski E. How medical errors took a little girl's life. *The Baltimore Sun.* December 14, 2013.
5. Foundation NPS. *Free From Harm: Accelerating Patient Safety Fifteen Years After To Err Is Human.* Boston, MA: National Patient Safety Foundation; 2015.
6. Wu AW. Medical error: the second victim. *The doctor who makes the mistake needs help too.* 2000;320(7237):726-727.
7. Chassin MR, Loeb JM. High-Reliability Health Care: Getting There from Here. *The Milbank Quarterly.* 2013;91(3):459-490.
8. Kwaan MR, Studdert DM, Zinner MJ, Gawande AA. Incidence, patterns, and prevention of wrong-site surgery. *Arch Surg.* 2006;141(4):353-357; discussion 357-358.
9. Neily J, Mills PD, Eldridge N, et al. Incorrect surgical procedures within and outside of the operating room. *Arch Surg.* 2009; 144(11):1028-1034.
10. Schmid F, Goepfert MS, Kuhnt D, et al. The wolf is crying in the operating room: patient monitor and anesthesia workstation alarming patterns during cardiac surgery. *Anesth Analg.* 2011; 112(1):78-83.
11. Schmid F, Goepfert MS, Reuter DA. Patient monitoring alarms in the ICU and in the operating room. *Crit Care.* 2013;17(2):216.
12. Hines S, Luna K, Lofthus J, et al. *Becoming a High Reliability Organization: Operational Advice for Hospital Leaders.* Rockville, MD: Agency for Healthcare Research and Quality; 2008.
13. Chassin MR, Becher EC. The wrong patient. *Annals of Internal Medicine.* 2002;136(11):826-833.
14. Reason J. Understanding adverse events: human factors. *Quality in Health Care.* 1995;4:80-89.
15. Reason JT. *Managing the risks of organizational accidents.* Brookfield, VT: Ashgate; 1997.
16. Civil Air Navigation Services Organization (CANSO). *Safety Culture Definition and Enhancement Process.* Hoofddorp, the Netherlands, CANSO: 2008.
17. Leape LL, Shore MF, Dienstag JL, et al. Perspective: a culture of respect, part 1: the nature and causes of disrespectful behavior by physicians. *Academic medicine: journal of the Association of American Medical Colleges.* 2012;87(7):845-852.
18. Leape LL, Shore MF, Dienstag JL, et al. Perspective: a culture of respect, part 2: creating a culture of respect. *Academic medicine: journal of the Association of American Medical Colleges.* 2012;87(7):853-858.
19. Riskin A, Erez A, Foulk TA, et al. The Impact of Rudeness on Medical Team Performance: A Randomized Trial. *Pediatrics.* 2015;136:487-495.
20. American Medical Association. The sick physician. Impairment by psychiatric disorders, including alcoholism and drug dependence. *JAMA.* 1973;223(6):684-687.
21. Beaudin CL, Pelletier LR, Quality NAfH. *Q Solutions: Healthcare Safety.* Chicago, IL: National Association for Healthcare Quality; 2012.
22. Wachter R. *Understanding Patient Safety, Second Edition.* New York: McGraw-Hill; 2012.
23. Rice S. More hospitals screen aging surgeons to make sure their skills are still sharp. *Modern Healthcare.* 2016. Available online at: http://www.modernhealthcare.com/article/20160611/MAGAZINE/306119988. Accessed March 12, 2017.
24. Williamson A, Feyer A. Moderate sleep deprivation produces impairments in cognitive and motor performance equivalent to legally prescribed levels of alcohol intoxication. *Occupational and Environmental Medicine.* 2000;57(10):649-655.
25. Peets A, Ayas NT. Restricting resident work hours: the good, the bad, and the ugly. *Crit Care Med.* 2012;40(3):960-966.
26. Black N. Is hospital mortality higher at weekends? If so, why? *The Lancet.* 2016;388(10040):108-111.
27. Zhou Y, Li W, Herath C, et al. Off-Hour Admission and Mortality Risk for 28 Specific Diseases: A Systematic Review and Meta-Analysis

of 251 Cohorts. *Journal of the American Heart Association.* 2016; 5(3):e003102.

28. Baldisseri MR. Impaired healthcare professional. *Crit Care Med.* 2007;35(2 Suppl):S106-S116.

29. Magnavita N. The unhealthy physician. *J Med Ethics.* 2007; 33(4):210-214.

30. Haerkens MHTM, Jenkins DH, van der Hoeven JG. Crew resource management in the ICU: the need for culture change. *Ann Intens Care.* 2012;2(1):39-39.

31. Schamel J. How the pilot's checklist came about. *Officer Review Magazine.* 2010;50(5):16.

32. Pronovost P, Needham D, Berenholtz S, et al. An intervention to decrease catheter-related bloodstream infections in the ICU. *N Engl J Med.* 2006;355(26):2725-2732.

33. Gawande A. *The Checklist Manifesto: How to Get Things Right.* New York: Henry Holt and Company; 2010.

34. Frakes MA, Van Voorhis S. Effectiveness of a challenge-and-respond checklist in ensuring safety behavior compliance by medical team members at a rotor-wing Air Medical Program. *Air Med J.* 2007;26(5):248-251.

35. Anthes E. Hospital checklists are meant to save lives - so why do they often fail? *Nature.* 2015;523(7562):516-518.

36. Brunsveld-Reinders AH, Arbous MS, Kuiper SG, de Jonge E. A comprehensive method to develop a checklist to increase safety of intra-hospital transport of critically ill patients. *Crit Care.* 2015;19:214.

37. Winters BD, Gurses AP, Lehmann H, Sexton JB, Rampersad CJ, Pronovost PJ. Clinical review: Checklists—translating evidence into practice. *Crit Care.* 2009;13(6):210-218.

38. Catchpole KR, de Leval MR, McEwan A, et al. Patient handover from surgery to intensive care: using Formula 1 pit-stop and aviation models to improve safety and quality. *Paediatr Anaesth.* 2007;17(5):470-478.

39. Association AMP. *Safe Handoff of Care in Air/Ground Medical Transport.* Salt Lake City, UT: Air Medical Physician's Association; 2012.

40. Greenberg CC, Regenbogen SE, Studdert DM, et al. Patterns of communication breakdowns resulting in injury to surgical patients. *J Am Coll Surg.* 2007;204(4):533-540.

41. Solet DJ, Norvell JM, Rutan GH, Frankel RM. Lost in translation: challenges and opportunities in physician-to-physician communication during patient handoffs. *Acad Med.* 2005;80(12):1094-1099.

42. Starmer AJ, Spector ND, Srivastava R, et al. Changes in medical errors after implementation of a handoff program. *N Engl J Med.* 2014;371(19):1803-1812.

43. Flanigan M, Heilman JA, Johnson T, Yarris LM. Teaching and Assessing ED. Handoffs: a qualitative study exploring resident, attending, and nurse perceptions. *West J Emerg Med.* 2015;16(6): 823-829.

44. Meisel ZF, Shea JA, Peacock NJ, et al. Optimizing the patient handoff between emergency medical services and the emergency department. *Ann Emerg Med.* 2015;65(3):310-317.e311.

45. Panchal AR, Gaither JB, Svirsky I, Prosser B, Stolz U, Spaite DW. The impact of professionalism on transfer of care to the emergency department. *J Emerg Med.* 2015;49(1):18-25.

46. Grissinger M. The five rights: a destination without a map. *Pharmacy and Therapeutics.* 2010;35(10):542-542.

47. Institute for Safe Medical Practices (ISMP). *2016-2017 Targeted Medication Safety Best Practices For Hospitals.* Horsham, PA: Institute for Safe Medication Practices; 2016.

48. American Academy of Pediatrics, et al. Joint policy statement—guidelines for care of children in the emergency department. *J Emerg Nurs.* 2013;39(2):116-131.

49. American College of Clinical Engineering. *Impact of Clinical Alarms on Patient Safety.* Plymouth Meeting, PA: American College of Clinical Engineering Healthcare Foundation; 2006.

50. Katz S, Falk J. Misplaced endotracheal tubes by paramedics in an urban emergency medical services system. *Ann Emerg Med.* 2001; 37(1):32-37.

51. Jemmett M, Kendal K, Fourre M. Unrecognized misplacement of endotracheal tubes in a mixed urban to rural emergency medical services setting. *Acad Emerg Med.* 2003;10(9):961-965.

52. Kue R, Brown P, Ness C, Scheulen J. Adverse clinical events during intrahospital transport by a specialized team: a preliminary report. *Am J Crit Care.* 2011;20(2):153-162.

53. MacDonald R, Banks B, Morrison M. Epidemiology of adverse events in air medical transport. *Acad Emerg Med.* 2008;15(10): 923-931.

54. Papson J, Russell K, Taylor D. Unexpected events during the intrahospital transport of critically ill patients. *Acad Emerg Med.* 2007;14(6):574-577.

55. Indek M, Peterson S, Smith J, Brotman S. Risk, cost, and benefit of transporting ICU patients for special studies. *J Trauma.* 1988;28(7):1020-1025.

56. Orr R, Felmet K, Han Y, et al. Pediatric specialized transport teams are associated with improved outcomes. *Pediatrics.* 2009; 124(1):40-48.

57. Frakes M. Flight team management of in-place endotracheal tubes. *Air Med J.* 2002;21(6):29-31.

9

Operational Safety and Survival

JONATHAN D. GRYNIUK, RENEÉ SEMONIN HOLLERAN, AND SPECIAL CONTRIBUTIONS FROM GORDON WORLEY

"Safety does not just happen, it is not a specific event or a 'thing'—it is an attitude."

Dr. Ira Blumen and the UCAN Safety Committee, 2002[1]

COMPETENCIES

1. Identify the safety risks related to air and surface patient transport.
2. Integrate methods to reduce safety risks related to air and surface transport.
3. Knowledge of the medical transport industry's safety initiatives to improve safety and reduce accident rates.
4. Integrate escribed safe operations around helicopters, fixed-wing aircraft, and ground transport vehicles.
5. Identify and utilize the components of air medical resource management.
6. Correctly perform emergency procedures, including emergency egress air and surface vehicles.
7. Integrate and perform assigned components of a postaccident incident plan.
8. Knowledge of the priorities in a survival situation.
9. Integrate and perform basic survival skills, including shelter building, fire building, water procurement, and signaling.

Most chapters in this book contain information intended to help the air medical or ground transport crew member provide care for the critically ill or injured patient. This chapter is different; its purpose is to encourage the development of a safety attitude. It seeks to foster an active awareness and commitment to safety in every aspect of every mission. In short, it is devoted to taking care of the transport team member.

A safety culture exists within every transport program. Some safety measures are good and some are not. For a strong positive culture, each member of the program must accept that they contribute directly to a safe environment. Every individual, whether they are a nurse, paramedic, physician, respiratory therapist, emergency medical technician (EMT), pilot, mechanic, communication specialist, or administrator, must accept personal responsibility for safety and be a safety advocate.

Definition of Safety

Webster's dictionary defines *safety* as ". . . the state of being safe from the risk of experiencing or causing injury, danger or loss." Few human endeavors are completely safe from risk. The medical transport environment by its nature presents a wide range of potential risks. Medical transport exists at the unique interface of aviation, public safety, emergency medicine, and critical care medicine, all of which are complex technologic and human systems. In any complex system, human errors inevitably occur.[2] Effective risk management and safety programs recognize this and focus efforts on both reducing the rate of errors and, more importantly, reducing the consequences of the errors that do occur.

Safety may best be defined in the medical transport setting as identifying risks and managing them to eliminate or significantly reduce the possibility of accident or injury. The following sections explore some of the significant risks associated with air and ground medical transport and identify what has been, and is being, done to manage these risks and improve safety in the transport environment.

Air Medical Safety Survey

In 2015, Coons and Zalar[3] conducted an Air Medical Safety Survey, which was published in the *Air Medical Journal*.[3] The authors found the following:

- Three-fourths of the programs offer multimedical transport including helicopter, fixed-wing, and ground transport.
- Over half of the bases were staffed 24 hours a day with single-engine aircraft, and 37% were staffed 24 hours a day with twin-engine aircraft.
- Sixty percent of the aircraft have autopilot capabilities.
- The primary staffing configuration is nurse–paramedic.
- Sixty-four percent of the programs have a fatigue management system.
- Eighty-four percent of the respondent programs conducted formal air medical resource management (AMRM) programs annually.
- Respondents reported that 98% of the pilots and medical crew participate in a debriefing process.

- Sixty-three percent reported participation from communication specialists.
- Eighty-nine percent of the programs had a safety officer.
- Fifty-three percent of the programs used their Part 135 operator's safety management systems (SMS).
- Eighty-five percent of the programs did a preflight walk-around.
- Ninety-six percent of the programs report the use of night vision goggles (NVGs).
- Respondents reported that pilots can always cancel a flight; 99% of the time the crew cancels, 75% of the time the maintenance technicians cancel, 66% of the time operational control cancels, and 59% of the time the communication specialist cancels.

Hazards in the Transport Environment

The use of the term *accident* in the following discussion reflects its use by the National Transportation Safety Board (NTSB) for an event ". . . in which any person suffers death or serious injury, or in which the aircraft receives substantial damage."[4] This does not suggest that these tragic events are or were unavoidable. Most, if not all, of the accidents discussed had controllable factors that could have potentially prevented the occurrence or lessened the severity of the event.

Air Medical Accidents

The first hospital air medical program was established in 1972. Following that, the air medical industry underwent tremendous growth, from that one program in 1972, to 32 in 1980, to 101 by 1985.[5-8] With this growth came the realization that air medical helicopters had an accident rate far greater than that of helicopters engaged in general aviation.

From 1980 to 1985, the helicopter Emergency Medical Services (HEMS) industry had an estimated accident rate of 12.3 accidents per 100,000 patients transported. The accident rate for nonscheduled turbine-powered air taxi helicopter operators, a comparable non-HEMS population, was 6.9 accidents per 100,000 patients for the same time period.[1,6-8] In 1988, the NTSB released the results of its investigation of 59 EMS accidents that occurred between 1978 and 1986. The study concluded that weather-related accidents were the most common and most serious type of accident experienced by EMS helicopters.[1,6-8]

The 1990s showed continued growth in the air medical industry, from an estimated 174 HEMS programs operating 232 helicopters in 1990 to 225 programs operating 360 helicopters in 1999.[1,6-8] In 1990, one accident occurred with no fatalities. During the next 5 years, an average of 5.5 accidents per year occurred. In 1996 again only one HEMS accident was seen, but this one was fatal, and three were seen in 1997. From 1998 to 2001, the accident rate increased sharply to an average of 10.8 HEMS accidents per year.[1,6-8] A review of 121 air medical accidents from the late 1970s through the late 1990s found weather-related accidents to be the most common type, with an increase of 10% from the 1980s to the 1990s.[6-8]

In 2002, the Air Medical Physician Association (AMPA) released "A Safety Review and Risk Assessment in Air Medical Transport," which examined HEMS accidents from 1980 to 2001.[1] This report looked not only at the total yearly numbers of accidents but also at accident, injury, and fatality rates as functions of the number of EMS aircraft operating, the number of patients transported, and the estimated total flight hours for each year. The analysis showed a generally decreasing trend in number of HEMS accidents per 100,000 patient transports from the high in 1982 of 24.9 per 100,000 (a higher rate than that calculated by the NTSB in 1988) to a low in 1996 of 0.57 per 100,000. The average for the last 5 years of the study (1997–2001) was 4.6 per 100,000 patient transports. The most common recurrent factors in HEMS accidents were again found to be poor weather conditions and operations at night.

In 2003, the year after the publication of the AMPA study, there were 18 HEMS accidents, 4 of which were fatal. The year 2004 had 13 accidents, and 2005 had 17, with 6 fatal accidents each year. In January 2006, the NTSB released an "Aviation Special Investigation Report" that examined 55 EMS aircraft accidents that occurred between January 2002 and January 2005, 41 of which were helicopter accidents.[1-34] The investigation identified these recurrent safety issues:
- Less stringent requirements for EMS operations conducted without patients on board
- A lack of aviation flight risk evaluation programs for EMS operations
- A lack of consistent comprehensive flight dispatch procedures for EMS operations
- No requirements to use technologies such as terrain awareness and warning systems (TAWS) and night vision imaging systems (NVIS) to enhance EMS flight safety

Also in 2006, Baker et al.[2] reviewed HEMS accidents from 1983 to 2005 to determine the factors related to fatal outcomes. They concluded that accidents that occur at night or in bad weather or that result in a postimpact fire have a higher risk of being fatal.[2]

In 2006, a total of seven HEMS accidents occurred, three with fatalities, and in 2007, six accidents occurred, two of which were fatal. The year 2008 brought the worst year in the industry's history for fatal accidents, with a total of 12 HEMS accidents from January to November 2008, including the first-ever midair collision of two helicopter air ambulances (included in these totals as two accidents). Nine of these accidents were fatal, claiming a total of 29 lives, including five patients. Between 2009 and 2015 there were 55 air medical helicopter accidents, 22 of which involved fatalities, with 56 lives lost.[1] In 2015, there were 260 HEMS programs in the United States operating 864 helicopter bases and a total of 1045 helicopters.[9]

Fixed-wing air medical accidents have not been as well studied as HEMS accidents. In 2015, 111 air medical programs listed in the Atlas and Database of Air Medical Services operated a total of 362 fixed-wing aircraft.[4] Seventy of these programs operated both fixed-wing aircraft and helicopters. A review of accident data from 2002 to November 2008 showed a total of 14 accidents from 2002 to 2006, 6 of which were fatal. In 2007 six fixed-wing air medical accidents occurred, four of which were fatal; none were found in 2008.[4]

Blumen[1] conducted a focused analysis of accidents from 1998 to 2013 and found there were 197 HEMS accidents. Of the 197 accidents, 190 were dedicated HEMS and 61 of these 190 were fatal. The 197 accidents involved 574 people and 172 of these people were killed. Among the people who died, 142 were crew members, 6 were dual-purpose crew members, and 18 were patients.

Hon et al.[26] reported that from January 2003 to the end of July 2015 there were a total of 59 air medical incidents: fifty-two occurred with helicopters and seven with fixed-wing aircraft. There were 104 fatalities. Factors identified that contributed to incidents included impaired visibility, equipment failure, pilot error, weather, and undetermined causes. The researchers found that postincident fire was related to a higher incident of fatalities. They did note a significant decrease in the amount of accidents, but this was offset by an increase in fatalities. Table 9-1 summarizes an analysis for factors associated with fatal crashes or injury.

The data presented previously do not pretend to paint the whole picture of accident risk in air medical transport. The actual rates and the causes of air medical accidents are continuing topics of intense study and debate.[2] Although specific numbers and root causes may not always be clear, what is clear is that there continues to be accidents and that patients and flight crews continue to be injured and killed. Also clear is that recurrent factors continue to be involved in air medical accidents, most notably operations at night and in inclement weather. Air transport crews need to maintain a respect for these hazards and promote (and use) every tool and practice available to reduce the risks of flight in the air medical environment.

Ground Ambulance Accidents

The same level of attention paid to air medical accidents has not been paid to ground ambulance accidents. Unlike air medical accidents, which must be reported and are investigated by the NTSB, ground ambulance crashes are generally monitored on a state or local level, which makes consistent nationwide data difficult to obtain. In 2014 the National Highway Traffic Safety Administration (NHTSA) reported an estimated mean of 4500 motor vehicle crashes involving an ambulance between 1992 and 2011.[32] Sixty-five percent resulted in property damage only, 34% resulted in an injury, and less than 1% resulted in a fatality. Sixty-three percent of the fatalities were occupants in other vehicles. In both fatal and nonfatal crashes, the majority of crashes occurred while the ambulance was in emergency use.

NHTSA published the "Model Minimum Uniform Crash Criteria,"[34] which includes a uniform way for police to collect data about an ambulance crash. Examples of data collected should include the following:
- Emergency transport
- Nonemergency transport
- Emergency operation
  - Warning equipment in use
  - Warning equipment not in use
- Ambulance seating/positioning
- Crash location
- Weather conditions
- Contributing circumstances
- Roadway surface conditions
- Motor vehicle body type
- Vehicle configuration
- Air bag deployed
- Alcohol and drug testing
- Driver distracted by

These studies show that ground ambulance accidents also have recurrent contributing factors. Safety training programs should focus on the awareness of these risks, safe driving, and proper use of safety equipment, such as seat belts. Ground transport programs need to establish the same safety culture and have the same commitment to safety and risk reduction as air medical programs.

Reducing the Risks

Since the 1980s, efforts have been made to reduce the risks of flight in the air medical environment. These efforts at risk reduction have taken many forms, from safety policies and procedures to training and new technologies.

TABLE 9.1	Univariate Analysis for Factors Associated with Fatal Crash or Injury		
Category	No injury or fatality	Injury or fatality	Significance*
Abnormal weather conditions	1/9	21/50	P = 0.057
Impaired visibility	1/9	23/50	P = 0.035
Aircraft make/type			
Agusta model	0/7	7/7	
Bell model	5/21	16/21	
Eurocopter model	2/20	18/20	
Other helicopter	2/4	2/4	
Fixed-wing aircraft	0/7	7/7	P = 0.096
Post-incident fire	1/9	22/50	P = 0.045
Time of incident (7pm-6am)	2/9	35/50	P = 0.007

*Variables reaching statistical significance (P < 0.20) for inclusion in multivariate analysis.

From Hon H, Wojda TR, Barry N, et al. 2016. Injury and fatality risks in aeromedical transport: focus on prevention. J Surg Res. 2016;204(2):297–303.

Critical Thinking, Decision Making, and the Human Factor

The probable cause for many of the accidents described previously is listed as *pilot error*, which is another way of saying the pilot made a bad decision, or a series of bad decisions, which resulted in the accident. Decision making in the aviation environment is a complicated process, with many factors that need to be considered. To be able to make good decisions, pilots and flight crew members need to have training in critical thinking and decision making in the HEMS environment and have access to decision-making tools.[30,31] These tools may be technologies, policies, algorithms, or other processes. No single tool or practice ensures a good decision, but used together they can be effective in helping pilots and crews make safe decisions. The human factor, the ability of the pilot and crew to make informed safe decisions, remains the single most important factor in ensuring safety in the medical transport environment.

Weather Minimums

From the beginning of the industry, weather and impaired visibility (instrument meteorologic conditions [IMCs]) have been recognized as a significant cause of accidents.[35] The Commission on Accreditation of Medical Transport Systems (CAMTS) accreditation standards require that programs have minimum cloud ceiling and visibility limits for operations under visual flight rules (VFR). In November 2008, the Federal Aviation Administration (FAA) released draft revisions to operations specifications that pertained to HEMS operations. The revisions include higher VFR ceiling, visibility, and obstacle clearance requirements when a "flight or sequence of flights includes a Part 135 segment." These new operations specifications became effective in February 2009. Each program's weather minimums must comply with FAA regulations, meet CAMTS requirements, and address the specific needs and hazards of the program's operating area. Once a program's weather minimums have been established, they need to be followed; "pushing the envelope" on minimums has been implicated in many weather-related HEMS accidents.

Another weather-related concern noted in the 2006 NTSB report was the lack of reliable information regarding weather conditions in many areas in which HEMS programs operate, which increases the risk of an inadvertent entry into IMCs (IIMCs). In an effort to find ways to reduce this risk, representatives of the HEMS industry, the FAA, and the University Center for Atmospheric Research conducted a HEMS Weather Summit in 2006. One result of this summit was the development of the Aviation Digital Data Service (ADDS) experimental HEMS Low Altitude Flight Tool (https://www.aviationweather.gov/hemst). The FAA met again with industry representatives to fine-tune the tool in 2013. This online application is designed to enhance the safety of flight in the low-altitude environment used by HEMS aircraft. It provides a visual representation of ceiling, visibility, convection, radar information, and geographic information system data in areas between established weather-reporting sites.

Mission Planning and Risk Assessment

The safe completion of any medical transport mission starts with mission planning. The first step in mission planning is an assessment of the potential risks involved, which leads to a decision about whether or not the mission should be accepted. Once the decision has been made to accept the mission, other aspects of mission planning must occur, including weight and performance planning, fuel management, destination considerations, pilot and crew duty time, and clinical factors.

Operational risk assessment begins with a daily or shift evaluation, which takes into account factors that remain relatively constant during the day. These factors can include prevailing weather patterns, pilot and crew experience, and the availability of safety technologies (discussed subsequently). Another risk assessment should be performed at the time of each mission request, evaluating the time of day, current weather conditions, weather forecasts, pilot and crew fatigue, and other variables. Some programs have established operational control centers to assist pilots in assessing the risks of certain missions by having the mission request reviewed and any identified risks evaluated by another individual (typically a senior pilot) before the request is accepted. Fig. 9.1 shows an example of a risk assessment tool (Operations Compliance Form [Risk Analysis] courtesy of Life Flight, Salt Lake City, Utah).

Risk assessment should be a fluid, dynamic process. If conditions change as the mission progresses, then so should the risk assessment. Pilots and flight crews need to continuously observe and evaluate the mission environment and the potential risks. If changes in the mission environment can be anticipated, then decision thresholds and alternative plans can be discussed and decided on ahead of time.

Declined Missions

Although the pilot-in-command (PIC) has the ultimate responsibility for accepting or declining any mission request, all members of the transport team have the right, and the responsibility, to refuse to accept any mission in which there is a legitimate safety concern. This includes both air and surface transport. Each program should have a written policy for declining or aborting missions, so that individual crew members do not have to worry about disciplinary action or other negative action as a result of refusing to participate in a mission because of safety concerns. The safety culture of the program should support the "All to say go, one to say no" philosophy.

Air Medical Resource Management

AMRM is the operational practice of involving all members of the flight team (pilot and clinical crew members) in mission planning, decision making, and mission safety. It is the air medical industry's adaptation of *crew resource management* (CRM), which is used in the commercial aviation industry and by the US Air Force. CRM grew out of several significant accidents that resulted from poor decision making on the part of airline pilots, and in some cases over the

Operations Compliance Form (Risk Analysis)

GENERAL:

This form is used to comply with the requirements of 14 CFR 135.617 and 14 CFR 135.621.

INSTRUCTIONS:

General Information

1. Enter one or two digit day of the month in the DAY field.
2. Enter the three letter abbreviation for the month (ie, JAN, FEB, MAR, etc.) in the MONTH field.
3. Enter the time, in military format (ie, 0800, 1621, 1945, etc) that the form was completed.
4. Circle either "NA" or "YES" for each of the four major categories, as appropriate.
5. When required, enter the name of the person providing approval for the operation.
6. When required, enter the final risk score, as provided by the OCS.
7. Sign the form as shown.
8. The completed form must be kept at the base where the operation originated from for a minimum of 90 days. Lead pilots will organize and maintain a system for management of these forms at their respective bases.

Crew Briefing

The **PEOPLE** briefing is used to meet the requirement of 14 CFR 135.621 for medical personnel who have not been trained.

Additional Fields

1. Remaining fields are for administrative purposes only and are not required.

Operations Control Specialist (OCS) Entry Form

Also included is the OCS Entry Form, an Excel spreadsheet based form used by the OCS to determine risk scoring and level of approval.

Sample Pilot Form (front)

OPERATIONS COMPLIANCE FORM

RISK ANALYSIS

WEATHER (All Legs, Current and Forecast) **NA/YES**
Ceiling < 3,000' AGL **OR**
Visibility < 5 sm **OR**
Temp/Dewpoint Spread < 3 deg **OR**
Surface Wind > 20 kts

FLIGHT CONSIDERATIONS **NA/YES**
LZ Density Altitude > 8,000' **OR**
Unimproved LZ **OR**
MSCA > 7,000' MSL

AREA FAMILIARITY **NA/YES**
Unfamiliar Base (less than 20%) **AND**
Unfamiliar Destination / Scene (past yr)

HUMAN FACTORS **NA/YES**
SLEEPY (any element) **OR**
More than Two Flights **OR**
Personal Issues

Score | Approved by

CREW BRIEFING

P hysiology
Route / altitude / environmental

E mergency Procedures
In-flight / landing / evacuation

O perational Differences
Day / night / NVG

P atient
Type / loading / hot on-off

L Z Safety
Helipad / scene / general

E ffective Communications
CRM / sterile cockpit

Route / Notes

DAY

MONTH

TIME

Flight #:__________
Aircraft ID:__________
Call Arrive:__________
Dispatch:__________
Liftoff:__________
Patient Miles:__________
Total Miles:__________

Hobbs Stop:__________
Hobbs Start:__________
Total:__________

T/O	LDG

Pilot's Signature

Intermountain Life Flight *FQA-0103* *Rev 16-02*

• **Fig. 9.1** An example of a risk assessment tool: the Operations Compliance Form. (Risk Analysis). (Courtesy Intermountain Life Flight, Salt Lake City, Utah.)

FATIGUE SELF-EVALUATION

SLEEP More than two hours short?[1]

LOST SLEEP More than four hours in debt?[2]

EARLY MORNING Flying between 0200 and 0600?

EXTENDED DAY Awake longer than 16 hours?

PUSHING IT More than 5-7 straight shifts?

You personal signs of fatigue[3]

1 You likely need 8 hours every 24 hours
2 The difference between the sleep you need and the sleep you get accumulates over time. It takes two consecutive full nights of sleep to get out of debt.
3 Delayed reaction time, problems focusing, moodiness, fixation, inattention, feelings of sleepiness degraded judgment, missed cues, etc.

VFR MINIMUMS

Use 14 CFR 91.155 when more restrictive

	DAY		NIGHT	
	Clg	Vis	Clg	Vis
Local	800'	3 sm	1,000'*	3 sm
Non Local	1,000'			5 sm

*1,500' without NVGs

PRE / POST FLIGHT

W	**EATHER** Ceiling / Visibility / Winds MECA
A	**IRCRAFT & EQUIPMENT** Non-Std Conf (LR Med, Trauma, Neo) Final Equipment Requirement Check Fuel NVGs
I	**NDIVIDUALS** Pilot – Risk Assessment Medical Team – Concerns & Questions Patient – Status & Weight
T	**IME & TRACK** Confirm Destination Route / Altitude / Airspeed / ETE
S	**AFETY** As Briefed / Unexpected Reportable Concerns (QA Report?)
M	**EDICAL** Concerns (Crew/Referring or Receiving) QA Report?
A	**VIATION** Weather Maintenance Issues
C	**OMMUNICATIONS** Flight Team / Comm Center EMS/Outside Agencies
O	**THER**

Sample OCS Entry Form (with supporting point assignments)

ROTOR WING RISK ANALYSIS

EXPERIENCE
Low ☑

TIME OF DAY
Night Shift ☑

WEATHER (all points, current/forecast)
Ceiling < 3,000' AGL ☐
Visibility < 5 sm ☑
Temp/Dewpoint Spread < 3 degrees ☐
Surface Wind > 20 kts ☐

FLIGHT CONSIDERATIONS
LZ Density Altitude > 8,000' ☑
MSCA (Min Safe Cruise Alt) > 7,000' ☐
Unimproved LZ ☐
Reserve Fuel < 30 Minutes ☐

AREA FAMILIARITY
Outside Local Area ☑
Unfamiliar Base ☐
Unfamiliar Destination / Scene ☐

HUMAN FACTORS
Fatigue (SLEEPY) ☐
More than Two Flights (91/135) ☐
Health ☐
Distracting Life Events ☐
Other Stressors ☐

ADDITIONAL RISKS
Prior Turn Down (wx related only)* ☐
Complicated Flight ☐

*Prior Turn Down past 60 minutes is automatic Ops consult

25
Consult? **Ops Only**

NOTE: Are there contingencies that should be considered?

Mitigations: When Ops Controllers, pilots and managers consider high risk flights they should review mitigation strategies that would lower associated risks. For example, if human factors is deemed a high risk area, consider using another pilot who would not be subject to those same factors.
Or, if another program turned down the flight because their only available aircraft was at a location with IFR conditions but our own aircraft and the planned route were VFR, then the flight could be accepted.

Low Experience	1.5	Multiplier
Night Shift	1.3	Multiplier
Ceiling	5	
Visibility	5	
TempDew	5	
Wind	5	
DA	5	
MECA	4	
Unimproved LZ	6	
Fuel	4	
LocalArea	3	
UnfamiliarBase	5	
UnfamiliarDestination	5	
Fatigue	8	
TwoFlights	7	
Health	5	
Distractions	5	
OtherStressors	5	
PriorTurnDown	10	
ComplicatedFlight	5	
Second Pilot Consult	40	
Manager Consult	60	

• **Fig. 9.1,** cont'd

objections of other flight crew members. CRM involves communication skills, situational awareness, problem solving, decision making, and teamwork.

The PIC was traditionally the sole decision maker in an airline cockpit. The rest of the crew followed the PIC's instructions and did not offer input or question decisions. By encouraging crew members to pay attention, make suggestions, and voice concerns, CRM involves all of the crew members in the decision-making process. The PIC still has the ultimate authority and responsibility for the aircraft, but other crew members are able to offer suggestions or, more importantly, question decisions they feel are unsafe or unwise.

The essence of AMRM/CRM is teamwork, based on good communication between all crew members and the use of all available resources to maximize mission safety. Mutual respect, trust, and an organizational culture that supports safety provide the best environment for effective communication and use of AMRM. AMRM classes should be a part of initial and recurrent training and should involve all members of the transport team, including the medical transport team, specialty teams, program administration, maintenance technicians, and communication specialists.

Helicopter Shopping

Fatal HEMS accidents have occurred when an HEMS program has accepted a mission that had been declined by another provider. The International Association of Flight and Critical Care Paramedics (formerly the National Flight Paramedics Association) published a position paper in 2006 that addressed the problem of local agencies placing sequential requests to different air medical programs in an attempt to obtain a response to a mission request that had been declined by one provider (or multiple providers) for reasons of weather, landing zone (LZ) availability, or other safety factors. This practice in commonly referred to as *helicopter shopping*.

In 2011, the Emergency Nurses Association and the Air and Surface Transport Association (ASTNA) developed a position paper to address helicopter shopping. This collaboration assisted in expanding the responsibility of this dangerous practice to both the prehospital and hospital environments. The paper was revised in 2016.[22]

All programs need to educate the EMS agencies, dispatch centers, and hospitals in their service areas about the hazards of this practice and work with them to develop systems to prevent it. When any program declines a mission request, the reason should be clearly stated and communicated to any other program that may be asked to accept the mission. Air medical programs that serve the same areas should have interprogram communication pathways to permit each program to notify others when a mission is declined or to inquire whether another program has turned down a request. These pathways may include regional or national turndown reporting websites or formal interprogram notification systems. If the nature of a flight request (such as location) suggests that another program may have been contacted first, the dispatcher/communication specialist should inquire whether

any other programs were contacted about the flight and the reasons for any declines.

Safety Technologies

In 2014, the FAA released "Initiatives to Improve Air Ambulance Safety." The basic recommendations are focused on stricter flight rules and procedure, improved communications and training, and additional onboard safety equipment. These recommendations are summarized in Box 9.1.

All reviews of air medical accidents have identified the same two environments as significant contributing factors: operations at night and during bad weather. These two environments have one major factor in common: reduced visibility. A variety of technologies can reduce the risk of operating during reduced-visibility conditions by supplying additional information about potential hazards in the flight environment. One of the recurrent safety issues identified in the 2006 NTSB report was the lack of requirements that air medical aircraft make use of these safety technologies to enhance flight safety.

In the 2015 safety survey conducted by Coons and Zalar,[3] the use of the following equipment is advocated, based on the FAA's 2009 HEMS recommendations.[3]

Instrument Flight

Flight operations under *instrument flight rules* (IFRs) are a common practice for fixed-wing aircraft but have historically been less common in helicopter aviation. Many older helicopter models used in air medical transport were not approved for instrument flight, except in emergency conditions. Many newer HEMS aircraft are IFR capable, and more and more programs are using this added capability.

When operating under IFR, the pilot is flying under the guidance of the FAA air traffic control (ATC) system. The controller monitors the position of the aircraft on radar and provides routing instructions that keep the aircraft away from terrain and other air traffic.[36] IIMC is always an emergency situation, but for an IFR-capable aircraft and pilot, encountering reduced-visibility conditions can present less risk of unexpected entry into IMC because the pilot has the option of planning the flight under IFR or of transitioning to IFR flight en route.

Night Vision Goggles

NVGs, also called NVIS, use an electronic system to amplify visible light and provide improved visibility during night operations. NVGs have been used by the military for many years and have seen a rapid acceptance in the HEMS community recently. In 2008 the National EMS Pilots Association released a survey of 382 active HEMS pilots on the subject of NVG usage in the HEMS environment. The responses were overwhelmingly in favor of the use of NVGs in night HEMS operations.[1,2,5,10,15,30,37] In the 2015 safety survey, 96% of the programs that responded reported NVG use. In the majority of programs (64%), both the pilot and transport team members wear NVGs.

• BOX 9.1 **Summary of Federal Aviation Administration Recommendations for Helicopter Emergency Medical Services**

Recommendations	Year
January 2005	Publication of a notice providing guidance for safety inspectors to help operators review pilot and mechanics decision-making skills, procedural adherence, and crew resource management practices
August 2005	Guidelines issued to inspectors promoting improved risk assessment and risk management tools to all flight crews including medical staff
September 2005	Guidance issued to operators to establish minimum guidelines for Air Medical Resources Management training
	All personnel involved in operations are included: pilots, maintenance technicians, flight nurses and paramedics, medical directors, specialty team members, communication specialists, program directors, and any other identified transport team members
September 2005	Revised standards issued for inspection and surveillance of air ambulance operators with special emphasis on operations control, risk assessment, and facilities and training, especially at outer facilities away from the certified holder's principle base of operations
December 2005	The FAA-established On-Demand Training Center Branch to work the 135 and 142 policy issues
	Inspectors with "helicopter only" experience were hired
Formed in 2005	International Helicopter Safety Team to promote safety and prevent accidents worldwide
January 2006	LOC and CFIT handbook released with description of acceptable models to develop LOC and CFIT Accident Avoidance Programs
March 2006	Guidance issued to inspectors on surveillance and oversight of public aircraft operators for air ambulance operations
March 2006	Weather summit in Boulder, Colorado, hosted by the FAA and University Cooperation for Atmospheric Research
	Developed and implemented a graphical flight planning tool for ceiling and visibility assessment along direct flights in areas with limited available surface observations capability (revised in 2013)
June 2006	Special Committee to develop H-TAWSS
	In the 2015 Safety Survey 67% of the surveyed programs reported H-TAWSS installed in aircraft[3]
August 2006	Aeronautic Information Manual revised to provide guidance to pilots on assessing ambient lighting for night visual flight rules operations and/off airport/heliport landing operations
May 2008	FAA's Flight Standards Service issued an advisory highlighting "best practices" for establishing operational control centers and training their specialists
November 2008	FAA published a notice in the Federal Registry that advised operators of important mandatory changes to air ambulance flights including: encouraging the use of night vision goggles TAWSs; all air ambulance operators will comply with Part 135 weather minimums, including repositioning flights with medical crew onboard
	The flight crew was required to determine a minimum safe altitude and obstacle clearance before each flight
January 2009	FAA established a task group to focus on surveillance of large helicopter emergency medical services operators, which resulted in an increase of inspectors and the organization of these inspectors into operator-specific oversight teams

CFIT, Controlled flight into terrain; *FAA,* Federal Aviation Administration; *H-TAWSS,* helicopter terrain awareness and warning systems standards; *LOC,* loss of control. From *Federal Aviation Administration.* 2014. Fact Sheet-FAA initiatives to improve helicopter air ambulance safety. https://insurancenewsnet.com/oarticle/FAA-Initiatives-to-Improve-Helicopter-Air-Ambulance-Safety-a-463889; 2014 Accessed 16.7.10; Coons J, and Zalar, C. 2015 Air medical safety survey. *Air Med. J.* 2016;35:120-125.

Terrain Awareness and Warning Systems

One of the common scenarios in air ambulance accidents is loss of adequate visibility and subsequent controlled flight into terrain. A TAWS provides the pilot with a visual display of the terrain along the flight path and alert the pilot with visual and audible alarms if the aircraft flies too close to the terrain. Some of these systems also include a *traffic collision avoidance system,* which provides information about the location of other nearby air traffic.

Satellite Tracking and Position Reporting

Automated flight following with a satellite-based tracking system provides the flight communication center with up-to-the-minute information regarding the position and status of the aircraft. In the event of an emergency situation, the exact position of the aircraft is always known. Many of these systems also permit satellite-based voice and data communications.

Crashworthy Aircraft and Vehicle Systems

Design changes to improve the crashworthiness of the airframe, fuel system, and seats in US military aircraft have shown improved crash survival rates.[3] Newer civilian and military helicopters are equipped with crashworthy landing gear, crashworthy fuel systems, and crash-attenuating seats that absorb energy and reduce the g force applied to the occupant in a hard impact to improve occupant survival in a crash.[2] In November 2015 the Air Medical Operators Association, in cooperation with helicopter manufacturers Airbus Helicopters and Bell Helicopter, announced their commitment to the installation of crash-resistant fuel systems (CRFS) in all new aircraft and equipping current aircraft with CRFS as those products become available (http://aams.org/aams-position-on-crash-resistant-fuel-systems-crfs).

Changes in ground ambulance design to enhance safety have included improved seat and seat belt/harness restraint systems for occupants of the rear compartment, ergonomic interior designs that permit easier access to the patient and supplies while remaining restrained, padded ambulance interiors, and backup camera systems.

Industry Safety Initiatives

When the disturbing HEMS accident rates of the 1980s were identified, the air medical industry recognized the need to improve safety and reduce accident rates. A great emphasis has been, and continues to be, placed on improving air medical safety and risk management techniques. A number of organizations have launched programs and established standards designed to improve safety practices, enhance the safety consciousness of the industry, and reduce or eliminate errors of consequence.[1,2,4,5,10,11]

Air and Surface Transport Nurses Association[10]

ASTNA (formerly the National Flight Nurses Association or NFNA) has long been a safety advocate and has published a series of position papers related to air medical safety. ASTNA is a professional nursing organization with a membership that includes transport nurses from throughout the United States and Canada. In 1988 the NFNA (ASTNA) published the position paper "Improving Flight Nurse Safety in the Air Medical Helicopter Environment." In this paper, the organization endorsed many of the recommendations of the NTSB study published earlier the same year. NFNA stated that "available knowledge and technology which could significantly enhance [a] flight nurse's safety in the air medical helicopter environment is not consistently applied and utilized in all air medical transport programs." The position paper proposed several corrective measures. The proposals dealt with (1) crew scheduling and rest periods; (2) the right of flight nurses to refuse to participate in a flight as a result of concerns for personal safety; (3) the need for programs to develop written protocols for the use of physical and pharmacologic restraints when combative or potentially combative patients are transported; (4) the need for programs to critically evaluate hot-loading and unloading policies (loading and unloading while the rotors are still running) and procedures and to ensure personnel assigned to hot load or unload do so only after proper training; and (5) the adoption of measures to maximize safety and reduce the potential of serious injury with use of helicopter design changes such as energy-attenuating seats, addition of shoulder harnesses to lap belts at each position in the aircraft, and development and installation of CRFS in aircraft as soon as possible.

The 1988 the NFNA position statement also dealt with specific in-flight duties to be performed by flight nurses to ensure a safe aviation environment. These responsibilities included (1) securing equipment during flight, (2) use of seat belts and shoulder harnesses, (3) properly securing patients within the aircraft, (4) judicious use of night lighting, and (5) isolation of the pilot and controls from potential patient movement.

In 1998,[38-41] the NFNA position paper was updated and expanded to include the following recommendations that flight nurses

1. Interact more with the PIC, participate in recurrent safety, permission, and postmission briefings; be taught how to report aircraft position; and undergo crew member emergency training
2. Are taught the use of appropriate personal protective gear, including helmets, flame-resistant flight uniforms, and protective footwear
3. Attend stress-management programs to enhance flight nursing performance
4. Are shown how to use backup aircraft that are similar to the primary aircraft in the flight program These recommendations have since become part of routine operations for a large portion of the air medical industry.

In 2011 NFNA published a 48-page comprehensive revision of "Transport Nurse Safety in the Transport Environment."[10] This document addresses safety in both air and surface transport environments. The following components are included in this document:

- Improved performance through appropriate scheduling and provision for adequate rest
- Improved safety through nurse interaction with the pilot or driver in command to ensure a safe transport environment
- AMRM
- Hot loading/unloading an aircraft
- Personal protective gear for flight nurses
- Reporting of hazardous situations and safety issues
- Vehicle configuration and design to maximize safety and reduce the potential of serious injury to transport crews in the event of a crash
- Maximizing transport nurse familiarity with vehicle/aircraft specific emergency procedures and equipment
- Patient restraint
- Transport nurse refusal to participate in a transport as a result of safety concern
- Safety considerations specific to ground critical care

- Training in survival techniques and emergency equipment and procedures
- Creating healthy work environments designed to promote and sustain the transport nurse's well-being

A revision and update of this paper is planned for the fall of 2017.

The Commission for Accreditation of Medical Transport Systems

Since 1990, CAMTS has lead the way in transport safety. The CAMTS Board is composed of multiple representatives for those who are involved in patient transport. Members of CAMTS have actively participated with the FAA and other members of the transport industry to develop and implement safety standards.

Each transport program needs *safety management,* which includes an SMS and safety and environment.[9] CAMTS notes that management is responsible for the SMS, but the management and staff are both responsible for making operations safer. More information about safety management is discussed later in this chapter.

Vision Zero

In 2005, the Association of Air Medical Services (AAMS), in cooperation with many other organizations, launched the Vision Zero Initiative "to reduce and eliminate errors of consequence—those events within the transport medicine environment that result in serious injury or fatality" by 80% in 10 years (http://aams.org/vision-zero/). The Vision Zero Initiative is intended to foster communication and cooperation between all aspects of the medical transport industry (safety organizations, professional associations, trade organizations, and regulatory agencies) to develop voluntary and regulatory measures to achieve the stated goals.

The Vision Zero Initiative continues today sponsored by Airbus Helicopters. Its website promotes the sharing of safety initiatives based on the four pillars of safety systems: safety risk management, safety policy, safety promotion, and safety assurance. More information about this information is available at http://aams.org/vision-zero/toolbox/.

Voluntary Safety Reporting

Voluntary safety reporting systems encourage individuals, transport programs, and aviation certificate holders to voluntarily report safety issues, concerns, and events. By submitting voluntary reports, programs and individuals may identify safety issues that affect more than just their program or agency and permit others to learn from their experience. The CONCERN Network (http://concern-network.org) is a voluntary reporting system whose purpose is "to increase awareness of safety hazards in the medical transport community." Transport programs submit reports of accidents or incidents, and bulletins are then distributed via email to CONCERN Network subscribers and maintained in an online archive.

The CONCERN Network[14] also supports another type of report titled the Hazard Awareness Reporting Page (HARP). HARP's purpose is to provide a mechanism for sharing what precautions or lessons that have been learned from transport team members' experiences of hazardous situations that nearly or could have resulted in tragedy. HARP reporting can be found at http://www.concern-network.org.

Transport team members may also submit anonymous reports. The FAA's Aviation Safety Action Program is designed to improve safety throughout the aviation industry. It allows participants to submit confidential reports that "identify actual or potential risks throughout their operations." All of the parties involved can then work together to develop or update operational practices to reduce the risk of accidents and other safety-related events. More information is available at http://www.faa.gov/about/initiatives/asap.

Safety Management

An effective comprehensive SMS should be a major part of all transport programs. The commitment to safety must include ". . . all disciplines and processes of the organization."[15] Safety needs to be a core component of the organizational culture of every transport program, from the CEO to the newest front-line employee.

An SMS must be proactive in eliminating injuries to personnel and patients as well as damage to equipment. All members of the transport team must feel empowered to create and maintain a culture of safety. A safety committee should be formed with representatives of all transport disciplines. There should be evidence of action plans, evaluation, and loop closure. One of the primary and most important roles of a safety committee is communication to and from all who participate in the transport process.

The Accreditation Standards published by CAMTS list the components of an SMS, which include the following[15]:

- A statement of policy commitment from the accountable executive
- A risk identification process and risk management plan that includes a nonpunitive system for employees to report hazards, risks, and safety concerns
- A safety committee
- A system to track and document root cause analysis
- A system to track, trend, and mitigate errors or hazards
- A safety manual (electronic and hard copy)
- Operational risk-assessment tools
- Ongoing safety training for all personnel (including managers)
- A system to audit and review organizational policy and procedures
- A system of proactive and reactive procedure to ensure compliance

Safety Committee

The safety committee should be composed of representatives of all disciplines involved in the transport program: aviation, clinical, maintenance, communications, and administration. The committee should meet at least quarterly to address safety issues, practices, concerns, or questions. Reports of the committee's discussions and actions should be easily accessible and communicated to all who participate in the transport process.

The safety committee should be linked to the program's quality management committee as well as risk management. Aviation and surface-related events are identified and tracked to minimize risks. There should be a policy as to what safety issues or incidents should be reported and to what agency. The policy should also identify who would be responsible to report.

Safety Training

Operational Safety Training

All regular transport team members, as well as members of specialty teams who may also participate in transports, should receive regular operational safety training. Operational safety training should include AMRM, mission planning, use of the program's operational risk-assessment tools, aircraft and ground vehicle safety, emergency scene operations, and survival. In addition to scheduled didactic sessions, operational safety training should include regular aircraft or ground vehicle emergency drills.[1,10,11,13,16,17,19,23,25,27-29,31,33,42]

Clinical Safety Training

Clinical safety training should review flight physiology and the stressors of flight, hazardous materials and items (HAZMAT) recognition and response, infection control, and the management of combative or violent patients. These subjects are addressed in detail in other chapters of this textbook. Other safety training topics may include employee wellness, injury prevention, and specific topics required by state, federal, or local statutes.

Aircraft Safety Training[1,10,11,13,16,17,19,23,25,27-29,31,33,42]

All flight crew members must be familiar with the aircraft in use by their program, including all regular and backup aircraft operated by the program in which the crew member may be expected to fly. Specific items with which all crew members must be familiar for all aircraft include the following:

- Operation of seat belts or harness
- Operation of all doors and emergency exits
- Emergency egress procedures
- Emergency egress of patients both with and without a backboard
- Emergency engine shutdown
- Emergency communications
- Oxygen and medical gas shutoff
- Location and operation of onboard fire extinguishers
- Location and use of other onboard emergency equipment, such as the survival kit, personal flotation devices (PDFs), and aviation emergency oxygen systems
- Hot-loading and offloading procedures and policies

Ground Ambulance Safety Training

Ground ambulance safety should be a part of the training presented by both ground and air transport providers. Air medical crews often are expected to transfer patients from an airport or other landing site to the hospital via ambulance. Ground vehicle safety training should include the following:

- Driver training (where applicable)
- Use of seat belts by all crew members while the vehicle is in motion
- Avoiding standing or kneeling in the patient compartment
- Oxygen and medical gas shutoff
- When to use red lights and siren (RLS) response
- Securing equipment in the ambulance
- Gurney operations and back/lifting safety

Occupational and Workplace Safety Training

All crew members must be familiar with the safety procedures and requirements of the assigned workplace, whether in a hospital, at an airport, or at another location. Items with which all staff need to be familiar include the location and type of fire extinguishers; use of the fire extinguishers; the process for refueling aircraft or vehicles; HAZMAT or fuel spill response; electricity and gas shutoff; occupational injury or illness reporting; and site-specific procedures or practices, such as emergency evacuation routes.

Outreach Safety Education

Along with safety training for transport program staff, safety training and practice must be provided for first responders and hospital personnel as well as others who may be asked to work around EMS aircraft. These personnel may include fire service, law enforcement, EMS, and park rangers or game wardens.

Safety in the Transport Environment[1,10,11,13,16,17,19,23,25,27-29,31,33,42]

Personal Safety

Personal safety is an important aspect of the safety attitude. For the individual crew member, personal safety is the mindset, habits, and daily practices that keep that individual safe. Each member of the transport team also bears the responsibility for the personal safety of others, including partner, pilot, patient, and fellow responders. For the transport service, personal safety means providing a safe work environment, appropriate personal protective equipment, and safety training. It also involves establishing and following safety standards and policies. The best safety training and equipment in the world are of little value if not used properly, and safety standards cannot be effective if they are not followed.

Fitness Standards

The transport environment is physically challenging and requires that transport team members maintain a high personal level of both physical and emotional fitness. Requirements of each program vary, and no industrywide formal guidelines exist.[40] Minimal physical requirements of any person working in the medical transport environment should include the ability to work within the space limitations of the transport aircraft and vehicles operated by the program; to lift and carry a reasonable amount of weight; and to function in the typical work environments encountered by the program, such as scene calls. Transport team members must not have any pre-existing conditions that could interfere with flexibility, strength, or cardiovascular fitness. Transport team members also must not have any condition that could cause altered mental or neurologic function.[15,41]

Fatigue Policies[2,13,15,30,33]

Studies on the effects of fatigue on performance have shown that they are similar to the effects of alcohol. Fatigue has been found to be a factor in a significant number of aviation mishaps and accidents. It should be addressed in the same fashion as other risks, especially during night operations. Transport programs need to have policies in place to address crew fatigue. Crew members should have the right to call a time-out from any flight or ground transport duties if they or a fellow flight team member feel that continuing duty is unsafe because of fatigue, no matter what the shift length. No adverse personnel action or undue pressure to continue should occur.

Pregnancy[15,21]

Many women of childbearing age work in the transport setting. No existing industry standard is found regarding pregnancy employment policies. The effects of high altitude, high noise levels, and vibration and the increased risk for injury in mishaps have been identified as potential risks to the fetus and maternal health. Transport team members who are considering pregnancy should discuss these risks with their personal physician and program administration.

Personal Protective Equipment

The 1988 NTSB study recommended that air medical personnel who routinely fly EMS helicopter missions wear protective clothing and equipment to reduce the chance of injury or death in survivable accidents.[24] The ASTNA position papers have also endorsed the use of protective equipment, which consists of helmets, fire-resistant uniforms, and boots.

Helmets

In the military, the use of flight helmets has been shown to protect significantly against head injuries.[19] Despite the obvious advantages afforded by flight helmets, acceptance in civilian air medical programs was not initially widespread. Reasons cited for not wearing helmets included high cost, uncertain benefit, and negative public relations.[19] However, a survey performed to determine the public's perception of helmet usage found that patients and family members positively viewed the use of helmets by air medical personnel.[39] The use of helmets by EMS pilots and flight

crew members has become the accepted standard. CAMTS now requires that all helicopter transport team members wear a helmet, including specialty team members.[15]

The flight helmet must be approved for use in helicopters. The chinstrap should hold the helmet firmly in place, and the liner needs to fit comfortably. Some manufacturers use customized liners that are molded to the individual's head. The helmet visor should be kept in the down position as much as possible during flight.

Helmets should receive routine maintenance. They should also be routinely evaluated for appropriate fit.

Fire-Resistant Clothing

The goal of fire-resistant clothing is to minimize skin exposure to the intense heat of an aircraft fire. The uniform should have long sleeves and be made of a flame- and heat-resistant material such as Nomex. Flame-resistant fabrics are designed to withstand high temperatures for a brief period, usually less than 20 seconds, which permits the wearer to evacuate a burning aircraft or vehicle.[10,24] The fabric can reduce the risk or severity of tissue damage but does not prevent thermal injury to the skin.

Undergarments worn under the fire-resistant flight suit (including briefs, t-shirt, or long underwear) should be made of natural fibers, such as cotton, silk, or wool.[25] When exposed to flames, synthetic materials such as polyester or polypropylene melt and become embedded into the skin. The uniform should also fit to allow a 0.25 inch of air space between the flight suit and undergarments. Nomex gloves protect the hands and should be considered by persons who wear fire-resistant uniforms.

Protective Footwear

Boots should protect the foot from punctures, lacerations, and thermal injuries and provide stability to the ankle on rough or uneven ground. Boots should be constructed of leather, or leather and Nomex, and extend several inches above the ankle. The sole should be thick and oil resistant, and the boot should have a safety toe and shank. It should also have adequate ventilation to prevent moisture from being trapped.

Hearing Protection

The average sound level produced by a running helicopter is between 90 and 100 decibels (dB). The Occupational Safety and Health Administration regulations require employers to provide hearing-conservation programs for employees exposed to time-weighted average sound levels of 85 dB or greater. Hearing protection, such as earplugs, earmuffs, or the flight helmet, should be worn during high-decibel exposures such as engine startup, hot loading and unloading, extreme noise levels at some scenes, and around running aircraft at airports. Earplugs are smaller and less expensive, but noise protection varies with fit; custom-fitted earplugs provide the most noise reduction. Earmuffs offer more uniform protection but are more expensive, are not as easily carried or stored, and may be less comfortable than earplugs. A properly fitted flight helmet provides adequate hearing protection for most individuals and should be worn at all times while in flight. Active noise reduction (or noise canceling) circuitry or communications earplugs can be added to most flight helmets to provide further noise attenuation.

Patient Safety

Along with the safety of the transport team, the safety of the patient being transported must be ensured. The patient should be properly restrained in the transport vehicle and provided with appropriate hearing and thermal protection. All patient care should be performed in a safe manner. Clinical decision making, patient treatment, and error reporting are all discussed elsewhere in this textbook, but each has a significant impact on patient safety. Keeping the patient safe should be an equally important part of the safety attitude.

Operational Safety

Aircraft Safety

Helicopter Safety

The most obvious component of the helicopter that presents a risk is the rotor system. The main rotor blades turn at approximately 400 rpm, with the rotor tips moving at more than 500 mph. At full speed, the main rotor blades create a disk that can be seen above the cabin. When the main rotor is spinning at lower speeds, such as during the startup and shutdown phases, the blades can flap or sail with wind gusts, which may allow the blades to drop below shoulder level. The degree to which this presents a hazard varies by aircraft model and design, but the best precaution is to never approach or depart any helicopter during startup or shutdown. The crouch position is advised for anyone approaching or departing the aircraft at other times while the blades are turning. When a helicopter lands on uneven ground or on a slope, the rotor disk comes closer to the ground on the uphill side. In this situation the aircraft should always be approached and departed from the downhill side in the crouched position, with constant attention paid to the terrain and the rotor disk. Program policy dictates whether patients are loaded into the aircraft with the rotor system turning, which is commonly referred to as *hot loading*. When loading or unloading patients and equipment, nothing should ever be carried above the head.

The tail rotor is potentially the most hazardous component of the helicopter. At a speed greater than 2000 rpm, it is nearly invisible. Aircraft manufacturers have worked to reduce the risks presented by the tail rotor by developing safer designs, such as the shrouded fenestron and no-tail-rotor systems. A safety person should be designated at all unsecured landing sites to ensure that no one inadvertently walks near the tail rotor. Fig. 9.2 shows an example of an aircraft with a shrouded fenestron tail rotor.

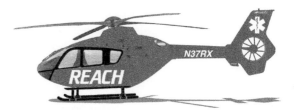

• **Fig. 9.2** Airbus Helicopters H-135 helicopter showing its shrouded fenestron tail rotor system. (Courtesy REACH Air Medical Services.)

All persons who approach the helicopter must do so in full view of the pilot and should not proceed under the rotor disk without the pilot's permission. The safest approach zone for most helicopters is from the sides, at the 3 o'clock or 9 o'clock position (12 o'clock is the nose of the aircraft; Fig. 9.3). Some aircraft models permit a safe approach from the front, depending on rotor or skid height and aircraft design. Flight crew members must be familiar with the safe approach zones for their program's aircraft. Those who work around the aircraft, such as EMS personnel, must be instructed to remain back from the aircraft after it lands and to approach only after being directed to do so by the pilot or a flight crew member and to never approach the aircraft from the rear.

The wind created by the moving rotor blades, referred to as *rotor wash,* can exceed 50 mph. In a hover and on the ground during the warm-up or cooldown stage, a rotor wash of approximately 25 mph can occur. Crew members should keep helmet visors down or wear protective glasses when operating around the running aircraft. All loose objects near the helicopter must be secured to prevent them from being blown away or ingested into the air intake of the helicopter's engine. Rotor wash also increases the windchill factor. An air temperature of 10°F combined with a 25-mph rotor wash creates a windchill temperature of −11°F.[16] Transport team members need to consider this and take steps to protect the patient before loading. Other hazardous areas that should be avoided include the engine exhaust ports (the exhaust temperature is approximately 400°C) and the pitot tubes, used to measure the aircraft's airspeed and heated to prevent ice formation, which presents a burn hazard.

Fixed-Wing Aircraft Safety

Fixed-wing aircraft have their own set of safety requirements. The propellers carry the same risk of injury as the rotors on a helicopter, and jet engines present risks from both the engine exhaust and the possibility of aspiration into the engine intakes. No one should be allowed to approach the aircraft until the engines have been shut down. Many fixed-wing aircraft used as air ambulances have pressurized cabins, which permit flight at higher altitudes. All crew members need to be familiar with how to ensure that the hatches are properly sealed and with emergency procedures in the event of cabin depressurization.

Ground Ambulance Safety

Study results of ground ambulance crashes described previously show that the high-risk environments for ground

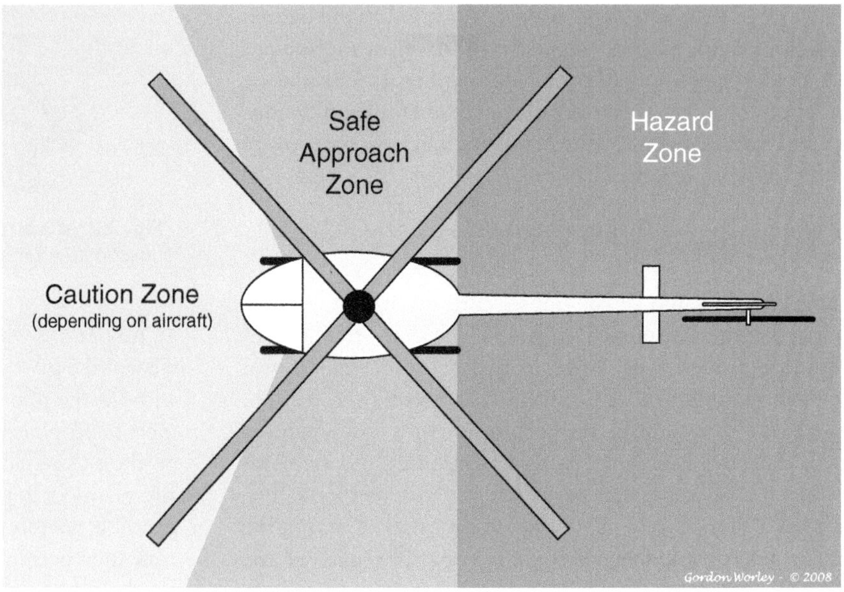

• **Fig. 9.3** Typical safe helicopter approach zones.

ambulance operations are emergency responses and inter-sections. Regulations for emergency response with use of RLS vary from state to state, but generally the decision is left to the transport team. In deciding whether or not an RLS response is necessary, the safety of all involved needs to be considered. Ground vehicle safety and driver training programs need to provide guidance regarding when to oper-ate in the RLS mode. Air transport programs should also educate their crews about when to use RLS in a ground vehicle. Use of proper safety equipment in ground vehicles should be just as important as in aircraft. Seat belts should be worn in both the front seat and the patient compart-ment, and all equipment should be properly secured.

Daily Preflight Procedures

At the beginning of each duty shift, the pilot and flight crew should complete an aircraft safety inspection. This inspec-tion should include an overall walk-around inspection of the aircraft and a check of onboard safety equipment. The pilot and flight crew should also perform their respective daily checklists and ensure that the aircraft is ready to re-spond. The daily risk assessment should be performed, and the pilot should brief the crew regarding weather, expected maintenance or other issues related to the aircraft, and any specific mission-planning needs.

Dispatch/Communications

The 2006 NTSB report recommended that air medical pro-grams be dispatched from a dedicated flight dispatch center, separate from any hospital or public safety dispatch center. The report also recommended expanding the role of the flight dispatcher/communication specialist to include specialized training in aviation weather, navigation, aircraft weight and balance planning, instrument approaches, and other aviation

topics. The intent of these recommendations was not to take any decision-making authority away from the pilot or flight crew but to provide a resource to the pilot for informed safe decisions. Communications and the role of the communica-tion specialist are discussed in detail in Chapter 6.

An important safety consideration during the dispatch of a mission is that the communication specialist should provide the pilot with the information needed to make the decision regarding whether or not the mission can be safely accepted but should not include any patient-specific infor-mation. The initial notification of the pilot should include the following:

- Nature of the request (scene call versus interfacility transfer)
- Location of the request
- Destination (if known)
- Patient weight (if known)
- Whether another aircraft or program has declined the request, and the reason for any such decline
- Known weather or other hazards

Once the pilot has evaluated the request and made the decision that the mission can be safely accepted, additional patient information may be communicated. An alternative method is to have the communication specialist contact the clinical crew separately and provide them with the patient information. The clinical crew should not discuss the pa-tient with the pilot until a decision has been made that the mission can be safely accepted. The clinical crew should under no circumstances pressure the pilot to accept a mis-sion on the basis of patient needs if the mission has been declined for safety reasons.

Helipad/Airport Safety

Hospital and off-site helipads should be designed to meet all applicable FAA and local regulations and should be able

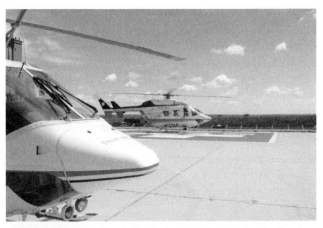

• **Fig. 9.4** Marked rooftop helipad with space for two aircraft. (Courtesy Air Care and Mobile Care, University of Cincinnati.)

to safely accommodate the weight and size of the largest helicopter expected to use the helipad (Fig. 9.4). Other helipad planning considerations include approach and departure routes, the location of the helipad relative to patient care areas, the provision of emergency exits, fire protection equipment, and helipad lighting. Provisions also need to be made for snow removal, fuel/HAZMAT/biohazard spills, and general cleaning. The helipad should be secured and monitored to prevent access by unauthorized persons. All flight crew members should be trained in fire safety and should know the location of fire alarm boxes and fire extinguishers. Smoking should be prohibited around or near the aircraft.

Crew members of aircraft based at airports need to be familiar with the safety and security requirements of the airport; the location of fire extinguishers and other emergency equipment at the base; and the methods of reporting an emergency to the FAA control tower (if present), airport administration, and local authorities. Other safety considerations at airports include access to restricted areas, awareness of runway/taxiway safety, and operations around other aircraft.

In-Flight Safety

In-flight safety begins with preliftoff checks of the aircraft to ensure that all doors and outside cowlings are secure, that engine and other covers/tie downs have been removed, that shoreline electric cords have been disconnected, and that the aircraft is ready for departure. It also includes the use of safety equipment such as helmets, seat belts, and shoulder harnesses during all phases of flight. At times, patient needs may necessitate that a crew member come "out of belt," but this should be done only while in level flight and with the approval of the pilot; the belts should be reapplied as soon as possible.

Situational Awareness

Situational awareness refers to the maintenance of an active awareness of all aspects of the flight environment. This awareness includes scanning for other aircraft, listening to radio traffic, maintaining a sterile cockpit during critical phases of flight, and observing for hazards on approach to scenes or other unfamiliar landing areas. Crew members should always advise the pilot when they need to be "eyes in," with their attention focused inside the aircraft for patient care or other reasons.

Crew members should scan for other air traffic as much as possible, especially when no patient is onboard. They need to report any obstacle or other air traffic, even though the pilot may have already seen it. Traffic or other hazards should be reported with use of clock position, with 12 o'clock being the nose of the aircraft and 6 o'clock being the tail. The location should further be identified as high, level, or low. One effective technique for scanning is the front-to-side method. This method involves starting with a fixed point in the center of the front windshield, slowly moving the field of vision leftward, returning to the center, refocusing, and then moving the eyes to the right. Other scanning techniques are available, and selection of one is a matter of preference, but the technique should involve some series of fixations. When the head is in motion, vision is blurred, and the mind does not register targets as easily.

The use of unmanned aerial vehicles (UAVs) and unmanned aerial systems (UAS) (also often called drones) has seen a significant increase over the last few years, and the growth is just beginning. The size of the drones can vary from as small as a hummingbird to as large as a regular aircraft. The FAA has issued regulations in the Small Unmanned Aircraft Rule (Part 107) about the use of drones. These regulations will take effect in August 2016. A summary of the regulations can be found at https://www.faa.gov/UAS/media/Part_107_Summary.pdf. Transport team members must always remain vigilant to prevent any potential incidents related to these aircraft.

Use of lasers in construction, speaker presentation, and general entertainment has presented a safety hazard to flight teams. Although it is illegal to point a laser at an aircraft, it still happens frequently. This can disorient the pilot and cause eye damage, especially when wearing NVGs. Programs should have policies in place to immediately report near UAV and laser hits to the local authorities and the FAA.

Sterile cockpit refers to restricting all nonessential communications over the aircraft intercom system. Federal aviation regulations (FAR 135.100) require the observance of sterile cockpit during all critical phases of flight, including taxi, takeoff, landing, and all other flight operations except cruise flight. Flight crew members should also attempt to maintain an awareness of the location of the aircraft along its flight path. Should a sudden emergency arise, quick communication of the aircraft's position may be necessary.

Flight Following

A crucial component of transport safety is having the location of the aircraft or vehicle known at all times, which is a process known as *flight following*. If an aircraft has any type of mishap that requires an emergency landing and the crew is unable to make a distress call, the flight following information permits the aircraft's position to be estimated with a high degree of accuracy. Typically, the communication specialist keeps abreast of the progress of the transport with periodic scheduled communications with the pilot or driver. Some programs use satellite-based real-time tracking systems that display the aircraft or vehicle location on a computer screen or map. Cellular telephones should not be used while in flight but may be used by ground transport teams to provide position/status reports.

When direct communications are not available, the pilot, driver, or crew should make contact with other transport program communication centers, emergency dispatch centers, airports, or hospitals along the flight or transport path and ask them to relay status reports. Flight following can also be requested from the FAA ATC system. Flight following with ATC has the added advantage of the aircraft being followed on radar by the controller.

Securing Patients and Equipment

The CAMTS[15] accreditation standards specify that patients must be secured with a minimum of three cross straps that restrain the patient to the litter at the chest, hips, and knees. Patients who are loaded head forward should also be restrained with a shoulder harness. The belts need to be adjustable to accommodate patients with specific needs or injury locations. The patient must also be secured in such a way that they are isolated from the pilot and the controls. Pediatric patients should be restrained with an appropriately sized securing device. If a car seat is used, it must have an FAA approval sticker.

Combative or potentially violent patients should be evaluated for the need for physical or chemical restraint before loading into the aircraft or vehicle. Physical restraints should be applied before takeoff. The use of physical or chemical restraints should be guided by program policies that are periodically reviewed and updated.

All bags and equipment must be secured while the aircraft or vehicle is in motion to prevent these objects from becoming projectiles and inflicting injuries to the patient or crew. Confirmation that all bags and equipment are properly secured should be a part of the preliftoff checks.

Scene Safety

The EMS scene call environment is one of the most potentially hazardous aspects of air medical operations.[1] The number of variables is huge, and the flight crew has direct control over only a small portion of the operation. Situational awareness, attention to detail, communications skills, critical thinking abilities, and knowledge of program and local EMS policies all come into play during each scene response. Flight crew members who operate in the scene call environment should be familiar with the Incident Command System (ICS, also called the Incident Management System) because it is used in their service area.[23]

Landing Zone Selection and Safety

Landing a helicopter at an unfamiliar location presents a variety of hazards. Each program should establish requirements for a suitable LZ for the program's aircraft. Generally, the LZ should be at least 75 × 75 feet for daytime use and 125 × 125 feet or larger at night. Larger is always better. A useful way to determine whether a proposed LZ is suitable is the mnemonic HOTSAW (hazards, obstructions, terrain, surface/slope/nature of the surface, animals, and wind/weather) (Box 9.2).

Although the pilot makes the ultimate decision about landing at any site, the initial selection and preparation of the LZ are often the responsibility of the local fire department or EMS

• BOX 9.2   HOTSAW: A Tool for Evaluation of Potential Landing Zones

Hazards

Potential Hazards within the Landing Zone
Rocks
Downed timber
Vegetation
Fences, loose debris
Vehicles

Obstructions

Overhead Obstructions along the Flight Path into or Out of the Landing Zone
Trees
Hills
Power lines
Flag poles
Buildings

Terrain

Nature of Landing Zone and nearby Terrain Features
Elevation
Uneven ground
Creeks or ditches
Surrounding terrain (mountains, cliffs, water, etc.)

Surface/Slope/Nature of Surface

Character of Surface
- Hard
- Soft/muddy (risk of landing gear sinking)
- Icy

Loose Surface Materials that May Blow in Rotor Wash
- Sand
- Snow
- Dirt
- Dry vegetation
- Slope of ground

Animals

Domestic animals (horses, cows, dogs, etc.)
Wild animals
Humans (bystanders and responders)

Wind/Weather

Wind speed and direction
Overall weather conditions (clouds, fog, height of cloud ceiling, precipitation, air)

provider. LZ selection and preparation should be a part of routine outreach education provided to first responders. Training should also include a discussion of radio and visual communications procedures, use of eye and hearing protection, hot-loading procedures, and an aircraft-specific orientation.

Two-way radio contact should be established with the LZ coordinator as early as possible before arrival. The usual preference is to use a dedicated air-to-ground frequency for LZ communications (one that is not in use for other on-scene radio traffic). If a hazard is identified during approach or landing, the LZ coordinator needs to be able to notify the aircraft immediately. The pilot should perform a high reconnaissance, followed by a low reconnaissance, which allows the pilot and flight crew to observe for hazards before the final approach. If the pilot or crew detect a problem with the LZ, the landing should be aborted and the LZ coordinator informed of the issue. If the concern can be immediately corrected, then the site may be used. If the situation cannot be easily resolved, then a new LZ may need to be chosen.

An awareness of activities in and around the LZ is important at all times when the aircraft is on approach, on the ground, and departing. Ground personnel should only be allowed to approach the aircraft when directed to do so by the pilot or a flight crew member. On departing the scene, the flight crew should provide the LZ coordinator with a final report. A "thank you" to the ground crew for their help is always a good idea.

Multiple Aircraft Response

When more than one helicopter is on scene, or other aircraft are expected to land, clear communications must be maintained between the pilots of all aircraft and with the LZ coordinator. All air medical personnel on scene should remain in communication with their own pilot via radio and with the pilot or crew of any other helicopter on scene via direct radio contact, relay via their own pilot, or hand signals. Crew members should never approach or pass under or near the rotor disk of another aircraft without the knowledge and approval of the pilot of that aircraft.

On-Scene Safety

Crew members must maintain an awareness of the hazards present in the prehospital setting. Unless specifically trained and authorized, transport team members should not participate in vehicle extrication or specialized rescue efforts. The extrication process should only be interrupted if immediate life-saving measures are needed, and then only if the procedure can be performed without unnecessary risk to the crew member or other rescuers. When responding to the scene of a violent crime, transport teams should always consult with law enforcement personnel to ensure the scene is safe before entering. When caring for a victim of a violent crime, care should be taken to disturb the scene no more than necessary to preserve possible evidence.

Hazardous Materials

Response to HAZMAT scenes must be done cautiously. The first priority is always the safety of the flight crew and aircraft.

The LZ should be upwind of the incident and at a safe distance. Air medical personnel should not participate in the decontamination process for HAZMAT-exposed cases, regardless of any skills or experience the individual crew members may possess. HAZMAT-exposed cases should never be placed onboard the aircraft until they have undergone complete decontamination by a qualified HAZMAT team.

Postmission Debriefings

A preflight briefing is an important part of mission safety. A postmission debrief is equally, if not more, important. It permits the crew to come together and review the mission and identify issues or concerns about any aspect of the flight, including adequacy and accuracy of mission planning, operational safety and decision making, and clinical care of the patient. Debriefings can help identify recurrent issues and mission-specific occurrences that need to be addressed. They may also identify risk factors that should be taken into account in the planning of subsequent missions.

When communication-related issues are identified, the communication center should also be included.

In-Flight Emergencies

An *in-flight emergency* is "a sudden unforeseen occurrence or incident requiring immediate action." These events can range from the catastrophic failure of a critical aircraft component to a malfunction in an aircraft system that does not present an immediate risk but indicates that prompt action must be taken to prevent further problems. A common aviation description of how to manage an in-flight emergency is to *aviate, navigate, and communicate.* The priorities are to maintain (or regain) control of the aircraft, decide on the next step, select an appropriate emergency landing site (if indicated), and then report the emergency to the program communication center, ATC, or the local emergency dispatch center.

The primary role of the transport team member in an in-flight emergency situation is to serve as a resource to the pilot. Once the pilot has announced an emergency, the crew members should[1,10,42]:

- Ensure sterile cockpit
- Assist the pilot as needed or requested
- Prepare self for an emergency landing: helmet strap tight, visor down, seat belts snug
- Prepare the patient for an emergency landing: position properly, secure/tighten seat belts
- Prepare the cabin for an emergency landing: secure equipment, shut off oxygen and inverter
- Look for suitable emergency landing sites
- Initiate emergency communications as directed by pilot

Training in emergency procedures should be part of the safety training program, and proficiency should be demonstrated annually. Regularly scheduled emergency drills permit practice and increase familiarity with emergency procedures.

Aircraft Mechanical Emergencies

Mechanical emergencies involve a malfunction in some aspect of the aircraft's systems. Sensors are located in all of the aircraft's important systems to provide the pilot with a visual or audible warning if a problem occurs in that system. Some of these conditions can be managed in flight, and others require that the aircraft land to ensure safety. The pilot should inform the crew as soon as a potential mechanical emergency situation is identified and advise them if an emergency landing is necessary.

Aircraft Fire Emergencies

Aircraft fires can be divided into two broad categories: those that involve the engines and fuel system and those that occur within the aircraft cabin. Engine fires usually trigger a warning light on the pilot's instrument panel and produce visible smoke. To confirm the presence of an engine fire on a helicopter, the pilot may put the aircraft into a gentle turn and ask the crew member on the side facing the inside of the turn to look back for a smoke trail. A confirmed engine fire is a serious emergency and requires that the affected engine be shut down. On twin-engine aircraft, emergency procedures should dictate that the pilot request visual confirmation from the crew that the correct engine is being shut down before actually doing so. Some aircraft have built-in fire extinguishers in the engine compartments.

Smoke from an aircraft cabin fire can fill the cabin quickly and potentially incapacitate the crew. Fire extinguishers should be located within easy reach of all crew members. On larger aircraft in which the medical crew is separated from the pilot, a fire extinguisher should be located in each compartment. In the event of a cabin fire, the crew members should shut off the oxygen source, turn off the inverter, and close the windows and vents to prevent acceleration of the fire. If the fire is caused by medical equipment plugged into the aircraft power supply, the equipment should be turned off and unplugged and the inverter turned off. If smoke and heat become excessive, the crew should open windows or doors with discretion, fight the fire aggressively with the fire extinguisher, and prepare for an emergency landing.[37] Aircraft fire extinguishers are typically filled with halon, an inert gas that extinguishes fire by displacing oxygen. Halon extinguishers present the risk of asphyxiation when discharged in a closed space and should only be used in ventilated spaces. Fire extinguishers should only be discharged in the aircraft cabin at the direction of the pilot.

Emergency Communications

Emergency communications are ultimately the responsibility of the pilot but may be delegated to a crew member, depending on program policy. If a crew member is expected to make emergency radio calls, this responsibility should be clearly defined in the program's emergency procedures. Emergency radio calls should only be made at the direction of the pilot. All members of the flight team should be familiar with radio operations.

In the event of an emergency landing as a result of a serious situation (engine fire, etc.), the term *Mayday* is used to ensure that the severity of the situation is clear to the receiving party and to indicate the need for additional assistance to respond to the emergency landing site (fire department, etc.). A Mayday call indicates immediate serious distress and should only be used in a true emergency situation. The typical way to declare an emergency over the radio is Mayday, Mayday, Mayday; (aircraft tail number/identifier) is making an emergency landing at (location) due to (nature of emergency).

In less serious situations that necessitate a precautionary landing, the appropriate description should be used, rather than a Mayday call. Include the location of the landing site and as much additional information as the circumstances dictate. In some situations, initial radio calls should be made to the local 911 emergency dispatch center, which may be easier to contact than the program's dispatch center and can rapidly mobilize any needed resources (fire department, ambulance, etc.).

Emergency Locator Transmitter

All EMS aircraft are required by the FAA to carry an emergency locator transmitter (ELT). The ELT is activated by an impact that exceeds $4g$ (four times the force of gravity) and broadcasts a signal on one of the universal distress frequencies: 121.5, 243, or 406 MHz. As of February 1, 2009, the COSPAS-SARSAT satellite system no longer monitors the 121.5 and 243 MHz frequencies. The 406-MHz ELTs transmit a digital signal that identifies the aircraft and contains global positioning system position information. The signal is received by the international COSPAS-SARSAT satellite system, and the information relayed to search and rescue (SAR) personnel. The 406-MHz ELTs also transmit a signal on the 121.5-MHz emergency frequency that may be used by radio direction-finding equipment to pinpoint the location of the beacon.[17]

Transport team members should know the location of the ELT on all of their program's aircraft and how to ensure that it has been activated. If an impact does not automatically activate the ELT, it can be activated manually by following the directions on the front of the unit. Each crew member should know the location and how to activate the ELT.

Emergency Landings

In an emergency or precautionary landing situation, in which a hard landing may be anticipated, flight crew members should assume the survival position before impact. They should sit upright with the knees together and feet approximately 6 inches apart. In forward-facing seats equipped with shoulder belts, one should hold the arms across the chest, forming an X with the forearms and grasping the shoulder harness. In forward-facing seats without shoulder belts, one should bend forward at the waist and encircle the knees with the arms. In aft-facing seats, one should sit upright with the head held against the seat head rest and the arms in an X across the chest. Crew members should keep a point of reference inside the cabin to maintain spatial orientation in case the aircraft comes to rest on its side or inverted.

Emergency Egress

All crew members need to be prepared to manage the emergency evacuation of the crew and patient from all of the aircraft used by their program. After an emergency landing, disorientation is common, particularly if the aircraft is not upright. The only available route of egress may involve climbing up to a door or window, into the cockpit, over seats, or over other occupants of the aircraft. One should make a quick survey to reestablish spatial orientation and assess the condition of the aircraft, other crew members, and the patient. In night conditions or in smoke-filled cabins, spatial orientation can be maintained with the hand-over-hand method, during which one hand is kept on a known reference point while a new reference point is selected with the other hand. After the aircraft has come to a complete stop, the aircraft should be exited by normal means when possible or by jettisoning doors, opening emergency exits, or using forcible means if necessary.[10,11]

Individual crew members should evacuate to a predesignated position away from the aircraft, typically the 12 o'clock position off the nose of rotor-wing aircraft and the 6 o'clock position off the tail for fixed-wing aircraft. Crew members should evaluate the risk of fire and other hazards before attempting the rescue of injured or entrapped fellow crew members or the patient. After a forced landing, a significant danger is fire. All crew members should be familiar with the emergency shutdown procedure for all aircraft in which they may be asked to operate and how to operate the fire extinguishers carried on the aircraft.

Emergency egress, aircraft evacuation, and emergency shutdown should be part of initial training for all crew members and should be practiced regularly. Crew members should keep in mind that they may need to perform postcrash emergency egress and evacuation when they are injured. Practice and drills should include consideration of how to open emergency exits or perform emergency shutdown with only one arm and with other possible disabilities.

Forced Water Landings

Air medical programs that frequently operate over large bodies of water need to ensure that all crew members are familiar with emergency egress procedures in the event of a forced water landing, or ditching. When flying over water, all flight team members should wear a PFD. Aircraft PFDs should have an attached strobe light that automatically activates on contact with the water. Flight team members may consider wearing additional survival gear and signaling devices in a vest system.

The ability to swim should be mandatory, and water egress procedures and open-water survival should be part of the training received by all flight team members. Each program should evaluate its risk of a water landing and provide specialized open-water survival equipment where appropriate.

In a ditching situation, jettisoning of doors and other emergency procedures should be performed under direction of the pilot. The sequence for emergency escape from an aircraft after a water landing is as follows.

Before Impact with the Water

1. Try to keep calm and concentrate on how you are going to get out.
2. Know which way the closest door is from your position.
3. Open or jettison doors as directed by the pilot.
4. Place one hand on a known reference point within the cabin.
5. Disconnect your ICS cable.
6. Place your other hand on the seat belt buckle (do not release).

After Impact with the Water

7. Do not attempt to exit the aircraft until the rotor or propeller has stopped moving.
8. Helicopters almost always capsize after striking the water; do not attempt to exit the cabin until the aircraft is upside down.
   - Wait for the helicopter to all but fully fill with water.
   - Take a deep breath.
   - Release your buckle; you will immediately float.
   - Pull yourself toward the closest door and out.
   - Do not swim or kick; this increases the chance of becoming entangled and you may unintentionally kick other crew members.
   - Exhale slowly during ascent to the surface to reduce the risk of pulmonary barotrauma.
   - If necessary, observe your air bubbles to determine which way is up.
9. Fixed-wing aircraft generally float for a few minutes.
   - Locate the safest exit route.
   - Open the appropriate door and crawl through.
   - Assist others in exiting.
   - Enter the water and move away from the fuselage before it sinks.
10. Do not inflate your life vest until outside and away from the aircraft.
11. If a helmet is worn, keep it on for insulation and visibility.

Open-water survival is discussed later in the chapter.

Ground Vehicle Emergencies

All persons riding in the front seat of a ground transport vehicle should wear their seat belts at all times. Everyone in the patient compartment should remain in seat belts as much as possible during patient care and stay in their seats with seat belts secured at all other times. Programs should have response plans to address ground vehicle accidents, as well as aircraft accidents. All vehicles should be equipped with fire extinguishers, and emergency egress and evacuation training should be a part of the annual training.

Postcrash Responsibilities

Crew Responsibilities

After any crash or other accident, the crew should first ensure the safety of all on board the aircraft or vehicle. Then, the crew members should attend to any injuries that have occurred and attempt to contact help. Help may be the local emergency dispatch center, the program communication center, or the FAA. A 911 call from a cellular phone may be the easiest and most expedient way to accomplish contact help, if a cellular signal is found.

Missing or Overdue Aircraft or Ground Vehicle Procedure

The practice of flight or ground transport following should be standard operating procedure in all transport programs. The communication specialist should maintain a constant awareness of the location of each aircraft or vehicle for which they are responsible. If a scheduled check-in is missed, or arrival is overdue, the communication specialist should initiate the *postaccident incident plan* (PAIP).

Postaccident Incident Plan

The PAIP is a program policy document that outlines the responsibilities of the communication specialist and program administration. CAMTS recommends that some elements of the following be in a transport program's PAIP[15]:

- Preplanned time frame to activate the postaccident/incident for overdue transport vehicle
- A method to ensure accurate information dissemination
- Coordination of transport of the injured transport team members
- Procedure to document communications and secure the information
- Procedures to release information to the press
- Resources for crisis management
- Method to determine whether program will remain in service

The PAIP must also contain the following related to the transport team and their families:

- List of personnel with current phone numbers and who to notify in case of an emergency.
- Other numbers for individuals who may need to be involved including sponsoring organization, risk management attorney, hospital administration, and human resources.
- Notification plans to include appropriate family members and support for family members.
- Family assistance should include coordination of family needs after the event, such as transportation, lodging, and food.
- Follow-through with the family and others who may have been involved with event.

The initial response to a missing or overdue aircraft or vehicle should be an attempt to locate the aircraft by contacting the FAA/ATC and EMS agencies, law enforcement agencies, other air medical programs, and airport facilities along the flight path. For other emergencies, the communication specialist should notify local fire and EMS resources of the incident and request a response to the emergency landing site. Provisions may be needed to continue the transport of the patient, in addition to management of the aircraft or vehicle emergency.

The PAIP should indicate which administrative personnel should be notified for each specific set of circumstances. In the event of an aircraft crash or another significant event, an administrative crisis team should be assembled. The members of this team and their duties should be clearly described in the PAIP.

Emergency drills should be conducted on a regular basis, including both day and night, and the PAIP should be reviewed and updated regularly.

Safety Attitude Revisited

The preceding sections of this chapter have discussed the historic and current safety records of the air medical industry and the initiatives, practices, and tools presently available to improve safety. These resources alone are not enough to prevent future tragedies. The vital component is the human factor. Every individual involved in medical transport must commit themselves to the development of a positive safety culture within their own program and throughout the industry. Each individual must stay informed about new safety practices and technologies and maintain an open mind about their use. Most importantly, all those involved in medical transport must make good, safe, informed decisions about every aspect of every mission as well as develop, maintain, and spread a safety attitude.

Ed MacDonald, an experienced HEMS pilot and safety advocate, in a paper titled "Dumb Down for Safety" published in the *Air Medical Journal* in 2008, summarized how to keep safe in the transport environment by following these three lessons[30]:

- Lesson 1: My crew and I are responsible for making good decisions that, above all, will cause no harm.
- Lesson 2: I will not operate in any conditions wherein I cannot see and avoid every hazard or have a way out.
- Lesson 3: Not dealing with internal and external pressure can push me to where I do not belong.

Survival Basics[11,12,17,18,20,23,25,28,32,35,41]

All medical transport crew members need to be prepared to face the possibility of a survival situation. The situation may result from an emergency landing in a remote location as a result of weather or mechanical issues or changes in the mission environment (such as weather deterioration while at a remote scene LZ). Ground transport vehicles may break down or be stranded by weather. Regardless of the cause, the essentials of survival remain the same.

The goal in a survival situation is survival until a rescue can be accomplished. Flight-following procedures provide the flight communication center with the general location of the incident. The ELT on the aircraft assists rescuers in locating the aircraft and crew. All air medical aircraft should be equipped with a complete survival kit, and all crew members should receive training in its use. Ground transport vehicles that operate in remote areas should also carry survival equipment. Crew members should be prepared to spend an unexpected 24 to 72 hours outdoors and be able to look after their own needs for that period.

Preparation and Priority Setting

Successful survival strategy is based on two equally important concepts: preparation and priority setting. In a survival situation, individuals who are both psychologically and physically prepared to survive and who can establish and address the priorities for their own survival needs have a much higher chance of surviving the situation.

Psychological Preparation

The biggest threat to survival in any emergency situation is panic. Panic reduces the mind's ability to respond properly to a threat and leads to actions that may worsen the situation. Fear, anxiety, anger, and denial are all normal reactions to an emergency situation, but they need not lead to panic. Preparing oneself psychologically for a survival situation means developing a positive attitude about one's own abilities to manage such a situation. Practice and familiarity with the tools and skills necessary in a survival situation help to build self-confidence and develop a positive "I can do this" attitude. The most valuable tool in one's survival kit is a mind that possesses a positive outlook.

Psychological preparation also involves preparing oneself for the possibility of being in a survival situation while injured or when others have been injured or killed in a crash. Practice and familiarity with survival skills, faith in the SAR system, personal beliefs, and introspection can all help crew members function and manage under such circumstances.

Physical Preparation

Physical preparation for survival consists of two primary areas: keeping oneself in good physical condition and the selection and carrying of the items needed for a survival situation. A good physical fitness routine is important for everyone, but the demands of a survival situation make good physical condition even more important.

Clothing and Personal Equipment

Clothing is the first line of defense against the environment and needs to be selected on the basis of the nature of that environment. Clothing should protect the wearer, be comfortable and practical, and meet the fire safety guidelines described previously. Garments should be layered; this method traps the most dead air, provides the best insulation, and allows adjustment as environmental conditions change. Even if the weather appears mild, a jacket should be taken on all transports. Gloves and a warm hat or cap should be carried during cold weather. Warm-weather clothing should protect against the sun. Long sleeves and pants legs, together with head and eye protection, diminish water loss and heat exposure.

Personal equipment includes a personal survival kit and other items carried by the crew member. The most well-designed and comprehensive aircraft or vehicle survival kit is not of much use if it is not accessible because of damage to the aircraft, fire, or injury.[41] Each crew member should carry basic survival items on their person (see Box 9.2).

Priority Setting

To establish the priorities in a survival situation, follow the *rule of threes.* The average person can survive 3 minutes without oxygen, 3 hours without shelter in extreme conditions, 3 days without water, and 3 weeks without food.[12] Once safety and immediate medical concerns have been addressed, the rule of threes should guide priority setting. The two biggest killers in the outdoors are inadequate thermoregulation (lack of shelter) and dehydration (lack of water).[12] With this in mind, the immediate priorities should be finding or creating shelter, building a fire, taking steps to maintain hydration, and signaling by whatever means possible.

Survival Skills

The subject of emergency survival cannot be covered fully in this brief section. Transport programs should conduct annual survival training to ensure that all crew members have the necessary knowledge and skills. Survival training should include hands-on practice with all of the items in the aircraft or vehicle survival kit and a review of survival strategies for a variety of environmental conditions, with emphasis on how to prepare for those that exist in the program's service area. Transport team members are encouraged to consult other sources of information to improve their individual survival knowledge and skills, including the references listed at the end of this chapter, other survival manuals, and outside survival classes.

Shelter

An emergency shelter should be as simple to construct as possible and provide protection from wind, rain, snow, sun, extremes in temperatures, and animals. It should be big enough to protect all survivors and their survival equipment but not large enough to be difficult to construct or to heat. Shelter building should be practiced during survival training.

The aircraft or vehicle should be the first choice for an emergency shelter. If the aircraft or vehicle is used for shelter, ensure that it is stable and will not roll or tilt on the terrain or during adverse weather. Any holes should be patched with sheets, tarps, or space blankets. All windows and exposed metal should be insulated to reduce heat loss. Avoid sleeping, or placing the injured on exposed metal or directly on the ground. Aircraft are usually poorly insulated; in cold weather, construction of a shelter near the aircraft that can be heated with a fire may be a better choice.[20]

If the aircraft or vehicle is not available or safe, a shelter must be located or constructed. Natural shelters such as caves, rock overhangs, or large trees may be available. Look for potential hazards such as dead trees or tree limbs that may fall in a strong wind, rock slides, caves with other inhabitants (such as bears, skunks, or cougars), and tall trees or rocks that may conduct lightning. If a shelter needs to be constructed, the first step is locating a suitable site. When selecting the site, attempt the following:

1. Stay as close to the aircraft or vehicle as possible.
2. Find a spot that is protected from the prevailing wind.
3. Avoid natural hazards such as overhanging tree branches, avalanche or rock fall chutes, and steep terrain.
4. Find a level spot that will stay dry; avoid dry streambeds that could flood.
5. Avoid low-lying areas that collect cold air.
6. Orient the door of the shelter toward the east so that the morning sun will warm the shelter.

Shelters can be constructed with a variety of natural materials, supplies from the survival kit, and items from the aircraft or vehicle. Examples are shown in Fig. 9.5. Natural materials that may be used for shelter construction include trees, branches, brush, logs, and rocks. In snow country, trench shelters are quick and easy to construct. Aircraft and vehicle parts that may be useful include doors (shelter panels), foam from seats or litters (insulation), and wiring (for tying or lashing). Large heavy-duty plastic trash bags are useful for constructing shelters. An individual can use one bag as a bivvy sack, or bags may be opened up and used as a tarp to build a lean-to. They can also be used to waterproof shelters constructed from brush or branches or to create a roof for a snow shelter. Mylar plastic space blankets are compact to store and effective at reflecting heat but tear easily and are noisy in windy conditions.[12,20] Corners, edges, and stress points on space blankets or plastic bags can be reinforced with duct tape.

Fire Building

A fire provides warmth, light, and a sense of security. If adequate clothing and shelter are available, a fire may not be needed for warmth. When the need is recognized, prepare the materials and start the fire before dark. Gather enough firewood to last through the night. Locate the fire so that it provides as much heat to the inside of the shelter as possible, and contain it within some type of boundary to prevent its spreading by accident. In high fire danger conditions, exercise caution when building any fire.

There are many methods of fire building and many ways to start a fire, including waterproof matches; lighters; and "metal matches," which create a shower of sparks when scraped with a steel edge (Fig. 9.6). Fire steels are available commercially. These consist of a steel rod $\frac{1}{4}$ to $\frac{1}{2}$ inch in diameter and a striker that can produce a shower of sparks and can work in wet conditions. At least two reliable methods of starting a fire

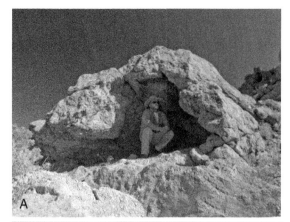
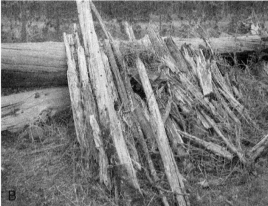
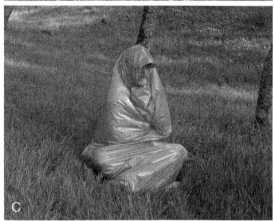
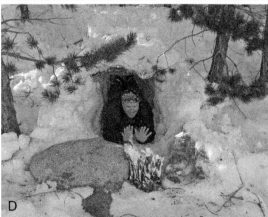

• **Fig. 9.5** Simple shelters. (A) Natural shelter: shallow cave in the desert. (B), Lean-to shelter made from natural materials. (C) Large heavy-duty plastic garbage bag may be used as a bivvy sack. (D) Snow trench shelter.

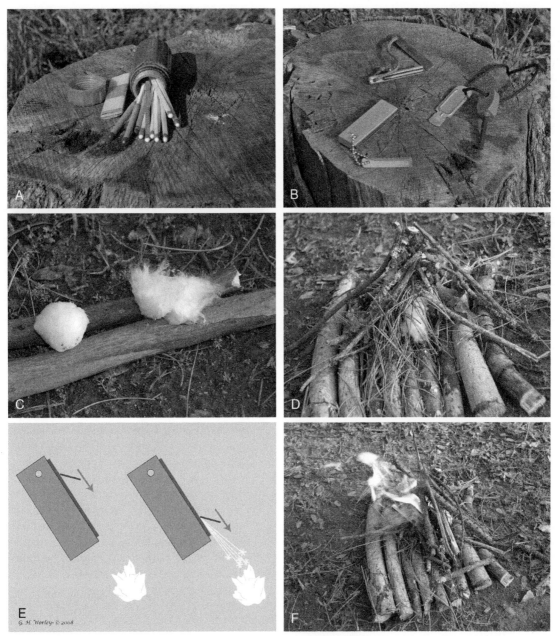

• **Fig. 9.6** Fire building. (A) Commercial stormproof matches *(left)* and strike-anywhere kitchen matches, waterproofed with clear nail polish *(right)*, in a waterproof match safe. (B) A variety of metal matches are available; all incorporate a piece of mischmetal that creates sparks when scraped with a steel edge. (C) A cotton ball smeared with petroleum jelly makes effective tinder *(left)*; six to eight will fit into a film can. To use, pull the cotton ball apart to expose the inner fibers *(right)*, which ignite easily. (D) Basic fire teepee with cotton ball tinder in the center. The tinder can be ignited with matches or a metal match. (E) Hold the tip of the metal match about an inch from the tinder and scrape the mischmetal insert with the striker, directing the shower of sparks onto the tinder. (F) As the fire builds, slowly add small and progressively larger kindling. (C, From Model minimum uniform crash criteria. <http://www.mmucc.us/>; 2016. Accessed 16.07.10.)

should be packed in the survival kit. Matches (even waterproof matches) should be stored in a waterproof match safe. Transport team members need to be familiar with the use of all of the fire-starting tools carried in the survival kit.

The simplest way to build a fire is to create a teepee of small sticks or kindling over a pile of fine dry tinder. On damp ground or snow, build the teepee on top of a platform of large dry sticks. Use the available fire-starting equipment to create a flame in the tinder. A few dry cotton balls and a few impregnated with Vaseline are excellent as fire starters and can produce a good flame for up to 8 minutes. As the tinder ignites and begins to set the small sticks on fire, slowly add small and progressively larger kindling to the fire. As the fire grows, larger pieces of wood may be added. Practice with the techniques of fire building should be a part of all survival training.

Hydration

Maintenance of adequate hydration is important in the survival setting. Each person should drink at least 1 to 1.5 L of water daily in temperate conditions. Extremes of temperature (hot or cold) and exertion can dramatically increase water requirements. A good rule of thumb is to drink enough water to produce at least 1 L of urine every 24 hours. Conserve available water stores by rationing until a water source is located. All surface water must be purified before drinking by boiling, filtration, or using water-purification tablets to prevent gastrointestinal (GI) infection from bacteria, viruses, or parasites. GI infections can lead to vomiting and diarrhea and cause significant water loss and worsening dehydration.

In woodland environments, water can be collected with a transpiration bag (Fig. 9.7). Place a plastic bag over a tree branch, ideally in the sun, with a small clean rock in one corner of the bag. The leaves or needles transpire water vapor, which then condenses and collects on the inside of the bag. Dew can be collected from leaves, plastic sheets, or the outside of the aircraft. If rain is expected, set up a method of catching the rainfall. Do not eat snow; this can cause substantial heat loss. Snow may be melted over a fire or by placing a canteen filled with snow in the sun or between the outer and inner layers of one's clothing. Protect water from freezing, keeping the container inside the shelter or under the outer clothing. In the desert, efforts to find and collect water may return less water than the amount that is lost in sweat. If rescue can be expected shortly, conserve water by resting in a shaded location and minimizing water loss from sweating.

Signaling

Once basic needs have been met, signaling becomes the next priority. As soon as an aircraft is reported overdue, SAR resources are mobilized. SAR aircraft initially search for transmissions from the aircraft radio and ELT. If the aircraft radio and the ELT are not operational, other methods of signaling must be used. Signals in groups of three are recognized internationally as distress signals.[17] Visual signals should have as much movement and contrast with the environment as possible.

1. *Portable radios and cell phones:* Aviation portable radios should be tuned to the last known ATC frequency or the emergency frequency (121.5 MHz). Conserve the batteries, turning on the radio to transmit only when an aircraft is heard. Cellular phone service now covers an extensive area in North America; a cellular signal may be obtainable even in remote locations.

2. *Smoke and fire:* In addition to providing warmth, the fire is a valuable signaling tool. At night, a fire can be visible for many miles. Smoke is an effective way to signal SAR aircraft during daylight. The addition of green leaves, grass, or water to the fire creates white smoke. The addition of oil, rubber, plastic, or pitchy wood creates black smoke. A can filled with sand and oil burns and generates black smoke for a long period of time. Use the color of smoke that provides the most contrast with the background.

3. *Flashlights, strobes, and flares:* A flashlight or a small light-weight strobe light can be an effective signal at night. Flares can be used if they are available in the aircraft but should be used with caution during high fire danger conditions. Many SAR aircraft are now equipped with NVG technology. Even the smallest light is visible for many miles to searchers with NVGs. It should be noted that "rescue lasers" are now approved by the FAA for the emergency signaling of searching aircraft and so forth. They are compact and battery operated.

4. *Signal mirror:* All crew members should practice signaling with the signal mirror. The preferred type of mirror is one made of laminated safety glass with a sighting hole in the center. Flash the mirror in the direction of any

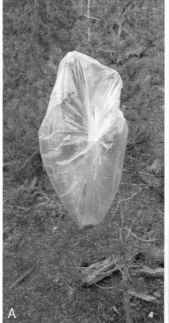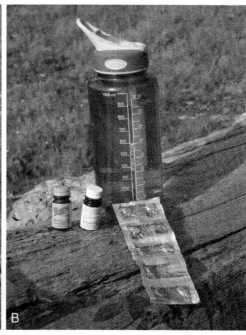

• **Fig. 9.7** Hydration. (A) Transpiration bag tied around a tree branch. (B) Water-purification tablets. Be sure to follow the manufacturer's instructions for each type.

A

B

aircraft that can be heard, even if it cannot be seen. Other shiny objects such as CDs, cans, foil, or aircraft parts may be used as improvised signal mirrors.

5. *Clothing and other colored objects:* Brightly colored parkas, space blankets, plastic garbage bags, signal panels, or other items that provide a contrast with the colors of the surrounding environment are useful signals. These may be placed on the ground in a geometric pattern or waved to create maximal visibility.
6. *Whistle:* A plastic whistle provides an effective way to signal ground SAR units. Use of a whistle is much more efficient than shouting. The standard signal is three blasts, pause, three more blasts, then listen for a reply.
7. *Ground-to-air signals:* Signals may be created by piling debris, digging trenches, or stamping out patterns in snow or sand. The most easily recognized patterns are a large X or the letters S-O-S.
8. *Dyes:* Dyes are effective in water and on snow. Fine dyes should be used downwind.

Food

The need for food is a low priority during a survival situation of fewer than 4 to 5 days. Although not a direct threat to survival in the short term, depleted energy stores can have other negative effects, including depression and diminished problem-solving capabilities. In cold weather, lack of calorie intake can increase the risk of hypothermia.

Overland Travel and Navigation

The first rule in a downed aircraft situation is to stay with the aircraft, because it is what searchers are looking for. Consider overland travel only in case of a clearly identified need, such as an injured person who needs immediate medical attention. Land navigation skills require training and practice. Cross-country travel should only be attempted by individuals who possess the necessary experience and skills and who have a clear picture of the route they need to follow to reach a location in which help may be obtained. Programs may want to consider adding a good compass to the survival kit to aid in land navigation. Personnel should be trained in their use.

If the decision is made to leave the aircraft, leave a detailed note listing the number of survivors, their condition, the intended route of travel, and the intended destination. Mark the outbound route with visible markers, such as strips of brightly colored cloth or surveyor's tape, to permit retracing the route of travel (if necessary) and aid searchers in following the trail. In most situations, the best decision is to stay put and devote one's energy to shelter building, water procurement, and signaling.[12,20]

Specific Environmental Considerations

Transport programs that operate in regions that have specific environmental conditions or seasonal weather patterns should conduct specialized survival training focused on those environments.

Water Landings and Open Water Survival

The process for emergency aircraft evacuation after a water landing was described previously. After impact with the water, the first priorities are to evacuate the aircraft, account for all persons who were on board, and move to a safe location away from the sinking aircraft. A prearranged rendezvous spot should be part of the emergency evacuation plan. If the accident occurs close to shore, consider swimming toward the shore. Distances can be hard to estimate, and one can easily become exhausted when swimming against waves or current.

If the distance does not seem to be within the survivor's capabilities to swim, or if one of the survivors is injured, the best option may be to minimize heat loss with the heat escape–lessening posture (HELP) shown in Fig. 9.8. Remain still and assume the fetal position, cross your arms over your chest, and bring your knees up to your chest. A PFD must be worn when assuming the HELP to stay afloat.[19] Surviving flight team members should huddle together to decrease heat loss. The flight helmet should be worn in the water because it provides insulation and improved visibility to searchers. Protect against salt and sun exposure by covering any exposed skin surface. Protection against hypothermia, care of the raft (if used), and signaling are the primary objectives in open-water survival.

Desert Survival

Desert areas can reach ambient temperatures of more than 120°F (50°C) during the day and drop to below freezing at night. Maintain an awareness of heat exposure and illness, minimize exertion, and rest in the shade as much as possible. Sheltering in the shade of the aircraft may be preferable to the interior during the daytime. Wear long sleeves and long pants, along with head and neck protection, sunglasses, and sunscreen. Water collection, hazardous plants and animals, and desert shelter construction should all be part of desert survival training.

Cold Weather Survival

Transport programs that operate in areas that have significant snowfall should conduct specialized winter survival training, including snow shelter construction, water procurement, fire

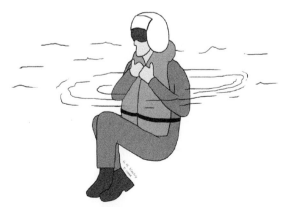

• **Fig. 9.8** Heat escape–lessening posture.

building in winter conditions, and the use of any specialized equipment in the survival kit (tents, snowshoes, etc.). Adequate clothing, sunglasses, and sunscreen should be worn or carried when operating in cold weather conditions.

International Survival Concerns

Transport teams who may cross international boundaries need to consider international survival concerns. Air medical team members should be aware of the climate and terrain of the areas that they fly over and of the final destination of the mission. Recognition of the need for additional survival equipment and food stores should be part of mission planning. In some countries, SAR resources are limited, and in many others, they are nonexistent.

Patient Care in a Survival Situation

In addition to looking after their own needs, a stranded transport team may also need to care for a patient or an injured team member. The first priority is to ensure the safety of everyone involved before starting medical care. Providing shelter and warmth for the injured should be a high priority and take precedence over everything except interventions to address life-threatening conditions. Ration patient care supplies, such as oxygen and intravenous fluids, and use battery-powered equipment to monitor the patient intermittently to conserve battery life. Mental and emotional preparation for an unfavorable patient outcome is also important, particularly if rescue is delayed.

Survival Equipment

Survival equipment should be carried on all air medical aircraft and on ground transport vehicles that operate in remote or severe weather settings. The specifics of the service area, climate, type of aircraft or vehicle, and time of year should all be considered in selection of survival equipment and supplies. The survival kit should be assembled and stored in a manner that affords easy access, ideally in the aircraft cabin. Transport team members should carry basic survival equipment on their persons, in case the aircraft survival kit is damaged or inaccessible. Box 9.3 lists recommended items to be included in personal and aircraft survival kits. Survival training should include hands-on use and practice of each item contained in the survival kit(s).

Summary

Safety should be the number-one priority of all transport services. Safety is a pervasive attitude that must be supported by all transport team members.

Just as transport team members must be safe, they must also be prepared to survive. The goal in a survival situation that involves a medical transport team and patient is to survive until a rescue can be accomplished.

This chapter has provided an overview of two important transport concepts. Every individual, whether nurse, paramedic, physician, respiratory therapist, EMT, pilot,

---

• BOX 9.3 Survival Kits

Basic Personal Survival Equipment (Minimum Recommended List)

Flashlight or headlamp
Water bottle
Knife
Nylon cord
Plastic whistle
Sunglasses
Waterproof matches in match safe or other reliable method of fire starting
Space blanket or large heavy-duty plastic trash bag
Compass
Energy bars

Basic Aircraft Survival Kit

Flashlight or headlamp
Water-purification tablets or water filter
Plastic whistle
Water container
Waterproof matches in match safe
Nylon cord or rope
Second reliable method of fire starting (metal match, etc.)
Space blankets or large heavy-duty plastic trash bags
Dry tinder (cotton balls/petroleum jelly)
Aluminum foil
Candle
Knife

Signal mirror
Compass
Signal flares
Maps
Ax or saw
Insect repellant
Duct tape
Sunscreen
Pocket survival guide or card

Additional Aircraft Survival Kit Items (Depending on Operating Environment and Aircraft Type)

Tent
Appropriate additional clothing
Sleeping bags and pads
Tarps or plastic ponchos
Cook kit
Snowshoes
Stove
Snow shovel
Foodstuffs
Inflatable raft
Handheld global positioning system unit
Fishing kit
Strobe light
Canned smoke or smoke flares

mechanic, communication specialist, or administrator, must accept personal responsibility for safety and be a safety advocate.

References

1. Blumen I. (Editor in chief). *Principles and Direction of Air Medical Transport*. 2nd ed. Salt Lake City, UT: Air Medical Physicians Association; 2015.

2. Baker SP, Grabowski JG, Dodd RS, et al. EMS helicopter crashes: what influences fatal outcome? *Ann Emerg Med*. 2006;47(4): 351-355.

3. Coons J, Zalar C. 2015 Air medical safety survey. *Air Med J*. 2016;35(2016):120-125.

4. Association of Air Medical Services. Atlas and database of air medical services (13th ed.). http://www.adamsairmed.org/pubs/ADAMS_Intro.pdf; 2015 Accessed 23.08.16.

5. Blumen I. HEMS accidents: reasons, rates, risks and recommendations, presented at the Critical Care Transport Medicine Conference Las Vegas. 2006.

6. Frazer R. Air medical accidents: a 20-year search for information. *Air Med J*. 1999;8(5):33.

7. Frazer R. Air medical accidents involving collision with objects. *Air Med J*. 2001;20(3):13.

8. Frazer R. Weather accidents and the air medical industry. *Air Med J*. 2000;6(6):49.

9. Aerossurance. *US HEMS Accident Rates 2006-2015*. http://aerossurance.com/category/air-accidents-incidents/; 2016 Accessed 23.08.16.

10. Air and Surface Transport Nurses Association. *Transport Nurse Safety in the Transport Environment*. http://c.ymcdn.com/sites/astna.org/resource/collection/4392B20B-D0DB-4E76-959C-6989214920E9/Transport_Nurse_Safety_in_the_Transport_Environment.pdf; 2011 Accessed 10.07.16.

11. Allen R, Cooper J. 776. Helicopter rescue and aeromedical transport. In: Auerbach IP, ed. *Wilderness Medicine*. 6th ed. Philadelphia: Elsevier Mosby; 2012:753-777.

12. Bowman WD, Kummerfeldt P. Essentials of wilderness survival. In: Auerbach P, ed. *Wilderness Medicine*. 6th ed. Philadelphia: Elsevier Mosby; 2012:777-804.

13. Clark J. Up all night. *Air Med J*. 2014;33(2):58-60.

14. Concern Network. http://www.concern-network.org/; 2017; Accessed March 18, 2017.

15. Commission on Accreditation of Medical Transport Services. *Accreditation Standards*. 10th ed. Sandy Springs, SC: CAMTS; 2015.

16. Cooper D. ed. *Fundamentals of Search and Rescue*. Sudbury, MA: Jones & Bartlett Publishers; 2005.

17. COSPAS-SARSAT. Farewell to 121.5 MHz. *COSPAS-SARSAT Bulletin*. 21. https://www.cospas-sarsat.int/images/stories/SystemDocs/Current/Bul%2021ENG_%2010Feb2009_small.pdf; 2009 Accessed 23.08.16.

18. Craighead FC, Craighead JJ. *How to Survive on Land and Sea*. 4th ed. Annapolis, MD: Naval Institute Press; 1984.

19. Crowley JS, Licina JR, Bruckart JE. Flight helmets: how they work and why you should wear one. *J Air Med Transport*. 1992;11(8):19.

20. Department of the Army. *Survival*, FM 3–05.70. Washington, DC: US Government Printing Office; 2002.

21. Drew K. Should a pregnant flight nurse be allowed to fly? *J Air Med Transport*. 1991;10(7):11.

22. Emergency Nurses Association and Air and Surface Transport Nurses Association. Joint consensus statement on "Helicopter Shopping." http://c.ymcdn.com/sites/astna.org/resource/collection/4392B20B-D0DB-4E76-959C-6989214920E9/2016_Joint_Consensus_Statement_on_Helicopter_Shopping.pdf; 2016 Accessed 10.07.16.

23. FEMA Emergency Management Institute. *IS-100 Introduction to Incident Command System*. Washington, DC. Available at https://training.fema.gov/emi.aspx; 2013 Accessed 10.07.16.

24. Hawkins M. Personal protective equipment in helicopter EMS. *Air Med J*. 1994;13(4):1123.

25. Holleran RS. Prehospital safety. In: Holleran RS, ed. *Prehospital Nursing: A Collaborative Approach*. St. Louis, MO: Mosby; 1994.

26. Hon H, Wojda T, Barry N, Macbean B, Anagnestakos J, Evans D, Thomas P, Stawicki S. Injury and fatality risks in aeromedical transport: focus on prevention. *J Surg Res*. 2016;204:297-303.

27. International Association of Flight Paramedics. *Position Paper on Helicopter Shopping*. Snellville, GA: IAFP; 2006.

28. Isakov AP. Souls on board: helicopter emergency medical services and safety. *Ann Emerg Med*. 2006;47(3):357-360.

29. Krebs MB, Guohua L, Baker SP. Factors related to pilot survival in helicopter commuter and air taxi crashes. *Aviation Space Environ Med*. 1995;66(2):99-103.

30. MacDonald E. Dumb down for safety. *Air Med Saf*. 2008; 27(6):273-275.

31. Mains R. Air medical resources management: Our last line of defense. *Air Med J*. 2015;34(2):79-81.

32. National Highway Traffic Safety Administration and Ground Ambulance Crashes. http://www.ems.gov/pdf/GroundAmbulanceCrashesPresentation.pdf; 2014 Accessed 10.07.16.

33. Nix S, Brunette S. Rest, Shift Duration, and Air Medical Crewmember Fatigue. *Air Med J*. 2015;34(5):289-291.

34. Model Minimum Uniform Crash Criteria. http://www.mmucc.us/; 2016 Accessed 10.07.16.

35. NOAA and National Weather Service. Aviation weather Testbed. http://new.aviationweather.gov/hems; 2016 Accessed 10.07.16.

36. Springer B. The IFR bullet: can it kill our accident rate? *Air Med J*. 2005;24(1):29-31.

37. National EMS Pilots Association November. *Helicopter Emergency Medical Services (HEMS) NVG Utilization Survey*, 2008. Available at http://www.nemspa.org; 2008. Accessed March 18, 2017.

38. National Flight Nurses Association. *Improving Flight Nurse Safety in the Air Medical Helicopter Environment*. Park Ridge, IL: NFNA; 1998.

39. Ryan T, Studebaker B, Brennan G. Patient impression of the use of helmets by HEMS personnel [abstract]. *J Air Med Transport*. 1992;11(10):65.

40. Wraa CE, O'Malley JO. Flight nurse physical requirements. *J Air Med Transport*. 1992;11(10):17.

41. Wolfe K, Reidy M, Robinson J. A crash experience proves need for personal rescue packs. *Air Med J*. 1994;13(10):429.

42. Mayberry RT. Medical air crew roles and responsibilities during aircraft emergencies. *Aero Med J*. 1988;3(4):16.

10

Patient Assessment

DENISE TREADWELL, CAROL RHOADES, AND RENEÈ SEMONIN HOLLERAN

COMPETENCIES

1. Obtain initial, focused, and comprehensive subjective and objective data through history taking, physical examination, and the review of records, pertinent laboratory values, and radiographic and other diagnostic studies.
2. Effectively communicate with the patient, bystanders, prehospital providers, referring personnel, and other health care providers.
3. Recognize and anticipate critical signs and symptoms related to the patient's illness or injury.
4. Perform critical patient interventions as indicated by the patient's illness or injury.
5. Anticipate potential situations that may arise associated with the patient's condition during the transport and prepare interventions accordingly.
6. Identify operations specific to air or ground transport that may impact the delivery of care and the safety of the patient and team.
7. Prepare the patient for transport via ground or rotor-wing or fixed-wing vehicle.
8. Identify and prepare for issues related to international transport.

The transport process begins with the identification of the need to transfer a patient. This step is usually initiated by members of the referring agency, such as prehospital care providers or health care providers in the transferring hospital.

Clear communication about the need for transport, the care the patient has already received, what will be needed from the transport team, and the specialty care available at the receiving facility should all be considered part of preparation for transport. This communication is initiated by the referring facility/agency, is confirmed and updated on transport team arrival, is included in the handoff report at the receiving facility, and concludes with providing patient follow-up information to the referring agency after the completion of the transport.[1-5]

Patient assessment provides the transport team with an opportunity to identify problems and interventions needed before transport. It also allows the transport team to anticipate and prepare for events that may occur during transport.

Patient assessment and preparation for transport are composed of multiple elements including primary and secondary assessment; prioritization and performance of critical interventions; anticipation and preparation of potential changes in the patient's condition that may occur during the transport; and treatment of specific problems, such as pain management.

The complex nature of the transport environment may not always permit the completion of a full patient assessment and all preparatory steps (Fig 10.1). The transport team must be familiar with all the components of a complete patient assessment and necessary preparation so that they can make appropriate decisions and perform the appropriate interventions for a safe and successful patient transport. Findings identified during the patient assessment may also be useful in determining the most appropriate receiving facility.[1-5]

Indications for Patient Transport

Currently, there exists no universal agreement regarding the indications for interfacility transport, specialty critical care transport, or air medical transport. Numerous research studies have identified reasons to transfer patients, and national organizations have suggested indications for air medical transport, particularly rotor-wing transport.[5-20] The need to transport a patient may be because of the lack of availability of necessary resources at the treating facility, availability of higher-level care with improved outcomes at other facilities, or the desire to move the patient to facilities closer to home or support systems for continued care. Identifying the need to transfer a patient, and determining the most appropriate mode of transport, is based on several factors, including the following:
- The severity of the patient's illness or injury
- Transport time, distance, terrain, and weather
- The need for nursing and medical expertise, diagnostic procedures, or other specialty services not available at the referring health care facility
- A request by the patient's family that the patient be transferred to another facility[21-24]

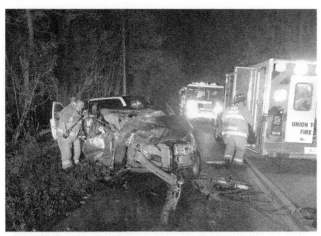

• **Fig. 10.1** Primary and secondary assessments can be difficult to perform depending on patient location. (Courtesy Air Care and Mobile Care, University of Cincinnati.)

Trauma Patient

Numerous guidelines for the air and surface medical transport of trauma patients are available. Air medical transport of trauma patients is a commonly accepted practice, probably because of the history of using helicopters to transport injured patients from the battlefield, and their subsequent use to transport trauma patients in the civilian population (see Chapter 1). In 2012 the Air Medical Physician Association (AMPA), the American College of Emergency Physicians (ACEP), the National Association of Emergency Medical Service Physicians, and the American Academy of Emergency Medicine published a joint position paper detailing guidelines for air medical transport.[4] Scoring systems have also been used to determine indications for patient transport. Some examples of these scoring systems are the revised trauma score; the trauma triage rule; the Glasgow Coma Score (GCS); the Glasgow Motor Score (score greater than 5); the Full Outline of UnResponsiveness score (FOUR Score); the Acute Physiology and Chronic Health Evaluation (APACHE) I, II, and III; the Prognostic Index; the Acute Trauma Index; and the vehicular trauma checklist.

The American College of Surgeons (ACS)[9,10,25,26] includes recommendations for the transfer of injured patients in both their Advanced Trauma Life Support course and their "Resources for the Optimal Care of the Injured Patient." In addition, the ACS recommends that the trauma patient should no longer be transferred to the closest hospital but to the closest appropriate hospital, preferably a verified trauma center.[9,10] Some of the recommendations of the ACS are listed in Box 10.1.

Patients with Cardiovascular, Cerebrovascular, and Medical Emergencies

Most of the earlier research related to the indications for transport involved trauma patients. Improved outcomes demonstrated by care provided in facilities specializing in stroke or cardiac care, such as primary stroke centers,

---

• **BOX 10.1** **American College of Surgeons Criteria for Consideration of Transfer from Level III Centers to Level I or II Centers**

1. Carotid or vertebral arterial injury
2. Torn thoracic aorta or great vessel
3. Cardiac rupture
4. Bilateral pulmonary contusion with PaO_2 to FiO_2 ratio less than 200
5. Major abdominal vascular injury
6. Grade IV or V liver injuries that necessitate >6 units of RBCs transfusion in 6 h
7. Unstable pelvic fracture that necessitates >6 units of RBCs transfusion in 6 h
8. Fracture or dislocation with loss of distal pulses
9. Penetrating injury or open fracture of the skull
10. Glasgow Coma Scale score <14 or lateralizing neurologic signs
11. Spinal fracture or spinal cord deficit
12. Complex pelvis/acetabulum factures
13. More than two unilateral rib fractures or bilateral rib fractures with pulmonary contusion (if no critical care consultation is available).
14. Significant torso injury with advanced comorbid disease (such as coronary artery disease, chronic obstructive pulmonary disease)

FiO₂, Fractional concentration of oxygen in inspired gas; *PaO₂*, partial pressure of oxygen in arterial blood; *RBC,* red blood cells.
Note: An injured patient may undergo operative control of ongoing hemorrhage before transfer if a qualified surgeon and operating room resources are promptly available at the referring hospital.
From American College of Surgeons. *Resources for Optimal Care of the Injured Patient.* Dallas, TX: American College of Surgeons; 2014.

---

comprehensive stroke centers, or regional cardiac centers, has prompted similar practices promoting timely transport of cerebrovascularly injured patients and cardiac patients to centers of excellence.[5,11,27] Assessment and determination of transport to a specialty facility bypassing local medical centers begins at the point of contact with Emergency Medical Service (EMS). Stroke protocols have been established jointly by the American Heart Association (AHA) and the American Stroke Association to minimize brain injury and to maximize the patient's recovery by rapidly identifying signs and symptoms of a stroke and transporting the patient immediately to specialized care. For cardiovascular patients, the American College of Cardiology and the AHA have developed parallel guidelines in support of rapid transport of patients suffering from acute coronary syndromes or other cardiac event to regional cardiac centers for more definitive care. Indications recognized for interfacility transfer of cardiac patients include the need for cardiac critical care that is not available at the referring facility, cardiac catheterization (such as percutaneous coronary intervention, which is also called cardiac catheterization), insertion of a balloon pump, mechanical assistance devices, experimental medications, and organ transplant.[28-30] Research and case reports have shown that patients with cardiovascular emergencies tolerate the transport process well and have benefited from it.[31-33] For other nontrauma cases, indications for interfacility

• BOX 10.2   Medical Classification Criteria Tool

Code Blue: Cardiopulmonary Arrest (Nontraumatic Source)

Class I: Life-Threatening Illness or Unstable Vital Signs

A. Unstable airway

Acute respiratory distress (i.e., acute pulmonary edema, unconscious patient, patient needs recent intubation)

B. Patient needs ventilatory support (oxygen saturation, <80% via pulse oximetry)

C. Circulatory instability

Clinical signs and symptoms of shock

Symptomatic hypotension, <90 mm Hg systolic

Symptomatic hypertension, >200 mm Hg systolic or >110 mm Hg diastolic

Unstable or symptomatic cardiac rhythms

Uncontrolled chest pain

Status post arrest

Therapies to include but not limited to the following:
- Transvenous pacer
- Intraaortic balloon pump
- External pacer
- Vasopressor administration

D. GCS, <8 (i.e., acute mental status changes, status epilepticus)

Class II: Potentially Life-Threatening Illness, but Vital Signs Currently Stable

A. Controlled pulmonary disease

B. Controlled or decreasing chest pain

C. Controlled acute cardiac dysrhythmias

D. Status post new-onset seizures

E. Vascular disorders

F. Thrombolytic therapy

G. Previously class I case that has been stabilized with treatment

H. GCS, 9–12

Class III: No Obvious Life-Threatening Illness and Vital Signs Stable

GCS, Glasgow Coma Scale.

From Loos L, Runyan L, Pelch D. Development of prehospital medical classification criteria. *Air Med. J.* 1988;17(1):14.

---

transfers are generally specific to the limited availability of specialty care and advanced equipment needed for the patient's condition at the referring facility.[5-7,34,35]

Loos et al.[36] developed a Medical Classification Criteria Tool modeled on trauma classification tools to assist in determining the severity of illness and what resources may be needed for appropriate transport. The advantages of this tool include enhancement of communication between the referring and receiving facility and advanced notification of the severity of the patient's illness so that the receiving facility can be appropriately prepared. This tool can also be used to monitor the appropriateness of medical transfers (Box 10.2).

The appropriateness of interfacility patient transfer is measured by comparing the benefits of the transfer with the patient and the risks. The APACHE, the Simplified Acute Physiology Score, and the mortality predication models scores are often used in the critical care setting as a predictor of the patient's mortality.[13,20,30,37-41]

Pregnant Women and Neonates

Other patients who may need transfer and transport include pregnant women and neonatal patients. The transport of these patients requires specially trained and specially equipped medical teams.[2-4,6,12,17,37] Indications for the transport of pregnant women include obstetric-related bleeding, hypertensive disorders of pregnancy, multiple gestation, fetal anomalies, preterm premature rupture of membranes, preterm labor, and medical–surgical conditions including trauma. Transfer is most commonly related to the need for neonatal tertiary care because it is preferable to transport the undelivered patient over neonatal transport. Indications for the transport of neonates include the age and weight of the infant and neonatal illness and injury that cannot be appropriately cared for at

the referring facility.[11,23] Teams must be able to monitor for maternal and fetal distress and have additional training and experience to manage those conditions during the transport. The care of these patients is discussed in more detail in Chapters 28 and 29.

Appropriate Patient Transfer

In 1986, Congress enacted the Emergency Medical Treatment and Labor Act (EMTALA) as a part of the Consolidated Omnibus Reconciliation Act (COBRA). This legislation, coupled with the 1990 Omnibus Reconciliation Act amendments to COBRA, furnishes guidelines, regulations, and penalties that govern patient transfer and transport. The implications of this law and its recent revisions are discussed in Chapter 32.[42]

With the transport of an ill or injured patient, transport services should provide (1) a transport team with the experience necessary to perform an initial assessment and stabilize the patient's condition before and during transport, (2) staff who can use the equipment and technology necessary to deliver care during transport to specific groups of patients, and (3) the ability to demonstrate that the transport will make a difference in patient outcome.[43]

The ACEP has developed guidelines for appropriate transfer and transport of ill or injured patients. These guidelines are summarized in Box 10.3. In addition, the American College of Critical Care Medicine has proposed its own recommendations for the transport of critically ill or injured patients. Box 10.4 contains a summary of these guidelines, which address both interhospital and intrahospital transport of patients. For more information and recommendations from AMPA for air medical transport in acute coronary syndromes and acute stroke syndromes, please visit www.ampa.org.

• BOX 10.3 American College of Emergency Physicians Guidelines for Transfer and Transport From Emergency Department to Another Facility

1. The optimal health and well-being of the patient should be the principal goal of patient transfer.
2. Emergency physicians and hospital personnel should abide by applicable laws regarding patient transfer. All patients should be provided an MSE and stabilizing treatment within the capacity of the facility before transfer. If a competent patient requests transfer before the completion of the MSE and stabilizing treatment, these should be offered to the patient and documented.
3. The transferring facility is responsible for informing the patient or responsible party of the risks and the benefits of transfer and documenting these. Before transfer, patient consent should be obtained and documented whenever possible.
4. The medical facility's policies and procedures and/or medical staff bylaws should identify the individuals responsible for and qualified to perform MSEs. The policies and procedures or bylaws must define who is responsible for accepting and transferring patients on behalf of the hospital. The examining physician at the transferring hospital will use his or her best judgment regarding the condition of the patient when determining the timing of transfer,

mode of transportation, level of care provided during transfer, and destination of the patient.
5. Payment for transport should not be retrospectively denied by insurance companies.
6. Agreement to accept the patient in transfer should be obtained from a physician or responsible individual at the receiving hospital in advance of transfer. When a patient requires a higher level of care other than that provided or available at the transferring facility, a receiving facility with the capability and capacity to provide a higher level of care may not refuse any request for transfer.
6. All pertinent records and copies of imaging studies should accompany the patient to the receiving facility or be electronically transferred as soon as is practical.
7. When transfer of patients is part of a regional plan to provide optimal care at a specialized medical facility, written transfer protocols and interfacility agreements should be in place.

MSE, Medical screening examination.
From American College of Emergency Physicians. *Appropriate Interhospital Patient Transfer.* Dallas, TX: American College of Emergency Physicians; 2016.

• BOX 10.4 Summary of American College of Critical Care Medicine Guidelines for the Transport of the Critically Ill or Injured Patient

1. The benefits of transferring the patient should outweigh the risks.
2. The practitioner needs to be aware of the legal implications of patient transfer and transport.
3. Before the patient is transported, physicians and nurses at the referring and receiving facilities should be in contact, a decision should be made about the mode of transportation to be used, and a copy of all medical records relevant to the patient's care should be secured.
4. Accompanying transport personnel should include a minimum of two patient care providers and a vehicle operator. At least one care provider should be a registered nurse.
5. The equipment (including monitors) and medications necessary to manage the patient's airway, breathing, and circulation

should be available. Communication equipment used during transport should also be available.
6. Continuous monitoring should take place during transport. At a minimum, ECG monitoring and monitoring of vital signs are required. Patients with specific problems may require additional monitoring, such as capnography and invasive monitoring.

ECG, Electrocardiogram.
Modified from the *Guidelines Committee of the American College of Critical Care Medicine Society of Critical Care Medicine and the Transfer Guidelines Task Force of the American Association of Critical Care Nurses.* Guidelines for the transport of the critically ill patient. <http://www.sccm.org>; 2004 Accessed 08.06.30.

The Emergency Nurses Association (ENA) developed a document in 1995, which was subsequently revised and updated in July 2015, that provides guidelines for the transport of ill or injured children. Unlike the documents previously mentioned, this document specifically addresses the needs of the ill or injured child. These guidelines are available from the ENA.[18]

Decision to Transport

Several factors must be considered by referring personnel when they decide to transport a patient. The first factor is the appropriateness of transport, as discussed previously. Identification of a suitable receiving facility is the second

factor that must be considered. When choosing a receiving facility, referring personnel must look at the resources available at the receiving facility, such as specialized care staff, equipment, bed availability, and expertise. Preplanning is an important step in any patient transfer. The existence of written policies and transfer agreements between receiving and referring agencies can speed up the transfer process and save time when it is the most precious. The location and accessibility of the receiving facility is also an important consideration. Those responsible for making the decision to transfer a patient should also consider the safety of the transport. Transport safety and the risks posed by "helicopter shopping," are discussed in Chapter 9.

Communication

Communication is probably one of the most important components in the preparation of the patient for transport. Communication center operations are discussed in Chapter 6. This discussion focuses on the communication process among personnel at the referring agency, including prehospital or health care facility and the receiving facility.

Communication begins before the transport team arrival. The initial communication may be made physician to physician, directly to the transport communication center, or via EMS dispatch centers. The transport communication center should have a written guideline regarding what information is required before launching a team. This information may include patient age, reason for transport, requested mode of transport, receiving facility and accepting physician, specialty equipment needed (such as balloon pump, pacer, and ventilator), patient weight, and whether family are requesting to travel with the patient. Referring personnel should follow their own guidelines of triage and transport and should align with EMTALA requirements. Transport teams can improve speed, efficiency, and safety with health care facilities through education regarding preparing a patient for transport, landing zone safety, and team capabilities.

When initial contact has been made by the referring agency, information that should be provided to the transport team includes the patient's chief symptom, the indications for transport, and the patient's current condition. The report should also include interventions already performed and their effects as well as measures that need to be taken to decrease the risks of deterioration during transport. There should be direct communication between the physician treating the patient and the accepting physician. The reason for the patient transfer, the treating physician's name and contact information, the accepting physician's name, bed assignment at the receiving facility, and all other pertinent contacts at both the referring and accepting facilities should be clearly identified and documented. Some transport programs require signed documentation by the treating or accepting physician to certify the need for transport before they transfer the patient because of recent reimbursement issues, particularly from Medicare.

When possible, there should be direct communication between the physician treating the patient and the accepting physician. Some communication centers can assist in finding an accepting physician if none has been identified and facilitate that connection. The reason for the patient transfer, the treating physician's name and contact information, the accepting physician's name, receiving hospital name and city, and all other pertinent contacts at both the referring and accepting facility, when available, should be clearly identified and documented. Physicians may accept a patient without knowing what the bed situation is at the hospital; thus a bed control, supervisor, or other hospital resource should be contacted and bed assignment verified. Some transport programs require signed documentation by the treating or accepting physician to certify the need for transport before they transfer the patient because of recent reimbursement issues, particularly from Medicare. The patient's diagnosis, age, and location must be identified so that an appropriately trained team is dispatched, and specialty members and equipment added before departure. Examples include patients with extracorporeal membrane oxygenation (ECMO), patients on an intraaortic balloon pump, neonates, maternal patients, and pediatric transports.[44] Critical care specialty transport teams and respiratory therapists may also be added to, or are part of, a regularly scheduled team. Teams must have at least enough information to determine whether additional equipment needs to be added. If not, crew members with knowledge of how to manage the equipment need to be added.

When the transport team arrives at the patient location, the team should identify the lead medical provider and ask if there are any immediate concerns. A report from the medical team at the referring facility or scene is obtained and should include the history of events, initial physical and diagnostic assessment, interventions provided, response to treatment, and concerns or outstanding needs identified. A structured handoff report can prove beneficial in capturing pertinent information in a potentially chaotic environment. Handoffs in patient care are a high-risk activity, providing opportunities for critical information to be lost or misunderstood.[21,45-47]

The transport team should be cognizant of how their interactions with referring personnel may be interpreted. The referring team is often invested in the care of the patient and may take offense at what they perceive as the transport team taking over and not communicating with them. Communicating directly, providing eye contact, asking for their input and concerns, and thanking them for the work they put in to prepare the patient for transport can go a long way in establishing a professional and respectful interaction.

Before departure from the referring location, any laboratory, radiographic, and diagnostic findings should be copied and sent with the patient. Radiographic and diagnostic study results may be transmitted electronically or by means of telemedicine before the patient leaves the receiving facility. If the patient has any valuables, then they must be accounted for. Valuables are sometimes easier left with a family member, whenever possible. Documenting what was transported with the patient and to whom it was given at the receiving facility is necessary to establish a chain of custody. Many hospitals require signed documentation of any valuables by both the transport team and the receiving personnel. Clothing or other valuables are sometimes considered evidence and should be treated as such based on evidence protocols.

Consent

Patients must consent to treatment and transfer after they have been informed of the risks and benefits involved.

Written or verbal consent for transport and for emergency treatment is not always possible to obtain directly from the patient or family. Consent for transport may be implied, particularly in the prehospital setting. Implied consent is granted in an emergency, when the patient is incapacitated and in a life-threatening situation and no family is available to provide consent.[14,48]

Although the patient's consent is implied, the transport team should always explain to the patient and available family members all procedures and the transport process. If family members are available, they may be able to provide consent for treatment. If consent forms are part of the transport documentation, the transport team should ensure that they are completed and transported with the patient. On interfacility transfers, the team may elect to leave a copy of the consent with the referring facility.

A Twenty-First-Century Patient Transport Challenge

During the last few years, the closing of rural and community hospitals, the decrease in nursing and other health care providers, the need to recognize critical access hospitals, and the lack of funds to provide health care has made the inter-hospital transfers of patients from rural and community hospitals to other facilities routine.[40,49,50] Many facilities that in the past accepted patients without question have now adopted diversion policies usually specific to select patient populations or acuity, which means a decrease in available beds, longer waits for transfer, longer transfer distances, refusal of some patients, transport of patients that were not typically transported in the past (psychiatric, ortho, etc.), and diversion. The ACEP has developed "Guidelines for Ambulance Diversion"[51] (Box 10.5).

Transport programs need to ensure that the patient is eligible for transfer based on the condition and capabilities of both the transferring and receiving facilities, has been

accepted at the receiving facility, and has a confirmed bed assignment and an accepting physician. Diversion notification should also include all services that provide patient transport to prevent any undue delay in patient transfer and transport.

Patient Assessment

Primary and secondary assessment, identification of patient problems, and initiation of critical interventions provide a framework for preparing a patient for transport. Each of these tasks must be performed in an organized, rapid, and complete manner. Patient assessment is a continuous process that occurs before, during, and after transport.

Prehospital Assessment

Assessment of the patient begins with assessment of the scene and whether the transport team responds directly to the patient or to another facility. The transport team should assess the surrounding environment for hazards, the number of patients present, and any clues to what has happened (number of vehicles, type of damage, etc.). Box 10.6 contains a summary of some of the hazards that may be encountered.[15]

On arrival at the referring facility, the transport team should survey the resources that are available to assist in preparing the patient for transport. In many cases the transport team brings a higher level of care on arrival to small or rural facilities. Equipment and supplies necessary for patient

---

• BOX 10.5   Guidelines for Ambulance Diversion

- Identify situations in which hospital resources are not available and temporary diversion is necessary.
- Notify EMS systems personnel and providers (out of hospital and hospital) of such occurrences.
- Provide for the safe, appropriate, and timely care of patients who continue to enter the EMS system during periods of diversion.
- Notify EMS systems personnel and providers (out of hospital and hospital) immediately when the situation that caused the diversion has been resolved.
- Explore solutions that address the causes of diversion and implement policies that minimize the need for diversions.
- Provide for the periodic review of policies and guidelines governing diversion.

EMS, Emergency Medical Service.
Modified from Brennan J. *Guidelines for Ambulance Diversion*. Irving, TX: American College of Emergency Physicians; 2012.

• BOX 10.6   Potential Environmental Hazards

Hazards at the Scene

Wires
Uneven ground
Vehicles
Accident itself
People
Signs
Light poles
Water
Loose debris
Hazardous materials (HAZMAT)
EMS rescue apparatus
Fire
Smoke
Weather hazards
Heavy machines or construction equipment
Unmanned aircraft
Lasers

Hazards at the Referring Facility

Buildings
People
Wires
Construction equipment
Shovels or other items used to clean landing zone area

EMS, Emergency Medical Service.

stabilization may be limited; thus the team may need to bring additional equipment.

The principles of patient assessment used by the transport team are no different than those used when patients are assessed within the walls of a hospital. However, the prehospital environment dictates that the assessment be organized, direct, and rapid. Adaptation and flexibility are necessary when patient assessment is performed outside the hospital. Confined spaces and lack of light, noise, and equipment that may or may not be functioning can present challenges to patient assessment in the prehospital care environment.[15]

Scene Assessment[15,26]

Initial assessment always begins with an evaluation of the area in which the aircraft or ambulance will be staged (i.e., on scene or at a facility). This is particularly important when in a helicopter, where hazards exist within the landing zone radius, debris may be present that can fly up in the rotor wash, and people on the ground can be unpredictable. The transport team should assess the surrounding environment for potential hazards. Box 10.6 contains a summary of some of the hazards that may be encountered. Refer to Chapter 9 for details about safety precautions and landing zone safety.

On arrival at the referring facility, the transport team should evaluate the available resources to assist in preparing the patient for transport. Equipment and supplies necessary for patient stabilization may have limited availability; thus the team should be independently supplied with the tools and knowledge to administer life-sustaining care until delivery to definitive care.

The principles of patient assessment used by the transport team are no different than those used when patients are assessed within the walls of a hospital. However, the prehospital environment dictates that the assessment be organized, direct, and rapid. Adaptation and flexibility are necessary when patient assessment is performed. Clinics and smaller hospitals may be limited in their diagnostic capabilities and resources. In the prehospital setting, confined space, lack of light, noise, hostile environment (such as weather extremes), and limited diagnostic equipment can present challenges to a thorough patient assessment.

History

Patient assessment begins with obtaining a history. The history of the events surrounding illness or injury, as well as comorbidities that may affect the condition, provides a guide for critical interventions and clinical decision making, raises the level of suspicion for occult issues, and helps in preparing the patient for transport. The history may also inform and prepare the transport team of the need for ongoing assessment and possible interventions related to the sequela associated with an illness or injury. For example, the history of a patient who has multiple rib fractures alerts the transport team to the potential of developing a tension pneumothorax or worsening oxygenation caused by pulmonary contusions.

Although the transport team may be given some patient information before arrival or while en route to the patient, it is often limited and can devolve before arrival. The team should be prepared to revise initial perceptions and course of action after their assessment.

General Principles of History Gathering

The transport team should keep in mind that the history provides the basis for everything that occurs afterward. It will guide treatment and transport decisions and can alert transport team members to potential problems that may develop during the transport. Henry and Stapleton stated,[53] "history is the patient's story of significant events related to and surrounding the present problem." It is important to follow an organized pattern when gathering a patient history.

The first step is to establish the patient's chief symptom or problem. If the patient is unable to provide this information, the transport team may obtain it from others at the scene (prehospital care providers, police, or bystanders), referring personnel (nurses or physicians), or any persons who may be with the patient. A survey of the scene by the transport team can also provide valuable information about what may have happened. Information about the mechanism of injury (MOI), such as vehicle damage or the height of a fall, can suggest possible injuries. If the patient is unconscious, the transport team should look for medical alert jewelry, syringes, medications, pill bottles, or information in the patient's wallet or purse.[15]

The history then progresses on to the history of the present illness or injury, a review of the pertinent body systems, and their general medical history. A common mnemonic used to collect history information is SAMPLE:

S: Signs and symptoms reported
A: Allergies, alcohol, or substance abuse
M: Medications, including immunizations, particularly in a pediatric history[54]
P: Past medical history, including illnesses and injuries
L: Last meal or intake
E: Events that led to the emergency and everything that has been done before the arrival of the transport team

If the patient's chief symptom or problem is related to pain, the PQRST method can be used to collect information for the history. PQRS[53,55-60]:

P: Provoking factors: What caused or causes the pain? Does anything relieve the pain or make it worse? What was the patient doing when the pain began?
Q: Quality of the pain: Some of the words used to describe the pain may provide the transport team member with clues to the origin of the pain. For example, patients who describe chest pain often use words such as "burning" or "crushing."

R: Region and radiation: The patient should be asked to point to the area in which the pain is felt. Pain patterns can provide the transport team with clues to the cause of the patient's pain and may help guide the management of the patient's pain.

S: Severity: A rating scale from 0 to 10 can be used to describe the severity of the pain.

T: Time: Determine the time of onset, the duration of the pain, if the pain has been constant or fluctuating, and/or what time of day it began.

As much information as possible should be collected and communicated with the receiving facility, particularly when the patient is transported from a referring facility. At other times, such as when patients are transported directly from the scene, information may not be as readily available. Obstacles such as the patient's inability to communicate because of their illness or injury, language barriers, the lack of witnesses to a particular event, or the absence of family members or significant others may limit the history information available.

Transport personnel should always assume that there are holes in the patient's history and that there may be potentially important pieces of information of which they are unaware. They may not be able to identify what these missing pieces are, but they should always have an awareness that in the chaos of a scene call or critical interfacility transport important pieces may be missing and always be on the lookout for new information.

The transport of a patient from a scene or health facility involves multiple transfers of patient care, also referred to as a patient pass-down or handoff. This has been identified as one of the highest risk aspects of emergency and critical care. It is very easy for important details about the patient's condition or other key bits of information to get lost in the chaos. It is important that the transport team follow an organized process for obtaining and subsequently relaying information. One simple step toward this is to write down as much as possible about the patient report.

Trauma History

Assessment of the traumatically injured patient includes gathering information on the MOI. Information on when, where, and how the patient was injured can guide the transport team in their assessment. A complete description of the event is often limited. However, a general idea of the MOI provides clues regarding additional injuries and complications associated with mode of injury. Box 10.7 describes predictable injuries that may occur because of motor vehicle crashes, which is an example of taking a trauma history.[15,47]

In recent years, instant photographs, video recorders, and digital cameras have been used to provide information about the MOI.[61] Rescuers must use caution when taking photographs of the scene and sharing these photos to prevent the violation of patient privacy laws or Health Insurance Portability and Accountability Act (HIPAA) regulations. Photographs should be of vehicles

---

> **• BOX 10.7** **Predictable Injuries that Result from Motor Vehicle Crashes**
>
> **Unrestrained Driver**
> Head injuries
> Facial injuries
> Fractured larynx
> Fractured sternum
> Cardiac contusion
> Lacerated liver or spleen
> Lacerated great vessels
> Fractured patella and femur
> Fractured clavicle
>
> **Restrained Driver**
> **Caused by a Lap Restraint**
> Pelvic injuries
> Spleen, liver, and pancreas injuries
>
> **Caused by a Shoulder Restraint**
> Cervical fractures
> Rupture of mitral valve or diaphragm
>
> Modified from McSwain NE, Frame S, Salomone J. *Basic and Advanced Prehospital Trauma Life Support.* 5th ed. St. Louis, MO: Mosby; 2003.

and property. Patient faces and deceased patients should generally not be photographed. Many transport services have strict HIPAA policies regarding disclosure of patient details, including the use of photographs and posting information and photos on social media outlets; therefore understanding of and strict adherence to company policies should be followed.

When obtaining the history of a trauma patient, the transport team should also gather information that describes the scene of the crash, particularly if they are first responders and there is no scene commander present. Did the collision involve multiple victims? Are all the victims accounted for? Were there fatalities? If the on-scene patients are unable to provide information about additional patients, the presence of schoolbooks, clothing, or toys may suggest that additional victims are present.[15]

For other types of traumatic injuries, information that should be obtained about the scene should include the height of a fall and the surface impacted, type and caliber of firearms (if known), size and type of a knife blade (again, if known), use of protective equipment such as helmets, and the size and weight of objects that may have fallen on or struck the patient.[21,47]

Diversity Assessment

Although the focus of patient care during the transport process is generally on critical needs, age, class, culture, beliefs, attitudes, customs, ethnicity, gender, nationality, race, religion, and sexual orientation influence response to illness and injury. The transport team must take into consideration these factors as well as the patient's concept of illness and health when providing care and respect and, when possible,

TABLE 10.1	Diversity Practice Model	
A	Assumption	What do we assume or take for granted about this individual or the community that they come from?
B	Beliefs or behaviors	How does my belief system affect the care I provide for this patient? Are my beliefs mirrored in the way I behave toward the patient? For example, will I view a patient who may not have bathed for a long period as homeless?
C	Communication	How does the patient communicate? Does the patient speak English? If not, is a translator available? Can the patient hear and/or see? Has the patient had an injury such as a stroke that impairs the ability to communicate or understand?
D	Diversity or identification of how the patient differs	Some diversity is visible, such as skin color, age, or ethnic background. Some is invisible, such as sexual orientation or class.
E	Education	Education involves learning about the patient's diversity
	Ethics	Ethical decisions are influenced by one's diversity

From *Emergency Nurses Association Diversity Task Force*. Approaching diversity: an interactive journey. https://www.ena.org/SiteCollection Documents/Position%20Statements/CulturalDiversity.pdf; 2012 Accessed 17.02.11.

adapt the care to include the impact of diversity on response to illness, injuries, and the need to be transported.[22]

Awareness and knowledge of all patient diversity is impossible. However, the transport process can be a little less stressful for the patient, the family, and the transport team when the multiple factors that influence a patient's response to illness and injury are not ignored.

In 1997, the ENA developed a diversity practice model that can assist in approaching patient diversity.[22] The components of this model are summarized in Table 10.1. The use of this model may offer some added patient care information and help providers recognize what makes us different and the same. Transport team members should become familiar with the patient populations they may interact with and learn about the special health care needs of these populations. This familiarity is often referred to as *cultural competence*.

Primary Assessment and Critical Interventions

The hands-on assessment of every patient begins with the primary assessment. This assessment may be done at the same time as the scene survey and obtaining the history. Primary assessment is a rapid assessment following the A-B-C-D-E mnemonic of the patient's airway, breathing, circulation, neurologic status (disability), and exposure of the patient to assess for all potential injuries. During the primary assessment, as patient problems are identified, critical interventions are initiated. The basic steps remain the same, whether at a scene or an interfacility transport. Recent guidelines recognized by the AHA stress the importance of recognizing signs of cardiac arrest in the cardiac patient and assessing the need for circulatory support before airway interventions by reordering of these priorities to circulation, airway, and breathing.[15,21,47]

Airway

The patient's airway is assessed to determine whether it is patent and maintainable. For any patient who may have a traumatic injury, cervical spine precautions should always be used while the airway is evaluated. Assessment of the patient's level of consciousness, in concert with assessment of the airway status, provides the transport team with an impression of the effectiveness of the patient's current airway status as well as potential for deterioration (Box 10.8).

If an airway problem is identified, the appropriate intervention should be initiated. The decision to use an intervention depends on the nature of the patient's problem and the potential for complications or deterioration during transport. Airway interventions are addressed in Chapter 11. Supplemental oxygen should be considered for all patients during transport. Generally hyperoxygenation is not indicated, except in preparation for intubation. Specific equipment, such as a pulse oximeter, CO_2 detector, or capnography, helps provide continuous airway evaluation during transport. The indications and the procedures for use of these devices are included in Chapter 12.

Pharmacologic Adjuncts for Airway Management Specific pharmacologic agents have been found to be useful in rapidly establishing an airway. These agents include those that provide sedation, amnesia, and neuromuscular blocking agents that facilitate intubation. An in-depth discussion of the use of these medications is provided in Chapter 11.

Neuromuscular blocking agents will eliminate a patient's ability to express pain or discomfort, and the transport team should always, with rare exception, provide sedation or analgesia in concert with the paralytic. The team should also

---

• BOX 10.8 Summary of Primary Airway Assessment

- Airway: Patent, maintainable, nonmaintainable
- Level of consciousness
- Skin appearance: Ashen, pale, gray, cyanotic, or mottled
- Preferred posture to maintain airway
- Airway clearance
- Sounds of obstruction

assess for signs of pain, such as elevated blood pressure (BP) and heart rate. Special care should be taken to ensure that the patient is positioned in a way that does not put pressure on extremities or pinch off circulation. Heat or cooling should be considered depending on environmental and patient condition.[46,65-67]

Breathing

The evaluation of breathing includes visual inspection of effort, rate, accessory muscle use, stridor, and equal rise and fall of the chest. Standing at the foot of the bed with the patient's chest exposed gives the best visual view of unequal chest rise. Palpation is useful in identifying subcutaneous air that may alert to the presence of a pneumothorax. A chest x-ray (CXR) will often not identify a pneumothorax, and subcutaneous air may be the first and only indication. Auscultation of the chest will identify adventitious breath sounds, absence of breath sounds, and equality across the lung fields. If the patient's breathing is compromised, intervention may be needed. The transport team must consider the immediacy of intervention and weigh it against complications and transport time. For example, if a chest tube is placed in a patient with severe chest trauma, they may require immediate blood transfusion for severe hemorrhage. Unless the team carries blood products, they may want to alert the trauma team to prepare for the procedure and transport rapidly. If the patient is apneic or in severe respiratory distress, immediate interventions are indicated. The transport team must identify the most likely cause of the compromise and proceed with the appropriate interventions. Emergent interventions may include basic life support (BLS) airway maneuvers, bag-mask ventilation, advanced airway management, and decompression of a suspected pneumothorax or insertion of a chest tube (Box 10.9). If a pneumothorax is suspected to be the cause of respiratory distress, a thoracostomy should be considered before intubation, because positive-pressure ventilation may push a simple pneumothorax into a tension pneumothorax. Ventilation interventions are discussed in Chapter 12.[46,62,63]

Circulation[1,8,9,47]

Active external bleeding should be quickly identified and controlled as a first step in circulatory assessment. Direct pressure should be applied immediately to accessible areas, such as the extremities. If this is unsuccessful in stopping the hemorrhage, one or two tourniquets should be applied above the bleeding site until no distal pulse can be palpated. For sites, such as joint junctions that are too high for a tourniquet, a hemostatic-type gauze can be successful in slowing or stopping the hemorrhage.

The transport team should observe the patient for indications of circulatory compromise. Skin color and temperature, diaphoresis, and capillary refill are appraised during circulatory assessment. Visual inspection of the skin detects paleness, mottling, diaphoresis, and distal discoloration that suggest hemorrhage or inadequacy of perfusion. Observation of the level of consciousness further evaluates the patient's cerebral perfusion (Box 10.10). Palpation of peripheral and central pulse for the presence of quality, rate, and bilateral equality should be assessed to both establish a baseline and identify perfusion competence. Delayed capillary refill identifies poor distal perfusion, whether from inadequate perfusion pressure or from hypothermia. Both central and distal color should be assessed and contrasted, looking for mottling, whiteness, or cyanosis and whether central, distal, or both. The temperature of the patient's skin, particularly cold and clammy, is another perfusion indicator and can be assessed along with the pulses.

Intravenous (IV) access is obtained for administration of fluid, blood, and medications. Depending on the patient's location and the accessibility of veins, peripheral, central, or intraosseous (IO) access may be used. Fluid resuscitation must be guided by the patient's response and should be administered with caution and consistent assessment in patients in hemorrhagic shock.

Disability: Neurologic Assessment[1,8,9,47]

Neurologic assessment includes assessment of the level of consciousness; the size, shape, and response of the pupil; and motor sensory function. The following simple method

---

• BOX 10.9 Summary of Primary Breathing Assessment

- Rate and depth of respirations
- Cyanosis
- Position of the trachea
- Presence of obvious injury or deformity
- Work of breathing
- Use of accessory muscles
- Flaring of nostrils
- Presence of bilateral breath sounds
- Presence of adventitious breath sounds
- Asymmetric chest movements
- Palpation of crepitus
- Integrity of chest wall
- Oxygen saturation measured with pulse oximetry

• BOX 10.10 Summary of Primary Circulation Assessment

- Pulse rate and quality
- Skin appearance: Color
- Peripheral pulses
- Skin temperature
- Level of consciousness
- Urinary output
- Blood pressure
- Cardiac monitor
- Invasive monitor

using the mnemonic AVPU may be used to evaluate the patient's level of consciousness:

A: Alert
V: Responds to verbal stimuli
P: Responds to painful stimuli
U: Unresponsive

Both the regular GCS and the pediatric GCS provide assessment of the patient's level of consciousness and motor function and serve as predictors of morbidity and mortality after brain injury.[1] The FOUR Score provides a more accurate assessment and prognosis of the intensive care or intubated patient's status in contrast to the GCS.[47]

If the patient has an altered mental status, the transport team needs to determine whether the patient has ingested any toxic substances, such as alcohol or other drugs, or may be hypoxic because of illness or injury. A patient with an altered mental status may pose a safety problem during transport. Use of chemical paralysis, sedation, or physical restraints may be necessary to ensure safe transport.[64]

Exposure[1,8,9,47]

With environmental conditions in mind, the body should be fully exposed for examination. Injury, rashes, bruising, and skin discoloration can be obscured by clothing, and important clues to underlying illness or injury can be missed. Although exposure for examination has been emphasized most frequently in the care of the trauma patient, it is equally important in the primary assessment of the patient with a medical illness to identify rashes, perfusion indicators, sources of infection, swelling/distention, and so forth. In addition, IV sites should be assessed for location, patency, and adequacy of securing for transport. Clothing can also hide bleeding that occurs because of thrombolytic therapy or rashes that may indicate potentially contagious conditions (Box 10.11).

Once patient assessment has been completed, the patient needs to be kept warm. Hypothermia can lead to cardiac arrhythmias, increased stress response, and hypoxia. Medications such as neuromuscular blocking agents interfere with the patient's ability to maintain a stable body temperature. If extended transport times are necessary, the team should reassess the patient's temperature during the transport.

Prevention of hypothermia should be considered a critical intervention, and methods to reduce heat loss should be initiated during the primary assessment. These interventions include the following[23,46,65-67]:

- Covering the patient with blankets or an insulated layer
- Limiting exposure when examinations are needed
- Preventing heat loss through conduction or convection by shielding the patient from the elements and out of the rotor wash, and away from metals, such as up against the aircraft doors, ambulance walls, or on a metal scoop stretcher
- Shielding the patient from wind and rotor wash
- Using warmed humidified oxygen and warmed IV fluids

Equipment Assessment

Although the concept of equipment assessment has not been routinely included in previous descriptions of primary assessment, it is an important step to ensure a safe transport. Before departure with the patient, the transport team should check that equipment, such as ventilators, pacers, infusions pumps, chest tube drainage systems, and so forth, are functioning correctly. All equipment should have airworthiness approval if transporting by rotor-wing or fixed-wing vehicle, or approved for transport outside of the hospital setting for ground transports. An adequate supply of oxygen should be calculated using patient demand, ventilator requirements, tank size, and transport time (including ground transitions) to ensure an adequate supply is available. The transport team should consider possible delays in transport in these calculations and factor in a buffer.

The transport team should be aware of the battery life of each piece of equipment in use and that backup batteries or a power source are available. For both oxygen and power requirements, the transitional phase of vehicle-to-handoff time should be considered.

Equipment secured to the patient, such as IVs, pacers, defibrillator patches, and ventilators, should be positioned and secured so they are accessible during transport and not easily disconnected or removed as patients are moved. Cervical collars should be appropriately sized, and the patient should be adequately secured and positioned so there are no pressure points. This assessment of equipment helps prevent complications during transport that could potentially leave the patient at risk of harm.[62]

Secondary Assessment

The ability to perform a secondary assessment is influenced by patient condition and transport time. If the illness or injury is time dependent, then the secondary assessment should occur during transport and not delay the departure from scene or bedside. However, space limitations, reduced lighting, and noise may interfere with the ability to perform a complete secondary assessment during transport.

Secondary assessment is done after the primary assessment is completed and involves a head-to-toe evaluation.[1,9,21,37,47] Patient data are collected by means of inspection, palpation,

---

• BOX 10.11 Summary of Exposure Assessment

- Appropriate tube placement: Endotracheal tubes, nasotracheal tubes, chest tubes, nasogastric or orogastric tubes, and urinary catheters
- Intravenous access: Peripheral, central, and intraosseous
- Identification of injury; active bleeding; indication of a serious illness such as presence of purpura

• BOX 10.12 Summary of Secondary Assessment

Skin

- Presence of petechiae, purpura, abrasions, bruises, scars, and birthmarks
- Rashes
- Abnormal skin turgor
- Signs of abuse and neglect

Head and Neck

- Presence of lacerations; contusions; raccoon eyes; Battle's sign; or drainage from the nose, mouth, and ears
- In the infant, examination of the anterior fontanel
- Gross visual examination
- Abnormal extraocular movements
- Position of the trachea
- Neck veins
- Swallowing difficulties
- Nuchal rigidity
- Presence of lymphadenopathy or neck masses

Eyes, Ears, and Nose

- Lack of tearing
- Sunken eyes
- Color of the sclera
- Drainage
- Gross assessment of hearing

Mouth and Throat

- Mucous membranes
- Breath odor
- Injuries to teeth

- Drooling
- Drainage

Thorax, Lungs, and Cardiovascular System

- Breath sounds
- Heart sounds

Abdomen

- Shape and size
- Bowel sounds
- Tenderness
- Firmness
- Masses (e.g., suprapubic mass)
- Femoral pulses
- Pelvic tenderness
- Color of drainage from nasogastric or orogastric tube

Genitourinary

- Blood at meatus
- Rectal bleeding
- Color of urine in catheter

Extremities and Back

- Gross motor and sensory function
- Peripheral pulses
- Lack of use of an extremity
- Deformity and angulation
- Wounds and abrasions
- Equipment is appropriately applied (e.g., traction splints)
- Vertebral column, flank, and buttock

---

and auscultation during secondary assessment. Whether the patient has had an injury or is critically ill, the evaluator should observe, touch, and listen to the patient.

Secondary assessment begins with an evaluation of the patient's general appearance. The transport team should observe the surrounding environment and evaluate its effects on the patient. Is the patient aware of the environment? Is there appropriate interaction between the patient and the environment?

Additional systems that should be assessed include the integumentary (color, presence of wounds, and temperature); head and neck (deformities, crepitus, and pain); eyes, ears, and nose (drainage); thorax and lungs (chest movement and heart and breath sounds); abdomen; genitourinary; and extremities and back (Box 10.12).

Pain Assessment

Determination of the amount of pain the patient has because of illness or injury is an important component of patient assessment. Physiologic indicators of pain include tachypnea, controlled respirations (splinting), tachycardia, hypotension, hypertension, nausea and vomiting, and diaphoresis. Behavioral indications of pain are crying, protective behavior, guarding, moaning, and self-focusing.

Baseline data are collected about the pain the patient has so that the effectiveness of pain management can be assessed during transport. Pain relief is one of the most important interventions for out-of-hospital patient care providers.[12,16,55,56,58,60]

Scoring Systems

Scoring systems were initially developed to identify patients who needed critical care that was not available at referring facilities,[8,9] such as patients who needed to be transported to a Level I trauma center. Scoring systems can be used in the field and for evaluation of patients who may need interfacility support. Scoring systems have routinely been used for the trauma patient, but are now used in the evaluation of critical patients, regardless of illness or injury. These systems include the Prehospital Index Score, CRAMS Scale Score, Triage-Revised Trauma Score, APACHE I, II, III, Prognostic Index, Acute Trauma Index, and the Baxt Trauma Triage Rule.

Preparing the Patient for Transport

This section summarizes patient preparation for transport. More in-depth discussions about patient preparation are contained in the clinical care sections of this book. The patient is prepared for transport based on information obtained from the primary and secondary assessment, mode of transport, transport time, and potential complications in relation to the patient's illness or injury during transport. Anticipating and planning for potential complications or worsening of patient condition will better prepare the transport team to either prevent or minimize complications and to facilitate rapid and efficient intervention should compromise occur.

Equipment used in transport has advanced over the last decade offering monitoring in transport that has not been previously available. Selection criteria should consider the cost and benefit to the patient in the transport setting. For advanced technology and improved processes, Continenza and Hill[17] recommended that the equipment should
- Be useful in the transport setting
- Be lightweight, portable, and perhaps fulfill several functions (Fig 10.2)
- Be easy to clean and maintain
- Have a battery life or power source that lasts the length of the transport
- Have the ability to be used both inside and outside the transport vehicle

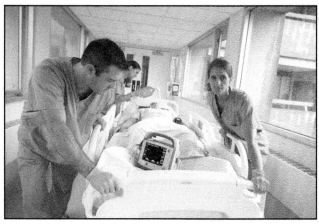

• **Fig. 10.2** Example of multifunctional monitor. (Courtesy Zoll Medical Corporation.)

- Be able to withstand the stresses of transport, such as movement, altitude changes, physical durability, water or fluid contamination, and temperature extremes

Box 10.13 contains a generic list of equipment that may be used during transport. The type of patient and the length of the transport dictate the amount and type of equipment carried by each service.

• BOX 10.13 **Equipment for Transport**

A comprehensive list of equipment that needs to be stocked by transport services consists of a core set of supplies. The following equipment list serves as a guide, but it must be upgraded for special patient considerations and streamlined in the event of cost constraints.

Airway Equipment

Resuscitation bags (infant, child, and adult)
All sizes of masks for bag-valve-mask ventilation
Nonrebreather masks
Pediatric
Adult
Nasal cannula
Oral and nasopharyngeal airways
Nebulizer setup
Portable suction unit
Tonsil suction
Suction catheters in the following sizes: 5/6F, 8F, 10F, 14F, and 18F
Magill forceps (pediatric and adult)
Laryngoscope handles (pediatric and adult)
Laryngoscope blades in the following sizes:
    Miller: 0, 1, 2, and 3
    MAC: 2, 3, and 4
Spare laryngoscope batteries and bulbs
Video laryngoscopy
Endotracheal tubes

Uncuffed		Cuffed		Endotrol
2.5	4.0	5.5	7.0	7.0
3.0	4.5	6.0	7.5	8.0
3.5	5.0	6.5	8.0	

Stylettes
Benzoin, adhesive tape, and tracheostomy tape

End-tidal CO_2 monitor
Positive end-expiratory pressure valve
Pulse oximeter
Ventilator and filter and spirometer (BiPAP capability)
Venturi mask
Aerosol mask for nebs
Heat and moisture exchangers
BiPAP mask
Alternate airways (laryngeal mask airway, Combitube, etc.)
Cricothyrotomy tray
Tracheostomy tubes
Needle cricothyrotomy setup
Gastric tubes in sizes 5 to 18
Catheter tip syringe
Surgilube

Cardiothoracic Equipment

Cardiac monitor and supplies, including extra batteries
Defibrillator and supplies, including adult and pediatric paddles
Defibrillator pads
Multipurpose pads (defibrillator/pacer)
External pacer and supplies
Transvenous pulse generator and cable
Noninvasive blood pressure monitor
Manual blood pressure equipment (pediatric, adult, and obese)
Doppler scan
Portable ultrasound
Pressure monitor and transducer and tubing kit
Thoracotomy tray and drainage system
Chest tubes in sizes 12–36F
Chest tube dressing
Needle decompression supplies
Pericardiocentesis setup
Multiple adapters (Sims, connectors, and small and large Y)

• BOX 10.13 Equipment for Transport—cont'd

Intravenous Access Equipment

Intravenous solutions based on local protocols
Blood tubing
Mini drip tubing
Extension tubing
Intravenous needles (24–14 gauge)
Butterfly needles (27–19 gauge)
Intraosseous needles (15 and 18 gauge)
Rapid-infusion catheters
Triple lumen catheter setup
Syringes of multiple sizes
Intravenous start packs
Razors
Arm boards
Laboratory blood tubes
Stopcocks
Pressure bag
Intravenous controllers or pumps and setup
Blood products and blood cooler

Medications

Advanced cardiac life support medications
Antianginal agents
Antiarrhythmics
Anticonvulsants
Antiemetics
Antihistamines
Antihypertensives
Diuretics
Local anesthetics
Narcotics
Nasal decongestant
Neuromuscular blocking agents
Steroids
Tocolytics
Vasopressor agents

Miscellaneous

Oxygen
Stethoscope
Standard precautions equipment
Infectious waste management receptacles
Sharp object safety boxes
Instruments
Bandage scissors
Trauma scissors
Hemostats
Ring cutter
Tape
Betadine solution

Dressing supplies (4 × 4s, elastic, bandages, and cravats)
Eye shields
Burn cable and electrodes
Cervical collars
Cervical immobilization device
Pediatric transport board
Car seat
Isolette
Obstetrics delivery tray
Cardiotocography and Fetal monitor
Bubble bag
Stockinette cap
Stuffed toys
Pediatric dosage calculation references
Soft or leather restraints
Linen, blankets, towels
Flashlight
Cellular telephone
Satellite telephones
Two-way radio
Thermometer
Camera (instant, digital, and video recorder)
Documents
Directions and map to receiving facilities

Additional equipment specific to a service may include the following:

Ambulance

Immobilization devices (because space and weight are less of a consideration in an ambulance than in a helicopter or fixed-wing aircraft)
Backboard
Traction splint
Vacuum splints

Helicopter

Ear protection for the patient and crew
Survival bag stocked with necessary equipment in the event of an emergency landing

Fixed-Wing Aircraft

Certain bulk supplies (because of extended transport times)
Intravenous solutions and medication
Food and drink for the crew
Patient comfort kit (e.g., bedpan, urinal, urinary catheter)

Survival Equipment

Life Rafts
Life Vests

Airway Management

Patient preparation begins with the assessment and management of the patient's airway. The team will first need to determine whether the patient can maintain his or her airway for the duration of the transport. The patient's neurologic status, facial or airway injury, swelling, and hemorrhage all influence airway maintenance.

Once need is determined, the best method of intervention given the patient's condition will need to be identified. These options are discussed in detail in Chapter 11. Factors that may influence the decision about when and how to manage the airway include the nature of the patient's illness or injury, the length of transport, space limitations in the transport vehicle, and the positioning of the crew in the transport vehicle.

Once intubation has been performed, tube placement and security should be evaluated. An unsecured endotracheal tube may be inadvertently dislodged. A tube that is positioned too high in the airway may also lead to dislodgement with patient movement or cause vocal cord damage if the balloon is inflated in the vocal cords. A tube that is too low, such as right-main stemmed, can lead to pulmonary injury from high airway pressures delivered to a single lung or collapse of the nonventilated lung. In addition, movement of the endotracheal tube can cause mucosal damage, induce gagging and coughing, and increase the patient's intracranial or intraocular pressure.[50,68,69]

Oxygen should be administered to maintain saturations or PaO_2 per clinical indication. Hyperoxygenation should not be used indiscriminately because of potential deleterious effects. Oxygen should be considered a medication and administered at the dose needed. Additional monitoring equipment such as a pulse oximeter, capnography, and apnea monitor should be used for continuous airway evaluation. These monitoring devices are discussed further in Chapter 12.

Ventilation Management

A rapid focused assessment of the patient's ventilatory status should be performed as the patient is prepared for transport. If a CXR has been obtained, it should be viewed to determine whether any pathology exists as well as appropriate positioning of devices. The transport team should assess the CXR using a systematic approach to interpretation. Interventions are based on clinical need and transport time. Breath sounds should be auscultated before transitioning to the transport vehicle when possible because of noise interference.

If a pneumothorax is suspected or is present on CXR, appropriate interventions should be initiated. It should be noted that a CXR, particularly supine, may not identify a pneumothorax, and other assessment should be used to support the need for chest tube placement. If a chest tube or tubes are already in place, the team should check that connections are secure; check that the tube is not kinked, occluded, or clamped; and assess for air leak and drainage as well as the adequacy of the system to evacuate air or fluid. The drainage system may need to be changed so that it continues to function during transport.

If an advanced airway is in place, a ventilator should be used for transport for consistent and safe delivery of ventilatory support. If the patient is on a ventilator when the transport team arrives, the team should identify and evaluate current settings, including minute ventilation, fractional concentration of inspired oxygen (FiO_2), positive end-expiratory pressure, tidal volume, and set, as well as spontaneous respiratory rate. If the patient is being bag ventilated, the team will need to select settings depending on clinical condition. Patients with severe respiratory compromise may take time to recover on transitioning to a transport ventilator because of alveolar derecruitment, and the team should resist the urge to remove the patient from the ventilator. Ventilation management and techniques to reduce derecruitment are discussed in Chapter 12.

Circulation Management

Initial care related to circulatory management is directed at controlling any active bleeding and support of cardiac function and output. Bleeding can be controlled with direct pressure with application of gauze pads and elastic tape or bandages or hemostatic gauze. The source, cause, and degree of the bleeding should be carefully evaluated before transport. The patient should be prepared for transport so that sheets or blankets do not inhibit regular visualization of wounds that may start, or restart, bleeding during transport. If blood is available and need exists, transfusion should be initiated. The receiving trauma center should be notified of uncontrolled hemorrhage potentially requiring damage control resuscitation and mass transfusion on arrival. After the clinical randomization of an antifibrinolytic in significant hemorrhage (CRASH-2) trial, interest in tranexamic acid to treat internal bleeding has risen. This is still controversial, and if used, strict guidelines set by the transport service in collaboration with ACS Trauma Center physicians should be followed.

Cardiovascular support by defibrillation, cardioversion, or cardiac pacing may be required to provide sufficient cardiac output during the transport. Patches can be placed before transport for easy and quick access in patients at risk. IV or IO access must be established, but it should not delay transport in patients with a time-dependent condition. Sufficient access to provide fluid replacement, blood infusions, and medication delivery may call for more than one IV. This is particularly important in patients dependent on IV therapy or who could deteriorate if an IV/IO line is lost during transport.

When medications are infused, infusion pumps may be used to ensure the appropriate delivery and titration of medication and are essential when vasoactive agents are used. Medication concentrations and dosages should always be double-checked when initiating or transitioning onto transport pumps. Infusion pumps should be equipped with concentration and dosing calculators. In an attempt to reduce error, the transport team may elect to mix its own infusions rather then transfer the medications mixed at the referring location. If invasive lines such as central, pulmonary, or arterial catheters are in place, the transport team needs to check the patency and functioning of these lines. The lines must be appropriately maintained and secured so that their functioning is not impaired and prevent accidental dislodgement. If a service transports patients with invasive lines, they should use a monitor that can monitor these readings. Air should be evacuated from all infusion bags not placed on an infusion pump with an air alarm. This is done to prevent air from entraining in the line when the bag is positioned in a nonupright position when moving the patient. This is particularly important in central and arterial line flush bags to prevent an accidental power flush of air directly into the circulation.

Urinary catheters must be appropriately placed and affixed so that they can drain and are not pulled or dislodged with patient movement. It is recommended that catheter bags are emptied before the patient leaves the referring facility. The amount of urine emptied from the bag and its color should be recorded.

Gastric Decompression

A gastric tube should be inserted to prevent the potential for aspiration and to provide gastric decompression during transport.[1] This procedure is not generally performed when a patient is transported directly from a scene, but it should be considered, particularly when the patient has undergone extended bag-valve-mask (BVM) ventilation.

As with the urinary catheter, the gastric decompression tube must be appropriately placed and secured to prevent it from being removed or repositioned outside the stomach. If the tube is not going to be placed on suction during transport, it should be capped so that it does not leak gastric contents. If not connected to suction on fixed-wing transports with potentially higher altitudes, opening the gastric tube to gravity at fixed intervals may be necessary to prevent gastric distention. When possible, the patient's stomach should be drained before the tube is plugged. The amount of the drainage and its color should be recorded.

When patients undergo treatment for extensive gastrointestinal bleeding, such as seen in a patient with liver disease, a specific type of gastric tube, such as the Sengstaken-Blakemore tube, may be in place. Traction must be maintained so that the tube continues to function properly. When this tube is present, the patient may be at risk for aspiration, asphyxia, gastric rupture, and erosion of the esophageal wall.[70] When the patient is transported with a gastric tube that may compromise the airway, the airway should be secured with intubation, and the transport team must be prepared to intervene if any complications occur and to provide continued traction on the tube.

Wound Care and Splinting

Wounds and splinting devices should be surveyed quickly, before the patient is moved. Hidden wounds may cause the patient discomfort and increase the risk of bleeding and long-term complications. Improperly placed splints or lack of splinting when indicated may cause additional injury.

Several types of splints and splint devices are available for transport. The transport team must be familiar with the type of equipment that is used. The team should be well practiced in the placement of the splint, potential complications of the device, and indications for removal. The neurovascular status of the extremity to which the splint is applied should be assessed and documented. Musculoskeletal, soft tissue and vascular emergencies are discussed in Chapter 17. Wound care is provided for patient comfort and protection. Dressing the wound helps control bleeding and keep it free of debris. If concern exists about additional bleeding or neurovascular compromise, the wound should be dressed in such a manner that continuous assessment is possible during transport. Any wet dressings are replaced with dry sterile dressings to prevent heat loss during transport. Care must be taken when changing dressings not to dislodge any clot that may have formed.

The need for infection control is important when tending the wounds of the patient being prepared for transport. Many patients being transported may have infected wounds that create a risk for the transport team and anyone else who may need to be transported in the vehicle. Appropriate personal protective equipment (PPE) and decontamination procedures should be followed for both the transport team members and the vehicles.[71]

Patient Safety[46]

Chapters 8 and 9 have been devoted to safety issues. In this section, the authors examine the safety measures that must be taken into consideration by the transport team when preparing the patient for transport. Placing a combative or psychologically unstable patient in a moving vehicle, in air or on ground, can pose a threat to team members and may require physical or chemical restraint to ensure the safety of all.

The Food and Drug Administration[64] has established guidelines for the use of restraints. These guidelines outline the need to clearly document the necessity of restraint use, the application of restraints, and ongoing monitoring requirements. Whenever restraints are applied care should be taken to ensure that skin integrity is not compromised; that the patient is positioned for comfort; and in the case of chemical restraint, the patient is assessed frequently for signs of pain or anxiety. All local and state laws regarding the use of restraints should be known and followed.

When transporting a child, the child's size, weight, and state laws necessitate that restraint systems appropriate for a child be used. Devices that may be used include care beds, car seats, restraint systems, and transport boards. Any equipment that is used during transport needs to meet both federal and state standards.

Pain Management

Pain management in the prehospital care environment is frequently not given priority consideration.[28] Several factors influence the use or lack of use of pain medications in the field, including the location of the patient, the nature of the patient's illness or injury, the possible masking of symptoms, and the effect of pain medications on the patient's vital signs. Movement, noise, changes in temperature, and fear may be contributing factors that cause or increase the patient's pain during preparation and transport.

Certain patient problems, such as chest pain related to myocardial infarction, has received the appropriate attention and treatment in the prehospital environment. However, acute pain, whether the result of trauma or other disease states, continues to be undertreated by health care professionals.[1,2,8,9,1,47]

To comply with guidelines set forth by The Joint Commission on Accreditation of Healthcare Organization, the transport team should assess and document a pain score appropriate to the patient population to measure the intensity of a patient's pain. The PQRST mnemonic previously described helps provide a baseline description of the patient's pain. If the patient received medication before the team's arrival, information about the medication used and its effect on the patient should be included in the pain assessment.

The World Health Organization (WHO) developed a pain relief ladder (available at http://www.who.int/cancer/palliative/painladder/en) outlining effective pain management guidelines intended for use in cancer patients. These guidelines involve a three-step approach to pain management advancing from nonopioid for mild pain ratings to strong opioids for moderate to severe pain ratings. These guidelines have been adapted for use in the emergency setting with many principles applicable to the transport environment.

Pain medications used for analgesia in the prehospital care environment need to be rapid in onset, short in duration, easy to administer, allow for multiple routes of administration, and easy to store. The IV route is the quickest method of administration and has a rapid onset. However, IV access may not always be available. The transport team needs to be familiar with specific medications that can be used during transport to provide analgesia and sedation. Adjuvant medications, such as antidepressants, antiemetics, anxiolytics, corticosteroids, and others, have been found to be effective in pain management when used in combination with analgesics. This knowledge must include appropriate medication dosage, possible drug interactions, adverse reactions, and management of these adverse reactions.

Also, during transport some patients may have received neuromuscular blocking agents for safe transport, management of specific problems, or both (although neuromuscular blocking agents should be used sparingly and not as a first step unless immediate safety precautions need to be implemented without delay). The transport team should pay attention to the needs of these patients for sedation and pain management because verbal and visual indicators of pain are eliminated.

Consideration of nonpharmacologic methods combined with conventional methods of pain management is also recommended for treatment of acute pain relief.[72] Nonpharmacologic methods that may be used by the transport team to help with pain management during transport include the following[1,2,8,9,21,47]:

- Distraction. Encourage patients to look out the window if they are alert enough to do so. A security object such as a stuffed toy may be of help to a child. Music via headset or built-in DVD players are also helpful distractors.
- Talk to the patient.
- Comfort: Attend to warmth, air, positioning, and nausea.
- Reduce fear: Describe everything that is going to occur. Wheels coming down, turbulence, loading/unloading,

and alarms may be routine to the medical team, but they may create anxiety and fear in patients and family.
- Allow a family member to accompany the patient.
- Therapeutic touch. Be cognizant that some people and cultures do not welcome touching.

Patient Preparation: The Family

Families react to trauma and acute illness of their loved one differently. Some families are resilient; however, others may feel overwhelmed because of high stress, ongoing burden, and limited resources that quickly deplete coping mechanisms. Culture, ethnicity, religious beliefs, and the patient's age may influence coping ability. The transport team should be supportive, nonjudgmental, and engage the family as much as possible given limited exposure time. They should provide some detail of the transport process and what they will experience when they arrive at the referring facility. They should instill a sense of safety and professional competence. Engaging the family can simply involve obtaining a patient history and asking a few personal questions, such as how the patient responds to heat or cold, or it may include taking a family member along on the transport whenever possible and as program policies allow. The transport team should recognize that the family's ability to retain information can be limited and should alert the receiving facility staff of the need for social service support.

A discussion about family needs, how to care for the family, and when transport of a family member is appropriate is contained in Chapter 32.

Cardiopulmonary Arrest During Transport[1-10,43,51]

A cardiopulmonary arrest during transport poses a unique challenge to the transport team. First, the team should confirm the patient's current code status with the referring physician and family, if present. The family should be apprised of the risks of transport and be aware of the condition of the patient before team departure. If there is a possibility of diversion to another facility, the team should make the family aware and get a phone contact number from them so the transport team can advise them of any changes.

The transport team must address four essential issues if a patient has a full cardiopulmonary arrest during the transport: (1) the service's policies and procedures for in-flight codes; (2) the decision to return, divert, or continue to proceed to the destination; (3) the availability of resuscitation equipment and medications; and (4) the endurance of the air medical personnel. After these issues have been weighed and deliberated, the transport team will make the final decision, in conjunction with medical direction or if unable to contact medical direction, policies, and procedures, on whether to continue resuscitative efforts.

Transport team members need to be well versed in the service's policies and procedures for cardiopulmonary arrest during transport. Every state has specific laws that deal with terminating resuscitation efforts in the prehospital arena. The program should have policies and procedures in place to direct the decision options and any medical control communication required should cardiopulmonary arrest occur.

In addition, legal aspects of interstate and international transport may complicate the decision to terminate resuscitation en route or before reaching the destination. Some locales require pronouncement of death be performed by provincially recognized licensed and credentialed professionals. Therefore some air medical services have a policy that a patient cannot be pronounced dead until the aircraft has landed and required notification of local authorities have been completed and documented, especially if the transport takes place outside the United States.[72-74]

Second, if the patient's condition deteriorates into a full arrest during any portion of the transport, the transport team must weigh distance and time factors to determine in which direction to transport. This decision may be based on the distance and time to return to the referring facility or to the closest appropriate facility, on the availability of ground ambulances, on resources at the referring facility (catheter laboratory for the patient with an ST elevation myocardial infarction [STEMI]), and on overall patient status. The question for the transport team is whether to divert the aircraft or continue to the destination after weighing all these factors.

The third essential issue relates to the service's available resuscitation equipment and medications. This equipment should at minimum include oxygen, endotracheal tubes, advanced cardiac life-support medications, fluids, and the battery power on life-support equipment. Given the limited supplies available in a transport vehicle, particularly long-distance transports, the transport team may need to make a decision based on exhausting all resuscitation supplies or medications.

Finally, the endurance of the personnel on the transport should be considered, especially for transports that also require extended ground times. The transport team may need to contact their medical director or when this not available, use preexisting protocols to recommend ceasing resuscitation efforts if the patient does not respond to medical therapy on a long transport.

"Do Not Resuscitate" or "Allow Natural Death" Orders

Transport services may provide do not resuscitate (DNR) or allow natural death (AND) transports at the family's request and not because of medical necessity. These transports are prescheduled with the service, and the transport team should be familiar with DNR or AND policies and procedures. Because various states have different definitions for DNR or AND patients, services that conduct these types of transports should provide policies and procedures for transport team members.

Documentation

Copies of any relevant documentation from the referring agency or EMS care providers should accompany the patient. If pictures of the scene of the accident are available, the transport team should bring them as well. Customized charting software for use with laptop computers and handheld devices provides an efficient and thorough way to document the patient assessment and record any changes or care provided during the transport. The documentation can then be downloaded into a centralized database that allows for storing and categorizing collected data. However, after the documentation is completed, the team must be able to provide copies to the staff of the receiving facility when the patient care is transferred.[75-77]

Copies of laboratory results, radiographic and diagnostic studies, and documentation by other health care providers should also accompany the patient unless they can be received electronically. Consent forms, reasons for transport, and any other pertinent papers should be placed in the transport vehicle so that the team does not forget them when the patient arrives at the receiving facility. Remember to maintain patient confidentially when transporting or reviewing patient records.[75-77]

Documentation by the transport team should reflect the reason the patient was transported; the interventions performed before, during, and after transport; and response to those interventions. Specific documentation may be required to maintain compliance with state EMS regulations, standards set by accrediting bodies, and sponsoring hospital requirements.[75-77]

Documentation of not only of what specific intervention was performed but also of how the decision was made and what diagnostic tools were implemented is important. For example, why was the decision made to perform rapid sequence induction to secure the patient's airway? If medications were administered for pain or arrhythmia management, did they influence the patient and what was that effect?[75-77]

The patient's chart is not only used to document interventions and their indications but also for continuous quality improvement and reimbursement of services. Documentation and data collection are an integral part of tracking and trending of quality metrics that may be used to identify quality practices, patient care, and improved patient outcomes. It must be clear, complete, and readable and allow for data collection and reporting.

What is documented and who does the documentation are determined by the transport service and the specific standards. Nurses and paramedics have standards that describe their practice and provide guidelines for documentation (e.g., Air and Surface Transport Nurses Association [ASTNA], formerly called the National Flight Nurses Association [NFNA]).[75-77]

Preparation for the Transport of the Bariatric Patient

Obesity is an unhealthy epidemic in the United States that is rapidly spreading to other parts of the world. A

TABLE 10.2	Weight Categories for Adults by Body Mass Index	
Category	**BMI (kg/m²)**	
Underweight	<18.5	
Normal	18.5–24.99	
Overweight	25–26.99	
Obesity	30	
Severe obesity	>35	
Morbid obesity	>40	
Weight Categories for Children by Age and Gender-Specific Percentile Calculations		
Obesity	>95th percentile of same age and gender	
Extreme obesity	≥120% of the 95th percentile of same age and gender	

BMI, Body mass index.

patient is considered overweight when their body mass index (BMI) is greater 25% and obese when their BMI is 30% greater than their calculated healthy weight range. Because of the increase in larger patients, the care of the bariatric patient has become an integral part of preparing a patient for transport. A bariatric patient includes patients who are overweight, obese, and morbidly obese and those who have had some sort of bariatric surgery. The American Association of Operating Room Nurses has developed weight categories by BMI (summarized in Table 10.2).[78-86] The transport team must consider several issues in the care and preparation for the transport of the bariatric patient.

Selection of an Appropriate Vehicle

The mode of transport is influenced by weight and balance of aircraft, as well as the ability to provide safe care given space limitations. Each transport program must have policies and procedures that address the weight and size of the patient that can be safely managed within the aircraft or ground vehicles. For example, a weight restriction may identify one limitation, but the girth of the patient can also impede safe and competent care in some transport vehicles.

It is imperative to comply with weight limitations for a helicopter or fixed-wing transport to maintain aircraft structural integrity and performance. Balance is also critical to address the center-of-gravity deviations in fully loaded helicopters that may change or affect handling characteristics. Operating within the aircraft weight and balance is a Federal Aviation Administration (FAA) requirement. Weight calculations include the weight of everything and everyone on board, and crew weights should be accurate and include any additional gear they carry, such as survival bags. All equipment, both standard on all transports as well as added in for mission-specific transports, need to be

included. Aircraft performance is also affected by temperature, altitude, and landing zone location.[87]

The transport team should be aware of and adhere to stretcher and loading ramp weight restrictions. The team must also assess the patient's physical limitations regarding mode of transport. For example, in a fixed-wing aircraft, rules and regulations require that a patient be flat for takeoff and landing and some patients may not be able to tolerate lying in a supine position for any period of time.

Patient Assessment and Intervention Differences in the Bariatric Patient

Given the current obesity epidemic, the transport team should understand the management challenges of the severely and morbidly obese patient in the acute care setting. They should be aware of and prepared for the comorbid conditions that may be exacerbated or emerge during acute illness. These factors and the implications for patient care are summarized in Table 10.3.[79-86]

The most challenging issues that transport members face when caring for an obese patient is the management of the patient's airway, breathing, and circulation.[79-86] The excess fatty tissue on the breast, neck, thoracic wall, abdomen, and in the mouth, pharynx, and around internal organs affects airway access, airway patency, and pulmonary function. Intubation, surgical airway, and ventilation require proper

TABLE 10.3	Comorbid Factors That May Accompany Obesity and Implications to Patient Care
Comorbid Factor	**Implications to Care**
Alveolar hypoventilation	Hypoxia may already be present in these patients
	Sedation and pain medication may increase hypoxia
Obstructive apnea	Patient may not be able to lay flat for loading or transport
	Preexisting hypoxia can be increased as well if the patient must be flat for transport
Gastroesophageal reflux	Patient is at greater risk for vomiting and aspiration
	Can be aggravated if patient must be flat for loading, unloading, and transport
Increased body tissue	Equipment may not obtain accurate readings
	Pulse oximeters may be unreliable because of increased finger thickness and poorly transmitted light waves
	Inappropriately fitting blood pressure cuffs do not provide accurate blood pressure readings
	Low QRS voltage interferes with cardiac monitoring

planning and preparation including positioning, preoxygenation, and intubation pharmacology selection. An obese patient can be difficult to ventilate with a BVM because of reduced pulmonary compliance, increased upper airway resistance, and abnormal diaphragmatic position.[79-80] The transport program should have developed and practiced difficult airway algorithms so they are prepared for complications and can respond effectively and efficiently. Mechanical abnormalities, increased airway resistance, and reduced lung compliance can all affect the management of ventilation in the morbidly obese patient. The advanced airway interventions and ventilation management of the bariatric patient are discussed in detail in Chapters 11 and 12.

Increased risk of gastroesophageal reflux will increase the risk of vomiting and aspiration with BVM ventilation. Even if a patient does not require intubation or BVM ventilation, the transport team should position the obese patient with the head elevated, as condition allows, for prophylaxis against aspiration and to ease spontaneous ventilatory efforts by reducing the effort needed to initiate a breath.

Several cardiovascular disorders in patients with significant obesity will affect clinical course and complicate management in the transport setting. The obese patient requires a higher blood volume to meet the perfusion needs of adipose tissue, and the heart compensates by increasing the stroke volume, without necessarily increasing heart rate, and subsequently results in an increase in cardiac output, left ventricular workload, and oxygen consumption. In addition, there is a decrease in the systemic vascular resistance. Pressure overload, increased blood viscosity, and hypertension make these patients more prone to left ventricular hypertrophy, which elevates the risk for systolic and diastolic dysfunction, congestive heart failure, cardiac dysrhythmias, and stroke. [79-86]

Fluid resuscitation and medication administration must be calculated and monitored. The transport team should be aware of whether the medication dosage of drugs they infuse or deliver are based on actual or predicted body weight.

Preparation for Transport

The transport team must be familiar with physical and physiologic changes related to the bariatric patient. Airway, ventilation, and circulation management must be approached with the appropriate training, equipment, and monitoring devices. Preparation is key for preventing complications.

Airway management must include equipment for a potential failed airway such as a laryngeal tracheal mask airway. Failed airway management is discussed in Chapter 11.

Excessive weight makes vascular access difficult. Alternative access, depending on skill and training, include IO access and central venous cannulation. Catheter length should be considered in all forms of venous access. Ultrasound-guided peripheral or central line access has become more common in the transport setting with the advancement of light-weight portable ultrasound devices.

Transport of the bariatric patient requires specialized equipment. Stretchers should be rated for the weight of the patient. These weight limits must be posted on the stretcher. In addition to the ability to support the patient's weight, securing devices, such as seatbelt extenders, should be available in all modes of transport to safety secure a patient to the stretcher. The stretcher must support the weight of the torso in the elevated head position. Obese patients are at higher risk of skin breakdown, particularly those with diabetes, and the ability to reposition during transport is often not reasonable. With that in mind, patients should be carefully positioned so the skin integrity is protected. Loading ramp limitations on fixed-wing aircraft must also be observed.

Adequate personnel must be available to get the patient both in and out of the transport vehicle. EMS crews, hospital personnel, or additional transport crew may be called on to assist with loading and unloading in all modes of transport. Consider the weight of the patient and what that translates to in lifting weight per each transport person. Several commercial devices are now available that have been found to ease patient transfer from beds to stretchers. Some transport companies also have specially equipped winch-capable vehicles to transport morbidly obese patients.

The care and transport of the bariatric patient presents unique challenges to the transport team. The primary key to safe and competent transport is identification of the physiologic changes related to obesity, provision of care based on these differences, and preparation for the transport.

Laboratory and Diagnostic Testing Interpretation

Laboratory Tests

Laboratory and diagnostic tests can provide additional information about patient illnesses and injuries that may necessitate interventions before and during transport. Select laboratory tests may be performed during the transport. For interfacility transports, the team should be prepared to review laboratory tests before transport at the transferring facility. Laboratory tests that may be of use to prepare for transport are summarized in Table 10.4. This list is not inclusive but does include some of the tests that may contribute to patient problems during the transport process.

Chest X-Ray Interpretation[1,24,66]

The CXR can identify important information to support or direct care during transport. A CXR assists in the confirmation of endotracheal tube placement, central line position, and chest tube effectiveness in evacuating air and/or blood. It may also identify pulmonary and cardiac abnormalities or thoracic injuries that may guide clinical decision making.

TABLE 10.4	Laboratory Tests Useful for Transport: Tests and Values	
Laboratory Test	**Normal Values**	
Arterial blood gases	pH: 7.36–7.44	
	PcO₂: 34–44 mm Hg	
	PO₂: 80–100 mm Hg	
	HCO₃: 22–26	
	O₂ saturation: 95% or greater	
Hemoglobin	Male: 14–18 g/dL	
	Female: 12–19 g/dL	
Hematocrit	Male: 40.7%–50.3%	
	Female: 36.1%–44.3%	
Internationalized normalized ratio	2.0–3.0 standard therapeutic range	
Platelet count	Adults: 150–400,000	
	Children: 150–450,000	
Potassium	3.5–5.0	
Sodium	135-145	
Lactate	2 mmol/L	
Troponin I	<0.01 ng/mL	

Altitude presents some risk of extension of a simple pneumothorax into a life-threatening tension pneumothorax, and the transport team should either perform or prepare for chest decompression (Fig 10.3).

CXR interpretation takes education and practice. Transport team members should take every opportunity to practice reading CXRs. They should be familiar with lung and thoracic anatomy. The Transport Professional Advanced Trauma Course provides an opportunity to interpret and discuss CXRs.

A systematic approach should be used to evaluate the CXR. There are many methods for systematic review, and the tool used is not as important as following a set structure

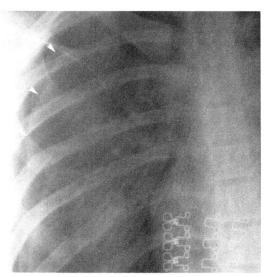

• **Fig. 10.3** Radiograph of pneumothorax. (From Mirvis SE, Shanmuganathan K. *Imaging in Trauma and Critical Care.* 2nd ed. Philadelphia, PA: Saunders; 2003.)

for interpretation. Once the film is identified for viewing, either electronically or in hard copy, proceed in a systematic fashion. Here is one example using the PQR-ABCDEFGHI method:

- *Position*: Position of the patient in relation to the radiographic beam should be noted. Is it a posterior-anterior (PA) upright film or is it an anterior-posterior (AP) film shot in an upright or a supine position? Is it a lateral view? An AP film will make the heart and great vessels look larger, limiting definitive interpretation for heart and mediastinal size.
- *Quality*: Technical quality of the film includes completeness of view, taken on full inspiration, and adequate penetration.
  - *Completeness of view*: The margins of all lung fields should be visible on the film. The top lung margin should extend to include the apices of the lungs. The bottom margins should include the costophrenic angle. The side margins should not crop off either side of the thoracic cage.
  - *Inspiration*: The CXR should be taken at full inspiration to give the best and most complete view of pulmonary structures. In full inspiration, the diaphragm should be found at the level of the 8th-10th posterior rib or 5th-6th anterior rib. A film taken on expiration may obscure heart borders or lower lung fields.
  - *Penetration*. Does the film have a white cast throughout (underpenetrated) or an overall dark hue throughout (overpenetrated)? A high-quality PA film should be able to barely identify the vertebral disk spaces through the heart shadow, but should lack bony detail. A sufficient film is one in which, at a minimum, the bronchovascular structures can be identified through the heart. An overpenetrated or underpenetrated CXR will obscure bone structure or soft tissues, respectively.
- *Rotation*: A rotated film may hide or make more prominent certain anatomic features. The quickest way to identify rotation is to locate the proximal ends of the clavicles and identify that they are equidistant from the vertebral bodies.
- *Airway*: This refers to the trachea position. It should be midline, but may be shifted away from a space-occupying pathology (air, blood, and fluid) or shifted toward collapse/atelectasis. Also, look for narrowing indicative of stenosis or edema.
- *Bones and tissue*: Examine clavicles, ribs, sternum, and thoracic spine. Look along the edges of the bone for interruptions that could indicate a break. Look in the surrounding soft tissue for evidence of subcutaneous air, suggesting a possible pneumothorax.
- *Cardiac*: Look at size, shape, and borders. The borders of the heart and mediastinum should be well defined. Familiarity with the structures that border the heart may suggest specific lung lobe abnormality. For example, if the right border of the heart is not clear or is obscured, then there is a suggestion of a right middle lobe abnormality. In relation to heart size, it should take up less

than half of the thoracic diameter (consider supine films that may make heart seem larger).

- *Diaphragm*: The outline of the diaphragm should be visible on both sides. The right hemidiaphragm should be slightly higher because of the location of the liver. Costophrenic and cardiophrenic borders should be visible. Haziness may indicate pleural effusion, and a deep costophrenic sulcus may be evidence of a pneumothorax. Absence of the diaphragm may indicate diagrammatic rupture. Look for air below the diaphragm, which may indicate bowel perforation.
- *Extraneous*: Tube and line placement identification.
- *Fields of the lung*: Examine the lung sections individually and as a whole. Look for bilateral symmetry, opacity, shadows, and vasculature. Vascular marking should be visible from the cardiac border to the chest wall. Loss of markings may indicate a pneumothorax. Assess for infiltrates, masses, air bronchograms, and increased vascularity
- *Gastric bubble*: Gastric air should be under the left hemidiaphragm. Gastric distension is noted and, if extreme, may affect cardiac function. A nasogastric (NG) tube should be placed whenever possible. An NG tube can be diagnostic in a CXR when it is seen in the chest cavity.
- *Hilum*: The hilum consists of the main bronchus and the pulmonary arteries. In the great majority of the population, the right side should be higher than the left. Space-occupying or space-eliminating pathologies can pull the hilum up or down. Increased congestion at the hilum is suggestive of pulmonary edema associated with cardiac failure.

Computed Tomographic Scan Interpretation[1,24,66]

The most common computed tomography (CT) scans evaluated by the transport team are cranial CT scans. CT scans of the head can assist with the diagnosis of neurologic injury and evaluation of seizures and stroke symptoms. Just as with CXR interpretation, evaluation of cranial CT scans takes education and practice. The CT scan should always be used in conjunction with a physical assessment.

A CT scan is created when radiographs pass through the body and are recorded in terms of different absorption values[1]; a denser body part absorbs more radiation. A CT scan can detect bleeding, fractures, and soft tissue injury.

CT scan interpretation requires familiarity with the basic anatomy of the part of the body that is being scanned. For example, a healthy head CT scan shows the skull as white and the brain as gray in color. Dark areas within the brain indicate areas filled with fluid. These areas include the ventricles, cisterns, and the sagittal and transverse tissues. The cisterns are four fluid spaces in the brain and are visible on the CT scan.

A systemic review to cranial tomography includes the following:

- Is this scan for the correct patient?
- Is this a contrast or noncontrast scan (contrast is the same density as blood and can obscure hemorrhage)?

- Is there artifact that may influence ability to interpret?
- Is the scout film available for overview?
- What window level (brain, soft tissue, and bone) is being viewed?

As with CXR interpretation, evaluation of the head CT should be systematic and a knowledge of cerebral anatomy is necessary. The following is one example of a systematic approach using the Blood Can Be Very Bad mnemonic.
Blood:

- Look for the *presence of blood*, which appears hyperdense (white) in the acute phase, and darkens with age as the clot retracts. The age of the hemorrhage can be estimated by whether it is hyperdense, isodense, or hypodense.
- *Evaluate for hemorrhagic lesions including* epidural, subdural, subarachnoid, intraparenchymal, intraventricular, and extracranial hemorrhage.
- Figs 10.4 to 10.6 show CT scans of a depressed skull fracture, an epidural hematoma, and a subdural hematoma, respectively.

Cisterns: Cisterns are structures that collect cerebrospinal fluid, which surrounds and protects the brain. Cisterns become effaced, fluid filled, and asymmetric with cerebral pathology such as edema.
Brain:

- Sulci and gyri: Look for effacement and asymmetry.
- Gray–white matter differentiation: Loss of differentiation is associated with cerebral edema.
- Areas of hypodensity (air and edema), hyperdensity (blood and calcification), and structural shift.

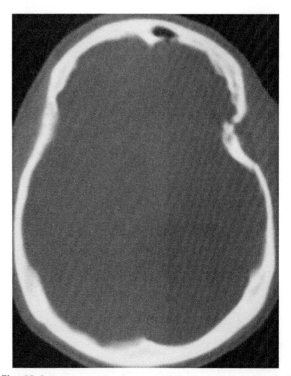

• **Fig. 10.4** Image reveals depressed left posterior frontal calvarial fracture. (From Mirvis SE, Shanmuganathan K. *Imaging in Trauma and Critical Care.* 2nd ed. Philadelphia, PA: Saunders; 2003.)

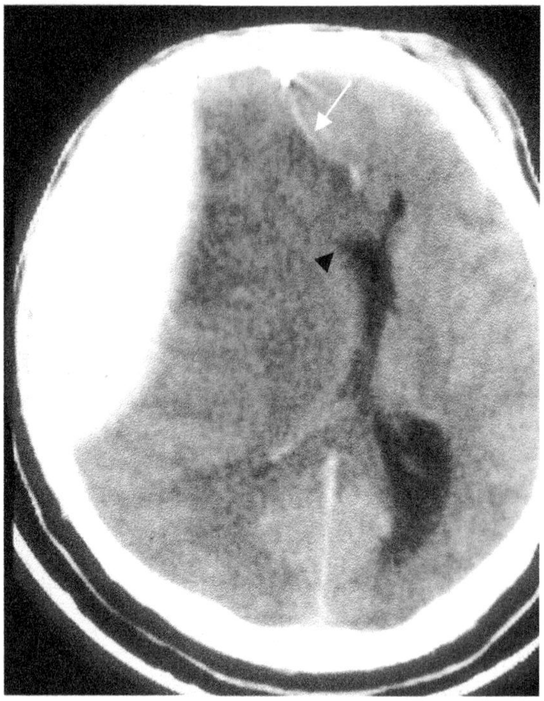

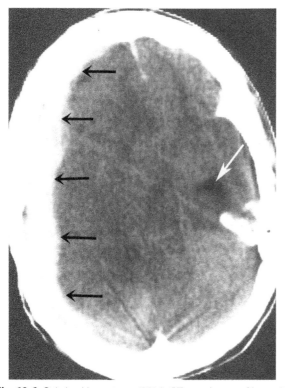

• **Fig. 10.5** Large right epidural hematoma. (From Mirvis SE, Shanmuganathan K. *Imaging in Trauma and Critical Care*. 2nd ed. Philadelphia, PA: Saunders; 2003.)

• **Fig. 10.6** Subdural hematoma (SDH). CT scan image of large right convexity SDH *(arrows)*. (From Mirvis SE, Shanmuganathan K. *Imaging in Trauma and Critical Care*. 2nd ed. Philadelphia, PA: Saunders; 2003.)

Ventricles:
- Examine the lateral, third and fourth ventricle for asymmetry, dilation, and effacement.

Bone:
- The bones of the skull are best viewed using the bony windows. Look for fractures.

Focused Assessment With Sonography[52]

Ultrasound is the ideal initial imaging modality because it can be performed simultaneously with other resuscitative cares, providing vital information without the time delay caused by radiographs or CT. Focused assessment with sonography (FAST) involves the use of bedside ultrasound to rapidly identify trauma injuries that are not apparent on the initial physical examination. Becoming more durable and cost-effective, ultrasound devices are now being used in the prehospital and transport environment to assist with nontrauma assessments and rapid identification and treatment of life-threatening conditions such as aortic aneurysms and fine asystole. Professionals, trained to practice in a variety of settings, can now use the FAST examination in a variety of different ways to guide clinical decision making. With trauma assessments, the primary purpose of the FAST examination was to rapidly identify free fluid in the peritoneal, pericardial, or pleural spaces and to detect specific emergencies with penetrating and blunt cardiac trauma, abdominal trauma, and chest trauma. The Association for Medical Ultrasound defined primary ultrasound windows to guide the FAST examination, which are included in Box 10.14.

Patient Assessment and Reassessment During Transport

The nature of the patient's illness or injuries and the initial interventions performed influence the assessment and management needed during air medical transport. Each of the clinical chapters in this textbook addresses the specific care needed during transport because of the patient's illness or injury. Some general principles of assessment and management during transport include the following:

- Transport team members should position themselves in the aircraft so that they can effectively manage the patient's airway, breathing, and circulation (ABCs).
- Airway equipment, including suction equipment, should be easily accessible.
- All IV, central, or IO lines should be accessible and functioning.
- All tubes and drainage systems should be functioning and secured to decrease the risk of dislodgement.
- If any question exists about cervical spine injury, the cervical spine should be immobilized for transport.

> **• BOX 10.14** **The Association for Medical Ultrasound Defined Primary Ultrasound Windows to Guide the Focused Assessment With Sonography Examination**
>
> - The right upper quadrant view uses the liver as an ultrasound window to interrogate the liver as well as the hepatorenal space for free fluid.
> - The left upper quadrant view uses the spleen as a window to interrogate the spleen and the perisplenic space above the spleen and below the diaphragm as well as the splenorenal recess.
> - The pelvic view allows for assessment of the most dependent space in the peritoneum for free fluid. Filling the bladder with fluid through an indwelling urinary catheter may help analysis for pelvic fluid.
> - The pericardial view uses the left lobe of the liver as an acoustic window for analysis of the heart.
> - The anterior thoracic view allows for identifying a potential separation of the pleura by a pneumothorax, which may be imaged typically in the second or third intercostal space.
> - The right and left pericolic gutter views through peritoneal windows inferior to the level of the ipsilateral kidney and next to the ipsilateral iliac crest may review free fluid surrounding the bowel.
> - The pleural space views may be investigated to identify abnormal fluid collections in the pleural space above the echogenic diaphragm. At times, fluid that may be hemorrhagic, proteinaceous, or infectious will appear more echogenic or complex.
> - The parasternal view allows visualization of the heart.
> - The apical view may allow visualization of the pericardial fluid.
> - The inferior vena cava views may be used as supplemental FAST views to aid in the assessment of the intravascular volume status and has shown to be useful in gauging fluid responsiveness in patients requiring volume resuscitation or transfusion of blood products.
>
> *FAST*, Focused assessment with sonography.
> Adapted from http://www.aium.org.

> **• BOX 10.15** **Patient Care Interventions**
>
> Airway management
> Electrolyte and acid–base management
> Drug management
> Neurologic management
> Respiratory management
> Physical comfort promotion
> Thermoregulation
> Tissue perfusion
> Psychological comfort promotion
> Crisis management
> Risk management
> Lifespan care
> Information management
>
> *BiPAP*, Bilateral positive airway pressure.
> (From McCloskey J, Bulechek G, Butcher H.: *Nursing Interventions Classification (NIC).*, St. Louis, MO: 2008, Mosby/Elsevier; 2008.)

- A combative patient should be properly restrained, physically and/or chemically, if indicated. If chemical restraint is chosen, the transport team needs to ensure that the patient receives adequate analgesia, sedation, and environmental control during the transport.
- All monitors should be placed within the transport team's field of vision.
- When indicated, wounds and injured limbs should remain exposed for inspection.

Assessment and preparation are the foundations of patient transport. Primary and secondary assessments provide initial information about the patient's current and potential problems. Based on these assessments, the transport team initiates appropriate interventions. Box 10.15 lists some of these interventions.[65]

Patient preparation includes not only obvious care but also anticipation of what may occur. In the prehospital care environment, resources are limited and anticipatory planning, safety, and prevention are key care interventions.

Ongoing reassessment is important for all patients. It allows the transport team to maintain an ongoing awareness of the patient's condition and response to interventions.

The nature and frequency of reassessment will be dictated by the patient's condition and the length of the transport.

Federal Aviation Regulations

Air medical services must actively participate in the daily aviation operations dictated by the FAA or national and international regulations specific to the operations of the air medical service in the country of residence, as applicable, to provide safety for all patients and care providers in the air transport environment. The fixed-wing and rotor-wing air taxi certificate holders must comply with the appropriate Federal Aviation Regulations (FARs). These regulations pertain to air traffic control, airports, visual flight rules (VFRs) and instrument flight rules (IFRs), and aircraft operations.[88-92] Most air medical services must comply with the appropriate FARs, depending on who possesses the air taxi certificate.

FAR Part 91 pertains to general operating and flight rules for aircraft flying in US airspace. FAR Part 135 provides specific rules for air taxi operators and commercial operators. Most air medical services are regulated under Part 135 of the FARs and hold air ambulance operation specifications because of the nature of transporting passengers or persons for compensation or hire.[18,25,26,88] In previous years, more than half of the fixed-wing transport programs in operation possessed their own FAR Part 135 certificate.[88-92] On the basis of an audit of their membership records conducted in 2008, the Association of Air Medical Services (AAMS) stated that approximately 23% of current AAMS members have voluntarily reported holding their own Part 135 US Air Carrier Certificate for either rotor-wing operations, fixed-wing operations, or combined. A brief explanation of weather minimums, weight and balance, the term *lifeguard*, and ambient temperatures as they relate to FARs gives the transport team an understanding of how they can assist the pilot in complying with FARs and ultimately with safety.[88-92]

Weather Minimums: Visual and Instrument Flight Rules

The FARs define explicit weather minimums and rules that must be in effect for an aircraft to operate within consistent safety standards. Under FAR Part 135, air medical services operate under either VFRs or IFRs.[88-92] The pilot of a fixed-wing aircraft must comply with the appropriate rules that define flying limitations in adverse weather conditions.

The *VFRs* govern the procedures for conducting flight under visual conditions as interpreted by the pilot. *Flight visibility* is defined by the distance forward into the visible horizon, and the ceiling (vertical boundary) is the height above the ground or water to the base of the lowest (broken) layer of clouds.[88-92] FAR Part 91.155 addresses the basic VFR weather minimums that are maintained for the corresponding altitude and class airspace for all aircraft.[88-92]

The *IFRs* govern the procedures for conducting instrument flight when weather conditions do not meet the minimum requirements for flight under VFRs.[88-92] IFRs indicate that the pilot intends to navigate via instrumentation for at least a portion of the flight. Most programs that operate fixed-wing aircraft have the capability to operate under IFRs. However, IFRs pose other limitations, such as the need to land at approved airports when instrument approaches are used; compliance with restrictions for takeoff, approach, and landing minimums; and identification of a contingency plan in the event an unanticipated need arises to land at an alternate approved airport.

Weight and Balance

Weight and balance requirements are important for rotor-wing and fixed-wing aircraft as specified in the airplane or rotorcraft flight manual. The manual contains aircraft performance data regarding maximum certified gross weights, center-of-gravity limits, and runway lengths that fixed-wing aircraft use for takeoff. Because fixed-wing airplanes (depending on the model) have fewer weight restrictions and more cabin space than do rotor-wing aircraft,[88-92] family members and other persons frequently accompany patients on fixed-wing aircraft transports.

Per FAR Part 91.605, the pilot must ensure that the aircraft is always loaded within weight and balance limits.[88-92] Because the gross weight of the aircraft is predetermined by the airplane flight manual, the pilot is responsible for determining the daily operational weight, which is the weight of the aircraft, fuel, pilot, air medical personnel, and equipment. These calculations must be completed before taking off on a medical transport. Therefore when in contact with the referring facility, air medical personnel should attempt to obtain the weights of patients and persons who will ride along. The pilot can benefit from early notification of the patient's weight, especially for the patient who weighs more than 300 lb, and the weight of any additional passengers that may accompany the patient or any additional equipment that may be brought on board. The pilot has final authority for weight limitations and may decide that family members or other persons may not accompany the patient. In addition, the pilot may decide to decrease fuel loads, rearrange the seating of passengers, unload unnecessary equipment, leave behind unnecessary passengers and air medical personnel, or depart from an airport with a longer runway.

A second important weight and balance requirement is that aircraft should be loaded within the center-of-gravity range or limitations.[88-92] Once the maximal weight has been determined, the weight distribution, or where the weight is placed in an aircraft, is critical for aerodynamic performance and safety while the aircraft is in flight.[88-92] The weight must be properly loaded fore and aft of the center of gravity, per the manufacturer's airplane flight manual.

Lifeguard Status

Air ambulance services may declare *lifeguard* status for priority flights in the air traffic control system. Lifeguard affords the airplane priority when taking off or landing and should be used with extreme discretion. This status is only "intended for those missions of an urgent medical nature" (i.e., when a patient's condition is deteriorating or in full arrest) when a patient is on board or for the "portion of the flight requiring expeditious handling."[88-92] Lifeguard status is filed with a flight service station. Although landing and departing time differences are minimal at small airports, lifeguard status often achieves a tremendous time advantage at metropolitan and international airports. An air medical aircraft that is on lifeguard status may be allowed to take off or land ahead of multiple commercial and private aircraft, but this causes delays for these aircraft or extends their holding pattern time, costing thousands of dollars. Therefore an air medical service must reserve lifeguard status for those times when it is absolutely necessary. Lifeguard status does not negate the need to comply with Transportation Security Administration reporting requirements.[69,88-92]

Ambient Temperatures

Several aircraft temperature considerations should be addressed before a flight commences, because temperature can present potential problems in the air medical environment. The first consideration is the amount of time the aircraft will spend on the ground, because air conditioning or heating cannot be left on for more than a few minutes during this time unless an auxiliary power unit is used. Unfortunately, auxiliary power units are usually not available at smaller airports, in which most fixed-wing transports originate.

A second temperature consideration is evident at higher altitudes, at which the ambient temperature decreases. As the altitude increases, temperature decreases to the *tropopause,* which is the location at which the temperature reaches its lowest point and remains constant. The fuselage circumference of most air medical aircraft tends to be relatively small, and insulation of the walls is such that the walls and floor feel cool. The cumulative effect of these factors is often a cooler environment in a fixed-wing aircraft.

A third temperature consideration is encountered when descending into tropical or humid climates. On descent, windows become fogged and other types of condensation occur inside the aircraft.

Additional Considerations

Based on investigative findings of recent air ambulance aviation incidents and accidents, the National Transport Safety Board has published recommendations to enhance safe operations. Furthermore, the FAA has issued similar guidance.[88-92] Air ambulance services are encouraged to operate all flights within the regulations governing the 14 Code of Federal Regulations (CFR) Part 135 flights, including positioning flights, especially when operated with VFRs as opposed to IFRs.[88-92] *Positioning flights* refers to flights that are conducted under 14 CFR Part 91 to optimally situate the aircraft. Weather minimums and crew rest requirements differ between Part 135 and Part 91 regulations, with Part 135 requirements being more restrictive. Part 91 flights may be done with medical team members on board, but flights with patients on board must be conducted in compliance with Part 135 regulations.

The recommendations and guidance also advocate air ambulance operators to develop flight risk evaluation programs. The programs should be part of the decision-making process and provide a methodology by which risks such as inclement weather, nighttime flight operations, lack of visual cues commonly used along possible flight routes, lack of familiarity with landing zones or sites, pilot training and expertise, and compelling factors that influence the decision to take the flight are systematically evaluated before acceptance of each flight. Coupled with the flight risk evaluation program, comprehensive flight dispatch and flight-following procedures performed by personnel with aviation experience may minimize undue risks and further enhance safe operations. Furthermore, because of these recommendations, air ambulance operators are required to establish an operational control center and train specialists to evaluate operational risks and approve each flight before the pilot and team are allowed to accept the transport request. Additionally, the FAA issued guidance to operators to establish minimum guidelines for air medical resource management training. The training emphasizes the specific needs of each team member from the pilot and medical crew to the mechanics, program directors, and communication specialists.[46]

The proposed use of available technology, namely terrain awareness warning systems (TAWSs), traffic collision avoidance systems (TCASs), and night vision imaging systems (NVISs), including but not limited to night vision goggles, may greatly reduce the incidents or accidents experienced in EMS operations resulting from controlled flight into terrain. Conversely, the use of NVISs requires special training and is not considered practical in more ambient lighted areas such as populated or urban areas.[88-92] The addition of TAWS and TCAS units may be costly and weight and space prohibitive for some older airframes in operation.

Fixed-Wing Patient Transport

In fixed-wing aircraft patient transport, the transport team must pay critical attention to preflight preparation because of long periods of time typically spent on the ground and in flight. Fixed-wing aircraft transports usually entail lengthy periods of patient care; thus detailed preflight information must be obtained so that air medical personnel can make appropriate preparations for the transport. The aircraft should not depart to pick up the patient until all preflight preparations are complete. In addition to preparation for the medical aspects of the flight, the logistics and itinerary must be worked out, and any other preflight information needed by the pilots must be obtained. The transport team and pilots should collaborate in gathering this preflight information and in coordinating the entire flight to ensure appropriate safe and quality patient care.

In this section of the chapter, issues encountered by care providers in the fixed-wing transport environment are discussed. The following topics are covered: preflight preparation, federal aviation regulations, preparation for patient transport, patient "packaging," in-flight factors that influence patient care, air medical personnel resources, in-flight codes, and safety and emergency procedures. In addition, issues related to international transports and escort flights are highlighted.

Preflight Preparation

Fixed-wing aircraft flight times are usually much longer than rotor-wing aircraft flight times and may vary greatly from service to service. Fixed-wing aircraft flight times may be as brief as 40 minutes within the state or as long as 3 to 6 hours within a particular region, across the country, or across international borders. In addition, transport distances may range from 150 to 500 miles for a propeller or turbopropeller aircraft to more than 500 miles for a jet. Preplanning by air medical personnel and the pilot is necessary if the patient transport is to go smoothly.

Once the patient transfer has been confirmed by a receiving physician and facility, the transport team should begin gathering information such as physicians' names, telephone numbers, and an accurate account of the patient's diagnosis and condition. This information will, it is hoped, ensure that the skills of the air medical personnel and the medical equipment available during transport are appropriate for the anticipated medical needs of the patient. In addition, logistic information such as patient and luggage weights, the number of family members who will ride along and their weights, and the "do not attempt resuscitation" (DNAR) status of the patient must also be obtained.

Preflight preparation also entails coordination of information with the pilot and appropriate authorities (e.g., Transportation Safety Administration, Customs and Immigration, State Department, and Department(s) of Public Health).[68,69,93] Issues to be discussed should include location of airports, refueling and restroom stops, weight and balance issues, in-flight times to and from airports, ground ambulance times to referring and receiving facilities, ground unit resources, nutritional and fluid requirements, notifications needed depending on the patient condition or diagnoses, and disposal of wastes. The transport team must consider in-flight and ground times when calculating the amount of IV fluids, medications, medical supplies, and oxygen that will be needed and when checking to ensure that medical equipment is fully charged.[41,48,45,71,88-92,94-96]

Preparation for Patient Transport

Transferring and Accepting Physician and Facility

The transport team must ensure that an appropriate referral is arranged for the fixed-wing transport. Because additional time is usually available to preplan for an interfacility fixed-wing transport, the names of both the referring and the accepting physician should be documented for the transfer.

In 1985, Congress enacted COBRA, which was amended in July and November 1990. COBRA protects indigent uninsured patients from being denied access to emergency care by hospitals or from being transferred inappropriately between hospitals based on the patient's ability to pay. This legislation requires that the referring hospital assume liability for the adequacy of stabilization before transfer. COBRA also requires documentation that the receiving hospital and accepting physician have been verified before patient departure. If a transfer is necessary for a patient whose condition is not yet stabilized, COBRA states that various conditions are to be met, including the following: (1) the physician certifies in writing that, in his or her professional opinion, the benefits of the transfer outweigh the risks; (2) the transferring hospital treats the patient within its capacity, which minimizes the risks to the patient; (3) the receiving facility agrees to accept the patient and has available space and qualified personnel to provide appropriate medical treatment; (4) the transferring hospital sends to the receiving facility all medical records (copies) available at the time of transfer; and (5) the transfer is affected through qualified personnel and transportation equipment.[41,48,45,71,88-92,94-96]

The transport team must often validate transfer information from the communication center. This information must be validated because these patients are transferred from towns, cities, and states in which air medical personnel are not necessarily familiar with the hospitals and physicians involved in the transfer.

Oxygen Requirements

Determination of in-flight and ground ambulance times from the referring to the receiving facility assists the flight nurse in calculating the amount of oxygen needed to meet the needs of the patient. The transport team must ensure sufficient oxygen to deliver 1.0 FiO_2 or to operate a ventilator, if needed, for 1 to 1.3 times the entire length of the patient transport. In some patient transports, more time is

TABLE 10.5	Calculation of Oxygen Cylinder

$$Time = \frac{(Pcylinder \times CF)}{V}$$

Cylinder	Conversion Factor
D	0.16
Jumbo D	0.25
E	0.28
G	2.41
H	3.14
K	3.14
M	3.14

CF, Conversion factor; *Pcylinder*, total pressure in cylinder is 500; *V*, flow rate in liters per minute.
From Oakes D. *Clinical Practitioner's Pocket Guide to Respiratory Care.* Philadelphia, PA: Health Educator Publications; 2006.

spent on the ground than in flight. Time spent on the ground may be 90 minutes or longer. Therefore all fixed-wing aircraft should carry a portable backup oxygen tank in case the main system fails or the ground ambulance has no oxygen available. Some foreign countries do not carry oxygen in their ambulances (Table 10.5).[41,48,45,71,88-92,94-96]

Patient Medical Equipment Requirements

Air medical services are advancing fixed-wing aircraft standards by providing dedicated aircraft with custom medical configurations, which allows services to hard-mount ventilators, heart monitors, and other patient medical equipment. Equipment that is needed may be chosen based on the mission and the scope of care provided by the air medical service. For example, a service whose mission is critical care for children and adults should have appropriate transport equipment readily available. This equipment may include a heart and hemodynamic monitor, a noninvasive BP monitor, a pulse generator (if the patient's condition requires it), IV pumps, a pulse oximeter, an onboard suction device, a transport ventilator, diagnostic devices such as ultrasound and handheld blood analyzers, an isolette, and a transport intraaortic balloon pump.

With the improvement of medical transport equipment in recent years, the most critical patients who need the support of several different pieces of medical equipment may now be transported without difficulty. Transport equipment, including IV pumps, ventilators, intraaortic balloon pumps, fetal heart monitors, ECMO equipment, and other devices, has been designed and tested for the transport environment.

Medical equipment that requires battery power should also have auxiliary power capabilities that can connect to the aircraft's inverter. The transport team should verify that the inverter power source on the aircraft and ground ambulance works properly in case batteries fail. Because many ground ambulances outside the United States do not have inverters, the transport team should have enough spare batteries available to complete the transport.

A portable suction unit should also be included in the standard equipment for fixed-wing transports. This unit provides the team with backup equipment should the main suction system fail. The portable suction unit is also valuable during transport once the patient is transitioned from the aircraft to areas or vehicles without functional or compatible power sources.

Finally, transport services must comply with state licensure requirements for air medical aircraft, which include specifications about medical equipment that must be placed on the aircraft. Because these requirements vary from state to state, some aircraft may be required to carry additional equipment per state regulations.

Patient Care Supplies and Medications

The fixed-wing aircraft must be stocked with sufficient medical supplies and medications to deliver necessary patient care for the full duration of transport. The medical bags should include equipment and medications for a wide range of patient conditions and accommodate for anticipated as well as unanticipated events. For example, patient condition may require continuous nebulizer treatments during transport. If this information was available before transport, the medical team should carefully consider the need to add to their medication stock before departure, particularly if the transport period is long. However, the patient condition could deteriorate between receiving patient information before transport and on arrival. As much as reasonably possible given space constraints, the volume of medications regularly stocked should consider these possibilities. Most referring facilities are very accommodating in providing the team with additional medications needed for transport, but this cannot always be relied on because of smaller hospital medication stock limitations. For long-distance transports, supplies and medication availability (including oxygen) should be carefully calculated.

Bedding and Linens

Because fixed-wing flights involve longer periods of patient care, comfort becomes a major issue. The traditional fixed-wing aircraft stretcher pads are hard, thin, and narrow and have limited flexibility. The transport team can plan ahead and attempt to use bedding, egg crates, or blankets on top of the stretcher to provide extra padding and create a softer surface. If an air mattress is to be used, air must be able to be released to prevent the mattress from rupturing in flight because of gas expansion at higher altitudes.

In addition, the transport team may stock extra pillows and egg crates for use in supporting the head, neck, back, and knees and for positioning between knees and elbows and elevating extremities and feet. On longer flights, the team must pay greater attention to the patient's position. Patients, especially those who are comatose or paralyzed, may need to be turned to prevent skin breakdown. The patient may be placed on a "turn" or "draw sheet" so that

air medical personnel can reposition the patient more easily in flight. Passive range-of-motion exercises also decrease the risk of blood pooling, deep vein thrombosis (DVT), pulmonary embolus (PE), and additional skin injury from immobility.

The transport team should also pay attention to their own immobility on long flights. Stretching exercises and increased fluid intake can help prevent circulatory problems (see Chapter 34).

Nutrition and Fluid Requirements

Adequate nutrition and fluids should be provided for all persons on board the aircraft. Depending on the transport time and the time of day, food may be catered for the patient, family, pilots, and air medical personnel at planned refueling stops. The team must choose the proper food or provide the specialized diet (e.g., a low-fat or diabetic diet) needed by the patient. Proper storage of the food and fluids is necessary. In addition, an adequate stock of fluids, such as juice, and plenty of water for the entire length of the transport should be available. Because of the longer in-flight times, higher altitudes, and stresses of flight, the team should provide sources for replenishing energy and preventing dehydration for all persons on board the aircraft. Emphasis should be placed on taking care of oneself in addition to the patient and other passengers during the transport.

Disposal of Contaminated Wastes

All air medical personnel must comply with Occupational Safety and Health Administration (OSHA) regulations regarding occupational exposure to blood-borne pathogens.[91] The medical transport service must have an exposure-control plan. Policies, procedures, and equipment must be addressed in the plan to comply with these regulations and protect employees from infectious disease exposure. Transport personnel must follow infection control policies by observing standard precautions and stocking extra PPE, supplies, and cleaning agents for these long flights. Depending on the flight distance and in-flight patient care times, the team must plan for the containment and disposal of contaminated needles, dressings, empty IV fluid bags, and human wastes per OSHA regulations. The team must also plan for providing care and properly disposing of wastes should the patient have a bowel movement. Multiple large red isolation bags may be used to dispose of wipes, bedpans, and urinals.[97]

Medical transport personnel, pilots, and family members should plan to use restroom facilities before departure and during fuel stops. Some fixed-wing aircraft may have toilet facilities.

Required Ground Ambulance Capabilities

For fixed-wing transports, the transport team can never assume that a ground ambulance unit is available. The team must investigate the capabilities and resources of the ambulance that arrives at the airport to include safety considerations such as available fire extinguishers and access to other safety equipment. If the patient requires multiple medical devices, inverter power should be available on the ambulance to power the equipment. The transport team should also assess the resources of the ambulance service to determine whether it can provide the appropriate BLS or advanced life support (ALS) services. In some countries, no resources may be available in the ambulance, in which case *all* medical equipment with adequate battery power, medications, and oxygen needed for the patient must be provided by the transport team.

Patient "Packaging" for Transport

Preparation

Preparation of a patient for a fixed-wing transport follows along the same lines as discussed previously regarding a thorough assessment, stabilization, and preparation process. Because of the longer transport times with the associated stressors of flight, the potential to deteriorate over the length of the transport should be assessed. If risk for decompensation is considerable, the transport team should look at risk versus benefit of intervening before departure. In rare cases, such as in time-dependent conditions or when transfer is on the tarmac, the transport team may "swoop and scoop" the patient. Most of the time, however, the team performs a rapid assessment at the referring facility and initiates patient care. Thorough communication before the team's arrival and a preflight plan help minimize the amount of time spent on the ground before departure.

Loading Considerations

After ground transport to the aircraft, air medical personnel must plan to transfer the patient into the aircraft and secure the medical equipment. Because most aircraft doors are relatively narrow, the team must make the patient package as slender as possible. Many air ambulance operators have recognized patient loading and unloading guidelines with predefined team member roles for optimal patient loading. Once on the aircraft, equipment must be secured per FAA regulations and placed in a position that permits continuous assessments while maintaining tubes and catheter patency and accessibility.

Numerous manufacturers provide equipment for loading a patient into fixed-wing aircraft. Because of an increase in fixed-wing transports, these companies have developed and marketed stands, lifts, slides, and sleds to assist with loading and unloading patients through narrow fixed-wing aircraft doors. These loading devices have significantly eased the loading procedure, but more importantly, they assist with preventing excessive movement and potential injury to the patient during loading and unloading and work-related injuries for the pilot and air medical personnel.

Immobilization Equipment

Immobilization devices present unique challenges for loading a patient through a fixed-wing aircraft door and positioning the patient in the aircraft. Some aircraft doors are too narrow to accommodate standard backboards for loading patients into aircraft. For this reason, tapered backboards are suggested. The team must also prepare for patients who have other immobilization devices, such as a traction splint, in place. Loading the patient on the aircraft may be difficult because of the length of the splint. In addition, positioning the patient can present challenges, especially for transports involving greater distances and longer periods of time inside the aircraft.

Bulky dressings, splints, and the need to maintain a position of comfort for an injured extremity may make transfer of the patient smoothly through the aircraft door difficult. In addition, the patient needs to be positioned in the aircraft so that the extremity can be supported while optimal positioning is maintained and access for care is allowed.

As discussed previously, if air-filled splints are used on fixed-wing transports, the transport team must closely monitor distal circulation during flight and must be able to release air from the splint as needed to prevent patient injury because of gas expansion at higher altitudes.

In-Flight Factors That Influence Patient Care

Limited Space

Just as with rotor-wing and some ground transport vehicles, fixed-wing transport team members must consider several issues that may not be factors in rotor-wing aircraft transport. Space may vary greatly from one aircraft to another. Propeller and turbopropeller aircraft tend to be more spacious than some of the jet models, which can be extremely important when patients need large ALS equipment or immobilization devices or when family members desire to accompany the patient.

Air Conditioner and Heater

In-flight climate-control systems may not meet most caregiver expectations. The thin walls and floor of the fuselage do not allow much space for thermal insulation. Therefore the air conditioning may not adequately cool the airplane to the desired temperature on extremely hot summer days; in the winter, some aircraft cabins may still feel cool when heaters are performing at maximum capacity. During fuel stops, most aircraft are dependent on the availability of a ground power unit to maintain comfortable cabin temperatures. Measures should be implemented to monitor and manage temperature extremes to prevent untoward patient outcomes and detrimental effects on medical equipment, pharmaceuticals, and supplies.

Extended Flight Times

Fixed-wing transports may involve longer flight times than generally appreciated with helicopter transfers. The patient should be assessed for risks related to the development of DVT, PE, and pressure ulcers often experienced with extended flight exposure. The effects of altitude combined with immobility places the patient at a greater risk for these complications. For any flights that involve lengthy flight times, the transport team should initiate measures to prevent the patient's development of these conditions, such as passive range-of-motion exercises, frequent repositioning, and the use of antiembolic stocking. There are patients who may be ill or at great risk of a DVT or a PE that may require pharmacologic agents for anticoagulation during transport. These decisions should be discussed in the preflight planning of the fixed-wing transport with the medical director or the referring physician.

Diversions

Because fixed-wing transport times are often longer than other types of patient transport, the potential for diversion of the flight is increased. Diversion can be prompted by mechanical problems, weather, or even a significant deterioration in the patient's status. Contingency plans must be in place before transport to address diversion so that patient care is not jeopardized.

Air Medical Personnel Resources

One of the most critical factors for fixed-wing transports is the team's knowledge of available resources and how these resources can be accessed. The transport team must be familiar with medical control policies and procedures. Medical control may be extremely helpful to those involved with political situations, a patient whose condition is deteriorating, cardiac arrests that occur during the flight, interstate transports, and flights outside of the United States. The transport team must ensure that the air medical service has policies and procedures in place and must know how to contact the medical control to deal with these situations. In addition, the transport team must be able to access communication center resources to contact the program director, clinical supervisor, or medical director as needed to assist with patient decisions and coordination of the patient transfer in emergency situations.

Medical Control

Most air medical services receive medical control services from the medical director and the designated medical control physicians. As discussed previously, most fixed-wing aircraft flights are interfacility transports. Therefore a physician referral has been made to transfer the patient to an accepting physician and facility. Before departure from the referring facility, a nurse may contact a medical control physician via telephone to discuss a patient's medical condition and request further orders as needed. Once the team is in the ground ambulance or in flight, the opportunities for telephone communication may be limited to satellite services, two-way pagers, or less than reliable cellular services.

Communication

The transport team should be familiar with all the communication devices available to them to contact the communication center, hospitals, and EMS agencies. The team should be able to contact medical control or the receiving facility while in flight should they need medical support.

Use of flight or satellite telephones is legal during flight, whereas use of cellular telephones or two-way pagers is illegal when airborne. Flight telephones are licensed and regulated by the Federal Communication Commission. Satellite telephones use global satellites for connection rather than the traditional cellular sites. When a flight or satellite telephone is available, the transport team can contact medical control during in-flight medical emergencies.

Safety and Emergency Procedures

Safety is the number-one priority for any patient transport. In the fixed-wing aircraft transport environment, the transport team should receive initial and annual ongoing education regarding fixed-wing aircraft operations, regulations, and unscheduled aircraft emergencies. Per FAR 91.505 and 135.331, all flight crew members should receive emergency training for each aircraft type and model. Because air medical personnel are considered passengers and not flight crew, an air medical service may not provide all the crew member emergency training requirements. All air medical personnel should receive safety education in potential in-flight emergencies and procedures appropriate for each kind and model of aircraft flown, which allows the air medical personnel to understand and assist the pilot with various procedures. According to ASTNA, the ability to function appropriately in an emergency is dependent on repetitive training and education with equipment and procedures. At a minimum, education should be provided for dealing with the following emergencies: (1) fire during the flight; (2) electrical failure; (3) hydraulic failure; (4) slow or rapid decompression; (5) water ditching, if flying over water; (6) rapid egress procedures; and (7) survival procedures, survival packs, personal survival gear, and other available equipment. For further review of emergency procedures and survival, see Chapter 9.[29,94]

International Transport Issues
Air Medical Service International Transports

The discussion of air medical transport no longer focuses only on domestic transports. International transports continue to expand for patients who need medical transport between countries. Although similarities exist between domestic and international air medical transports, there are many unique differences. This section focuses on some of the issues and obstacles that may be encountered with international transports, such as preflight preparation and logistics, documentation, language barriers, patient locations, ground ambulance times and resources, pilot and air medical personnel duty times, and medical equipment and supplies.[72,73]

Preflight Preparation and Logistics

Preflight preparation is critical for international air medical transports. As with long-distance fixed-wing transports, extensive logistical planning must be completed by the entire team because of the extensive transport times. Preflight plans must include customs, immigrations, international weather briefings, landing permits, refueling stops, ground handling, international travel risk assessments, oxygen requirements, catering arrangements, medical equipment needs, and rest requirements. Inadequate preparations or failure to notify the appropriate authorities only frustrate the air medical team and create significant delays. In addition, meticulous attention should be given to obtaining as much accurate patient information as possible to prepare for the medical needs of the patient.[28,44,65,75,76] Because international transports of critically ill and injured patients may not be accomplished on commercial airlines because of patient transport restrictions, some air medical services have expanded their profile to conduct international transports. These programs have dedicated jets that are medically configured, including redundant medical equipment and systems. These jets also offer lavatory facilities and auxiliary power units for maintaining a comfortable cabin environment and charging medical equipment during the ground time portion of the transport.[72,73] Many aviation companies can assist an air medical service in preparation for international transport.

Documentation

Air medical personnel and pilots should always have the appropriate documentation for customs and immigration requirements on their person. This documentation includes passports, entry and exit visas, and immunization records for not only the destination location, but may also be required for locations traversed en route to or from the destination. International guideline charts are available to explain requirements for different countries.[72,73] The State Department can advise on the specific customs and immigration requirements for a country.

The Centers for Disease Control and WHO publish guidelines for required and recommended immunizations for each country. The patient and all accompanying passengers should also have the required customs and immigration papers. The transport company is held responsible for any fines or citations incurred from the lack of these required documents.

When planning for the flight, the appropriate documentation must also be verified for the patient and any passengers. Frequently the pilot organizes this information when filing the flight plan and making arrangements with customs.

As discussed previously, the team must document all assessment findings, care administered during the transport, and the patient's status throughout the transport as part of the medical record. Documentation must be done in a manner that allows the nurse to leave a copy of the chart with the patient when care is transferred to the receiving facility.

Language Barriers

When attempting to obtain an accurate patient diagnosis and discover the patient's medical condition and care needs,

air medical personnel may deal with language barriers from the referring facility, physician, or family members that may require the use of a translator. Many long-distance telephone companies and hospitals now offer translators fluent in multiple languages. The use of a medical professional translator is preferred. Allowing family members to provide translation is less than optimal but may be used if other options are not available. In addition, insurance companies, travel assistance companies, and air ambulance providers that coordinate these international flights often have multilingual professionals available for translating patient information.

The medical director or clinical supervisor and the transport team involved with the flight must use the necessary resources to obtain patient information that is as accurate as possible, even if this delays the transport. This information ensures that the skills of the air medical personnel and the available medical equipment are appropriate for the anticipated medical needs of the patient.

The air medical personnel must also plan for language barriers when arriving at the patient location and during the flight. An interpreter may be needed at the referring hospital or clinic to translate the medical terms, current treatment, and patient care needs.[47] In addition, the air medical personnel on the flight benefit from learning specific medical terms and words related to caring for the patient during the flight (e.g., terms related to current chest pain status and restroom needs).

Patient Location

International air medical transports may involve patients who are located not only in hospitals but also in clinics, private homes, infirmaries, first-aid stations, trailers, hotels, physician offices, cruise ships or docks, and other locations that may never have been encountered. The stability of the patient's condition on arrival may be unpredictable and the initial information provided inaccurate; therefore the transport team must be prepared for the worst-case scenario. Patients may arrive at the airport via taxi with minimal initial medical treatment. The air medical personnel may be the first ALS providers to assess the patient and should be prepared, with skills and supplies, to initiate a higher level of medical assessment and intervention.

Transport preparations should include a visit to the patient by the medical team at the referring facility before transport. This time should involve a patient evaluation, obtaining medical records, and completing final arrangements. Each team member must always practice professional courtesy and obtain permission before entering the patient care area, examining the patient, and reviewing medical records. The transport team must keep in mind that medical care and local customs may influence their approach to the patient and the referring facility.

Ground Transport Times

Preflight planning must include an accurate calculation of the distance and ground times between the patient's location and the airport and from receiving city airport to the receiving hospital.

Information such as traffic and road conditions may also be sought.[28,44,65,75,76] This information is extremely important for calculating oxygen requirements; the battery life of equipment; and necessary supplies, such as medication infusions, to safely complete the transport from starting point to end.

Ground Ambulance Resources

Whether the patient is transported to the airport or the team is transported to the patient, the resources of the ground unit may be limited. The ground transport vehicle may be a private car, a taxicab, a suburban vehicle, a travel trailer or camper, a pickup truck with a camper shell, or an ambulance unit. Some ambulances may be stripped to an empty unit with no oxygen source or suction equipment, whereas others may be elaborately stocked with supplies and medical equipment. In addition, the skills of the ambulance personnel that accompany the team and patient may vary widely, from a driver with no medical knowledge to emergency medical personnel, nurses, or physicians with varying degrees of skills.

Finally, one must consider the safety issues of the ground transport to and from the airplane. Road conditions, driving skills and compliance with traffic laws, the inability to secure equipment, and the lack of familiarity with the ground transport unit and local area by the medical team are a few of the concerns that may be faced during the ground transport. These issues contribute additional stresses to the international transport of patients (see Chapter 34 for how to manage the stresses of transport).

Pilot and Air Medical Personnel Duty Times

Duty and rest times must be considered for each international transport for the pilot and air medical personnel. This issue is already addressed for pilots because they must comply with FAR Part 135.267 flight time limitations and rest requirements.[70] Therefore during the preflight preparation, rest requirements must be calculated into the plan and arrangements made for relief pilots to assume flight duties at appropriate fuel stops or at the destination.

When making preflight preparations, air medical personnel should determine the length of the flight and patient care times and use judgment in scheduling adequate team breaks. Depending on the duty times of the flight and medical crew members, an overnight stay may be necessary to comply with crew rest and FAA requirements. This stay may involve the acquisition of lodging for each team member. Many times these arrangements are easily facilitated with use of a handling agent in the country to which the patient is transferred; this agent can assist with hotel arrangements, aircraft refueling, catering, ground transportation, and any other needs of the team.

Rest for air medical personnel may be accomplished during the flight depending on available rest areas on board the aircraft, with members of the team resting in a rotation in which the transport nurse, paramedic, physician, or other medical team member is always monitoring and managing patient status and needs. For extremely long transports, the air medical service may send a relief team of air medical personnel to a scheduled fuel stop to assume patient care. Programs should have policies that define when rests occur and when relief medical teams are required.[88-92]

Medical Equipment and Supplies

As with preflight preparations for any fixed-wing aircraft transport, the transport team must ensure that plans are complete for international transports. The transport team must be meticulous in planning and arranging for adequate oxygen, medical equipment, batteries, supplies, pharmaceuticals, bedding and linens, nutrition and fluids, and disposal of contaminated wastes. A greater potential for unexpected delays exists for these transports because of customs coordination, ambulance delays, and refueling stops. In addition, international transports may be of longer duration than other transports and to destinations with no or limited medical supplies or supplies that are incompatible with that of the air medical personnel. Therefore air medical personnel should stock enough medical supplies and medications for twice the predicted time of transport.

Many countries require special permits or have adopted specific requirements for the transport of certain medications. These requirements should be identified before the team's arrival to prevent any delays or confiscation of the medications needed to care for the patient. Medications should be kept in kits or medical packs, identified as medications needed for patient care, and never carried in the team members' personal luggage.

Finally, the compatibility of medical equipment with foreign electrical current may need to be considered. The team may need to obtain several types of foreign adapters to convert the current so that monitors and suction units can be properly charged. The equipment manufacturer should be consulted on the ability to fully charge the equipment on differing hertz, or cycles per second, of foreign electrical currents.

Escort and Medical Assist Transports on Commercial Airliners

One more form of patient transport, called a commercial medical *escort flight* or *medical assist transport,* should be discussed. Escorts may be either domestic or international transports. These transports are referred to as *commercial medical escorts.* A commercial medical escort is defined as the escort of a patient with a stable condition on a contracted aircraft or a commercial airliner with the airline's approval with only one attendant who may be an emergency medical technician (EMT), EMT-paramedic, registered nurse, or medical doctor.[46] These flights may involve transporting a patient at the BLS level who needs medical assistance, a critically ill or injured patient, or one who needs ALS or extensive nursing care.[92] The number and expertise of the accompanying attendants needed depends on the patient's condition, the ability to ambulate, and the length of the transport. In addition, when determining the medical escort team configuration, the requirements of the commercial airline must also be considered.[46]

Regarding preflight preparation and logistics for this type of transport, the transport professional should ensure that all arrangements are complete and plan to address several unique obstacles. These issues include not only commercial air carrier regulations, documentation, airline oxygen requirements, oxygen adapters, and electrical power, but also privacy, wheelchair or other assistance as needed for transfers through airports and terminals during plane changes, and accommodations during layovers or delays. Because transport of a patient on a commercial airliner requires approval of the escort by the air carrier's medical desk and coordination that is not under the control of the air medical service, these arrangements may take several days to an entire week to complete.

Commercial Air Carrier Regulations

Regulations for transporting a patient on an airliner vary, depending on the patient's designated level and condition. Many commercial air carriers allow a patient in stable condition who needs limited care to sit in the first-class or business-class section for transport.[46] With these cases, the patient must be able to sit upright during taxi, takeoff, and landing. On the other hand, transfer of a critically ill patient may necessitate the purchase of multiple seats (6–12) in the business-class section or in the rear coach compartment of the airplane so that the litter can be secured and patient can be safety restrained in a supine position during critical times of flight. Many airlines prohibit stretcher-bound patients. Most of the airliners that can accommodate patients that are unable to travel in a seated position have a dedicated patient litter that rests above the folded passenger seats and is bolted to the seat tracks.[46] Special arrangements should be made with each commercial airline because each carrier has a different patient litter, loading and securing procedures, and quantity of medical oxygen available. The transport team should plan for the logistics of these escorts to ensure that the transport is completed smoothly.

In addition, provisions must be made for transporting medical equipment and supplies in such a way that they are readily available for the patient and yet secured per the FARs. The equipment should also be organized so that it can be easily transferred and checked by customs and immigration authorities.

Documentation

Air medical personnel must organize all the paperwork necessary for the entire transport, including airline tickets, passports, itinerary, and customs documents. This documentation for the air medical personnel, patient, and family members must be readily available for customs and immigration authorities. Air medical personnel should always keep this paperwork on their person.

As with other transports, patient documentation must be completed and copies of the medical record must be left with the patient at the receiving facility.

Airline Oxygen Requirements

Each air carrier has a different procedure for obtaining oxygen and securing the oxygen tanks. The oxygen tanks routinely provided by most airlines deliver only 2 to 4 L/min. Therefore arrangements must be made to have extra oxygen tanks available for patients who require 100% O_2, a ventilator, or an oxygen concentrator. A minimum of 24 hours of notice is necessary, but frequently several days are needed to make such arrangements.[46] Many airlines charge additional fees to provide medical oxygen and may restrict the amount that can be secured because they have limited capacity to accommodate and secure larger oxygen tanks. In addition to having oxygen provisions during flight, the availability of oxygen within the terminals during layovers and plane changes must be considered. The commercial airline may not have the ability to provide oxygen outside the aircraft and gate area.[46]

Oxygen Adapters

Particular attention should be given to the oxygen adapters and regulators available on each airliner. Most of this equipment is not compatible with air medical transport ventilator fittings. In addition, oxygen flow meters are often irregular.

Electrical Power and Adapters

The commercial air carrier's electrical power sources must be assessed and coordinated to power the medical equipment to include adapters, voltage output, and amperage. A power source may be needed for transport ventilators, heart monitors, IV pumps, and suction equipment. As previously mentioned, the appropriate adapters must be obtained to convert the current in these foreign airplanes.

Privacy

Most commercial airline have various rules pertaining to patients in critical condition. Their presence may disturb or upset other passengers. Some airlines provide privacy for the patient by installing temporary curtains, but most of the time they are inadequate. Other airlines may require the patient be transported in a private medical suite.[46] Additional sheets or drapes may be necessary to provide adequate privacy for the patient.

Nonstop Flight or Flight With Minimal Plane Changes

Every attempt should be made to make reservations on a nonstop flight or to minimize the number of plane changes and layovers for the patient transport.[46] Decreasing the number of stops or delays eliminates the frustrations of making additional arrangements to get on and from the airplane, to transfer the patient, and to provide documentation for customs and immigrations officials. In addition, plans must be made to organize all the medical equipment, patient and family belongings, and luggage of air medical personnel for each transfer.

Summary

Although many general principles of practice and patient care are identical in the transport environment and process, whether by air or surface, differences do exist. The complex nature of the transport environment provides many challenges. Preparation for transport requires education and training, preplanning, and intuition. All members of the transport team must be able to deliver safe and competent patient care in the transport environment in which they practice.

References

1. Air & Surface Transport Nurses Association. *Transport Provider Advanced Trauma Course.* 6th ed. Aurora, CO: ASTNA; 2014.
2. Air & Surface Transport Nurses Association. *ASTNA Standards for Critical Care and Specialty Transport.* Centennial, CO: Cottrell Printing; 2015.
3. Air & Surface Transport Nurses Association. *Transport Nurse Safety in the Transport Environment.* Aurora, CO: ASTNA; 2015.
4. Air Medical Physicians Association. *Appropriate and Safe Utilization of Helicopter Emergency Medical Services.* Salt Lake City, UT: AMPA; 2013.
5. Air Medical Physicians Association. *Appropriateness of Medical Transport in Acute Stroke Syndromes.* Salt Lake City, UT: AMPA; 2012.
6. American Heart Association and Alterman D. Consideration in pediatric trauma. *eMedicine, Medscape J.* http://www.emedicine.com; 2015 Accessed 07.09.16.
7. American College of Emergency Physicians. *Appropriate Interhospital Patient Transfer.* Dallas, TX: ACEP. https://www.acep.org/MobileArticle.aspx?id=29114&parentid=748; 2016 Accessed 07.09.16.
8. American College of Emergency Physicians. *Interfacility Transportation of the Critical Care Patient and Its Medical Direction.* Dallas, TX: ACEP; 2012.
9. American College of Surgeons. *Advanced Trauma Life Support Program for Doctors.* Chicago, IL: ACS; 2012.
10. American College of Surgeons. *Resources for Optimal Care of the Injured Patient.* Chicago, IL: ACS; 2014.
11. American Heart Association/American Stroke Association. *Guidelines for the Early Management of Adults with Ischemic Stroke.* Dallas, TX: American Heart Association; May 2007.
12. Aoki B, McClosky K. *Evaluation, Stabilization, and Transport of the Critically Ill Child.* St. Louis, MO: Mosby; 1992.
13. Bosk E, et al. Which patients, and where: A qualitative study of patient transfers from community hospitals. *Med Care.* 2011; 49(5):592-598.
14. Burney R, et al. Evaluation of hospital based aeromedical programs using therapeutic intervention scoring. *Aviat Space Environ Med.* 1988;59:563-566.
15. Campbell J, Alson, R. *International Trauma Life Support.* 8th ed. Upper Saddle River, NJ: Pearson Prentice Hall; 2016.
16. Chalfin D, et al. Impact of delayed transfer of critically ill patients from the emergency department to the intensive care unit. *Crit Care Med.* 2007;35(6):1477-1483.
17. Continenza J, Hill K. Transport of the critical child. In: Blumer J, ed. *Pediatric Intensive Care.* St. Louis: Mosby; 1990.
18. Emergency Nurses Association. *Facilitating the Interfacility Transfer of Emergency Care Patients.* Des Plaines, IL: ENA; 2015.
19. O'Malley RJ, Watson-Hopkins M. Monitoring the appropriateness of air medical transports. *AirMed J.* 1994;13(8): 323-325.
20. Petri D, et al. Medically appropriate use of helicopter EMS: the mission acceptance/triage process. *Air Med J.* 2007;26(1): 50-54.
21. Emergency Nurses Association. *Emergency Nurse Pediatric Course (ENPC).* 4th ed. Des Plaines, IL: ENA; 2012.
22. Emergency Nurses Association. *Cultural Diversity in Emergency Care.* Des Plaines, IL: ENA; 2012.
23. Husum H, et al. Preventing post-injury hypothermia during prolonged prehospital evacuation. *Prehosp Disaster Med.* 2002; 17(1):23-26.
24. Mirvis SE. *Imaging in Trauma and Critical Care.* 2nd ed. Philadelphia, PA: Saunders; 2003.
25. Emerman C, Shade B, Kubincanek J. Comparative performance of the best trauma triage rule. *Am J Emerg Med.* 1992;10(4): 294-297.
26. Falcone RJ, et al. Is air medical scene response for illness appropriate? *Air Med J.* 1993;12(6):191, 193-195.
27. Jauch EC, Saver JL, Adams HP Jr, Adams H, Bruno A, Connors J, Demaerschalk B, et al. Guidelines for the early management of patients with acute ischemic stroke: A guideline for healthcare professionals from the American Heart Association/American Stroke Association. *Stroke.* 2013;44(3):870-947.
28. Hatlestad D, Van Horn J. Air transport of the IABP patient. *Air Med J.* 2002;21(5):42-48.
29. National Highway Traffic Safety Administration. *Guide for Interfacility Patient Transfer.* Washington, DC: NHTSA; 2003.
30. Rapsang A, Shyam D. Scoring systems in the intensive care unit: a compendium. *Indian J Crit Care Med.* 2014;18(4):220-228.
31. Sethi D, Subramanian S. When place and time matter: how to conduct safe inter-hospital transfer of patients. *Saudi J Anaesth.* 2014;8(1):104-113.
32. Surgenor S, et al. Survival of patients transferred to tertiary intensive care from rural community hospitals. *Crit Care.* 2001; 5(2):100-104.
33. Warren J, et al. Guidelines for the inter-and intrahospital transport of critically critical care. *Med.* 2004;32(1):256-262.
34. Gabram S, Piancentini L, Jacobs L. The risk of aeromedical transport for the cardiac patient. *Emerg Care Q.* 1990;2:72.
35. Holdefer WF, Treadwell D, Tolbert JT. International air medical transport, program profile. *Int Air Amb.* 1998;7:36.
36. Loos L, Runyan L, Pelch D. Development of prehospital medical classification criteria. *Air Med J.* 1998;17(1):13.
37. Brink LW, et al. Air transport, transport medicine. *Pediatr Clin North Am.* 1993;40(2):452.
38. Crippen D. Critical care transportation medicine: new concepts in pretransport stabilization of the critically ill patient. *Am J Emerg Med.* 1990;8(6):551-554.
39. Ohning B. Transport of the critically ill newborn. *eMedicine, Medscape.* http://emedicine.medscape.com/article/978606-overview; 2015 Accessed 30.10.16.

40. Ridley S, Carter R. The effects of secondary transport of critically ill patients. *Anesthesia.* 2007;44(10):822-827.

41. Sanders MJ. *Mosby's Paramedic Textbook.* 4th ed. Burlington, MA: Jones & Bartlett Learning; 2011.

42. United States Code: *Consolidation Omnibus Budget Reconciliation Act (COBRA) of 1985 (42USC139dd)*, as amended by the Omnibus Budget Reconciliation Acts (OBRA) of 1987, 1989, and 1990.

43. American College of Emergency Physicians. *EMTALA.* Available at https://www.acep.org/news-media-top-banner/emtala/; 2014 Accessed 18.08.16.

44. Hart M, et al. Air transport of the pediatric trauma patient. *Emerg Care Q.* 1986;3:21.

45. Clark K, Doyle J, Duco S, Lattimer C. *Transitions of Care: The Need for a More Effective Approach to Continuing Patient Care.* (Issue brief). Washington, DC: Joint Commission; 2012.

46. Commission on Accreditation of Medical Transport Systems (CAMTS). *Standards.* 10th ed. Anderson, SC: CAMTS; 2015.

47. Emergency Nurses Association. *Trauma nursing core course (TNCC).* 7th ed. Des Plaines, IL: ENA; 2014.

48. Association of Air Medical Services, Medevac Foundation, Survivors Network. *Air Medical Accident/Incident Preparation, Response, and Recovery: Lessons from Crash Survivors.* 1st ed. Alexandria, VA: Association of Air Medical Services; Oct 2012.

49. US Department of Transportation. *Guide for Interfacility Patient Transfer.* Washington, DC: NHTSA EMS Division; 2003.

50. Velianoff G. Overcrowding and diversion in the emergency department. *Nurs Clin North Am.* 2002;37(1):59-66.

51. American College of Emergency Physicians. *Ambulance Diversion.* Dallas, TX: ACEP; 2012.

52. Association for Medical Ultrasound. *Focused Assessment With Sonography for Trauma (FAST) Examination.* Laurel, MD: AIUM; 2014.

53. Henry M, Stapleton E. *EMT Prehospital Care.* Philadelphia, PA: Saunders; 2006.

54. McCloskey K, Orr R. *Textbook of Pediatric Transport Medicine.* St. Louis, MO: Mosby; 1995.

55. Baharuddin K, et al. Assessing patient pain scores in the emergency department. *Malays J Med Sci.* 2010;17(1):17-22.

56. Benevilli W, Thomas S, Brown D, et al. Safety of fentanyl during transport of trauma patients. *Air Med J.* 1995;14(3):156.

57. Frakes M, et al. Efficacy of fentanyl analgesia for trauma in critical care transport. *Am J Emerg Med.* 2006;24(3):286-289.

58. Mirski M, Hemstreet M. Critical care sedation for neuroscience patients. *J Neurolog Sci.* 2007;261(1):16-34.

59. Stewart R. Analgesia in the field. *Prehosp Disaster Med.* 1989; 4(1):31.

60. US Department of Health and Human Services. *Acute Pain Management: Operative or Medical Procedures.* Washington DC: USDHHS; 1992.

61. Sharp D. Flight crews' use of digital cameras. *Air Med J.* 2002; 21(5):24-27.

62. Baptiste A. Technology solutions for high-risk tasks in critical care. *Crit Care Nurs Clin North Am.* 2007;19:177-186.

63. Oakes D. *Clinical Practitioner's Pocket Guide to Respiratory Care.* Philadelphia, PA: Health Educator Publications, Inc; 2006.

64. Benson J. *FDA Safety Alert: Potential Hazards With Restraint Devices.* Rockville, MD: Food and Drug Administration; 1992.

65. Hatfield ML, Lang A, Han ZQ, et al. The effect of helicopter transport on adult patients' body temperature. *Air Med J.* 1999; 18(3):103-106.

66. York Clark D, Stocking J, Johnson J. *Flight and Ground Transport Nursing Core Curriculum.* Denver, CO: Air and Surface Transport Nurses Association; 2006.

67. Zecca, et al. Endotracheal tube stabilization in the air medical setting. *J Air Med Transport.* 1991;10(3):7-10.

68. US Department of Transportation. *Safety Alert for Operators SAFO 0600.* Washington, DC: Flight Standards Service; 2006.

69. US Transportation Safety Administration. *Standard Security Program: 3(12-5).* Washington, DC: TSA; 2007.

70. Treger R. Sengstaken-Blakemore tube placement. *eMedicine, The Medscape J.* http://emedicine.medscape.com/article/81020-overview; 2016 Accessed 30.10.16.

71. Treadwell D. *The Commercial Carry-on, Insurance Journal Supplement: 17.* Bristol, UK: Voyageur Publishing & Events LAD; 2007.

72. Holdefer WF, et al. International air medical transport, part II: results and discussion. *J Air Med Transport.* 1990;9(8):8-11.

73. Holdefer WF, Diethelm AG, Tolbert FT. International air medical transport, part I: methods and logistics. *J Air Med Transport.* 1990;9(7):6-8.

74. Holdefer WT, Treadwell D, Moore S, et al. International air medical transport ventilator dependent patients. *Int Air Amb.* 1999;9:22.

75. Harrigel DJ, Carroll M, Fanning C, Steinberg MB, Parikh A, Usher M. Interhospital transfer handoff practices among U.S. tertiary care centers: A descriptive survey. *J Hosp Med.* 2016; 11(6):413-417.

76. Hart M. Patient assessment, preparation and care. *US Department of Transportation: Air Medical Crew National Standard Curriculum.* Washington, DC: US Department of Transportation; 1988.

77. MedEvac Foundation International. *Air Medical Services: Critical Component of Modern Healthcare Systems.* Alexandria, VA: MedEvac; 2011.

78. Binks A, Pyke M. Anaesthesia in the obese patient. *Anaesth Intens Care Med.* 2008;9(7):299-302.

79. Brunette DD. Resuscitation of the morbidly obese patient. *Am J Emerg Med.* 2004;22(1):40-47.

80. Bushard S. Trauma in patients who are morbidly obese. *AORN J.* 2002;76(4):585-589.

81. Centers for Disease Control. *Defining Adult Overweight and Obesity.* Atlanta, GA: CDC; April 2012.

82. Drake D, Dutton K, Engelke M, et al. Challenges that nurses face in caring for morbidly obese patients in the acute care setting. *Surg Obesity Related Dis.* 2005;1(5):462-466.

83. Fencl J, Walsh A, Vocke D. The bariatric patient: an overview of perioperative care. *AORN J.* 2015;102(2):116-131.

84. Ide P, Farber E, Lautz D. Perioperative nursing care of the bariatric surgical patient. *AORN J.* 2008;88(1):30-58.

85. McCullough P, Silver M, Kennard E, et al. Impact of body mass index on outcomes of enhanced external counterpulsation therapy. *Am Heart J.* 2006;151(1):139.

86. Szczensiak SL. Trauma in the bariatric patient. In: McQuillan K, Makic MBF, Whalen E, eds. *Trauma Nursing: From Resuscitation Through Rehabilitation.* 4th ed. Philadelphia, PA: Saunders Elsevier; 2009.

87. Forgey WW. *Wilderness medicine: Beyond First Aid.* 6th ed. Guilford, CT: Falcon Guides; 2012.

88. Federal Aviation Administration. *Code of Federal Regulations: Title 14, Aeronautics and Space, Parts 91 and 135.* Washington, DC: US Department of Transportation; 2008.

89. Federal Aviation Administration. *Code of Federal Regulations: Subpart F 135.261-269.* Washington, DC: US Department of Transportation; 2008.

90. Federal Aviation Administration. *Code of federal regulations: subpart F 135.271-273.* Washington, DC: US Department of Transportation; 2008.

91. Federal Aviation Administration. *Public Helicopter Emergency Medical Services (HEMS) Operations Notice N 8000.318.* Washington, DC: US Department of Transportation; 2006.

92. Federal Aviation Administration. *Fact Sheet—FAA Initiative to Improve Helicopter Air Ambulance Safety.* Washington, DC: US Department of Transportation; 2014.

93. US Government Accountability Office. *Aviation Safety: System Safety Approach Needs Further Integration into FAA's Oversight of Airlines,* in Report to Congressional Requisiters. Washington, DC: US Government Accountability Office; 2005.

94. National Flight Nurses Association. *Practice Standards for Flight Nursing.* St. Louis, MO: Mosby; 1995.

95. National Transportation Safety Board. *NTSB Adopts EMS Special Investigation Report and Issues New Recommendations.* Washington, DC: NTSB; 2006.

96. Treadwell D. In case of emergency: selecting a qualified air ambulance provider. *URMIA J.* 2007;61-66.

97. US Department of Labor. *Occupational Safety and Health Administration: Occupational Exposure to Bloodborne Pathogens,* 29 CFR part 1910.1030. Washington, DC: US Department of Labor, Occupational Safety and Health Administration; 2006.

11

Airway Management

MICHAEL A. FRAKES AND DAVID J. OLVERA

COMPETENCIES

1. Describe the process of primary and secondary assessment in airway management.
2. Identify the indications for basic and advanced airway management.
3. Describe and use the universal emergency airway algorithm for airway management.
4. Identify the indications and contraindications for specific airway interventions.
5. Formulate plan to decide approach on advanced airway management.
6. Demonstrate the ability to perform alternative airway management.
7. Describe the pharmacology of advanced airway management.

Maintaining a patent airway is the first priority in patient care, and airway management may account for some of the most difficult clinical situations encountered by transport personnel. The most common errors in airway management are failures to anticipate the need for airway management and failure to prepare the patient, provider, and team for the procedure.

Although many skills and a great deal of equipment are needed for control of the airway, the essential component of the airway management skill set is critical thinking. The transport team must know when to intervene, when not to intervene, how to intervene, and how to avoid complications. Critical thinking and technical skills are developed through quality education, practice, and repetition, all of which must be developed in concert. It is foolish to practice technical skills without attention to the critical thinking and decision-making criteria that accompany their use.

Technical perspectives are woven into the critical thinking approach defined in this chapter, which will address patient and airway assessment, considerations in planning the approach to airway management, techniques to optimize preparation, strategies to optimize procedural success, and strategies to prevent procedural and physiologic complications.

Patient Assessment

The assessment associated with airway management falls into four broad categories: primary assessment, secondary assessment, indications for management, and evaluation of the patient's anatomy and physiology related to an indicated procedure. The history, mechanism of injury, and progression of illness may also provide subjective and objective data and assist the transport team in the determination of a course of action.

Primary and Secondary Assessment Surveys

All patient care begins with an evaluation of the primary assessment—ensuring that the airway is patent and that the patient is breathing adequately. If either of these conditions are not met, a basic life support intervention is life-saving. Airway patency can almost always be reestablished with basic interventions such as patient positioning, unless precluded by injury involving the cervical spine, by the use of a suction device, and by the use of oral and/or nasal airway adjuncts. Patients who have a patent airway but inadequate or ineffective spontaneous ventilations should have ventilatory assistance with some kind of a bag-valve-mask (BVM) device, such as a self-inflating or a flow-inflating bag. Those who require basic life support interventions for their airway or breathing for more than a few minutes will almost always require more advanced interventions for longer-term management. The circulatory portion of the primary survey can also offer useful information because skin color, temperature, moisture, and the heart rate can suggest hypoxia or shock states.

The secondary survey can provide anatomic and physiologic indications that may indicate the need for an intervention, even in the face of a satisfactory primary examination. Look again at color; pallor, rather than cyanosis, is an indicator of shock. Sympathetic nerve stimulation causes blood to shunt from minor to major organs, and the skin is considered a minor organ. Cyanosis does not occur until approximately 5 g of hemoglobin per 100 cc of capillary blood is deoxygenated.[1] This makes cyanosis a late indicator of hypoxia, although an earlier one in patients with profound anemia. Like pallor suggests shock from decreased peripheral perfusion, mental status change suggests decreased oxygen delivery to the brain. Patients with mental status changes should be presumed to have a brain oxygenation defect until it is ruled out.

Working caudally, inspect the neck for obvious injuries and for an expanding hematoma, edema, and jugular vein distention. Palpate for subcutaneous emphysema and the position of the trachea. Look at the patient, the neck, and the chest for the use of accessory muscles, nasal flaring, and the position the patient assumes. Auscultation identifies absent or decreased breath sounds, which suggest pneumothorax, hemothorax, other effusion, obstruction, infection, or consolidation. Auscultation may also reveal grunting, wheezing, or stridor. Upper airway problems usually involve a barking cough or strider, whereas wheezing and grunting breath sounds are associated with lower airway disease or obstruction. Adventitious breath sounds provide indications about pathology in lower airway structures and lung parenchyma.

Palpate the chest wall for tenderness, crepitus, subcutaneous air, and symmetry of movement. Particularly in noisy environments, palpation can help identify equal rise and fall of the chest. Percussion, like palpation, can provide excellent information about the status of the underlying thoracic structures. The normal lung sound is resonant, a hemothorax is dull, and a tension pneumothorax is hyperresonant.

When evaluating the airway, consider the anticipated clinical course of the patient: Is the patient maintaining his or her airway? Will the patient be able to maintain it during transport? Is there a chance that the mechanism of injury or illness will lead to a need to intervene during transport? Also consider the range of resources and expertise available at the present location, at nearby locations, and during the transport. At times it may be reasonable to seek assistance with a difficult or potentially difficult airway from the resources at a local hospital before proceeding with airway interventions at the scene or before beginning transport.

Indications for Airway Management

The indications for airway management, whether noninvasive or invasive, can be generally summarized as "five Ps":

- Protection of the airway: Indication for patients who do not have adequate protective airway reflexes to manage secretions. Classically, these are patients who cannot swallow, follow basic commands, or who have a Glasgow Coma Score that has dropped below 9 from their original baseline of a normal score.
- Positive pressure: Indication for patients with insufficient ventilatory effort.
- Partial pressure of oxygen (PO_2): Indication for patients who will benefit from a higher FiO_2 or mean airway pressure to maintain a saturation above 93% or, in rare circumstances, whatever higher target is required. Additionally, when a patient is in shock, an imbalance exists

between oxygen supply and demand. As oxygen consumption increases linearly with work of breathing and respiratory efficiency declines as the work of breathing increases, external ventilator support can reduce that oxygen demand while increasing oxygen delivery. Particularly in patients with septic or hypovolemic shock, early intubation may be extremely beneficial.[2]
- Pulmonary toilet: Indicated when it is necessary to access the airway to remove blood, secretions, infection, or foreign bodies.
- Patient progression: Indicated for patients who are likely to develop difficulties with protection, effort, oxygenation, or ventilation during the course of the transport.

For the transport provider, a sixth "P," protection, may also be a factor. The management of aggressive behavior in the transport environment, particularly the air transport environment, may necessitate the use of sedation so deep that it leads to respiratory depression or the inability to protect an airway.

Physical Examination in Anticipation of a Procedure

When the goal of airway management interventions is to improve the patient's hemodynamic and physiologic status, it is important not to cause deterioration in oxygenation, ventilation, or vital signs. Accordingly, if the primary and secondary examinations suggest the need for intervention in the airway, the third critical phase of the patient assessment is for factors that suggest the potential for difficulty or complications with the airway management procedure, physiology, or postprocedure management.

A number of mnemonics can help remember factors that are associated with difficulty in performing various basic and advanced procedures.

Difficult Bag-Valve-Mask Ventilation: ROMAN

R: Radiation/restriction. The term *stiff lungs* refers to patients who have difficulty and resistance in ventilation and require high-ventilation pressures. These patients usually have airway obstruction or reactive airway disease. More commonly it is noted that patients with chronic obstructive pulmonary disease (COPD), acute respiratory distress syndrome, advanced pneumonia, or term pregnant patients are susceptible to stiff lungs. It can also be noted if a patient snores when they sleep or has sleep apnea, which could result in difficulty with ventilation.

O: Obesity/obstruction/obstructive sleep apnea. Patients who are obese (body mass index [BMI] >26 kg/m^2) are often difficult to ventilate adequately by bag and mask. Women in their third trimester of pregnancy also can have an increase in body mass. Both types of patients could lead to decreased compliance in bag-valve ventilation. Similarly, obstruction caused by angioedema, Ludwig angina, upper airway abscess, epiglottis, and other similar conditions will make BVM more difficult.

M: Mask seal/male sex/Mallampati. Consider facial features such as bushy beards, blood, and disruption of the facial anatomy as issues that may cause difficulty providing a proper mask seal. Both male sex and a Mallampati class 3 or 4 airway can appear also to be independent predictors of difficult BVM. The Mallampati score describes the ability to see structures in the oropharynx. Classically, the patient sits up, opens the mouth maximally, and protrudes the tongue maximally without phonating. In a class I airway, the soft palate, uvula, fauces, and tonsillar pillars are visible. In a class II airway, the tonsillar pillars disappear, but the soft palate, uvula, and fauces are visible. In a class III airway, only the base of the uvula and soft palate are visible. In a class IV airway, none of the soft palate is visible. The Mallampati classes are illustrated in Fig. 11.1.

A: Age. Diminishing muscle tone with advancing age, particularly over age 55, can lead to difficulty in bag mask ventilation. Pediatric patients under 3 can also be considered difficult because their muscle tone has not yet fully developed.

N: No teeth. It may be difficult to provide a proper seal on edentulous patients because of diminished structure of the airway. If a patient has dentures, consider leaving the dentures in place during application of BVM and removing them for instrumentaiton.[3]

Difficult Direct Laryngoscopy: LEMONS

L: Look externally. Evaluate normal face and neck anatomy, face and neck pathology, face shape, sunken cheeks, protruding front teeth, and a receding mandible. Include an evaluation for a beard, which reduces the ability to get a seal for mask ventilation, and consider neck circumference. Increasing neck circumference is an independent predictor of intubation difficulty, the risk of which increases from about 5% with a 40-cm neck to 35% with a 60-cm neck.[4]

E: Evaluate the 3-3-2 rule. Direct laryngoscopy (DL) requires the ability to line up oral, pharyngeal, and laryngeal axes, and the 3-3-2 rule identifies patients in whom the ability to achieve that alignment is more likely to be difficult. Patients should be able to place three of their own fingers between the upper and lower incisors of a fully opened mouth, three fingers along the mandible from the tip of the chin posteriorly, and two fingers from the laryngeal prominence to the floor of the mouth.

M: Mallampati score. The Mallampati score describes the ability to see structures in the oropharynx. Intubation is typically not difficult in class I and class II airways. In a class III airway, DL is predicted to be moderately difficult. In a class IV airway, DL is unlikely to be successful (see Fig. 11.1).

O: Obstruction. Evaluate for potential mechanical obstruction from a foreign body, tumor, swelling, expanding hematoma, or abscess.

N: Neck mobility. The neck should flex freely and the head should extend freely so the patient can assume the classic sniffing position.

S: Saturation. Attempting to preoxygenate or maintain saturations above 93% during intubation attempt.[3]

Difficult Extraglottic Device: RODS

R: Restricted mouth opening. Ensuring the patient can open the mouth enough to allow access of rescue device.

O: Obstruction/obesity. Assess if it is possible to pass the extraglottic device into the mouth to allow adequate oxygenation or if there is an obstruction caused by increased extraglottic tissue.

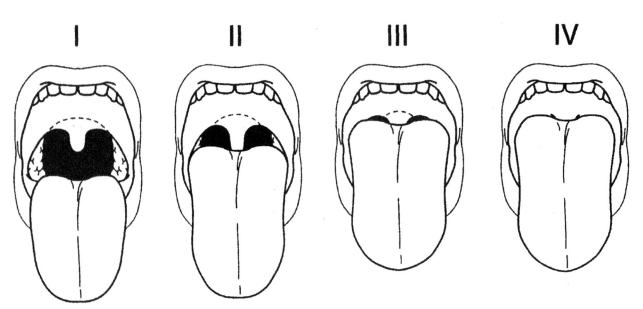

I   **II**   **III**   **IV**

• **Fig. 11.1** Mallampati classes. (From Karan SB, Bailey PL. *Techniques in Gastrointestinal Endoscopy.* St. Louis, MO: Elsevier; 2004.)

D: Disrupted/distorted airway. When placing the extraglottic device, will it be able to be seated in a correct manner or is the airway disrupted or distorted?

S: Stiff lungs. Is there a resistance to ventilation caused by airway resistance (asthma, COPD) or issues with pulmonary compliance?[3]

Difficult Cricothyrotomy: SMART

S: Surgery (recent or remote). After surgery it could be noted that the anatomy might not be in correct alignment, and it might be difficult to find landmarks. Another consideration is the scar tissue after surgery; it might be more difficult to access the membrane.

M: Mass. A hematoma or mass over the cricothyroid membrane might make access to the surgical airway more difficult.

A: Access/anatomy. With populations having increasing BMI it is noted that identifying landmarks might become more difficult because of the extra tissue. Other challenges might include a patient wearing a C-collar or a patient with a short neck.

R: Radiation (and other deformity or scarring). A patient with a history of radiation may have distortion and scarring.

T: Tumor. Access to the airway either from outside or inside the airway when a tumor is present can lead to increased bleeding and difficulty identifying landmarks.[3]

These preparation guidelines can be helpful memory aids and triggers. At the same time, the accuracy of any prediction rule for difficult airway management is limited. Even among professional anesthesia providers, 93% of patients with difficult airway were unanticipated, and some of the rules can be difficult to apply in emergency situations.[5,6] It is most prudent to approach each patient with the idea that the airway will prove to be difficult.

Physiologic Examination and Considerations Associated With Airway Management

The assessment must include not only physical findings associated with technical procedures but also factors suggesting peri-intubation physiologic deterioration. Three classic physiologic risk factors should be considered in airway evaluation and preparation: hypoxia, hypotension, and severe metabolic acidosis.[7] Additionally, patients who have complex cardiovascular physiology that affects right ventricular function (such as chronic pulmonary hypertension, massive pulmonary embolism, or right-sided myocardial infarction) or patients with altered cardiac anatomy from repair of congenital heart defects will require particular thought and care in the development of an induction and intubation plan.

Hypoxemia

Hypoxemia is a failure to maintain adequate arterial oxygenation and often represents one of the triggers for both invasive and noninvasive airway management. Intubation, particularly intubation facilitated by medications that suppress spontaneous ventilation, creates a risk for desaturation. The goal is to prolong the duration of the safe period of hypoventilation before desaturation below a peripheral oxygen saturation (SpO_2) of 90%. It is impossible to predict how long the period of desaturation will last. In patients with hyperdynamic conditions, with high oxygen demands, or with poor oxygen delivery capabilities, hypoxia develops more quickly. Children normally have twice the metabolic demand of adults, along with a smaller reserve capacity, so they commonly desaturate more quickly than adults, as do pregnant women and patients with a higher BMI.

Patients who are about to have invasive airway management procedures performed on them should have optimal preoxygenation before the procedure begins and should have passive oxygenation throughout the procedure. Raising the head of the bed 30 degrees during ventilation helps with oxygenation, and any patient requiring ventilatory support or being prepared for airway management should have head elevation. Even a trauma patient on a backboard can be placed in reverse Trendelenburg position. Physiologically, head elevation lowers the gastric bubble below the cardiac sphincter, increases functional residual capacity (FRC), improves dynamic compliance by removing weight from the chest, and increases lung volumes. Almost 50% of lung volume is lost when the patient is laid flat.[7,8]

With the patient's head elevated, apply high-flow oxygen through a tight-fitting face mask with high-flow oxygen to maximize the oxygen saturation, partial pressure of oxygen, and exchange nitrogen in the residual capacity of the lungs for oxygen. In light of this, preoxygenation should get the SpO_2 as close to 100% as possible and ideally persists for at least 3 minutes. Remember that it is possible to preoxygenate many patients who have reduced ventilation if there is effective tidaling, and positive-pressure ventilation (PPV) may not be required.[7,8]

For patients whose oxygen saturation cannot be raised above 93% with supplemental oxygen, consider the use of positive pressure through a continuous positive airway pressure (CPAP) or bilevel positive airway pressure (BiPAP) device or with a bag-valve device. If positive pressure is used, there should be at least 5 cm H_2O of positive end expiratory pressure in the system for any positive-pressure device.[8] Some experts suggest the use of a "delayed-sequence" intubation technique, in which sedation improves the ability to use positive pressure to improve saturation before an airway procedure.[7] In planning such an approach, pay attention to the patient's protective airway reflexes; inadequate airway protection is an indicator for invasive airway management and a contraindication to noninvasive ventilation.[2,8]

At the start of the invasive airway procedure, begin passive oxygenation. This technique, first described more than 50 years ago and well known to critical care practitioners in conjunction with brain death examinations, capitalizes on the ability of hemoglobin to take up oxygen by diffusion. Even without lung expansion, oxygen diffuses into the blood at least 12 times as fast as carbon dioxide accumulates in the alveoli. Extension of this concept to emergency intubation can prolong the duration of safe hypoventilation without desaturation. The requirements for oxygen uptake are a patient airway for oxygen delivery and a high oxygen concentration gradient. For emergency intubation, the easiest method is to place a nasal cannula on patients during their preparation for intubation and to begin 15 L/min of oxygen flow through the cannula as the patient becomes obtunded.[8]

During the procedure it is important monitor pulse oximetry continuously. Airway procedures must be aborted before the patient desaturates below 93% and the patient is reoxygenated with a positive-pressure device. Remember that the value of pulse oximetry is a lagging indicator; finger pulse oximetry reflects oxygen saturation changes by a mean of about 2 minutes after arterial blood gas samples change in healthy patients. Probe location, physiologic state, and body temperature affect the delay.[9]

Hypotension

Approximately 25% of patients develop transient hypotension after emergent intubation and transition to PPV.[10] Sedative and anxiolytic medications as well as many induction agents have vasodilatory and negative inotropic qualities, and the conversion from negative pressure (spontaneous) to PPV changes preload and afterload.

Patients should be evaluated for current hemodynamic stability and their risk for postprocedure deterioration. In particular, make an effort to make the patient euvolemic and be prepared to administer a crystalloid fluid challenge. An elevated shock index may help identify patients at risk for intraprocedure hypotension who will benefit from volume administration.[7,11-13] If the patient has a tenuous blood pressure or cardiac function, it makes sense to have a vasopressor infusion such as norepinephrine prepared: mixed, on an infusion pump, and attached to a functional intravenous (IV) therapy for immediate use, or perhaps even running at a very low dose before administering the induction agents.

In a practice extrapolated from the operating room (OR), in which most induction agents and vapor anesthetics are vasodilators, some nonanesthesia providers will use so-called "push-dose pressors" to temporarily stabilize hemodynamics in the peri-intubation patient. The practice is well discussed in popular literature but not well reported in the scientific literature. There is little doubt that small IV doses of epinephrine or phenylephrine will most often improve blood pressure, both through vasoconstriction and epinephrine by increasing heart rate and contractility.[14-16]

The approach and timing appear to be nonstandardized.[14] The individualized approach, unfamiliar dilutions and doses, and need for providers to dilute the agents themselves create some patient safety risk that teams considering implementation should address.[14,16] Bolus doses of infusion agents are indicated for transient hypotension related to the properties of induction agents. They are no substitute for adequate preprocedure preparation or for the appropriate use of continuous infusion vasopressor agents.

Severe Metabolic Acidosis

For patients with severe metabolic acidosis, one of the physiologic compensatory mechanisms is hyperventilation. Accordingly, the period of hypoventilation associated with a medication-assisted intubation can disrupt that compensatory effort, as can careless postprocedure ventilator management. In these patients, it may be reasonable to avoid intubation, if possible, or to intubate the patient while maintaining spontaneous respiration. Once the patient is intubated, postprocedure management must include a minute ventilation that matches the preintubation ventilation volume.[7]

Intervention

Basic Life Support Airway Interventions

In patients with a history of trauma, all airway interventions must be performed with consideration of the cervical spine. The airway should be opened, all blood or emesis suctioned, and foreign bodies removed. The need for ready access to a working suction machine throughout transport cannot be overemphasized. The tongue may be displaced from the oropharynx through placement of an airway adjunct or use of a modified jaw thrust. If the patient's mandible is not intact, the tongue can be protracted directly.

The addition of a simple mechanical adjunct can maintain the patient's airway. When properly positioned, both oral and nasal airways rest in the lower posterior pharynx and can improve the effectiveness of mask ventilation or free the provider to perform other activities. The appropriate size for both oral and nasal airways is obtained by comparing the length of the airway device with the distance from the nares or mouth to the angle of the mandible (Figs. 11.2 and 11.3).

In patients with intact airway reflexes, placement of either device may precipitate vomiting, gagging, or laryngospasm. An incorrectly placed oropharyngeal airway may worsen airflow or create an airway obstruction where none existed that is created by the tongue being pushed posteriorly against the pharyngeal wall or the epiglottis being pushed against the laryngeal opening.

Nasopharyngeal airways may be used in patients with marginal stupor or coma who need assistance in maintaining an open airway and cannot tolerate an oral airway, but it should be avoided for any patient with suspected head or facial trauma.[17] Selection of the appropriate size of nasal airway is important because traumatic insertion may cause severe epistaxis or adenoid bleeding, especially in children. Lubricant use facilitates insertion, and the airway is initially placed with the beveled edge along the nasal septum. When the left nostril is used, the nasopharyngeal airway must be inserted upside down to maintain the beveled edge against the septum and then rotated once the airway tip is in the

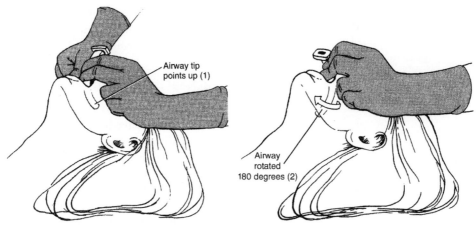

Airway tip
points up (1)

Airway
rotated
180 degrees (2)

• **Fig. 11.2** Insertion of oropharyhgeal airway. (From Lynn-McHail D, Carlson K, editors. *AACN Procedure Manual for Critical Care,* ed 4. Philadelphia, PA: Saunders; 2001.)

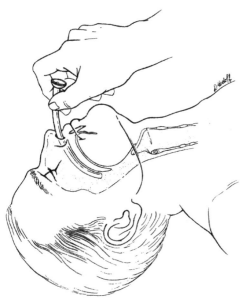

• **Fig. 11.3** Correct placement of nasopharyngeal airway. (From Proehl J. *Emergency Nursing Procedures,* 4th ed. Philadelphia, PA: Saunders; 2009.)

posterior pharynx. If significant resistance is met, the other nostril should be tried. In a nonfacial trauma patient, the tip of the nose can be lifted to allow for direct passage of the nasopharyngeal airway.

Proper position for both adjuncts must be confirmed with assessment of airflow and efficacy of ventilation. Breath sounds must be assessed after placement to ensure airway patency has not been compromised; likewise, head position must be optimized to ensure obstruction has not occurred. Where indicated, the cervical spine must be protected.

For patients with hypoxia, provide supplemental oxygen to achieve saturations above 93%. Good BVM skills are essential for the transport professional. Ventilatory assistance is indicated for patients with apnea, severe hypoventilation, or for patients who need positive pressure to improve saturation. Delivered tidal volumes vary with bag type, hand size, and patient body characteristics; the transport team must evaluate the effectiveness of BVM ventilations. The addition of an oral or nasal airway improves the effectiveness of manual ventilation, and placement is a mandatory step in the process of using a BVM on any patient in whom use is not contraindicated. Again, raising the head of the bed 30 degrees during ventilation helps with oxygenation and ventilation. Any patient requiring ventilatory support or being prepared for airway management should have head elevation. Pulse oximetry should be available to aid in oxygen desaturation detection, and if end-tidal CO_2 capnography is available, a regular waveform with exhalation should be noted.

The ROMAN mnemonic, described earlier, identifies patients who are at risk for being difficult to ventilate with a BVM device. Additionally, in patients who are edentulous, leaving the teeth in place to give the cheeks structure and then removing them just before intubation often aids ventilation. After BVM ventilation is begun in a patient with the head elevated and an oral or nasal airway in place, evaluate for effective chest rise. If there is no effective chest rise, or if there is persistent or new desaturation, the mnemonic MR. SOPA describes interventions to improve the effectiveness of mask ventilation:

M: Mask is tightly applied to the face
R: Reposition the head into the "sniffing" orientation
S: Suction the nares and the pharynx
O: Open the mouth
P: Pressure of PPV can be increased to a maximum of 40 cm H_2O
A: Alternate airway plan and consideration.[18]

Proceed to two-person BVM technique if the effectiveness of manual ventilations is in doubt. One or two providers can maintain a proper mask seal while another squeezes the bag reservoir. The use of the thenar eminence or two-hand technique may be useful (Fig. 11.4). This technique is achieved by placing the thenar eminence of the hand on the mask, wrapping the mask on the face, and then placing the fingers

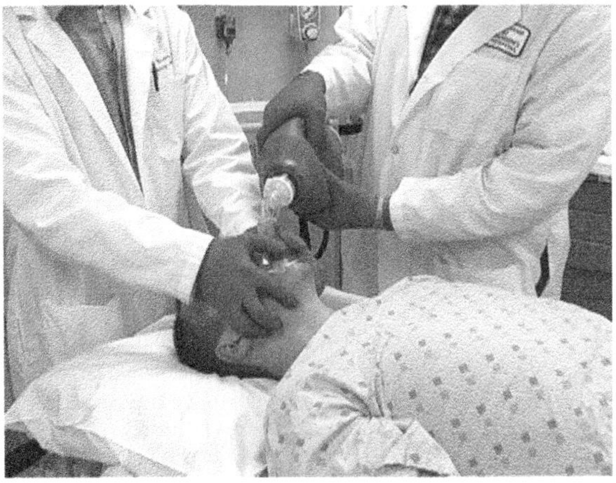

• **Fig. 11.4** The two-hand thenar eminence technique of bag-mask-ventilation. (From Reardon RF, Mason PE, Clinton JE. *Clinical Procedures in Emergency Medicine*. Philadelphia, PA: Elsevier; 2010.)

under the prominent line of the jaw, avoiding any soft tissue because it might occlude the airway.[19]

Advanced Airway Management Techniques

Although intubation is a life-saving procedure, it is not without the potential for the development of serious complications. These include soft tissue injuries to the mouth, dental injury, vocal cord injury, tracheal injury, endotracheal tube (ETT) misplacement, aspiration, pneumothorax, cardiac dysrhythmias, vital sign deterioration, and hypoxia. Complications can also occur with the use of neuromuscular blocking agents (NMBAs), anxiolytics, and sedative hypnotics that are used to facilitate intubation.[20]

The use of a checklist in high-stakes operations is a well-proven strategy to improve safety. In medicine, checklists have improved the safety and reduced complications for various procedures in various settings.[21,22] The risk of an intubation-related complication for patients intubated in the emergency department (ED) is approximately 12%.[23] Although a number of factors to consider in predicting difficulties in airway management have been described, predicting difficult mask ventilation and intubation is a fool's errand. Even among professional anesthesia providers, 93% of patients with difficult airway were unanticipated, and only 25% of those predicted were actually difficult.[6] Accordingly, particularly in the emergency and transport environments, where ad hoc teams come together at critical times, the use of a preintubation checklist to aid in team and equipment preparation is intuitively a best practice. In the limited available literature, the use of a checklist improved preparation and reduced patient complications by up to 84%, without increasing preparation time or time to intubation.[24,25]

Development of a checklist is a complicated venture and likely will need to be individualized to each practice group. Generally, factors related to preparing primary and backup equipment, primary and backup medication and procedure plans, preparing the patient physiologically, reviewing team roles, and reviewing critical decision points should be included.

Tracheal Intubation
Anatomy

Intubation of the trachea is considered the gold standard for artificial airway support, providing protection against aspiration, allowing for controlled ventilation, and offering a method of emergency drug administration. In addition, intubation protects the airway in situations of potential upper airway closure from the progression of processes such as epiglottitis, airway burns, soft tissue trauma, or infections. Orotracheal intubation is the most common method of invasive airway management for all age groups. The procedure requires finesse and psychomotor skills.

Few, if any, true contraindications to orotracheal intubation exist in the emergency setting. However, circumstances that create challenges to effective mask ventilation are relative contraindications. Similarly, conditions that will make a surgical airway difficult should give the transport team pause before inducing hypoventilation or apnea in a patient for intubation.

Endotracheal intubation is generally successful, with variability linked to context. The incidence of failed intubation is about 1 per 2000 in elective surgery, 1 per 300 in obstetric anesthesia, and under 1 per 100 in the ED.[23,26] The Ground Air Medical Quality Transport Quality Improvement Collaboration collects information specific to critical care transport and reports intubation, ventilation, and airway management performance data.[27,28]

The ability to perform advanced airway maneuvers begins with knowledge of normal anatomy. Endotracheal intubation entails manipulation of the anatomy to allow passage of an ETT through the larynx. An understanding of the relationship of the cartilage of the larynx and its relative position helps with faster and more confident intubation. This knowledge is especially important when structures are only partially visible or are displaced as a result of injury. Familiarity with the anatomic differences between the adult and pediatric airway is also helpful.

The larynx, or voice box, is an intricate arrangement of nine cartilages, three single and six paired, connected by membranes and ligaments and moved by nine muscles. From above, it attaches to the hyoid bone and opens into the laryngopharynx, and on the inside it is continuous with the trachea. In an adult it extends from the level of the fourth to the sixth cervical vertebrae.

The three single cartilages—the thyroid cartilage, cricoid cartilage, and the epiglottis—form the basic boxlike structure of the larynx and provide the major external landmarks. The thyroid cartilage, commonly known as the Adam's apple, is formed by the fusion of two curving cartilage plates and is typically larger in men than in women because of the growth-stimulating influence of male sex hormones during puberty. The ring-shaped cricoid cartilage is sandwiched between the thyroid cartilage above the first tracheal ring and connected to the thyroid cartilage by the cricothyroid membrane. That membrane is the desired location for a cricothyrotomy.

The upper free edge of the cricothyroid membrane forms the vocal cords. Because of the attachment of the vocal cords to the cricoid ring and the cricoid ring to the thyroid cartilage, external laryngeal manipulation (ELM) may help bring the vocal cords into view during intubation. The Sellick maneuver (posterior pressure on the cricoid cartilage designed to occlude the esophagus and prevent aspiration) is a part of medical history. Sellick's original study was a nonrandomized case series of head-down patients.[29] There is no evidence clearly demonstrating a benefit or a harm in the routine use of cricoid pressure to prevent regurgitation or aspiration.[30,31]

The third single cartilage is the epiglottis, which is a spoon-shaped structure that lies directly over the glottic opening and prevents anything other than air from entering the tracheal inlet. The epiglottis is the major visual landmark for performance of tracheal intubation (Figs. 11.5–11.7).

The most important paired cartilages of the larynx are the arytenoids. They are pyramid shaped and anchor the vocal cords in the larynx. The remaining two pairs of cartilages, the cuneiform and corniculate, form the posterior wall of the larynx. Committing these structures to memory assists the laryngoscopist in quickly identifying the glottic opening; when the opening is obscured from view, the ETT can be steered into position with the structures in view as reference points.

The vocal cords look pearly white because of their avascular nature. At rest, the vocal cords lie partially separated or abducted. Excessive secretions or aspiration stimulate the airway and activate the defense reflexes. Laryngospasm, or spasmodic closure of the vocal cords, is the most severe form of airway closure and can totally prevent ventilation and the passage of an ETT. If a tube is forced through the cords with excessive pressure, an arytenoid can be dislocated and permanent hoarseness can result.

Cormack and Lehane quantified the ability to visualize the glottic opening during laryngoscopy (Fig. 11.8). In the Cormack-Lehane scale, grade I is visualization of the entire glottic opening, grade II is just the arytenoids cartilages or posterior glottic opening, grade III is only the epiglottis, and only the tongue is visible in grade IV. Grade I and II views are associated with high intubation success rates, and grade III and IV views are linked with lower success rates.

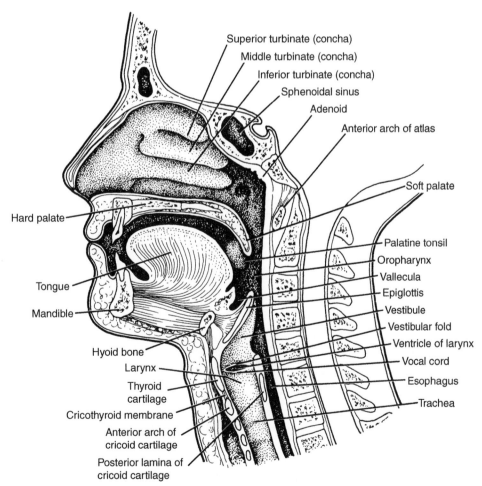

• **Fig. 11.5** Sagittal view of airway. (From Rosen P, et al. *Emergency Medicine: Concepts and Clinical Practice,* vol 1, 2nd ed. St. Louis, MO: Mosby; 1988.)

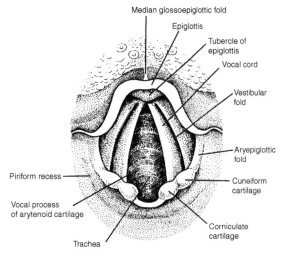

• **Fig. 11.6** Laryngoscopic view of airway. (From Rosen P, et al. *Emergency Medicine: Concepts and Clinical Practice,* vol 1, 2nd ed. St. Louis, MO: Mosby; 1988.)

Median glossoepiglottic fold
Epiglottis
Tubercle of epiglottis
Vocal cord
Vestibular fold
Aryepiglottic fold
Cuneiform cartilage
Corniculate cartilage
Trachea
Vocal process of arytenoid cartilage
Piriform recess

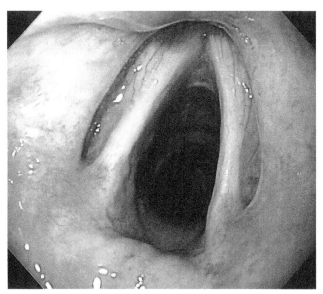

• **Fig. 11.7** View of the vocal cords. (From Wilcox MD. *Atlas of Clinical Gastrointestinal Endoscopy,* 3rd ed. Philadelphia, PA: Saunders; 2012.)

Other operators simply describe the percent of glottic opening that is visible during the laryngoscopy.[3]

Potential Complications

Complications of oral and nasal endotracheal intubation can be both significant and disastrous (Box 11.1). The need for first-pass success is imperative because the incidence of airway and hemodynamic adverse events correlates with the number of intubation attempts. Even a second attempt at intubation can increase the complication rate close to 47%, and the rate rises to 63% with a third attempt. The American Society of Anesthesiologists Task Force on the Management of the Difficult Airway suggests limiting laryngoscopic attempts to three.[20,32] Other experts suggest that a fourth attempt by a more experienced colleague is permissible.[33] It is interesting that self-reported rates of airway management complications underreport those confirmed by direct observation of the procedure.[34]

Unsuccessful intubation or a missed inadvertent esophageal intubation may lead to prolonged hypoxia and result in long-term injury or death. Oxygenation must be maintained throughout airway management attempts, and other means of oxygenation and ventilation must be used if a patient cannot be intubated. Intubation predisposes the patient to a number of harmful physiologic responses, including laryngospasm, bronchospasm caused by airway irritability or aspirated secretions, hypertension, and dysrhythmias unrelated to hypoxia.[20] The stimuli of DL and endotracheal intubation produce a sympathetic response that increases mean arterial pressure above baseline by up to 44%, heart rate by up to 36%, and intracranial pressure (ICP) by up to 22 mm Hg.[35,36] Unrecognized right mainstem bronchus intubation is a complication that may lead to inadequate ventilation and left lung atelectasis. Trauma to the teeth, soft tissues of the mouth, posterior pharynx, or vocal cords caused by improper use of the laryngoscope blade or by forcing an ETT is a complication of oral intubation.

The safety of inline immobilization of the trauma patient's cervical spine with a gentle laryngoscopy is well established. Once the patient has become properly obtunded with pharmacologic agents, have an assistant hold the cervical spine

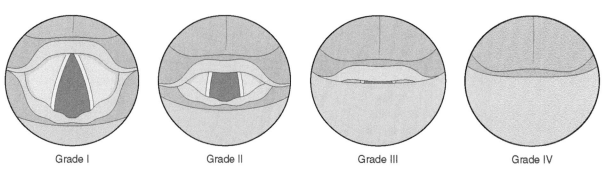

Grade I   Grade II   Grade III   Grade IV

• **Fig. 11.8** Cormack Lehane grades. (From Miller RD, Pardo M. *Basics of Anesthesia,* 6th ed. Philadelphia, PA: Saunders; 2012.)

• BOX 11.1   Complications of Intubation

Early Complications That Occur During the Intubation Procedure

1. Neck

Cervical strain: subluxation/dislocation, fracture, and neurologic injury

2. Mouth

Soft tissue injury that results in abrasion and hemorrhage involving lips, tongue, buccal mucosa, and pharynx

Temporomandibular joint subluxation/dislocation

Dental injury

3. Airway/respiratory

Arytenoid: dislocation and avulsion

Vocal cord: spasm, avulsion, and laceration

Pyriform sinus perforation that results in pneumothorax and pneumomediastinum

Tracheal and bronchial rupture

Right mainstem bronchus intubation, with atelectasis and respiratory compromise

Bronchospasm

4. Gastrointestinal

Esophageal: intubation and perforation

Vomiting and aspiration

5. Cardiovascular

Hypertension, tachycardia, bradycardia, and dysrhythmias

Cardiac arrest and interruption of CPR

Late Complications That Occur After Tube Is in Place

1. Airway/respiratory

Tube obstruction: secretions, blood, and kinking

Accidental extubation and endobronchial intubation

Vocal cords: ulceration

Trachea: ulceration, ischemic necrosis, and paralysis

Pneumothorax and pneumomediastinum

Aspiration and atelectasis

Cough that results in increased intrathoracic, intracranial, and intraocular pressures

2. Gastrointestinal

Esophageal intubation

Tracheoesophageal fistula

3. Cardiovascular

Tracheoinnominate artery fistula

4. Infections

Sinusitis, pneumonia, tracheobronchitis, mediastinitis, and abscess

5. Tube dislodgment

and remove the anterior part of the C-collar during the intubation attempt to maintain spinal motion restriction while still allowing the mandible to be displaced anteriorly, facilitating mouth opening and a satisfactory glottic view. On completion of the intubation, replacing the anterior part of the collar is necessary to maintain correct position.

The ETT cuff pressure should be measured. Although no ideal pressure has been defined, most recommendations are between 20 and 30 cm H_2O. High cuff pressures can cause complications including tracheal ischemia and fistula formation, and mucosal damage can begin to occur within 14 minutes.[37,38]

Direct Laryngoscopy

When using DL, a direct line of sight is used to perform the intubation. Laryngoscope blades come in curved shapes, such as the MacIntosh, or straight shapes, such as the Miller, Phillips, or Wisconsin. Generally speaking, the wide flange of the curved blade aids in controlling the tongue, considered the primary obstacle to intubation, better than the straight blade. The ability of the flanged curved blade to control the tongue also leaves more room on the right side of the mouth to manipulate the endotracheal blade into place. In addition, the curved blade follows the natural curvature of the anatomy better than the straight blade, which often must be inserted in a stepwise fashion of lifting, relaxing, and advancing.

The straight blade, although more difficult for control of the tongue, has an advantage in viewing the glottic opening of patients who are considered to have an anterior positioned larynx. Such is the case in pediatric patients, patients with receding chins, and patients with short muscular necks. In these patients, the larynx is located more forward, and curved blades often do not provide an adequate view. If the laryngoscopist secures a good view of the cords with a straight blade, but without totally maintaining the tongue to the left of the blade, the tongue may lap over the blade and prevent manipulation of the tube through the cords.

The curved tip of the MacIntosh is inserted into the vallecula, the space between the base of the tongue and the pharyngeal surface of the epiglottis. Lifting the blade lifts the hypoepiglottic ligament and indirectly lifts the epiglottis to expose the larynx (Fig. 11.9). The straight Miller blade is passed so that the tip lies beneath the laryngeal surface of

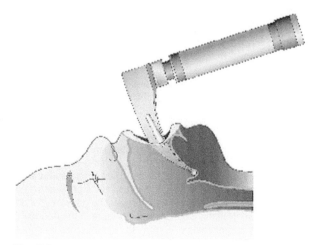

• **Fig. 11.9** Use of a curved laryngoscope blade. (From Donoghue AJ, Walls RM. *Pediatric Emergency Medicine.* Philadelphia, PA: Elsevier; 2008.)

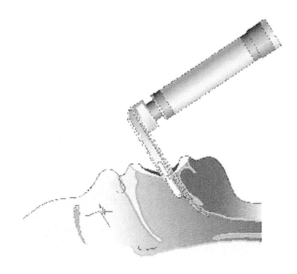

• **Fig. 11.10** Use of a straight laryngoscope blade. (From Donoghue AJ, Walls RM. *Pediatric Emergency Medicine*. Philadelphia, PA: Elsevier; 2008.)

the epiglottis. The epiglottis is then directly lifted to expose the vocal cords (Fig. 11.10). Steps for orotracheal intubation are included in Box 11.2.

When the laryngoscopist uses a hand to improve laryngeal visualization, the method is also referred to as ELM. ELM from an assistant or with the laryngoscopist's free right hand may also assist the intubator in visualizing the laryngeal inlet. Use some caution with pressure directed posteriorly, because too much cricoid pressure may worsen the laryngeal view and reduce airway patency.[39] There is no good evidence in favor of, or in favor of rejecting,

---

• BOX 11.2 Steps for Orotracheal Intubation

1. Position the patient. Nontrauma patient: Flex the neck forward and extend the head backward, creating a sniffing position. Trauma patient: Maintain in-line traction.
2. Preoxygenate the patient.
3. Hold the laryngoscope in the left hand, and open the patient's mouth with the right hand.
4. Insert the blade into the right side of the mouth, sweep the tongue to the left, and advance to the appropriate landmarks. The Miller (straight) blade tip goes beyond the epiglottis; the MacIntosh (curved) blade tip enters the vallecula.
5. Pull the laryngoscope blade at a 45-degree angle; avoid twisting the laryngoscope handle. Visualize the epiglottis and vocal cords. Apply cricoid pressure.
6. Insert the ETT from the right corner of the mouth, and watch the tube pass through the vocal cords. Use the largest tube possible. Remove the stylet.
7. Inflate the tube cuff with 5 to 10 mL of air or to minimal occluding volume. (Minimal occluding volume is determined by placing the hand over the mouth and noting cessation of air leak with ventilation.) Capillary flow pressure in the tracheal mucosa is approximately 25 mm Hg, so cuff pressure should be less than that.
8. Confirm tube placement
9. Secure the tube in place.

---

the routine use of the Sellick maneuver to prevent passive regurgitation.[30,31]

MacIntosh, the British anesthesiologist who developed the MacIntosh laryngoscope blade, is credited with developing the *endotracheal tube introducer* (ETI) in the 1940s. The ETI is 60 cm long and is curved 35 degrees at the end. The tip permits it to be steered behind the epiglottis and into the glottic opening, even when only the posterior arytenoids or the epiglottis are visualized during the intubation attempt.

To use the introducer, often referred to as a "bougie," perform laryngoscopy in the usual manner. Hold the ETI in the right hand and advance it toward the epiglottis, or where the cords are presumed. If the introducer goes blindly down the trachea, the laryngoscopist receives confirmation by way of feeling "clicks" as the curved tip of the introducer slides over the tracheal rings or "holdup" where the introducer reaches the carina or the right or left mainstem bronchus and cannot be further advanced. If holdup is noted, which may or may not be accompanied with clicks, it is nearly 100% confirmation that the introducer is in the trachea. Clicks are confirmed in 90% of tracheal intubations with the ETI. Holdup may possibly occur in a patient with esophageal stenosis with a false-positive result or with cricoid pressure. If the introducer is advanced without clicks or holdup, it has likely gone down the esophagus. This route is confirmed when the laryngoscopist literally realizes that the entire introducer has been inserted with only a few centimeters left in the hand. In this situation, pull back on the introducer until the curved tip is seen again and redirect it.

Once the intubation specialist is confident the ETI has entered the trachea, with positive holdup, click, or both signs, an assistant places an ETT over the introducer. The intubation specialist then advances the tube, similar to the Seldinger technique, over the introducer while holding the laryngoscope in the left hand. Maintaining the laryngoscope in place facilitates sliding the tube over the introducer. The assistant can stabilize the introducer by holding the free end above the ETT as the intubation specialist advances the it.

At times, the ETT may resist passing through the cords. If this should occur, back the tube out slightly and rotate the tube 90 degrees to the left (the Murphy eye is now in the upright position), and then advance. If this maneuver is unsuccessful, rotate the tube to the right 90 degrees and advance. In rare situations, the tube may need to be rotated 180 degrees to pass through the cords. Once the ETT passes through the cords, remove the introducer and confirm placement in the usual manner.

Video-Assisted Intubation

With the advancement of video-assisted laryngoscopy, the need for direct visualization is assisted with the use of a video-transmitting device on the tip of the laryngoscope blade. The video transmits an image to a monitor via a camera element located on the laryngoscope blade. The views obtained with the video-assisted laryngoscope can be enhanced via magnification and wide-angle view. The improvement of the ability to visualize the airway is due to both the placement of the video camera and the angulation of the laryngoscope blade.[40]

Video devices often have blades with increased angulation, from traditional MacIntosh curvature to hyperangulated blades with a 60-degree angulation. Hyperangulated blades look around the curvature of the tongue very effectively and can facilitate procedure success when the anatomy is "anterior." However, their perspective (looking upward at the glottic opening from the base of the tongue) can lead to difficulty in tube delivery. If the blade is inserted too deeply, the video-imaging element gets very close to the larynx. In this instance, the view will be great, but the extreme angle of approach will create difficulty passing the tube because of the angle, the shortened delivery area, and the decreased field of view on the screen. Additionally, operators must be careful to look in the mouth while inserting an ETT on a hyperangulated stylette to avoid injury to the soft palate, tonsils, or hypopharynx.[41]

Reported advantages over DL include a better view of the larynx with no need for head extension in patients with limited cervical spine motion, improved ability to visualize the larynx when anatomic disruption is present, and a faster learning curve for inexperienced intubators.[42,43] The mnemonic HEAVEN can help illuminate the choice between video and DL:

H: Hypoxemia. DL is faster, although video laryngoscopy (VL) may be easier with anatomic difficulty.
E: Extremes of size. VL (out to in) uses a slow, controlled advancement toward the epiglottis, and DL (in to out) advances into the airway with slow removal of the laryngoscope blade until the airway comes into sight. In pediatrics a straight blade will lead to increased success.
A: Anatomic disruption/obstruction. The process is VL out to in and DL in to out.
V: Vomited blood or fluid in airway. Use DL if bloody or uncontrollable vomiting.
E: Exsanguination. DL is faster, but use VL with anatomic difficulty.
N: Neck mobility. VL is gentler.[44]

The approach to the airway with an indirect tool is slightly different than with DL. The patient should be in a supine, neutral position, compared with the classic sniffing position. Malposition, along with a small mouth opening, are known predictors of difficult VL.[45] Follow the curvature of the specific blade when forming the ETT and stylette. The blade is inserted to the midline or slightly to the left of midline, rather than along the right side. Once an attempt is started slowly, walk the blade down the tongue until exposure of the uvula, then lift to expose the epiglottis. Once the epiglottis is found, position the device and obtain a glottis view. A Cormack-Lehane grade II view might be more successful than a grade I because it allows the camera to work in a further recessed manner, which will allow more room for manipulation of the ETT to pass through the cords. Once the tube is at the entry to the vocal cords, continue to advance the tube through the cords while a partner removes the stylette. Some video-assisted devices, particularly those without a hyperangulated blade, allow for a "crossover" technique, in which the operator can use the same tool for either direct or video-assisted laryngoscopy.[40]

Intubation Without a Device

With the widespread use of medication-assisted intubation techniques and indirect laryngoscopy, there has been a decrease in the use of intubation without a device. However, when necessary, the use of nasotracheal and digital intubation may be an option.

Nasotracheal Intubation

Nasotracheal intubation is referred to as a blind procedure because the larynx is not visualized as in the orotracheal method. Once considered an ideal technique for intubation of the patient with suspected cervical spine injury, the nasotracheal intubation technique has since been replaced with inline cervical immobilization together with rapid sequence intubation (RSI) and oral intubation. All blind techniques can produce airway trauma that includes laryngeal and glottic damage, esophageal intubation, and significant bleeding that leads to a "can't ventilate, can't intubate" situation.

Today, the nasotracheal technique has few true indications. The only absolute contraindication to the standard blind nasotracheal technique of intubation is apnea. Relative contraindications include the following:
- Suspected basilar skull fracture
- Acute epiglottitis
- Severe nasal or maxillofacial fractures
- Upper airway foreign body, abscess, or tumor
- Anticoagulation therapy or other coagulopathies

Nasotracheal intubation puts the patient at risk for the development of meningitis or encephalitis, so special consideration must also be given to the patient for whom bacteremia would be particularly detrimental, such as those who are immunocompromised or have cardiac valve disease or a prosthetic valve.[3]

In patients with spontaneous respirations and limited oral access, such as angioedema or other obstructive oral processes, nasotracheal technique with a cooperative patient and an experienced provider is a reasonable alternative to a surgical airway. Other patients who might potentially benefit from a nasotracheal intubation include patients with severe dyspnea who cannot tolerate lying supine, such as those with pulmonary edema, congestive heart failure, or COPD exacerbation. Patients with dyspnea often have breath sounds that are easily heard and a glottis that tends to remain open, making nasotracheal intubation relatively easy provided the patient is well prepared. For successful performance of the blind method of tracheal intubation, the patient must have spontaneous respirations. A directional-tip ETT can assist in successful performance of this rare procedure as well as the use of a whistle device to amplify the sound of spontaneous respirations.[46]

Digital Intubation

Digital or tactile orotracheal intubation is another blind intubation technique that was the original method of intubation beginning in the mid-1700s. With the invention of the laryngoscope, the technique became obsolete and is of limited usefulness in clinical practice. However, digital intubation can be helpful when other conventional methods have failed or in an austere setting in which limited equipment, lighting, or space is problematic. Digital intubation requires that the patient is completely unconscious and that the mouth be opened widely without fear of the patient biting. This technique relies on the ability of the intubation specialist to guide the tip of the tube through the glottic opening with the middle and index fingers of the nondominant hand. The primary limitation of this technique is the length of the intubation specialist's fingers in relation to the patient's oral and upper airway anatomy.

Extraglottic Devices

The category of extraglottic covers a spectrum of devices separated into two subclasses: supraglottic devices and retroglottic devices. Extraglottic devices traditionally were thought to be used as "rescue" or "backup devices"; however, they are properly used as primary devices or temporizing devices in proper situations, particularly when preprocedure airway assessment suggests that DL might be difficult. Uses for extraglottic devices can be summarized as follows:

- An airway rescue device when intubation has failed.
- A "single-attempt" rescue device preformed simultaneously with preparation for cricothyrotomy in the "*can't intubate, can't oxygenate*" failed airway.
- An easier and more effective alternative to BVM in the hands of basic life support providers or nonmedical rescue personnel.
- An alternative to endotracheal intubation by advanced life support providers.
- An alternative to endotracheal intubation for elective airway management in the OR for appropriately selected patients.
- A conduit to facilitate endotracheal intubation, such as an intubating laryngeal mask airway (LMA).[3,33]

Two concerns with extraglottic devices are compression of the carotid artery with impaired cerebral blood flow and the stability of the device. There is some disagreement in the literature about whether extraglottic devices impair carotid blood flow in patients, either in cardiac arrest or at all.[47,48] The Combitube is the airway appliance that is most difficult to dislodge, and other common supraglottic devices, the LMA and King airway, are removed with force similar to an ETT.[49]

Supraglottic Airway Devices

Supraglottic devices surround the area around and above the glottis. Examples of supraglottic devices are LMAs, or the I-gel.

Laryngeal Mask Airway

The first-generation LMA was developed by the British anesthesiologist Archie Brain and introduced in 1988. The device comes in appropriate sizes for all patients, including neonates to large adults, and LMAs reliably provide rescue ventilation in cases when difficult airways are encountered.[50] The LMA consists of an airway tube, a mask, and a mask inflation tube. It provides for ventilation by forming a seal over the larynx above the cords. The tip of the LMA rests in the esophagus, and there are two rubber bars that cross the tube opening at the mask end to prevent herniation of the epiglottis into the LMA tube. Sizing is based on patient weight. Insertion of the LMA is shown in Fig. 11.11. Typical first-time insertion success rates range between 90% and 95%, with insertion times between 30 and 50 seconds.[51]

The LMA is also available in several variations, including versions with the addition of a port to allow for gastric decompression, with a more rigid shape to facilitate insertion, and with an improved seal pressure up to 40 cm H_2O. The intubating LMA allows for ventilation while providing a conduit for blind passage of a specially designed ETT for intubation.

A classic concern about the LMA is that it does not offer a definitive defense against regurgitation and aspiration, so it leaves the airway less protected than one secured by a cuffed ETT. A meta-analysis of 547 published studies on the LMA, however, concluded that "(p)ulmonary aspiration with the LMA is uncommon and comparable to that for outpatient anesthesia with the face mask and tracheal tube."[52]

All air-filled devices, including cuffed ETTs and the cuffs of supraglottic devices, may expand at altitude and pressures should be monitored with changes in altitude.

I-Gel

The I-gel is the newest supraglottic airway. Unlike previous devices, it does not use inflatable cuffs to achieve a seal of the esophagus and pharyngeal structures. The I-gel is produced from an entirely synthetic medical-grade thermoplastic, which gives it a gel-like feel and is anatomically designed to fit snugly into the perilaryngeal structures, essentially mirroring the supralaryngeal anatomy. Current available sizes allow use in patients who weigh between 2 and 100 kg. It is easily placed with 98% success on one or two attempts, sustains a peak airway pressure of 30 mm Hg, and incorporates into its design a bite block and a gastric channel that allows for passage of a gastric tube up to 14 French in size.[53] The I-gel is the least studied of the supraglottic devices.

Retroglottic Devices

Retroglottic, or esophageal tube, airways are blind-insertion devices designed with high-volume, low-pressure cuffs that occlude the esophagus and posterior oropharynx, directing PPVs through the esophagus. The pharyngeal balloon may also tamponade oral bleeding and prevent aspiration of blood into the trachea. The oropharyngeal balloon does not prevent aspiration of teeth or other oral debris, and the oropharyngeal balloon can migrate out of the mouth anteriorly,

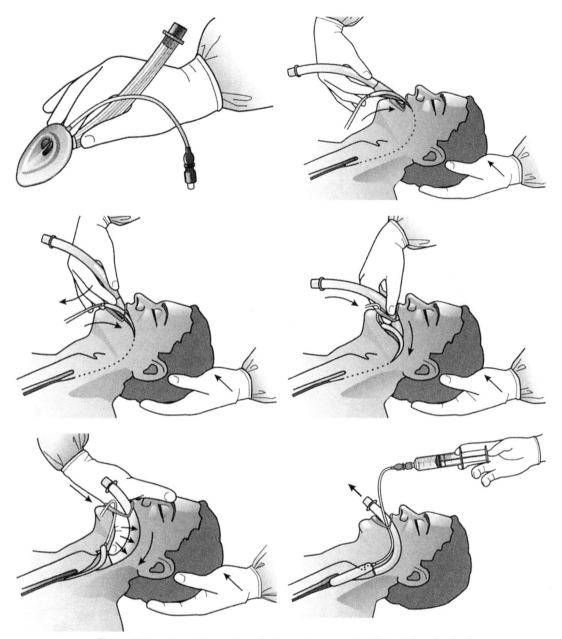

• **Fig. 11.11** Insertion of laryngeal mask airway. (Courtesy of LMA North America, Inc.)

partially dislodging the airway. Retroglottic airways are contraindicated in patients who are awake and semiobtunded. They cannot be used in patients with known esophageal injury or in situations of caustic ingestion.

Retroglottic devices can be used with blind insertion, but it is recommended to use a laryngoscope blade with insertion to help facilitate smooth insertion and prevent any folding of the distal tip of the device. If an esophageal tube airway is inserted and ventilation is not possible, then it is generally because the placement is too deep, and stepwise withdrawal of the device with attempted ventilation should result in successful ventilation

For the King LT version, the device will sustain a peak pressure of 60 mm Hg and pediatric sizes are available. Proper sizing is essential to successful use (Box 11.3).

Surgical Airway

In rare cases, it is necessary to use a percutaneous approach to secure the airway. The procedure is rare across the spectrum of emergency medical service, transport, and hospital care, but it has a high success rate.[23,54-56] A firm understanding of the anatomy of the neck is needed to facilitate success in these cases (Fig. 11.12).

Needle Cricothyrotomy

Needle cricothyrotomy involves the insertion of an over-the-needle cannula through the cricothyroid membrane into the trachea. Conceptually, the needle cricothyrotomy is quicker and easier to perform than a surgical cricothyrotomy and is

• BOX 11.3	King-LT Sizing Guide				
Size	2	2.5	3	4	5
Connector Color	Green	Orange	Yellow	Red	Purple
Patient Criteria	35-45 inches (90-115 cm) Or 12-25 kg	41-51 inches (105-130 cm) or 25-35 kg	4-5 feet (122-155 cm)	5-6 feet (155-180 cm)	Greater than 6 feet (>180 cm)

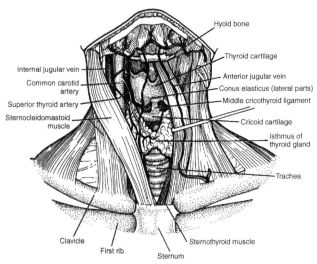

• **Fig. 11.12** Anterior aspect of neck with relative anatomic structures. (From Rosen P, et al. *Emergency Medicine: Concepts and Clinical Practice*, vol 1, 2nd ed. St. Louis, MO: Mosby; 1988.)

an alternative technique for practitioners unable to perform a cricothyrotomy. The procedure is performed infrequently, with reported success rates between 37% and 100% and some papers reporting significant complications.[56-59]

Steps for this procedure are included in Box 11.4. The use of a kink-resistant catheter with a 10-gauge, 14-gauge, or 16-gauge cannula is recommended. The needle is removed, and the cannula is left in place. Commercially available cannulas are designed with side holes in addition to the

• BOX 11.4	Steps for Needle Cricothyrotomy

1. Stabilize the patient's head in a neutral position.
2. Identify the cricothyroid membrane and prepare the skin.
3. Stabilize the cricoid and thyroid cartilages with the nondominant hand.
4. Insert a 12-gauge or 14-gauge over-the-needle intravenous catheter into the membrane at a 45-degree angle caudally (toward the feet). On passage into the trachea, the needle is removed, and the cannula is advanced caudally.
5. The hub of the needle is connected, preferably to a jet ventilator capable of delivering oxygen at a pressure of 50 psi. Otherwise, the connector is removed from a 3.0-mm ETT and attached to the intravenous catheter. It is then connected to a bag-valve-mask device. This method is temporary until other means of airway securement can be achieved.

distal port and incorporate a flange that aids securement of the catheter. The additional holes decrease pressure-related mucosal damage.

When used in an adult, the cannula must then be connected to an oxygen-delivery device capable of delivering short bursts of oxygen from a high-pressure source of 50 psi. When used in pediatric patients, a pressure regulator set at a maximal pressure of 20 to 30 psi should be used to decrease the risk of barotrauma. This method of ventilation is known as *translaryngeal jet ventilation*, and it provides emergency oxygenation and ventilation by passive recoil of the chest wall and exhalation by way of the upper airway. In situations in which complete upper airway obstruction is suspected, a needle cricothyrotomy does not allow for exhalation and barotrauma results. In such a situation, a cricothyrotomy is the airway of choice.[3]

The ventilatory rate should be from 12 to 20 breaths per minute (bpm) with an insufflation time of about 1 to 2 seconds. In young children less than 5 years old, an alternative method to the use of the jet ventilator allows for the connector from a No. 3 ETT to be connected to the cannula, which is then connected to a resuscitation bag. This technique meets oxygen requirements. However, ventilation is minimal at best, and respiratory acidosis quickly results. The respiratory acidosis that results generally limits ventilation in this manner to approximately 30 minutes. The use of a resuscitation bag is at best a temporary measure, whereas jet ventilation is considered a true PPV technique.[3]

Surgical Cricothyrotomy

Surgical cricothyroidotomy is performed when other forms of airway management have failed and the patient cannot be adequately ventilated and oxygenated with a bag and mask. The indication for surgical airway is the patient who cannot be ventilated or oxygenated by other means. Airway inaccessibility may be the result of trauma, which can cause abnormal anatomy or profuse bleeding, obscuring visualization of the glottic opening, or the result of a foreign body, mass lesion, or edema. There is no absolute contraindication because the alternative is hypoxic death. Relative contraindications include the inability to locate the correct landmarks, primary laryngeal injury, and coagulopathy. As a surgical airway is a possibility with every airway management plan that includes suppressing spontaneous ventilations, such an approach should be planned with extreme caution in patients who have the relative contraindications.

There are three variations of the surgical cricothyrotomy technique: classic surgical, Seldinger, and rapid four step (Boxes 11.5–11.7). Generally, a vertical incision over the midline is recommended for minimization of bleeding. If the incision is too small, identification of the structures is more difficult. The nondominant hand should be used for

---

• BOX 11.5 Steps for Surgical Cricothyrotomy

1. Stabilize the patient's head in a neutral position.
2. Identify the cricothyroid membrane and prepare the skin.
3. Stabilize the cricoid and thyroid cartilages with the nondominant hand.
4. Make a vertical incision 5 to 7 cm through the skin.
5. Identify the cricoid membrane, and insert the tracheal hook. Use the tracheal hook, now in the nondominant hand, to stabilize the thyroid. Apply upward traction (45-degree angle) on the inferior margin of the thyroid cartilage.
6. Use the tip of a no. 11 blade to create a horizontal incision through the cricoid membrane. Avoid insertion of the blade too deeply and injury of the posterior wall of the trachea or the esophagus.
7. Insert a Trousseau dilator and spread vertically to enlarge the diameter of the cricoid space. Mayo scissors may be used to help enlarge the space in the transverse direction.
8. Remove the tracheal hook.
9. Place a cuffed ETT or tracheostomy tube through the dilator.
10. Remove the dilator. Secure the tube, and verify proper position in the usual manner.

• BOX 11.6 Rapid Four-Step Cricothyrotomy Technique

1. **Palpation** (Fig. 11.13A). To perform the procedure, one should position oneself at the patient's left shoulder and palpate the cricoid membrane with the index finger of the left hand, allowing the thumb and middle finger to palpate and stabilize the trachea.
2. **Incision** (Fig. 11.13B). With the right hand, a No. 20 scalpel is used to make a horizontal incision into the inferior aspect of the cricothyroid membrane. The scalpel is pushed through the membrane at a 60-degree angle to create a 2.5-cm horizontal incision. The scalpel is *not* removed; it is held in place.
3. **Traction** (Fig. 11.13C). A tracheal hook is held perpendicular to the longitudinal axis of the patient. With the left hand, the tracheal hook is placed flush against the caudal surface of the scalpel blade and slid down along the trachea. The tip of the hook is rotated 90 degrees in the inferior direction, and ventral/caudal traction is applied to the superior margin of the cricoid cartilage. The scalpel is then removed, and traction is maintained on the trachea by placing the left hand on the patient's sternum.
4. **Intubation** (Fig. 11.13D). This step is similar to orotracheal intubation. A cuffed endotracheal tube or tracheostomy tube is placed with the right hand. Tube placement is confirmed, and the hook is removed. If an endotracheal tube is used, the beveled side initially should be facing cephalad during insertion to decrease advancement of the tube superior to the vocal cords.

• BOX 11.7 Cricothyrotomy: Seldinger Technique

1. Position the patient and identify appropriate landmarks.
2. Insert a small locator needle into the cricothyroid membrane. Aspirate air to confirm needle placement into the trachea.
3. Pass a soft-tipped wire through the needle and thread it into the trachea. Keep control of the wire at all times to prevent wire aspiration.
4. With a No. 11 blade, cut a small incision adjacent to the needle to facilitate passage of the airway device.
5. Place the airway tube with its internal dilator over the wire through the tissue into the trachea. If resistance is met, extend or deepen the skin incision. A gentle screwing motion may also facilitate passage.
6. Confirm tube placement.

---

grasping and stabilization of the larynx from the beginning of the skin incision until the airway is secured. This keeps structures in midline and in place. A 6.0-cuffed ETT or #4 Shiley tracheostomy tube is placed through the incision and into the trachea. The angle and rounded tip of the tracheostomy tube can make inserting that tube more difficult than a standard ETT.

For the traditional open technique, a modification is to place a bougie or ETI in the trachea after the incision is made, assisting with securing the airway as well as preventing intubation of a false passage.[33] The rapid four-step cricothyrotomy technique was developed for use in the prehospital environment. This technique relies on palpation rather than direct visualization of the cricothyroid membrane, which decreases the need for suction and additional light (Fig. 11.13). Studies suggest the rapid four-step technique aids in establishing an airway quicker than the traditional technique but may be associated with a higher complication rate.

Circumstances in which identification of the anatomy for surgical airway is difficult represent a contraindication to inducing apnea for intubation. If the anatomy of the neck is distorted, the trachea can be identified with slow advancement of a needle connected to a syringe through the skin and attempted aspiration of air. Once air has been aspirated, signaling entrance into the trachea, the needle and syringe should be left in place and the tissues cut down over the needle.

Pediatric Management

The pediatric airway differs from the adult until about the age of 8 years when the larynx resembles that of the adult in structure and position. The greatest differences exist in the child who is 2 years or less, and patients between the years of 2 and 8 represent a transitional period.

An infant's head is much larger in proportion to the rest of the body and results in a natural sniffing position. As a result, neck flexion is not necessary to attain the sniffing position and bag-mask ventilations. In infants and some young children, the sniffing position is too pronounced,

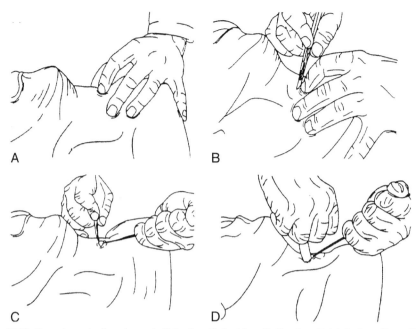

• **Fig. 11.13** Four-step cricothyrotomy: A, Palpation. B, Incision. C, Traction. D, Intubation. (From Brofeldt BT, Osborn MI, Sakles JC, et al. Evaluation of the rapid four-step cricothyrotomy technique: an interim report. *Air Med J.* 1998; 17(3):127.)

and the transport team provider may need to place a towel under the infant's shoulders to raise the rest of the body and straighten the airway, improving airflow.

The infant is also an obligate nose breather, and secretions or edema in this area can cause airway compromise more easily than in adults. Infants and small children have tongues that are large in relation to the size of the oropharynges, which makes the tongue, as it is in the adult, the most common cause of airway obstruction. The relatively small size of children's mouths also makes intubation more difficult. Because of the small size of the pediatric airway, minimal edema can create a life-threatening obstruction. An infant's airway, normally 4 mm in diameter, decreases to 2 mm with 1 mm of circumferential edema caused by secretions or trauma caused by intubation. In comparison, the adult airway, normally 8 mm in diameter, decreases to 6 mm with 1 mm of circumferential edema (Fig. 11.14). The result is only a 25% decrease in diameter in the adult compared with a 50% decrease in the infant with an equal amount of swelling.

The vocal cords of a young child are more pliable than those of the adult and are easier to damage, resulting in potential obstruction. The presence of hypertrophied tonsils and adenoid tissues can cause rapid development of upper airway obstruction and is a significant source of bleeding when traumatized. In addition, the larynx is situated higher in relation to the cervical spines than in the adult. In the infant, the glottic opening is at C1; as the child ages, the glottic opening moves down to the level of the adult at C4 to C5. The anterior position of the larynx in the infant and young child leads to more frequent intubations of the esophagus. In a situation in which the laryngoscopist

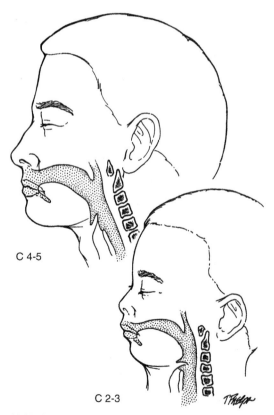

C 4-5

C 2-3

• **Fig. 11.14** Comparative anatomy of adult and infant airways. (From Nichols DG, et al, eds. *Golden Hour: The Handbook of Advanced Pediatric Life Support,* 2nd ed. St. Louis, MO: Mosby; 1996.)

recognizes no landmarks, a likely indication is that the laryngoscope blade has been passed too far and needs to be withdrawn until structures are recognized.

The anatomic differences between the pediatric and adult airways are illustrated in Fig. 11.11 and can be summarized as follows:

1. A child's larynx lies more cephalad than an adult's larynx.
2. A child's epiglottis is at an angle of 45 degrees to the anterior pharyngeal wall, whereas an adult's larynx lies parallel to the base of the tongue.
3. A child's epiglottis is large, stiff, and U-shaped, whereas an adult's epiglottis is flattened and more flexible.
4. The larger tongue of infants and children and the position of the hyoid bone depress the epiglottis.
5. The cricoid ring is the narrowest portion of a child's airway.

In addition to the anatomic differences noted, the critical care transport team members must be aware of the physiologic differences between children and adults. Of critical importance is the recognition that infants and children experience oxygen desaturation much quicker than adults. This faster desaturation time after apnea is the result of the higher metabolic oxygen consumption rate compared with the adult. The infant and child's oxygen consumption rate is twice that of an adults, and the FRC is significantly less.

Lungs can easily be overdistended, and barotrauma induced by overzealous PPV can develop. Ventilation should be limited to the amount of air needed to cause the chest to rise. Excessive volumes exacerbate gastric distention and increase the risk of pneumothorax. When possible, a self-inflating bag-valve ventilation system should be used, optimally with a pop-off valve. Resuscitation bags are available for neonates (delivering volumes of 500–600 mL) and adults (delivering volumes of 1.0–1.5 L). An oxygen reservoir should be used to enhance the oxygen concentration. Initial respiratory rates used for controlled ventilation should approximate normal spontaneous respiratory rates based on age.

The proper ETT size can be determined in several ways. An indispensable tool in assisting with and reducing medication dosing errors is the use of the Broselow–Luten resuscitation tape system. The Broselow tape was initially designed to assist in the estimation of weight in cases of pediatric trauma. Since that time, information on equipment sizes and medications has been added, greatly reducing the anxiety of caregivers who primarily treat adult patients. Additionally, the tube size can be estimated by age. For neonatal patients, the gestational age (in weeks) divided by 10 and rounded down defines the tube size. For older children, the formula

$$\left(\frac{\text{Age in years}}{4}\right) + 4 = \frac{\text{internal diameter of ETT (mm)}}{\text{for uncuffed tubes}}$$

$$\left(\frac{\text{Age in years}}{4}\right) + 3.5 = \frac{\text{internal diameter of ETT (mm)}}{\text{for cuffed tubes}}[60]$$

The ETT depth is estimated as three times the inside diameter of the tube size. This rule of thumb applies to premature infants and to adults when the appropriately sized tube for the patient's age is in place.

A part of airway management for children is the placement of a gastric tube. A child's stomach is relatively larger than an adult's stomach and may contain food and a significant amount of air. Children tend to swallow air when crying (aerophagia). If full, the stomach may impinge on the diaphragm and decrease vital capacity. If a postintubation chest radiograph is available, the tip of the ETT should be at the T2 to T3 vertebral level or at the level of the lower edge of the medial aspect of the clavicle.

Medication-Assisted Airway Management

Since the 1980s, the use of sedation and NMBAs to facilitate advanced airway management before and during transport has evolved. It is clear that the use of NMBAs facilitates improved success and patient safety in emergency airway situations.[61,62] There are two approaches available: rapid and delayed sequence intubation.

RSI of anesthesia was introduced for patients with a full stomach to protect the airway from potential aspiration of the gastric contents. The practice includes preoxygenation, administration of a predetermined induction drug dose, the use of NMBAs, and then tracheal intubation when relaxation has occurred. In the early 1980s, the technique of rapidly gaining control of the airway with the same drugs as in the OR became known as RSI when done in the ED. The practice is identical in both situations. Whether performed in the ED or outside the hospital, the procedure calls for avoidance, when possible, of PPV, which results in gastric distention. If the situation warrants, neuromuscular blockade may be maintained with the administration of a longer-acting NMBA after confirming and securing the ETT.

Delayed sequence intubation is a "procedural sedation, where the procedure is preoxygenation," and is designed to permit activities that improve preoxygenation and subsequently extend the duration time of safe apnea. In contrast to RSI, the technique of delayed sequence intubation temporally separates administration of the induction agent from the administration of the muscle relaxant to allow adequate preoxygenation, which might not otherwise be tolerated by the patient. To accomplish this, the sedative agent must not induce hypoventilation (ketamine is often a recommendation). When the desired level of preoxygenation is achieved, the muscle relaxant is given, and the procedure progresses.[63,64]

Premedications

The stimuli of DL and endotracheal intubation produce a well-documented sympathetic response that increases mean arterial pressure, heart rate, and ICP. This sympathetic response may be particularly detrimental to patients with cardiovascular disease and head injury. Pretreatment medications can be administered in situations where the sympathetic response to intubation must be controlled.[36,65,66]

Opioids provide anesthesia and analgesia and decrease sympathetic tone. Compared with morphine, fentanyl has greater lipid solubility and causes less histamine release, which gives it a faster onset, shorter duration, and greater hemodynamic stability. Accordingly, it is preferred for use in induction. Doses of 5 mcg/kg effectively minimize the reflex sympathetic response to laryngoscopy but at an increased risk of premature apnea. More moderate doses of 2.5 to 3 mcg/kg decrease adverse effects while still blocking roughly half of the sympathetic response. Blood pressure moderation is more effective than heart rate control.[36,65,67,68] Fentanyl can cause a chest wall muscle rigidity that makes ventilation impossible. Muscle rigidity appears to be related to dose and to administration rate. The likelihood of chest wall rigidity is rare in doses of 5 mcg/kg or less in adults, but the risk, even at traditional doses, is real in neonatal and pediatric patients.[36,65]

Esmolol, a unique beta blocker with an ultrashort onset and half-life, is used in the OR as a pretreatment option for patients with a particular need for sympatholysis during intubation. It is rarely used outside of that environment. Single bolus doses of up to 200 mg (in adults) reduce some of the sympathetic effect, with better control of heart rate than blood pressure. A combination of 2 mcg/kg of fentanyl with 2 mg/kg of esmolol effectively limits both heart rate and blood pressure increases, allowing only about a 12% rise in either parameter.[36,65,67-69]

Atropine is used to counterbalance the cholinergic effects of succinylcholine, which can produce significant bradycardia, especially in children, young adults, and in patients given a repeat dose of succinylcholine. Any child who is to receive succinylcholine should receive pretreatment with atropine due to the pronounced vagal effect from airway manipulation that occurs in this age group, combined with cholinergic effects of succinylcholine. Atropine also decreases oral secretions, which can be a benefit to the intubation specialist.

There is no good evidence that premedication with intravenous lidocaine, once a common practice with RSI, is helpful.[65,68,70]

Sedation

Induction agents are given to render the patient unconscious during intubation. Administer an induction agent to all patients, even those with apparent unconsciousness, unless the patient is in full arrest. Common induction agents in use today are etomidate, propofol, and ketamine.

Etomidate is a barbiturate-like derivative without the adverse effects of the barbiturates. It acts rapidly, producing hypnosis in less than 30 seconds at a dose of 0.3 mg/kg, and recovery is prompt. Cardiovascular stability is characteristic of patients receiving etomidate, with little or no decreases in mean arterial pressure in normovolemic patients and in patients with limited cardiac reserve. Blood pressure changes are more likely to occur in hypovolemic patients. Etomidate decreases cerebral blood flow, cerebral metabolic oxygen demand, and ICP. Etomidate does not suppress the sympathetic response to laryngoscopy.[66,71]

Disadvantages of etomidate administration include pain during injection, involuntary skeletal muscle movements, and adrenocortical suppression. During this time the adrenal cortex is not responsive to adrenocorticotrophic hormone. This may be detrimental to patients on long-term steroid replacement therapy, or other forms of adrenal suppression, or patients in septic shock.[66,71]

Propofol is a lipid-soluble induction agent that combines rapid onset with rapid awakening. Unconsciousness and excellent amnesia occur within 30 seconds following a dose of 2 to 2.5 mg/kg. The awakening from propofol is more rapid and complete than from any other induction agent. Propofol, however, is a direct myocardial depressant that also blunts compensatory tachycardia. Accordingly, in patients with cardiac disease or hypovolemia, propofol may be a suboptimal choice for induction.

Ketamine is a phencyclidine derivative that produces dissociative anesthesia. Anesthesia and analgesia come from dissociation between the thalamus and limbic system. Patients appear to be in cataleptic states in which the eyes remain open with a slow nystagmic gaze. Ketamine is unique among induction agents because it is the only induction agent that provides amnesia and analgesia. Induction in 60 seconds is achieved following a dose of 1 to 2 mg/kg IV or within 2 to 4 minutes following an intramuscular dose of 5 to 10 mg/kg.

Ketamine administration triggers the release of centrally mediated catecholamines and inhibits their reuptake, producing an indirect sympathomimetic effect that is believed to preserve hemodynamic stability and which may be beneficial in patients with reactive airway disease. As with all of the induction agents, this drug does not perform perfectly. Postprocedure hypotension is reported in up to one-quarter of patients who have ketamine induction for intubation, with a greater risk in hypovolemic patients. An elevated shock index may help identify those at risk for hypotension.[72] Skeletal muscle tone remains intact, which helps maintain a patent upper airway; however, the presence of protective upper airway reflexes should vomiting or regurgitation occur cannot be assumed.

There are some adverse effects with the drug. Ketamine-induced cardiac stimulation may adversely increase myocardial oxygen demands in patients with ischemic heart disease. Caution should be taken in patients involved in a hypertensive crisis because administration of ketamine can cause an increase in blood pressure. Airway secretions are increased by ketamine and may precipitate laryngospasm, which can be attenuated with the use of an anticholinergic agent, such as atropine, as a premedication.

Historically, ketamine was contraindicated in patients involved in severe head injuries; however, further research shows no evidence that it causes harm in traumatic brain injury patients.[73] Awakening from ketamine anesthesia may be associated with unpleasant visual, auditory, and proprioceptive illusions that may progress to delirium. Administration of benzodiazepines can decrease the incidence of emergence reactions associated with ketamine.

Neuromuscular Blocking Agents

All *NMBAs* work at the level of the neuromuscular end plate, disrupting neurotransmitter (acetylcholine [ACh]) function and preventing effective contraction of skeletal muscle (Fig. 11.15). These agents do not produce analgesia, anesthesia, or amnesia, and reports exist of patients with total recall and pain perception who received NBAs without sufficient anesthesia during operations and procedures. Therefore sedation of the patient is essential before and during extended periods of use of NBAs.

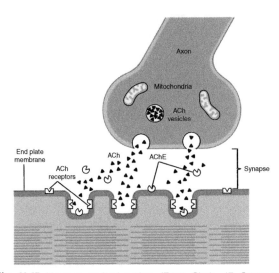

• **Fig. 11.15** Neuromuscular junction. (From Clark, JB Queener SF, Karb VB. *Pharmcologic Basis of Nursing Practice,* 4th ed. St. Louis, MO: Mosby; 1993.)

NMBAs can be classified in three ways: type of block produced (depolarizing versus nondepolarizing), duration of action (ultrashort, short, intermediate, or long), and structure (ACh-like, benzylisoquinolinium compound, or aminosteroid compound). Table 11.1 compares common NBAs.

Succinylcholine

Succinylcholine, the only depolarizing NMBA in use, is effectively two joined ACh molecules. When Ach receptors are activated, they open and then close voltage-sensitive sodium channels, which inactivates them. In the interval until the membrane potential is reset, junctional neuromuscular transmission is blocked and the muscle is flaccid. The use of succinylcholine produces many side effects and clinical considerations. Because of succinylcholine's structural resemblance to ACh, the primary parasympathetic neurotransmitter, it stimulates cholinergic receptors at other sites in addition to those at the neuromuscular junction. The stimulation of nicotinic receptors in the sympathetic and parasympathetic nervous system and muscarinic receptors in the sinoatrial node of the heart can produce bradycardia and lead to hypotension. Associated bradycardia is more pronounced in children and adults who receive repeated doses and is attenuated by the use of atropine as a pretreatment drug.

Fasciculations signal the onset of paralysis by succinylcholine. They are the result of uncoordinated motor unit contractions that may be clinically important.[74,75]

Succinylcholine-induced hyperkalemia is rare but continues to be reported in the literature and is associated with cardiovascular instability, hyperkalemic dysrhythmias, and death. Normal muscle releases enough potassium during succinylcholine-induced depolarization to raise serum

TABLE 11.1	**NMBAs**			
NMBAs	Intravenous dosage (mg/kg)	Onset (min)	Duration (min)	Comments
Depolarizing				
Succinylcholine	Adult dose: 1.0-1.5 Pediatric dose: 1.5-2.0	1.5-2.0	4-6	Pretreat with atropine in children and adolescents; many adverse effects.
Nondepolarizing				
Pancuronium	00.04-0.01	3-5	60-100	Stimulate heart rate and cardiac output; no histamine release.
Atracurium	0.4-0.5	2-3	20-45	Metabolism independent of kidney or liver function; histamine release.
Rocuronium	0.5-1.0	1-2	20-40	Shortest onset of all nondepolarizing NMBAs; no histamine release.
Vecuronium	0.1	2-3	20-40	Minimal cardiovascular effects; no histamine release.
Mivacurium	0.15-0.25	2-3	12-20	Shortest duration of all nondepolarizing NMBAs; histamine release. No longer available in the United States.

potassium by 0.5 to 1.0 mEq/L. Pathologic conditions with potential for hyperkalemia with succinylcholine include upper or lower motor neuron defect; prolonged chemical denervation with muscle relaxants or clostridial toxins, direct muscle trauma, tumor, or inflammation; thermal trauma; disuse atrophy; and severe infection.

In denervation injuries, ACh receptors develop outside the neuromuscular junction, which is referred to as upregulation. These extrajunctional receptors allow succinylcholine to affect widespread depolarization and extensive potassium release. The higher the upregulation is, the more profound is the hyperkalemia. The potential for severe hyperkalemia with succinylcholine can occur as early as 4 to 5 days of immobilization and can persist as long as the condition that induced it continues to present. Quadriplegics and paraplegics with persistent paralysis, therefore, could have the potential for succinylcholine hyperkalemia throughout life

A common belief is that the use of succinylcholine for induction in patients with open globe injuries is contraindicated. Physiologically, succinylcholine is associated with an increase in intraocular pressure (IOP). However, when an open globe injury occurs, it is often associated with crying, forceful blinking, and rubbing of the eyes, all of which create a much larger rise in IOP than that associated with the use of succinylcholine. The belief that succinylcholine caused vitreous extrusion has been perpetuated for nearly 50 years and relied on anecdote rather than documented case reports.[76]

Succinylcholine is known to be a trigger for malignant hyperthermia (MH) in susceptible patients. MH is a hypermetabolic disorder of the skeletal muscles. Classic signs include hyperthermia, tachycardia, increased carbon dioxide production, increased oxygen consumption, acidosis, muscle rigidity, and rhabdomyolysis. If untreated, the syndrome is fatal. Early detection is essential and relies on observed increases in end-tidal carbon dioxide and body temperature, followed by laboratory confirmation of acidosis. The incidence of MH in adults is rare; however, children are known to be at higher risk, with more than 50% of all cases of MH appearing in children less than 15 years of age. MH is treated with dantrolene sodium administered in doses of a 2.5-mg/kg bolus followed by additional doses up to 10 mg/kg. Further treatment is aimed at cooling the patient, treatment of arrhythmias (avoid calcium channel blockers), aggressive fluid therapy to maintain urine output, and monitoring for coagulation abnormalities. Patients should be monitored for 48 to 72 hours after the initial event because as many as 25% of patients have a recurrence of symptoms.

Nondepolarizing Agents

The South American arrow poisons known as curares were described by the explorers of the new world as early as the 16th and 17th centuries. Investigations into these poisons led to the development in 1943 of the first nondepolarizing drug tubocurarine, which was used as a muscle relaxant during surgical anesthesia.

Unlike succinylcholine, which binds to the muscle receptor and acts as an agonist, nondepolarizing muscle relaxants bind to the receptors and prevent depolarization with ACh. Therefore nondepolarizing NMBAs are referred to as competitive antagonists. Nondepolarizing agents as a rule have a slower onset of action and maintain neuromuscular blockade longer than succinylcholine. Although succinylcholine is associated with numerous undesirable side effects, the nondepolarizing NMBAs are not considered a substitute in RSI because of their slow onset of action and prolonged recovery time. The onset of action of these medications may be increased with a higher dose of the drug, but a greater risk exists of triggering cardiovascular side effects, such as tachycardia, and prolonging the duration of paralysis in a "can't intubate, can't ventilate" situation, which could have disastrous consequences.

The search for a nondepolarizing muscle relaxant with the onset of action equal to that of succinylcholine and with minimal side effects led to the development of rocuronium, which is a steroidal nondepolarizing agent with intermediate duration. When dosed in the range of 1.0 to 1.2 mg/kg, rocuronium produces intubation conditions similar to succinylcholine in a similar time frame.[77,78] The agent's onset and duration are dose dependent, and pediatric patients seem to experience a shorter time of relaxation. There are suggestions in the literature that rocuronium has a favorable hemodynamic profile and may have a beneficial effect on mortality compared with succinylcholine. Currently, there is no consensus that a meaningful difference exists or on the potential mechanisms that would contribute to such variability.[74,77,79-81]

Vecuronium is also a steroidal, nondepolarizing NMBA. The normal dose is 0.1 mg/kg. It is not possible to achieve intubating conditions with vecuronium in a time similar to rocuronium or succinylcholine. Even when the vecuronium dose is tripled, the speed of onset is still around 90 seconds.[78,82] With the slow onset of intubation conditions, operators use more of the safe apnea time waiting for the development of good intubating conditions. Because of this they have less time to do the procedure and, potentially, there is a greater likelihood of multiple attempts and the need to interpose mask ventilation because of desaturation. Both increase the risk of adverse events.[20]

Medications, disease processes, and physiologic conditions may interfere with the effectiveness of NMBAs. Neurologic diseases such as myasthenia gravis can prolong paralysis. Hyperthermia and hypothermia may have an impact on the pharmacology of selected NMBAs. Electrolyte imbalances such as hypermagnesemia may also prolong paralysis.

Monitoring Airway Patency During Transport

There is no single perfect way to ensure that an airway appliance is properly placed. Physical examination alone is insufficient, and even direct visualization of the ETT can be imperfect in the context of an airway that is difficult to visualize. A combination of physical examination and mechanical detection techniques must be used on every patient and reused throughout the episode of care.[83] The rate of undetected ETT misplacement in the out-of-hospital environment is significant.[84]

End-Tidal Carbon Dioxide Detection

End-tidal CO$_2$ detection is the most accurate and easily available method to monitor correct ETT position and ventilator circuit integrity in patients who have adequate tissue perfusion, and it is highly reliable in pulseless patients with high-quality cardiopulmonary resuscitation. Continuous end-tidal CO$_2$ detection is the standard of care for any patient with an airway appliance during transport.[85-87]

Disposable qualitative end-tidal CO$_2$ detectors evaluate proper ETT placement by incorporating a nontoxic, pH-sensitive chemically treated indicator that changes color in the presence of carbon dioxide. False-negative results (color remains purple despite correct tracheal placement) can occur during cardiac arrest, severe airway obstruction, and pulmonary edema and in severely hypocarbic infants. In low-perfusion states, such as occur in cardiac arrest, the colorimetric end-tidal CO$_2$ can produce a detectable color change. In a study of 566 prehospital intubations of patients in cardiac arrest, a color change occurred in 95.6%, with only one false-positive result. In addition to verification of endotracheal placement after intubation, the device can also be used to monitor tube placement during transport.

Capnometry is the measurement of end-tidal CO$_2$ values with each breath. The instrument works by emitting an infrared light beam through a gas sample either located immediately distal to the ETT (mainstream capnometry) or by analyzing a gas sample from the breathing circuit (sidestream capnometry). A capnogram is a time-scaled graphic representation of the capnometry values.

Similar to the way that an electrocardiogram adds helpful information about the pulse rate, the waveform of a capnogram adds valuable information about the presence of CO$_2$ or even the capnometry value.[85] A sudden decrease in CO$_2$ to zero with no waveform indicates a dislodged ETT, a kinked or obstructed ETT, or a ventilator disconnect. An incremental decrease in CO$_2$ may indicate sudden and severe hypotension or cardiac arrest. An incremental increase in CO$_2$ can indicate hypoventilation or a partial endotracheal obstruction and can occur with sodium bicarbonate administration or rising body temperature. A sudden and dramatic rise in end-tidal CO$_2$ is one of the clinical indicators of MH. However, as with any piece of equipment, caution should be exercised when capnography is used to ensure the clinical picture matches the readings: carbon dioxide present in the exhaled gas indicates that alveolar ventilation has transpired but does not necessarily mean that the ETT is in the trachea. A tube positioned in the pharynx also provides normal readings (Figs. 11.16 and 11.17).

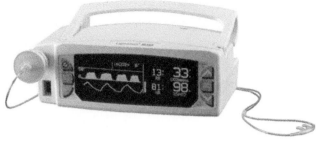

Normal capnogram

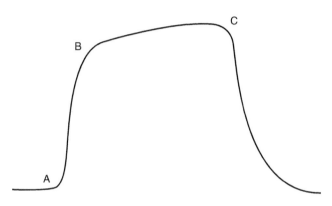

A: Exhalation begins
B-C: Plateau = outflow of alveolar gas
C: End-tidal CO$_2$

• **Fig. 11.16** End-tidal carbon dioxide waveform. (From Dean JA, *McDonald and Avery's Dentistry for the Child and Adolescent,* 10th ed. St. Louis, MO: Elsevier; 2016.)

It is important to emphasize that the end-tidal CO$_2$ value and the arterial partial pressure of CO$_2$ are not reliably related. The end-tidal value is a function of metabolic rate, minute ventilation, and cardiac output, and not just gas exchange. Accordingly, any alteration in metabolism, minute ventilation, or cardiac output affects the end-tidal value, whereas only changes in minute ventilation affect the arterial value. Arterial partial pressure can be higher or lower than the exhaled value, and the difference between the two varies with patient position, disease state, and medication use.[85,88-98]

Esophageal Aspiration Devices

The negative pressure test, with a specially designed syringe or a self-inflating bulb, may be helpful in determining ETT position.[87] After intubation, either device can be connected to the ETT, and the plunger is pulled back, in the case of the syringe, or the self-inflating bulb is compressed and then attached to the end of the ETT. Because of the rigid support provided by the cartilaginous rings, when the plunger of the syringe is pulled back, air is aspirated without resistance if the ETT is placed in the trachea. The easy aspiration of approximately 20 mL of air is a positive result for tracheal intubation. If resistance or negative pressure is

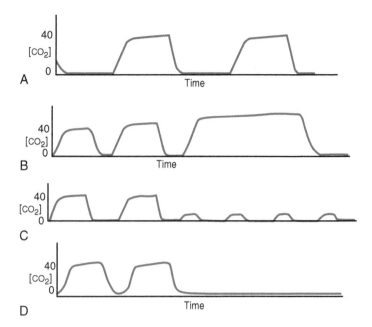

• **Fig. 11.17** Normal and abnormal end-tidal carbon dioxide waveforms. A, Normal waveform. B, Decreasing respiratory rate, preserved tidal volume. C, Hypoventilation from decreased tidal volume. D, Loss of waveform from apnea or extubation. (From Nagler J, Krauss B. Capnography: a valuable tool for airway management. *Emerg Med Clin North Am.* 2008; 26(4):881-897.)

encountered when the plunger is pulled back, the esophagus has been intubated.

Pulse Oximetry

In the ED or critical care unit, health care providers rely on arterial blood gases or, more specifically, the partial pressure of oxygen tension (PaO_2) drawn on an intermittent basis to guide therapy. Oxygen in the blood is dissolved in the plasma or is bound to hemoglobin. The oxygen dissolved in the plasma is referred to as the partial pressure of oxygen

(PO_2). The normal value ranges from 80 to 100 mm Hg. The PO_2 accounts for only 1% to 2% of the total oxygen content. The vast majority of oxygen is carried bound to hemoglobin molecules and is reported as the oxygen saturation (SaO_2 or SpO_2). Total oxygen-carrying capacity of the blood (CaO_2) is $(1.39 \times Hb \times SpO_2/100) + (0.003 \times PO_2)]$.[2] In arterial blood, the normal value of oxygen saturation (SaO_2) ranges from 95% to 97.5%.

Pulse oximetry provides a reliable and continuous evaluation of oxygenation. The relationship between the PaO_2 and SaO_2 is displayed in Fig. 11.18 in the oxyhemoglobin

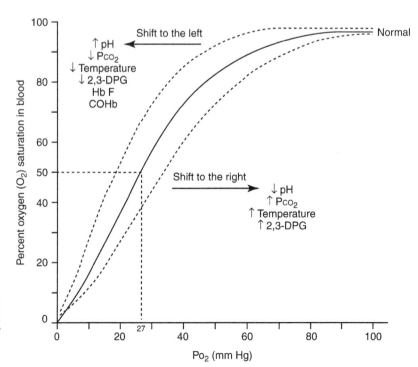

• **Fig. 11.18** Oxyhemoglobin dissociation curves: normal and shifted. (From Schick L, Windle P. *PeriAnesthesia Nursing Core Curriculum: Preprocedure, Phase I and Phase II PACU Nursing,* 3rd ed. St. Louis, MO: Saunders; 2016.)

dissociation curve. The relationship is not a linear one. The upper portion of the curve shows a compensatory mechanism of the body. In a healthy adult, more oxygen than necessary is carried. A drop in the PaO_2 from 100 to 80 mm Hg shows a minimal change in the SaO_2. The steep portion of the curve shows a rapid decline in SaO_2 with small decreases in PaO_2. When the SaO_2 falls to less than 90%, a rapid decline is seen in the oxygen content.

There is a time lag, referred to as latency, between a change in arterial oxygen tension and the change in pulse oximetry values. This time lag can be up to 3 minutes. Accordingly, it is important to think of pulse oximetry as reporting the history of oxygen saturation and not necessarily the current state.[9,99]

Pulse oximeters use a light source and photo-detector device. Accordingly, successful use depends on good alignment between the light source and detector in the sensor and on the placement of the sensor over a good pulse site. Thus the accuracy of pulse oximetry may be affected by clinical conditions, such as hypotension, hypothermia, or during vasopressor therapy, as a result of vasoconstriction. Oximetry signal reliability is affected by motion, hypothermia, dyshemoglobinemias, and intravenous dye.

Summary

Assessment and management of the patient's airway is the primary role of the transport team. Knowledge of when and how to perform basic and advanced airway management is critical in the transport environment. When in doubt, it is best to go back to using a strong basic technique to help prepare for advanced airway management. Good clinical judgment, skill, and familiarity with the pharmacology of airway management are necessary so that patients receive competent care and complications that can occur in the care of the critically ill or injured patient are prevented.

References

1. Martin L, Kahil H. How much reduced hemoglobin is necessary to generate central cyanosis. *Chest.* 1990;97(1):182-185.
2. Society of Critical Care Medicine. *Fundamental Critical Care Support.* 5th ed. Mount Prospect, IL: Society of Critical Care Medicine; 2012.
3. Brown C, Sakles J. *Walls Manual of Emergency Airway Management.* 5th ed. Philadelphia: Wolters Kluwer; 2017.
4. Brodsky JB, et al. Morbid obesity and tracheal intubation. *Anesthesia & Analgesia.* 2002;94(3):732-736.
5. Levitan RM, Everett WW, Ochroch EA. Limitations of difficult airway prediction in patients intubated in the emergency department. *Ann Emerg Med.* 2004;44(4):307-313.
6. Norskov AK, et al. Diagnostic accuracy of anaesthesiologists' prediction of difficult airway management in daily clinical practice: a cohort study of 188 064 patients registered in the Danish Anaesthesia Database. *Anaesthesia.* 2015;70(3):272-281.
7. Mosier J, et al. The physiologically difficult airway. *West J Emerg Med.* 2015;16(7):1109-1117.
8. Weingart S, Levitan R. Preoxygenation and prevention of desaturation during emergency airway management. *Ann Emerg Med.* 2012;59(3):165-175.
9. MacLeod DB, et al. The desaturation response time of finger pulse oximeters during mild hypothermia. *Anaesthesia.* 2005; 60(1):65-71.
10. Kim WY, et al. Factors associated with the occurrence of cardiac arrest after emergency tracheal intubation in the emergency department. *PLoS One.* 2014;9(11):e112779.
11. Berger T, et al. Shock index and early recognition of sepsis. *West J Emerg Med.* 2013;14(2):168-174.
12. Montory K, et al. Shock index as a mortality predictor in patients with acute polytrauma. *J Acute Dis.* 2015;4(3):202-204.
13. Mutschler M, et al. The shock index revisited—a fast guide to transfusion requirement? A retrospective analysis on 21,853 patients derived from the TraumaRegister DGU. *Crit Care.* 2013;17:1-9.
14. Panchal AR, et al. Efficacy of bolus-dose phenylephrine for peri-intubation hypotension. *J Emerg Med.* 2015;49(4):488-494.
15. Weingart S. Push-dose pressors for immediate blood pressure control. *Clin Exp Emerg Med.* 2015;2(2):131-132.
16. Tilton LJ, Eginger KH. Utility of push-dose vasopressors for temporary treatment of hypotension in the emergency department. *J Emerg Nurs.* 42(3):279-281.
17. Ellis DY, Lambert C, Shirley P. Intracranial placement of nasopharyngeal airways: is it all that rare? *Emerg Med J.* 2006; 23(8):661-661.
18. Weiner GM, Zaichkin J, eds. 7th ed. *Textbook of neonatal resuscitation.* Elk Grove Village, IL: American Academy of Pediatrics; 2016: 326.
19. Gerstein N, et al. Efficacy of facemask ventilation techniques in novice providers. *J Clin Anesth.* 2013;25(3):193-197.
20. Mort T. Emergency tracheal intubation: Complications associated with repeated laryngoscopic attempts. *Anesth Analg.* 2004; 99(2):607-613.
21. Hales BM, Pronovost PJ. The checklist—a tool for error management and performance improvement. *J Crit Care.* 2006;21(3): 231-235.
22. Gawande A. *The Checklist Manifesto: How to Get Things Right.* New York: Henry Holt and Company; 2010.
23. Brown CA 3rd, et al. Techniques, success, and adverse events of emergency department adult intubations. *Ann Emerg Med.* 2015;65(4):363-370.e1.
24. Smith K, et al. A preprocedural checklist improves the safety of emergency department intubation of trauma patients. *Acad Emerg Med.* 2015;22(8):989-992.
25. Long E, et al. A randomised controlled trial of cognitive aids for emergency airway equipment preparation in a paediatric emergency department. *Scand J Trauma Resusc Emerg Med.* 2016; 24:8.
26. Cook TM, MacDougall-Davis SR. Complications and failure of airway management. *Br J Anaesth.* 2012;109(Suppl 1): i68-i85.
27. Schwartz HP, et al. Quality metrics in neonatal and pediatric critical care transport: a national delphi project. *Pediatr Crit Care Med.* 2015;16(8):711-717.
28. Collaborative GQ. Available from: http://gamutqi.org/; 2016 September 28.
29. Sellick B. Cricoid pressure to control regurgitation of stomach contents during induction of anesthesia. *Lancet.* 1961;2(7199): 404-406.
30. Algie CM, et al. Effectiveness and risks of cricoid pressure during rapid sequence induction for endotracheal intubation. *Cochrane Database Syst Rev.* 2015(11):Cd011656.
31. Bhatia N, Bhagat H, Sen I. Cricoid pressure: Where do we stand? *J Anaesthiol Clin Pharmacol.* 2014;30(1):3-6.

32. Sakles J, et al. The importance of first pass success when performing orotracheal intubation in the emergency department. *Acad Emerg Med.* 2013;20(1):70-78.

33. Frerk C, et al. Difficult Airway Society 2015 guidelines for management of unanticipated difficult intubation in adults. *Br J Anesth.* 2015;115(6):827-848.

34. Kerrey BT, et al. Rapid sequence intubation for pediatric emergency patients: higher frequency of failed attempts and adverse effects found by video review. *Ann Emerg Med.* 2012;60(3):251-259.

35. Wadbrook P. Advances in airway pharmacology. *J Emerg Med Clin North Am.* 2000;18(4):767-788.

36. Frakes M. Esmolol: A unique drug with ED applications. *J Emerg Nurs.* 2001;27(1):47-51.

37. Sengupta P, Sessler D, Maglinger P. Endotracheal tube pressure in three hospitals and the volume required to produce an appropriate cuff pressure. *BMC Anesthesiol.* 2004;4(1):8.

38. Tollefsen W, et al. Endotracheal tube cuff pressures in pediatric patients intubated before aeromedical transport. *Pediatr Emerg Care.* 2010;26(5):361-363.

39. Levitan RM, et al. Laryngeal view during laryngoscopy: a randomized trial comparing cricoid pressure, backward-upward-rightward pressure, and bimanual laryngoscopy. *Ann Emerg Med.* 2006;47(6):548-555.

40. Olvera D, et al. *Implementation of CMAC PM device and focused airway management training to improve first pass success (Abstract), in Critical Care Transport Medicine Conference.* Charlotte, NC: 2015.

41. Phelan MP, Dhimar J. Techniques for improving video laryngoscopy with a hyperangulated blade. *Acad Emerg Med.* 2016;23(8):e15.

42. Griesdale DE, et al. Glidescope video-laryngoscopy versus direct laryngoscopy for endotracheal intubation: a systematic review and meta-analysis. *Can J Anaesth.* 2012;59(1):41-52.

43. Sakles JC, et al. Learning curves for direct laryngoscopy and glidescope video laryngoscopy in an emergency medicine residency. *West J Emerg Medi.* 2014;15(7):930-937.

44. Olvera D, et al. Prospective validation of a novel difficult airway prediction algorithm for emergency airway management (Abstract), in World Airway Management Meeting. 2015.

45. Aziz MF, et al. Predictors of difficult videolaryngoscopy with GlideScope or C-MAC with D-blade: secondary analysis from a large comparative videolaryngoscopy trial. *Br J Anaesth.* 2016;117(1):118-123.

46. Levitan RM, Technologies AC. *Airway Cam Guide to Intubation and Practical Emergency Airway Management.* Wayne, PA: Airway Cam Technologies; 2004.

47. Segal N, et al. Impairment of carotid artery blood flow by supraglottic airway use in a swine model of cardiac arrest. *Resuscitation.* 2012;83(8):1025-1030.

48. White JM, et al. Radiographic evaluation of carotid artery compression in patients with extraglottic airway devices in place. *Acad Emerg Med.* 2015;22(5):636-638.

49. Carlson JN, Mayrose J, Wang HE. How much force is required to dislodge an alternate airway? *Prehosp Emerg Care.* 2010;14(1):31-35.

50. Parmet JL, et al. The laryngeal mask airway reliably provides rescue ventilation in cases of unanticipated difficult tracheal intubation along with difficult mask ventilation. *Anesth Analg.* 1998;87(3):661-665.

51. Flaishon R, et al. Laryngeal mask airway insertion by anesthetists and nonanesthetists wearing unconventional protective gear: a prospective, randomized, crossover study in humans. *Anesthesiology.* 2004;100(2):267-273.

52. Brimacombe JR, Berry A. The incidence of aspiration associated with the laryngeal mask airway: a meta-analysis of published literature. *J Clin Anesth.* 1995;7(4):297-305.

53. Middleton PM, et al. Higher insertion success with the I-gel supraglottic airway in out-of-hospital cardiac arrest: a randomised controlled trial. *Resuscitation.* 2014;85(7):893-897.

54. Furin M, et al. Out-of-hospital surgical airway management: does scope of practice equal actual practice? *West J Emerg Medi.* 2016;17(3):372-376.

55. Marcollini E, et al. A standing order protocol for cricothyrotomy in prehospital emergency patients. *Prehosp Emerg Care.* 2004;8(1):23-28.

56. McIntosh S, Swanson E, Barton E. Cricothyrotomy in air medical transport. *J Trauma.* 2008;64(6):1543-1547.

57. Hubble MW, et al. A meta-analysis of prehospital airway control techniques part II: alternative airway devices and cricothyrotomy success rates. *Prehosp Emerg Care.* 2010;14(4):515-530.

58. Cook TM, Woodall N, Frerk C. Major complications of airway management in the UK: results of the Fourth National Audit Project of the Royal College of Anaesthetists and the Difficult Airway Society. Part 1: anaesthesia. *Br J Anaesth.* 2011;106(5):617-631.

59. Peterson GN, et al. Management of the difficult airway: a closed claims analysis. *Anesthesiology.* 2005;103(1):33-39.

60. de Caen AR, et al. Part 12: Pediatric Advanced Life Support. 2015 American Heart Association Guidelines Update for Cardiopulmonary Resuscitation and Emergency Cardiovascular Care. *Circulation.* 2015;132(18 suppl 2):S526-S542.

61. Wilcox SR, et al. Neuromuscular blocking agent administration for emergent tracheal intubation is associated with decreased prevalence of procedure-related complications. *Crit Care Med.* 2012;40(6):1808-1813.

62. Kociszewski C, et al. Etomidate versus succinylcholine for intubation in an air medical setting. *Am J Emerg Med.* 2000;18(7):757-763.

63. Weingart SD. Preoxygenation, reoxygenation, and delayed sequence intubation in the emergency department. *J Emerg Med.* 2011;40(6):661-667.

64. Weingart SD, et al. Delayed sequence intubation: a prospective observational study. *Ann Emerg Med.* 2015;65(4):349-355.

65. Feng CK, et al. A comparison of lidocaine, fentanyl, and esmolol for attenuation of cardiovascular response to laryngoscopy and tracheal intubation. *Acta Anaesthesiol Sin.* 1996;34(2):61-67.

66. Masoudifar M, Beheshtian E. Comparison of cardiovascular response to laryngoscopy and tracheal intubation after induction of anesthesia by Propofol and Etomidate. *J Res Med Sci.* 2013;18(10):870-874.

67. Gupta S, Tank P. A comparative study of efficacy of esmolol and fentanyl for pressure attenuation during laryngoscopy and endotracheal intubation. *Saudi J Anaesth.* 2011;5(1):2-8.

68. Ugur B, et al. Effects of esmolol, lidocaine and fentanyl on haemodynamic responses to endotracheal intubation: a comparative study. *Clin Drug Investig.* 2007;27(4):269-277.

69. Miller DR, et al. Bolus administration of esmolol for controlling the haemodynamic response to tracheal intubation: the Canadian Multicentre Trial. *Can J Anaesth.* 1991;38(7):849-858.

70. Robinson N, Clancy M. In patients with head injury undergoing rapid sequence intubation, does pretreatment with intravenous lignocaine/lidocaine lead to an improved neurological outcome? A review of the literature. *Emerg Med J.* 2001;18(6):453-457.

71. Bergen J, Smith D. A review of etomidate for rapid sequence intubation in the emergency department. *J Emerg Med.* 1997;15(2):221-230.

72. Miller M, et al. Hemodynamic response after rapid sequence induction with ketamine in out-of-hospital patients at risk of shock as defined by the shock index. *Ann Emerg Med.* 2016;68(2):181-188.

73. Cohen L, et al. The effect of ketamine on intracranial and cerebral perfusion pressure and health outcomes: a systematic review. *Ann Emerg Med.* 2015;65(1):43-51.e2.

74. Patanwala AE, et al. Succinylcholine is associated with increased mortality when used for rapid sequence intubation of severely brain injured patients in the emergency department. *Pharmacotherapy.* 2016;36(1):57-63.

75. Schreiber JU, et al. Prevention of succinylcholine-induced fasciculation and myalgia: a meta-analysis of randomized trials. *Anesthesiology.* 2005;103(4):877-884.

76. Murgatroyd H, Bembridge J. Intraocular pressure. *Contin Educ Anesth Crit Care Pain.* 2008;8(3):100-103.

77. Perry JJ, et al. Rocuronium versus succinylcholine for rapid sequence induction intubation. *Cochrane Database Syst Rev.* 2008(2):Cd002788.

78. Chatrath V, et al. Comparison of intubating conditions of rocuronium bromide and vecuronium bromide with succinylcholine using "timing principle." *J Anaesthesiol Clin Pharmacol.* 2010;26(4):493-497.

79. Taha SK, et al. Effect of suxamethonium vs rocuronium on onset of oxygen desaturation during apnoea following rapid sequence induction. *Anaesthesia.* 2010;65(4):358-361.

80. Tang L, et al. Desaturation following rapid sequence induction using succinylcholine vs. rocuronium in overweight patients. *Acta Anaesthesiol Scand.* 2011;55(2):203-208.

81. Lyon RM, et al. Significant modification of traditional rapid sequence induction improves safety and effectiveness of pre-hospital trauma anaesthesia. *Critical Care.* 2015;19(1):134.

82. Magorian T, Flannery KB, Miller RD. Comparison of rocuronium, succinylcholine, and vecuronium for rapid-sequence induction of anesthesia in adult patients. *Anesthesiology.* 1993;79(5):913-918.

83. Rudraraju P, Eisen LA. Confirmation of endotracheal tube position: a narrative review. *J Intensive Care Med.* 2009;24(5):283-292.

84. Wang H, Yealy D. Out of hospital endotracheal intubation: Where are we? *Ann Emerg Med.* 2006;47(6):532-541.

85. Gravenstein JS, et al. *Capnography.* Cambridge, UK: Cambridge University Press; 2011.

86. Anesthesiologists ASO. Standards for basic anesthetic monitoring. Available from: http://www.asahq.org/sitecore%20modules/web/~/media/modules/digital%20briefcase%20apps/asa%20practice%20management/standards%20guidelines%20statements/anesthesia%20care/standards-for-basic-anesthetic-monitoring.pdf#search=%22standards basic anesthetic monitoring%22; 28 Oct 2015.

87. Takeda T, et al. The assessment of three methods to verify tracheal tube placement in the emergency setting. *Resuscitation.* 2003;56(2):153-157.

88. Anderson C, Breen P. Carbon dioxide kinetics and capnography during critical care. *Crit Care.* 2000;4(4):207-215.

89. Crobo J, et al. Concordance between capnography and arterial blood gas measurements of carbon dioxide in acute asthma. *Ann Emerg Med.* 2005;46(4):323-327.

90. Cantineau J, Merck P, Lambert Y. Effect of epinephrine on end-tidal carbon dioxide pressure during prehospital cardiopulmonary resuscitation. *Am J Emerg Med.* 1994;12(3):267-270.

91. Deakin C, et al. Prehospital end-tidal carbon dioxide concentration and outcome in major trauma. *J Trauma.* 2004;57(1):65-68.

92. Drew K, et al. End-tidal carbon dioxide monitoring for weaning patients. *Dim Crit Care Nurs.* 1998;17(4):127-134.

93. Falk J, Rackow E, Weil M. End-tidal carbon dioxide concentration during cardiopulmonary resuscitation. *N Engl J Med.* 1988;318(10):607-611.

94. Guthrie B, Adler M, Powell E. End-tidal carbon dioxide measurements in children with acute asthma. *Acad Emerg Med.* 2007;14(12):1135-1140.

95. Lee J, et al. Relationship between arterial and end-tidal carbon dioxide pressures during anesthesia using a laryngeal tube. *Acta Anaesthesiol Scand.* 2005;49(6):759-762.

96. Remond C, Jimeno M, Dubouloz F. Measurements of end-tidal carbon dioxide in extrahospital transport. *JEUR.* 1998;11(4):179-186.

97. Shankar K, Moseley H, Kumar Y. Arterial to end-tidal carbon dioxide tension difference during cesarean section anesthesia. *Anesthesia.* 1986;41:698-702.

98. Shankar K, Moseley H, Kumar Y. Arterial to end tidal carbon dioxide tension difference during anesthesia for tubal ligation. *Anesthesia.* 1987;42:482-486.

99. Schallom L, et al. Comparison of forehead and digit oximetry in surgical/trauma patients at risk for decreased peripheral perfusion. *Heart Lung.* 2007;36(3):188-194.

12

Mechanical Ventilation

ERIC BAUER

In today's critical care transport environment, advanced airway management with endotracheal intubation is the standard of care. The industry has garnered new techniques based on research aimed at making this life-saving procedure more successful, with first-pass success without hypoxia being the ultimate goal. However, once the endotracheal tube (ETT) is secured and confirmation with quantitative end-tidal carbon dioxide ($EtCO_2$) waveform capnography is maintained, ventilating a patient becomes the next primary focused task. Gone are the days of ventilating patients in the critical care environment with a bag-valve-mask (BVM). The decision is not based on *whether* one should use a mechanical ventilator but more on *how* mechanical ventilation will assist in providing the highest quality care for the patient. It is then essential to have an in-depth understanding of transport ventilation and its application in the transport environment.

Mechanical ventilation has many advantages over conventional BVM ventilation, with mechanical ventilators able to provide consistent and uninterrupted ventilation. This is of significant importance when transporting patients with time-sensitive critical illness. Even a brief interruption of bag-mask ventilation can potentially lead to adverse effects, which could negatively alter the patient's clinical course. Additionally, patients with unstable conditions who need multiple interventions during transport are best served when all crew members are available to efficiently and quickly provide the care needed. The use of a ventilator eliminates the need for one crew member to manually ventilate, allowing all crew members to address other issues of care. It is important for the transport team to constantly monitor the patient and the ventilator for alarms or changes that need to be addressed.

The advent of smaller, lighter, and more sophisticated ventilators extends the capability and flexibility available to the critical care transport provider. The type of ventilator chosen and its capabilities depend on the mission profile, weight and space restrictions, along with the specific population served. Regardless of the ventilator selected, the critical care transport provider must understand the terminology (Table 12.1), modes, strategies, and complications. Appropriate selection of alarm parameters, the ability to troubleshoot problems, and analysis of blood gas values, along with other data are imperative in ventilator management.

Transport Ventilator Selection

Multiple resources are available to programs researching the purchase of a transport ventilator. In the United States the Food and Drug Administration (FDA) is the regulatory agency that must approve all medical equipment, including transport ventilators, before utilization in practice. Transport teams can also look to the American Society of Testing and Materials (ASTM) for established minimum specifications for safety and performance requirements on ventilators. In addition, programs should verify airworthiness testing, which analyzes equipment for electromagnetic disturbances (radio transmission) and for functionality with exposure to vibration and environmental extremes.

Transport ventilators can be broadly classified as automatic resuscitators or sophisticated ventilators. *Automatic resuscitators* are rudimentary devices with minimal or no monitoring and alarm capabilities. The fractional concentration of oxygen in inspired gas (FiO_2) is generally fixed, and set parameters are limited to rate and tidal volume (Vt). They are intended for the prehospital setting and to be used by medical personnel with limited exposure to ventilation management. There has been a paradigm shift in the prehospital transport environment to include the understanding of critical care concepts and advanced mechanical ventilation strategies. *Simple ventilators* offer greater choices in modes of ventilation, rate, volume, and FiO_2. They offer demand flow for spontaneously breathing patients, more alarm features, and minimal monitoring options. These ventilators are also intended for use in the prehospital setting. *Sophisticated ventilators* supply multiple modes of ventilation—for example, bi-level non-invasive positive pressure ventilation (NiPPV), continuous positive airway pressure (CPAP), synchronized intermittent mandatory ventilation (SIMV), pressure-regulated volume-controlled ventilation (PRVC), and airway pressure release ventilation (APRV), to list a few.[1,2] These ventilators are equipped with a full complement of alarms and monitoring capabilities.[3] Trained medical personnel proficient in ventilation

TABLE 12.1   **Terminology Related to Ventilators**

Term	Definition
ALI	Pulmonary condition characterized by acute hypoxemic respiratory failure, diffuse bilateral pulmonary infiltrates on CXR, pulmonary wedge pressure <18 mm Hg, and PaO_2/FiO_2 ratio of <300
ARDS	Severe form of ALI differentiated by a PaO_2/FiO_2 ratio <200
Asynchrony	Incongruity between patient's respiratory effort and ventilator breath delivery; increases work of breathing
Auto-PEEP	Gas trapped in alveoli at end of expiration caused by insufficient expiration time, bronchospasm, or mucous plugging; causes dynamic alveolar hyperinflation and increases work of breathing; also referred to as intrinsic PEEP
Barotrauma	Damage to lung tissue from high airway pressures; alveolar rupture may lead to pneumothorax, pulmonary interstitial edema, and pneumomediastinum
Cyclic atelectasis	Repeated opening of alveoli on inspiration and collapsing on expiration
Derecruitment	Collapse of open alveoli
Dynamic alveolar hyperinflation	Increase in lung volume at end of expiration caused by incomplete exhalation
Extrinsic PEEP	Mechanical application of PEEP (see PEEP)
FiO_2	Fraction of inspired oxygen ranges from 0.21 (21%) to 1.0 (100%); normal ambient air FiO_2 is 0.21
FRC	Volume of air remaining in lungs at end of normal expiration
IBW	Expected weight of person based on gender and height; used to base targeted Vt in adult population
Male	IBW = 50 kg + 2.3 kg for each inch over 5 feet
Female	IBW = 45.5 kg + 2.3 kg for each inch over 5 feet
I:E ratio	In normal conditions, expiratory phase is passive and twice as long as the active inspiratory phase (1:2)
Inspiratory flow	Rate at which breath is delivered on ventilator (it is measured in liters per minute); the higher the flow, the faster the breath is delivered; flow is equal to Vt divided by inspiratory time
Intrinsic PEEP	See auto-PEEP
P_{aw}	Average pressure to which lungs are exposed over one inspiratory/expiratory cycle
PaO_2/FiO_2 ratio	Calculation used to quantify the degree of hypoxemia and oxygenation abnormality in patients with acute respiratory failure; PaO_2 derived from arterial blood gas is divided by the fraction of inspired oxygen (normal is 500); patients with ALI are at <300, and patients with ARDS are at <200; the lower the number, the greater the degree of pulmonary abnormality; for example, a patient on 60% FiO_2 has a PaO_2 of 70 mm Hg (70/0.6 = 115)
PEEP	Positive pressure maintained at end of expiration; therapy used in mechanical ventilation to increase volume of gas remaining in lungs at end of expiration (FRC)
Permissive hypercapnia	Lung-protective ventilation strategy that uses low Vt or lower rates to reduce lung injury associated with high volumes and alveolar overdistension; carbon dioxide is allowed to rise as a consequence
PIP	Measurement in lungs at peak of inspiration
Plateau pressure	Pressure exerted on small airways and alveoli; measured by holding inspiratory pause during ventilator delivered inspiration; plateau pressures >30 mm Hg have been associated with alveolar overdistension lung injury
Recruitment	Refers to opening of collapsed alveoli; alveolar recruitment maneuvers refer to increasing PEEP, for short durations, to open collapsed alveoli and improve oxygenation; level of PEEP, duration, and frequency of this maneuver is determined by the clinician
tI	Time over which Vt is delivered or pressure maintained (depending on mode); set as I:E ratio or inspiratory flow
Tidal volume	Volume of gas inspired or expired in one breath
Trigger sensitivity	Measure of amount of negative pressure or inspiratory flow that must be generated by the patient to trigger the mechanical ventilator into the inspiratory phase
VE; MV	Volume of air that moves in and out of the lungs in 1 minute; it is the product of tidal volume and respiratory rate: VE = Vt × R
V/Q ratio	High V/Q = dead space ventilation; alveoli are ventilated, but perfusion to lungs is impaired; examples are pulmonary embolus and hypotension Low V/Q = shunt ventilation; alveoli are perfused, but there is impaired aeration; examples are ARDS and pneumonia
Volutrauma	Volume-related overdistension injury of alveoli inflicted by mechanical ventilation

ALI, Acute, lung injury; *ARDS*, acute respiratory distress syndrome; *CXR*, chest x-ray; *FiO₂*, fraction of inspired oxygen; *FRC*, functional residual capacity; *IBW*, ideal body weight; *I:E*, ratio of inspiratory time to expiratory time; *MV*, minute ventilation; *P_aw*, mean airway pressure; *PEEP*, positive end-expiratory pressure; *PIP*, peak inspiratory pressure; *R*, rate; *tI*, inspiratory time; *VE*, minute ventilation; *V/Q*, ventilation/perfusion ratio; *Vt*, tidal volume.

management use them for scene and interfacility transports alike.

The choice of a ventilator varies with program profile. The following are some factors that should be considered.

Program Considerations

Mission Type

Great consideration needs to be taken when evaluating a program's choice of transport ventilator. Whether a program transports adult, pediatric, or neonatal patients or all of the above, decision makers need to evaluate the best choice that fits the demographics transported by the program. Pediatric patients need ventilators capable of delivering lower Vt. For example, a 10-lb (4.5-kg) 2-month-old ventilated with a Vt of 6 mL/kg needs a ventilator to deliver volumes as low as 27 mL. However, most transport ventilators do not have the ability to deliver volumes below 50 mL in a volume mode of delivery. These patients will need to be placed on a pressure control or pressure-regulated volume-targeted mode of delivery for Vt less than 50 mL. Decisions like this should guide the program in making a ventilator selection that meets the primary transport demographics. If the program transports critically ill neonates or newborn patients, a ventilator that has the capabilities, modes, and features that allow for ventilation in this age demographic is warranted and optimal. However, if programs transport the full spectrum of patients from newborns to adults, the selection needs to be based on a ventilator that fits any potential patient population.

In today's large critical care transport industry, it's essential that all critical care transport teams have a sophisticated ventilator that allows for optimal treatment in both interfacility and scene missions. Transport teams need to be able to effectively ventilate a patient involved in a severe motor vehicle accident that has had subsequent traumatic brain injury (TBI) and associated chest injuries, or a patient in septic shock with associated adult respiratory distress syndrome (ARDS). Both of these patient types pose challenges in oxygenation and ventilation, even with highly sophisticated ventilators. Another important consideration in the selection of transport ventilators revolves around the overall efficiency in oxygen consumption and the battery life.

Budget

In addition to the outright cost of the ventilator, consideration of clinical engineering availability for preventative maintenance and repairs should be weighed. Warranty coverage, loaner availability, manufacturer support, service record, and turnaround time for major repairs should also be explored.

Ventilator Considerations

Guidelines

The American Association of Respiratory Care has established a consensus statement on the essentials of mechanical

TABLE 12.2	Transport Ventilator Guidelines	
Essential	**Recommended**
Set Parameters	
Positive pressure ventilation	Flow or I:E ratio
100% FiO$_2$	Spontaneous breath modes
PEEP	Triggering mechanism
Mandatory rate	
Monitoring Capabilities	
Peak airway pressure	Expired Vt
PEEP pressures	Expired spontaneous volume
	I:E ratio
	Mechanical rate
	Spontaneous rate
Alarms: Level 1 (Immediately Life-Threatening)	
Power failure	
Loss of gas source	
Absence of gas delivery (apnea)	
Excessive gas delivery	
Exhalation valve failure	
Timing failure	
Alarms: Level 2 (Potentially Life-Threatening)	
Battery power loss	
Circuit leak	
Blender failure	
Circuit occlusion	
Loss or excessive PEEP	
Autocycling	

FiO$_2$, Fraction of inspired oxygen; *I:E*, ratio of inspiratory time to expiratory time; *PEEP*, positive end-expiratory pressure.
From the *Consensus Statement of the Essentials of Mechanical Ventilators* from the American Association of Respiratory Care. 37(9):1000–1008, 1992.

ventilators. Components are classified as either essential or recommended (Table 12.2). Manufacturers of sophisticated transport ventilators are guided by these recommendations.

Durability and Safety

Transport ventilators should be compact, lightweight, and easy to secure; have proper electromagnetic shielding; and tolerate vibration, altitude changes, and extremes of temperatures. Some monitor screens are difficult to see in the sunlight or dim lighting. Contrast adjustments should have a wide range, with alarms having visual and loud audible alerts. Ventilator settings and alarm buttons or dials should not be easy to inadvertently reposition, with most ventilators having a feature that locks the controls.

Oxygen Consumption

In addition to the patient-delivered gases, some ventilators use a gas source to drive the pneumatics, increasing the gas consumption of the ventilator during operation. A wide range of oxygen consumption exists between transport ventilators that should be compared with the transport range within a program.

Power

Battery life is of particular concern to programs that cover large geographical areas in which transports occur over hours rather than minutes. Lithium ion batteries have one of the best energy-to-weight ratios and a longer shelf-life as a result of a slower loss of charge when not in use. They have no memory effect, which causes rechargeable batteries to lose charge capacity over time. They are also the most expensive. NiCad batteries are particularly susceptible to memory effect. Battery life on transport ventilators can range from less than 2 hours to 14 hours.

Selection Process

An organized selection process should be used in the search for a transport ventilator. The following is one suggested evaluation tool:

1. With the mission profile in mind, have the members of the flight team list and rank desired ventilator criteria. Indicate required components versus "nice-to-haves." Is the team more comfortable with volume-controlled or pressure-controlled ventilators, or does the ventilator provide both options?
2. Recruit respiratory therapists and medical directors in the criteria-listing process.
3. Gather a list of ventilators that best meet the criteria.
4. Rule out any ventilators on the list that do not meet airworthiness testing criteria or regulatory approval.
5. Search for published bench-testing reports.
6. Bring the ventilator into a clinical engineering bench test to verify that the ventilator functions as per published specifications. Some of the other considerations might be ease of use, safety, durability, portability, power usage, oxygen consumption, and functionality.
7. Use clinical engineering to assess for preventative maintenance, parts availability, and field repairs.
8. Use the ventilator on patients. If possible, trial it on patients in the hospital before field-testing.
9. Rank the ventilators from most desired to least desired.
10. Use the program's budgetary process to assist with financial negotiations.
11. The evaluation team makes the final recommendation on the basis of the team criteria, clinical use, and financials.
12. Make a recommendation to management.

Training

Mechanical ventilators require initial and ongoing training. The more sophisticated the ventilator, the more specialized training is required. Highly sophisticated ventilators are the standard of care in the critical care environment. Becoming safe and proficient in ventilator management during critical care transport requires extensive initial and ongoing training. Safe operation of today's sophisticated ventilators requires training beyond just an overview of what knobs to turn or buttons to push to change a specific parameter. Critical care flight crew members must have a good understanding of pulmonary pathophysiology as well as what effect the ventilator changes they make will have on the patient based on their disease process. When transporting critical, ventilated patients, it would be optimal to staff every transport vehicle and aircraft with a registered respiratory therapist skilled in ventilation management, but the reality is that most transport programs are staffed with nurses and paramedics. Because these crew members may not have a great deal of experience managing mechanical ventilators, their initial training and orientation program should include a significant portion of time devoted to pulmonary pathophysiology, arterial blood gas (ABG) interpretation, and ventilator management strategies. It is essential for all programs to maintain a rigorous quality management program to ensure their crew members are using safe, effective ventilation strategies.

Ventilator-Induced Lung Injury

Ventilator-induced lung injury (VILI) is damage inflicted on the lung as a direct result of mechanical ventilation. Patients with acute lung injury (ALI), ARDS, chronic obstructive pulmonary disease (COPD), and asthma are particularly prone to VILI associated with high transpulmonary pressures, high Vt, and cyclic atelectasis, which compounds the difficulty in ventilation management. *Transpulmonary pressure* is the pressure difference across the lung calculated by subtracting the pleural pressure from the alveolar pressure. Alveolar pressure is most closely approximated in ventilated patients by the end-inspiratory plateau pressure (Pplat). The Pplat is believed to be a better indicator of alveolar overdistension than the peak inspiratory pressure (PIP) because it is not influenced by upper airway resistance or ventilator equipment.[1,4] The crew measures the Pplat by performing an inspiratory hold maneuver while in the volume mode, or by pressing the inspiratory pause button for 0.5 second and taking a pressure reading. It is important to know that the patient's Pplat will always be the lower pressure compared with the PIP. The Pplat should be evaluated once the patient is placed on the mechanical ventilator and trended every 10 to 15 minutes or based on the patient's presentation. To get an accurate Pplat, the patient must be well sedated. If the patient actively attempts to exhale during the inspiratory hold maneuver, it will result in an erroneous reading.

Barotrauma

Barotrauma is the damage to lung tissue that causes alveolar rupture and migration of air into the extrapulmonary space. Historically, this has been attributed to high airway pressure. Barotrauma may lead to pneumothorax, tension pneumothorax, pneumomediastinum, air embolus (rare), and subcutaneous emphysema. Whether high PIPs are a direct cause of barotrauma or just a marker of severe lung disease is not clear.[1] In a retrospective study of patients enrolled in the ARDS Network trial of low Vt ventilation, mean airway pressure and plateau pressure were not predictive indicators of barotrauma.[1,4]

Volutrauma

In years past, Vt ranges had been initiated on patients between 10 and 15 mL/kg. This was based on the idea that larger Vt would prevent atelectasis. In 1994 a group of researchers came together and established the ARDS Network. Their landmark study, published in May 2000, proved that lower Vt led to a decrease in mortality and established a new norm for mechanical ventilation Vt of 6 to 8 mL/kg of ideal body weight (IBW). Based on this and subsequent studies, attention has been placed on ventilator-induced injury caused by high volumes and *alveolar overdistension,* also referred to as *dynamic hyperinflation.* The stretch of alveoli causes microvascular injury, high permeability pulmonary edema, accumulation of fluid in the interstitial and alveolar space, disruption of surfactant function, and alveolar collapse.[3] Monitoring and controlling the Pplat is one strategy used to prevent or minimize the excessive alveolar stretch associated with VILI. The ARDS Network study demonstrated that maintenance of the Pplat at or less than 30 cm H_2O was associated with a statistically significant decrease in ventilator days and improved mortality rates.[5] The ARDS Network ventilation protocols set a goal plateau pressure of less than 30 cm H_2O and recommend it be checked after each change in positive end-expiratory pressure (PEEP) or Vt. Some controversy exists regarding the need to reduce Vt if the Pplat is greater than 30 cm H_2O; however, a secondary analysis of the ARDS Network trial suggested that a beneficial effect was seen in Vt reduction from 12 mL/kg IBW to 6 mL/kg, regardless of the Pplat before the Vt was reduced.[3] In the case of high Pplat greater than 30 cm H_2O, the transport team needs to take steps in reducing the Pplat to less than 30 cm H_2O. Those primary steps are outlined in the following:

1. Identify the pathophysiology behind the potential high Pplat. Attempt to correct problems, i.e., pneumothorax, tension pneumothorax, gastric distension (orogastric/nasogastric tube placement).
2. Reduce the patient's Vt to the lower levels of the lung-protective strategy. Volume will cause transiently high alveolar pressures. Lower the Vt in 1-mL/kg increments until the Pplat is less than 30 cm H_2O or 4 mL/kg is reached. At this point the provider starts sacrificing volume and overall minute ventilation. In addition, while lowering the Vt to achieve a desired Pplat of less than 30 cm H_2O, the same minute ventilation needs to be maintained. This requires increasing the respiratory rate to match the starting minute ventilation if possible. A certain degree of elevation in the arterial PCO_2 level is acceptable while attempting to maintain a pH greater than 7.30. See the ARDS.net protocol card that shows the recommendations from the May 2000 study (Fig. 12.1).

Patients with ARDS/ALI are not the only individuals at risk for VILI with high-volume ventilation. In a retrospective cohort study of 332 patients, 24% who did not have ALI at the initiation of mechanical ventilation developed injury within 5 days.[3] One of the primary risk factors for the development of ALI was high Vt (>9 mL/kg IBW) ventilation, which suggests that high Vt may lead to the development of ALI in patients at risk. It was then recommended that the lung-protective strategy be delivered on all patients at a range of 4 to 8 mL/kg, with the recommended starting range being 6 to 8 mL/kg.

Overdistension injury is not only associated with high Vt. A normal Vt delivered to a diseased lung with large areas of low compliance can cause overdistension of available alveoli. Large segments of alveoli may be closed in patients with ARDS/ALI, leaving a small portion of the lung to receive the full Vt, which results in high pulmonary pressures and increasing susceptibility to volutrauma.[1,3]

Cyclic Atelectasis

Cyclic atelectasis is the opening of alveoli on inspiration and collapsing on expiration. Animal models have shown that this repeated opening and closing causes the release of cytokines and development of local and systemic inflammatory response,[2] further extending lung injury. PEEP is used to curtail the collapsing of lung units on expiration, particularly in low Vt strategies. It is important to remember that Vt is the key to alveolar recruitment. However, PEEP is needed to maintain alveolar recruitment during the exhalation process. Alveoli that suffer from repeated cyclic atelectasis will eventually not reinflate, and atelectasis trauma ensues.

Oxygen Toxicity

High levels of oxygen over a prolonged period of time have been shown to produce cytotoxic effects, presumably as the result of free radical production.[1,3] How this relates to the clinical care of patients with acute respiratory failure is still being researched. In a recently published 2013 study in the *AANA Journal,* the authors found that 90% of healthy adults that were given medications for airway induction and ETT placement reported pulmonary atelectasis, which lasted for up to 24 hours after airway induction and subsequent mechanical ventilation. It is thought that causes of pulmonary atelectasis stem from three different mechanisms: airway closure resulting from reduced functional residual capacity (FRC), mechanical lung compression, and absorptive atelectasis, respectively. The pathophysiology behind this phenomenon is related to the high concentrations of oxygen. During normal breathing, atmospheric air is made up of multiple gases, primarily nitrogen at 78% and oxygen at 21%. Nitrogen is a very heavy, dense gas that does not diffuse easily. Its job is to stay in the alveolar sacs and act as a "pillow" or "intrinsic PEEP." In times of 100%

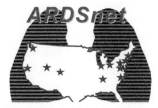

NIH NHLBI ARDS Clinical Network
Mechanical Ventilation Protocol Summary

INCLUSION CRITERIA: Acute onset of
1. $PaO_2/FiO_2 \leq 300$ (corrected for altitude)
2. Bilateral (patchy, diffuse, or homogeneous) infiltrates consistent with pulmonary edema
3. No clinical evidence of left atrial hypertension

PART I: VENTILATOR SETUP AND ADJUSTMENT
1. Calculate predicted body weight (PBW)
   Males = 50 + 2.3 [height (inches) - 60]
   Females = 45.5 + 2.3 [height (inches) -60]
2. Select any ventilator mode
3. Set ventilator settings to achieve initial V_T = 8 ml/kg PBW
4. Reduce V_T by 1 ml/kg at intervals $\leq$ 2 hours until V_T = 6ml/kg PBW.
5. Set initial rate to approximate baseline minute ventilation (not > 35 bpm).
6. Adjust V_T and RR to achieve pH and plateau pressure goals below.

pH GOAL: 7.30-7.45
Acidosis Management: (pH < 7.30)
   If pH 7.15-7.30: Increase RR until pH > 7.30 or $PaCO_2$ < 25 (Maximum set RR = 35).

If pH < 7.15: Increase RR to 35.
   If pH remains < 7.15, V_T may be increased in 1 ml/kg steps until pH > 7.15 (Pplat target of 30 may be exceeded).
   May give $NaHCO_3$
Alkalosis Management: (pH > 7.45) Decrease vent rate if possible.

I: E RATIO GOAL: Recommend that duration of inspiration be $\leq$ duration of expiration.

PART II: WEANING
A. **Conduct a SPONTANEOUS BREATHING TRIAL daily when:**
   1. $FiO_2 \leq 0.40$ and PEEP ≤ 8 OR $FiO_2 \leq 0.50$ and PEEP ≤ 5.
   2. PEEP and $FiO_2 \leq$ values of previous day.
   3. Patient has acceptable spontaneous breathing efforts. (May decrease vent rate by 50% for 5 minutes to detect effort.)
   4. Systolic BP $\geq$ 90 mmHg without vasopressor support.
   5. No neuromuscular blocking agents or blockade.

OXYGENATION GOAL: PaO_2 55-80 mmHg or SpO_2 88-95%
Use a minimum PEEP of 5 cm H_2O. Consider use of incremental FiO_2/PEEP combinations such as shown below (not required) to achieve goal.

Lower PEEP/higher FiO2

FiO₂	0.3	0.4	0.4	0.5	0.5	0.6	0.7	0.7
PEEP	5	5	8	8	10	10	10	12

FiO₂	0.7	0.8	0.9	0.9	0.9	1.0
PEEP	14	14	14	16	18	18-24

Higher PEEP/lower FiO2

FiO₂	0.3	0.3	0.3	0.3	0.3	0.4	0.4	0.5
PEEP	5	8	10	12	14	14	16	16

FiO₂	0.5	0.5-0.8	0.8	0.9	1.0	1.0
PEEP	18	20	22	22	22	24

PLATEAU PRESSURE GOAL: $\leq$ 30 cm H_2O
Check Pplat (0.5 second inspiratory pause), at least q 4h and after each change in PEEP or V_T.
If Pplat > 30 cm H_2O: decrease V_T by 1ml/kg steps (minimum = 4 ml/kg).
If Pplat < 25 cm H_2O and V_T< 6 ml/kg, increase V_T by 1 ml/kg until Pplat > 25 cm H_2O or V_T = 6 ml/kg.
If Pplat < 30 and breath stacking or dys-synchrony occurs: may increase V_T in 1ml/kg increments to 7 or 8 ml/kg if Pplat remains $\leq$ 30 cm H_2O.

B. **SPONTANEOUS BREATHING TRIAL (SBT):**
If all above criteria are met and subject has been in the study for at least 12 hours, initiate a trial of UP TO 120 minutes of spontaneous breathing with FiO2 $\leq$ 0.5 and PEEP $\leq$ 5:
   1. Place on T-piece, trach collar, or CPAP $\leq$ 5 cm H_2O with PS $\leq$ 5
   2. Assess for tolerance as below for up to two hours.
      a. $SpO_2 \geq$ 90: and/or $PaO_2 \geq$ 60 mmHg
      b.   Spontaneous $V_T \geq$ 4 ml/kg PBW
      c.   RR $\leq$ 35/min
      d.   pH $\geq$ 7.3
      e.   No respiratory distress (distress= 2 or more)
         ➤ HR > 120% of baseline
         ➤ Marked accessory muscle use
         ➤ Abdominal paradox
         ➤ Diaphoresis
         ➤ Marked dyspnea
   3. If tolerated for at least 30 minutes, consider extubation.
4. If not tolerated resume pre-weaning settings.

Definition of UNASSISTED BREATHING
(Different from the spontaneous breathing criteria as PS is not allowed)

1. Extubated with face mask, nasal prong oxygen, or room air, OR
2. T-tube breathing, OR
3. Tracheostomy mask breathing, OR
4. CPAP less than or equal to 5 cm H_2O **without pressure support or IMV assistance.**

• **Fig. 12.1** Mechanical ventilator protocol card. (From NIH-NHLBI ARDS Network.)

oxygen delivery, the nitrogen gets washed out and replaced by oxygen. In contrast, oxygen is extremely soluble in blood and will diffuse into the pulmonary capillaries very quickly, leaving the alveoli without any gas left for that pillow effect (intrinsic PEEP).

Administration of 100% oxygen to patients is reasonable during emergencies and resuscitation, but should be weaned down during transport if the patient's oxygen saturations allow. The American Heart Association recommends weaning oxygen down to the lowest levels while maintaining

SpO_2 greater than 94% during post cardiac arrest care. Life-threatening hypoxia should always be treated with 100% oxygen delivered via facemask, ETT, or tracheotomy.

Some patients may be more susceptible to high levels of oxygen; for example, preterm neonates are at risk for long-term retinal damage and bronchopulmonary dysplasia (BPD). Also susceptible are children with congenital cyanotic and partially repaired cyanotic-heart lesions who are at risk of hemodynamic instability as a result of oxygen-induced excess pulmonary blood flow.[1] The newest Neonatal Resuscitation Program (NRP) guidelines have recommended preductal oxygen saturation parameters beginning at 1 minute after birth and going to 10 minutes, with 1-minute preductal oxygen saturation goals of 60% to 65%, and a 10-minute goal of 85% to 90%. Treating neonates with supplemental oxygen should only occur if their preductal oxygen saturation is less than the recommended parameters from NRP and should only be treated until their oxygen saturations reach the recommended levels based on minutes since birth. Any neonate with bradycardia, despite the oxygen saturation, will be treated with positive pressure ventilation and supplemental oxygen.

Classification of Positive Pressure Ventilation

No universal consensus exists on classification of ventilators or ventilation modes, and descriptions vary with the literature. The elements in classification that are most pertinent to transport teams are volume control ventilation, pressure control ventilation, and CPAP. No research exists to suggest improved outcomes between volume-controlled and pressure-controlled ventilation strategies. Within these categories, ventilation modes can be described as mandatory, assisted, or spontaneous, depending on the dynamic necessary to initiate an inspiratory breath.

- *Mandatory:* Mandatory breaths are initiated, controlled (volume or pressure), and terminated by the ventilator. No synchronizing of the ventilator breaths occur with patient-initiated breaths. Example: continuous mandatory ventilation (CMV).
- *Assisted:* Spontaneous breaths are initiated by the patient but controlled and ended (assisted) by the ventilator. Example: assist-control (AC).
- *Spontaneous:* Spontaneous breaths are initiated, controlled, and terminated by the patient. Example: CPAP.

Volume Ventilation

Volume-controlled pressure-variable ventilation is the most common mode of ventilation used on transport ventilators. The Vt is preset and delivered during the set inspiratory time of the ventilatory cycle. Once that Vt is reached, inspiration ends and exhalation begins. The inspiratory pressure varies depending on the compliance and resistance of the

lung, with higher pressures associated with greater lung resistance or low compliance. The advantage of this form of ventilation is the guarantee of minute ventilation (respiratory rate multiplied by the tidal volume, Vt × R). On the other hand, the potential for lung injury exists when high pressures are required to deliver the set Vt in patients with low lung compliance. To mitigate against ventilator-induced barotrauma or lung injury, pressure limits are set. If the high-pressure limit is reached during the delivery of the set Vt, the inspiration is terminated, even if the targeted Vt has not been achieved. Volume ventilation can be delivered using CMV, AC, or SIMV, with or without pressure support (PS), depending on the brand of ventilator.

Pressure Ventilation

Pressure-controlled ventilation delivers an inspiratory breath to a preset pressure limit. The inspiratory cycle is terminated when the rise time interval is met and the inspiratory time, set on the ventilator by the clinician, has been reached. The clinician sets the base ventilatory rate, the inspiratory pressure, and the inspiratory time. The Vt delivered varies depending on the compliance and resistance of the lung. For example, smaller volumes are delivered in patients with low pulmonary compliance or high airway resistance. The advantage of this mode of ventilation is that it limits the distending pressure of the lung, reducing the risk of VILI. The disadvantage of this mode is the absence of guaranteed minute ventilation with the potential for hypoventilation or hyperventilation. Most modern ventilators are capable of delivering pressure ventilation using AC or SIMV.

Pressure-Regulated Volume-Controlled Ventilation

PRVC is a relatively new mode of ventilation that attempts to blend the best of volume and pressure ventilation modes. The clinician sets a Vt and a high-pressure limit. After a test breath, the ventilator software will adjust the inspiratory flow wave pattern to attempt to deliver the set Vt within the pressure parameter that has been set. If it is unable to do so, inspiration continues (until the set inspiratory time has been reached), but the ventilator will begin to limit the Vt once the PIP has reached 5 cm H_2O below the set high-pressure limit. In pure pressure ventilation, the Vt can increase significantly when resistance and compliance falls, but in PRVC if a patient's airway resistance or lung compliance improves, the Vt will not exceed what has been set. This helps protect against overinflation and maintains consistent minute ventilation.

Continuous Mandatory Ventilation

CMV is a volume-initiated or pressure-initiated mode of ventilation in which the Vt and ventilatory rate are set. Spontaneous respiratory effort by the patient is ignored, and no patient triggering is possible. This method of ventilation is uncomfortable and is not recommended or used much anymore. If used, the patient would need to be primarily chemically paralyzed, sedated, and treated for pain. This mode may be used for patients who have no spontaneous respiratory effort. *CMV-assist* is a term used by some ventilator manufacturers to refer to AC ventilation; however, the primary transport ventilators used in the critical care environment, including the Drager-Oxylog 3000 plus, LTV 1200, ReVel, and Hamilton T-1, do not use this language and designate just AC.

Assist-Control Ventilation

With *AC ventilation*, the clinician sets a base ventilatory rate; however, the patient is allowed to breathe faster than the set rate. Every breath, whether patient or ventilator initiated, receives the full set Vt. This mode of ventilation requires minimal work from the patient and is often used during the early hours and days after intubation to allow the patient to rest while the underlying cause of respiratory failure is addressed.

AC can be either volume-controlled or pressure-controlled. In volume mode AC, both the ventilatory rate and Vt are set parameters. Parameters also set by the clinician on more sophisticated transport ventilators include either inspiratory flow rate or inspiratory time, waveform, and trigger sensitivity. Patient hyperventilation may occur in this mode; therefore, minute ventilation should be monitored. Historically, AC has been the primary mode seen in the hospital setting, but in the transport environment this mode can cause additional issues with ventilation. Ambulance and aircraft vibration and simple movements by the transport crew can cause autotriggering to occur. This can cause added discomfort, air trapping, and subsequent auto-PEEP. Patients need to be monitored closely for these potential problems during transport.

Synchronized Intermittent Mandatory Ventilation

SIMV can be used in either volume or pressure ventilation modes. The primary distinction between SIMV and AC ventilation is how the ventilator contributes to spontaneous respiratory effort. Similar to AC, SIMV mode provides breaths at a set rate and set Vt (or pressure), which will give a guaranteed minimum minute ventilation. However, unlike AC, spontaneous respiratory efforts do not receive an assisted Vt at the set mandatory Vt level. During the respiratory time interval, the ventilator will deliver a mandatory breath or allow a spontaneously triggered breath by the patient. During the next respiratory time interval, if the patient has not triggered another spontaneous breath, the ventilator will then give a mandatory breath. As noted earlier, the patients' spontaneous breath can be augmented with the addition of PS. The main goal of PS is to reduce the work of breathing only during spontaneous breaths initiated by the patient. The patient is able to initiate spontaneous breaths based on the sensitivity (trigger setting)

level set by the clinician, and positive pressure is delivered through the ventilator circuit to help overcome the resistance of the ETT and ventilator circuit. PS levels are commonly set at 5 to 10 cm H_2O over PEEP.

Pressure Support Ventilation

Pressure support ventilation (PSV) is an assisted mode of ventilation in which the patient initiates a breath, triggering the ventilator to deliver a preset level of inspiratory pressure. The patient determines the respiratory rate, inspiratory time, and Vt.[1] Because the patient triggers all breaths, this mode is only effective in the spontaneously breathing patient. The higher the PS is set, the less ventilatory workload for the patient. PSV can be combined with other modes of ventilation, such as SIMV and CPAP, but is not active in AC. It is sometimes used in weaning patients from the ventilator by progressively decreasing the degree of PS. A minimal amount of PSV (5–10 cm H_2O) should be provided to overcome the resistance to the ETT and ventilatory circuit. If the intent is to provide complete ventilatory support, then PSV should be set relatively high (15–20 cm H_2O). Minute ventilation should be closely monitored when used in patients with susceptibility to respiratory depression.

Invasive Continuous Positive Airway Pressure

CPAP is neither volume-controlled nor pressure-controlled ventilation, although it can and should be augmented with PS. Patients breathe spontaneously at their own rate and Vt via an artificial airway with a continuous level of elevated baseline pressure. This has the same effect as PEEP in opening collapsed alveoli and increasing FRC. This mode is primarily used to assess the patient's ability to ventilate and oxygenate before extubation. It is also used in patients without oxygenation or ventilation abnormalities who need only airway protection (e.g., patients who are alert and awake but have laryngeal edema or airway compression). This mode should be used with caution in patients who have the potential to decompensate neurologically or hemodynamically. For this reason, in the setting of the critical care transport environment, CPAP is rarely used for acutely ill patients.

Choosing a Mode

There are many different perspectives regarding which mode of ventilation is better for the highly critical patients transported in the critical care environment. In a hospital setting with quiet environments, little patient movement, and better ventilators that can stop autotriggering, AC may be a great mode of ventilation. In contrast, the transport environment brings many different dynamics that may cause transport ventilator autotriggering if used incorrectly. Considering the standard dynamics that transport teams encounter, including patient movement, ambulance and aircraft vibrations, and the new industry standard of attempting to maintain patients on pain management and sedation only while withholding long-acting paralysis, some clinicians feel that SIMV may offer added benefits during transport. Others, however, feel that in the early stages of acute illness, AC is the preferred mode because it provides the most support for the patient. There is no clinical evidence proving one mode is superior to another, so many transport programs follow the preferences of their medical directors or pulmonologists at the receiving tertiary care facility in their region.

Noninvasive Positive Pressure Ventilation

Noninvasive positive pressure ventilation (NiPPV) refers to mechanical ventilatory support provided without an endotracheal or tracheostomy tube. It is applied with a face or nasal mask, mouthpiece, high-flow nasal cannula, or nasal prongs, although generally it is used with a snug-fitting nasal or facial mask.[2] This method is useful in both chronic and acute disorders and is discussed here as it relates to acute respiratory failure or acute exacerbation of a chronic respiratory condition.

When successful, NiPPV can eliminate the need for intubation and its complications, while preserving the ability to speak, cough, and swallow. It decreases the work of breathing, increases alveolar ventilation, allows rest for respiratory musculature, and improves gas exchange. The strongest evidence of support for the successful use of NiPPV is in patients with acute exacerbation of COPD and in patients with acute cardiogenic pulmonary edema.[1,2] It may also be used in patients who refuse intubation. NiPPV is contraindicated for patients who need emergent intubation because of cardiac or respiratory arrest and for patients with hemodynamic instability, inability to control the airway (high risk for aspiration), upper airway obstruction, facial trauma or deformity, unstable arrhythmia, or organ failure unrelated to respiratory failure. Patients who have difficulty breathing in the supine position, especially when related to obesity, should be carefully considered before transport via NiPPV.

NiPPV can be delivered via CPAP and volume-cycled or pressure-limited modes. CPAP delivers a constant positive pressure during inspiration and expiration. Volume-cycled ventilators are often not well tolerated because masks cause a loss of Vt leading to constant alarms set off by the ventilator. Pressure-limited modes include PS, pressure-control, and bilevel positive airway pressure (BiPAP). BiPAP ventilation delivers both inspiratory positive airway pressure and expiratory positive airway pressure (similar to CPAP and PEEP). The patient triggers each breath. In the event of apnea, alarms and backup rates should be set.

Success of NiPPV is associated with user expertise, familiarity of equipment, and patient selection.[1,2] NiPPV, more than any other method of ventilation, requires a clinician skilled in the art of mechanical ventilation because the patient is awake and alert and only lightly sedated (or not sedated at all). Patient comfort and cooperation are the key

to success, so it is important that the clinician understand the advanced ventilator adjustments that can make a big difference in patient comfort and ventilator synchrony. When initiating NiPPV, a properly fitting mask must be selected. Applying the mask gently (or allowing the patient to hold the mask if they are able) until the patient is comfortable and in sync with the ventilator, before securing the straps, improves patient comfort.

CPAP, as opposed to PSV or BiPAP, may be selected when hypoxemia from cardiogenic pulmonary edema or upper airway obstruction from underlying obstructive sleep apnea is contributing to respiratory failure. CPAP can be delivered effectively using widely available lower-tech products with no mechanical ventilator required. CPAP devices consist of a tightly fitting facemask and a flow and CPAP generator or PEEP valve. PSV or BiPAP modes are chosen when ventilatory failure is a component, and positive pressure ventilation is needed to support failing respiratory muscles, such as in COPD exacerbation or neuromuscular disease. BiPAP requires a mechanical ventilator designed for noninvasive ventilation and flight crew members trained in its use.

The efficacy of NiPPV in the transport setting has not been clearly defined. Programs should develop specific criteria that involve not only proper patient selection but also the practicality of use in the medical transport environment. The use of NiPPV in acute hospital and home settings is steadily increasing. Requests to transport patients already successfully managed on NiPPV are on the rise. Critical care transport crew members need to be aware that patients being successfully managed in a hospital on sophisticated hospital noninvasive ventilators may not always tolerate the change to the transport ventilator. Transport ventilators often cannot match the inspiratory flow capabilities of the hospital ventilators and may increase the work of breathing on a patient already on the brink of needing intubation. Noninvasive ventilation requires high oxygen flow rates and will deplete a portable ventilator's battery faster than conventional ventilation, so crew members also need to be aware of their vehicle's oxygen capacity and have a power source readily available. Compliance with the aviation provider's protocols regarding electromagnetic interference must be maintained when considering use of a patient's personal NiPPV device in an aircraft.

Advanced Ventilatory Modes

Airway Pressure Release Ventilation

APRV was designed to be an effective, safe alternative for difficult-to-oxygenate patients with ALI or ARDS. During APRV, the ventilator applies a relatively high level of CPAP for a prolonged time to maintain alveolar recruitment with intermittent timed releases, which help to eliminate CO_2. The high, prolonged CPAP level is referred to as P-high. P-low is the pressure level during the release phase (usually 0–5 cm H_2O). The time spent at P-high is called T-high, and the short time spent at P-low is called T-low. P-high is usually set at a level between 20 and 30 cm H_2O, whereas P-low is set between 0 and 5 cm H_2O. APRV has been referred to by some as a form of inverse ratio ventilation because inspiration (T-high) is usually 4 to 6 seconds, whereas expiration (T-low) is just 0.2 to 0.8 seconds long.[6] The key difference is that in APRV, the patient is allowed to breathe spontaneously during P-high.

Spontaneous breathing plays a very important role in APRV, allowing the patient to control his or her respiratory frequency during P-high, thus improving patient comfort and patient-ventilator synchrony with reduction in the amount of sedation necessary. APRV requires a sophisticated ventilator with an active internal exhalation valve so the patient can breathe spontaneously at the high CPAP level. APRV was developed for ARDS patients and should not be used in patients with obstructive lung disease.

High-Frequency Ventilation

High-frequency ventilation (HFV) modes provide alveolar ventilation with Vt that are less than or equal to dead space volume by delivering them at supraphysiologic frequency. The goal of HFV therapy is to produce adequate alveolar ventilation at low Vt with preservation of end-expiratory lung volume to minimize volutrauma and barotrauma.[5,7,8] This form of ventilation is more commonly used for newborn and pediatric patients than adults. In practice, the high-frequency devices most often used are high-frequency oscillatory ventilation (HFOV) and high-frequency jet ventilation (HFJV).

Indications for HFV include disease states such as bronchopleural fistulas and airway injuries, patients at risk for pulmonary barotrauma (i.e., those with mean airway pressures [P_{aw}] >18–20 cm H_2O or plateau pressures >35 cm H_2O), and patients with diffuse alveolar disease (i.e., ALI, ARDS), in which a major therapeutic goal is to preserve end-expiratory lung volume while limiting end-inspiratory lung overdistension.

HFV requires complicated, specialized equipment, and it is strongly recommended that trained respiratory therapists, with experience using these devices, be part of the transport team if patients are being transported on HFV.

High-Frequency Jet Ventilation

HFJV delivers inspiratory gas through a jet injector, near the carina, at high velocity. This is accomplished with a specific ETT with a jet injector or an in-line jet injector adapter that is added to the existing ETT. HFJV is most often used simultaneously with a conventional ventilator that is able to provide PEEP and Vt breaths (10 mL/kg) to the patient to preserve end-expiratory lung volume.

- Rates of 100 to 600 beats/min are delivered with a Vt of 3 to 5 mL/kg.
- Risks include airway injury from the jet flow of gas positioned near the carina and air trapping.
- Expiration is passive.
- HFJV is generally limited to patients less than 8 years of age because of limitations in minute ventilation support.

High-Frequency Oscillatory Ventilation

HFOV is the most widely used HFV technique in clinical practice today. High-frequency oscillatory ventilators maintain lung recruitment by delivering a relatively high distending pressure (i.e., P_{aw}) while providing ventilation through superimposed, piston-generated, sinusoidal pressure oscillations (delta P [ΔP]) at a frequency of 3 to 15 Hz (180–900 oscillations per minute). Adequate oscillatory pressure (ΔP) generally produces visible chest vibration ("wiggle") from the clavicles to the lower abdomen or pelvis.

HFOV uses a relatively high P_{aw} to improve oxygenation. When transitioning to HFOV, the initial P_{aw} is generally set 3 to 5 cm H_2O above the P_{aw} on conventional ventilation immediately before transition. After the transition, the clinician should titrate the P_{aw} in 1- to 2-cm H_2O increments until oxygenation improves enough to allow a reduction in FiO_2 below 0.6 and global lung recruitment to a level at which both hemidiaphragms project at the level of the 8th to 10th posterior ribs on a chest x-ray.[5,7,8]

- Ventilation is primarily determined with oscillatory pressure amplitude (ΔP). Increase the ΔP in 2- to 3-cm H_2O increments to improve CO_2 clearance. The chest wiggle is attained by adjusting the ΔP on the ventilator.
- Ventilation is also influenced by the oscillation frequency, because frequency is inversely related to delivered Vt in HFOV. Although ventilation, at higher frequencies, generally delivers Vt of 1 to 3 mL/kg, physiological Vt that approach those used in typical conventional ventilation strategies can be produced at the low end of the frequency spectrum.[7,8]
- HFOV is the only mode of mechanical ventilation in which expiration is active rather than passive.

Inhaled Nitric Oxide

Inhaled nitric oxide (iNO) is a naturally occurring vasodilator administered as an inhaled gas for selective pulmonary vasodilation, without associated systemic hypotension. As iNO diffuses across the alveolar-capillary membrane, the smooth muscle cells in the adjacent pulmonary vasculature relax, decreasing pulmonary vascular resistance (PVR). Oxygenation improves as the vessels that perfuse ventilated alveoli are dilated, redistributing blood flow and reducing intrapulmonary shunting. iNO in the bloodstream is bound to hemoglobin and is rapidly deactivated, causing little effect on systemic vascular resistance and blood pressure.

Therapy indications include pulmonary hypertension and isolated right heart failure. iNO can be administered through a nasal cannula or ventilator circuit at a dose of 5 to 40 parts per million (ppm), with a typical starting point of 20 ppm. Once therapy is started, do not abruptly discontinue or disconnect a patient from iNO without specific medical orders from a physician. PVR could significantly increase and cause acute hypoxia and right ventricular dysfunction.

The most common patient population placed on iNO therapy are newborns with meconium aspiration and pulmonary hypertension. It has also been used with mixed results on adult patients with severe ARDS.

Methemoglobinemia and alveolar cytotoxicity are rare adverse reactions reported with iNO therapy. Monitor methemoglobin levels with blood gas samples if available.

Helium-Oxygen Mixture

Helium-oxygen mixture (Heliox) is a biologically inert gas with a much lower density than oxygen-nitrogen. With inhalation, resistance to airflow is reduced and areas of turbulent flow through obstructions may be converted to a streamlined nonturbulent (laminar) flow, improving the work of breathing.

Clinical indications for Heliox include upper airway obstruction associated with edema (postextubation stridor or croup), obstruction from compression, respiratory processes with high airway resistance or obstructive pathology (bronchiolitis or status asthmaticus), or respiratory distress syndrome. Heliox may also be used for children with BPD (to decrease the work of breathing), for augmentation in the delivery of nebulized bronchodilators to obstructed lower airways, and to allow time for the onset of therapeutic medications or the resolution of the disease process. If successful, it may negate the need for intubation. The benefits are usually evident in several minutes. Administration consideration includes the following:

- Usually administered with 30% oxygen through a tight-fitting mask.
- Commercially available in helium:oxygen concentrations of 80:20 or 70:30.
- Do not administer pure helium, always administer with oxygen. If manually blending helium and oxygen, place an in-line oxygen concentration device to ensure adequate oxygen mix.

Positive improvement has been reported in the adult population in patients treated for upper airway obstructions as a result of thyroid masses, radiation injury, lymphoma, cancer, or angioedema.[1,9]

Ventilator Settings

Selection of ventilator mode and settings are determined by clinical assessment, degree of alteration in oxygenation or ventilation, disease pathophysiology, institutional or physician preference, and capabilities of the transport ventilator.

Tidal Volume

Tidal volume (Vt) is set in volume-controlled ventilation modes. To reduce the likelihood of alveolar overdistension and high airway pressures, the Vt should be based on IBW rather than actual body weight in adult patients. In the past, high Vt of 10 to 15 mL/kg have been used to maintain normocapnia and pH, and to prevent atelectasis-related hypoxemia. However, adverse effects of barotrauma and volutrauma have led to recommendations for lower Vt, which are said to be lung protective. The benefit of a low Vt ventilation strategy was shown in the landmark ARDS Network randomized controlled multicenter trial of 861 patients that compared the use of low Vt (4–6 mL/kg IBW and plateau pressure <30 cm H_2O) with traditional Vt (12 mL/kg IBW and plateau pressure <50 cm H_2O) in ARDS patients. The trial was stopped early after interim analysis results showed a 23% reduction in mortality rates in the low Vt group.[5,10]

In light of the study outcomes, Vt should be initiated at 6 mL/kg IBW in patients with ARDS/ALI. Adjust the respiratory rate to achieve the desired partial pressure of carbon dioxide in arterial blood ($PaCO_2$) or pH. Low Vt ventilation often requires acceptance of a degree of respiratory acidosis and is discussed in more depth in the section Ventilation Strategies (permissive hypercapnia).

Patients with obstructive disease, such as COPD and asthma, benefit from lower Vt of 6 to 8 mL/kg IBW to reduce lung inflation and extend exhalation time.[2,7] In most other patients, use of a Vt greater than 8 mL/kg is rarely necessary (and may be harmful), and a starting volume of 6 to 8 mL/kg with ventilator adjustments to meet the pH and $PaCO_2$ targets is reasonable.

Peak Inspiratory Pressure

PIP is set in pressure-targeted modes. When initiating pressure-control ventilation, the target pressure should initially be set to give the patient a measured exhaled Vt of 6 to 8 mL/kg IBW, with peak pressures of 16 to 24 cm H_2O commonly required. As stated previously, Vt and minute ventilation are not static, but they change dynamically with lung compliance, which warrants close monitoring.

In volume-cycled modes, PIP is a dynamic value reflective of a combination of patient and ventilator variables. Vt, PEEP, and inspiratory time are ventilator settings that contribute to inspiratory pressures. On some ventilators, inspiratory time is not a set parameter but is determined by the set respiratory rate and ratio of inspiratory time to expiratory time (I:E ratio). PIP increases or decreases as lung compliance worsens or improves.

Rate, Breaths per Minute, and Frequency

During initial selection of the rate, consider the patient's age (pediatric, newborn, and adult), minute ventilation, and Vt. *Minute ventilation,* or minute volume, is equal to the respiratory rate multiplied by the tidal volume (Vt × R), with a normal range of 4 to 9 L/min. Adjustments to the rate depend on the clinical goal and disease process to meet the desired pH or $PaCO_2$ range. When Vt of 10 to 12 mL/kg were used, ventilator rates of 12 beats/min were common for adults. However, with Vt now appropriately set at 6 to 8 mL/kg of IBW, initial rates of 14 to 16 are more appropriate. Pediatric rates often range from 20 to 30 beats/min, depending on the age of the child. Generally, increasing the rate decreases the $PaCO_2$ and increases the pH. Conversely, decreasing the rate increases the $PaCO_2$ and decreases the pH. With assisted ventilation modes in spontaneously breathing patients, care must be taken to monitor for hyperventilation and auto-PEEP.

Fractional Concentration of Oxygen in Inspired Gas

If the partial pressure of oxygen in arterial blood (PaO_2) is unknown, the *fractional concentration of oxygen in inspired gas* (FiO_2) is typically set at 100% on initiation of mechanical ventilation but should be reduced as soon as possible and as tolerated by PaO_2 or pulse oximetry. FiO_2 is used in combination with PEEP to maintain the PaO_2 or peripheral oxygen saturation (SpO_2) above the minimum threshold. The oxygenation goals set by the ARDS Network for patients with ALI/ARDS are PaO_2 of 55 to 80 mm Hg or SpO_2 of 88% to 95%.[5,10] The Brain Trauma Foundation recommends that PaO_2 be maintained at more than 60 mm Hg or SpO_2 at more than 90% in patients with TBIs.[4,10] The American Heart Association advises that oxygen saturations be maintained at 94% to 99% in patients with cardiac compromise.[3] If high levels of FiO_2 do not reverse hypoxia, then PEEP can be added incrementally to achieve oxygenation goals.

The FiO_2 selections may be limited by the transport ventilator's blending or air entrainment capabilities.

Positive End-Expiratory Pressure

PEEP exerts pressure in the patient's airway above the atmospheric level throughout the respiratory cycle, increasing the FRC by opening collapsed alveoli. The FRC is the air that remains in the lungs at the end of passive expiration; it is reduced with loss of chest wall mobility (obesity) or lung compliance.[1,11] The increase in FRC through the addition of PEEP is referred to as *recruitment* and decreases intrapulmonary shunting of blood through lung regions with collapsed alveoli, improving ventilation to perfusion ratio matching. The ideal PEEP setting prevents cyclic atelectasis and overdistension injury while optimizing oxygenation. When possible, the overall goal should be to use the lowest PEEP setting necessary to acquire an acceptable PaO_2 with an FiO_2 of less than 0.60. Most patient's benefit from the addition of 5 cm H_2O PEEP to overcome the decrease in FRC as a result of the airway resistance caused by the ETT. Unless otherwise indicated, initial ventilator settings should include a PEEP of 5 cm H_2O.

In several circumstances, PEEP should be used with caution because it increases intrathoracic pressure, reducing venous return and preload. However, it has been shown that it may be better to apply more PEEP and reduce FiO_2 in an attempt to optimize oxygenation, and at the same time limit the oxygen toxicity potential. In addition, many patients may suffer from refractory hypoxia and require the added PEEP. In these cases it may be necessary to augment

the additional PEEP with vasopressors so optimal oxygenation and mean arterial pressure can be achieved.

In patients with unilateral lung disease, preferential distribution of minute ventilation and PEEP may be directed to areas of healthy lung (least resistance) and do little for the injured or diseased lung. This can cause alveolar overdistension injury of healthy alveoli and compress the vasculature surrounding the alveoli, worsening the shunt. When possible, placement of patients into a lateral position with the good lung in the dependent position may help improve blood flow and gas exchange to healthy tissue.

Auto-PEEP, also termed *intrinsic PEEP*, refers to air trapped in the alveoli at end expiration. Causes include high minute ventilation, mechanical expiratory flow limitation (foreign body obstruction and mucous plug), and physiological expiratory resistance (asthma and COPD). Large Vt or high respiratory rates increase the minute ventilation and reduce exhalation time. A new breath is delivered before full exhalation occurs and traps air in the alveoli. Similarly, patient-generated rapid respiratory rates in assisted ventilator modes caused by agitation, patient-ventilator asynchrony, or low sensitivity thresholds can lead to subsequent incomplete exhalation and auto-PEEP. Patients with obstructive lung disease are particularly vulnerable to air-trapping as a result of airway collapse or narrowing. Auto-PEEP can lead to hypotension, barotrauma, and increasing ventilator-patient dyssynchrony. Modern transport ventilators can measure auto-PEEP with an expiratory hold maneuver, so it should be monitored and efforts made to minimize the occurrence, especially in asthma and COPD patients.

Inspiratory-to-Expiratory Time Ratio and Flow Rate

The normal I:E ratio is 1:2 or 1:3. An increase in the flow rate, or how fast a breath is given, causes a decrease in the inspiratory time, which allows for a longer period of expiration. The I:E ratio may be adjusted for disease pathology. The inspiratory time can be adjusted directly on most transport ventilators. If there is no inspiratory time adjustment, the inspiratory flow rate, Vt and respiratory rate can be used to affect the I:E ratio. Patients with reactive airway disease, or asthma, benefit from a longer expiratory time of 1:4, 1:5, or greater. Patients with hypoxia may benefit from a longer inspiratory time, reflective of an I:E ratio of 1:2. In some cases, I:E ratios of 1:1 can be attempted; however, these ratios may lead to hemodynamic compromise from auto-PEEP and contribute to volutrauma.

For most adults, flow rates of 50 to 60 L/min are usually adequate, although higher flow may often be needed to produce adequate ventilation, particularly in patients with obstructive lung disease.[2] Some transport ventilators are not equipped with the ability to adjust flow, and longer expiratory times are adjusted through the I:E ratio or inspiratory time settings. The flow limitations of some transport ventilators limit extension of the expiration time and shortening of the inspiration time. In this situation, an inadequate time for expiration in patients with obstructive disease may lead to auto-PEEP, high plateau pressures, overdistension, and barotrauma. Clinicians can overcome this to some extent by decreasing the Vt or respiratory rate. This decrease may require some degree of respiratory acidosis to prevent lung overdistension from air trapping. However, patients tend to do better being in a state of hypercapnia compared with hypocapnia, and the maintenance of mild respiratory acidosis may be warranted at times.

Flow Pattern

Some transport ventilators allow the clinician to select flow patterns, which dictate how an inspiratory flow is delivered. Flow pattern advantage depends on the patient's lung compliance, chest wall elasticity, airway resistance, and transport ventilator capability. Determination of which pattern optimizes ventilation-perfusion is not always predictable and is often an exercise of trial and error.[9,11]

Trigger Sensitivity

An assisted breath (AC ventilation, pressure-controlled ventilation, or PSV) can be triggered by either pressure or flow. *Flow triggering* detects a change in the flow of gas with spontaneous effort. A base (or bias) flow continually moves past the patient. When the patient makes an inspiratory effort, the ventilator detects a deviation in the flow and is triggered to deliver a supported breath. A bias flow of 5 to 10 L/min is often used with a trigger sensitivity threshold of 2 L/min.[5] This means that most transport ventilators use flow trigger as their primary trigger. However, each ventilator is different and every user should always identify their manufacturer's guide for correct understanding and application of the trigger. The flow trigger works off the bias flow. The bias flow is the amount of volume moving through the ventilator circuit during exhalation. When the trigger is set at a level of 3, it is setting a trigger at 3 L/min out of the total bias flow. This 3 L/min needs to be reduced to its simplest form to understand how the patient uses this for triggering. First, convert 3 L to 3000 mL and 1 minute to 60 seconds. This allows simplification into a smaller number that makes sense; dividing 60 s/3000 mL gets 50 mL/s. This means that the patient has to have an effort of 50 mL to trigger a breath on a sensitivity level of 3, respectively. This same method also can be applied to sensitivity settings of 4 to 9. One negative to the transport ventilators being primarily flow triggered stems from the low threshold for autotriggering.[5] As the previous example illustrated, a sensitivity level of 3 has the patient taking a minimum effort of 50 mL/s to trigger a breath. By simply grabbing the ventilator circuit, the flight crew can easily simulate this and cause an autotriggered breath to be given if the ventilator is in the AC mode, for example. It is for this reason that the flight team should always start at a higher sensitivity level than in a normal stationary patient environment, with 3 to 5 being a good starting point.

Pressure triggering requires a demand valve that senses a negative airway pressure generated by the patient during initiation of a spontaneous respiratory effort. The demand valve sensitivity is set at a level that allows the patient to easily take a breath but not so sensitive that it interprets artifact, such as patient movement, air leak, or water in the ventilator circuit, as an attempted breath. This could cause unintended hyperventilation, respiratory alkalosis, and auto-PEEP. If the sensitivity is set too high, the ventilator does not trigger a breath when the patient makes a spontaneous effort and increases the patient's work of breathing. The usual threshold is set at −2 to −3 cm H_2O in the transport environment. For example, the ReVel ventilator has a feature that allows flight crew members to move from the standard default flow trigger to a pressure trigger by turning the trigger setting knob counterclockwise until "P" is seen. This is then in a pressure trigger mode, with a default trigger of −3 cm H_2O. This is a great feature and useful if difficulties arise in transport with autotriggering in the standard flow trigger setting.[5]

Changing one ventilator parameter may affect other ventilator variables and should be reassessed after adjustments are made. For example, inspiratory time (tI) is equal to Vt divided by flow (tI = Vt/flow). Changing these parameters changes the other parameters. Likewise, on some ventilators, alteration in the FiO_2 may change the flow enough to alter the delivered Vt. Clinicians should be familiar with ventilator capabilities and limitations. Know the parameters that are automatically adjusted by the ventilator to compensate for changes made by the user.

Ventilation Strategies

Obstructive Lung Disease

Care needs to be taken in patients intubated for severe asthma and acute exacerbations of COPD to minimize air trapping and auto-PEEP and to avoid overventilation. As such, arterial CO_2 levels of greater than 100 mm Hg are common and can be alarming in these patients. However, attempting to quickly lower those CO_2 levels with high set ventilator rates can lead to catastrophic consequences, such as bilateral pneumothoraces. The goal for these patients is to provide adequate oxygenation and ventilation support while allowing the other treatment modalities to take effect. The CO_2 level will eventually improve. Vt of 6 to 8 mL/kg with slower rates than normal (10–12 breaths/min in adults), higher inspiratory flow rates, and shorter inspiratory times all allow for the longer exhalation times required in these patients. I:E ratios of 1:4, 1:6, or even 1:8 may be necessary to minimize air trapping.[5]

ARDS

ARDS patients are managed with lower Vt (4–6mL/kg) and higher respiratory rates. Vt is decreased to maintain Pplat less than 30 cm H_2O. Oxygenation is usually the primary problem for these patients, so high FiO_2 and high PEEP levels are commonly required. The ARDS Net organization provides a detailed protocol card that is helpful in managing these patients.[3]

Permissive Hypercapnia

Ventilating with slower rates for obstructive lung disease patients and lower Vt for ARDS patients can result in hypercapnia. *Permissive hypercapnia* is a lung-protective strategy aimed at decreasing alveolar ventilation to prevent lung injury. The use of small Vt or lower rates produces higher $PaCO_2$ and lower pH levels. In permissive hypercapnia strategies, acidemia is tolerated to a pH of 7.20 to 7.25 mm Hg or lower. Hypercapnia and acidemia are not the goal of this approach, but rather the tolerated consequence. Acidosis at this level is generally well tolerated when achieved gradually. The small Vt and/or slower respiratory rates associated with permissive hypercapnia may be uncomfortable and will require sedation and sometimes paralysis to offset the increased respiratory drive and agitation associated with discomfort. The high $PaCO_2$ in permissive hypercapnia causes cerebral vasodilation and increased intracranial pressure (ICP), so this approach is contraindicated in patients with head injuries or cerebral hemorrhage.

Trauma Patients

Hypoventilation and hyperventilation are both harmful for trauma patients (especially head trauma patients). The goal of mechanical ventilation for these patients is physiological normal ABG values. Hyperventilation is effective at decreasing ICP, but it does so at the expense of cerebral perfusion and has been associated with worse outcomes. This strategy is no longer practiced, with $PaCO_2$ ranges being targeted at 35 mm Hg. The only role for hyperventilation of head trauma patients may be as a short-term measure in a patient that is experiencing severely increased ICP or acute brainstem herniation due to a surgically correctable cause, with hyperventilation being able to buy time to get this type of patient to surgery.

Troubleshooting

Monitoring

Patients on mechanical ventilation need vigilant and continuous monitoring of ventilator parameters and clinical assessment. Oxygen saturations and $EtCO_2$ should be monitored and their limitations in clinical use well understood. Pulse oximetry does not detect saturations below 83% with the same degree of precision or accuracy as it does at higher saturations, nor does it perform well in low perfusion states. Many errors made in pulse oximetry readings are related to artifact. The pulse oximetry waveform should be compared with the patient's heart rate to ascertain accurate readings.

$EtCO_2$ monitors have been shown to be accurate in both the prehospital and hospital settings. In normal conditions, the $EtCO_2$ reads 3 to 5 mm Hg lower than the $PaCO_2$.

However, it is important to understand that $EtCO_2$ in hypoperfusion states (hypovolemia, hypotension, and reduced cardiac output), or in patients with ventilation-perfusion abnormalities, will be significantly (and unpredictably) lower than the patient's arterial CO_2. $EtCO_2$ reflects a patient's perfusion status as well as ventilation, and a drop in the $EtCO_2$ reading may be one of the first indicators that a patient is going into pulseless electrical activity. Additionally, it is important to know that the $EtCO_2$ will never be higher than the patient's $PaCO_2$. In cases in which transport teams do not have access to the most recent ABG, $EtCO_2$ can be used to predict $PaCO_2$. One must understand that there is a gradient as stated earlier and that this gradient is not 100% accurate. In patients with increasing dead space or perfusion states related to treatment or worsening condition, the gradient between $PaCO_2$ and $EtCO_2$ will widen. Although $EtCO_2$ monitoring is an excellent tool for transport, and is the standard of practice for determining proper ETT placement, decisions regarding mechanical ventilator setting adjustments should take the entire clinical picture into account, not just the $EtCO_2$ values.

Many transport programs have point-of-care testing capability during transport. If available and time allows during longer transports of critically ill ventilated patients, obtaining an ABG sample can be extremely valuable in guiding ventilator management decisions.

A baseline minute ventilation and $EtCO_2$ value should be determined before a patient is transferred from a referring facility ventilator to a transport ventilator, particularly when ventilation modes are changed, to help guide adequacy in matching ventilation. Monitoring of minute ventilation values also assists in the detection of hyperventilation or hypoventilation and contributes in the reevaluation of treatment, ventilation mode, and ventilator settings.

Ventilator Alarms

Alarm limits should be set to warn transport crews of mechanical and physiological problems. Silencing alarms or changing limits without carefully considering the cause can be deleterious to the patient. Additionally, setting alarms should not give the transport team a false sense that the ventilator will warn of potential adverse situations. Continuous monitoring of the ventilator should take place throughout the patient interaction.

Because peak inspiratory and plateau pressures are associated with VILI, high-pressure alarm limits particularly should be tightly controlled and assessed. Increased PIP without changes in the plateau pressure is indicative of increased airway resistance, such as a kinked ETT, secretions, bronchospasm, or obstruction. Elevated peak *and* plateau pressures are associated with decreased compliance such as pulmonary edema, pneumothorax, pleural effusions, abdominal distension, or auto-PEEP.

Ventilator alarms are difficult to hear in the transport setting. They should be turned to maximal volume, and the machine should be positioned so that flashing alarm lights can be visualized. Airway status should be evaluated

---

• BOX 12.1 | Indications for Endotracheal Intubation
Problem: Failure or Anticipated Failure to Protect the Airway

- Obtunded or comatose with loss of gag reflex
  - Traumatic brain injury
  - Overdose
  - Anoxia
  - Cerebral insults (cerebrovascular accident, aneurysms, etc.)
- Obstruction
  - Edema related to trauma
  - Inhalation injury
  - Foreign body aspiration
  - Congenital anomaly
- Pharmacological therapy: Profound sedation or analgesia used to treat or diagnose certain conditions, such as:
  - Status epilepticus
  - Increased intracranial pressures
  - Diagnostic procedures in combative patients
  - Elective procedures

Problem: Failure to Oxygenate

- Shunt ventilation: Alveoli are perfused but not ventilated
  - Pneumonia
  - Acute lung injury
  - Pulmonary hemorrhage or contusion
  - Atelectasis
  - Congenital cardiac disease
- Dead space ventilation: Alveoli are ventilated but not perfused
  - Pulmonary embolus
  - Hypotension
  - Low cardiac output states

- Diffusion abnormalities: Obstruction or restriction of gas exchange across the capillary-alveolar membrane
  - Pulmonary edema
  - Pulmonary fibrosis
- Oxygen extraction: Inability to extract oxygen
  - Sepsis
  - Carbon monoxide poisoning
  - Cyanide poisoning

Problem: Failure to Ventilate

- Neurological
  - Spinal cord injury or disease
  - Brain injury or disease
  - Overdose
  - Guillain-Barré syndrome
- Muscular
  - Myopathies
  - Myasthenia gravis
- Anatomical
  - Pleural effusions
  - Hemothorax or pneumothorax
  - Abdominal compartment syndrome
  - Bronchospasm, reactive airway disease
  - Congenital anomalies
- Infectious
  - Botulism
  - Respiratory syncytial virus
  - Pertussis

• BOX 12.2 | DOPE

D: Displaced endotracheal tube
O: Obstructed endotracheal tube
P: Pneumothorax
E: Equipment (ventilator) failure

---

immediately with any patient deterioration. The DOPE acronym (D, displaced ETT; O, obstructed ETT; P, pneumothorax; E, equipment [ventilator] failure) is a useful tool to remember possible causes of airway compromise (Boxes 12.1, 12.2). If any question exists as to the cause of deterioration, the patient should be disconnected from the ventilator and manually ventilated until all possibilities are considered. Common ventilator alarms are listed in Table 12.3.

Ventilator Asynchrony

Ventilator asynchrony occurs when disparity is found between patient respiratory effort and ventilator delivery, often described as "fighting the ventilator." Ideally, to decrease the work of breathing and reduce respiratory distress, the ventilator should cycle with the patient's intrinsic respiratory rhythm.[1,4,9] Anxiety and discomfort are often associated with mechanical ventilation. Sedation and pain management

should be evaluated, treated, and reassessed for adequacy. Initial ventilator settings can be adjusted after connecting the patient to the ventilator and assessing the patient's breathing pattern and demand.

The patient's respiratory effort and triggering sensitivity should be assessed in assisted and spontaneous modes of ventilation, whether volume limited or pressure limited. If the sensitivity threshold is set too high, the patient's respiratory efforts are not recognized and the ventilator is not triggered to provide a breath. Alternately, if set too low, the ventilator autotriggers or delivers breaths in response to extrinsic stimuli (ambulance or aircraft vibrations and movement) or water in the circuit.

One problem related to volume-limited ventilators is inadequate flow of gas, which causes patients to feel like they are not getting enough air and to attempt to extract more gas out of the ventilator.[4,9] This situation is uncomfortable for patients, and many transport ventilators only have the option of adjusting inspiratory time, or I:E ratio, and not flow directly. However, some ventilators allow the user to adjust flow via the *Rise Time* profiles found in the extended features menus of many ventilators. By adjusting to a quicker *Rise Time (0.1 seconds)*, you then allow for more flow and a corresponding increase in Vt. Patients with poor lung compliance or obstructive disease need high inspiratory flow rates to receive full Vt support during the set inspiratory time. Lengthening the inspiratory time compromises

TABLE 12.3   Troubleshooting Ventilator Alarms

Initial assessment:
Airway: Is the ETT in the correct position? Check ETT insertion depth, check EtCO$_2$, and check breath sounds.
Breathing: Check breath sounds, look for chest excursion, check pulse oximetry, and check patient color.
Circulation: Check the pulse, ECG, and blood pressure.
Remove patient from the ventilator and manually use a resuscitation bag if any compromise is found.

Alarm	Cause	Management
Apnea	Insufficient spontaneous breathing by patient in CPAP or pressure support mode	Switch ventilator mode to one that provides set rate
High airway pressure	ETT obstruction: sputum, kink, biting	Suction airway
	Decreased compliance or increased resistance	Treat cause of resistance
		Adjust mode or settings
	Circumferential burns	Rule out hypoxia before treating agitation
	Bronchospasm, lung collapse, pneumothorax, endobronchial intubation, worsening of lung process	CXR analysis
		Change ventilator mode to one that is better tolerated or provide sedation/analgesia
	Anxiety/fear/pain/fighting of ventilator	
Low airway pressure	Ventilator disconnect	Ensure that all connections are intact and tight
	Leak in ventilator system	
	Cuff leak	Troubleshoot ETT cuff
	Inadvertent extubation	BVM if ETT was dislodged
Oxygen pressure low	Oxygen cylinder is empty	
	Cylinder valve is closed	
	Unit not connected to wall terminal	
	Aircraft/ambulance oxygen flow in off position	

BVM, Bag-valve-mask; *CPAP*, continuous positive airway pressure; *CXR*, chest x-ray *ECG*, electrocardiogram; EtCO$_2$, end-tidal CO$_2$; *ETT*, endotracheal tube.

the long expiratory time needed by these patients who are already prone to air trapping and auto-PEEP.

Patient oxygenation and ventilation requirements may exceed the capabilities of some transport ventilators and may require deep sedation or neuromuscular blockade to complete some patient transports. This is not the absolute norm, and each patient should be given continuous aliquots of pain and sedation medications while attempting to limit long-acting paralysis, if at all possible. This strategy should be undertaken after careful consideration of the cause of asynchrony, the ventilator capabilities, and alternative means of transport. More sophisticated transport ventilators and ventilation strategies often require the skill and knowledge of a respiratory therapist and the transport from a larger ambulance or fixed-wing aircraft.

Summary

This chapter provided an overview of mechanical ventilation in the transport environment. The topic of mechanical ventilation and application of ventilation strategies will be one of the most challenging learning aspects for critical care providers. The transport team must be familiar with indications for mechanical ventilation, pulmonary physiology, and the equipment that is used during patient interaction. It is essential to continually broaden your understanding of mechanical ventilation so you are prepared for the highly critical patients you will be asked to transport.

References

1. Cairo J. *Pilbeam's Mechanical Ventilation: Physiological and Clinical Applications.* 6th ed. St. Louis: Mosby; 2015.
2. Esquinas A. *Noninvasive Mechanical Ventilation: Theory*, Equipment, and Clinical Application. 2nd ed. New York: Springer; 2016.
3. Elie M, Carden D. *Acute Respiratory Distress Syndrome.* Williston, VT: Morgan and Claypool Life Sciences; 2013.
4. Hess D, Kacmarek R. *Essentials of Mechanical Ventilation.* 3rd ed. New York: McGraw-Hill; 2014.
5. Bauer E. *Ventilator Management: A Pre-Hospital Perspective.* 2nd ed. Scottsville, KY: FlightBridgeED, LLC; 2015.
6. Daoud EG. Airway pressure release ventilation: annals of thoracic medicine. *Ann Thorac Med.* 2007;2(4):176-179.
7. Remensberger P. *Pediatric and Neonatal Mechanical Ventilation.* New York: Springer; 2015.
8. Walsh B. *Neonatal and Pediatric Respiratory Care.* 4th ed. St. Louis, MO: Elsevier; 2015.
9. Chang D. *Clinical Application of Mechanical Ventilation.* 4th ed. Clifton Park, NY: Delmar Cengage Learning; 2013.
10. Davis D, Aguilar S, Smith K, et al. Preliminary report of a mathematical model of ventilation and intrathoracic pressure applied to pre-hospital patients with severe traumatic brain injury. *Prehospital Emergency Care.* 2014;19(2):328-325.
11. Nourbakhsh E, Nugent K. *A bedside guide to mechanical ventilation.* Lubbock, TX: Texas Tech University Health; 2011.

13

Shock

MICHAEL A. FRAKES

S hock, the "rude unhinging of the machinery of life," is a cellular-level imbalance between oxygen supply and demand. It is common in critical care, affecting about one-third of critical care patients.[1-3] The oxygen utilization defect comes from one or more of four potential, but not necessarily exclusive, mechanisms: hypovolemia, structural or functional cardiac failure, obstruction to cardiac filling or return, and abnormal intravascular volume distribution. Septic shock, a form of distributive and hypovolemic shock, is the most common. In one report of intensive care unit (ICU) patients with pressor-dependent shock, septic shock occurred in 62% of patients, cardiogenic shock in 16%, hypovolemic shock in 16%, other types of distributive shock in 4%, and obstructive shock in 2%.[4]

Physiology

When oxygen demand exceeds oxygen supply, no matter the mechanism, cellular respiration shifts to anaerobic metabolism, with decreased energy availability, increased carbon dioxide production, and the accumulation of lactic acid and other toxic by-products. An understanding of shock, therefore, requires an understanding of both cellular respiration and oxygen delivery.

Cellular Respiration

The processes of cellular respiration break down one glucose molecule into carbon dioxide and water. The final results of the three processes (glycolysis, the Krebs cycle, and oxidative phosphorylation) also generate adenosine triphosphate (ATP; Fig. 13.1).

In glycolysis, glucose is ultimately converted into two molecules of pyruvate, and a small amount of ATP is created. A transition reaction in the mitochondrial matrix, pyruvate oxidation, converts the pyruvate to acetyl coenzyme A. The Krebs, or citric acid cycle, is an eight-reaction series that will occur only in the presence of oxygen. In the cycle, glucose is oxidized to carbon dioxide, carbon dioxide is released, and two molecules of ATP and both NADH and $FADH_2$ are produced.[5]

It is in the process of oxidative phosphorylation that the majority of ATP is produced. Electrons are released from NADH and $FADH_2$ as they are passed along a series of enzymes. The ions then flow back through special pores in the mitochondrial membrane, driving ATP synthesis with a net yield of 34 ATP molecules and 6 water molecules per glucose molecule.[5]

In the absence of oxygen, there is a significant reduction in ATP creation. The absence of this cellular energy source impairs normal processes including active transport, muscle contraction, and protein synthesis. It also decreases energy available for energy-dependent functions, including carbohydrate, lipid, and protein metabolism.

Oxygen-Carrying Capacity and Delivery

Oxygen delivery (DO_2) is the total amount of oxygen delivered to the tissues per minute, irrespective of blood flow distribution. Oxygen delivery can be calculated as $DO_2 = CaO_2 \times CO$, where the oxygen content is $CaO_2 = (1.39 \times Hb \times SpO_2/100) + (0.003 \times PO_2)$. In the context of shock, this emphasizes that decreased oxygen delivery is a function of one or more of anemia, hemoglobin (Hb) desaturation, or low cardiac output. Cardiac output is $CO =$ Stroke Volume $\times$ Heart Rate, and stroke volume is determined by preload, afterload, and contractility, which essentially leaves six variables for oxygen delivery: Hb, Hb saturation, preload, afterload, heart rate, and contractility (Fig. 13.2).[2,5,6]

In the oxygen delivery equation, it is worth noting that oxygen-carrying capacity is over 450 times more dependent on oxygen saturation than on partial pressure. The S-shaped oxyhemoglobin dissociation curve allows blood to unload oxygen where it is needed most: small changes in PaO_2 lead to large changes in the saturation, which benefits peripheral tissues. Shifts of the oxyhemoglobin dissociation curve result from changes in pH, temperature, 2,3-diphosphoglycerate, and type of Hb (Fig. 13.3). Except in cases of profound anemia, there is essentially no gain, and there may be physiologic harm, in increasing the PaO_2 above the level at which the Hb saturation is 99%. An oxygen saturation of 94% may be sufficient for most patients.[5-8]

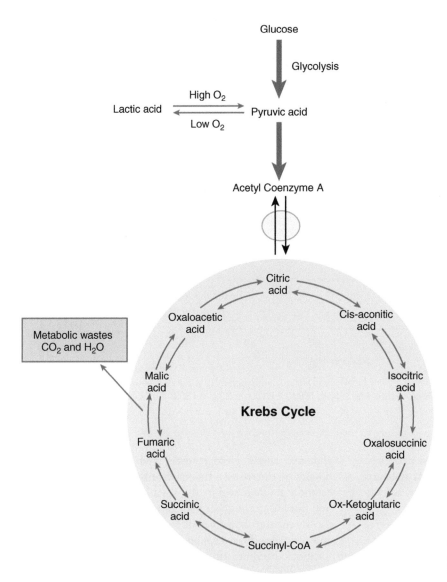

• **Fig. 13.1** Krebs Cycle. (Modified from Sanders M. *Mosby's Paramedic Textbook,* ed 3, Philadelphia: Mosby; 2007.)

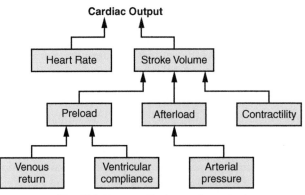

• **Fig. 13.2** Factors affecting cardiac output.

Global oxygen consumption (VO_2) measures the total amount of oxygen consumed by the tissues per minute. Body oxygen consumption is the difference between oxygen delivery and consumption: $DO_2 - VO_2$. It can be measured directly or derived from the Fick equation using cardiac output and arterial and venous oxygen measures: $VO_2 = CO \times (CaO_2 - CvO_2)$. Measures of oxygen saturation in the pulmonary artery or superior vena cava provide objective data on the balance between oxygen supply and consumption. The normal range is 60% to 80%. [5,6]

Physiologic Response to Shock

The physiologic response to shock also describes the body's compensatory mechanisms for the underperfused or underoxygenated states. The vasomotor centers in the pons and medulla control the immediate response, which are triggered when baroreceptors in the carotid bodies and aortic arch detect falling pressure. Those inhibitory centers normally maintain systolic blood pressures at an individual's physiologic set point somewhere between systolic pressures of about 50 and 180 mm Hg. Chemoreceptors, also

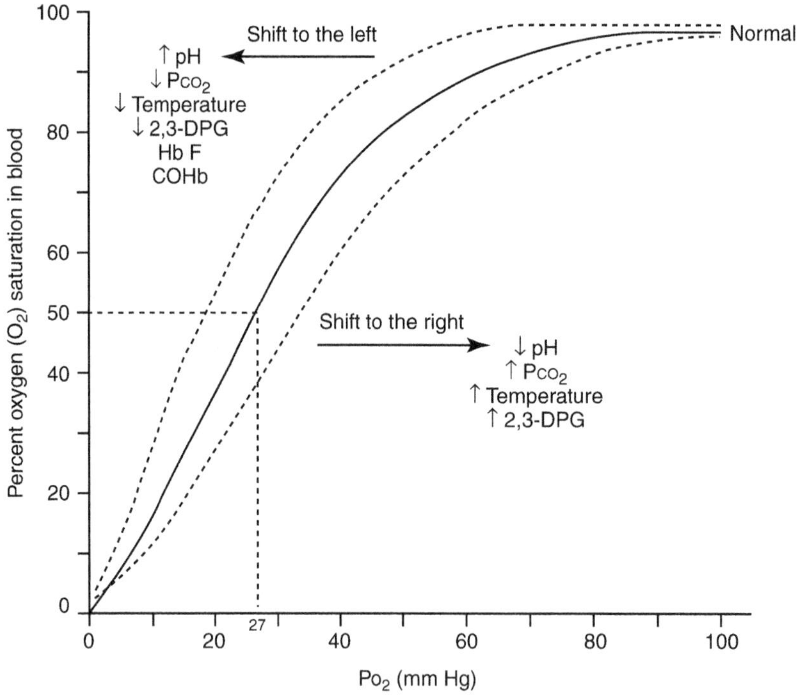

• **Fig. 13.3** Oxyhemoglobin dissociation curves: Normal and shifted. (From Schick L, Windle P. *PeriAnesthesia Nursing Core Curriculum: Preprocedure, Phase I and Phase II PACU Nursing*, ed 3, St. Louis, MO: Saunders; 2016.)

located in the carotid sinus and aortic arch, sense decreased oxygenation from decreased carrying capacity or delivery, and hypoxia triggers the same vasomotor center activity that hypotension does.[2,6]

The sympathetic response to hypoperfusion is the release of norepinephrine and epinephrine, which increases heart rate and myocardial contractility; constricts peripheral vasculature, particularly in the arterioles and venules; and increases minute ventilation. In the lungs, hypoxic vasoconstriction shunts blood away from even underventilated areas of the lung to improve gas exchange. The aim of these hemodynamic changes is to maintain perfusion to essential organs. Interestingly, other areas in the brain, including the hypothalamus and cerebral cortex, can also trigger the same vasomotor center activity in response to psychological and physical stimuli such as strong emotions, pain, or cold.[2,6]

Fluids within the body are located in the vascular, interstitial, and intracellular spaces. Movement of fluid between spaces is regulated by solute concentrations and pressure gradients. Neurohormonal changes in response to decreased perfusion states redistribute fluid to the intravascular spaces. Low atrial filling pressures trigger increased arginine vasopressin levels, reaching a maximal antidiuretic effect in about 2 hours. At the same time, renal detection of low circulating blood volume causes the release of renin, triggering the release of angiotensin I, subsequently converted to angiotensin II and stimulating aldosterone release. Aldosterone increases renal sodium retention, decreasing urinary water losses. This takes 12 to 24 hours to reach full effect. There is also an increase in serum blood glucose through a combination of gluconeogenesis, glycogenolysis, and inhibition of glucose uptake by the tissues. This relative hyperglycemia shifts the osmotic gradient within the vascular space in an effort to pull fluid from the other two compartments. Early in shock, the vasculature is primed for increased calcium sensitivity and reactivity (Figs. 13.4 and 13.5).[2,5,6]

Shock becomes decompensated when natural mechanisms fail to maintain perfusion, and hypotension develops. Normally, sodium and potassium are moved against concentration gradients to maintain a slightly negative intracellular charge. Moving these ions against a concentration gradient requires energy. With depleted energy sources, the energy-dependent sodium-potassium pump begins to fail. Normal cell membrane potential also fails, and sodium and water move into the cells, further decreasing microvascular perfusion. Cellular edema causes cell membrane disruption, which releases lysosomal enzymes, injuring surrounding cells.[2] As shock progresses, vascular reactivity and calcium sensitivity begin to decline. Endothelial dysfunction associated with decreased nitric oxide formation and release will also develop, creating an inability for endothelium and smooth muscle to counteract increased sympathetic tone, creating areas of persistent hypoperfusion. This may be one of the links in the progression from inflammation to tissue infarction. An example of this dysfunction is observed in an extremity mottled from shock-induced vasoconstriction, which does not display the normal blanching and reflow, or "reactive hyperemia," seen when pressure is put on a capillary bed (Figs. 13.6 and 13.7).[2,6]

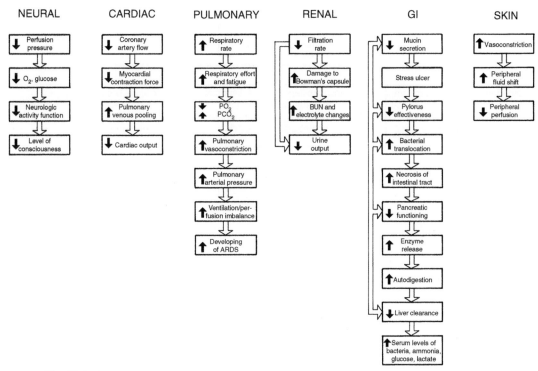

• **Fig. 13.4** Major organ system changes associated with hypoxia and shock. (Modified from Kitt S, et al. *Emergency Nursing,* Philadelphia: Saunders; 1995.)

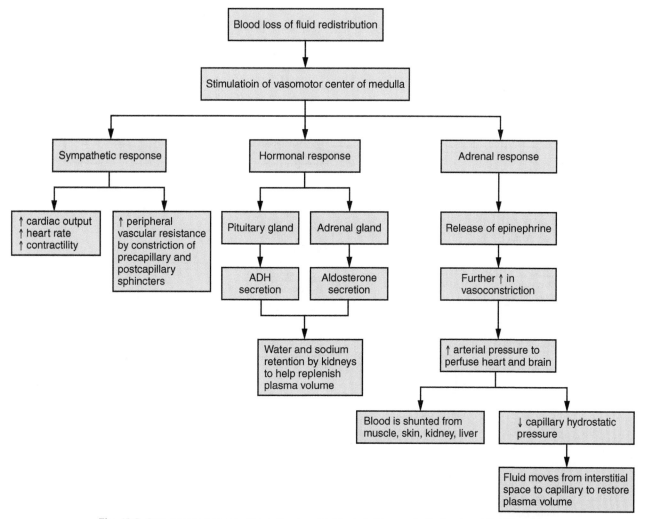

• **Fig. 13.5** Compensated shock. (From Sanders M. *Mosby's Paramedic Textbook,* ed 3, Philadelphia: Mosby; 2007.)

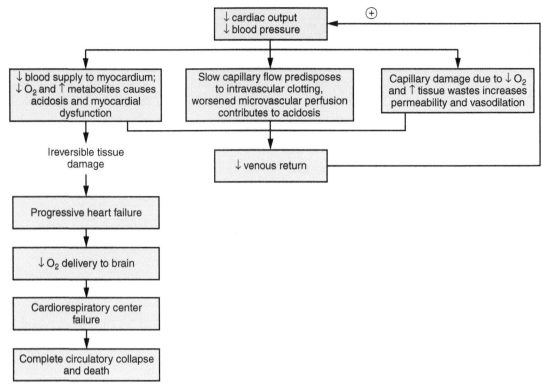

• **Fig. 13.6** Uncompensated shock.

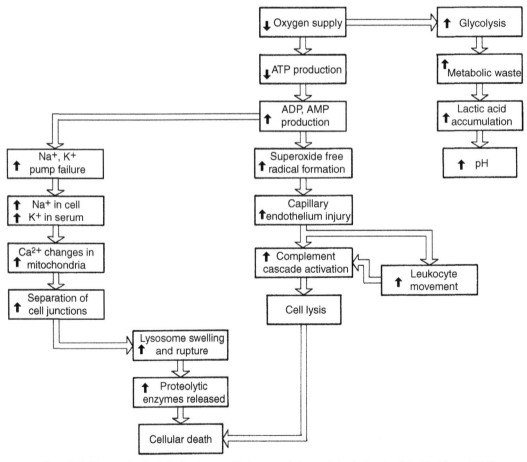

• **Fig. 13.7** Micropathophysiologic changes that occur during cellular ischemia. (Modified from Kitt S, et al. *Emergency Nurisng,* Philadelphia: Saunders; 1995.)

In shock states in which there is vascular endothelial damage or a trigger to the immune system, the linked inflammatory and coagulation cascades are activated. Prolonged cellular hypoxia can also trigger inflammation. The localized inflammatory response is designed to facilitate leukocyte and monocyte migration toward the trigger, augmented by chemotaxis, lymphocyte and macrophage function, lysosome activity, reactive oxygen species (ROS), and superoxide anions. Inflammation generates ROS that, along with other inflammatory mediators, alters the microcirculation. Neutrophil apoptosis may be inhibited, enhancing the release of inflammatory mediators. In other cells, apoptosis may be augmented, increasing cell death, thus, worsening organ function. Permeability changes in an underperfused gastrointestinal tract can permit translocation of enteric bacteria, potentially contributing to systemic infection. Septic shock may be more proinflammatory than other forms of shock because of the actions of bacterial endotoxins.[2,5,6]

Coagulopathy always accompanies bleeding or inflammation. Normally, local inflammation and coagulation are protective. With systemic inflammation and decreased microvascular circulation, widespread platelet aggregation and fibrin deposition create distributed microthrombi and simultaneously consume platelets and fibrinogen. This alters the usual balance between procoagulant and anticoagulant processes and stimulates a widespread procoagulant imbalance (Fig. 13.8).[2,5,6]

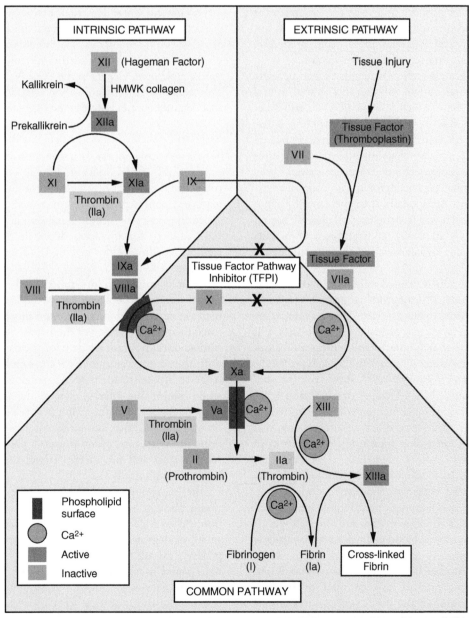

• **Fig. 13.8** The Coagulation Cascade. (From Mitchell RN. Hemodynamic disorders, thromboembolic disease, and shock. In Urden LD, Stacy KM, Lough ME. *Critical Care Nursing,* ed 7. St. Louis, MO: Mosby; 2014.)

Diagnosis

A diagnosis of shock is based on clinical, hemodynamic, and biochemical signs, which can broadly be summarized into three components: physical examination findings, vital signs, and laboratory values. Physical signs of shock reflect the compensatory mechanisms for shock and the effects of hypoxia. Organs with high metabolic demands will demonstrate altered function most rapidly with the onset of ischemia, whereas those with lower demand will show altered function only if ischemic time is prolonged. Accordingly, three organ systems are most affected: cutaneous (skin that is cold and clammy, with vasoconstriction and cyanosis), renal (urine output of less than 0.5 mL/kg of body weight per hour), and neurologic (altered mental state, which typically includes obtundation, disorientation, and confusion).[2]

The type and cause of shock may seem obvious from the medical history and physical examination. This should not preclude a full physical examination to avoid premature diagnostic closure and missed clinical information.

Vital sign changes also reflect attempts to compensate: heart rate and respiratory rate will increase, as well, unless precluded by other factors, including medications and other physiologic insults. Blood pressure will ultimately decrease if the shock state is untreated. This decline in blood pressure is considered the point at which compensatory mechanisms have failed and the shock becomes "uncompensated."

All vital signs must be considered in the context of expected values for age. Additionally, the appearance of hypotension can also be masked in patients with chronic hypertension who can be markedly underperfused at arterial pressures that are not hypotensive for those with normal autoregulation.

The shock index (SI) is defined as heart rate divided by systolic blood pressure, with a normal range of 0.5 to 0.7 in healthy adults. First introduced in 1967 to measure hypovolemia in patients with hemorrhagic or septic shock, it appears to be an earlier and more helpful indicator of shock than the vital sign measures in isolation. Physiologically, the SI is inversely related to cardiac index, stroke volume, and mean arterial pressure (MAP).[9] Values over 0.9 or 1.0 are associated with worsened outcomes in patients with circulatory failure, trauma, and septic shock, and increasing SI is also associated with increasing transfusion requirement in traumatic shock.[10-13]

Serum lactate or base deficit measures can help identify patients in shock and assess the response to resuscitation. The lactate produced as a product of anaerobic metabolism is an indirect marker of oxygen debt, and the base deficit values derived from arterial blood gas measures are similarly sensitive and specific. A normal serum lactate is under 2 mmol/L and a normal base deficit is between +2 and −2 mEq/L.[2] Either measure can be used to improve clinical decision making in any shock state. In an example from trauma patients, the addition of a cellular marker of perfusion to vital sign measures nearly doubles the sensitivity in predicting major injury. Normotensive trauma patients with hyperlactatemia from cellular hypoperfusion have a 4.2 times greater chance of death than normotensive patients with a normal serum lactate. In patients with shock, the degree of lactate or base deficit derangement correlates closely with mortality, and the progression toward normal demonstrates resuscitation success as reliably as trending improvements in mixed or central venous oxygen saturation.[11,14-16]

It is important to note that there are causes for hyperlactatemia other than shock, particularly excessive muscle activity, including seizures, metformin ingestion, thiamine deficiency, malignancy, liver failure, and mitochondrial disease.[17]

Management

Early detection of shock states and early intervention is necessary to prevent worsening organ dysfunction. The cellular effects of an oxygen supply and demand imbalance are consistent across all etiologies of shock, so it is not necessary to clarify the diagnosis before resuscitation begins: initial management is problem oriented. Generally, the "three Vs" (volume resuscitation, attention to ventilation, and consideration of vasopressors) identify the triad of early interventions.

Volume

Where oxygen delivery is a function of oxygen-carrying capacity and cardiac output, cardiac output is related to preload and contractility, and volume status can affect preload and contractility, properly timed and properly balanced intravascular volume expansion is an essential part of the treatment for any form of shock. Even patients with cardiogenic shock may benefit from carefully monitored and titrated fluid boluses.

Properly controlled and timed fluid administration improves outcomes, whereas excess fluid administration can increase shock morbidity and mortality.[18-24] The goal is to reach the plateau portion of the Frank–Starling curve where cardiac output is independent of preload, although this is difficult to assess clinically, by using some style of fluid challenge technique to identify the patient's response (if any), while minimizing adverse effects. The technique used for most patients is administering 5 to 10 mL/kg over 15 to 30 minutes and then evaluating for a favorable physiologic response (heart rate, blood pressure, pulse pressure, or perfusion signs) and for adverse effects such as a change in heart or lung sounds.[25]

The "passive leg raise" (PLR) may be beneficial in identifying patients who will benefit from volume administration. Beginning with the patient semirecumbent (head elevated 45 degrees), then lowering the upper body flat and passively raising the legs 45 degrees, about 300 mL of venous blood is relocated from the lower body to the right heart. An increase in cardiac output or a derivative, such as end-tidal carbon dioxide ($EtCO_2$), indicates a patient who will have a beneficial cardiac output effect from fluid administration.[20] A PLR-induced increase in $EtCO_2$ greater than or equal to 5% predicted a fluid-induced cardiac index change over 15% with 71% sensitivity (95% confidence interval: 48–89%) and 100% specificity.[26]

Ventilation

Administer supplemental oxygen to achieve a peripheral saturation of 94% or greater. Remember that the oxygen-carrying capacity equation demonstrates almost no benefit from supplemental oxygen once the saturation is at 99%, and the literature suggests a possibility of harm from hyperoxemia.[5,7] In addition to improving oxygen delivery, mechanical ventilation reduces the oxygen demand from respiratory muscle work, and the increased intrathoracic pressure decreases left ventricular (LV) afterload. Accordingly, endotracheal intubation is helpful in resuscitation for patients with persistent hypoxemia, persistent or worsening acidemia, and markedly increased work of breathing. Patients with shock are not good candidates for noninvasive ventilation.[2]

A clinical pearl linking volume resuscitation and mechanical ventilation is that an abrupt decrease in blood pressure following either the initiation of positive pressure ventilation or an increase in positive end-expiratory pressure suggests that the increased intrathoracic pressure is decreasing preload. Clinicians should include an evaluation for hypovolemia, and possibly a thoughtful fluid challenge, in the differential diagnosis for the blood pressure decline.[2]

Vasopressors

If hypotension persists despite fluid administration, the use of a vasopressor is indicated. Adrenergic agonists are the first-line vasopressors because of their rapid onset of action, high potency, and short half-life, which allows easy dose adjustment. Stimulation of each type of adrenergic receptor has potentially beneficial and harmful effects that must be considered when choosing an agent.[25] The administration of vasopressor agents through peripheral intravenous lines, particularly in short-term, early resuscitation situations, is safe.[27,28]

Norepinephrine is an excellent initial choice for most adult patients. It has mixed α- and β-adrenergic properties that benefit both peripheral vasomotor tone and cardiac output. Dopamine also has both α and β properties, but is associated with worse outcomes in many patients. In patients with cardiogenic shock, dopamine induced more arrhythmias and was associated with worsened mortality. It was also associated with worsened outcomes in patients with septic shock.[3,4,29] Unless the adult patient is bradycardic, dopamine is probably not a good first-line vasopressor agent.

Epinephrine has predominantly β effects at low doses and α effects that increase at higher doses. It can be effective as an added agent for refractory shock states.[30] The addition of low-dose vasopressin to a catecholamine infusion may be associated with a survival benefit for some shock patients requiring a second agent. It should not be used at doses higher than 0.04 U/min, and it should be administered only in patients with a high level of cardiac output.[25,31,32]

So-called "renal-dose" dopamine, doses under 3 μg/kg/min, may selectively dilate the hepatosplanchnic and renal vasculature and has long been thought to be beneficial for renal protection. Controlled trials have shown no benefit and have suggested the possibility of harm. The concept of renal-dose dopamine in critical care has been relegated to folklore.[29,33,34] Dopaminergic stimulation may also have undesired endocrine effects on the hypothalamic-pituitary system, resulting in immunosuppression, primarily through a reduction in the release of prolactin.[3,25,29]

Hypovolemic Shock

Hypovolemic shock can be hemorrhagic or nonhemorrhagic. *Hemorrhage,* loss of plasma and red cell mass from the vascular system, can be either internal or external. Normal blood volume is approximately 7% of the ideal adult body weight (approximately 70 mL/kg) and up to 90 mL/kg in children.[35] Physiologic response varies with volume loss. Changes in blood pressure at times may not be seen until 30% to 40% of the total blood volume is lost, so attention to physical examination findings and other vital signs are important in detecting impending shock.[2,36,37] Remember that an elevated SI is associated with a need for transfusion in hemorrhagic shock.[12,13]

Intrathoracic and intraabdominal bleeding are well recognized as causes of hypovolemia in trauma. Significant losses from noncavitary causes (pelvic fracture, skin laceration, and multiple long bone fractures) may also cause a severe shock state. For example, an isolated closed femur fracture can result in a blood loss of up to 2 L. The mortality rate in pelvic fracture is up to 15%, and up to 70% of those deaths are attributed to blood loss.[38]

Not all hemorrhagic shock patients have traumatic hemorrhage. Obstetric hemorrhage is the leading cause of maternal mortality worldwide, and patients with gastrointestinal bleeding and large vessel disruption are also common triggers for large-volume resuscitation.

When available, blood products are optimal for patients with hemorrhagic shock. Current guidelines generally support the early administration of platelets, fresh frozen plasma, and, perhaps, cryoprecipitate when more than two units of packed red blood cells will be rapidly transfused. There appears to be an advantage to approximating a 1:1:1 ratio between packed red blood cells, plasma, and platelets in the context of massive transfusions.[39,40] Out-of-hospital considerations in hemorrhagic shock resuscitation are presented in Box 13.1.[41-46]

Severe anemia is associated with worsened outcomes in critical care patients, but evidence dating back to the last century demonstrates that a liberal transfusion strategy to reverse anemia is not beneficial.[47-49] Transfusion to a Hb of 7 g/dL in adult patients improves outcomes, or is at least not inferior, compared with transfusion to a higher target in critical care patients, both overall and in the subgroups of patients with cardiovascular disease, traumatic head injury, and mechanical ventilation.[47,50-52] The administration of

• BOX 13.1 **Considerations in Out-of-Hospital Hemorrhagic Shock Resuscitation**

With respect to resuscitation from traumatic hemorrhagic shock, there is little value to prehospital fluid resuscitation. In a large United States registry study, unadjusted mortality was significantly higher in patients who received prehospital IV fluids, an outcome reproduced in subgroups of penetrating trauma, hypotensive patients, patients with severe brain injury, and patients undergoing immediate surgery.[41] A large European trial similarly found that increasing prehospital intravenous fluid volumes in trauma patients increased the risk of mortality, particularly in patients without severe brain injury.[42] Massive crystalloid resuscitation is clearly associated with coagulopathy, increased hemorrhage, and the development of the abdominal compartment syndrome.[43] Similarly, there is no evidence that the prehospital administration of plasma and packed red blood cells to trauma patients offers an outcome benefit over usual care, even in sophisticated transport systems.[44,45,46]

blood products carries real risk to the patient, which should factor into the decision to transfuse (Box 13.2).[53-75]

The role of tranexamic acid is unclear. The drug, used extensively in obstetric and orthopedic settings, inhibits intrinsic hyperfibrinolysis, a phenomenon particularly associated with trauma-associated coagulopathy. The therapeutic benefit appears to be time dependent, specifically within the first 3 hours of injury. The literature is not well settled, but this may be a reasonable option for prehospital and resuscitation bay providers managing patients with traumatic hemorrhagic shock, in addition to the established use in severe maternal hemorrhage.[76-79]

Patients with hemorrhagic shock and associated resuscitation are at risk for falling into the synergistic and self-perpetuating "bloody vicious cycle" or "triad of death" of acidosis, coagulopathy, and hypothermia (Fig. 13.9). This phenomenon, and a thoughtful approach to management,

• BOX 13.2 **Adverse Effects of Blood Transfusion**

Acute Reactions

Acute Hemolytic Transfusion Reactions
A hemolytic transfusion reaction is one in which red cell destruction follows transfusion. Symptoms appear within minutes. The interaction of recipient antibodies with donor red cell antigens results in destruction of transfused cells. Rarely, transfusion of ABO-incompatible plasma or platelets also can cause red cell hemolysis. The incidence of acute hemolytic reaction is about 1 per 76,000 transfusions, with a mortality of 1 per 1.8 million transfused units.[53,54]

Febrile Nonhemolytic Transfusion Reactions
Febrile nonhemolytic transfusion reactions are characterized by an otherwise unexplained rise in temperature of at least 1°C during or shortly after transfusion. Antipyretic premedication may mask the fever, but it does not prevent the cytokine-mediated chills and rigors. Other causes of fever should be excluded before making a diagnosis. These reactions are seen more often after a transfusion of platelets (up to 30% of platelet transfusions) than red blood cells, because platelets are stored at room temperature, which promotes leukocyte activation and cytokine accumulation.[54,55]

Allergic Reactions
Urticaria is the mildest form of an allergic reaction, with an incidence of 1% to 3%.[53,56] Anaphylaxis occurs in 1 per 20,000 to 50,000 transfusions.[57] The identification and management of anaphylactic shock are discussed elsewhere in this chapter.

Transfusion-Related Acute Lung Injury
Transfusion-related acute lung injury (TRALI) is an important cause of transfusion-associated morbidity and mortality, with a reported incidence between 0.41 and 1 case per 5000 component units transfused. TRALI is the new (within 6 hours) onset or worsening of hypoxemia (PaO_2/FiO_2 <300 mm Hg), with a chest x-ray consistent with pulmonary edema. Lung injury is most often transient: approximately 80% of patients will improve within 96 hours.[53] The pulmonary edema in TRALI is noncardiogenic and is not improved by diuretic therapy.[58-60]

TRALI is believed to be an antigen–antibody mediated reaction. Antibodies can be formed after exposure to foreign antigens by pregnancy, transfusion, or transplantation, and

transfusion may lead to neutrophil activation and resultant pulmonary endothelial damage, capillary leakage, and pulmonary edema.[61]

All plasma-containing components have been implicated in TRALI, with the risk greatest for platelets, followed by plasma, then packed red blood cells. Products donated by females, particularly by multiparous females, appear to be more likely to trigger reactions. It may also be that products donated by younger donors carry a greater risk for adverse outcomes. Other risk reduction strategies include using packed red blood cells with storage times under 2 weeks and platelet products with storage times under 2 days, because reactive compounds may accumulate during storage.[59-62]

Transfusion-Associated Circulatory Overload
Transfusion-associated circulatory overload may precipitate acute pulmonary edema within 6 hours of transfusion. Management is consistent with the management of other pulmonary edema patients: fluid restriction, diuresis, and consideration for positive pressure ventilation.[63,64]

Citrate Toxicity
When large volumes of blood components containing citrate are transfused rapidly, the increased plasma citrate chelates calcium and magnesium ions, resulting in hypocalcemia and hypomagnesemia. The transfusion rate must be high: over 6 units per hour (35 mL/min) of blood must be transfused to precipitate a reduction in ionized calcium levels. Citrate toxicity/hypocalcemia is more likely in patients with hypothermia, hepatic failure, alkalosis, and pediatric patients.[65,66]

Disorders of Potassium
Extracellular potassium in transfused blood rarely causes problems because of rapid dilution, redistribution into cells, and excretion.[53] An infusion rate of about 120 mL/min is probably required.[66] Irradiated cells have greater potassium leakage. Interestingly, hypokalemia is more common than posttransfusion hyperkalemia because donor cells reaccumulate potassium intracellularly, and citrate metabolism causes further intracellular movement. Catecholamine release and aldosterone urinary loss can also trigger hypokalemia in the setting of massive transfusion.[54]

Delayed Reactions: Occurring After 24 Hours

Alloimmunization

Antibodies are produced in response to immunization by antigen-positive red cells following transfusion, organ transplantation, or fetal–maternal hemorrhage during pregnancy. Up to 3% of patients exposed to foreign red cells will form ABO antibodies, with more in some patient groups: up to 40% of sickle cell anemia patients and 9% of thalassemia major patients have ABO antibodies. An acute life-threatening hemolytic anemia, described earlier, can occur in alloimunized patients when they are transfused.[67,68]

Transfusion-Associated Immunomodulation

Transfusion-associated immunomodulation (TRIM) is the down-regulation of a recipient's cellular immune response as a result of allogenic blood transfusion. This downregulation increases the chances of postoperative infections, hospital-acquired infection, cancer recurrence, and possibly a transfusion-related multiple organ dysfunction syndrome. It is believed to be leukocyte mediated. The use of autologous blood or leukocyte-reduced blood can mitigate the adverse effects of TRIM.[69-71]

Storage Lesion

There is some suggestion that the storage time for blood products may be linked to adverse effects, or the so-called "storage lesion" of blood. The proposed mechanism for this is multifactorial, including decreased deformability with resultant decreased ability to circulate through the microvasculature, depletion of 2,3-diphosphoglycerate, and increased adhesiveness and aggregation. However, recent trials and recent meta-analyses of the available literature are equivocal.[54,72-75]

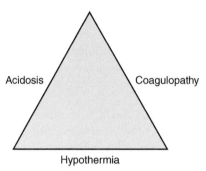

Acidosis   Coagulopathy

Hypothermia

• **Fig. 13.9** The "Triad of Death."

have been described for over two decades.[80-84] As described earlier, metabolic acidosis is a key physiologic derangement in shock. Systemic adverse effects seem to occur when the pH declines below 7.2 and include impaired cardiac output, contractility, ability to maintain vasomotor tone, and impaired platelet function.[85]

Hypothermia in shock is multifactorial, with contributors including exposure for resuscitation, administration of relatively cold fluids, medications that reduce normal thermoregulatory mechanisms, and reduced metabolic substrate to power heat generation. Reduced temperature decreases tissue oxygen delivery by shifting the oxyhemoglobin dissociation curve to the left, contributing to acidosis. Hypothermia impairs clotting factor function and creates an imbalance between thromboxane and prostacyclin that impairs platelet function, and clotting factor function also predictably declines with temperature.[86]

Shock resuscitation, then, involves attention not only to appropriate efforts to restore hemodynamic function appropriately but also to preventing hypothermia and to the possibility of developing coagulopathy. In trauma, the idea of "damage control surgery," in which hemostasis is achieved through temporizing measures, such as intraabdominal packing and definitive repair, is delayed until temperature, vital signs, and coagulation are managed is a classic and effective demonstration of this.[84] The concepts extend to all states of shock.

It is fairly easy to measure vital signs and temperature. Measurements of pH and perfusion measures such as lactate are also fairly straightforward and can even be completed at the bedside. Clotting factor function evaluation typically requires some delay for laboratory measurement and is limited: it does not show platelet dysfunction or hyperfibrinolysis. Because laboratory studies are processed at normal body temperature, the results do not reflect the impact of hypothermia.[87]

Thromboelastography (TEG) provides rapid, real-time, and more specific measures of coagulation system function than do traditional laboratory tests. Very simply, TEG measures the strength of fibrin-platelet bonds in whole blood. A small (0.36-mL) whole-blood sample in a heated cup is rotated at six times per minute to mimic venous circulation and activate coagulation. The cup has a central pin and connecting torsion wire that measure the speed and strength of fibrin formation and fibrin-platelet binding, which then convert that information to numeric values and a graphical representation of the complete hemostatic process including coagulation, platelet function, and fibrinolysis.[88]

Nonhemorrhagic volume loss usually rises from vomiting, diarrhea, excessive sweating (such as from heat emergency), polyuria, and loss of denuded skin from the body surface area. Patients can also translocate fluid into the "third space" or extravascular space, particularly with sepsis or intraabdominal injury. The shift is caused by direct vessel injury, mediator-driven increases in capillary permeability, and osmotic shifts as plasma proteins move into the interstitial space. Significant edema may be noted either in the affected areas or systemically as these fluid shifts occur. Patients with this third spacing–induced hypovolemia may particularly benefit from the addition of large molecule-containing fluids, such as proteins or starches, to their volume repletion to improve the intravascular osmotic tone.[2]

Distributive Shock

Vasomotor dysfunction results in either high/normal arterial resistance with expanded venous capacitance, or low arterial resistance. This dysfunction causes a relative hypovolemia as blood is sequestered in either the arterial or venous beds. The absolute blood volume does not change, but an increase in vascular space results in a decrease of effective blood volume and tissue perfusion. Septic shock and neurogenic shock are classic forms of distributive shock.

Septic Shock

Septic shock is a subset of sepsis in which underlying circulatory and cellular/metabolic abnormalities are profound enough to substantially increase mortality. As described earlier, sepsis involves organ dysfunction, indicating a pathobiology more complex than infection plus an accompanying inflammatory response alone.[2,6,89]

Even a modest degree of organ dysfunction when infection is first suspected is associated with an in-hospital mortality in excess of 10%. Patients with suspected infection who are likely to have a prolonged ICU stay or to die in the hospital can be promptly identified at the bedside with a validated scoring tool called Quick Sequential Organ Failure Assessment (qSOFA), which is a subset of the full inhospital Sequential Organ Failure Assessment score. These high-risk adult patients have two or more of the following: alteration in mental status (Glasgow Coma Scale <15), systolic blood pressure less than or equal to 100 mm Hg, or respiratory rate greater than or equal to 22/min. Positive qSOFA criteria should also prompt consideration of possible infection in patients not previously recognized as infected. Patients with septic shock can be identified with a clinical construct of sepsis with persisting hypotension requiring vasopressors to maintain a mean MAP greater than or equal to 65 mm Hg and having a serum lactate level greater than 2 mmol/L (18 mg/dL) despite adequate volume resuscitation. With these criteria, hospital mortality is in excess of 40%.[89] For the management of septic shock, a protocolized approach with a goal of effective resuscitation in the first 6 hours is well known to improve results. Care is addressed at volume resuscitation to euvolemia; early support of the MAP to at least 65 mm Hg using vasopressors, if needed; and early appropriate antimicrobial therapy.[2,4,90,91] Norepinephrine is the most commonly used vasopressor and is the better initial choice in most patients. Early use of vasopressin in the face of escalating norepinephrine doses may be a useful approach, and the use of epinephrine as an initial or second-line vasopressor agent is reasonable. Although the role of steroids in the care of patients with septic shock is unclear, the administration of a single dose of a mineralocorticoid steroid for septic shock patients who require a second vasopressor for blood pressure support is also a reasonable intervention.[30-32,90,92,93] There is robust and interesting debate about whether all of the components of the groundbreaking early goal-directed sepsis therapy bundle are necessary, but there is agreement on these core elements and the benefit of early therapy.[94-96]

Lactate or base deficit levels are useful in identifying patients with shock and are helpful in trending the success (or failure) of resuscitative measures.[15-17]

Neurogenic Shock

A patient with acute spinal cord injury may present with or develop neurogenic shock, suggested by hypotension and a variable heart rate response. This occurs secondary to sympathetic denervation, resulting in arteriolar dilation and pooling of blood in the venous compartment, and interruption of cardiac sympathetic innervation, particularly above the T6 level. Loss of supraspinal control of the sympathetic nervous system leads to unopposed vagal tone with relaxation of vascular smooth muscles below the level of the cord injury, resulting in decreased venous return, decreased cardiac output, hypotension, loss of diurnal fluctuations of blood pressure, reflex bradycardia, and peripheral adrenoreceptor hyperresponsiveness.[97-100]

The same physiologic disruption contributes to the autonomic dysreflexia sometimes seen in postacute patients with spinal cord lesions, in which sympathetic-mediated vasoconstriction is induced by afferent peripheral stimulation below the level of the lesion. For example, stimuli such as urinary catheterization, dressing changes, or surgical stimulation can lead to severe blood pressure spikes out of proportion to the stimulus.

Management is first aimed at ensuring euvolemia. Subsequently, vasomotor tone is restored, using an agent that minimizes bradycardia. The appropriate resuscitation end point and optimal mean arterial blood pressure for maintaining spinal cord perfusion is not known; there may be a benefit to maintaining MAP at a minimum of 85 mm Hg for the first 7 days following injury.[97,101] There is no role for steroids in the treatment of neurogenic shock caused by spinal cord injury.[102]

Anaphylaxis

Anaphylaxis is an acute systemic allergic reaction that results from the release of chemical mediators after an antigen–antibody reaction. The reaction is mediated by immunoglobulin E (IgE), which rests on the surface of mast cells and basophils in the body, especially in respiratory and gastrointestinal system cells. A reaction results in the release of mediators including histamine, kinins, and the slow reactive substance of anaphylaxis, which cause three major effects: (1) vasodilation, (2) smooth muscle spasm, and (3) increased vascular permeability with edema formation (Fig. 13.10).[103,104]

Anaphylactoid reactions are clinically indistinguishable from anaphylactic reactions, but are not IgE mediated and do not require prior sensitization; rather, they occur via direct stimulation of mast cells or by complement activation. They are caused most often by drugs, such as iodinated radiograph contrast, nonsteroidal antiinflammatory agents, blood transfusion, some antibiotics, and opiates.[104]

Symptoms of anaphylaxis are usually sudden in onset and can progress in severity over minutes to hours. Patients at risk of severe anaphylaxis include those with peanut and tree nut allergy, preexisting respiratory or cardiovascular disease, previous biphasic anaphylactic reactions, and advanced

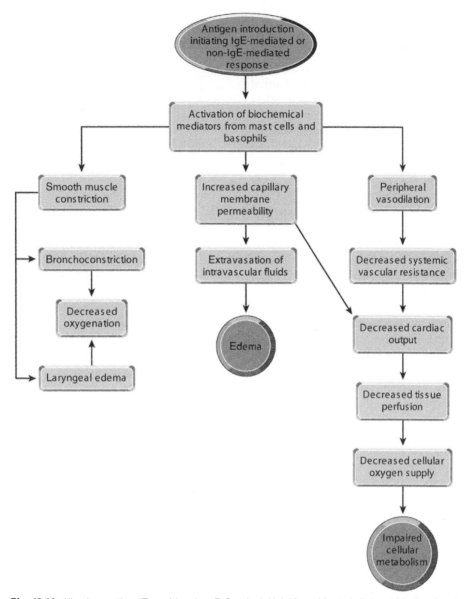

• **Fig. 13.10** Allergic reaction. (From Monahan F, Sands J, Neighbors M, et al. *Phipps' Medical-Surgical Nursing*, ed 8, Philadelphia: Elsevier; 2008.)

age. Interestingly, most patients with fatal or near-fatal anaphylaxis do not have a history of severe reactions. [103,104]

The broad spectrum of anaphylaxis presentations requires an index of suspicion and good clinical judgment, because early recognition prevents progression to a more serious outcome. Typically, at least two of the four organ systems are involved: cardiovascular, respiratory, gastrointestinal, or skin. Although most cases of anaphylaxis include cutaneous manifestations, their absence does not exclude the diagnosis. Similarly, anaphylaxis frequently presents without hypotension.

The life-saving therapy in anaphylactic shock is epinephrine, administered initially as an intramuscular (IM) injection in the anterolateral thigh. There are no randomized controlled studies of epinephrine during anaphylaxis; there is agreement on a recommended dose of 0.01 mg/kg (maximum dose, 0.5 mg) IM, repeated every 5 to 15 minutes,

as needed. For patients who do not respond to IM epinephrine injections, administer intravenous or intraosseous epinephrine. Crystalloid volume resuscitation and other vasopressors, as adjuncts to epinephrine administration, may be helpful. [103,104]

There is no substitute for epinephrine in the treatment of anaphylaxis. Administration of H_1 and/or H_2 antihistamines and corticosteroids should be considered adjunctive therapy. [103,104]

Cardiogenic Shock

Cardiogenic shock is hypoperfusion caused by cardiac failure. The classical diagnostic factors include hypotension, reduced cardiac index (<1.8 L/min/m² without support or under 2.2 L/min/m² with cardiovascular support), and elevated ventricular filling pressures. Myocardial infarction (MI) with LV failure is the most common cause, affecting 5% to 8% of hospitalized ST elevation MI (STEMI) patients and up to 2.5% of non-STEMI patients. Although LV failure is the most common physiologic cause, about 5% of cardiogenic shock patients have right ventricular (RV) failure. Mechanical complications such as ventricular wall rupture, papillary muscle rupture, and valve failure are potential causes of, or contributors to, cardiogenic shock, as are infectious sources (endocarditis and myocarditis), structural cardiomyopathies, and blunt or penetrating cardiac injury.[25,105]

Treatment is aimed in two directions: resolution of the cause and supportive therapy. For patients with STEMI, time-sensitive recanalization is clearly associated with improved outcomes: each 15-minute time reduction saves 6.3 lives per 1000 treated patients.[106] Support until revascularization and recovery from the damage caused before revascularization or the resolution of other causes is permitted by supportive therapies, including pharmacologic and mechanical support. For cardiogenic shock, even more so than for other forms of shock, norepinephrine favors improved outcomes over dopamine.[4] The intraaortic balloon pump is a common mechanical aid in cardiogenic shock, putatively improving coronary artery perfusion and reducing afterload. Interestingly, there is still some room for debate on the efficacy of the balloon pump. A series of individual trials and several meta-analyses suggest that it is equivocal or perhaps helpful in most patient groups; most agree that it does not worsen outcomes.[107-111] Other devices to decompress and support the left ventricle exist, as do more robust circulatory support devices. All of these increasingly common approaches are covered elsewhere in this book.

Obstructive Shock

Obstructive shock is an obstruction to cardiovascular flow resulting in impaired diastolic filling or significantly increased afterload. The mechanisms for this are pulmonary embolism (PE), pericardial tamponade, tension pneumothorax, and, in pediatric patients, a structural lesion.

Pulmonary Embolism

Acute PE interferes with both the circulation and gas exchange. RV failure caused by pressure overload is considered the primary cause of death in severe PE. Pulmonary artery pressure increases only if more than 50% of the total cross-sectional area of the pulmonary arterial bed is occluded. A PE is considered massive when accompanied by shock or hypotension (either relative or absolute).[112]

The patient history is important in making the diagnosis. Major trauma, surgery, lower limb fractures, joint replacements, spinal cord injury, and cancer are common predisposing factors for PE. Oral contraceptive use is the most frequent predisposing factor in women of childbearing age, and PE is a major cause of maternal morbidity and mortality, particularly in the third trimester and extending out to three postpartum months after delivery. Infection and blood transfusion are also associated with PE.[112]

Pulmonary embolism is 76% likely in the presence of three or more of the following electrocardiographic features:
1. Incomplete or complete right bundle branch block
2. S wave in leavds I and aVL >1.5 mm
3. A shift in the transition zone in the precordial leads to V5
4. Q wave in leads III and aVF, but not in lead II
5. Right-axis deviation, with a frontal QRS axis
6. A low-voltage QRS complex <5 mm in the limb leads
7. T wave inversion in leads III and aVF or leads V1 to V4

Because PE is known as the "great masquerader," the diagnosis should be considered in patients with shock and elevated central venous pressure not readily explained by another diagnosis, such as MI, arrhythmia, or other forms of obstructive shock. Symptoms are vague (dyspnea, pleuritic chest pain, and cough are the three most common) but still occur in 50% or fewer patients.[112]

The electrocardiogram (ECG) has low sensitivity and specificity, but it can be helpful in evaluating clot burden and RV dysfunction. In the classic PIOPED study, 30% of patients had a normal ECG, but 49% had nonspecific ST segment or T wave changes.[113] Inverted T waves in leads V1-V4 may be present and may correlate with disease severity.[114] Box 13.3 describes one helpful, multifinding, ECG interpretation rule for use in detecting PE.[115] It is important to note that the classic S1Q3T3 pattern is not a significant finding in the cited studies.

D-Dimer testing can be useful in excluding the diagnosis of PE. The use of an age-adjusted threshold of 500 μg/L or 10× patient age in years, whichever is higher, is safe and improves accuracy.[116]

Management of the patient with massive PE is first directed at supporting the right ventricle. Acute RV failure is the leading cause of death in patients with massive PE. Volume resuscitation in fluid-responsive patients is reasonable; however, aggressive volume resuscitation without hemodynamic response is of no benefit. Vasopressor support, particularly norepinephrine, is indicated in hypotensive patients. Patients with suspected PE should be rapidly anticoagulated. For those with hemodynamic instability, use of systemic fibrinolysis is associated with a mortality reduction.[112]

Cardiac Tamponade

Cardiac tamponade occurs when blood or effusion accumulates in the closed and relatively noncompliant pericardial sac. The heart is unable to fill, which leads to decreased cardiac output. Acute changes usually become symptomatic rapidly, and surprisingly large chronic accumulations can be well tolerated. The most common causes of larger pericardial effusions are neoplastic, uremic, and idiopathic. Effusions as a complication of MI, coagulopathy, chest radiation, and instrumentation are also common. The treatment is decompression of the pericardial space. Optimization of preload and support of the right ventricle can help temporize the patient until invasive management is possible.[117]

Tension Pneumothorax

Tension pneumothorax results in a complete collapse of one or both lungs with compression on mediastinal vessels and organs. This impairs venous return to the heart and increases afterload. Air under tension should be evacuated emergently by a needle and followed by a chest tube.[36] There is more discussion about this in the Trauma section.

Conclusion

The physiology, presentation, and management of shock is simultaneously complex and simple. Transport teams should be vigilant for the development of the oxygen supply and demand imbalance common to all shock states and should be prepared to intervene before significant vital sign changes are present. The oxygen utilization defect comes from one or more of four, not necessarily exclusive, mechanisms: hypovolemia, cardiac failure, obstruction to cardiac filling or return, and abnormal intravascular volume distribution, and the cellular effects are consistent across all etiologies of shock. For initial resuscitation, it is not necessary to clarify the diagnosis, and the initial problem-oriented management generally follows the triad of volume resuscitation, attention to ventilation, and consideration of vasopressors.

References

1. Cairns CB. Rude unhinging of the machinery of life: metabolic approaches to hemorrhagic shock. *Curr Opin Crit Care*. 2001; 7(6):437-443.
2. Dries D, ed. *Fundamental Critical Care Support*. 5th ed. Mount Prospect, IL: Society of Critical Care Medicine; 2012.
3. Sakr Y, Reinhart K, Vincent, L. Does dopamine administration in shock influence outcomes? Results of the sepsis occurrence in acutely ill patients (SOAP) study. *Crit Care Med*. 2006;34(3):589-597.
4. De Backer D, Biston P, Devriendt J. Comparison of dopamine and norepinephrine in the treatment of shock. *N Engl J Med*. 2010;362(9):779-789.
5. Hall JE. *Guyton and Hall Textbook of Medical Physiology*. 13th ed. St. Louis, MO: Elsevier; 2016.
6. Bonanno FG. Physiopathology of shock. *Journal of Emergencies, Trauma and Shock*. 2011;4(2):222-232.
7. Helmehorst H, Roos-Blom M, van Westerloo D, deJonge E. Association between arterial hyperoxia and outcome in subsets of critical illness: A systematic review, meta-analysis, and meta-regression of cohort studies. *Crit Care Med*. 2015;43(7):1508-1519.
8. Link MS, Berkow LC, Kudenchuk PJ, et al. Part 7: Adult Advanced Cardiovascular Life Support: 2015 American Heart Association Guidelines Update for Cardiopulmonary Resuscitation and Emergency Cardiovascular Care. *Circulation*. 2015; 132(18 suppl 2):S444-S464.
9. Rady MY, Nightingale P, Little RA, Edwards JD. Shock index: a re-evaluation in acute circulatory failure. *Resuscitation*. 1992; 23(3):227-234.
10. Berger T, Green J, Horeczko T, et al. Shock index and early recognition of sepsis. *West J Emerg Med*. 2013;14(2):168-174.
11. Callaway D, Shapiro N, Donnino M, et al. Serum lactate and base deficit as predictors of mortality in normotensive elderly blunt trauma patients. *J Trauma*. 2009;66(4):1040-1044.
12. Montory K, Charry J, Calle-Toro J, Nunez L, Poveda G. Shock index as a mortality predictor in patients with acute polytrauma. *J Acute Dis*. 2015;4(3):202-204.
13. Mutschler M, Nienaber U, Munzbert, et al. The shock index revisited—a fast guide to transfusion requirement? A retrospective analysis on 21,853 patients derived from the TraumaRegister DGU. *Crit Care*. 2013;17(4):R172.
14. Donnino M, Andersen L, Giberson T, et al. Initial lactate and lactate change in post-cardiac arrest: a multicenter validation study. *Crit Care Med*. 2014;42(8):1804-1811.
15. Jansen T, van Bommel J, Schoonderbeek F. Early lactate-guided therapy in intensive care unit patients: a multi-center, open-label, randomized controlled trial. *Am J Respir Crit Care Med*. 2010; 182(6):752-761.
16. Jones A, Shapiro N, Trzeciak S, et al. Lactate clearance vs. central venous oxygen saturation as goals of early sepsis therapy: a randomized clinical trial. *JAMA*. 2010;303(8):739-746.
17. Andersen L, Mackenhauer J, Roberts J, et al. Etiology and therapeutic approach to elevated lactate levels. *Mayo Clin Proc*. 2013; 88(10):1127-1140.
18. Boyd JH, Forbes J, Nakada TA. Fluid resuscitation in septic shock. A positive fluid balance and elevated central venous pressure are associated with increased mortality. *Crit Care Med*. 2011;39(2):259-265.
19. Bundgaard Nielsen M, Secher N, Kahlet H. Liberal vs. restrictive perioperative fluid therapy. *Acta Anaesthesiol Scand*. 2009; 53(7):843-851.
20. Cherpanath T, Hirsch A, Geerts B, et al. Predicting fluid responsiveness by passive leg raising: A systematic review and meta-analysis of 23 clinical trials. *Crit Care Med*. 2016;44(5):981-991.
21. Holte K, Kehel H. Fluid therapy and surgical outcomes in elective surgery. *J Am Coll Surg*. 2006;202(6):971-989.
22. Holte K, Klarskov B, Christensen D. Liberal versus restrictive fluid administration to improve recovery after laparoscopic cholecystectomy. *Ann Surg*. 2004;240(5):892-899.
23. Nisanevich V, Felsenstein I, Almogy G. Effect of intraoperative fluid management on outcome after intra-abdominal surgery. *Anesthesiology*. 2005;103(1):25-32.
24. Wiedemann H, Wheeler A, Bernard G. Comparison of two fluid management strategies in acute lung injury. *N Engl J Med*. 2006; 354(24):2564-2575.
25. Vincent J, DeBacker D. Circulatory shock. *N Engl J Med*. 2013; 369(18):1726-1734.
26. Monnet X, Batallie A, Magalhaes E, et al. End-tidal carbon dioxide is better than arterial pressure for predicting volume responsiveness by passive leg raising. *Intensive Care Med*. 2013;39(1):93-100.
27. Cardenas-Garcia J, Schaub K, Belchikov Y, et al. Safety of peripheral intravenous administration of vasoactive medication. *J Hosp Med*. 2015;10(9):581-585.
28. Ricard J, Salomon L, Boxer A, et al. Central or peripheral catheters for initial venous access of ICU patients. *Crit Care Med*. 2013;41(9):2108-2115.
29. Bellomo R, Chapman M, Finfer S, et al. Low-dose dopamine in patients with early renal dysfunction. *Lancet*. 2000;356(9248): 2139-2143.
30. Levy E, Perez P, Perny J, Thivilier C, Gerard A. Comparison of norepinephrine-dobutamine to epinephrine for hemodynamics,

lactate metabolism, and organ function variables in cardiogenic shock. *Crit Care Med*. 2011;39(3):450-455.

31. Russell J, Walley K, Gordon A. Interaction of vasopressin infusion, corticosteroid treatment, and mortality of septic shock. *Crit Care Med*. 2009;37(3):811-818.

32. Russell J, Walley K, Singer J. Vasopressin versus norepinephrine infusion in patients with septic shock. *N Engl J Med*. 2008; 358(9):877-887.

33. Jones D, Bellomo R. Renal-dose dopamine: from hypothesis to paradigm to dogma to myth and, finally, superstition? *J Intensive Care Med*. 2005;20(4):199-211.

34. Lauschke A, Teichgraber UK, Frei U, Eckardt KU. 'Low-dose' dopamine worsens renal perfusion in patients with acute renal failure. *Kidney Int*. 2006;69(9):1669-1674.

35. Hazinski M. *Nursing Care of the Critically Ill Child*. ed 3. St. Louis, MO: Elsevier; 2012.

36. ATLS Subcommittee, American College of Surgeons' Committee on Trauma, International ATLS Working Group, et al. Advanced trauma life support (ATLS(R): the ninth edition. *J Trauma Acute Care Surg*. 2013;74(5):1363-1366.

37. Bonanno FG. Hemorrhagic shock: The "physiology approach." *Journal of Emergencies, Trauma, and Shock*. 2012;5(4):285-295.

38. American College of Surgeons, Committee on Trauma. *Advanced Trauma Life Support for Doctors Student Course Manual*. 8th ed. Chicago: American College of Surgeons; 2008.

39. Napolitano L, Kuzek S, Luchette F, et al. Clinical practice guideline: red blood cell transfusion in adult trauma and critical care. *Crit Care Med*. 2009;37(12):3124-3157.

40. Spahn D, Bouillon B, Cerny V, et al. Management of bleeding and coagulopathy following major trauma. *Crit Care*. 2013; 17(2):R76.

41. Haut E, Kalish B, Cotton B, et al. Prehospital intravenous fluid administration is associated with higher mortality in trauma patients: A National Trauma Data Bank analysis. *Ann Surg*. 2011; 253(2):371-377.

42. Hussemann B, Heuer M, Lefering R, et al. Prehospital volume therapy as an independent risk factor after trauma. *BioMed Research International*, 2015;2015:354367.

43. Madigan M, Kemp C, Johnson J, Cotton B. Secondary abdominal compartment syndrome after severe extremity injury. *J Trauma*. 2008;64(2):280-285.

44. Holcomb J, Donathan D, Colton B, et al. Prehospital transfusion of plasma and red blood cells in trauma patients. *Prehosp Emerg Care*. 2015;19(1):1-9.

45. Miller B, Du L, Krzyaniak M, Gunter O, Nunez T. Blood transfusion: In the air tonight? *J Trauma Acute Care Surg*. 2016; 81(1):15-20.

46. Smith I, James R, Cietzke J, Midwinter M. Prehospital blood product resuscitation for trauma: a systematic review. *Shock*. 2016;46(1):3-16.

47. Carson J, Noveck H, Berlin J. Mortality and morbidity in patients with very low postoperative hemoglobin levels who decline blood transfusion. *Transfusion*. 2002;42(7):812-818.

48. Hebert P, Wells G, Blajchman M. A multicenter, randomized, controlled clinical trial of transfusion requirements in critical care. *N Engl J Med*. 1999;340:409-417.

49. Shander A, Javidorozi M, Naqvi S. An update on mortality and morbidity in patients with very low postoperative hemoglobin levels who decline blood transfusion. *Transfusion*. 2014;54(10):2688-2695.

50. Hebert P, Blajchman M, Cook D. Do blood transfusions improve outcomes related to mechanical ventilation? *Chest*. 2001;119(6):1850-1857.

51. Hebert P, Yetisir E, Martin C. Is a low transfusion threshold safe in critically ill patients with cardiovascular disease? *Crit Care Med*. 2001;29(2):227-234.

52. McIntyre LA, Fergusson DA, Hutchison JS, et al. Effect of a liberal versus restrictive transfusion strategy on mortality in patients with moderate to severe head injury. *Neurocrit Care*. 2006;5(1):4-9.

53. Mazzei C, Popovsky M, Kopko P. Noninfectious complications of blood transfusion. In: Roback JB, Combs M, Grossman BB, eds. *Technical Manual*. 16th ed. Bethesda, MD: American Association of Blood Banks; 2008:715-749.

54. Sahu S, Hemlata VA. Adverse events related to blood transfusion. *Indian Journal of Anaesthesia*. 2014;58(5):543-551.

55. Heddle NM, Klama L, Meyer R, et al. A randomized controlled trial comparing plasma removal with white cell reduction to prevent reactions to platelets. *Transfusion*. 1999;39(3):231-238.

56. Hennino A, Berard F, Guillot I, et al. Pathophysiology of urticaria. *Clin Rev Allergy Immunol*. 2006;30(1):3-11.

57. Domen R, Hoeltge G. Allergic transfusion reactions. *Arch Pathol Lab Med*. 2003;127(3):316-320.

58. Bux J, Sachs U. The pathogenesis of transfusion related acute lung injury. *Br J Haematol*. 2007;136(6):788-799.

59. Goldberg AD, Kor DJ. State of the art management of transfusion-related acute lung injury (TRALI). *Curr Pharm Des*. 2012; 18(22):3273-3284.

60. Kim J, Na S. Transfusion-related acute lung injury; clinical perspectives. *Korean J Anesthesiol*. 2015;68(2):101-105.

61. Toy P, Gajic O, Bacchetti P, et al. Transfusion-related acute lung injury: incidence and risk factors. *Blood*. 2012;119(7):1757-1767.

62. Chassé M, Tinmouth A, English SW, et al. Association of blood donor age and sex with recipient survival after red blood cell transfusion. *JAMA InternMed*. 2016;176(9):1307-1314.

63. Agnihotri N, Agnihotri A. Transfusion associated circulatory overload. *Indian J Crit Care Med*. 2014;18(6):396-398.

64. Clifford L, Jia Q, Yadav H, et al. Characterizing the epidemiology of perioperative transfusion-associated circulatory overload. *Anesthesiology*. 2015;122(1):21-28.

65. Dzik WH, Kirkley SA. Citrate toxicity during massive blood transfusion. *Transfus Med Rev*. 1988;2(2):76-94.

66. Sheridan R, Lhowe L, Brown B, et al. *The Trauma Handbook of the Massachusetts General Hospital*. Philadelphia, PA: Lippincott, Williams, & Wilkins; 2004.

67. Alves VM, Martins PRJ, Soares S, et al. Alloimmunization screening after transfusion of red blood cells in a prospective study. *Rev Bras Hematol Hemoter*. 2012;34(3):206-211.

68. Yazdanbakhsh K, Ware RE, Noizat-Pirenne F. Red blood cell alloimmunization in sickle cell disease: pathophysiology, risk factors, and transfusion management. *Blood*. 2012;120(3):528-537.

69. Blajchman MA. Transfusion immunomodulation or TRIM: what does it mean clinically? *Hematology*. 2005;10(Suppl 1): 208-214.

70. Sparrow RL. Red blood cell storage and transfusion-related immunomodulation. *Blood Transfusion*. 2010;8(Suppl 3):S26-S30.

71. Vamvakas EC, Blajchman MA. Transfusion-related immunomodulation (TRIM): an update. *Blood Rev*. 2007;21(6):327-348.

72. Kim-Shapiro DB, Lee J, Gladwin MT. Storage lesion: role of red cell breakdown. *Transfusion*. 2011;51(4):844-851.

73. Koch CG, Li L, Sessler DI, et al. Duration of red-cell storage and complications after cardiac surgery. *N Engl J Med*. 2008; 358(12):1229-1239.

74. Lacroix J, Hébert PC, Fergusson DA, et al. Age of transfused blood in critically ill adults. *N Engl J Med*. 2015;372(15): 1410-1418.

75. Steiner ME, Ness PM, Assmann SF, et al. Effects of red-cell storage duration on patients undergoing cardiac surgery. *N Engl J Med*. 2015;372(15):1419-1429.

76. Cole E, Davenport R, Willet K, Brohl K. Tranexamic acid use in severely injured civilian patients and the effects on outcomes. *Ann Surg*. 2015;261(2):390-394.

77. Morrison J, Dubose J, Rasmussen T, Midwinter M. Military application of tranexamic acid in trauma emergency resuscitation. *Arch Surg*. 2012;147(2):113-119.

78. Roberts L, Shakur H, Coats T. The CRASH-w trial: a randomised controlled trial and economic evaluation of the effects of tranexamic acid on death, vascular occlusive events, and transfusion requirement in bleeding trauma patients. *Health Technol Asssess*. 2013;17(10):1-79.

79. Wafaisade A, Lefering R, Bouillon B, et al. Prehospital administration of tranexamic acid in trauma patients. *Critical Care*. 2016;20(1):143.

80. Duchesne J, McSwain N, Cotton B, et al. Damage control resuscitation: the new face of damage control. *J Trauma Acute Care Surg*. 2010;69(4):976-990.

81. Kashuk J, Moore E, Millikan J, Moore J. Major abdominal vascular trauma: a unified approach. *J Trauma*. 1982;22(8):672-679.

82. Mikhail J. The trauma triad of death: Hypothermia, acidosis, and coagulopathy. *AACN Clin Issues*. 1999;10(1):85-94.

83. Moore E. Staged laparotomy for the hypothermia, acidosis, and coagulopathy syndrome. *Am J Surg*. 1996;172(5):405-410.

84. Rotondo M, Zonies D. The damage control sequence and underlying logic. *Surg Clin North Am*. 1999;77(4):761-777.

85. Dunn E, Moore E, Breslich DJ. Acidosis induced coagulopathy. *Surg Forum*. 1979;30:471-473.

86. Djadetti M, Fishman P, Beressler H, Chaimoff C. pH induced platelet ultrastructural alteration. *Arch Surg*. 1979;114(6):707-710.

87. Holcomb J, Watts S, Hodgets T. Damage control resuscitation: directly addressing the early coagulopathy of trauma. *J Trauma Acute Care Surg*. 2007;62(2):307-310.

88. Brazzel C. Thromboelastography-guided transfusion therapy in the trauma patient. *AANA J*. 2013;81(2):127-132.

89. Singer M, Deutschman C, Seymour C, et al. The third international consensus definitions for sepsis and septic shock. *JAMA*. 2016;315(8):801-810.

90. Dellinger RP, Levy MM, Rhodes A, et al. surviving sepsis campaign: international guidelines for management of severe sepsis and septic shock: 2012. *Critical Care Med*. 2013;41(2):580-637.

91. Liu VX, Morehouse JW, Marelich GP, et al. Multicenter implementation of a treatment bundle for patients with sepsis and intermediate lactate values. *Am J Respir Crit Care Med*. 2016;193(11):1264-1270.

92. Annane D. Corticosteroids for severe sepsis: an evidence-based guide for physicians. *Ann Intensive Care*. 2011;1(1):7.

93. Avni T, Lador A, Lev S, et al. Vasopressors for the treatment of septic shock: systematic review and meta-analysis. *PLoS ONE*. 2015;10(8):e0129305.

94. ARISE Investigators, ANZICS Clinical Trials Group, Peake SL, et al. Goal-directed resuscitation for patients with early septic shock. *N Engl J Med*. 2014;371(16):1496-1506.

95. Mouncey PR, Osborn TM, Power GS, et al. Trial of early, goal-directed resuscitation for septic shock. *N Engl J Med*. 2015; 372(14):1301-1311.

96. Rivers E, Nguyen B, Havstad S, et al. Early goal-directed therapy in the treatment of severe sepsis and septic shock. *N Engl J Med*. 2001;345(19):1368-1377.

97. Consortium for Spinal Cord Medicine: Early acute management in adults with spinal cord injury: a clinical practice guideline for health-care professionals. *J Spinal Cord Med*. 2008;31(4):403-479.

98. Gondim F, Lopes A, Oliveira G, et al. Cardiovascular control after spinal cord surgery. *Curr Vasc Pharmacol*. 2004;2(1):71-79.

99. Guly H, Bouamra O, Lecky F. The incidence of neurogenic shock in patients with isolated spinal cord injury in the emergency department. *Resuscitation*. 2008;76(1):57-62.

100. Krassioukov A, Claydon V. The clinical problems in cardiovascular control following spinal cord injury: An overview. *Prog Brain Res*. 2006;152:223-229.

101. Ryken TC, Hurlbert RJ, Hadley MN, et al. The acute cardiopulmonary management of patients with cervical spinal cord injuries. *Neurosurgery*. 2013;72(suppl 2):84-92.

102. Hurlbert RJ, Hadley MN, Walters BC, et al. Pharmacological therapy for acute spinal cord injury. *Neurosurgery*. 2013; 72(Suppl 2):93-105.

103. Simons FE. Anaphylaxis pathogenesis and treatment. *Allergy*. 2011;66(Suppl 95):31-34.

104. Campbell R, Li J, Nicklas R, Sadosty A. Emergency department diagnosis and treatment of anaphylaxis: a practice parameter. *Ann Allergy Asthma Immunol*. 2014;113(6):599-608.

105. Reynolds H, Hochman J. Cardiogenic shock: Current concepts and improving outcomes. *Circulation*. 2008;117(5):686-697.

106. Nallamothu B, Bradley E, Krumholz H. Time to treatment in primary percutaneous coronary intervention. *N Engl J Med*. 2007;357(16):1631-1638.

107. Fan ZG, Gao XF, Chen LW, et al. The outcomes of intra-aortic balloon pump usage in patients with acute myocardial infarction: a comprehensive meta-analysis of 33 clinical trials and 18,889 patients. *Patient Prefer Adherence*. 2016;10:297-312.

108. Porier Y, Volsine P, Piourde G, et al. Efficacy and safety of preoperative intra-aortic balloon pump use in patients undergoing cardiac surgery: A systematic review and meta-analysis. *Int J Cardiol*. 2016;15(207):67-79.

109. Romeo F, Acconcia MC, Sergi D, et al. The outcome of intra-aortic balloon pump support in acute myocardial infarction complicated by cardiogenic shock according to the type of revascularization: a comprehensive meta-analysis. *Am Heart J*. 2013;165(5):679-692.

110. Thiele H, Zeymer U, Neumann FJ, et al. Intraaortic balloon support for myocardial infarction with cardiogenic shock. *New England Journal of Medicine*. 2012;367(14):1287-1296.

111. Zhang J, Lang Y, Guo L, et al. Preventive use of intra-aortic balloon pump in patients undergoing high-risk coronary artery bypass grafting: a retrospective study. *Med Sci Monit*. 2015; 21:855-860.

112. Konstantinides S, Torbicki A, Agnelli G, et al. 2014 ESC Guidelines on the diagnosis and management of acute pulmonary embolism. *Eur Heart J*. 2014;35(43):3033-369.

113. Stein P, Terrin M, Hales C, et al. Clinical, laboratory, roentgenographic, and electrocardiographic findings in patients with acute pulmonary embolism and no pre-existing cardiac or pulmonary disease. *Chest*. 1991;100(3):598-603.

114. Ferrari E, Imbert A, Chevalier T, et al. The ECG in pulmonary embolism. *Chest*. 1997;111(3):537-543.

115. Sreeram N, Cheriex EC, Smeets JL, et al. Value of the 12-lead electrocardiogram at hospital admission in the diagnosis of pulmonary embolism. *Am J Cardiol*. 1994;73(4):298-303.

116. Righini M, Van Es J, Den Exter PL, et al. Age-adjusted D-dimer cutoff levels to rule out pulmonary embolism: The ADJUST-PE study. *JAMA*. 2014;311(11):1117-1124.

117. Sagrista-Sauleda J, Merce AS, Soler-Soler J. Diagnosis and management of pericardial effusion. *World J Cardiol*. 2011; 3(5):135-143.

14

General Principles of Trauma Management

ROBERT L. GRABOWSKI AND ALLEN C. WOLFE, JR.

COMPETENCIES

1. Demonstrate the ability to perform scene safety and trauma triage.
2. Perform a primary and secondary assessment of the injury.
3. Initiate critical interventions for the injured patient before and during transport.
4. Predict injury patterns based on the mechanism of injury.

Trauma is defined as injury to human tissue and organs caused by the transfer of energy from an external source. Injuries are caused by some form of energy beyond the tissue's resilience to tolerate.[1,2] Regardless of gender, race, or economic status, unintentional injury is the fourth leading cause of death for all ages in the United States, surpassing stroke in the last few years,[3] and the leading cause of death for those aged 1 to 44 years.[1-3] In 2013, 130,557 deaths were reported as the result of trauma.[3] Traumatic events are rarely accidental, and most are actually preventable.[4] Thus the term *accident* is no longer used in the trauma literature. Unintentional injuries are a major source of morbidity and mortality. For this reason, injury prevention has become a major public health goal.[5]

The cost of trauma-related injuries exceeds $400 billion annually in the United States.[6] These costs include treatment costs, both medical and subsequent psychological; lost wages; benefits; and other productivity losses.[6]

Injury Dynamics

The time elapsed from the actual injury to initiation of definitive care is a key factor in patient morbidity and mortality. One of the most important factors that have historically reduced morbidity and mortality rates in trauma patients is rapid transport. However, the addition of highly trained medical personnel has brought critical care management

outside the trauma center to the rural hospital or the scene of the trauma, further reducing the patient's time to meaningful intervention.

The transport of the patient with multiple injuries requires in-depth knowledge and skills as well as expert prioritization and organizational skills. A thorough understanding of the mechanisms of injury and the kinematics of trauma are essential for any transport team member caring for injured patients. Knowledge of these principles helps guide appropriate assessment and treatment to ensure the best possible outcome.

History

One of the first steps in caring for a patient with multiple injuries is obtaining a history of events, both preceding and following the trauma. With interfacility transfers, this information is most commonly obtained from other nurses, physicians, and family members. The history at a scene response generally comes from many individuals, including law enforcement, firefighters, other emergency medical services (EMS) personnel, and bystanders.

When responding via rotor-wing aircraft to the scene of a trauma, an aerial view of the situation helps the transport team begin data collection about the patient, mechanism of injury, and other potential circumstances (Fig. 14.1). The transport team has the advantage of evaluating the entire scene, the damage sustained to the vehicles or the buildings, the extent of impact, and the objects thrown or blown out of the central area of impact.

A thorough history is vital to direct the patient's care. Because time is a critical factor for survivability, the history should be obtained while gaining access to the patient or while simultaneously performing the primary assessment. At the scene, life-threatening injuries are always top priority, and a detailed history may be impractical initially, in certain cases. If the patient has an altered level of consciousness, then the only history obtained may be from the

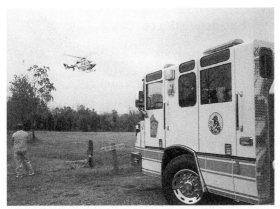

• **Fig. 14.1** When approaching a scene from the air, the transport team begins collecting information about the incident.

hospital or emergency personnel present, who may not be going to the receiving hospital. Therefore the history should be elicited during concurrent patient assessment because the team may not get another chance to obtain this much-needed information. When appropriate, the mnemonic AMPLE may be used to help elicit a history from the patient:

A: Allergies
M: Medications currently used
P: Past illness or Pregnancy
L: Last oral intake (including food, alcohol, drug use, etc.)
E: Events leading up to, or Environment factors related to the injury

Additional important information includes time of incident, mechanism of injury, use of any safety devices, any alteration in the patient's level of consciousness, and the patient's medical history.

A more detailed history may be obtained from the patient during the secondary survey as time and patient condition allow, and can be routinely performed in the transport vehicle.

Mechanism of Injury

Injuries occur when external forces are applied to the body. The type and amount of force applied and the tissues' response to the force determine the extent of injury.[2] When the body's tissue cannot withstand any additional force, destruction occurs, as seen in common forms of injuries, such as fractures, lacerations, ruptured internal organs, etc. A complete understanding of a force and the way it is applied is necessary to predict potential injuries and adequately care for the injured patient.

Newton's first law of motion states that a body at rest tends to remain at rest, and a body in motion tends to remain in motion, until acted on by an outside force. When the body contacts an object, energy is transferred, and damage occurs (Fig. 14.2).

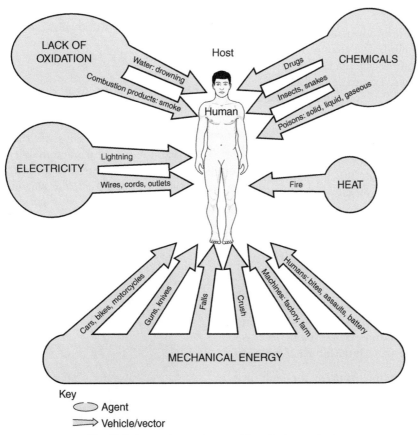

• **Fig. 14.2** Energy forces that can affect the human body.

Force is a result of energy transference, which can be explained by the laws of physics:
1. Energy can be neither created nor destroyed; it can only change form.
2. Kinetic energy = (Mass $\times$ Velocity^2)/2
3. Force = Mass $\times$ Acceleration

Because energy is neither created nor destroyed, only transferred, its transference is dependent on the mass of the object multiplied by its speed squared over a common denominator of two.

This same force is applied to destruction of the body. Energy is transferred from the automobile to the human occupants in the vehicle. Several factors determine the amount of energy the human absorbs, including the following:
1. The amount of energy absorbed by the objects that initially collide (e.g., the telephone pole and the automobile)
2. The amount absorbed by protective factors, such as seat belts, helmets, padded steering wheels, dashboards, and airbags

The forces involved in the impact cause varying degrees of destruction. The more slowly the force is applied, the less energy transference and the lower the degree of destruction. The extent of injury is also dependent on which body part(s) receive the impact[7]; for example, the skull can take more force before damage occurs, compared with the abdomen.

Force can be delivered via compression, acceleration, deceleration, or shearing.[7]

Compression: Direct pressure on a structure is the most common type of force applied. The amount of injury sustained is dependent on the amount of force, length of time of compression, and the area compressed.[7]

Acceleration/deceleration: Acceleration is the increase in the velocity of a moving object. Deceleration is the decrease in velocity of an object.[7] In an automobile crash, the body is thrown forward (accelerates) by the impact and decelerates as it comes into contact with the steering wheel, seat belt, or dashboard. The internal organs initially also accelerate and decelerate as they come into contact with internal structures such as ribs, which causes destruction to the tissues and vasculature.

Shearing: Shearing forces occur when tissues, organs, or both are pushed ahead of underlying or overlying structures. This commonly occurs at sites of junction between differently weighed, or affixed versus nonaffixed structures. An example of this is in acceleration/declaration trauma, when a nonaffixed portion of the aorta is forced anterior while the affixed portion is more or less stable. These opposing forces then cause a tear in the intima of the vessel.

The viscoelastic properties of tissues in the body help absorb energy. When the energy delivered is below the limit of injury, the energy is absorbed and causes no damage. When the forces applied deliver more energy than the body can absorb, strains occur.[7] Strains may be classified as tensile,

TABLE 14.1 Characteristics of Strains

Type	Reaction	Examples
Tensile	Stretching	Bony fractures, aortic tears
Shearing	Movement of tissue in opposite directions	Brain injuries, lacerations/avulsions
Compressive	Crushing force	—

shearing, or compressive. Table 14.1 displays the characteristics and examples of each type of strain.

Kinematics of Trauma

Injury patterns can be predicted by evaluating the mechanism of injury that has occurred and the estimated amount of force generated. Although all patients should be evaluated individually, certain injuries are common to certain forces and mechanisms of injury. Prediction of these injuries is referred to as *kinematics*. Age, buffers, or preventive measures taken, and velocity are factors in the alteration of injury patterns, and the caregiver should consider these factors in evaluation of a patient.[8]

Blunt Injuries
Motor Vehicle Crashes

Motor vehicle crashes are the leading cause of injuries and traumatic deaths worldwide, accounting for over 1 million deaths per year and an estimated 20 to 50 million significant injuries (Fig. 14.3).[6]

Head-On Collisions As an automobile collides with another automobile, or with any object head on, energy is transferred to the vehicle and subsequently, its occupants. The front of the vehicle routinely stops less than one-half second after impact. The rear of the automobile continues to move forward until all the energy is dispersed. Although the front end of the car is destroyed, the rear of the vehicle causes the

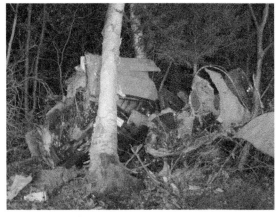

• **Fig. 14.3** Motor vehicle crash.

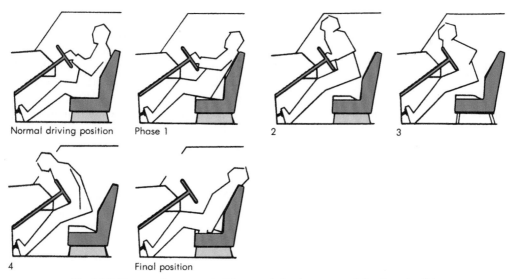

Normal driving position   Phase 1   2   3

4   Final position

• **Fig. 14.4** Phases of movement of the unrestrained occupant during frontal collision.

destruction by its continued forward movement. The same principle of injury occurs with the body during a head-on collision. The initial impact occurs in the front of the vehicle. The unrestrained driver hits the steering wheel with the thorax, the head may hit the windshield, and the knees contact the dashboard (Fig. 14.4). Predictable injuries from initial impact are fractured ribs, pneumothorax, or hemopneumothorax; concussion/traumatic brain injury, skull fractures, patella and femur fractures; dislocated hips; and acetabular fractures. The progression of injury proceeds, as does the automobile, and the person's internal organs are thrown from the rear forward until all energy is dispersed. Common internal injuries include ruptured spleen (direct compression from the steering wheel), lacerated liver (stretching of hilum until the tensile strength is exceeded), and ruptured thoracic aortas (heart and aorta are forcibly thrown forward and opposing sections stretch and tear).

The restrained driver in a head-on collision has much of the energy absorbed by the seat belt and air bag, if present. The seat belt may impose a load 20 to 50 times as great as the body weight. The only portion of the human body capable of incurring this load is the pelvis. Unless the patient has the belt properly applied securely over the pelvis, direct compression of the abdomen may occur. The first indicator of these injuries is often the presence of abrasions over the abdomen from the seat belt. Other injuries associated with seat belt use include sternal fractures, breast injuries, and lumbar vertebral body fractures. As seen with abdominal seat belt injuries, abrasions, ecchymosis, or both are important indicators. Lap belts should be worn with a diagonal shoulder strap to stop forward movement of the upper body. Diagonal straps worn alone can cause severe neck injuries, including decapitation. Air bags cushion forward motion only. They are effective in a first collision, but because they deflate immediately, they are not effective in multiple-impact collisions. When the air bag deploys, it can produce injury to the patient. The most common injuries seen are abrasions of the arms, chest, and face, which can include injuries caused by the patient's eyeglasses.[7,9,10]

Rear-End Collisions An automobile that sustains a rear impact rapidly accelerates, causing the car to move forward under the patient. Predictable injuries are to the back (T12-L1 is the most common area of injury), legs (femur, tibia/fibula, and ankle fractures), and neck (cervical strain and cervical fractures caused by hyperextension), if the head restraint is not in the proper position. If the automobile undergoes a second collision by striking a car in front of it, the predictable head-on injuries also need to be evaluated.

Side Impact An automobile struck on the side routinely causes lateral injuries to the patient. An unrestrained occupant sitting on the same side that sustained most of the impact may have initial injuries to the side of the body that received the impact; these may include the clavicle, ribs, femur, and tibia/fibula. Abdominal injuries, such as a ruptured spleen, are seen in these crashes, usually because of the fractured lower lateral ribs, but also because of direct compression on the abdomen.[7] Secondary injuries occur when the patient is propelled to the other side of the car, which causes injuries to the opposite side.

Rollovers Predictable injuries caused by vehicle rollovers are more difficult to define (Fig. 14.5). The unrestrained

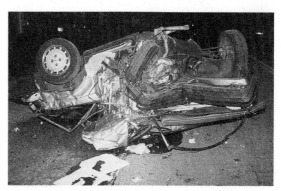

• **Fig. 14.5** Rollover motor vehicle crash.

patient tumbles inside the vehicle, and injury occurs to the impacted areas of the body. The caregiver should always care for these patients judiciously, realizing the potential for multiple-system injuries.

Motorcycle Crashes

Because motorcycles offer minimal or no initial energy transference, energy is directly absorbed by the rider, and injuries can be substantially more severe than with other motor vehicle crashes. The predicted injuries during a motorcycle crash, like those during other motor vehicle crashes, depend on the type of collision that occurs.

Head-On Collisions For accurate prediction of injuries that involve the motorcycle rider, an understanding of the design of a motorcycle is helpful (Fig. 14.6). The center of gravity is located in front of the driver's seat. As the cycle strikes an object head on, the rear (or lighter) portion tips upward from the weight under the handlebars, which prevents the driver, who is propelled over the handlebars, from total ejection. Associated injuries with this type of crash are fractured femurs, tibias, and fibulas (from the handlebars); chest and abdominal injuries (from direct compression against the handlebars or tire); and head and neck injuries (from impact with the tire or any object in front of the cycle). Any motorcycle crash can cause the rider to be ejected, but ejection is most common during head-on collisions. As with ejection from any vehicle, the head acts as the missile. Suspicion of, and intervention for, major head and cervical spine injuries are imperative with any ejected patient.

Side Impact Injuries associated with side-impact motorcycle crashes are related to the body parts crushed between the motorcycle and the second object. Most commonly seen injuries involve the leg and foot on the impact side. Open fractures of the femur, tibia/fibula, and malleolus are predictable.

Laying Down the Motorcycle Motorcycle riders have learned the technique of laying down the motorcycle and

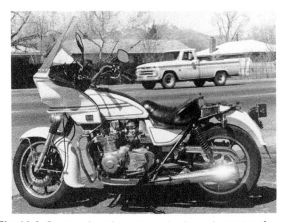

• **Fig. 14.6** Construction of a motorcycle places the center of gravity in front of the driver's seat. Head-on collision causes the cycle to tip up and throw the occupant over the front.

sliding off to the side before colliding with another object. The energy transference is a result of sliding away from the bike. Commonly seen are abrasions on the affected side. Fractures may occur if the patient hits the road hard or comes in contact with another object. Protective clothing and gear, such as leather jackets, pants, gloves, boots, and helmets, absorb more energy than average clothing. In this type of impact, patients may prevent abrasions and more serious injuries.

Falls

Falls from heights greater than 15 to 20 feet are associated with severe injuries. In predicting injuries associated with falls, caregivers should understand the following:

1. The average roof of a one-story house is approximately 15 feet off the ground; a two-story fall is approximately 30 feet.
2. With a fall greater than 15 feet, adults usually land on their feet. At less than 15 feet, adults land as they fall; that is, if they fall head first, they land on their head.
3. Because small children have proportionally larger heads, no matter what the distance, they tend to fall head first.

The caregiver must estimate the distance fallen as well as determine the surface on which the patient landed. A soft landing surface, such as dirt or sand, absorbs much more energy than a hard surface, such as concrete.

Three predictable injuries are seen in falls. The forces involved are deceleration and compression. The first injury, calcaneus fractures, is caused by compression of the feet on impact. Second, the energy dissipates after impact and the top of the body pushes down toward the point of impact, and this increased axial pressure load can lead to compression fractures to the thoracolumbar spine, commonly T12-L1. Finally, as the body moves forward and the patient puts out both arms to complete the fall, bilateral wrist fractures can occur.

Penetrating Trauma

All objects that cause injury from penetration deliver the same two types of force: *crushing* and *stretching*.[11-13] Depending on the velocity and size of the penetrating object, the resulting wound can be small or massive.

Stab Wounds

Stab wounds are considered low velocity and produce damage by crushing tissues as the penetrating object enters. An object that is narrow at the beginning and thicker at the end crushes the tissues as it enters and stretches them apart as the thicker part is inserted. The area of injury inflicted by stab wounds is typically localized to the area of insertion. The penetrating instrument may still be embedded in the patient. If this is the case, embedded objects should be stabilized with bandages for transport and not removed (Fig. 14.7).

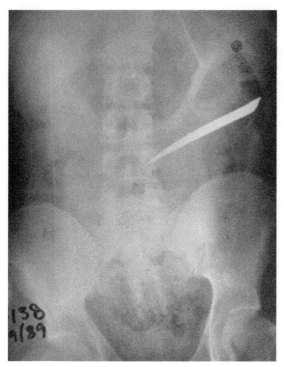

• **Fig. 14.7** Knife with the handle broken off embedded in a patient. Object was discovered when the radiograph was taken.

Firearm Injuries

Bullet wounds are caused by four different mechanisms: (1) direct contact by the missile, (2) crushing force in the immediate vicinity of the missile, (3) temporary cavity formation, and (4) collapse of the temporary cavity.[12,14]

The severity of the wound depends on the amount of energy transferred from the bullet to the body. This transference of energy is dependent on several factors: the type of weapon used, the type of bullet, the distance from which the weapon was fired, and the body part penetrated.

Firearms can be handguns, rifles, or shotguns. Handguns and some rifles are considered medium energy, and assault rifles and hunting rifles are high energy. The greater the amount of gunpowder in the cartridge, the greater the speed of the bullet, and the greater the kinetic energy.[7] The degree

of damage caused by the penetrating missile is influenced by the following factors:

Yaw and tumbling: Yaw is deviation of the bullet up to 90 degrees from a straight path, and tumbling is rotation of the bullet 360 degrees. Both cause increased crushing and stretching of tissue, resulting in greater damage.

Deformation of a bullet when striking tissue: Certain bullets are constructed of soft lead and flatten on impact. Others have hollow points that cause a mushrooming effect on impact. Hollow-point bullets are also known as expanding bullets. The increased diameter of these bullets increases tissue destruction.

Fragmentation: Each fragmented portion of the missile causes damage in its path. Increased velocity increases the potential of fragmentation.

Explosive effect: Explosive bullets are intended to cause massive damage with a single shot. The bullet is composed of black powder and lead shot. On impact, detonation of the powder causes explosion and disintegration of the bullet casing, which further propels the lead shot.[7]

The closer to the target the bullet was when fired, the greater the amount of kinetic energy transferred to the tissues, causing more widespread destruction. For this reason, firing distance is important to ascertain during the history taking.

Cavitation occurs with all penetrating objects. The permanent cavity is formed from the crushed tissue produced by the object. Temporary cavity formation occurs from transfer of kinetic energy from the missile to the tissue. The velocity, size, shape, and ballistic behavior of the missile and the biophysical properties of the tissue determine the extent of the temporary cavity. As a missile strikes tissue, temporary cavitation occurs forward of and lateral to the missile. Relatively elastic tissues, such as lung, bowel wall, and muscle, tolerate the stretch of the temporary cavity much better than the solid nonelastic organs, such as the liver and spleen.[8] The literature has estimated temporary cavity formation as large as 30 times the missile diameter.[15] Studies have indicated that temporary cavitation is usually no more than 10 to 20 times the missile diameter for high-velocity missiles, especially involving relatively inelastic tissues. (Fig. 14.8).[8,16]

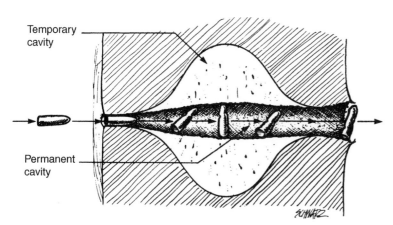

Temporary cavity

Permanent cavity

• **Fig. 14.8** Effects of yaw and temporary and permanent cavitation from a missile. Permanent cavity is caused by necrotic muscle tissue. Temporary cavity is caused by stretching of soft tissue. (From Weiner SL, Barrett J. *Trauma Management for Civilian and Military Positions.* Philadelphia, PA: Saunders; 1986.)

Pathophysiologic Factors

Trauma causes severe stress to the human body and is associated with a flux of hormones and physiologic reactions (Table 14.2). The degree of metabolic and hormonal changes depends on the severity of injury, the effectiveness of resuscitation, and the preinjury condition of the patient. Generally, metabolic response to shock from injury in the early stage differs from that in the late stage (Table 14.3).

In the early stage, the body responds to hypoperfusion as a stress to the body. Many of the changes that are mediated through the sympathetic nervous system occur rapidly. The

TABLE 14.2 Major Pathophysiologic Changes in Shock

Change	Effect
Early Stage (Compensatory/Nonprogressive)	
Increased epinephrine and norepinephrine α-Adrenergic and β-adrenergic receptors stimulated	Increased cardiac output to increase blood flow to tissues
α-Adrenergic effects: skin and most viscera	Vasoconstriction and decreased blood supply
β-Adrenergic effects: heart and skeletal muscles	Vasodilation and increased blood supply and heart rate
Renin–angiotensin response	Vasoconstriction and secretion of aldosterone; sodium and water retention, which supports intravascular volume; potassium loss
Increased glucocorticoids and mineralo-corticoids	Sodium and water retention to increase intravascular volume; potassium loss
Hypoxemia	Hyperventilation and bronchodilation; provides more oxygen to tissues; may cause respiratory alkalosis
Decreased hydrostatic fluid pressure	Fluid shifts from interstitial space to intravascular space to increase vascular volume
Late Stage (Noncompensatory/Progressive)	
Decreased blood flow to heart	Impaired cardiac pumping ability (decreased cardiac output); blood pressure decreases
Anaerobic metabolism	Acidosis; decreased adenosine triphosphate; failure of cellular sodium-potassium pump (potassium leaves cell, sodium and water enter cell); cellular damage
Arteriolar dilation and venule constriction	Fluid shift from intravascular to interstitial space, reducing blood pressure
Decreased blood flow to kidneys with acute tubular necrosis	Decreased kidney function (oliguria or anuria, retention of nitrogenous waste products and potassium)
Decreased blood flow to pancreas	Production of myocardial depressant factor

From Phipps WJ, Sands JK, Marek JF. *Medical-Surgical Nursing: Concepts and Clinical Practice.* 6th ed. St. Louis, MO: Mosby; 1999.

TABLE 14.3 Comparison of Signs and Symptoms in Early and Late Shock by Body System

System	Early Shock	Late Shock
Respiratory system	Hyperventilation; ↑ minute volume; ↓ $PaCO_2$; normal PaO_2; bronchodilation	Respirations shallow; breath sounds may suggest congestion; ≠↑ $PaCO_2$; ↓ PaO_2; pulmonary edema; ↓ pulse oximetry
Cardiovascular system	Blood pressure normal to slightly lowered; ↑ diastolic pressure; narrowed pulse pressure; tachycardia; cardiac output normal in hypovolemic shock, slightly decreased in cardiogenic shock, and increased in septic shock; mild vasoconstriction in hypovolemic and cardiogenic shock; vasodilation in septic shock ↓ blood pressure; ↓ cardiac output; tachycardia continues; vasoconstriction worsens in hypovolemic, cardiogenic, and septic shock	↓ Blood pressure; ↓ cardiac output; tachycardia continues; vasoconstriction worsens in hypovolemic, cardiogenic, and septic shock
Renal system	Decreased urine output; ↑ urine osmolarity; ↓ urine sodium concentration; hypokalemia	Oliguria or complete renal shutdown; hyperkalemia; buildup of waste products
Acid-base balance	Respiratory alkalosis	Metabolic acidosis; respiratory acidosis
Vascular compartment	Fluid shift from interstitial space to intravascular compartment; thirst	Fluid shift from intravascular to interstitial and intracellular spaces, causing edema

TABLE 14.3	Comparison of Signs and Symptoms in Early and Late Shock by Body System—cont'd	
System	**Early Shock**	**Late Shock**
Skin	Minimal to no changes in hypovolemic and cardiogenic shock; warm flushed skin in septic shock	Cool clammy skin in hypovolemic, cardiogenic, and septic shock; cool mottled skin in neurogenic and vasogenic shock
Hematologic system	Release of RBCs from bone marrow to increase vascular volume; platelet aggregation	DIC; ↓ hematopoiesis leading to ↓ white blood cells, ↓ hemoglobin, ↓ hematocrit, ↓ platelets
Mental-neurologic system	Restless; alert; confused	Lethargy; unconsciousness
GI-hepatic system	No obvious changes	Perfusion decreases; bowel sounds diminished; gastric distention; nausea, vomiting

DIC, Disseminated intravascular coagulation; *GI*, gastrointestinal; *PaCO2*, arterial carbon dioxide pressure; *PaO$_2$*, arterial oxygen pressure; *RBC*, red blood cell.
From Phipps WJ, Sands JK, Marek JF. *Medical-Surgical Nursing: Concepts and Clinical Practice.* 6th ed. St. Louis, MO: Mosby; 1999.

overall effect is an increase in systemic vascular resistance and a decrease in cardiac vagal impulse, which leads to an initial increased heart rate and systolic blood pressure (SBP). A response is mediated through the renin–angiotensin system that occurs more slowly. The response is again to vasoconstrict and to increase blood volume via retention.[17,18]

In the early stage, the compensatory mechanisms are beneficial because the heart and brain receive adequate blood supply, but this is done at the expense of the kidneys and other abdominal organs. If the underlying cause of shock is corrected, then the patient may do well. If the cause is not corrected, the compensatory mechanisms are not able to continue to perfuse vital organs well enough, and the mechanisms themselves become deleterious to the body. The shock then progresses to the late stage.[18]

During late-stage shock, blood flow to all body tissues is impaired, cellular metabolism fails, and acidosis and energy deficiency results. Without enough energy, the cell functions fail, and lysosomes are damaged, spilling digestive enzymes into the rest of the cell and destroying it. As the enzymes come into contact with adjacent cells, these cells also are destroyed, and eventually, the cellular death leads to tissue death, which can progress to organ death. Shock is a dynamic process; at some point, a cycle begins that cannot be stopped, and an irreversible stage of shock can develop.

One syndrome is seen after a severe physiologic insult with initial successful resuscitation of the patient. This syndrome has been termed *multiple organ dysfunction;* the belief is that the local injury from trauma and hypoperfusion causes a local inflammatory response. The response is probably a result of endothelial injury, platelet activation, the release of inflammatory mediators, and activation of the clotting cascade. This response leads to the development of a hyperinflammatory state and a hypermetabolic state, with increases in oxygen consumption and demand. The lung is usually the first organ to fail, followed by the kidneys, immune system, gastrointestinal tract, and liver, resulting ultimately in sepsis, cardiovascular collapse, and death. Evidence suggests that the gastrointestinal tract plays a strong role in the initiation and continuation of the syndrome. Patients who are subjected to

circulatory shock may sustain mild ischemia to the gut, which may lead to necrosis of the superficial mucosa, with loss of epithelial barrier function. Once the barrier function is lost, bacterial translocation is facilitated. This release of bacteria, endotoxin, and other luminal factors is thought to contribute to a systemic inflammatory response.[19]

A critical concept to understand when caring for the bleeding trauma patient is the triad of hypothermia, acidosis, and coagulopathy. Hypothermia may be caused by the environment or by caregiver interventions. When patients are disrobed for assessment, infused with room-temperature intravenous fluids and refrigerated blood products, a significant drop in core temperature will follow if measures are not taken to prevent this occurrence, such as using warmed intravenous fluids, administering blood using a heated infuser, or keeping the transport vehicle or resuscitation bay at a warm temperature. Autoregulation of body temperature requires a much greater than normal amount of oxygen and energy in the already hypermetabolic state of the ill and injured. Not only does hypothermia result in increased energy and oxygen use; it also worsens bleeding. Many reactions within the coagulation cascade are temperature dependent; therefore a drop in temperature will lead to platelet dysfunction and prolonged coagulation.

Acidosis in the injured patient is most commonly caused by hypoperfusion of the tissues, producing lactic acid as a result of anaerobic metabolism, and hypoventilation, caused by a myriad of reasons, such as traumatic brain injury. Severe acidosis can lead to myocardial dysfunction, worsening hypoperfusion, and worsening coagulopathy; reactions within the coagulation cascade decrease significantly in an acidotic environment.

Coagulopathies, or bleeding disorders, can be caused by hypothermia and/or acidosis, but they can also be caused or exacerbated by a previous genetic bleeding disorder, massive hemorrhage (loss of clotting factors), dilution (massive intravenous fluid administration and diluting circulating clotting factors), and prior medication use (i.e., antiplatelets such as aspirin; vitamin K antagonists such as warfarin; herbal supplements such as garlic, ginger, and ginkgo biloba). All three factors of the triad affect each other and should each be considered in concert whenever caring for the hemorrhaging trauma patient.

These factors emphasize the importance of the amount of physiologic stress the patient receives and the need for rapid assessment and transport of the trauma patient to definitive care.

Primary and Secondary Assessment

In development of a systematic approach for assessment of trauma, caregivers must intervene in life-threatening injuries, discover occult injuries, and prioritize care. In the prehospital setting, scene evaluation is important and includes an assessment of safety. Every transport team member is responsible for recognizing all possible dangers and ensuring that none still exist. No caregiver should become a victim. They should evaluate the scene and, if necessary, move the patient to a safe area before initiation of treatment. The transport team is challenged by many factors while performing a detailed assessment. Three of the most common factors are time, noise level, and the inability to fully disrobe a patient. The transport team is responsible for evaluating each patient situation individually to determine the best approach for conducting an assessment. For example, transport of a patient via helicopter from the scene of the accident may routinely require that the team performs the primary assessment on the scene, loads the patient, and performs the secondary assessment in the aircraft or ground vehicle, avoiding delay of definitive care. However, the auscultation of breath sounds and bowel sounds is not possible during rotor-wing transport and should be performed before liftoff and out of the normal assessment sequence.

Primary Assessment

The focus of the primary assessment is evaluation and identification of life-threatening conditions (Fig. 14.9). Problems identified during this portion of the evaluation are managed by the transport team immediately and simultaneously. The mnemonic ABCDE is used to complete the primary assessment[20-22]:

A: Airway and cervical spine stabilization
B: Breathing and ventilation
C: Circulation with hemorrhage control
D: Disability (neurologic status)
E: Exposure (the patient is undressed)[4,22]

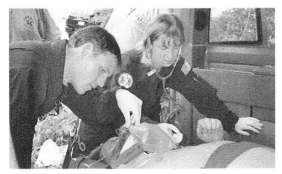

• **Fig. 14.9** Transport nurses performing a trauma assessment.

Airway

A secure, patent airway is the first priority. The airway is always assessed immediately for patency, protective reflexes, foreign body, blood/secretions, and injury. While the airway is assessed, the cervical spine should be protected simultaneously. Basic maneuvers should be instituted, including suctioning and opening of the airway with a chin-lift or jaw-thrust technique. The chin-lift technique should be avoided in patients with potential for cervical spine injury; instead, use a modified jaw-thrust maneuver in this patient population.[23] A patient with a head injury or facial fractures risks loss of airway patency, and the transport team should always be prepared to manage the airway before it occludes. Frequent suctioning is often indicated, and the equipment should be at hand. Endotracheal intubation allows for optimal, definitive control of the airway. The transport team must be able to recognize the indications for airway management and perform the type of intervention (basic or advanced) that is optimal for the situation and clinical condition. Patients with a Glasgow Coma Scale (GCS) of 8 or less are at increased risk for aspiration and hypoventilation. A definitive airway should be considered for patients with a GCS of 8 or less.

Breathing

Breathing is assessed by evaluating the patient's respiratory rate, depth, and effort of inspiration. Breath sounds should be auscultated bilaterally in all fields. Pulse oximetry and end-tidal carbon dioxide monitoring are the gold standard for monitoring the intubated patient during transport. Most life-threatening injuries are in the chest and affect breathing (Box 14.1). Recognition of these injuries is imperative to effective management of ventilation. Once a patent airway is established, the caregiver must determine the effectiveness of air exchange. Observation of the rise and fall of the chest alone is not sufficient for the caregiver to determine the status of breathing. The caregiver should assess the rate of ventilation, use of accessory muscles, and for the presence of circumoral cyanosis (a late sign in adults). If spontaneous breathing is inadequate or absent, the crew should initiate positive-pressure ventilation via a bag-valve device and appropriate airway adjuncts. For patients who do not need bag-valve-mask–assisted ventilations, high-flow oxygen via a nonrebreather mask can be effective to augment oxygenation. All patients with multisystem trauma should receive empiric

---

• **BOX 14.1** **Indicators of Immediate Life-Threatening Chest Injury**

1. Open pneumothorax
2. Flail chest
3. Massive hemothorax
4. Tension pneumothorax
5. Cardiac tamponade
6. Penetrating cardiac wounds
7. Air embolus

supplemental oxygen during transport, regardless of whether or not they are symptomatic; however, it should be titrated down as soon as the patient is stabilized, maintaining an SpO_2 greater than 94% in stable patients is appropriate.[6]

Portable ultrasound is becoming more readily available in the transport environment. Point-of-care ultrasound may be used as an adjunct in the primary survey to assess for lung sliding as a highly sensitive and specific means to identify pneumothoraces. Dependent on the user's experience and training, using ultrasound to assess for lung sliding can be more sensitive and specific in identifying pneumothoraces than a standard anterior-posterior chest radiograph.[24] A skilled user may also use ultrasound to appreciate intrathoracic fluid, combined with clinical correlation, to assess for hemothoraces.

Circulation

Evaluation of circulation is accomplished with assessment of the patient's mental status, skin color, temperature, and pulse rate and quality. Quick palpation of radial pulses may be sufficient for the caregiver to determine effective circulation in the unconscious patient. If a radial, femoral, or carotid pulse is not palpable, then chest compressions should be initiated. The patient should be placed on a cardiac monitor as soon as possible/practical.

Rapid assessment for massive or uncontrolled hemorrhage should be performed at this part of the assessment. If found, the spectrum of escalating forms of hemorrhage control should be applied: direct pressure to wound; concurrent elevation (if applicable); manual compression of the proximal arterial pulse point; and, if no manual control, application of a tourniquet proximal to the injury site. If the patient is noted to have massive hemorrhage from an extremity, not controlled by manual means, the care provider should not hesitate to apply a proximal tourniquet. Prehospital, both military and civilian, use of tourniquets has shown to significantly decrease death by exsanguination rates, and is associated with low complication rates.[6,22] There has been an increased prevalence of hemostatic dressings in the prehospital environment. These dressings are typically gauze bandages that are impregnated with different types of compounds to help accelerate clotting and/or seal the wound. Definitive studies are still being performed; however, current evidence suggests these hemostatic dressings to be more efficient than standard gauze dressings alone, especially in the coagulopathic patient, and have a desirable safety profile.[25,26]

The crew who performs airway, breathing, and cervical spine control at the scene and gains vascular access en route may best treat patients who need immediate surgical intervention. This process allows minimal delay for the patient who needs immediate surgery. The concept that an intravenous line is supportive, rather than restorative, care to the patient is important to remember. Unlike intubation and ventilation of the patient, an intravenous line cannot correct a problem. It only provides supplemental therapy until the underlying condition is corrected, and should not delay transport to definitive care. However, when intravenous access is necessary for immediate medication administration,

i.e., for rapid sequence induction, or blood product administration, i.e., in the periarrest exsanguinating patient, vascular access should be secured before/during transport.

Vascular access may be needed to administer medications to secure the airway and to provide pain management during transport. Advanced training and technology has provided transport teams with a variety of new ways to gain vascular access. Intraosseous devices such as the intraosseous line have proven to be simple quick ways to gain vascular access in both the conscious and unconscious patient, both pediatric and adult. Cannulation of the internal/external jugular, subclavian, and femoral veins has been used by transport teams to gain vascular access; however, the transport team needs to carefully evaluate whether a delay may occur with multiple attempts in gaining vascular access on scene.

Choices of intravenous fluids for resuscitation may include crystalloid, colloid, and blood products. Initial fluids should be crystalloids such as normal saline solution or lactated Ringer's solution. Patients who do not respond to 1 to 2 L of crystalloid resuscitation, or who appear to be in hemorrhagic shock, should be infused with type O uncross-matched blood.[27] Because red blood cells are not independently lost during hemorrhage, a multiproduct transfusion protocol should be considered if available. The best ratio for administration of blood products is 1:1:1 (red blood cells:plasma:platelets). The prehospital administration of plasma in the traumatically injured patient is still under investigation. Although not a true aspect of the primary survey, the use of tranexamic acid (TXA) should be considered whenever encountering the patient with massive hemorrhage and/or receiving blood transfusion. TXA is a medication that binds to plasminogen, preventing the conversion to plasmin, which prevents the breakdown of fibrin and the breakdown of clots that have formed. Studies have shown that, if given within 3 hours of injury, administration of intravenous TXA has significantly reduced mortality, with minimal adverse effects.[28,29]

Again, point-of-care ultrasound may be used here as an adjunct to the primary survey. The focused assessment with sonography for trauma or FAST examination can be rapidly performed to identify hemoperitoneum (free blood between the inner abdominal wall and internal organ) and pericardial effusion/cardiac tamponade (fluid/blood collection between the pericardial sac and the musculature of the heart). The ultrasound can then also be used to help the care provider safely perform an ultrasound-guided pericardiocentesis to relieve the tamponade.

Disability/Neurologic

A rapid neurologic examination establishes the patient's level of consciousness. The mnemonic *AVPU* (Alert, responds to Verbal stimuli, responds to Painful stimuli, or Unresponsive), the GCS, pupillary response and symmetry, the presence of extremity movements, and lateralizing motor findings can be used by the caregiver to assess disability. The GCS and the gross motor and sensory status of all four extremities should be determined and noted; this is especially important to assess before administration of sedating and neuromuscular blocking agents because this information will need to be reported to the receiving facility. The AVPU scale may also provide a quick assessment of the patient's level of consciousness and assist the transport team in determination of whether critical interventions, such as airway management, may be needed before transport. Consideration for blood glucose testing should be made in the disability assessment of the patient with altered mental status, because hypoglycemia can be present or have been a causative factor in the traumatic injury.

Exposure/Environmental Control

The patient should be disrobed and evaluated for any life-threatening injuries. Environmental control involves assessment of the core body temperature and prevention of hypothermia. Exposure is particularly important in the patient with a traumatic mechanism of injury in which failure to identify a second or third injury may result in an inaccurate clinical picture. This is especially true for the patient with potentially multiple sites of penetrating trauma, i.e., multiple gunshot wounds.

Exposure of the chest is essential for evaluation of life-threatening injuries, and exposure of the abdomen is crucial for proper examination, and both should be done in all trauma patients. All restrictive clothing, such as belts or bras, should be removed or cut away. While exposing the patient during the assessment, attention must be given to keeping the patient warm. Blankets should cover the body areas not being examined at the time. Hypothermia yields deleterious effects to the traumatically injured patient.

Secondary Assessment

The secondary assessment is a complete examination of the patient from head to toe. A more complete and traditional history and physical examination is performed. The secondary assessment is not to be performed until after the primary assessment has been completed and all life threats stabilized. If during the secondary assessment the patient begins to deteriorate, then the primary assessment is to be repeated and the patient stabilized before moving on. It is common to not complete the secondary assessment on the seriously injured patient in the field, when there is a short transport time, before arriving to the hospital because of multiple interventions to stabilize life threats found in the primary assessment.

The secondary assessment proceeds in a systematic fashion from head to toe to reveal all injuries the patient has sustained. During this assessment, the caregiver strictly adheres to assessment of the patient and does not intervene for specific injuries. To avoid missed injuries, the caregiver must develop a routine when performing the secondary assessment. Inspection, auscultation, palpation, and collection of information the patient offers are the keys to performing this assessment. When proficient, the transport team should be able to perform the secondary assessment in approximately 60 seconds. Focusing on obvious injuries is easy during this assessment, but the challenge is to discover occult injuries that may have an adverse effect on the

patient's morbidity or mortality and may cause major problems for both the patient and the team during transport.[30]

After completion of the secondary assessment, the caregiver can focus on the patient's specific injuries to determine their severity and to intervene when necessary, for example, by splinting an extremity. Remember the importance of protection from hypothermia when exposing areas for assessment. Also, reporting all information regarding the patient to the receiving trauma team is important, especially any episodes of hypotension or loss of consciousness that the patient may have had. The mnemonic *FGH* can be used to complete the secondary assessment.

Full Set of Vital Signs, Focused Adjuncts, and Family Presence

The *F* in the FGH mnemonic stands for full set of vital signs, focused adjuncts, and family presence. A full set of vital signs should include blood pressure, pulse rate, respiratory rate, oxygen saturation, and temperature. This should be obtained before initiation of the head-to-toe assessment. Focused adjuncts can include attaching necessary equipment, placing an indwelling urinary catheter, and inserting a gastric tube for the patient with intubation. Family presence can assist the transport team with language or cultural barriers, medical history, and events surrounding the injury.

Give Comfort Measures

The *G* of the FGH mnemonic is a reminder to the transport team to provide comfort measures. These measures may include reassuring the patient, providing warmth, sedation/anxiolysis, and analgesia to the conscious or unconscious patient.

History

The *H* of the FGH mnemonic stands for history. This information obtained may be prehospital information from EMS caregivers or patient-generated information.

The primary and secondary assessments, along with the treatment of life-threatening injuries, are the most important aspects of trauma care the transport team can deliver. They direct the priorities of care during transport and for the staff at the receiving hospital and are the cornerstone for optimal outcome of the patient with multiple injuries.

Inspect the Posterior

Inspection of the posterior is generally not done in the transport process, but should be performed if able to do so without a delay in transport and without unnecessarily undoing spinal motion restriction measures. This is more clinically significant in the initial evaluation of the patient with a multiple penetrating trauma.

Scoring of Trauma Patients

Numeric scoring for determination of the severity of injuries is common practice. Scoring provides a potential outcome classification for trauma patients, through single-system injuries, multisystem injuries, or the patient's physiologic condition. A variety of injury-severity scores exist, but none are 100% accurate, and their questionable reliability should be considered with their use. Common prehospital scoring systems and accepted retrospective scores are discussed in the following subsections.

Prospective Scoring

A goal of emergency response personnel has long been to develop a numeric score to determine the severity of a patient's injuries at the accident scene. Use of such a score would mean rapid verification of trauma patients and appropriate triage to a trauma center; thus appropriate resources could be used, and morbidity and mortality rates could be significantly decreased.

Numerous prehospital scoring indexes have been developed, and two have gained national support.

Trauma Score

The *Trauma Score* is a physiologic index composed of five categories: SBP, respiratory rate, respiratory expansion, capillary refill rate, and score on the GCS (Fig. 14.10). The score is a number between 1 and 15. Associated with each score is a probability of survival for that score. The lower scores are associated with higher mortality rates. To increase the reliability of the outcome predictions, the *Revised Trauma Score* has been developed. It includes the GCS, SBP, and respiratory rate (Table 14.4), but both capillary refill rate

	Rate	Codes	Score
A. Respiratory rate	10-24	4	
Number of respirations in 15	25-35	3	
seconds: Multiply by 4	>35	2	
	<10	1	
	0	0	A. _____
B. Respiratory effort	Normal	1	
Retroactive: Use of accessory	Retractive	0	
muscles or intercostal retraction			B. _____
C. Systolic blood pressure	≥90	4	
Systolic cuff pressure: Either arm,	70-89	3	
auscultate or palpate	50-69	2	
	>50	1	
No carotid pulse	0	0	C. _____
D. Capillary refill			
Normal: Forehead or lip mucosa			
color refill in 2 seconds	Normal	2	
Delayed: More than 2 seconds			
capillary refill	Delayed	1	
None: No capillary refill	None	0	D. _____
E. Glasgow Coma Scale	Total GSC points	Score	
1. Eye opening			
Spontaneous _____ 4	14-15	5	
To voice _____ 3	11-13	4	
To pain _____ 2	8-10	3	
None _____ 1	5-7	2	
	3-4	1	E. _____
2. Verbal response			
Oriented _____ 5			
Confused _____ 4			
Inappropriate words _____ 3			
Incomprehensible			
sounds _____ 2			
None _____ 1			
3. Motor response			
Obeys commands _____ 6			
Purposeful move-			
ments (pain) _____ 5			
Withdraw (pain) _____ 4			
Flexion (pain) _____ 3			
Extension (pain) _____ 2			
None _____ 1			
Total GCS points (1 + 2 + 3) _____		Trauma Score _____	

(Total points A + B + C + D + E)

• **Fig. 14.10** Components of the Trauma Score.

TABLE 14.4 Revised Trauma Score Variable Break Points				
Glasgow Coma Scale Score	Systolic Blood Pressure (mm Hg)	Respiratory Rate (breaths/min)	Coded Value
13–15	>89	10–29	4
9–12	76–89	>29	3
6–8	50–75	6–9	2
4–5	1–49	1–5	1
3	0	0	0

and respiratory expansion have been removed because of subjectivity.[14] The major limitation of the Trauma Score remains is that it measures physiologic response. As long as the patient compensates, or is supported by mechanical ventilation, the score does not accurately reflect condition.[31]

Mechanism, Glasgow, Age, and Arterial Pressure The mechanism, Glasgow, age, and arterial pressure (MGAP) is a scoring system similar to the Revised Trauma Score, but it integrates mechanism of injury and age and removes the respiratory component. The score (out of 29) is determined by totaling values for the following: GCS score; SBP: +5 for SBP greater than 120 mm Hg, +3 for SBP 60 to 120 mm Hg, 0 for SBP less than 60 mm Hg; mechanism: +4 if blunt trauma; and age: +5 if less than 60 years old (Table 14.5). Initial studies for this scoring system identified three groups: low risk (23–29 points), intermediate risk (18–22 points), and high risk (<18 points). Suggested approximate mortality rates for these groups were 2.8%, 15%, and 48%, respectively.[32]

Retrospective Scoring

Attachment of a numeric score to each diagnosed injury is the concept of retrospective scoring.

TABLE 14.5 Mechanism, Glasgow Coma Scale, Age, and Arterial Pressure	
Mechanism	Measured Score
Blunt trauma	+4
Penetrating trauma	0
Glasgow Coma Scale	
+ (GCS Score)	
Age	
<60 years	+5
>60 years	0
Systolic Blood Pressure	
>120 mm Hg	+5
60−120 mm Hg	+3
<60 mm Hg	0

Abbreviated Injury Scale

The *Abbreviated Injury Scale* (AIS), published by the American Association for Automotive Medicine, categorizes injuries into six body regions (head, neck, thorax, abdomen, spine, and extremity and external) and assigns an individual score to each injury (Box 14.2). Scores are integers from 1 to 6, according to severity. The lower the score is, the less severe the injury.[33] The AIS method was designed to determine the severity of motor vehicle injuries. In the 1985 revision of the AIS, penetrating injuries were addressed in all body regions, but the scale is still considered more sensitive to blunt injuries. The AIS allows determination of individual injury severity but does not take into account multisystem injuries.

Injury Severity Score

The *Injury Severity Score* (ISS) quantifies multisystem injury by use of the AIS scores. The ISS is determined by adding the squares of the highest AIS scores in the three most severely injured body systems (Table 14.6). The ISS is a number between 1 and 75, with 1 being a minor injury and 75 being largely nonsurvivable. A patient who receives a score of 6 in any AIS category is automatically scored as having an ISS of 75. Any patient with an ISS greater than 15 is widely considered to be a major trauma patient.

• BOX 14.2 Abbreviated Injury Scale
0 = No injury
1 = Minor
2 = Moderate
3 = Severe
4 = Serious
5 = Critical
6 = Maximum; virtually nonsurvivable

TABLE 14.6 Injury Severity Score			
Region	Injury Description	Abbreviated Injury Scale	Squared Top 3 Scores
Head and neck	Hemorrhagic contusion	3	9
Face	No injuries	0	
Chest	Multiple rip fractures	4	16
Abdomen	Grade V splenic laceration	5	25
Extremity	Bilateral femur fractures	3	—
External	No injuries	0	—
	Injury Severity Score = 50		

Trauma and Injury Severity Score

The *Trauma and Injury Severity Score* method is a statistical equation that ties together the revised trauma score, ISS, age, and type of injury to determine the probability of survival for the patient.[31,34]

With the focus on percentage of mortality, the injury scoring systems have yet to address the probable morbidity associated with physiologic response and actual injuries. Despite years of experience and research, none of these scoring systems have been found to be significantly superior to the others.[35] However, a recent study has suggested the MGAP scale to be more accurate in predicting mortality than the revised trauma scale.[36]

Field Triage

Use of field triage to determine whether to take a patient to a trauma center is a necessary skill for caregivers in many parts of the United States. Proper identification of patients who meet trauma center criteria is routinely based on physiologic criteria, such as blood pressure lower than 90 mm Hg; anatomic criteria, such as two long-bone fractures; and a field triage score, such as the revised or pediatric trauma score.[1] Fig. 14.11 displays the standard field triage criteria for delivery of a patient to a trauma center.

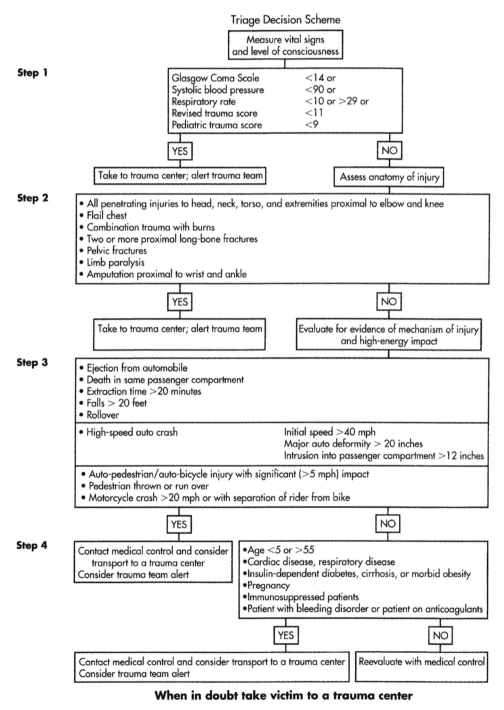

• **Fig. 14.11** Trauma triage decision making. (From Committee on Trauma, American College of Surgeons. *Resources for Optimal Care of the Injured Patient*. Chicago: American College of Surgeons; 1993.)

When in doubt take victim to a trauma center

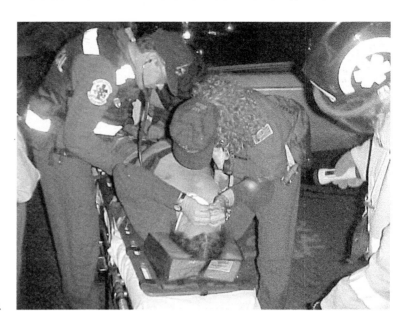

• **Fig. 14.12** Transport team performing field triage.

Triage Patient Transport

Care of the patient with multiple injuries during transport is aimed at maintaining adequate airway; breathing; and circulation, continued stabilization, and constant monitoring of the patient. The success of the transport depends on the caregiver's ability to anticipate the patient's progression and expect the unexpected (Fig. 14.12).

Emerging Trends in Trauma Care

Already discussed in this chapter has been the increased use of hemostatic agents (dressings and TXA), tourniquets, prehospital ultrasound, and prehospital blood product administration. New trends in resuscitation goals have also been seen in the "damage control resuscitation" scheme.

Damage control resuscitation is the concept of treating hemorrhagic shock in which the provider performs early transfusion of packed red blood cells (PRBCs), plasma, and platelets in a 1:1:1 ratio, while restricting crystalloid fluids, using the goal of a SBP of 80 to 100 mm Hg (in adults), and while preventing/correcting coagulopathy and hypothermia.[37] A key component of this concept is immediate damage control surgery, which is the strategy of performing exploratory or hemorrhage control surgery with the aim of stopping internal bleeding and restoring physiologic function, but not anatomic normality. An example of this would be in the multisystem trauma patient, on which the surgeon would perform an open laparotomy, control all sources of bleeding, pack the abdomen and cover with a temporary dressing, and admit the patient to the Intensive Care Unit (ICU). Once the patient stabilizes in the ICU, the surgeon would then take the patient back to the operating room for definitive repair of the remaining injuries and surgical wound closure, generally 1 to 2 days after the initial surgery.[38]

It should be noted that there is currently no literature to support the use of this goal of permissive hypotension and damage control resuscitation in pediatric patients.[39] Also, this strategy should be avoided in the patient with traumatic brain injury, because hypotension in this population can lead to a significant worsening of morbidity and mortality.

Another emerging treatment strategy is using nonoperative strategies, such as those performed in interventional radiology: balloon occlusion of bleeding vessels, transarterial embolization (purposeful clotting off of a given artery), and stent grafts. Nonoperative management strategies have become the standard of care in the hemodynamically stable patient with blunt abdominal trauma and some vascular injuries. Recent studies have demonstrated the beneficial outcomes of using a nonoperative strategy in select hemodynamically stable patients with penetrating injuries.[40-42]

Resuscitative endovascular balloon occlusion of the aorta (REBOA) is another nonsurgical procedure, which is used for hemorrhagic shock patients. REBOA involves percutaneously placing an endovascular balloon through the femoral artery and threading it up into the aorta. The balloon is inflated in the aorta to augment afterload and decreasing flow to the hemorrhage site, while increasing pressure and flow to proximal vital organs such as the heart and brain. Although generally performed in the emergency department or operating room, REBOA is being further investigated and slowly moving into the prehospital environment.[43,44]

Summary

The members of the transport team provide a critical level of knowledge and expertise of care for the patient with multiple injuries in the prehospital setting. By understanding the kinematics of trauma, performing a thorough assessment, and delivering care in an organized manner, the transport team has a positive effect on decreasing morbidity and mortality rates of such patients.

CASE STUDY

Multiple Trauma

The transport team was dispatched to a multiple-victim scene in a rural area, 30 minutes from the hospital. Reports were that two victims were dead and one other was severely injured. Initial responders performed the initial basic care practice. On arrival, the flight crew's aerial view of the scene revealed a single car that had been split in half. Rescuers were attending to the victim, and two bodies lying near the wreckage were covered with sheets.

The patient had been thrown from the vehicle over the guardrail, approximately 15 feet. The patient was a 19-year-old girl whose left leg had been amputated above the knee. Bleeding was not being controlled despite application of a pressure dressing before arrival. She had multiple abrasions and lacerations on her face and chest. Her GCS score was 7 (eyes, 1; verbal, 1; motor, 5). She was pale and diaphoretic. She had a palpable femoral pulse of 130 beats/min and a respiratory rate of 8 beats/min. She was immobilized on a backboard, with cervical collar and head blocks in place. She had one intravenous line in place.

The transport team elected to intubate the patient because of her low GCS score and her advanced level of shock. While gathering equipment for intubation, hemorrhage control was obtained by applying a tourniquet to the patient's thigh. Appropriate rapid sequence induction was initiated, and the patient was intubated without difficulty. During the intubation, a member of the rescue squad placed a second intravenous line. A palpable systolic pressure of 70 mm Hg was ascertained. One liter of 0.9% sodium chloride had already been infused. The transport team carried PRBCs and rapidly began transfusing the patient. She was loaded into the aircraft and secured. En route to the hospital the patient's SBP increased to 110 mm Hg. The crew initiated a slow bolus of 1 g of TXA and provided appropriate postintubation sedation and analgesia.

During the 15-minute transport to the trauma center, the patient's condition remained mildly hypotensive (SBPs between 90 and 110 mm Hg) and tachycardic (100–115 beats/min). No additional neuromuscular blocking agent was administered. The patient was admitted to the shock resuscitation unit, and a report was given to the resuscitation team.

References

1. National Center for Health Statistics (NCHS). *Health, United States, 2005 with Chartbooks on Trends in the Health of Americans.* Hyattsville, MD: NCHS; 2005.

2. Anderson RN, Smith BL. Deaths: leading causes for 2002. *Natl Vital Stat Rep.* 2005;53(17):1-10.

3. Xu J, Murphy S, Kochanek K, Bastian B. *Deaths: Final Data for 2013. National Vital Statistics Reports.* Vol 64 no 2. Hyattsville, MD: National Center for Health Statistics; 2016.

4. Emergency Nurses Association. *Trauma Nursing Core Course Provider Manual.* 6th ed. Des Plaines, IL: Emergency Nurses Association; 2007.

5. US Centers for Disease Control. *Harvard School of Public Health: U.S. Burden of Disease and Injury Study, Preliminary, Unpublished Results.* Atlanta, GA: Centers for Disease Control; 2000.

6. Bergen G, Chen L, Warner M, Fingerhut L. *Injury in the United States: 2007 Chartbook.* Hyattsville, MD: National Center for Health Statistics; 2008.

7. National Association of Emergency Medical Technicians. *Prehospital Trauma Life Support.* 8th ed. St. Louis, MO: Mosby; 2014.

8. *Trauma Nursing Core Course (TNCC): Provider Manual.* 7th ed. Des Plaines, IL: Emergency Nurses Association; 2014.

9. Weninger P, Hertz H. Factors influencing the injury pattern and injury severity after high speed motor vehicle accident—A retrospective study. *Resuscitation.* 2007;75(1):35-41.

10. Abbas AK, Hefny AF, Abu-Zidan FM. Seatbelts and road traffic collision injuries. *World J Emerg Surg.* 2011; 6(1):18.

11. Maiden N. Ballistics reviews: mechanisms of bullet wound trauma. *Forensic Sci Med Pathol.* 2009;5(3):204-209.

12. Cone DC, Brice JH, Delbridge TR, Myers JB. *Penetrating Trauma in Emergency Medical Services: Clinical Practice and Systems Oversight.* Chichester: John Wiley & Sons; 2015.

13. Kuhajda I, Zarogoulidis K, Kougioumtzi I, et al. Penetrating trauma. *J Thorac Dis.* 2014;6(Suppl 4):S461-S465.

14. Copes W. *Major Trauma Outcome Study: Letter to MTOS Participants.* Chicago, IL: American College of Surgeons; 1988.

15. Garner J. Mechanism of wound production. In: Smith J, Greaves I, Porter KM, (Authors). *Oxford Desk Reference—Major Trauma.* Oxford: Oxford University Press; 2011:410.

16. Part 1: Guidelines for the Management of Penetrating Brain Injury. *J Trauma.* 2001;51(2):S3-S6.

17. Kassavin DS, Kuo YH, Ahmed N. Initial systolic blood pressure and ongoing internal bleeding following torso trauma. *J Emerg Trauma Shock.* 2011;4(1):37-41.

18. Lewis S. *Medical-Surgical Nursing: Assessment and Management of Clinical Problems.* 9th ed. St. Louis, MO: Elsevier/Mosby; 2013.

19. Keel M, Trentz O. Pathophysiology of polytrauma. *Injury.* 2005; 36(6):691-709.

20. Legome E, Shockley LW. *Trauma: A Comprehensive Emergency Medicine Approach.* Cambridge: Cambridge University Press; 2011.

21. Pepe P, Fowler R. Prehospital care of the patient with major trauma. *Emerg Med Clin North Am.* 2002;20(4):953-974.

22. American College of Surgeons. *Advanced Trauma Life Support Student Course Manual.* 9th ed. Chicago: American College of Surgeons; 2012.

23. National Association of Emergency Medical Technicians. *Prehospital Trauma Life Support.* 8th ed. Burlington, MA: Jones & Bartlett; 2016.

24. Fox JC. *Atlas of Emergency Ultrasound.* Cambridge: Cambridge University Press; 2011.

25. Inaba K, et al. Tourniquet use for civilian extremity trauma. *J Trauma Acute Care Surg.* 2015;79(2):232-237.

26. Grotenhuis R, et al. Prehospital use of hemostatic dressings in emergency medical services in the Netherlands: A prospective study of 66 cases. *Injury.* 2016;47(5):1007-1011.

27. Gabrielli A, Layon AJ, Yu M, et al. *Civetta, Taylor, & Kirby's Critical care.* 4th ed. Philadelphia, PA: Lippincott Williams & Wilkins; 2008.

28. Rembe JD, et al. Comparison of hemostatic dressings for superficial wounds using a new spectrophotometric coagulation assay. *J Transl Med.* 2015;13:375.

29. Binz S, et al. CRASH-2 study of tranexamic acid to treat bleeding in trauma patients: a controversy fueled by science and social media. *J Blood Transfusion.* 2015;2015:874920.

30. Nishijima DK, Simel DL, Wisner DH, Holmes JF. Does this adult patient have a blunt intra-abdominal injury? *JAMA.* 2012; 307(14):1517-1527.

31. Chawda M, Hildebrand F, Pape H, Giannoudis P. Predicting outcome after multiple trauma: which scoring system? *Injury.* 2004;35(4):347-358.

32. Bouzat P, et al. Prediction of intra-hospital mortality after severe trauma: which pre-hospital score is the most accurate? *Injury.* 2016;47(1):14-18.

33. Copes WS, et al. The Injury Severity Score revisited. *J Trauma.* 1988;28(1):69.

34. Singh J, Gupta G, Garg R, Gupta A. Evaluation of trauma and prediction of outcome using TRISS method. *J Emerg Trauma Shock.* 2011;4(4):446-449.

35. Gjerde Andersen N, Rehn M, Oropeza-Moe M, Petter Oveland N. Pre-hospital resuscitative endovascular balloon occlusion of the aorta. *Scand J Trauma Resusc Emerg Med.* 2014;22(Suppl 1):P19.

36. Chawdaa M, Hildebrand F, Pape H, Giannoudis P. Predicting outcome after multiple trauma: which scoring system? *Injury.* 2004;35(4):347-358.

37. Napolitano L, et al. Tranexamic acid in trauma: How should we use it? *J Trauma Acute Care Surg.* 2013; 74(6):1575-1586.

38. Zalstein S, Pearce A, Scott D, Rosenfeld J. Damage control resuscitation: A paradigm shift in the management of haemorrhagic shock. *Emerg Med Australas.* 2008;20(4):291-293.

39. Lamb CM, MacGoey P, Navarro AP, Brooks AJ. Damage control surgery in the era of damage control resuscitation. *Br J Anaesth.* 2014;113(2):242-249.

40. Hughes NT, Burd RS, Teach SL. Damage control resuscitation: permissive hypotension and massive transfusion protocols. *Pediatr Emerg Care.* 2014;30(9):651-656.

41. Gould J, Vedantham S. The role of interventional radiology in trauma. *Semin Intervent Radiol.* 2006;23(3):270-278.

42. Raza M, et al. Non operative management of abdominal trauma—a 10 years review. *World J Emerg Surg.* 2013;8:14.

43. Como J, et al. Practice management guidelines for selective nonoperative management of penetrating abdominal trauma. *J Trauma.* 2010;68(3):721-733.

44. Tsurukiri J, et al. Resuscitative endovascular balloon occlusion of the aorta for uncontrolled haemorrahgic shock as an adjunct to haemostatic procedures in the acute care setting. *Scand J Trauma Resusc Emerg Med.* 2016;24(1):13.

15

Neurologic Trauma

ROBERT L. GRABOWSKI AND ALLEN C. WOLFE, JR.

COMPETENCIES

1. Perform a neurologic assessment.
2. Provide critical interventions for the patient with neurologic trauma to achieve maximal potential for recovery.
3. Use guidelines in the management of traumatic brain or spinal cord injury during transport.

Traumatic neurologic emergencies involve disorders of both the central and the peripheral nervous systems. In one way or another, most of these disorders ultimately affect the respiratory system; thus airway management is crucial. However, depending on the patient's condition, specific treatment may be instituted to lessen the impact of emergencies with which the transport team has to contend. The ultimate result of the disorders may be a progression to coma, often in association with increased intracranial pressure (ICP) or spinal cord injury (SCI). Therefore the transport team must understand the causes of increased ICP and the neurologic syndromes discussed subsequently in this chapter.

Traumatic Brain Injury

Traumatic brain injury (TBI) statistics are staggering. TBIs are the leading cause of death related to trauma. Estimates are that both fatal and nonfatal TBIs in the United States occur in 715 of 100,000 emergency department visits and in 91 of 100,000 that require hospital admission.[1] Seventy-four percent of all head TBIs occur in patients 25 years old or younger; however, those 65 years of age and older were most likely to die of TBI, at a rate of 45%.[2] During the past 20 years, United States involvement in the Middle East wars has shown the devastation of TBI. The cost of care for people who survive neurologic injuries is in the millions of dollars.[1] Head injury is the major cause of death related to motor vehicle crashes. The primary solution to the death and devastation caused by neurologic trauma is prevention.

The outcome for a patient who has sustained a TBI may be determined by the severity of the injury and the time elapsed before the patient receives adequate medical attention; thus the need is for rapid evaluation, assessment, and transfer of the patient to an appropriate-level care facility by the transport team. The transport team must possess a basic knowledge of the principles of pathophysiology of TBI to apply appropriate diagnostic and therapeutic methods and perform a thorough and ongoing systemic evaluation of the patient.

When trauma to the head occurs, the skin and subcutaneous tissues provide some dampening effect on impact. However, the brunt of the blow is delivered to the skull, which can flatten, indent, fracture, or dislocate when struck with a blunt object. The maximal depression occurs instantly and is followed within a few milliseconds by several oscillations. A severe blow to the skull actually causes a generalized deformation by flattening in the direction of the impact, with a corresponding widening of the diameter at right angles to the impact line.[3]

The skull travels faster under impact than does the brain. Although the unbending skull often contuses the brain at the site of impact, severe brain injuries occur when the brain is hurled against the skull's rough bony prominence, the crista galli, the major sphenoid wings, or the petrous bones. It is not uncommon for the frontal and temporal poles to be injured. The undersurface of the temporal poles and, less often, the occipital poles are contused or pulped as a result of the unbending skull. Similar damage can also be caused by the edges of the relatively unyielding falx cerebri and tentorium. So-called coup–contrecoup lesions develop in opposite areas of the brain on impact.[4]

Damage may result from direct injury or from compression, tension, or shearing forces caused by the particular injury. In addition, secondary complications result from the TBI. Cerebral edema and subsequent ischemia may ensue. An immediate increase in ICP seems to occur on impact; however, a secondary increase also occurs several minutes after the injury. The increase in ICP at the time of impact results from acceleration and deceleration of the head and deformation of the skull, the former being more significant than the latter.[3]

During impact, cerebrospinal fluid (CSF) may offer some protection to the brain. However, this protective layer is insufficient in the subarachnoid space around the frontal and temporal lobes, which are the most frequent sites of contusion.[5]

Types of Traumatic Injuries: Pathologic and Clinical Considerations

TBI may exist in isolation; however, various combinations of injuries usually occur. Each component of concurrent injuries contributes in a different degree to the overall severity and outcome of the injury.[5]

Skull Fracture

The skull is composed of three layers: an outer layer, a middle cancellous layer, and an inner layer that is half as thick as the outer layer and contains grooves that have large vessels. Whether a fracture actually occurs in the area of impact depends on the type of injury. The more concentrated and focused the impact tends to be, the greater the likelihood of a fracture.

Most skull fractures are linear. A *linear skull fracture* produces a line that usually extends toward the base of the skull. Impact can produce a single linear fracture or multiple fractures, referred to as linear stellate fractures, which radiate outward from the compressed area. Although linear fractures may look benign, they can cause serious complications. One such complication is infection. If the fracture line is open a few millimeters at the time of impact, debris such as hair, dirt, and glass may travel into the cranial vault. Linear fractures may also lead to epidural hematoma formation if the fracture line crosses a groove in the layer of the skull that houses the middle meningeal artery. Another complication occurs when the dura, which is strongly attached to the skull, tears at the fracture site.

Diastatic and Basilar Skull Fractures *Diastatic fracture* involves a separation of bones at a suture line or a marked separation of bone fragments; both are usually visible on computed tomographic (CT) scans. Facial fractures may also play a role in head injuries. A blow to the lower jaw when the jaw is closed can cause the mandibular condyles to displace upward and backward against the base of the skull, leading to a concussion or a basilar skull fracture. Another type of facial fracture, which may or may not involve the cranium, is an orbital blowout fracture, which usually involves the floor of the orbit and is caused by blunt impact to the orbit and its contents.

Basilar skull fractures can occur when the mandibular condyles perforate into the base of the skull, but they most often result from extension of fractures of the calvaria. Basilar fractures often produce Battle's sign (an oval-shaped bruise over the mastoid) or raccoon eyes (ecchymotic areas around the eyes).

Depressed Skull Fracture The presence of depressed elements of a fracture may warrant specific diagnostic and therapeutic measures. If the depressed fracture is closed, the rationale for surgical correction is to evacuate any local mass if present, repair any dural lacerations to prevent cerebral herniation through the defect, and correct any cosmetic disfigurement caused by the depression. Generally, if the

depression on the tangential view of the skull is greater than the thickness of the skull, the dura is probably lacerated, and surgery is recommended. A compound depressed skull fracture usually requires surgical debridement, whereas depressions of a lesser degree, unless over the forehead, rarely necessitate surgical exploration.

Skull fractures can be the source of various complications, including intracranial infections, hematomas, and pneumocephalus (air within the cranium), as well as meningeal and brain tissue damage. Traumatic pneumocephalus may occur if the frontal, ethmoid, or sphenoid sinuses or the mastoid processes are fractured. Air is then able to enter the skull collecting in the epidural, subdural, subarachnoid, interventricular, or intercerebral space. Pneumocephalus seldom produces symptoms unless it is under tension, producing compression of the underlying brain tissue. The incidence rate of pneumocephalus and CSF rhinorrhea with sella turcica fractures is small, but a high incidence rate of infection exists if this condition is present. Associated palsies of the oculomotor, trochlear, trigeminal, or abducens nerves may also be present.[5] The transport providers should instruct the pilot that the patient has a condition that requires flying at a low altitude. The pilot will determine the safe altitude.

Generally, temporal bone fractures can cause pneumocephalus if dural tearing occurs in conjunction with injury to the eustachian tube, the middle ear, or the mastoid process. The patient may have sensory neurologic hearing loss, otorrhagia, or CSF rhinorrhea in the presence of a temporal bone fracture.

Hemorrhage

Subdural Hematoma A *subdural hematoma* is a collection of blood in the potential space between the arachnoid mater and the dura. It may occur as a result of a contusion or laceration of the brain with bleeding into the subdural space, tearing of the veins that bridge the subdural space, or an extension of an intercerebral hematoma through the brain surface into the subdural space. Subdural hematomas have a tendency to be crescent shaped in appearance on radiologic examination because they follow the layer of the dura and are not affected by the suture lines of the skull (Fig. 15.1). They can also be unassociated with skull fractures.[3,6]

Subdural hematomas are classified as acute, subacute, or chronic, depending on the time elapsed between the injury and the appearance of signs and symptoms of neurologic dysfunction. As with other types of TBI, the time course of development and the degree and rate of neurologic dysfunction depend on many factors. As a general rule, if dysfunction occurs within 24 hours, the hematoma is acute; if it occurs between 2 and 10 days, it is subacute; and if it occurs after 2 weeks, the hematoma is chronic. This particular classification is partially pathologic. The location of the hematoma and the amount of mass effect play important roles in determination of the timing of surgical intervention.

Elderly patients may have larger subdural hematomas with slowly developing symptoms because they have larger

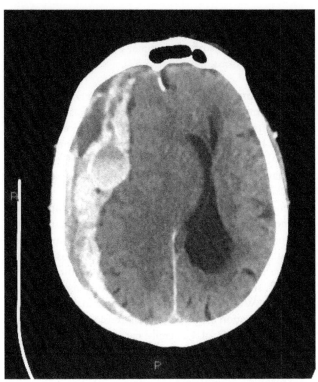

• **Fig. 15.1** Subdural hematoma on computed tomographic scan. (From Dr. Derek Smith, Radiopaedia.org.)

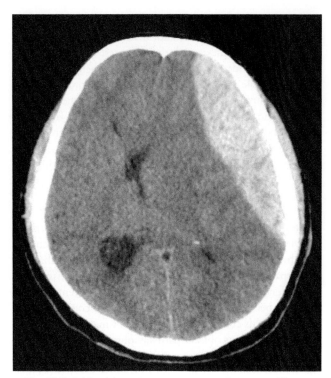

• **Fig. 15.2** Epidural hematoma on computed tomographic scan. (From Dr. David Cuete, Radiopaedia.org.)

potential subdural spaces as a result of cerebral atrophy. In contrast, symptoms may be displayed rapidly, and marked increases in ICP may develop in a younger patient with a smaller subdural hematoma.

Subdural hematomas that occur in children under the age of 2 years have signs and symptoms that include a bulging fontanel and a large head (because of separation of the sutures), as well as retinal hemorrhages (because of increased ICP). In the infant patient, a shocklike state may also develop because a relatively large blood volume loss may be caused by a subdural hematoma.

Acute subdural hematomas are usually associated with high morbidity and mortality rates. These rates can usually be estimated by the patient's presenting Glasgow Coma Scale (GCS) score. A GCS score of less than 8 has an associated mortality of 50% to 90%. Patients with a GCS score of 9 to 12 have associated 21% to 46% mortality, and those with a score greater than or equal to 13 have a mortality rate reported as low as 0%.[6] This potentially high mortality rate reflects the usually severe nature of the associated injuries and the not infrequent association of rapidly rising ICP resulting from the mass effect and development of cerebral edema. Two separate related pathophysiologic problems are cerebral contusion and edema and the presence of blood in the subdural space. The CT scan is valuable in the determination of whether surgical intervention may be indicated. If the major problem contributing to poor neurologic status is the mass effect, then surgical intervention may be necessary. If the major problem is the cerebral injury, then corrective treatment should be directed toward ICP management.

Epidural Hematoma An *epidural hematoma* is the collection of blood, usually arterial, between the skull and the dura. Epidural hematomas are classified as acute or subacute. An acute epidural hematoma that is arterial in origin generally produces symptoms within a few hours. On radiologic examination, acute epidural hematomas follow the outer layer of the dura, are usually limited by the suture lines of the skull, and take on a lenticular shape (Fig. 15.2). Subacute epidural hematomas are generally venous in origin and take a longer time to produce symptoms. These hematomas are associated with linear skull fractures in 90% of patients, but they may also occur as a result of blunt injuries in which no evidence of fracture is seen.[7-8] The classic symptoms displayed with epidural hematoma are transient loss of consciousness, recovery with a lucid interval during which neurologic status returns to normal, and the secondary onset of headache and a decreasing level of consciousness. As a result of the initial injury, the middle meningeal artery may tear and cause traumatic unconsciousness. Spasm and clotting then occur in the middle meningeal artery, and the bleeding stops. During the next several hours, the artery gradually bleeds, and a hematoma is formed. As pressure accumulates, the dura is stripped from the inside of the skull. Once a headache with a decreasing level of consciousness becomes obvious, the secondary rise in ICP has already occurred, and distortion of the brain with significant mass effect occurs. Because compensatory mechanisms of the inner cranial space have already been exhausted, the patient's neurologic status rapidly deteriorates. The patient experiences a downhill course, usually with dilation of the ipsilateral pupil because of third-nerve compression by the herniating temporal structures; progressive unconsciousness with weakness or decerebration of either the contralateral extremities or the ipsilateral extremities; Cheyne–Stokes respirations; and, if no treatment is initiated, loss of pupillary reflexes, caloric responses, bradycardia, and death. Thus on identification of the epidural hematoma in the earliest possible stage, when a headache and drowsiness are the only symptoms, transfer of the patient for immediate neurosurgical intervention is extremely important.[6-8] The classic history and clinical progression, however, is only seen in one-third of patients with epidural hematomas. Another third are unconscious from the time of injury, and the final third are never unconscious. In children, bradycardia and early papilledema may be the only warning signs.

Subarachnoid Hemorrhage A subarachnoid hemorrhage (SAH) refers to blood collecting between the arachnoid membrane and the pia mater (brain surface). This subarachnoid space is generally occupied by connecting tissue and CSF. Hemorrhage into the intraventricular system can also be seen, because these are communicating compartments. Because of this communication, an SAH may lead to hydrocephalus by means of CSF pathway obstruction or blockage of arachnoid granulations (projections that absorb CSF into the venous system). In addition to the risk for hydrocephalus, and increased ICP by that obstructive mechanism, SAH may also increase ICP secondary to space-occupying hemorrhage or edema. SAH also yields a risk for seizures and cerebrovascular spasm related to hemorrhaged blood degradation on the surface of the brain and around vasculature.[7-9]

SAH is one of the most common CT findings in TBI, and is found in approximately 40% of all cases of TBI, but reported as widely as 11% to 60% (Fig. 15.3). Generally,

traumatic SAH has a better prognostic outcome than does spontaneous SAH. However, it is important to consider if the SAH is a result of the trauma, or if the SAH was the *cause* of the trauma.[9]

Cerebral Contusion *Cerebral hemorrhagic contusions* frequently occur in patients, particularly adults, after TBI. Of the patients who die of TBI, 75% have contusions found on autopsy. Hemorrhagic contusions are infrequently seen in children, but areas of localized decreased density on a CT scan may represent nonhemorrhagic contusions, or possibly local ischemia.[4]

Generally, no surgical intervention is recommended in the treatment of cerebral contusions because brain tissue cannot be removed from areas of the brain that control motor, sensory, or visual functioning. If, however, the contusion occurs over the frontal or temporal lobes, with significant edema and shift, surgical removal of contused portions of the brain is feasible. When a temporal lobe contusion is present and signs of herniation are seen, surgical excision of the temporal lobe may be beneficial. Generally, patients with contusion are treated with medical control of elevated ICP.

Intracerebral Hematoma Movement of one section of brain tissue over or against another section causes tears in blood vessels, which leads to contusions or *intracerebral hematomas,* also known as *intraparenchymal hematomas.* Most intracerebral hematomas are found in the frontal and temporal lobes, are usually very deep, and are associated with necrosis and hemorrhage. The anatomic relationship between these areas and irregularities of the skull has already been discussed. Intracerebral hematomas are readily identified on CT scan (Fig. 15.4). The clinical picture may vary from no neurologic defect to deep coma, depending on the location and severity.

Traumatic Brain Injury: Diffuse Axonal Injuries

Diffuse axonal injury (DAI) occurs when the delicate axons of the brain are stretched and damaged as a result of rapid movement of the brain. Mechanisms of injury associated with acceleration and deceleration forces, like those that occur with high-speed motor vehicle crashes or ejection from a vehicle, can cause this type of diffuse brain injury. Because the axons have been damaged, interference with neural transmission is seen, and multiple neurologic deficits can range from headache and amnesia to severe deficits that include deep coma, posturing, and respiratory compromise. Severe DAI is usually associated with a high mortality rate.[8,10] Although there are several treatment strategies currently under investigation, there is no curative treatment to DAI; current goals are aimed at supportive care.

Penetrating Injuries

Gunshot Wounds When a person is shot at close range, evidence of soot or gunpowder may be visible on the skin. When the muzzle of the gun is somewhat farther from the scalp but still close, evidence of powder burns may exist.

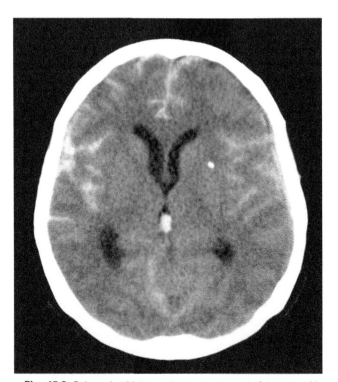

• **Fig. 15.3** Subarachnoid hemorrhage on computed tomographic scan. (From Dr. David Cuete, Radiopaedia.org.)

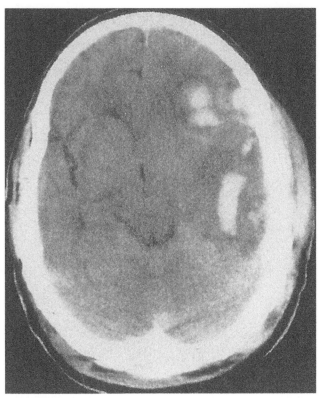

• **Fig. 15.4** Intracerebral hematoma (intraparenchymal hematoma). (From Ellenbogen RG, Abdulrauf SI, Sekhar LN. Principles of Neurological Surgery. Philadelphia: Saunders; 2012.)

A bullet striking the skull can cause great destruction of the underlying brain tissue.

Although some of the bullet's kinetic energy may be dissipated on impact by transfer to the bone and soft tissues, the impact on the brain after a bullet penetrates the skull is still great. The bullet's ability to destroy tissues is directly related to its kinetic energy at the moment of impact. The degree of damage to the brain depends primarily on the muzzle velocity of the bullet and the distance between the gun and its target, as previously discussed in Chapter 14.

A bullet that passes through the head produces a larger defect on the inner table of the skull than that produced on the outer table. High-velocity bullets cause extensive injury to the brain and cranium. The entrance wound is usually smaller than the exit wound, but a great deal of variation in size may be seen. Multiple linear fractures that radiate from either the entrance or exit wound are common. Some fractures may be far away from the trajectory of the bullet, particularly in thin bones. The transport team should describe the wounds but not attempt to determine whether they are entrance or exit wounds.

Injuries to the major cerebral arteries, veins, or venous sinuses can occur in any of the bullets' intracranial passages. Cerebral injuries cause an immediate, but transitory, increase in ICP. The eventual ICP depends on the degree of intracranial bleeding, which may be profuse even in the absence of injury to major vessels. Secondary cerebral edema causes a delayed increase in ICP. Damage to the hemisphere causes loss of cerebral autoregulation, decreased cerebral blood flow, an increase in cerebral blood volume and ICP, and eventually brain death.

Intracranial hematomas are frequently associated with penetrating wounds to the brain. If the bullet passes close to or transverses the ventricle, an intraventricular hematoma may result.

Infection is seen often in injuries caused by shell fragments because these fragments are more likely than bullets to carry dirt, hair, and bone fragments into the brain. Infections develop most often from retained bone fragments, improper closure of the scalp and dura, and delay of definitive surgery beyond 48 hours.

Whenever the skull has been penetrated, a risk of intracranial infection exists. The injury should be managed to minimize that risk. All patients with penetrating injuries should receive tetanus prophylaxis and intravenous antibiotics.[11,12]

Most stab wounds are caused by assaults with sharp instruments such as knives, scissors, and screwdrivers or when the patient (often a child) falls on a stick or sharp toy. The best method is to transport the patient with a stab wound with the object immobilized, secured, and left in place.

If the penetrating object has been removed, determination of exactly where penetration of the skull occurred may be difficult, particularly if entry occurred at the eyelid or sclera. When the patient arrives at the hospital, the area of injury is explored and debrided, as with an open injury.

Physical Assessment: Traumatic Brain Injury

Examination of a patient who is unconscious requires integration of information from several systems: mental status, pupils, other cranial nerves, motor system, and respiratory function (Table 15.1).

Level of Consciousness

The best indicator of changes in ICP, especially from a mass lesion, is a patient's level of consciousness.[4,7] *Consciousness* is a mental state in which the person is stimulated by the environment and can react appropriately to it. A useful way of describing the conscious state is to divide it into alert, lethargic, or obtunded stages (Box 15.1).

The *alert* patient readily responds to the examiner, although, depending on the state of the central nervous system (CNS) injury, some confusion, speech disturbance, and motor deficits may be seen. The *lethargic* patient appears to be drowsy or asleep but can be aroused easily and can respond reasonably appropriately to the examiner's questions. However, if left alone, the patient slowly returns to an apparent sleep state or lack of attentiveness. The *obtunded* patient is extremely drowsy, arouses with greater difficulty than a lethargic patient, rarely answers in complete sentences, and certainly does not volunteer information. During the active questioning period, the examiner may have to repeatedly stimulate the patient to gain attention.

Deterioration beyond the obtunded level results in the unconscious state. This state may be classified as either stupor or coma. The *stuporous* patient does not verbalize

TABLE 15.1 **Physiologic Disturbance Correlated With Anatomic Level of Lesion**

Parameters	Cerebral Cortex	Diencephalon	Thalamus	Midbrain	Pons	Medulla
Mental status	Awake, alert, lethargic, obtunded	Light stupor	Deep stupor	Coma	Coma	Coma
Motor response	Appropriate	Focal response to pain	General response to pain	Decerebrate posturing, decorticate posturing	Flaccid	Flaccid
Pupil response	Normal size and reactivity	Small	Small	Midposition	Small	Small
Oculocephalic, oculovestibular reflex	Not testable	Normal response	Normal response	Abnormal	Abnormal	Abnormal[a]
Respiratory Status	Variable	Variable	Cheyne–Stokes	Central neurogenic hyperventilation	Apneustic pattern	Apnea

[a]May be normal with isolated medullary injury.

• BOX 15.1 | **Stages in Progression From Consciousness to Unconsciousness**

Conscious State

Alert: Patient responds readily but may have some confusion, speech disturbance, or motor deficit.

Lethargic: Patient appears drowsy or sleepy but can be aroused to respond to questioning.

Obtunded: Patient is extremely drowsy, is difficult to arouse, and rarely answers in complete sentences; examiner may have to repeatedly stimulate to gain patient's attention.

Unconscious State

Stuporous: Patient does not verbalize appropriately or coherently; may moan and groan or utter monosyllables; responds to painful stimuli by moving extremities.

Comatose: Patient gives no evidence of awareness.

---

appropriately or coherently. Two distinct levels of activity can characterize this state. The patient in a lightly stuporous state may moan and groan in response to stimulation or may utter an occasionally recognizable monosyllabic word, often a slang or curse word. The patient who is in a light stuporous condition responds to pain by moving all extremities, unless a primary motor system injury exists, and appears to crudely localize the site of the pain. However, a patient who is in a deeply stuporous state does not appear to localize and protect against pain. The patient who is in true *coma* may have decorticate posturing, decerebrate posturing, or flaccid motor response.

During examination of the pattern of motor response, the examiner must be aware of the possibility of primary motor system injury. For example, a left cortical lesion or a lesion in the left internal capsule may cause a contralateral hemiparesis that, even in the awake patient, may distort the motor response.

The comatose state is roughly divided into three levels of reflex motor activity: decorticate posturing, decerebrate posturing, and flaccidity. These allow the use of clinically descriptive terms rather than more precise neurophysiologic descriptions. The patient in a *decorticate state* is unconscious and gives no evidence of awareness. Painful stimulation causes extensor rigidity in the lower extremities combined with a flexor posture of the upper extremities. Depending on the extent of the underlying damage to the motor system, this posturing may occur spontaneously or after painful stimulation and may be more prominent on one side than the other. *Decerebrate posturing* is exhibited by extensor rigidity in all four extremities. The patient who is *flaccid* has no motor response to painful stimulation.

For consciousness to be present, a stimulus must be presented to the CNS and must pass through the brainstem (with the exception of visual stimulation) to the diencephalon. From there, the stimulus must reach the cerebral cortex, where it is recorded. The patient must have sufficient cortical function so that the stimulus can excite associations through memory, which lets the patient acknowledge the presence of the stimulus and make use of that stimulus to relate appropriately to the external environment.

For example, when an intracranial mass lesion develops after head trauma and unconsciousness does not initially result, the patient may be expected, as the mass lesion increases, to progress systematically through the various levels and stages just described. The mass lesion may be a hematoma or significant cerebral edema. A patient with a TBI resulting in a primary upper brainstem lesion might be unconscious and may immediately present in a comatose state without ever having had cortical or diencephalic deterioration. A person who survives a near-drowning or delayed cardiopulmonary resuscitation may have severe bilateral cortical injury and may not progress significantly. A person with a spontaneous hemorrhage in the brainstem, particularly in the region of the pons or midbrain, is expected to become suddenly comatose with no evidence of an orderly progression through the stages noted previously.

Examination of the Pupils

The pupils are innervated by both the parasympathetic (third cranial nerve) and the sympathetic systems, with the former causing constriction and the latter causing dilation. The size of the pupil depends on the degree to which each system influences the pupil at the time of examination. The normal pupil constricts promptly to light. Examination of the pupils consists of assessment of the relative size of the two pupils and their reactivity to light. Injury to the parasympathetic system results in pupillary dilation caused by unopposed sympathetic response.

Injury to the parasympathetic system may occur within the midbrain at the origin of the parasympathetic contribution to the third nerve, or it may occur outside the brainstem in which the third nerve exits and proceeds forward beneath the brain into the region of the cavernous sinus. The sympathetic innervation begins in the posterior hypothalamus, descends the length of the brainstem and cervical cord, and exits in the lower cervical upper thoracic area, where it proceeds up the neck in the cervical sympathetic chain to the base of the skull and then out to the orbit where innervation occurs.

Injury to the sympathetic system results in pupillary constriction because of the actions of the unopposed third nerve. The sympathetic system can be injured within the CNS anywhere along its pathway and during its course through the chest and neck. Because of the relatively small size of the structures involved, lesions within the brain or brainstem are unlikely to affect either the parasympathetic or the sympathetic systems unilaterally. Therefore we can assume that if bilateral pupil abnormalities are seen, a lesion in the brain or brainstem has affected the nerve supply to the pupils. For example, bilaterally small pupils may very well be caused by a lesion within the brainstem that affects both descending sympathetic tracts. On the other hand, a unilaterally affected pupil can be expected to be caused by a lesion of the tracts outside the brain or brainstem (extraaxial). A unilaterally dilated pupil may be caused by compression of the third nerve by a herniating temporal lobe after it has exited the midbrain and as it crosses the floor of the skull. A unilateral small pupil that results from sympathetic denervation reacts more sluggishly to light. Bilaterally dilated and fixed pupils are generally caused by global hypoxia or by bilateral temporal lobe herniation from central cerebral edema with bilateral third-nerve compression. Bilaterally constricted pupils may be caused by central herniation of the posterior hypothalamus at the site of origin of the sympathetic fibers through the tentorial notch or by bilateral involvement within the brainstem, such as from a pontine hemorrhage. Midbrain lesions that affect the parasympathetic bilaterally yield pupils that are in midposition and are nonreactive to light. Examination of other cranial nerves is helpful because they can reveal the competency of brainstem function including the III, IV, and VI cranial nerves.

Brainstem and Cranial Nerves

The integrity of the brainstem can be evaluated with examination of certain cranial nerves, especially those related to conjugate gaze. In the patient who is awake, conjugate gaze is controlled by visual input through the complex system that coordinates the function of the extraocular muscles by way of cranial nerves III, IV, and VI. In the patient who is unconscious, however, visual input gives way to vestibular input to control conjugate gaze. This is best evaluated with examination of the oculocephalic or oculovestibular reflexes.[7,8,13,14]

The oculocephalic reflex is demonstrated by stimulating the vestibular system through movement of the head in reference to the neck. While the patient lies supine on the ground, stretcher, or bed, the person performing the assessment opens the patient's eyelids. In normal circumstances, the eyes should stare at the sky or ceiling. The nurse then rotates the head briskly but gently to one side or the other. In normal circumstances, the eyes may momentarily remain in their position in the orbits but immediately track conjugately to the side opposite the direction of the movement so that the eyes are directed once again toward the sky or ceiling. If conjugate activity cannot be observed (e.g., if one eye tracks and the other one does not or if neither eye tracks, also known as "doll's eyes"), this signals an abnormality and suggests a disturbance of the brainstem. This maneuver should never be performed in a patient with a TBI or multiple trauma until the cervical spine has been determined to be without injury.

The oculovestibular reflex is demonstrated by cold caloric stimulation, in which cold saline solution is irrigated into the external auditory canal. In a few seconds, the eyes conjugately deviate to the side of the irrigation and remain in that position from several seconds to several minutes. If this response is not seen, an abnormality is present in the brainstem involving the medial longitudinal fasciculus, the vestibular system, or both.

The midportion of the pons may be evaluated by the presence or absence of the corneal reflex. The corneal reflex can quickly be assessed by lightly touching the cornea with the corner of a soft gauze dressing and observing whether a blink reflex occurs.

Motor Examination

The motor system is best examined in conjunction with an examination of the patient's mental status or level of consciousness. The awake patient can be asked to perform certain motor tasks, such as moving the legs or gripping. If the patient is unconscious, motor activity in response to pain is a good way to determine the level of unconsciousness, as previously described.

Respiratory Pattern

Most patients with significant head injuries have hypoventilation early after the injury. Later, the respiratory pattern may vary, depending on the level of the lesion. Patients with decorticate posturing often have an accompanying Cheyne–Stokes pattern of respiration with a regular crescendo–decrescendo change in the volume of inspiration, with the rate remaining rather regular. The patient with decerebrate posturing may have central neurogenic hyperventilation. Patients with brainstem lesions may have varying rates and depths of respiration, and an ataxic element is often noted. With lower brainstem lesions, the rate becomes more irregular, more shallow, and less frequent, until medullary lesions result in respiratory paralysis. Often the transport team needs to intubate the patient for respiratory control.

Glasgow Coma Scale

The GCS, as shown in Table 15.2, is widely used to measure the severity of coma in patients and is therefore an indicator of prognosis. However, eye-opening response may not be accurately assessed in the patient with severe maxillofacial injuries whose airway is mechanically supported. In addition, in a patient with a contralateral mass lesion, the best motor response may not depict progressing hemiparesis. When examining a patient, the GCS results are best recorded in the narrative record that goes to the receiving health care providers.

Reexamination

Successful acute management of the comatose patient depends on frequent examination of the patient to determine the level of neurologic function and rate of deterioration. The information provided in Table 15.2 can be helpful in this analysis.

When the transport team sees the injured patient for the first time, a baseline neurologic evaluation should be performed. Findings during subsequent examinations provide the transport team with an understanding of the intracranial injury. When a focal mass lesion such as a hematoma or focal contusion develops in a patient, the patient shows steady progression in depth of coma through the various levels depicted in Table 15.2. For example, when the initial examination of a patient results in findings compatible with a diencephalic level of coma, the coma is determined to have deteriorated to a midbrain level if the patient is subsequently found to have decerebrate posturing, midposition pupils, and central neurogenic hyperventilation. If the insult is unilateral, hemiparesis and an ipsilateral dilated pupil are seen before bilateral motor signs of herniation are seen.

TABLE 15.2 **Glasgow Coma Scale**

Circle the Appropriate Number and Compute the Total

Best eye opening response:		_____Right	_____Left
	Never		1
	To pain		2
	To verbal stimuli		3
	Spontaneously		4
Best verbal response:	No response		1
	Incomprehensible sounds		2
	Inappropriate words		3
	Disoriented and converses		4
	Oriented and converses		5
Best motor response:		_____Right	_____Left
	No response		1
	Extension abnormal (decerebrate rigidity)		2
	Flexion abnormal (decorticate rigidity)		3
	Flexion withdrawal		4
	Localizes pain		5
	Obeys commands		6
	Total: _____3–15		
Neurologic evaluation	Record on GCS sheet		
	Repeat evaluation frequently		
	A score of 15 is normal; below 7 indicates coma; 3 signifies brain death		
	Vital signs:		
	Level of consciousness		
	GCS		
	Pupillary size and reactivity		
	Right _____		
	Left _____		
	Focal weakness		
	Present _____		
	Absent _____		

GCS, Glasgow Coma Scale.

If the patient initially shows signs of coma resulting from a primary brainstem injury, which is a static lesion, a further deterioration in the level is not demonstrated within the next few hours, other than what is normally seen with a developing mass lesion.

Interventions and Treatment

The management of TBI is based on both national and international guidelines that are now evidence based (Box 15.2).[15] Each transport team should have developed protocols to manage these patients. The primary focus of the transport team should be prevention and treatment of hypoxia, hypotension, and increased ICP, while optimizing cerebral perfusion pressure (CPP).[7,8,15]

CPP is the pressure gradient representing the flow of blood to the brain (cerebral blood flow). CPP is defined as the difference of the mean arterial pressure (MAP) minus the ICP.[15]

$$CPP = MAP - ICP$$

• BOX 15.2 Summary of the Guidelines for the Management of Severe Traumatic Brain Injury That Affect Patient Transport

Initial Resuscitation

Complete and rapid physiologic resuscitation is the first priority, and no treatment should be directed toward intracranial hypertension in the absence of indications of deterioration in neurologic status or signs of impending herniation. However, when signs of neurologic deterioration are present, aggressive management must be initiated and should include:
- Hyperventilation
- Administration of intravenous mannitol or HTS
  Sedation, analgesia, and neuromuscular blockade must be used in a discretionary manner.

Resuscitation of Blood Pressure and Oxygenation

Hypotension defined as a systolic blood pressure of less than 90 mm Hg or mean arterial pressure of 65 mm Hg must be avoided or aggressively managed.
At Pao_2 <60 mm Hg, apnea should be managed by securing the patient's airway and maintaining adequate ventilation.

Intracranial Pressure Treatment Threshold

Interpretation and treatment of ICP based on any threshold should be corroborated by frequent clinical examination and monitoring.

Controlled Hyperventilation

Avoid hyperventilation during the first 24 hours because reduced blood flow compromises cerebral perfusion.
Ventilation managements should be aimed at an end-tidal CO_2 goal of 35 to 40 mm Hg.

Use of Mannitol or Hypertonic Saline

Administration of mannitol or hypertonic saline may occur before initiation of ICP monitoring with signs of transtentorial herniations or deterioration of neurologic status.

ICP, Intracranial pressure.

The goals of preventing hypotension and preventing/treating raised ICP are to, ultimately, optimize CPP. Current consensus of the literature suggests maintaining a CPP of 60 to 70 mm Hg after TBI in adult patients.[15]

Management is based on the severity of the injury, which is usually measured by the patient's GCS. The following classification with the GCS has been suggested to identify the gravity of the patient's injury[4,8,15]:
- Mild GCS: 14 to 15
- Moderate GCS: 9 to 13
- Severe GCS: 3 to 8

Because the transport team may not always know the patient's primary diagnosis (i.e., subdural hematoma, epidural hematoma), management of patients based on GCS and the related physical examination results assists the team in providing the appropriate care to these patients.

The transport team's highest priority is establishing an adequate airway, providing oxygenation, and preventing or managing hypotension.[15] The awake patient should be placed on 100% oxygen. If the patient is unable to maintain the airway or the transport team anticipates the potential for deterioration during transport, the patient should be intubated. Care must be taken to maintain cervical spine protection while gaining access to the airway. A gastric tube should be inserted with care to prevent aspiration. Pulse oximetry and end-tidal CO_2 ($EtCO_2$) devices should be used throughout the transport process to monitor the patient's oxygenation and perfusion.

If the patient is restless or agitated, hypoxia should be suspected until a specific cause can be found. Most patients with head injuries have sustained other injuries that cause pain. Even in the patient who is inattentive or stuporous, hypoxia rather than pain should be considered the cause of restlessness until this is proven otherwise.

Choice of medications used for rapid sequence intubation (RSI) of the patient with TBI requires a great deal of clinical experience, gestalt, and review of current literature.

Lidocaine as a pretreatment agent for patients undergoing RSI was in theory thought to be ideal for those who are at risk for increased airway resistance (i.e., asthma) or increased ICP (i.e., intracranial hemorrhage). However, there is no high-quality evidence that directly addresses whether pretreatment with lidocaine effectively reduces the rise in ICP caused by laryngoscopy and endotracheal intubation. What little evidence exists consists of small trials that have reached contradictory conclusions.[15,16]

Fentanyl, another common pretreatment agent, is thought to decrease potential elevated ICP and cardiovascular disease exacerbations by sudden elevations in blood pressure. This drug should be avoided if the patient is hemodynamically unstable. No data exist regarding the effects of fentanyl alone on the ICP of patients with acute head injuries undergoing RSI.[16]

There has been off-label use of "push dose" vasopressor therapy in air medical transport practice, but there are no major studies supportive of this practice improving outcomes. The theory is supporting the hemodynamic status of the hemodynamically unstable patient by pushing a specific dose before RSI to offset the potential drop during intubation and postintubation.

The intubated patient who is restless or resists ventilatory support is increasing their ICP, which may be extremely critical. These patients should be managed with pharmacologically appropriate doses of sedation, analgesia, and neuromuscular blocking agents.[10,17-19] Because of the effects of analgesic and sedation agents on the patient's hemodynamic status, the effects of these medications must be closely monitored by the transport team. However, pain can be a powerful stimulus to increasing physiologic metabolism and oxygen consumption, and its effects on the patient's ICP must be considered. Analgesia and sedation should be adequately provided before considering prolonged neuromuscular blockade, which should be avoided in patients at risk for posttraumatic seizures to maintain clinical assessment for seizure activity.

Generally, hypertension and bradycardia may develop in patients who have increased ICP. Hypotension and tachycardia are not signs of intracranial injury, except in a patient with herniation. However, small children may become hypovolemic from scalp lacerations associated with head injuries and should be monitored and treated accordingly with volume replacement.

Patients with head injuries may lose cerebral autoregulation (Fig. 15.5). If this is the case, cerebral perfusion is directly related to mean systemic arterial pressure. Thus hypotension may lead to underperfusion, and hypertension may lead to vascular congestion and mass effect. Both extremes should be avoided.

Hypotension has been found to contribute to significant mortality and morbidity of patients with head injuries.[15,20,21] Fluids and blood products should be administered to maintain systolic blood pressure greater than 90 mm Hg. Rapid transport for surgical intervention may be the only definitive management for some hemorrhagic hypotension. Hypotension is rarely seen in isolated head injuries. When hypotension is seen in the multisystem trauma patient, hypovolemia/hemorrhage should always be ruled out and treated. Hypotension in these patients is most often secondary to acute hemorrhage, impaired autonomic nervous system control, iatrogenically from medication use, or less commonly from

SCI or subacute diabetes insipidus. If euvolemia does not correct hypotension, infusions of norepinephrine or phenylephrine should be considered to maintain an adequate MAP and CPP.[15,20]

Posttraumatic seizures that develop during transport should be promptly treated because they produce hypoxia, increase cerebral metabolic demand, risk rebleeding of vessels, and cause increased ICP. Intravenous administration of benzodiazepines is indicated for initial seizure management. Prophylactic use of antiepileptic medications may be considered, especially if the patient is receiving neuromuscular blocking agents[14-16]; however, data concerning the use of prophylactic antiepileptics in the post-TBI patient is controversial. Phenytoin and levetiracetam have been suggested to be equally beneficial in reducing early seizure rates. However, this reduction of seizures has not yet been shown to be beneficial to the patient's outcome. Also, these medications, especially phenytoin, are known to have adverse drug effects, including a potentially adverse effect on neurocognitive outcomes.[6,13,22,23] Unconscious patients or those who have a depressed level of consciousness associated with seizure activity should be intubated for maximal control of the airway. Because an adequate airway is of paramount importance, the airway should be secured immediately.

Hyperthermia also increases ICP and is associated with worse outcomes; thus normal body temperatures should be maintained with the use of acetaminophen suppositories or cooling techniques. Shivering should be controlled because it increases ICP, metabolism, and oxygen consumption.

If neuromuscular blocking agents are used, close monitoring of the patient's temperature is important for the presence of hypothermia, because of the inability of the patient to shiver, or for evidence of malignant hyperthermia, particularly in children.

Routine hyperventilation is no longer recommended in the initial management of the patient with a TBI. However, it may be acutely indicated with signs and symptoms of herniation. Signs of herniation may include the following[8,19,24]:
- Unilateral or bilateral pupillary dilation
- Asymmetric pupillary reactivity
- Motor examination results that show either extensor posturing or no response
- Other evidence of deterioration of the neurologic examination, such a known midline shift or impending herniation on the CT scan results

The patient's CO_2 level should be maintained between 35 to 40 mm Hg throughout the transport. During the first 24 hours of TBI, cerebral blood flow is reduced by 50%. A CO_2 less than 30 will impede cerebral perfusion and is associated with worsened neurologic outcomes.[8] With hyperventilation, the patient's $PaCO_2$ decreases, triggering cerebral vasoconstriction. This cerebral vasoconstriction leads to decreased cerebral blood volume, decreasing ICP; however, this decrease in cerebral blood volume can lead to cerebral ischemia, especially in the patient with a poor perfusion state postinjury. The fourth edition of the *Traumatic Brain Injury Guidelines* (2016) state studies have shown that after severe TBI, cerebral metabolic rate is not always low and can be variable. Cerebral ischemia has been documented in

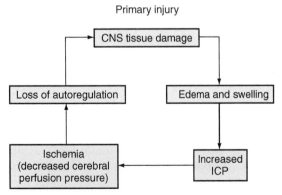

Primary injury

• **Fig. 15.5** Sequence of pathophysiologic events initiated by primary injury.

a number of studies after severe TBI, changing long-standing recommendations concerning ventilation therapy.

$EtCO_2$ waveform capnography monitoring is the most appropriate method to monitor $EtCO_2$ in TBI patients. It is the standard of care for monitoring $EtCO_2$ in any intubated patient during transport. The transport team must pay careful attention when manually assisting an intubated patient with head injury. The patient should be placed on mechanical ventilation as soon as practically able and should not be transported via manual ventilation because of increased risk of CO_2 fluctuations. Aggressive ventilations can also cause additional injury.[21,25]

Hyperosmolar therapy, such as mannitol or hypertonic saline (HTS), may be used to treat increasing ICP, manifested by deterioration in the patient's neurologic status. Mannitol is an osmotic diuretic that decreases the patient's ICP by increasing the patient's serum osmolarity, creating an osmotic gradient in which water is drawn into the serum from the brain tissue. This act of cerebral dehydration reduces brain volume (reducing ICP), transiently increases plasma volume (until diuresed), and decreases blood viscosity (increasing cerebral blood flow). This mechanism requires an intact blood-brain barrier (BBB) to draw fluid across. In theory, if the BBB is severely disrupted, or after multiple doses of mannitol (which can contribute to breaking down the BBB), mannitol can leak into the parenchyma and cause a reverse gradient, worsening cerebral edema. Mannitol should be administered through an intravenous filter.[4,7,15,25-27] It has been the "go-to" medication for this indication for decades; however, HTS has been under investigation for a potential replacement or alternative to this long-standing drug.[21]

HTS, available in a wide array of tonicities (3, 7.5, 23.4%, etc.), has been under investigation for a couple of decades. Initially, research suggested there is no difference in effect when compared with mannitol. The latest research, however, suggests that HTS is just as effective, and potentially more effective, at lowering ICP than mannitol.[21,28] Although there is literature to support one treatment being superior to the other in reducing ICP, there is no literature to support a difference in outcomes based on choosing one agent over the other. HTS uses a similar mechanism as mannitol; it increases serum osmolarity and creates an osmotic gradient to decrease water content in the brain, reducing brain volume, and subsequently ICP. HTS has also been shown to dehydrate endothelial cells, in turn increasing internal vessel diameter; this, coupled with an increase in plasma volume, yields an improved blood flow. The key difference between HTS and mannitol is the diuretic effect. Because mannitol is an osmotic diuretic, one should consider avoiding this agent in the hypovolemic, multisystem trauma patient, and/or the hypotensive patient. HTS would likely be a better agent in this role, because its effects are less transient, and it does not cause an eventual loss of needed fluid volume.[21,28]

Invasive technology for TBI and increased ICP has greatly advanced in the last several years. Although there are a myriad of devices available for treatment and monitoring,

all devices are designed to either indirectly or directly measure brain perfusion and/or reduce ICP. Transport care providers are less likely to see these devices in practice, because the facilities that have the resources available to perform and use these devices are likely the facilities to which the patients are being transported to and not from. However, it is important to understand the purpose and utility of these devices. A few common devices include the following:

External ventricular drainage (EVD) catheter: A burr hole is drilled through the skull and a catheter is placed directly into the anterior horn of the lateral ventricle. The EVD is the gold standard in ICP management because it has the ability to directly measure ICP, and can drain CSF to reduce ICP as needed.

Subdural bolt: A hollow, fluid-filled screw is drilled through the skull to just below the inner table of the skull (the dura). Similar to other invasive pressure-monitoring devices, the fluid-filled screw is zeroed and transduced to measure the pressure within the cranial vault. Bolts are easier to place than EVDs and are less likely to become infected; however, a bolt can only measure ICP, but cannot perform any therapeutic action on it.

Lumbar drainage catheter: A catheter is placed in the subarachnoid space via needle puncture between lumbar vertebrae, similar to a lumbar puncture ("spinal tap"). This catheter can measure pressures within the space and drain CSF. These drains can be particularly helpful if there is a contraindication or hindrance to EVD placement, or as temporizing measure.[29-31]

Brain tissue oxygen pressure ($PBtO_2$) monitoring: A small hole is drilled through the skull and a thin filament probe is placed directly into parenchymal tissue. This probe helps measure focal oxygen stores and their use to the area being measured. Because of the focalized area of measure, there has been controversy as to where the device should be placed; it may be seen in healthy tissue to estimate general, whole-brain oxygenation, or adjacent to the site of injury to determine spread of the injurious lesion. There have been significant improvements in outcomes using this measure to guide therapies.[15]

It is important to remember when transporting a patient with a CSF drain that these drains are transduced to a particular level, affected by gravity, and changes in position can dramatically alter the amount of CSF being drained. For this reason, CSF drains should be clamped (stopcock to the "off" position) during movement and repositioning and reopened after motion is completed.

Finally, when ICP is refractory to medical management, a decompressive craniectomy or craniotomy may be performed. A craniectomy involves surgically removing a large segment of the skull to reduce pressure within the cranial vault. In certain cases, the bone flap removed can be stored for an attempt to later replace the segment after a significant period of time when all physiology has returned to baseline. A small craniotomy, or burr hole, is a hole that is drilled into the skull to provide, generally temporizing, relief of pressure. This is most commonly indicated for large epidural or subdural hemorrhages. A craniectomy is a much more definitive treatment and may be used in a wide variety of conditions, compared with the burr hole, and has been shown to improve refractory ICP. It has yet to conclusively demonstrate significant improvement in long-term outcomes. A craniectomy must be performed in the operating room by a neurosurgeon, whereas a Burr hole may be performed in an emergency department by a trained, nonsurgeon provider. This is generally only indicated if the patient is acutely deteriorating or neurosurgical intervention is several hours away.[15]

Maxillofacial Trauma

Trauma to the face can occur by many mechanisms. Most frequently it is seen in sports injuries, recreational activities, and more seriously in motor vehicle collisions and assaults. Treatment of these injuries is generally best performed at a trauma center, because these injuries typically require the involvement of numerous specialty services. Injuries to the face can impact the patient's mortality as well as heavily impacting psychosocial aspects and activities of daily living. Changes in the way we eat, speak, laugh, kiss, see, smell, and overall experience the world can cause a terrible detriment to the patient's psychological health. Also, alterations to one's face can cause a significant change to a person's identity, because the face is associated with who a person is. However, in the acute phase of injury, and during transport, attention should be focused on immediate life threats.

Injuries to the face and jaw can produce significant airway compromise. Complications such as blood, bone, dirt, and debris in the upper airway can cause immediate or delayed obstruction and subsequent hypoxia, followed by death or disability. When caring for the patient with maxillofacial trauma, the care provider should be hypervigilant in assessing for airway compromise. These injuries can lend themselves to a need for prompt airway management and may require atypical approaches. The patient that presents after a shotgun injury to the lower face, or after a fall from 40 feet, face down, onto cement may not be easily intubated by traditional laryngoscopic technique. Adjuncts and alternatives such as the gum elastic bougie, fiber-optic or video-assisted laryngoscopy, retrograde intubation, and so forth may need to be used. Much less frequently performed is a nasotracheal intubation, and this should be avoided in the patient without radiologic clearance from basilar skull fracture. A critical skill to have when caring for patients of maxillofacial trauma is that of the surgical cricothyrotomy. A surgical airway is needed in approximately 5% of patients suffering gunshot wounds or blast injuries to the face, especially when affecting the jaw or lower third of the face.[4]

Facial fractures can lead to multiple issues. In addition to airway obstruction, facial fractures can cause significant pain, damage to facial or cranial nerves, or lacerate a multitude of facial vessels. This can lead to significant hematoma formation, or even exsanguination in extreme cases. Formation of hematomas in key areas can be devastating. One such example

includes a retrobulbar hematoma (blood accumulating posterior to the eye), which causes the optic nerve to become stretched and impede optic vasculature. A retrobulbar hematoma is ophthalmic emergency and can lead to blindness if pressure is not rapidly, surgically relieved. Rapid transport to a provider, or bringing a skilled transport provider, to perform an emergent lateral canthotomy is essential to salvaging the patient's sight. Significant force facial fractures should also lead the provider to consider the patient at high risk for intracranial injuries, and appropriate precautions should be applied. These patients should be transported to a trauma center for evaluation, including those with complicated facial fractures, such as Le Fort–type fractures.

Spinal Cord Injury

All trauma patients, especially those with a head injury, are suspect for SCI and should be treated accordingly.[32,33] The transport team should perform a baseline evaluation of the patient with a spine injury before transfer and should monitor the patient closely for changes in neurologic status during the transfer process. These patients should be transferred supine on a firm surface with the spine in good alignment. Studies suggest that logrolling of patients with spine injuries is destabilizing at the fracture site and should be avoided if possible. A scoop stretcher may be used to transfer the patient onto the rigid transport stretcher to avoid the torsion effects produced by the logrolling maneuver.[13,32-34]

Current literature and recommendations are challenging the ingrained practices of emergency medical services (EMS) regarding spinal immobilization. It is reported that over 5 million patients are immobilized in the prehospital/transport arena in the United States each year; however, the incidence of SCI is only about 12,000 patients per year, including cervical spine injuries, which would be protected by a rigid cervical collar alone.[33] Use of a long backboard is not without harm. Adverse effects of backboard use include pain, induced discomfort leading to unnecessary radiologic imaging, respiratory compromise, and pressure sores.[33,34] Because of the low incidence, adverse effects, and lack of proof of benefit, the empiric use of backboards is under scrutiny. Many EMS systems are beginning to institute protocols to avoid use of backboards, except for during extrication, or for those patients at high risk for injury on assessment. Decline in use is especially seen in the patients with penetrating trauma and those that were ambulatory on scene without significant pain.[14,34] The National Association of EMS Physicians and American College of Surgeons Committee on Trauma have released a position statement stating that the full immobilization with use of a long backboard should be reserved for patients with the following:

- Blunt trauma and altered level of consciousness
- Spinal pain or tenderness
- Neurologic complaint (numbness or motor weakness)
- Anatomic deformity of the spin
- High energy mechanism of injury *and:*
- Drug or alcohol intoxication;

- Inability to communicate; and/or
- Distracting injury.[14]

When appropriate and delineated by established guidelines, patients with cervical spine injury may be transported in traction. Proper equipment, such as a spring-loaded scale system, is necessary because the use of hanging weights is inappropriate in the transport setting.

Etiology and Incidence Rate

The incidence rate of SCIs that result in paralysis or debilitating weakness as a consequence of trauma to the spinal cord has been analyzed statistically in many different ways in many different countries. An estimated 12,000 cases of SCIs occur per year in the United States.[1,2,35]

The age distribution of acute SCIs peaks in the 15- to 24-year-old age group. Frequency decreases in the middle-age group, with a second peak occurring at about the age of 55 years.[1-3,35] The incidence rate in women is lower for all age groups. Traffic accidents continue to be the most frequent cause of SCIs in all age groups. Motorcycles and bicycles cause 10% to 12% of SCIs. Excessive consumption of alcohol is a factor in one-third of cases involving accident victims with SCIs.[1-3,35]

More than half of work-related SCIs are caused by falls, and falls are the primary cause of SCIs in the home, particularly among the elderly, who fall down steps, fall from chairs, or fall off ladders.

Approximately 7% of SCIs are caused by accidents that occur during sporting and recreational activities and most commonly occur as a result of diving into shallow water. The increasing number of women involved in sports is reflected in the rise of injuries for that group.[1-3,35]

Initial Assessment

Management of spinal cord trauma begins with the realization that the patient may have an unstable spine. Whether at the accident scene or at a local referring hospital, the transport team should conduct a rapid, thorough primary and secondary assessment of the patient with an SCI before transfer. This assessment provides a baseline for serial assessments and reveals additional injuries and commonly associated complications, such as aspiration, neurogenic shock (bradycardia and hypotension), and poikilothermy.[1,3,4,8]

Airway

The patient's airway should be checked for patency and cleared of foreign matter or secretions. With the spine protected, the upper airway in a patient with an altered mental status should be opened with use of the modified jaw-thrust maneuver to allow spontaneous or assisted ventilation.[4]

Breathing

Breathing may be absent or inadequate in patients with high cervical cord injury (C4 or above), which results in loss of both diaphragmatic and intercostal phrenic nerve intervention and paralysis of these respiratory muscles. In such cases, assisted ventilation with a bag-valve-mask and tracheal intubation with oxygen supplementation is indicated. RSI with judicious spine immobilization may be necessary for airway and ventilation control. Regardless of the method chosen to manage the patient's airway, the transport team must ensure proper consistent protection of the entire spine.

Circulation

As with all critically injured patients, intravenous access is mandatory for patients with SCIs. Intravenous lines may be inserted on the scene or en route, depending on the patient's condition, distance of transfer, and existing protocols. Isotonic solutions such as lactated Ringer's solution or normal saline solution are preferred. The rate and volume of infusion is based on the patient's cardiovascular response. Neurogenic shock may be present in patients with cervical or high thoracic spine injury. Interruption of sympathetic outflow below the level of injury results in loss of autoregulation, a decrease in vascular tone, and the inability of the heart to increase its intrinsic rate. With passive vasodilation and a normal or bradycardic state, the patient becomes hypotensive.[4] The transport team should differentiate this shock state from hypovolemia and infuse crystalloids and/or blood products accordingly. MAP should be maintained at 85 to 90 mm Hg, although clinical research validating this goal is lacking.[20] If the patient's condition is hemodynamically unstable, administration of a vasoactive drug such as norepinephrine or dopamine may be indicated. Phenylephrine should be reserved for nonbradycardic, purely vasogenic, spinal shock. Risk versus benefit should be weighed when adding vasopressor therapy to augment MAP in SCI when there is concurrent TBI, as previously discussed. This can cause overelevation of CPP and lead to cerebral edema and increased ICP. Hypovolemia must be ruled out before vasopressor therapy is started.[7,15]

This loss of sympathetic tone or injury-induced sympathectomy produces poikilothermy. In this state, the patient loses the ability to vasodilate and sweat in hot environments and the ability to vasoconstrict and shiver in cold environments. Thus the patient's core body temperature often reflects the environment and must be considered if warming or cooling techniques are withheld.[15]

Vasovagal reflex with tracheal suctioning must also be considered for these patients. Preoxygenation is important to prevent vagal stimulation and severe bradycardia, which could lead to a decrease in CPP, which could be deleterious in a patient with concomitant TBI. It may even cause cardiac arrest.[15]

Secondary Assessment

Once the primary survey has been completed, critical interventions have been initiated, and the patient's condition has been stabilized, the transport team can perform a secondary assessment. This includes performing a baseline neurologic evaluation; obtaining a history of the incident and history of allergies, medications, previous illnesses or injuries; time of the patient's last meal; and completely exposing and examining the patient. Data about the mechanism and time of injury are valuable. To help expedite the transfer, this information can be obtained during the head-to-toe assessment.

Examination of the patient with an SCI should be performed with the patient maintained in a neutral position and the entire spine protected. A sensory and motor assessment helps the transport team determine the level and extent of injury. Autonomic function such as anal sphincter control can be assessed, and if sacral sparing is present, the injury should be considered incomplete.[4]

Unless the cervical spine area has been already immobilized before arrival, the transport team should visually inspect and carefully palpate it to determine the presence of deformity, crepitus, pain, and muscle spasm, which are frequently associated with cervical spine injury. A priapism will indicate a traumatic SCI, which is caused by a pooling of blood from a decrease in systemic vascular resistance. A second team member should maintain cervical spine in-line stabilization while this is performed and until an immobilization collar is applied.

Lower Spine Injuries

The patient should be asked to wiggle their toes. If the patient can move the toes of both feet, he or she should be asked to raise each leg slightly, one at a time. The patient's legs should not be raised if the prior examination revealed no movement or association. If the patient shows any obvious weakness, injury to the spinal cord must be assumed.

Cervical Spine Injuries

The patient should be asked to wiggle their fingers. If the patient can do so, the patient should be asked to raise each arm, one at a time. Again, substantial active movement of the upper extremity should be avoided if evidence exists of obvious fractures of the spine or extremity. The transport team should ask the patient to squeeze two fingers with both hands. In addition, the transport team should ascertain the patient's dominant hand and cross over, matching the team member's dominant hand to the patient's dominant hand. The strength of the patient's grasp should be similar. If the patient cannot move his or her fingers and arms or has obvious weakness, SCI in the cervical region should be assumed.[4]

Patients with cervical spine injuries are at high risk for neurogenic or spinal shock and respiratory compromise. As mentioned earlier, these patients may require vasopressor and/or inotropic support; however, hypovolemia and hemorrhagic shock are significantly more common in the trauma patient. This should always be ruled out before initiating these drugs in the trauma patient. These patients should be transported with cervical immobilization, cardiac and blood pressure monitoring, and respiratory function monitoring; nasal cannula $EtCO_2$ monitoring lends itself to significantly more rapid means of detecting respiratory decline than does SpO_2 monitoring.[15,25]

Sensory Examination

The presence of a sensory deficit confirms the suspicion of a cord or nerve-root injury. The transport team should test the patient's ankles and wrists and ask the patient if he or she can feel the touch. In the event that the patient cannot feel the touch in one or more places or reports numbness or tingling, SCI can be assumed. Particular sets of clinical presentations on sensory examination can lead the transport clinician to a higher suspicion of a given type of SCI pattern, otherwise known as spinal cord syndromes.

Spinal Cord Syndromes

Anterior cord syndrome: Paraplegia below the level of injury, with loss of pain and temperature sensation

Central cord syndrome: Motor impairment with some sensory impairment, usually to a worse degree in the upper extremities than the lower

Brown-Séquard syndrome: Loss of motor function on ipsilateral side of injury, with sensory impairment to contralateral side of injury

Complete cord transection: Complete loss of motor and sensory function below the level of injury; high-level injuries can be associated with spinal shock

Neurologic Examination of the Unconscious Patient

The condition of an unconscious patient's spinal cord should be checked by pricking the skin lightly on the soles of the feet or ankles with a sharp object. If no spinal cord damage has occurred, the painful stimulus triggers an involuntary muscle reflex and the extremities move, unless the patient is in a profound coma. If the cord is damaged, no such response will be seen. The lack of response to pinpricks in the upper extremities indicates damage to the spinal cord in the cervical region. Failure of only the lower extremities to respond indicates SCI in the thoracic or lumbar regions.

The degree of functional loss with sudden spinal cord transection depends on the level of the injury. The higher the injury, the more function is lost. Complete sudden cord transection results in complete flaccid paralysis below the level of injury; areflexia (spinal shock) below the level of injury; urinary retention; and occasionally, in the male patient, priapism.

Incomplete sudden cord transection results in varying degrees of paralysis and sensory loss below the level of injury, areflexia (below the level of injury), and varying degrees of bladder or bowel paralysis. Box 15.3 can be used as a guide for evaluation of muscle strength and motor function.

Interventions and Treatment

The patient with SCI frequently has other traumatic injuries and may have varying degrees of stability. Judicious airway assessment and management is needed for the patient with SCI when injuries are found in the cervical region. In the absence of hypovolemia, intravenous fluids should be monitored closely and maintained at a rate that prevents pulmonary overload. The transport team may potentially initiate steroids if the injury is at L1 or above, time from injury is within 8 hours, and the team has received authorization to do so. Methylprednisone previously has been recommended as

• BOX 15.3   Muscles to Be Tested for Evaluation of Motor Strength

Actions to be Tested	Muscles	Cord Segment
Abduction of the arm	Deltoid	C5
Flexion of the forearm	Biceps	C5, C6
Extension of the forearm	Triceps	C7
Flexion of digits 2–5	Flexor digitorum and profundus	C8
Opposition of meta-carpal of thumb	Opponens pollicis	C8, T1
Hip flexion	Iliopsoas	L12
Knee extension	Quadriceps femoris	L3-L4
Dorsiflexion of foot	Deep peroneal	L5
Dorsiflexion of big toe	Extensor hallucis longus	L5
Plantar flexion of foot and big toe	Gastrocnemius flexor	S1

one of the methods of treatment for the patient with an isolated blunt SCI. The Consortium for Spinal Cord Medicine Member Organizations does not recommend routine use of high-dose steroids in the prehospital care environment. Despite four prospective blinded randomized controlled trials investigating the effect of methylprednisone in acute SCI, there exists no Class I medical evidence of any beneficial effect.[15] The administration of high-dose steroids should only be performed after consultation with a neurosurgeon. If the patient's potential spine injury has not been appropriately ruled out, the transport team must ensure that the patient remains immobilized or in motion restriction until arrival at the receiving facility. Alternative methods of immobilization and motion restriction, such as vacuum mattresses, are being introduced that hopefully will decrease the risk of skin breakdown when a patient must remain immobilized for long transports.[32]

Classification of Cervical Spine Injuries by Mechanism of Injury

Flexion Injuries

Anterior subluxation (Box 15.3) is a flexion lesion characterized by disruption of the posterior ligament complex (Fig. 15-.6). Because the anterior longitudinal ligament remains intact and the disk is not completely disrupted, this lesion is stable at the time of injury and is difficult to see radiographically.[14,32]

Physicians disagree on whether bilateral interfacetal dislocations result from hyperflexion or a combined flexion and rotary force. Unilateral and bilateral *interfacetal dislocations* involve soft tissue injury of the posterior ligament complex, and CT scans frequently reveal an unstable injury with a high incidence rate of cord damage.[4,14,32]

The stability of a *simple wedge fracture* depends on associated posterior ligament disruption. This flexion injury usually results from a compressive force on the anterior portion of the vertebral body with stretching of the posterior ligament complex. These fractures are generally in the mid or lower cervical segments and are considered stable fractures because of maintenance of posterior and anterior ligaments and the integrity of the interfacetal points.[14,32]

Teardrop hyperflexion fracture dislocations are seen as a result of diving or traffic accidents and falls. This type of fracture is extremely unstable because the vertebra is displaced posteriorly as the person strikes an object, and displacement disrupts the apophyseal joint capsule disk below. The anterior margin of the vertebra fractures in a teardrop-shaped fragment, and the fractured vertebra remains displaced posteriorly. Although often severe, the degree of neurologic deficit depends on the severity of hyperflexion compression. Patients who sustain teardrop flexion fractures frequently have acute anterior cervical cord syndrome. Immediate quadriplegia, loss of anterior cord senses (pain and temperature), and retention of posterior cord senses (position, motion, and vibration) result.[14,32]

Flexion-Rotation Injuries

Fractures that result from *flexion-rotation* are characterized by the displacement or fracture of one or more vertebrae. Fractured vertebrae may produce a unilateral facet dislocation with corresponding nerve-root compression. Severe distraction forces, those forces that cause separation of bone fragments, may cause an anterior displacement of the upper cervical body greater than 50%, which can result in bilateral locked facets and major cord injury, such as quadriplegia.[4,14]

Extension-Rotation Injuries

Pillar fractures, usually caused by motor vehicle accidents and falls, are the most common combined injury of the cervical spine. The mechanism of injury results in a force concentrated on the apophyseal joints of the mid and lower cervical segments and resultant vertical fractures of a lateral mass. A distraction of the fracture elements is probably caused by rebound flexion of the head and neck.[4,14]

Vertical Compression

Compression cervical spine injuries include the Jefferson fracture of the atlas and the bursting fracture of the lower cervical vertebrae. Compression fractures of the cervical spine are uncommon because the injury must occur from force transmitted vertically through the skull and occipital condyles of the spine at the precise moment the spine is straight.[7,8,14]

Extension Injuries

Most *hyperextension* injuries result from contact with a windshield or other structure in the interior of an automobile. Extension injuries can be of three types. The *extension*

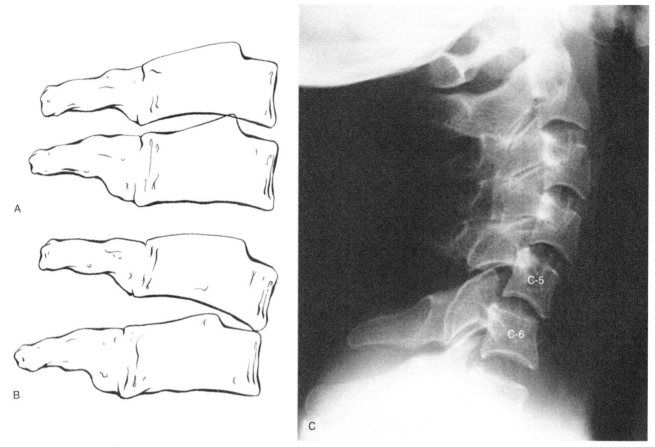

• **Fig. 15.6** A, Normal alignment of the cervical vertebrae in the lateral view. B, Subluxated position with narrowing of the intervertebral disk, anterior angulation, and widening of the space between the spinous processes. C, C5-C6 subluxation. Note the widened space between the spinous processes. (From Eiff PM, Hatch R. *Fracture Management for Primary Care*. ed 3. Philadelphia: Elsevier Saunders, 1998.)

teardrop fracture is a rare extension injury that involves the anterior corner of the axis, the second cervical vertebra. This type of fracture is usually associated with preexisting degenerative arthritis of the cervical spine. The *hangman's fracture* is an unstable bilateral fracture of the pedicles of the axis. This fracture is often associated with dislocation of the C2 or C3 cord segment and prevertebral soft tissue swelling.[7,8,14] *Hyperextension fracture-dislocation* injuries are associated with direct force backward or a backward and upward force without an axial loading force. The typical hyperextension-dislocation injury is accompanied by the following triad of signs: (1) midface skeletal or soft tissue injury, (2) varying degrees of central cord syndrome, and (3) a lateral cervical spine radiograph that appears normal with the exception of diffuse prevertebral soft tissue swelling (Fig. 15.7).[7,8] This type of extension injury is believed to be responsible for the quadriplegia in the rare patient whose cervical spine films appear normal. The probable mechanism of injury is cord compression between the posterior vertebral body, lamina, and ligamentum flavum during extension.

Thoracic and Lumbar Spine Injuries

Injuries to the thoracic and lumbar spine vary in severity from muscle strains and ligamentous strain to fractures of the vertebral body, fractures of the dorsal elements, dislocation of the facets, and complex combination fracture dislocations. The spinal cord and the nerve roots may be injured by an encroachment into the spinal canal. Patients with stable compression fractures may sustain concomitant injury to the spinal cord, and patients with grossly unstable comminuted fractures may escape neurologic injury. Generally, the more comminuted, displaced, and unstable the spine fracture, the greater the likelihood of severe cord damage.[4,6-8,13,36]

Direct injuries to the spine and the spinal cord may occur as a result of a direct blow, such as from a falling tree limb or other heavy object, a stab wound, or a gunshot wound. Most injuries are caused by indirect trauma to the vertebral column resulting from energy generated by forces applied to the head, shoulders, trunk, or pelvis. These forces may contain an axial load as the main force with varying degrees of lateral bending, flexion, extension, or torsion.

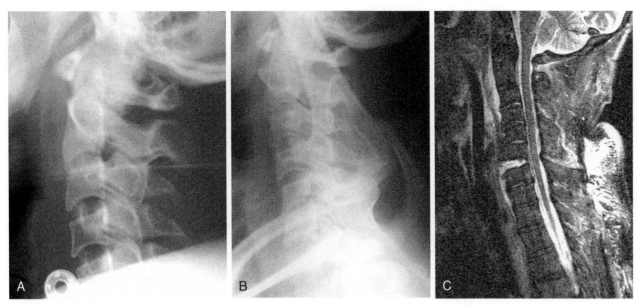

• **Fig. 15.7** Hyperextension dislocation (hyperextension sprain). (From Hart, BL. *Spine Surgery*. Philadelphia: Elsevier; 2005.)

The thoracic and lumbar spine are most commonly injured by the kinetic energy produced by the person's body traveling through space and a sudden deceleration of the shoulders, upper trunk, or buttocks against an immovable object, with the vector of forces concentrated in an area of the thoracic or the lumbar spine. The most common area is that of the thoracolumbar junction, with specific patterns of vertebral body fractures and dorsal-element dislocation at T11 and T12, rotational-flexion fractures of both body and dorsal elements at T12 to L1, and bursting fractures of the body of L1. Fractures of the midthoracic spine usually occur at the T5 or T6 level.

The most common site of lumbar fractures is L2 or L3. Chance fractures, a specific type of flexion-distraction injury, occur when a person is restrained by a seat belt and experiences sudden deceleration, which causes sudden flexion and distraction centered at the midlumbar spine. Patients with these fractures often escape spinal cord cauda equina damage, and the fracture may be overlooked in the presence of TBI or associated small intestinal injuries. Hence, presence of these fractures may increase the chance of intraabdominal injury. Any person who has pain after being in an automobile accident in which a seat belt was worn must be examined specifically for the presence of a spinal fracture.

The thoracic spine is protected from injury by the rib cage, the sternum, and the chest wall. These bony structures permit little flexion and extension motion of the upper and midthoracic spine; however, a normal rotation motion does occur. The lumbar spine allows for more flexion, extension, and lateral motion because it lacks the previously mentioned supporting structures.

Midthoracic spine injuries are usually caused by acute flexion, rotation, and axial load forces at the midthoracic region, resulting in either a simple compression fracture of the vertebral bodies or a complex fracture dislocation in which the vertebral body and the dorsal elements are fractured.

Most injuries at the thoracolumbar junction are caused by a combination of flexion, rotation, and axial load. An injury that is centered at T11 to T12 frequently causes a dislocation without fracture of the posterior facets and a slice fracture through the upper portion of the T12 vertebral body.

Rotational forces are commonly associated with fracture dislocations of the T12 to L1 levels. If the injury has more of an axial load than a rotational force, the body of L1 suffers a burst injury. In this type of injury, the posterior elements of the lamina, spinous process, and facet joints may be intact or may also be fractured. An example would be the lover's fracture, or jumper's fracture, where concomitant fracture of the calcaneus and burst fracture of a thoracolumbar vertebrae are seen, after the patient has fallen from a significant height, feet first.

Summary

The management of all neurologic traumatic emergencies includes rapid assessment, airway management with spinal protection, and serial examinations throughout the assessment and transfer phases. On completion of the transfer, the receiving caregivers must be provided with a thorough report of events, including the time of the incident, the mechanism of injury or preceding events, care rendered by the referring facility and the transport team, response of the patient to care initiated, medical history of the patient, and observed changes in the patient's condition. This thorough report provides the receiving caregivers with information to guide their management and ensure continuity of care for the patient with the best possible chance for a positive outcome.

CASE STUDY

Neurologic Trauma

A 22-year-old male unrestrained driver struck the back end of a parked car. He was thrown 25 feet from the vehicle. Because of the mechanism of injury, the local emergency medical services agency called the transport team directly to the scene so that the patient could be transferred to a level I trauma center.

The transport team found on arrival that the patient was unresponsive with a Glasgow Coma Scale of 5. He had facial abrasions and swelling with palpable crepitus.
1. Eye opening: 1
2. Verbal response: 1
3. Motor response: 3

He was being ventilated via bag-valve-mask device, and his jaws were clenched. He was successfully intubated with appropriate rapid sequence induction) on the first attempt. He was placed on the ventilator, and the minute volume was titrated to yield an end-tidal CO_2 (EtCO$_2$) of 35 to 45 mm Hg. He had strong peripheral pulses, and the monitor showed a sinus tachycardia at a rate of 120 beats/min. One intravenous line had been established before arrival, a second intravenous line was placed, and the patient was appropriately immobilized and packaged for transport. He was provided appropriate postintubation sedation and analgesia.

During transport, the patient's blood pressure was measured at 180/128 mm Hg. His heart rate decreased to 48 beats/min. His right pupil became fixed and dilated.

Discussion

The patient's change in vital signs reflected increasing intracranial pressure. Based on his blood pressure, pulse rate, and fixed dilated pupil, the transport team initiated controlled hyperventilation at a rate of 30 breaths per minute to achieve an ETCO$_2$ of 35 to 40 mm Hg and administered a 3% hypertonic saline bolus en route. These acute changes in the patient's neurologic status were clear indications for aggressive management to decrease the intracranial pressure.

On arrival to the receiving facility, the patient's blood pressure had decreased to 160/100 mm Hg, and his heart rate had increased to 100 beats/min. He was taken for an emergent computed tomographic scan, which showed a large epidural hematoma with mass effect on the left. He was then taken to the operating room for decompression.

References

1. Centers for Disease Control and Prevention, National Center for Injury Prevention and Control, Division of Unintentional Injury Prevention. Rates of TBI-related Emergency Department Visits, Hospitalizations, and Deaths—United States, 2001–2010. Retrieved from http://www.cdc.gov/traumaticbraininjury/data/rates.html; 2016, January 22 Accessed 17.10.16.
2. Centers for Disease Control and Prevention, National Center for Injury Prevention and Control, Division of Unintentional Injury Prevention. Rates of TBI-related Emergency Department Visits by Age Group—United States, 2001–2010. Retrieved from http://www.cdc.gov/traumaticbraininjury/data/rates_ed_byage.html; 2016, January 22 Accessed 17.10.16.
3. Huang K, et al. The neurocritical and neurosurgical care of subdural hematomas. *Neurocrit Care.* 2016;24:294-307.
4. Mattox K, Moore E, Feliciano DV. *Trauma.* New York, NY: McGraw-Hill; 2013.
5. Haddad S, Arabi Y. Critical care management of severe traumatic brain injury in adults. *Scand J Trauma Resusc Emerg Med.* 2012;20:12.
6. Dunn J, Smith M. Critical care management of head injury. *Anaesth Intensive Care Med.* 2008;9(5):197-201.
7. Jallo JI, Loftus CM. *Neurotrauma and Critical Care of the Brain.* New York: Thieme; 2009.
8. Abelson-Mitchell N. *Neurotrauma: Managing Patients with Head Injury.* Chichester, UK: Wiley-Blackwell; 2013.
9. Wu Z, Li S, Lei J, et al. Evaluation of traumatic subarachnoid hemorrhage using susceptibility-weighted imaging. *AJNR Am J Neuroradiol.* 2010;31(7):1302-1310.
10. El-Orbany M, Connolly L. Rapid sequence induction and intubation: current controversy. *Anesth Analg.* 2010;110(5):1318-1325.
11. Shackford S, et al. Gunshot wounds and blast injuries to the face are associated with significant morbidity and mortality: results of an 11-year multi-institutional study of 720 patients. *J Trauma Acute Care Surg.* 2014;76(2):347-352.
12. Enam S, Kazim S, Tahir M, et al. Management of penetrating brain injury. *J Emerg Trauma Shock.* 2011;4(3):395.
13. McQuillan KA, Thurman PA. Traumatic brain injuries. In: McQuillan KA, ed. *Trauma nursing: from resuscitation through rehabilitation.* 4th ed. Philadelphia, PA: Saunders; 2009.
14. Guidelines for the Management of Acute Cervical Spine and Spinal Cord Injuries. *Neurosurg.* March 2013;72(suppl 2):1-259.
15. Guidelines for the Management of Severe Traumatic Brain Injury. 4th ed. https://braintrauma.org/guidelines/guidelines-for-the-management-of-severe-tbi-4th-ed#/; September, 2016 Accessed 19.10.16.
16. Zeiler FA, Sader N, Kazina CJ. The impact of intravenous lidocaine on ICP in neurological illness: a systematic review. *Crit Care Res Pract.* 2015:ID 485802.
17. Kirkman MA, Smith M. Intracranial pressure monitoring, cerebral perfusion pressure estimation, and ICP/CPP-guided therapy: a standard of care or optional extra after brain injury? *Br J Anaesth.* 2014;112(1):35-46.
18. Robinson N, Clancy M. In patients with head injury undergoing rapid sequence intubation, does pretreatment with intravenous lignocaine/lidocaine lead to an improved neurological outcome? A review of the literature. *Emerg Med J.* 2001;18(6):453-457.
19. Stevens RD, Lazaridis C, Chalela J. The role of mechanical ventilation in acute brain injury. *Neurol Clin.* 2008;26(2):543-563.
20. Hawryluk G, et al. Mean arterial blood pressure correlates with neurological recovery after human spinal cord injury: analysis of high frequency physiologic data. *J Neurotrauma.* 2015;32(24):1958-1967.
21. Bhardwaj A, Ulatowski JA. Hypertonic saline solutions in brain injury. *Curr Opin Crit Care.* 2004;10(2):126.
22. Consortium for Spinal Cord Medicine Member Organizations. *Early Acute Management in Adults with Spinal Cord Injury: A Clinical Practice Guideline for Health Care Professionals.* Washington, DC: Paralyzed Veterans of America; 2008.

23. Hurlbert JR, Hadley MN, Walters BC, et al. Pharmacological therapy for acute spinal cord injury. *Neurosurgery*. 2015; 72(suppl 2): 93-105.

24. Armin SS, Colohan ART, Zhang JH. Vasospasm in traumatic brain injury. *Acta Neurochir Suppl*. 2008;104(13):421-425.

25. Richardson M, et al. Capnography for monitoring end-tidal CO2 in hospital and pre-hospital settings: A Health Technology Assessment [Internet]. *Canadian Agency for Drugs and Technologies in Health*. 142, 2016.

26. Jones K, et al. Levetiracetam versus phenytoin for seizure prophylaxis in severe traumatic brain injury. *Neurosurg Focus*. 2008; 25(4):E3.

27. Kirmani B, Mungall D, Ling G. Role of intravenous levetiracetam in seizure prophylaxis of severe traumatic brain injury patients. *Front Neurol*. 2013;4:170.

28. Kamel H, Navi BB, Nakagawa K, Hemphill JC 3rd, Ko NU. Hypertonic saline versus mannitol for the treatment of elevated intracranial pressure: a meta-analysis of randomized clinical trials. *Crit Care Med*. 2011;39(3):554-559.

29. Speck V, et al. Lumbar catheter for monitoring of intracranial pressure in patients with post-hemorrhagic communicating hydrocephalus. *Neurocrit Care*. 2011;14(2):208-215.

30. Feyen BF, Sener S, Jorens PG, Menovsky T, et al. Neuromonitoring in traumatic brain injury. *Minerva Anesthesiol*. 2012;78(8):949-958.

31. Jiang JY, et al. Efficacy of standard trauma craniectomy for refractory intracranial hypertension with severe traumatic brain injury: a multicenter, prospective, randomized controlled study. *J Neurotrauma*. 2005;22(6):623-628.

32. Morrissey J. Research suggests time for change in prehospital spinal immobilization. *J of Emerg Med Services*. 2013;38(3): 29-39.

33. National Spinal Cord Injury Statistical Center. *Facts and figures at a glance*. Birmingham, AL: University of Alabama at Birmingham; 2013.

34. White CC, et al. EMS spinal precautions and the use of the long backboard - resource document to the position statement of the National Association of EMS Physicians and the American College of Surgeons Committee on Trauma. *Prehosp Emerg Care*. 2014;18(2):306-314.

35. Centers for Disease Control and Prevention, National Center for Injury Prevention and Control, Division of Unintentional Injury Prevention. Rates of TBI-related Deaths by Age Group—United States, 2001–2010. Retrieved from http://www.cdc.gov/traumaticbraininjury/data/rates_deaths_byage.html; 2016, January 22 Accessed 17.10.16.

36. Bullock MR, Povlishock JT. Guidelines for the management of severe traumatic brain injury. *J Neurotrauma*. 2007;24(S1): 1-106.

16

Thoracoabdominal Trauma

CLYDE GENTRY AND ALLEN C. WOLFE, JR.

COMPETENCIES

1. Identify clinical indications of thoracoabdominal injuries.
2. Recognize signs and symptoms of life-threatening thoracoabdominal injuries.
3. Perform appropriate critical interventions to manage thoracoabdominal injuries.

Trauma remains the number one cause of death for Americans between 1 and 46 years old, and it is the number one cause of death overall. Its economic impact exceeds $671 billion annually. Each year more than 192,000 people lose their lives to trauma.[1]

Injuries to the chest and abdomen are common in trauma patients. Blunt trauma may be isolated to a specific location in the abdomen or involve a single organ, such as the liver. Frequently injuries involve both compartments, and it is difficult in the field to differentiate exactly where the patient is injured or where is the source of bleeding. The diaphragm separates the thoracic and abdominal compartments and can be compromised itself, as in the case of a ruptured diaphragm.

Penetrating injuries can easily involve both the chest and abdomen. The challenge remains: early assessment, recognition, and intervention by first responders. Rapid transport with advanced critical care teams providing diagnostic tools and life-saving interventions reduces time to the operating room and definitive care.

Thoracic trauma continues to be a leading cause of death in those younger than 40 years. Thoracic injury is seen in nearly 50% of multiple trauma patients. With approximately 150,000[2,3] deaths per year in the United States alone, thoracic trauma is a common and potentially deadly injury that in many cases can be corrected with tube thoracostomy and volume resuscitation. Rapid recognition and early intervention is the key. For the critical care transport team, special consideration is given to these patients regarding altitude changes as gas expands. Many transport teams are not the first at the scene of an incident. It is imperative that emergency medical services (EMS) is familiar with these injuries so that rapid recognition and early interventions are started and augmented on arrival of the critical care transport team. Outreach education by critical care transport teams will assist EMS and provide expert seamless care to the nearest trauma center equipped to care for these patients.

Thoracic injuries are classified as either blunt or penetrating. Blunt injuries are associated with direct compressive force and/or rapid deceleration forces. A common mechanism could be an automobile traveling at 70 mph that strikes a telephone pole. There are three types of impacts: car versus pole, interior versus occupant, and internal organs versus chest. In this scenario there could be multiple injuries to the lung, great vessels, and mediastinum. Blunt injuries are also seen in falls, assaults, and sports. Penetrating trauma occurs as a result of gunshot wounds (GSWs), stab wounds, impalements, and bomb fragments. GSWs and blast injuries are ever-increasing in frequency leading to an injury pattern that is challenging to treat in the field and during transport.

Thoracic injury can be categorized into what many in the field refer to as the "deadly dozen": airway obstruction, open pneumothorax, tension pneumothorax, hemothorax, flail chest, cardiac tamponade, myocardial contusion, traumatic aortic rupture, tracheal or bronchial tree injury, diaphragmatic tears, esophageal injury, and pulmonary contusion.

The ABCDEs of resuscitation continue to serve as a framework for the management of thoracic injuries. The primary survey can quickly help detect life-threatening injuries and initiate rapid interventions.

Airway Obstruction

There is no more important and critical intervention than recognition and proper treatment of airway obstruction or respiratory failure. In many cases simple airway maneuvers such as a jaw thrust or proper positioning will alleviate an airway obstruction.

Assessment

Maintenance of the airway is a priority in the trauma patient. Inadequate ventilation can lead to hypoxia and delivery of oxygen to tissue. Position of the tongue is important because of the potential for it to migrate backward and block the larynx in the unconscious person. Swelling of the oral cavity, laryngeal spasm or foreign bodies, fluids, and broken teeth are potential hazards to airway maintenance.

Intervention

Correct and appropriate bag-valve-mask technique is crucial to ventilation and oxygenation. Patients requiring intubation should be managed in a sequential organized approach optimizing success. All providers performing intubation and rapid sequence induction should be under strict medical control, and skills should be monitored and tracked. Intubation in the field has been associated with poor success rates in providers who are not properly and regularly trained. Utilization of advanced airway equipment (videoscopic devices), end-tidal CO_2 ($EtCO_2$) detection, and pulse oximetry are the rule rather than the exception.

Open Pneumothorax

Open or "sucking" chest wounds can lead to an accumulation of air inside the pleural space. Closed pneumothorax leads to an escape and accumulation of air inside the pleural space.

Assessment

Dyspnea, tachypnea, tachycardia, hyperresonance on the injured side, decreased or absent breath sounds on the injured side, and an open sucking wound may be heard on inspiration. If available, ultrasound examination will show no lung sliding.

Intervention

In the prehospital setting, the wound should be covered with an occlusive dressing taped on three sides. This type of dressing will have a flutter valve effect; air can leave but cannot get back into the wound. Do not tape the dressing on all four sides. A tension pneumothorax can be created because air is being prevented from leaving the pleural space. If a tension pneumothorax develops, the dressing should be removed immediately and a needle thoracostomy should be executed (Figs. 16.1 and 16.2).

Continuous Assessment and Evaluation

Constant monitoring of the patient's vital signs, pulse oximetry, and end-tidal capnography are essential. Assessing for increasing dyspnea, subcutaneous emphysema, tracheal deviation, and changes in neurologic status alerts the transport team to critical changes and interventions required for treatment.

Tension Pneumothorax

Both blunt and penetrating thoracic trauma can cause a tension pneumothorax. Air progressively accumulates

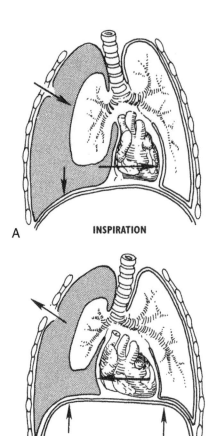

• **Fig. 16.1** Sucking chest wound. (A) Inspiration. (B) Expiration. (From Marx JA et al. *Emergency Medicine: Concepts and Clinical Practice.* 7th ed. Philadelphia, PA: Mosby; 2010.

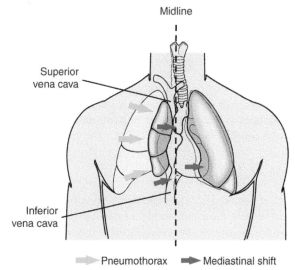

• **Fig. 16.2** Tension pneumothorax. (From Sole ML, Klein D, Moseley M. *Introduction to Critical Care Nursing,* 4th ed. Philadelphia, PA: Saunders; 2004.)

to such a degree that it applies pressure to the heart, great vessels, and opposite lung and displaces the trachea and mediastinum. The pressure increases to a point at which it precipitates circulatory collapse and subsequent cardiac arrest.

Assessment

Severe respiratory distress, tachypnea, tachycardia, hypotension, hyperresonance of the affected side, absent breath sounds on the injured side, chest pain, distended neck veins (may be flat in severely hypovolemic patients), increased pulmonary inspiratory pressure (PIP), tracheal deviation, and cyanosis are all signs and symptoms of tension pneumothorax. These patients, if conscious, may be agitated and anxious.

Interventions

This is a critical situation for which the life-saving intervention is rapid decompression of the pleural space. A large-bore needle (such as a 14-gauge or 16-gauge 2-inch needle) should be placed in the second intercostal space, midclavicular line on the affected side or lateral midaxillary line at the fourth or fifth intercostal space. The needle should be placed superior to the rib margin to avoid the intercostal artery. A "rush" of air may be present on insertion. If done in air transport, the rush of air may not be heard; instead, improvement in the patient's symptoms and a return to hemodynamic stability should be seen.[4] A 2016 study by Laan et al. found that the lateral midaxillary approach for a needle decompression has the lowest predicted failure rate of needle decompression effectiveness in multiple populations.[4] If the tension pneumothorax reoccurs, a simple thoracostomy (finger thoracostomy) may be warranted. The procedure is the only way to know for sure you got into the thorax and relieved the tension physiology.

As soon as possible, a tube thoracostomy must be performed. This is considered definitive care. Large-bore intravenous (IV)/intraosseous access should be initiated as soon as possible to provide fluids and/or blood for resuscitation.

Continuous Assessment and Evaluation

Constant reevaluation of the patient's cardiopulmonary status is warranted. If the chest tube is placed and a persistent air leak occurs, the presence of tracheobronchial disruption must be considered.

Massive Hemothorax

Blunt or penetrating injury causes bleeding into the pleural space. This is most commonly caused by rib fractures or parenchymal injuries, or venous injuries. Bleeding from arterial injuries is less common. The rapid and massive accumulation of blood and fluid in the pleural space can result in severe hemodynamic compromise.

The compliant lung offers very little resistance to large amounts of blood in the pleural space and hypovolemic shock results (Fig. 16.3).

Assessment

Dyspnea, tachypnea, chest pain, signs of shock, tracheal deviation, decreased breath sounds to the injured side (blood does not conduct sound), and dullness to percussion

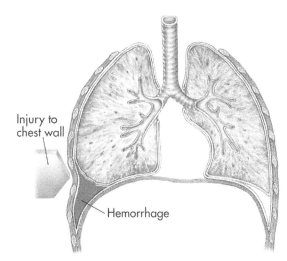

• **Fig. 16.3** Hemothorax. (From Seidel HM. *Mosby's Guide to Physical Examination,* 7th ed. St. Louis, MO: Mosby; 2011.)

are signs and symptoms of a massive hemothorax. Neck veins are typically flat because of hypovolemia. In transport, ultrasound can readily detect hemothorax.

Interventions

Most hemothoraces simply need drainage with a chest tube. First, secure the airway if needed. Large-bore IV lines should be initiated for fluid resuscitation with warm fluids. Fluids should be carefully monitored. Excessive fluids in the presence of thoracic trauma can lead to hypoxemia, especially in the presence of concurrent pulmonary contusions. Blood should be initiated as soon as possible if warranted. The recent introduction of tranexamic acid (TXA) therapy should be initiated. Chest tube drainage greater than 200 ml/h for 4 to 5 hours should have the chest tube clamped. Reexpansion pulmonary edema is a rare complication resulting from rapid emptying of air or liquid from the pleural cavity. Although this is infrequent, mortality may occur in up to 20% of cases and is attributed to the abrupt reduction in pleural pressure, especially as a result of extensive pneumothorax drainage or when there is long-term pulmonary collapse.[5] Continued output will require surgical intervention, such as a thoracotomy, which is based on initial chest tube drainage, hemodynamic status, and rate of ongoing blood loss. Surgery is usually likely for outputs of more than 1500 ml or 200 ml/h for 4 to 5 hours.

Continuous Assessment and Evaluation

Constant monitoring of ventilator, hemodynamic, and neurologic status is critical. Constant update to the receiving facility also is critical so resources can be made available on arrival of the patient.

Flail Chest

Flail chest is usually caused by blunt trauma. Multiple rib fractures and flail segments can cause instability in the chest wall. Flail chest usually involves the anterolateral chest because of heavy posterior muscles and because the scapula protects the posterior chest wall. Paradoxical chest movement interferes with the normal function of the thoracic cage, causing inadequate gas exchange. The instability of the chest wall and pain from rib fractures lead to hypoventilation and subsequent hypoxemia. The possibility of an underlying pulmonary contusion further contributes to hypoxia.

Assessment

Observation of the chest wall excursion is important. Taking a second to watch respirations at the foot of the bed of the patient will pick up most flail chests, because the flail segment will move in the opposite direction from the rest of the thoracic cage. The patient will have respiratory distress, cyanosis, grunting, and use of accessory muscles. The patient will be in pain, so judicious use of pain-relieving medications is warranted.

Interventions

The first intervention is airway management, if needed. Severe hypoxemia may be present, and advanced airway management is highly suggested. Oxygen, IV access, and pain management are warranted. Stabilization of the affected side is accomplished with a gauze pad. No sandbags or IV fluids bags are needed.

Evaluation

Constant monitoring of the cardiopulmonary status is required. Pulse oximetry and EtCO$_2$ will assist in ventilator management. Pain control should be considered for patient comfort (Fig. 16.4).

Cardiac Tamponade

Cardiac tamponade is the result of an accumulation of blood in the pericardial sac from a medical condition or a blunt or penetrating trauma. The collection of blood within the thick, fibrous pericardial sac causes pressure against the heart, decreasing function and cardiac output.

Assessment

The patient with acute cardiac tamponade shows signs of decreased cardiac output, such as altered mental status, cool clammy skin, tachycardia, and falling blood pressure. Beck's triad consisting of narrowed pulse pressure, jugular venous distention (JVD), and muffled heart sounds may be present. However, if the patient is severely hypovolemic, JVD may not be present. Decreased voltage of electrocardiogram (ECG) complexes may be present. Fluid will be identified in pericardial sac with ultrasound (Fig. 16.5).

Interventions

Aggressive IV fluid management is used to keep systolic blood pressure at 90 to 100. This is to ensure the volume inside the ventricles does not overcome the fluid accumulated in the pericardial space. An emergent pericardiocentesis may be required. The catheter, preferably a 18G, 7 to 9 cm or bariatric 12 cm, is introduced through the left xiphocostal angle. The needle is at a 15- to 30-degree angle with the abdominal wall. The needle should be aimed toward the left shoulder and be advanced slowly while continuously aspirating. If no fluid is aspirated, the needle should be withdrawn promptly

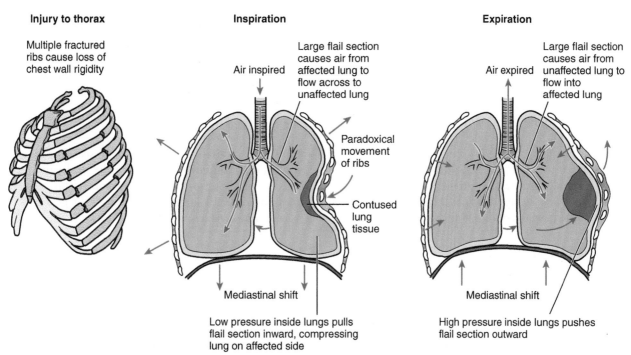

| Injury to thorax | Inspiration | Expiration |

Multiple fractured ribs cause loss of chest wall rigidity

Air inspired

Large flail section causes air from affected lung to flow across to unaffected lung

Paradoxical movement of ribs

Contused lung tissue

Mediastinal shift

Low pressure inside lungs pulls flail section inward, compressing lung on affected side

Air expired

Large flail section causes air from unaffected lung to flow into affected lung

Mediastinal shift

High pressure inside lungs pushes flail section outward

• **Fig. 16.4** Flail chest. **(A)** Normal lungs. **(B)** Flail chest on inspiration. **(C)** Flail chest on expiration. (Modified from Aehlert B. *Mosby's Comprehensive Pediatric Emergency Care,* 2nd ed. St. Louis, MO: Mosby; 2007.)

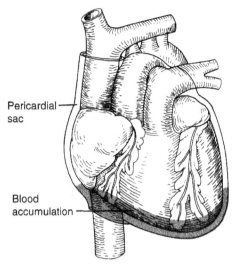

• **Fig. 16.5** Cardiac tamponade. (From Sheehy SB. *Emergency Nursing: Principles and Practice*. 4th ed. St. Louis, MO: Mosby; 1992.)

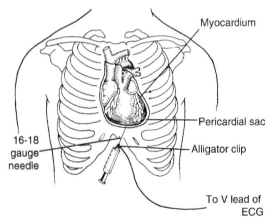

• **Fig. 16.6** Pericardiocentesis. (From Sheehy SB. *Emergency Nursing: Principles and Practice*. 4th ed. St. Louis, MO: Mosby; 1992.)

and redirected. A needle is placed into the pericardial sac to aspirate blood. Improvement in the patient's condition usually follows with improved function of heart and cardiac output. Ultrasound guidance has made pericardiocentesis even more successful (Fig. 16.6).

Evaluation

Aggressive management and continued monitoring of hemodynamics guide therapy. It is possible pericardiocentesis may have to be repeated during long transports.

Myocardial Contusion

Direct or indirect blunt trauma to the myocardium cause hemorrhage and inflammatory changes within cardiac tissue. These lesions may vary in size from small areas to large contusions and necrosis of the myocardium. One can think of myocardial contusions as an acute myocardial infarction (MI) from a traumatic origin. Signs and symptoms are very similar.

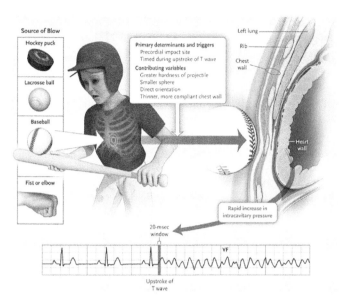

• **Fig. 16.7** Myocardial contusion. (From Contaragyris C, Peytel E. Sudden death caused by a less lethal weapon chest-wall injury (Commotio cordis). *Anaesthesia Critical Care & Pain Medicin.* 2012;31:5.)

Assessment

If the patient has had a direct blow to the chest, he or she may have chest pain, hypotension, tachycardia, dysrhythmias, changes in heart tones, rales from pulmonary edema, heart failure, and cardiogenic shock. There may be ST segment changes on ECG. On ultrasound there may be wall motion abnormalities (Fig. 16.7).

Interventions

Management is similar to that for an acute MI—oxygen and IV access. Follow advanced cardiac life support protocol for acute coronary syndrome/ST elevation MI and dysrhythmias. Administer judicious IV fluids and inotrope administration if needed. Give diuretics if in heart failure, with severe pulmonary edema, or for prolonged transport times. Use nitroglycerin for afterload reduction if there are signs and symptoms of heart failure or pulmonary edema.

Aortic Disruption

Rupture, laceration, transection, or dissection of the aorta lead to extravasation of blood into the mediastinum. This can be from blunt or penetrating trauma. This is the most common cause of immediate death and is generally from falls or motor vehicle accidents (MVAs).

Assessment

The patient may not exhibit any signs of external trauma. Hypotension, decreased level of consciousness, hypertension of the upper extremities, decreased quality of femoral pulses compared with upper extremities, parascapular/upper back pain, chest pain, left apical cap due to pleural blood above apex of the left lung, and large hemothorax with widened mediastinum are all symptoms of aortic disruption. Fracture of the first rib and deviation of the trachea to the right indicate a high suspicion for aortic disruption.

Interventions

Secure the airway, and insert two large-bore IV lines for fluid and/or blood administration. Do not over fluid resuscitate. Keep low normal blood pressure less than 120 systolic. Keep the heart rate below 100 after adequate resuscitation. Consider a short-acting antihypertensive. Insert a chest tube for hemothorax and consider TXA. Facilitate rapid transport to appropriate trauma center.

Tracheobronchial Injuries

Tracheobronchial disruptions are infrequent, but a life-threatening percentage of blunt thoracic chest trauma injuries are most likely in the cervical trachea area.[6] Injury to the trachea or large airways causes rupture or perforation. Blunt ruptures or tears of the lower trachea or mainstem bronchus are generally caused by a dashboard, steering wheel, or clothesline injuries. Penetrating injuries are rare and usually occur in the proximal trachea.

Assessment

Dyspnea, subcutaneous emphysema with blunt trauma and fluctuating in size with penetrating tracheobronchial injuries, hoarseness, recurrent pneumothorax, pneumomediastinum, decreased or absent breath sounds, and a continuous air leak with chest tube drainage are all signs of tracheobronchial injuries. Hemoptysis may not be present, but it is not a reliable finding.[6]

Interventions

Avoid intubation if possible. If intubation is needed, fiberoptic bronchoscopy maybe helpful. It is desirable to go lower than the injury. At times, one-lung ventilation may be necessary. The patient will need surgical repair for large tears or if clinically unstable.

Esophageal Injuries

Blunt trauma injury to the esophagus is rare, but if it does occur, it is usually caused by a direct blow against a hyperextended neck. Both blunt and penetrating esophageal injuries have a high mortality and morbidity. Gastric contents and bacteria leaking into the mediastinum can lead to mediastinitis and to sepsis. Perforation also results in massive fluid loss and possibly hypovolemic shock.

Assessment

Hematemesis, dysphagia, upper abdominal pain, subcutaneous emphysema, mediastinal air, bloody nasogastric (NG) drainage, and particulate matter in a chest tube may be seen. Saliva exiting through penetrating esophageal injuries assists in the diagnosis.

Interventions

Advanced airway management, nothing by mouth (NPO), NG tube, antiemetics, IV fluids, antibiotics, and possible chest tube placement may be used if gastric contents are in the pleura. These patients usually require surgical repair of the defect.

Diaphragmatic Injury

Blunt or penetrating trauma can cause a traumatic defect in the diaphragm. The diaphragm separates the thoracic and abdominal cavities and is responsible for changes in intrathoracic pressures that cause respiration. Herniation of abdominal contents into the thoracic cavity causes compression of the ipsilateral lung and displacement of the mediastinal structures. Cardiopulmonary insufficiency results, causing significantly reduced respiratory efficiency.

Assessment

The patient may show signs of dysphagia, dyspnea, and abdominal pain. Sharp epigastric pain radiating to the left shoulder (Kehr's sign) also occurs. There may be bowel sounds present in the chest, decreased breath sounds on the affected side, and possibly a scaphoid abdomen caused by loss of abdominal contents into the chest.

Interventions

Interventions include advanced airway management, making the patient NPO, establishing an IV and NG tube for decompression, and eventually surgical repair.

Pulmonary Contusion

Pulmonary contusion occurs from blunt trauma. It is a direct injury to the parenchyma resulting in edema and hemorrhage. Hypoxia is caused by loss of the ability to exchange gases at the cellular level. This is one of the most problematic issues, especially for the long-term patient. These patients can spend weeks on ventilatory support and are complex to manage. Using advanced ventilators is desired in the transport of these patients.

Assessment

These patients usually exhibit dyspnea, tachycardia, hemoptysis, hypoxia, and respiratory insufficiency. They may also have chest pain from chest wall contusions or abrasions. Pulse oximetry and $EtCO_2$ may also be affected with negative readings.

Interventions

Provide advanced airway management and pulmonary toilet as needed. If intubation is needed, expect higher pressures and increased positive end-expiratory pressure. The use of bilevel positive airway pressure and continuous positive airway pressure has shown to be beneficial, especially if the patient is awake and cooperative. Judicial use of IV fluids is recommended. If faced with fluid overload, consider diuretics.

Resuscitative Endovascular Balloon Occlusion

Internal hemorrhage requires rapid recognition and surgical intervention. Aortic occlusion is part of thoracic management and allows for an opportunity for definitive hemorrhage control. Resuscitative endovascular balloon occlusion involves placement of an endovascular balloon in the aorta to control hemorrhage and to augment afterload in traumatic arrest and hemorrhagic shock states. The London Air Ambulance services were the first in the world to perform the procedure in 2014. It is similar to open cross-clamping of the aorta during emergency thoracotomy in the emergency department or operating room. The procedure has not been used in the United States prehospital world (Fig. 16.8).

Abdominal Trauma

The mechanism of abdominal injury is the same as that of thoracic trauma. Abdominal injury is the most frequent cause of potentially preventable death. The abdominal cavity can hold large amounts of blood and may or may not be distended. Blunt trauma results from compression after being crushed between solid objects such as a steering wheel and vertebrae or a shearing force causing a tear or rupture at points of attachment of involved organs. Penetrating trauma can be caused from stab wounds, GSWs, or foreign objects. A far more common mechanism of injury (MOI) is now blast injuries from explosions. The military has experienced this MOI for years, and now it is seen in incidents such as the Boston Marathon bombing. Abdominal trauma is subtle, and signs and symptoms are difficult to detect. Classic signs of injury include decreased bowel sounds (blood and fluid are poor conductors of sound) and pain or guarding on assessment over the specific injured area. Organ injuries are associated with location and MOI. In recent years the use of ultrasound has enhanced detection of abdominal injuries. The most recent ultrasound machine is much more compact and lightweight than its predecessors. A focused assessment with sonography examination, or FAST, on patients, especially the unconscious patient, can reveal critical data influencing aggressive management and care. Another advantage of ultrasound is to assist with the location and cannulation of venous access in the compromised patient.[7-9]

Patients with abdominal injuries can have symptoms that vary from altered mental status and tachycardia to shock and a distended abdomen. Any patient with profound shock without obvious cause should be suspected of having a significant intraabdominal injury, and aggressive management should be instituted. Securing the airway with spinal precautions and providing ventilator support, wound management, IV access, fluids, and rapid transport to definitive care remains critical to optimal outcome.

Specific Abdominal Injuries

Diaphragm

The diaphragm separates the thoracic cavity from the abdominal cavity. It is one of the strongest muscles in the human

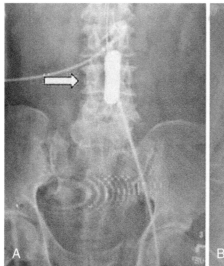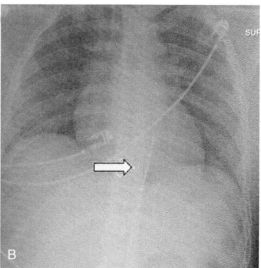

• **Fig. 16.8** Resuscitative endovascular balloon occlusion (REBOA) with saline and contrast, **(A)** with saline only, **(B)** in pelvic trauma. (From Brenner ML, Moore LJ, DuBose JJ, et al. A clinical series of resuscitative endovascular balloon occlusion of the aorta for hemmorhage control and resuscitation. *J Trauma Acute Care Surg.* 2013; 75(3):506-511.)

body. Typically blunt trauma exerts tremendous force on the diaphragm, resulting in rupture. These tears or ruptures are usually on the left side because the spleen is smaller than the liver and is less protected. Herniation of bowel contents into the thoracic cavity can cause respiratory compromise. Intestinal strangulation may also develop.[2,7]

The transport team may have difficulty in diagnosing a diaphragmatic tear. On chest x-ray there may only be an irregularity in the level of the diaphragm. If abdominal contents have migrated into the thoracic cavity, there may be absent breath sounds on the effected side or bowel sounds may be heard if the abdominal contents are present. Respiratory distress is common with herniation because of decreased tidal volume and pain.

Treatment for a suspected diaphragmatic tear with possible herniation should focus on airway management, oxygenation, and ventilation because of decreased tidal volume. As in any patient with respiratory failure, rapid intervention of intubation and ventilation should be executed. All patients that are intubated should have an NG tube placed. This will decrease gastric dilatation and the possibility of aspiration.

Spleen

The spleen is the most commonly injured organ from blunt (25%) and penetrating (7%) trauma. Forty percent of all spleen injuries have no symptoms. They may exhibit Kehr's sign or referred shoulder pain from left hemidiaphragm irritation.[10-12] Patients may exhibit signs of hemorrhagic shock such as altered mental status, tachycardia, delayed capillary refill, and hypotension. The abdomen may be tender to palpation over the left upper quadrant or may be distended and painful.

Liver

The liver is the largest organ in the abdominal cavity and the second most commonly injured intraabdominal organ in blunt trauma. It is extremely vascular and at any time holds 30% of the cardiac output. Liver injuries are usually from direct trauma to the liver itself causing fractures to the liver tissue. Deceleration forces may avulse vasculature-supplying blood flow to the liver, resulting in significant bleeding.[11] Penetrating trauma to the liver accounts for 37% of injuries and carries a 10% mortality rate. Any penetrating injury below the fourth intercostal space may have directly injured the liver and or spleen.

Assessment

Patients with blunt and penetrating injuries can have symptoms that vary from altered mental status and tachycardia with slight abdominal distention to profound shock and a markedly distended and taut abdomen. A distended abdomen may indicate severe bleeding from either liver and/or spleen. When these patients are assessed, inspection and palpation of the abdomen should be done to locate contusions, abrasions, and pain. Other injuries, such as rib and scapular fractures, are associated with liver trauma. The

amount of force in blunt abdominal injuries and the mechanism of injury and location of wounds in penetrating trauma are important indicators of liver injuries. Ultrasound findings include fluid in Morrison's pouch.

Pancreas and Duodenum

Lying in the retroperitoneal space, the pancreas and duodenum are in close proximity to each other and are typically injured together. The rate of injury is low with less than 3% of all abdominal injuries.[13,14] Complications of infection, fistula formations, gastrointestinal disorders, and pancreatitis contribute to the majority of deaths in these injuries.

Assessment

Symptoms of isolated blunt pancreatic and duodenal injuries may be difficult to observe in the prehospital environment. If duodenal digestive juices and blood are contained within the peritoneal space, the patient may not have any abdominal symptoms. Assessment usually shows tenderness over the area of the pancreas and absence of bowel sounds. The patient may be hemodynamically stable, with symptoms associated only with peritonitis or no symptoms at all. These injuries are difficult to diagnose, but careful history taking can assist in identification. Other possible symptoms include persistent emesis, inability to tolerate oral diet, and increasing amylase.

Treatment

The transport treatment for these patients includes a high index of suspicion for injury when the patient has vague abdominal symptoms after trauma. Treatment includes any procedures necessary for patient stabilization and supportive care for the patient's respiratory and cardiovascular status if the patient remains stable. If duodenal injury is suspected, gastric tube insertion reduces the gastric and duodenal juice infiltration of the peritoneal space. Outlying hospitals may transfer these patients several days after injury when isolated pancreatic and duodenal symptoms occur.

Colon and Small Intestine

Colon and small intestine damage usually occurs more frequently in penetrating than in blunt trauma. In many cases the liver, spleen, and other organs are injured. Ninety percent of colon injuries are caused by penetrating trauma.[2,15,16] The small intestine is the most commonly injured organ in penetrating injuries because of the volume it occupies in the abdomen. Blunt injury to the small intestine occurs with crushing of the bowel against the spinal column. Improper use of seat belts, steering wheel impact, or blunt object applied to the abdomen can produce the crushing effect. If the victim has a transverse bruise across the lower abdomen from a lap belt, rupture of the small intestine should be considered. Bowel evisceration may occur with penetrating trauma or blast injuries. Bowel contents should be covered with sterile saline solution during transfer.

Assessment

A thorough assessment for abdominal trauma should be done for any suspected intestinal injury. It is important to inspect, locate, and identify all wounds from penetrating trauma. Remember that documentation should focus on the location of "holes" and not to classify them as entrance and exit wounds. This should be done by other experts to prevent conflicts in legal findings. For interfacility transports, transport crews may find paper clips covered with tape to identify the location of holes to determine projection. Examination of the back, buttocks, and perineum (small-caliber bullets can bounce and travel anywhere) is essential. Evisceration of bowel may be found with penetrating and blast injuries. The color and size of the protruding bowel should be noted on initial examination.

Symptoms of isolated colon injury are associated with peritoneal irritation from blood and fecal matter. Blood is extremely irritable to the peritoneum. Pain on palpation and guarding may be present on examination. If a peritoneal lavage has been done, there may be fecal matter present. Abdominal radiographs may reveal free air in the peritoneum or a loss of psoas shadow. Symptoms of small bowel injury include tenderness, patient's reluctance to change position, rebound tenderness, and guarding. Radiographic films may reveal free air in the peritoneum or a small bowel ileus.

Treatment

Most injuries of the intestine are associated with more life-threatening injuries, and transport management should be prioritized accordingly. While airway and cardiovascular systems are being stabilized, saline solution dressings should be applied to any eviscerated bowel or dry dressings to open wounds. The amount of blood loss should be noted at the scene. Most complications of bowel injuries occur later in the patient's course of recovery. The major factors related to morbidity and mortality are sepsis, abscess formation, wound infection, and intraabdominal peritonitis.

Gastroesophageal Trauma

Injuries to either the stomach or esophagus are uncommon. Both are well protected within the upper abdominal cavity. The pliability of the stomach does reduce the chances of injury. However, if the stomach is full during blunt trauma, it is more likely to rupture. Most injuries to these structures arise from penetrating trauma. Peritoneal signs will be present on assessment. Gastric tube drainage may be blood tinged or frank blood may be present. Radiologic studies may show free air in the abdomen.

Abdominal Vascular Injuries

Penetrating abdominal wounds account for 90% to 95% of all abdominal vascular injuries.[11] In blunt vascular injuries the mechanism of injury is usually compressive or deceleration forces that result in avulsion of small vessels from larger vessels and intimal tears in the larger vessels. Intimal tears can result in thrombus formation, and avulsions can result in exsanguination. Penetrating injuries result in lacerations of tissues and free bleeding. The major vessels include the aorta and vena cava and the renal, mesenteric, and iliac arteries and veins. Vascular system injuries are a primary cause of death in patients with GSWs and stab wounds to the abdomen. Mortality rates are high even if the patient presents with no signs of shock.

Assessment

Assessment of patients who have a vascular injury to the abdomen may have no active external bleeding but show signs of severe shock. Bleeding can be profuse and not respond to fluid bolus or replacement. With arterial injuries, the femoral pulse may not be present on the affected side. Major venous injuries may produce profound shock, but signs may be delayed up to 30 minutes after injury. Bleeding from these injuries may be controlled with direct pressure to the area or compression.

Treatment

Rapid transport to surgical intervention is key in the survival of abdominal vascular injuries. The use of TXA and blood and blood products in transport has gained momentum because of the experience the military gained while dealing with patients with multiple injuries.

Genitourinary Trauma

Genitourinary trauma includes injuries to the kidneys, bladder, ureters, urethra, and genitalia. Although not usually immediately life-threatening like the injuries previously discussed, these have specific causes for concern for the transport team. Because of the position of the urinary and reproductive organs within the abdominal cavity, a high index of suspicion for trauma to the genitourinary organs should be maintained when regions of the abdomen and/or back are injured.

Renal and Ureter Trauma

Renal trauma is frequently associated with abdominal injury; the kidney is the third most commonly injured abdominal organ. Injuries sustained from blunt mechanisms such as MVAs, falls, contact sports, and assaults account for 70% to 80% of all renal trauma, and 5% of patients with renal trauma may eventually lose renal function.[11,17] Blunt injures sustained from sudden deceleration or acceleration can result in the stretching of the ureters and renal arteries and veins with the weight of the kidneys. Contusions are generally from a direct blow to the flank. Of all renal and ureter blunt traumas, 85% are minor contusions; the remaining 15% consist of vascular injury, deep cortical lacerations, or shattered kidneys.

Penetrating injuries are usually caused by GSWs or stabbings to the back and/or abdomen, with 80% incidence rate of associated injury to other abdominal organs. Low-velocity bullet injuries are more common than high-velocity injuries (79% versus 8%); the damage is typically parenchymal laceration. Often, high-velocity GSW injury results in nephrectomy because the kidney explodes on impact or passage of the bullet. Most renal injuries (80%–85%) are minor and consist of contusions and minor lacerations, and 10% are major and extend into the medulla, collecting system, or both with possible result of extravasation of urine. Vascular injuries occur in 1% to 3% of renal injuries, and retroperitoneal hematoma formation is likely.

Urethral injury, although rare, is generally a result of penetrating trauma such as GSWs or stab wounds. Rapid deceleration injuries may result in avulsion of the ureter from the renal pelvis.

Assessment and Symptoms

During the secondary assessment, any contusions, abrasions, or stab penetrations to the back or flank area should alert the transport team to the possibility of renal trauma. The patient may have flank pain. Kidney damage should always be suspected with GSWs to the abdomen. Hematuria is a marker for both renal and extrarenal abdominal injuries after blunt trauma. All patients with gross hematuria should be evaluated after transfer for both renal and associated abdominal injuries. In addition, patients in shock or with a history of shock and microscopic hematuria after blunt trauma should be suspected of abdominal injuries. Studies show that patients with microscopic hematuria but no shock do not have any major renal injury and are treated conservatively without surgical intervention. Patients should be adequately hydrated to assure clear urine to prevent acute kidney injury (AKI).

Treatment

Because renal injuries are not usually immediately life-threatening, the transport team should give supportive care and identify the patient's risk for kidney injury when other life-threatening injuries are absent. If a urinary catheter is present, the transport team should transport with gravity drainage and monitor urinary output. Ureter injury will probably not be diagnosed until full evaluation is completed in the trauma center; therefore no specific intervention exists in transport. At the receiving center, surgery may be indicated for major kidney injuries, urethral tears, or renal vascular damage. Many of these injuries are managed without surgical intervention.

Bladder and Urethral Trauma

Blunt trauma to the bladder is commonly associated with pelvic fracture (90% of cases). The bladder lies within the pelvic girdle, and bone fragments from the pelvis can penetrate the bladder. This can result from the compressive and/or shearing forces seen in blunt trauma. Rupture occurs with a direct blow to the lower abdomen. A distended or full bladder increases the risk of bladder rupture during blunt trauma. Rupture of the bladder can cause extravasation of urine into the peritoneal cavity. Although urine is sterile, no symptoms may be noticed for several days. Ultrasound may be able to detect bladder rupture, and injury may be identified sooner. Urethral injuries are associated with bladder rupture and pelvic fractures. These injuries occur much more frequently in men than women because of the length of the urethra. The urethra may be torn at the level of the prostate gland by pelvic fractures. Straddle injuries such as horseback riding, bicycle riding, and gymnastics as well as direct penetrating trauma may cause injuries to the lower or more external urethra.

Assessment

Identification of patients at risk is the best way for the transport team to determine bladder and urethral injuries in the field. Subjective symptoms that are common in both bladder and urethral injuries are lower abdominal pain, groin tenderness, and the inability to void. Hematuria is likely in bladder trauma. Shock is usually associated with other visceral or vascular injuries. Blood at the meatus is the single most important sign of urethral injury.

Treatment

Transport treatment of patients with bladder and urethral injuries should emphasize a high index of suspicion for their injuries, and life-threatening injuries should take priority. Urinary catheters should not be inserted when blood is found at the meatus until after a urethrogram has confirmed an intact tract. Further damage can be done with the insertion of a Foley catheter. If transport times are prolonged and a full bladder is suspected, controlled insertion should be accomplished. Autonomic hyperreflexia is a serious complication of prolonged bladder distention. It can cause hypertension, bradycardia, and increased intracranial pressure. The transport team should keep these symptoms in mind when transporting patients diagnosed with urethral tears and inability to void. Transport to trauma centers should be done without delay. Further diagnosis and treatment will be accomplished with retrograde cystography for bladder trauma and retrograde urethrography for urethral injuries (Fig. 16.9).

Genital Trauma

Genital trauma is more common in men than in women. The female reproductive tract is well protected within the pelvis. Injuries to female genitalia are infrequent with either blunt or penetrating trauma. Bone fragments from a pelvic fracture may pierce female reproductive organs. Injuries to the external female perineum from straddle accidents can result in hematoma formation. In men,

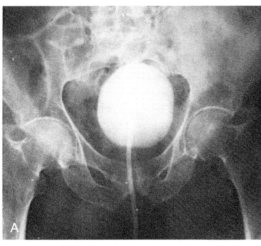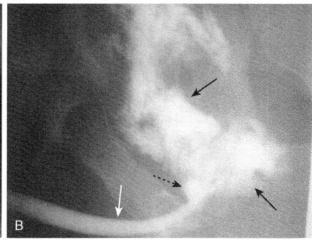

• **Fig. 16.9 (A)** Cyctogram. **(B)** Urethral trauma. Contrast instilled retrograde through the penile urethra *(solid white arrow)* is seen to leak from the posterior urethra secondary to a performation *(dotted black arrow)* and collects outside of the urinary system in the perineum and extraperitoneal bladder spaces *(solid black arrows)*. (A, From Herring, W. *Learning Radiology: Recognizing the Basics*. Philadelphia, PA: Saunders Elsevier; 2012. B, From Ehrlich RA, McCloskey ED, Daley JA. *Patient Care in Radiopgrahy: With an Introduction to Medical Imaging*. St. Louis, MO: Mosby; 2004.

penetrating trauma to the penis and scrotum is caused most often from GSWs. Urethral disruption may accompany these injuries. Other causes of blunt injury are MVA, industrial accidents, and assault. Of scrotal injuries, 50% are caused by blunt trauma, and patients usually have contusions, hematomas, avulsions, laceration, or testicular rupture on examination.

Assessment

Assessment of the patient with genital injury includes a thorough history and visual inspection. Reports of the event can be a source of embarrassment to the patient, so the transport nurse must listen without judgment. Discrepancies between the history and mechanism of injury should be noted and reported. On physical examination, visually inspect the perineal area hematoma formation anywhere on the perineum, scrotum, or penis. If the scrotum is swollen and painful, ruptured testis should be suspected. Rectal injury can be identified when the perineum is examined. The transport nurse should look for any signs of injury and document any lacerations or avulsions, including the presence and amount of any vaginal bleeding. Menstrual history is important for female patients.

Treatment

Unless bleeding is profuse, injuries to the genitals are not immediately life-threatening. Treatment should consist of saline-soaked gauze to the avulsion and lacerations, particularly those to the scrotum. Ice packs to the scrotum and penile hematomas help reduce swelling and pain; direct pressure should be applied to areas of penile injury. In the case of penile or scrotum amputation, the recovered parts should be transported in saline-soaked gauze on ice without direct contact between the ice and tissue.

Vaginal bleeding is difficult to control, and a pressure dressing should be applied if possible. Exsanguination can occur with major vaginal tears because of the rich blood supply. When severe bleeding and shock are present, transport to the nearest center capable of treating gynecologic emergencies should be the first priority. Impaled objects should be left in place and immobilized. The success rate of repair of genital injuries is high, even penile reimplantation has been successful with microvascular surgery.

Bariatric Considerations

Classified at a body mass index greater than 35, the bariatric trauma patient presents some unique characteristics in patient management when the thoracic or abdomen is injured. The chest wall compliance is decreased because of increased abdominal cavity contents, which makes location for insertion of a chest tube challenging. The transport provider may have to insert the chest tube higher than normal to avoid hitting abdominal structures. Because of the declining functional capacity due to size, lung volume is lost in patients who lie flat. Therefore "ramping" or reverse Trendelenburg position is encouraged during preoxygenation and intubation if sitting up is contraindicated. The effects of preoxygenation markedly decrease with obesity. Significant soft tissue injuries may occur because of excessive tissue, and injuries may hide in folds. In the bariatric patient, the ultrasound waves have farther to travel and are attenuated along the way. In resuscitation of the hypotensive episodes, bariatric patients are under resuscitated.[18]

Summary

The transport of the thoracoabdominal trauma patient presents many challenges to the critical care transport team. These injuries can be potentially lethal. The transport team must maintain a high index of suspicion for occult injuries as well as injuries that are obvious on examination. Sources of bleeding in both the thoracic and abdominal cavities may make it difficult to assess just how much blood a patient has lost. The use of blood and TXA and rapid transport to an appropriate trauma center is vital. Early recognition, aggressive management, integration of technology (ultrasound if available), and rapid transport to qualified trauma centers has proven to enhance patient survival and the return as a productive member of society.

CASE STUDY

Impaled Object

The transport team was dispatched to the scene for a 30-year-old male who had fallen approximately 30 feet from the roof of a barn onto a sledgehammer that was standing upright on grass-covered ground. On EMS arrival the patient was awake and talking with labored respirations. His Glasgow Coma Scale was 14. Vitals were blood pressure 110/60, pulse 125, and respirations 30. The patient was immobilized with a C-collar, backboard, and head blocks. Two large-bore IV lines were started and O2 15 L by nonrebreather mask was applied. EMS reported that the sledgehammer had entered the patient's scrotum and had traveled into his abdomen and chest.

On arrival the transport team found the patient to be in severe pain, but answered questions appropriately. He was tachypneic at a respiratory rate of 30. O2 saturation was 95% with an end-tidal CO2 of 24. Blood pressure was 110/60, and pulse was 128. Skin was cool and clammy, and capillary refill was 3 seconds. Trachea was midline. Breath sounds were slightly diminished on the left side. The sledgehammer's handle was thought to be all the way up into the left chest to the left clavicle.

The abdomen showed hypoactive bowel sounds with pain on palpation over both the upper and lower left quadrants. The sledgehammer's handle could be seen underneath the skin and subcutaneous tissue. The entrance of the hammer was just left and inferior to the scrotum. There was minimal bleeding, and it was controlled.

The long bones appeared to be intact with no deformities with good neurovascular function.

The patient continued to speak full sentences and rated his pain to be at 9 on a 1 to 10 scale. He was given fentanyl 75 μg IV, which made significant improvement in his pain. The decision not to intubate the patient was made after the patient's respiratory status improved with pain control. The patient was loaded into the aircraft.

In flight the patient became hypotensive, and a fluid bolus was given. After minimal improvement, a unit of packed red blood cells was initiated and tranexamic acid was given. The patient was transferred to the trauma bay after a 15-minute flight to the nearest trauma center.

Outcome

After evaluation in the trauma bay the patient was taken to the operating room where the sledgehammer was carefully removed. Injuries included ruptured bladder, small bowel laceration, a ruptured diaphragm, and small left pneumothorax. After a 2-day ICU stay, the patient was transferred to the surgical floor with rehabilitation and subsequent discharge. He has had a good recovery, is back working, and is the proud father of two children.

EMS, Emergency medical services; IV, intravenous.

CASE STUDY

Abdominal Evisceration

The transport team was requested to a small community hospital to transport a pipe bomb blast victim. Report was taken en route to the hospital that said an 18-year-old male was making a pipe bomb when it accidently went off in his lap. Both his upper and lower extremities were destroyed, and his abdomen was totally eviscerated. The patient was awake and talking on EMS arrival. The EMS unit started bilateral external jugular IVs, immobilized the cervical spine, and placed him on a backboard. The abdomen was covered with saline-soaked abdominal pads, and immediate transport to the hospital was begun. En route to the hospital, the patient became hypotensive and tachycardic. The patient's mental status deteriorated, but he was arousable on arrival to the ED.

On the transport team's arrival the patient was receiving two units of blood along with normal saline at a wide open rate. The blood pressure was 90/48, heart rate 130, respiratory rate 24, and O2 saturation was 90 on 15 L by nonrebreather mask. Neurologically, the patient was awake but confused. Glasgow Coma Scale was 12. Pupils were 5 to 2, reactive, and brisk.

Trachea was midline with good bilateral breath sounds. There were minor abrasions to the chest wall. The abdomen was eviscerated with bloodstained dressings in place. There were no extremities.

The transport team decided to manage the airway with as little sedation as possible. He was intubated and the airway secured. The O2 saturations improved to 96%. The ED readied four more units of blood for transport. The patient was quickly prepared for transport and covered with warmed blankets to reduce heat loss.

In flight the patient continued to receive blood and fluids for hemodynamic support. The patient required no further sedation after intubation. His systolic blood pressure remained near 100.

On arrival to the trauma bay, a rapid assessment was done. The patient was then taken to the operating room where surgical repair of the abdomen was done. All extremities were lost and close amputation of the remaining tissue was performed. The patient was transferred to the ICU and expired 2 days later. His course was complicated by disseminated intravascular coagulation and adult respiratory distress syndrome.

ED, Emergency department; EMS, emergency medical services, IV, intravenous.

References

1. American College of Surgeons Committee on Trauma. *Thoracic Trauma: Advanced Trauma Life Support for Doctors*. 9th ed. American College of Surgeons: Chicago, IL; 2012.

2. Pollack AN: *Critical Care Transport*, 2nd ed. Burlington, MA: Jones and Bartlett; 2017.

3. Marx JA, Hockberger RS, Walls RM, et al. *Rosen's Emergency Medicine: Concepts and Clinical Practice*. Philadelphia, PA: Mosby/Elsevier; 2010.

4. Laan DV, Vu TD, Thiels CA, et al. Chest wall thickness and decompression failure: a systematic review and meta-analysis comparing anatomic locations in needle thoracostomy. *Injury*. 2016;47(4):797-804.

5. Dias OM, Teixeira LR, Vargas FS. Reexpansion pulmonary edema after therapeutic thoracentesis. *Clinics*. 2010;65(12):1387-1389.

6. Mattox KL, Moore EE, Feliciano DV. *Trauma*. New York: McGraw-Hill Medical; 2013.

7. Gould J, Vedantham S. The role of interventional radiology in trauma. *Semin Intervent Radiol*. 2006;23(3):270-278.

8. Raza M, et al. Non operative management of abdominal trauma—a 10 years review. *World Journal of Emergency Surgery*. 2013;8:14.

9. Como J, et al. Practice management guidelines for selective nonoperative management of penetrating abdominal trauma. *J Trauma*. 2010;68(3):721-733.

10. McQuillan KA, Makic MB, Whalen E. *Trauma Nursing: From Resuscitation through Rehabilitation*. St. Louis, MO: Saunders/Elsevier; 2009.

11. American College of Surgeons. *Advanced Trauma Life Support: Student Course Manual*. Chicago: American College of Surgeons; 2012.

12. Gurney D. *Trauma Nursing Core Course (TNCC): Provider Manual*. Des Plaines, IL: Emergency Nurses Association; 2014.

13. Hardy M, Snaith B. *Musculoskeletal Trauma: A Guide to Assessment and Diagnosis*. Edinburgh: Churchill Livingston; 2011.

14. Smith WR. *Management of Musculoskeletal Injuries In The Trauma Patient*. New York: Springer-Verlag; 2016.

15. Zalstein S, Pearce A, Scott D, Rosenfeld J. Damage control resuscitation: a paradigm shift in the management of haemorrhagic shock. *Emergency Medicine Australasia*. 2008;20(4):291-293.

16. Lamb CM, MacGoey P, Navarro AP, Brooks AJ. Damage control surgery in the era of damage control resuscitation. *Br J Anaesth*. 2014;113(2):242-249.

17. Hughes NT, Burd RS, Teach SL. Damage control resuscitation: permissive hypotension and massive transfusion protocols. *Pediatr Emerg Care*. 2014;30(9):651-656.

18. Uppot RN. Impact of obesity on radiology. *Radiologic Clinics of North America*. 2007;45(2):231-246.

17

Musculoskeletal and Soft Tissue Trauma

ANTHONY BACA

COMPETENCIES

1. Compare and contrast assessment findings consistent with arterial and venous bleeding.
2. Distinguish between compressible and noncompressible bleeding.
3. List hemorrhage control measures to stop compressible bleeding.
4. Demonstrate appropriate assessment steps for the injured extremity.
5. Identify and treat potential complications related to musculoskeletal emergencies.

Soft tissue and orthopedic injuries can be life-threatening, resulting in rapid exsanguination and death; fortunately, most of these types of injures are not life-threatening. However, a simple soft tissue injury, fracture, or dislocation can become a devastating injury resulting in severe, permanent disability. Even a moderate sprain, if inadequately treated, can result in an unnecessarily extended disability and can lead to recurrent injuries.

The hands of a pianist, the elbow of a pitcher, and the legs of a dancer are all vital to each of these people. Although soft tissue and musculoskeletal injuries are rarely fatal, they often result in long-term disability that accounts for millions of dollars lost to the economy each year.[1] The first care provided to a patient with a fracture, dislocation, or severe sprain often determines the ultimate results that occur as a consequence of the injury.[1] The transport team can often prevent permanent disability with a prompt temporary measure, such as hemorrhage control, basic wound care, immobilization, or splinting, especially in patients with multiple traumas when more definitive management must be postponed until life-threatening injuries have been taken care of adequately.

Musculoskeletal System and Soft Tissue

A basic understanding of the composition and function of musculoskeletal and soft tissues are essential to proper management of traumatic emergencies and ultimately to the welfare of the patient as a whole. *Soft tissue* structures include tissues that connect, surround, or support the bones and organs of the body, including skin, fascia, blood vessels, nerves, and fat. The term *soft tissue* also encompasses the nonbone tissues of the musculoskeletal system including tendons, ligaments, and muscle. The *musculoskeletal system* is composed of bones, ligaments, muscles, joints, tendons, blood vessels, and nerves. The function of the musculoskeletal system is to allow movement, provide support, and protect internal organs.[1-3]

Various soft tissues have differing functions, but all share a number of commonalities. Soft tissues are innervated with blood supply and nerves and rely on nervous tissue for sensation and direction as well as vasculature for continuous blood supply. As a result, soft tissue disruption results in pain and hemorrhage.

Bone is a living structure with its own neurovascular innervation and capacity to heal. It is a specialized connective tissue with a calcified collagenous intercellular substance and is either cancellous or compact. The calcium content of bone depends on many factors such as parathyroid hormone and estrogen, dietary intake, and stress. An acid-base balance with a slight decrease in pH can cause bone demineralization.[1-3]

Definitions

Orthopedic injuries, or injuries to the axial skeleton, are not typically an emergency but do require urgent care. However, some fractures in isolation can cause life-threatening hemorrhage. Pelvic and femur fractures can result in massive blood loss. Isolated open fractures with significant collateral vessel damage and external hemorrhage can also be life-threatening, and the individual blood loss associated with multiple fractures can culminate in life-threatening hemorrhage. The blood lost associated with fractures can vary based on the location. According to the American College of Surgeons in 2012, rib fractures typically account for 125 mL of blood lost, radial and ulna fractures 250 mL to 500 mL, humerus

500 mL to 750 mL, tibia or fibula 500 mL to 1000 mL, femur 1 L to 2 L, and pelvic fracture greater than 1 L.

Soft tissue and orthopedic injuries associated with underlying organs increase injury burden. For example, rib fractures with underlying pulmonary contusion or liver injury result in a more complex course and higher injury burden than the same rib fractures without underlying injury. Even among extremity injuries, a fracture or dislocation of the knee or elbow can cause permanent damage to nerves and vessels distal to the injury if not taken care of immediately. Table 17.1 lists various orthopedic injuries with possible complications.

A soft tissue *injury* is any injury that results in disruption of soft tissue. Soft tissue injuries can be categorized as open and closed. Examples of closed injuries include contusions, sprains, and strains; and open injuries include lacerations, punctures, abrasions, avulsions, amputations, and burns.

Mechanisms of Injury

Multiple mechanisms may cause injury to the musculoskeletal system or soft tissue, including motor vehicle collisions (one of the most common); falls, particularly to the elderly; sports, such as football and soccer; and routine activities, such as cleaning around the house. Either accelerating or decelerating forces may cause injury to bones or soft tissue. An important point to remember is that when a force is applied to the musculoskeletal system and causes an injury, the surrounding tissue and organs may be injured along with the bones and muscles.[3-5]

TABLE 17.1	Urgent Complications of Orthopedic Injuries
Injury	**Possible Complications**
Clavicle fractures	Brachial plexus compression or damage; pneumothorax or hemothorax
Humerus fractures	Injury to brachial artery or radial nerve
Pelvic fractures	Injury to bladder, urethra, rectum
Distal femoral shaft fractures	Femoral or popliteal vessel injury
Proximal tibia fractures	Compression of the anterior tibial compartment; tibial nerve injury
Clavicular head dislocation	Compression of trachea, subclavian, and carotid arteries
Posterior elbow dislocation	Compression of brachial artery
Posterior hip dislocation	Aseptic necrosis of the femoral head and sciatic nerve damage
Knee dislocation	Compression of the popliteal vessel
Ankle dislocation	Compression of the pedal artery

From Perdue P. Abdominal injuries and dangerous fractures. *RN.* 1981; 44(7):35,84.

Hemorrhage Management

Soft tissue injury management must start with immediate identification of the presence or absence of active bleeding. If active bleeding is present, it must be categorized as life-threatening or non–life-threatening bleeding. Life-threatening bleeding may be the result of bright red pulsatile arterial blood flow, but it can also occur as a result of brisk continuous darker venous bleeding. Early exposure of the patient's entire skin surface is critical to ensure that a source of major bleeding is not missed.

Historically, trauma resuscitation has been taught in a stepwise paradigm with the first focus on airway, then breathing, followed finally by circulation assessment and management (which includes assessment for life-threatening hemorrhage). This classic ABC approach to priority identification and management has changed. More recent opinions advocate a major paradigm shift toward assessment for major hemorrhage before ABC assessment. Reducing the risk of hypothermia is also an important part of resuscitation assessment.

Nearly half the patients that die of major trauma die in the first hour of injury. Of these patients, nearly half die of major hemorrhage. As a critical care transport clinician, it is critical to understand that all major bleeding must be stopped as fast as possible. It also is critical to understand that all major hemorrhages should be categorized as either compressible or noncompressible. This understanding should fundamentally impact resuscitation and transportation priorities. Noncompressible bleeding includes bleeding in the head, thorax, abdomen, retroperitoneum, or pelvis that requires surgical exploration for hemorrhage control. Examples of noncompressible hemorrhage include great vessel injuries, large liver lacerations, and life-threatening bleeding associated with major pelvic fractures. Patients with noncompressible bleeding require urgent transportation to a facility that can perform emergent surgical or endovascular hemorrhage control, and priority should be focused on movement toward surgical intervention. Resuscitative efforts should be aggressive, with a mean arterial pressure (MAP) of 65 or greater, especially with traumatic brain injury involvement. In the severely hypotensive multisystem trauma patient with multiple injuries and lack of complete advanced diagnostic imaging, critical care transport clinicians should assume that at least some element of total blood loss is the result of noncompressible injury.

In contrast, compressible life-threatening bleeding includes any major hemorrhage that occurs in a part of the body in which hemorrhage control can be achieved by direct compression, or by compression of the major vessels proximal to the injury site. Examples of compressible hemorrhage include major vascular injuries to the extremities and scalp. Patients with compressible injury foremost need immediate hemorrhage control. Although compressible hemorrhage patients also need rapid transport to a major trauma center, the rush to transport should not inhibit what the patients need most—aggressive, immediate hemorrhage control. If the focus on patient movement to a trauma center results in substandard hemorrhage control, further resulting in significant blood loss in transport, care is substandard.

Most bleeding can be stopped with a dry sterile dressing and dedicated attention to direct pressure on the bleeding surfaces of the wound. Commercial hemostatic dressings with impregnated chemicals that promote hemostasis may be preferable to simple dry sterile dressings. Commercial hemostatic dressings cost significantly more than regular dry sterile dressings, and there are continuing debates for and against the idea that commercial hemostatic dressings work better than plain dry sterile dressings for severe hemorrhage control. Current Tactical Combat Casualty Care and the American College of Surgeons Hartford Consensus Guidelines advocate for early use of hemostatic dressings in major hemorrhage. Historical recommendations to elevate an injured extremity and/or apply pressure to arterial pressure points in an attempt to control major hemorrhage have been largely abandoned and were thought to be futile. Failure to control compressible major extremity hemorrhage quickly with direct pressure should prompt immediate placement of a commercial tourniquet

In the prehospital environment, the critical care transport team may need to accomplish multiple priorities simultaneously with limited resources. Compressible major bleeding should be managed first with direct pressure if adequate resources are available to ensure undivided continuous direct pressure *in* the wound. Pressure on the surface of the skin while wound edges remain open will do little to stop major bleeding. Similarly, application of bulky dressings to the skin surface, or undedicated direct pressure, which becomes lost because of provider distraction, will have similar ineffective results. If a patient has major extremity hemorrhage, and inadequate personnel are available to dedicate adequate attention to correctly applied direct pressure, a tourniquet should be applied early. Once other priorities are managed (i.e., airway protection, ventilation, movement to transport vehicle), providers may be able to dedicate adequate resources to direct pressure.

When a tourniquet is used, it should be placed proximal to the sight of major bleeding but be mindful of reassessment to ensure there are no injuries under the tourniquet. The tourniquet should be tightened until it completely obliterates the distal pulse. If a single tourniquet is tightened to maximum capability, but distal pulses are still present or bleeding remains uncontrolled, a second tourniquet may be placed proximal to the first tourniquet. Tourniquets applied ineffectively may have a counterproductive effect for those patients who have also suffered a venous injury alongside an arterial injury. Initial application of a tourniquet to a conscious or semiconscious person causes extreme pain from the compression of the tourniquet. It is not uncommon for the patient to resist adequate tightening of the tourniquet. Tourniquet application should not be delayed until the patient is hypotensive or in shock; rather, it should be applied early on recognition of severe hemorrhage. After application, it is critical to reassess tissue distal to the tourniquet frequently for return of pulses or bleeding.

Ongoing resuscitation interventions may raise blood pressure to a point where the tourniquet no longer occludes distal blood flow. In this case the tourniquet may need to be tightened further.

Soft Tissue Wound Management

Local wound care is initiated by assessing the wound for evidence of hemorrhage or debris and the presence of bone ends protruding through the skin. These findings should be noted on the chart, and a dry sterile dressing should be applied. No attempt should be made to pull bones back beneath the skin. Open wounds without active hemorrhage but with significant contamination might require irrigation before dressing. Saline or tap water work equally well. Extensive irrigation, debridement, and exploration should be deferred until arrival at the receiving hospital. Patients with large wounds, especially those that may be tied to an open fracture, should receive early intravenous antibiotics including a first-generation cephalosporin (such as cefazolin 1–2 g) and an aminoglycoside (such as gentamicin 5 mg/kg). Good wound care is as important to a positive outcome as is good splinting. This technique should not be overlooked. Tetanus status should be noted at some point during patient care.

Traumatic Amputations

Complete *traumatic amputations* of extremities occur from time to time from various kinds of trauma, such as motor vehicle collisions, entanglements in farm or industrial machinery, or crushes caused by heavy objects or falls.

If bleeding is not a problem, then a transport clinician should flush the wound with crystalloid solution depending on the local protocols, apply a dry sterile dressing and mild pressure gauze wrap to the extremity, and immobilize and elevate the extremity. As the patient is taken into care, warmed, fluid resuscitated, and wrapped in Mylar or blankets, there is significant potential that vessels that have retracted into the amputation site, or spasmed closed, will reopen and hemorrhage will ensue. Traumatic amputations, specifically those amputations that are located more proximal to a joint, should be monitored closely by a dedicated crew member or have presumptive tourniquets applied proximal to the amputation site before lifting. Special care should be taken to remain vigilant in those transport airframes that have limited access to areas of the lower body if the lower extremities are involved.

The transport team should then flush the amputated part with crystalloid solution, wrap it in saline-moistened gauze (if unavailable, use a clean sheet), and place it in a plastic bag or container. Then, the severed part should be put in another container and cooled with another plastic bag that contains ice. Dry ice should not be used because it increases necrosis. As with any acute vascular injury, the expediency with which the patient and amputated part reach definitive care directly correlates with the success of reimplantation.

The decision of whether a patient is or is not a candidate for reimplantation should only be made by a surgeon capable of performing reimplantation.

Classification of Orthopedic Injuries

When force is applied to a limb, the energy of the impact dissipates to deform supporting structures. An excessive amount of force may damage more than one structure in the line of force.[4] This type of stress to the axial skeleton and its supporting structures can cause various types of injuries, including fractures, dislocations, sprains, tendon injuries, and strains.

Fractures

A *fracture* is defined as any break in the continuity of the bone or cartilage, and it may be either complete or incomplete, depending on the line of fracture through the bone.[4,6] Fractures generally are classified as closed or open. If the skin is unbroken, then the fracture is technically *closed*, regardless of the number of fractures. If the skin is broken, then the fracture is *open*, although it may be simple and minor in nature. Any broken skin in the area of a fracture must be included in the report. An open fracture is more serious because of the risk of infection. Fig. 17.1 illustrates nine different types of fractures as defined by radiographic appearance.

Fractures of the long bone may produce steady, slow bleeding and can result in 750 mL of blood loss from the humerus or tibia and 1500 mL of blood from each femur.[7-8] Ongoing blood loss from open bone ends poses a significant risk to the patient. Open long bone fractures that have been dressed before flight crew arrival or shortly after arrival should be closely monitored during transport. The risks for the development of significant hemorrhage from exposed long bone ends mirror those risks associated with nonbleeding traumatic amputation. As rewarming and fluid resuscitative efforts are undertaken, the patient is at high risk of significant hemorrhage. Wrapping bone ends in hemostatic dressings before bulky dressing application could be considered.

These patients must be watched closely for shock, and the long bone fracture should be immobilized for comfort. Another risk associated with fractures, even uncomplicated ones, is that of fat embolism, which can cause varying degrees of respiratory distress, including respiratory failure. Signs and symptoms of fat embolism are petechial rash, diffuse pulmonary infiltrates, hypoxemia, confusion, fever, tachycardia, and tachypnea. Patients at highest risk of fat embolism are those with long bone fractures of the lower extremity.[5,9,10]

Dislocations

A *dislocation* is the displacement of the normal articulating ends of two or more bones. A *complete dislocation* causes a tearing of the ligaments. A dislocation may also be described as *compound* when the joint is exposed to the outside air. Joints that are frequently dislocated are shoulders, elbows, fingers, hips, and ankles. Less frequently seen are dislocated wrists or knees. A dislocation is referred to as *subluxated* when the displacement is incomplete.

Assessment of an Orthopedic Injury

For adequate assessment data, a good history is important. This information can be obtained by talking to the first respondents on the scene or by reading the medical record. As previously discussed, an injury can often be anticipated by knowing the mechanism of injury and the circumstances under which it was sustained. To document a musculoskeletal assessment, certain orthopedic terms may be used. Box 17.1 lists common orthopedic terms.

Open fractures produce greater blood loss and risk of infection than closed fractures; thus they demand more immediate attention. However, closed fractures also must be carefully monitored.[10] The examination for fractures should be organized by body areas, with observation first for obvious deformities. If conscious, the patient should be asked to try to move each extremity. If a fracture or dislocation exists, movement or attempted movement is almost always painful, or extremely limited with a dislocation. Range of motion, or lack of it, needs to be recorded. The extremities should be palpated proximally to distally, with evaluation for pain, displacement, crepitus, and decreased or absent pulses. The transport team should gently press laterally inward on the iliac crests and also press gently down on the symphysis pubis to assess for increased pain and to determine pelvic stability,[11] and on the sternum and rib cage to determine stability of the ribs.

The classic signs of musculoskeletal trauma include deformity, localized swelling, pain, pallor, diminished or absent pulses, paresthesia, and paresis or paralysis.[7] If the patient is conscious, the transport team can ask about the patient's pain and its location. Peripheral pulses (especially those distal to the fracture site) should be checked bilaterally for presence and quality. Paresthesia should be checked in the conscious patient by touching or pinching the affected extremity and assessing for altered sensation. Always compare patient responses on each side.

Capillary refill should be monitored and skin temperature noted.[5,7,8] Paralysis at the time of the injury or ensuing paralysis on repeated examination may influence the transport location.

Joints above and below the fracture site or point of injury need to be evaluated. Neurovascular status assessments of the affected extremity should be done frequently, but especially before and after transport.

Children need special consideration when evaluating for musculoskeletal injuries. Because their bones are more flexible than those of adults, greater force is often necessary to cause a fracture. Therefore a child who has sustained even minor rib fractures must be assumed to have sustained serious internal injuries. The transport team should suspect

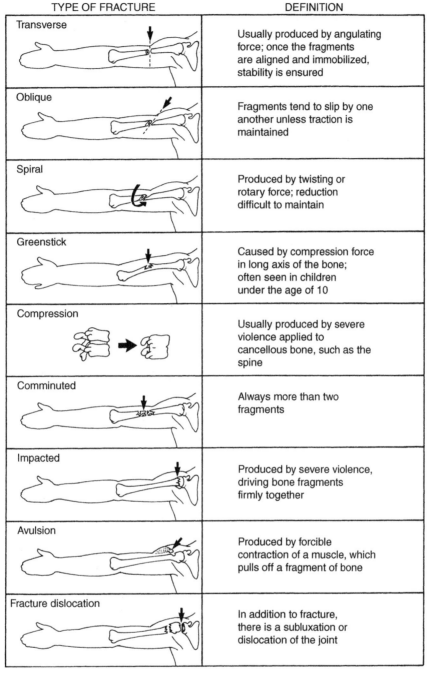

TYPE OF FRACTURE	DEFINITION
Transverse	Usually produced by angulating force; once the fragments are aligned and immobilized, stability is ensured
Oblique	Fragments tend to slip by one another unless traction is maintained
Spiral	Produced by twisting or rotary force; reduction difficult to maintain
Greenstick	Caused by compression force in long axis of the bone; often seen in children under the age of 10
Compression	Usually produced by severe violence applied to cancellous bone, such as the spine
Comminuted	Always more than two fragments
Impacted	Produced by severe violence, driving bone fragments firmly together
Avulsion	Produced by forcible contraction of a muscle, which pulls off a fragment of bone
Fracture dislocation	In addition to fracture, there is a subluxation or dislocation of the joint

• **Fig. 17.1** Fractures according to radiographic appearance.

splenic or diaphragmatic injury in a child with low rib fractures. Injury to the flexible skeleton of the young child may cause different results than in the adult patient.[5,7,8]

Management of Orthopedic Injuries

Improper handling of a patient with an injury to the musculoskeletal system may convert a simple problem into a much more serious one. The closed wound may become an open one, a clean wound may become grossly contaminated, or blood vessels and nerves may be seriously injured. The five basic principles for management of fractures and dislocations are to (1) avoid unnecessary handling; (2) immobilize; (3) apply clean dressings to wounds; (4) control hemorrhage with direct pressure; and (5) check for the "5 Ps" distal to the injury—pain, pulselessness, paresthesia, pallor, and paralysis.[1,5,7,8]

Splinting

Good emergency care rendered to a patient with any type of orthopedic injury decreases hospital stay, speeds recovery, and lessens the chance of serious complications. Because the extent of injury is difficult to assess initially, the best

Abduction: Movement of a body part away from the body's midline.
Adduction: Movement of a body part toward the midline.
Ankylosis: Decreased range of motion caused by stiffening of the joint.
Dorsiflexion: Movement of the hand or foot upward.
Eversion: Movement of the ankle outward.
Extension: Movement of the joint to open it or to maximally increase its angle.
External rotation: Outward rotation.
Flexion: Bending of the joint.
Hyperextension: Extension past neutral.
Internal rotation: Inward rotation.
Inversion: Movement of the ankle inward.
Kyphosis: Round back; increased flexion of the spine.
Lordosis: Sway back; increased hyperextension of the spine.
Plantar flexion: Movement of the foot downward.
Pronation: Movement of the forearm to place the palm downward.
Rotation: Movement of one bone turning on another.
Scoliosis: Lateral curvature of the spine.
Supination: Movement of the forearm to place the palm upward.
Torsion: Twisting of the bone on its axis.
Valgus: Deformity that causes an outward turning of the foot or toe (e.g., genu valgus or knock-kneed).
Varus: Deformity that causes an inward turning of the foot or toe (e.g., genu varus or bowlegged).

method is to assume a fracture is present and immobilize it until further evaluation can be made with radiography.

The primary objective of splinting is to prevent motion of fractured bone fragments or dislocated joints, preventing the following complications[1,5,7,8]:

1. Laceration of the skin by broken bones, which can increase the risk of contamination and infection
2. Damage to local blood vessels, which can cause excessive bleeding into surrounding tissue, ischemia, and even tissue death
3. Restriction of blood flow to an area as a result of pressure of bone ends on blood vessels
4. Damage to nerves by inadvertent excessive traction, contusion, or laceration, which can result in possible permanent loss of sensation and paralysis
5. Damage to muscles, with possible subsequent necrosis, scarring, and permanent disability
6. Increased pain associated with movement of bone ends
7. Hypovolemic shock
8. Delayed union or nonunion of fractured bones or dislocated joints

Some basic principles of management for any type of orthopedic injury must be considered in splint application. These include the following[1,5,7,8]:

1. Visualize the injured area by cutting off all clothing in the surrounding area, which is especially important when the size of the transport vehicle may challenge one's ability to easily see all of the patient during transport.
2. Check and document neurovascular assessment before applying the splint. Marking the location of a palpated

pulse makes consistent evaluation of the injured extremity easier.
3. If an extremity is extremely angulated and a distal pulse cannot be palpated, gentle traction may be applied to attempt to reduce the fracture. A fracture should never be forced.
4. All open wounds should be covered with a dry dressing.
5. A splint should be applied to immobilize the joint above and below the fracture.
6. Padding should be placed in the splint to prevent pressure against bony areas and the risk of additional injury to the skin.
7. Bone ends should never be pushed back into a wound. Bone ends should be padded and covered. Keeping an open fracture clean may assist in decreasing infection.
8. Rapid transport of a patient with an unstable condition may override any attempts to splint fractures.
9. If a possible injury is suspected, then apply a splint.
10. Reassess neurovascular status after the splint has been applied.

The transport team must address certain considerations, including the size of the transport vehicle, the transport vehicle's configuration, and altitude as it relates to the use of splints, when splinting a patient's injuries and preparing the patient for transport.

Soft Splint

A *soft splint* is one that has no inherent rigidity, such as a pillow or a rolled blanket. Both can provide considerable support when wrapped around an injured part and bandaged.

Rigid Splint

A *rigid splint* has inherent rigidity. It is placed along the side, front, or back of the injured extremity, and when used correctly, it immobilizes the fracture. Rigid splints are effective only when they are long enough to allow the entire fractured bone to be immobilized, are padded sufficiently, and are secured firmly to an uninjured part.[6,11]

Many items, such as rolled newspapers or pieces of wood, can be used to make a rigid splint. Whatever is used, however, must be long enough to immobilize the injured area one joint above and below the injured area, be strong enough, and be well padded enough to do the job (Box 17.2).

Traction Splint

Traction splints are also rigid splints. However, they are not used to reduce a fracture but to align it and immobilize the bone to prevent further damage during movement and transportation.[9] The traction splint immobilizes with a steady longitudinal traction pull exerted on the injured extremity. Traction splints should not be used on an injury to an upper extremity because of the danger of further damage

- Expose and examine the injured extremity. Look for a wound, tenting of the skin, or obvious discoloration that may indicate the presence of or potential for an open fracture.
- Support the body part.
- Remove jewelry and constrictive items of clothing.
- Assess and document sensory and circulatory status before immobilization. If no palpable distal pulse is found, medical control may recommend application of gentle traction along the long axis of the extremity (distal to the injury) until the distal pulse is palpable.
- Immobilize the extremity so that the splint includes the joints above and below the fracture or the bones above and below the dislocation. Avoid excessive movement of the body part. (Movement may increase bleeding into the tissue space, increase the risk of fat embolism, or convert a closed fracture to an open fracture.)
- *Note:* Immobilization requires a minimum of two rescuers.
- When applying splints to the hand or foot, leave the fingers or toes exposed to provide for inspection and evaluation of neurovascular status.
- Reevaluate and document sensory and circulatory status after immobilization. If a nerve or pulse deficit develops after splinting, remove the splint and place the extremity in its original position.

From Sanders MJ. *Mosby's Paramedic Textbook.* St. Louis: Mosby; 1994.

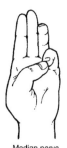 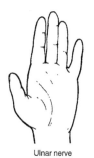 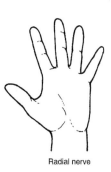

Median nerve Ulnar nerve Radial nerve

• **Fig. 17.2** Testing for neurologic function in the upper extremities.

little gross angulation occurs, and the arm may be splinted with a sling and swathe.[1,7,8]

Fractures of the midshaft of the humerus endanger the radial nerve. The transport team can check for damage to the radial nerve by observing the patient's ability to spread the fingers. If damage has occurred, pain on movement and tenderness at the fracture site is seen. If angulation is present, a transport clinician should use gentle constant traction, apply a sling, and, with traction still held, place a padded board along the outer border of the humerus. A swathe is applied around the sling, the padded board, and the injured arm, binding the arm to the chest. A fracture without angulation may be splinted in the same manner.

Fractures of the elbow endanger the radial, ulnar, and median nerves and the brachial artery. The transport clinician should check for a pulse, movement, and sensation (Fig. 17.2). The fracture should be splinted in the exact position found, with a rigid splint above and below the fracture. If possible, the arm should be bound to the side to offer additional support.

After gentle traction has been applied to any severe angulation of a fracture of the radius or the ulna, a rigid splint should be applied, immobilizing both the elbow and the wrist.

Fractures of the wrist without angulation should be splinted in the same manner as the radius and the ulna. Those fractures with severe angulation, however, should be splinted in the position found.

Severe hand injuries often involve both soft tissue and bone injury. In most cases, the hand should be splinted in the position of function, with the fingers slightly bent and a bulky fluff dressing in the palm of the hand. A rigid splint should also be used to immobilize the wrist.[7,8]

Splinting Dislocations of the Upper Extremities

When a shoulder is dislocated, the normal rounded appearance of the shoulder is flattened. The two basic types of shoulder dislocations are anterior and posterior. Most dislocations are anterior. In the anterior dislocation, the patient holds the arm away from the body, and a bony prominence is seen in the front of the shoulder.[7,8,12]

or impeding circulation. Traction splints are contraindicated with possible fracture of the pelvis, fractured knee, fracture or serious wound to the tibia/fibula, and severe injury in which a wound and loss of bone continuity exists. Examples of traction splints are the Thomas half-ring, the Hare traction splint, Kendrick traction device, and the Sager splint.[9] Traction splints immobilize by pulling on the distal portion of the entire extremity below the fracture. The time necessary to apply a traction splint should be weighed against the need for rapid transport.

Splinting Fractures of the Upper Extremities

Fractures of the clavicle usually occur at the middle and distal thirds of the bone from a blow to the shoulder. Pain, swelling, and deformity are generally evident. Supporting the arm in a sling and binding it against the chest with a swathe sufficiently immobilizes the fracture. However, injuries that occur in motor vehicle collisions may fracture the bone more medially, pushing it into the thoracic outlet and possibly injuring the long subclavian artery or vein or the brachioplexus.[1]

Fractures of the upper end of the humerus may or may not involve the shoulder joint. Pain and tenderness are seen, but severe angulation is less commonly observed. The goal in treatment of humeral fracture is to maintain shoulder function. This goal can best be achieved by treating the problem as a soft tissue injury that happens to involve bone.[9] If gross deformity is found at the fracture site, the arm should be splinted in the position in which it is found with padded boards and pillow splints. In most cases, however,

A pillow splint, and frequently the help of a second person to hold the arm, is used for maximal stability without changing the deformity. With a posterior dislocation, little deformity is evidenced, and the arm is held against the chest or abdomen. A sling and swathe are all that is necessary to maintain position. A rare inferior dislocation (the humerus is dislocated downward from the shoulder) may cause the patient to hold the arm above the head. The transport critical care transport clinician splints it in the position found. These patients should be transported in a sitting position when possible.

A dislocated elbow may appear as a posterior or anterior dislocation. With a posterior dislocation, which is more common, the arm is flexed. A long splint with the flexion maintained should be applied. A sling helps to maintain stability. This patient should also be transported in a sitting position if possible. With an anterior dislocation, the arm is extended and the joint immovable because of pain. Again, the transport team splints the injury in the position found.

A dislocated wrist has an obvious deformity, and a well-padded splint should be used. The index finger is the most commonly dislocated finger, with the deformity being obvious and the fingertip slightly cyanotic and cold. A splint helps to control pain. Immobilization is all that is needed for both injuries.

Splinting Fractures of the Lower Extremities

Fractures of the hip and proximal femur are anatomically divided into two types: fractures of the neck of the femur (transcervical) and fractures through the trochanters (intertrochanteric). Both appear the same clinically, with pain and swelling around the hip, pain on hip motion, and various degrees of shortening and external rotation.[9,12] The fractured hip is best splinted with pillows in the position found. In assessment of a hip injury, associated injuries to the knee and sciatic nerve as well as ipsilateral femoral shaft fractures may be seen.

With fractures of the shaft of the femur, a strong contraction of the gluteus medius muscle occurs, with a tendency to pull the proximal fragment of the femur outward as the adduction causes bowing at the fracture point.[12,13] These fractures should be splinted immediately with a traction splint and kept in the splint until definitive orthopedic care is rendered. Femoral shaft fractures can cause extensive blood loss that can lead to hypovolemic shock, so these patients should be carefully monitored for early signs of shock.

Fractures of the knee should be splinted as they are found, with no attempt made to correct any angulation. Checking for and reporting changes in pulse, movement, and sensation is especially important with any type of knee injury. Fractures of the patella are recognizable as swelling of the anterior knee with little or no resistance to extension of the joint. A transport clinician should splint this kind of fracture with a rigid splint and the patient's knee in extension.

Fractures of the tibia or fibula are managed with a rigid splint. The splint should immobilize both the ankle and knee joints and is best when carried as high as the groin. Great care must be taken with these fractures to prevent penetration of bone ends through the skin because the skin is thinner in this area of the leg.[8,9,13]

Severely angulated fractures of the ankle should be straightened with traction applied to the heel and forefoot. A rigid splint should then be applied to immobilize the foot and ankle. If any question of a sprain or fracture exists, the injury should be splinted until a diagnostic radiograph can be made.

Splinting Dislocations of the Lower Extremities

Differentiating between a dislocated hip and a fractured hip is often impossible, although with a dislocated hip the patient's thigh is sometimes flexed to some extent and turned slightly inward. Treatment for either one is the same. The transport team should splint, with pillows or sheets and blankets, in the position found. Because of the close proximity of the sciatic and femoral nerves, an immediate neurologic assessment of the affected limb is of the utmost importance (Fig. 17.3). A rapid reduction within 8 hours should be done by a physician to minimize avascular necrosis of the femoral head causing destruction of the hip joint.

Dislocations and fractures of the knee are treated the same. Any resistance to attempts to straighten an angulation indicates that it should be splinted in the position found, again paying heed to pulse, movement, and sensation. A rigid splint, preferably a padded board, should be used. All patients with a knee injury should be considered high risk for popliteal artery injury. Distal pulses, skin color, and capillary refill should be checked frequently. The ankle brachial index (ABI) can be measured by obtaining an upper extremity blood pressure, followed by a second blood pressure on the calf of the injured extremity just above the ankle. To determine the ABI, divide the lower extremity systolic blood pressure by the upper extremity systolic blood pressure. An ABI greater than 0.9 has been associated with low risk of popliteal artery injury.

Ankle dislocations rarely occur without associated fractures and should be aligned and splinted exactly the same as ankle fractures. Dislocation of the foot is rare but generally involves more than one joint. It also should be treated the same as a fracture of the foot. Toe dislocations are innately stable and need no splinting.[8]

Whenever possible after splinting a dislocation or a fracture, the transport team should elevate the affected extremity and apply ice to the injured part. This makes the patient more comfortable and can make the splinting of the extremity easier.

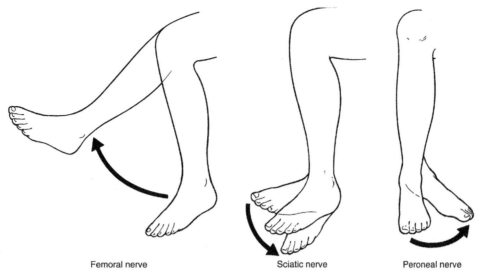

Femoral nerve   Sciatic nerve   Peroneal nerve

• **Fig. 17.3** Testing for neurologic function in the lower extremities.

Pelvic Fractures

A pelvic fracture can be one of the most serious injuries that a patient can sustain. Arterial injuries occur in 20% of patients with pelvic fractures; however, disruption of large venous structures in the pelvis frequently result in fatal hemorrhage. Posterior fractures are more likely than anterior fractures to cause hemorrhage. The major cause of death is hemorrhage from arteries and veins torn by the fracture or dislocation.[1,5,7,8]

The most common form of pelvic fracture results from a severe external force applied directly on the pelvis or from an indirect force transmitted upward along the shaft of the femur. Minor fractures of the pelvis include breaks of individual bones without a break in the continuity of the pelvic ring. These fractures are relatively stable and rarely necessitate hospitalization. Major pelvic fractures are generally fractured in at least two separate places, and a separation of one or both sacroiliac joints may be found. These fractures are commonly seen in patients with multiple traumas.

Approximately 60% of pelvic fractures should be considered major injuries because of the complications of injury to the structures lying within the pelvis.[1,5,7,8] Along with the danger of damage to the major blood vessels within the pelvic girdle, fractures of the pubic ramus may lacerate the urethra, fractures of the brim of the pelvis may disrupt the ureters, and the bladder itself may rupture.[1,5,7,8] Open fractures of the pelvis occur with direct communication between fracture fragments and a laceration of the skin, vagina, or rectum. This uncommon fracture is caused by a high-velocity injury, and subsequent massive hemorrhage occurs with a 50% mortality rate. Even small amounts of blood on vaginal or rectal examination should indicate the possibility of an open fracture.[1,5,7,8]

Control of bleeding is a top priority.[9,11] All patients with an unstable pelvis, and those with a significant mechanism of injury and pelvic pain on palpation, should be immobilized with a commercial pelvic binder. If a commercial binder is not available, critical care transport clinicians can use a sheet to bind the pelvis. The goal of pelvic binding is not so much to "splint" the fracture but to decrease the pelvic ring space, thus creating a smaller space for blood loss. The importance of pelvic binding cannot be overstated, because patients can and do die of pelvic hemorrhage in transport. A diagnosis of a pelvic fracture with hemodynamic instability should be treated aggressively with massive colloid resuscitation known as a massive transfusion protocol. In a large multicenter study, Lustenberger and colleagues found inaccuracies in the detecting of clinically unstable pelvic injuries in a prehospital environment.[14] Therefore, if a patient is hypotensive resistant to resuscitation and severely injured blunt trauma, you must assume a bleeding in the pelvis and apply a binder. Crossing or tying the legs together will also decrease the pelvic ring space by internal rotation. However, the pelvic binder is ideal but do not make the binder too tight; this may cause over reduction.

Fat Embolism

Fat embolism is a complication that may occur with large bone, pelvic, and rib fractures. It is generally not seen until 12 to 72 hours after injury. The transport team may encounter a patient with fat emboli, especially if it is a delayed transport.[7,8]

Clinical signs of fat emboli include respiratory failure, shock, and elevation in serum lipase levels. Thrombocytopenia can also occur, and patients may have multiple petechiae present. A low platelet count (<150,000) may be present also.

Long bone fractures should be appropriately immobilized. Patients should be closely monitored for respiratory distress, especially lack of improved oxygenation despite increasing the amount of FiO_2. If the patient in intubated, positive end-expiratory pressure may be used to maintain an adequate PO$_2$ during transport.[7,8]

Compartment Syndrome

Compartment syndrome develops with increased pressure within the compartment space of an extremity or other area of the body from bleeding, soft tissue swelling, fluid accumulation (such as in a burn injury), or because of external sources such as splinting.[7,8] Fractures, crush injuries, burns, and pit viper snake bites may put a patient at risk for compartment syndrome as well as prolonged compression of an extremity in a splint.

The diagnosis of compartment syndrome does not require advanced imaging or laboratory testing. Suspicion of compartment syndrome must be considered in any patient with extremity trauma and pain out of proportion to the injury. Patients often describe compartment syndrome pain as deep, burning, or unrelenting. Extreme pain with passive movement of the affected extremity is a hallmark symptom of compartment syndrome. Patients may also complain of neurologic symptoms such as paresthesia in the effected extremity. Clinical signs of compartment syndrome include pallor, cool skin, decreased capillary refill, and weak or absent distal pulses. These changes are suggestive of decreased blood flow and are very late signs of compartment syndrome.

If an external dressing or immobilization device contributes to compartment syndrome, then it should be removed. Ideally compartment splint pressure should be measured. If the compartment pressure is greater than 30 mm Hg, or is within 30 mm Hg of the patient's MAP, a fasciotomy may be indicated. Emergency fasciotomy must be done within 4 hours to prevent irreversible damage to muscles and nerves. However, the procedure should not be done without consultation with medical control.[9,13]

Fasciotomy is a sterile surgical procedure requiring in-depth knowledge of surgical anatomy to reach and release all affected compartments.

Summary

In most cases, orthopedic and soft tissue injuries are not life-threatening; however, the long-term outcome for patients who sustain these injuries is greatly influenced by the initial care that they receive. The transport team should approach soft tissue and orthopedic emergencies with these goals in mind: (1) identify life-threatening bleeding and aggressively manage major hemorrhage; (2) minimize the complications associated with fractures, both open and closed; (3) decrease complications of immobility caused by these injuries; (4) facilitate the general management of more definitive care; and (5) help to preserve and restore complete function of the affected extremity.[7,8]

CASE STUDY

Multisystem

A 17-year-old unrestrained female was riding in the front passenger seat of a car with her feet up on the dash. While traveling approximately 55 miles per hour, her brother (the driver of the vehicle), became distracted by a text message, and their vehicle struck the rear of a parked tractor trailer. On arrival, critical care transport team members found the patient on the ground being immobilized to a long spine board. Firefighters reported they just extricated the patient from the vehicle. Patient assessment revealed an approximately 60-kg lethargic teenage female with a pulse of 140, blood pressure of 70/40, respiratory rate of 24, SpO$_2$ of 97%, and an end-tidal CO$_2$ of 24. The patient had no evidence of head, chest, or abdominal injuries. An EFAST ultrasound examination did not reveal evidence of life-threatening thoracic trauma. Subdiaphragmatic examination was also negative for free fluid. Physical assessment revealed pelvic instability on palpation, obvious bilateral closed femur fractures, and an obvious open midshaft fracture of the tibia and fibula. Although extremely weak, distal pulses were palpable in all four extremities.

Critical care transport clinicians quickly assessed the patient and determined she required rapid transport to a Level 1 trauma center for control of major hemorrhage associated with multiple life-threatening fractures. Crew members initiated high-flow oxygen and then wrapped the pelvis with a commercial pelvic binder in an attempt to decrease pelvic bleeding. Because the patient had an unstable pelvis, crew members deferred traction splint placement, instead securing both lower extremities to the spine board. Right lower extremity external bleeding terminated after tourniquet placement. After departure, crew members initiated their program mass transfusion policy administering packed red blood cells and plasma. In transport the patient's level of consciousness improved as her heart rate decreased to 110 and her blood pressure rose to 92/58. On arrival at the trauma center the patient went to the interventional radiology laboratory emergently for pelvic hemorrhage control. Subsequently, she went to the operating room for repair of her pelvic, bilateral femur, tibia, and fibula fractures.

References

1. Smith WR. *Management of Musculoskeletal Injuries in the Trauma Patient.* New York: Springer-Verlag; 2016.
2. Skinner HB, McMahon PJ. *Current Diagnosis & Treatment in Orthopedics.* New York: McGraw-Hill Medical New; 2014.
3. Clarke S, Santy-Tomlinson J. *Orthopaedic and Trauma Nursing: An Evidence-Based Approach to Musculoskeletal Care.* Chichester, UK: Wiley Blackwell; 2014.
4. Hardy M, Snaith B. *Musculoskeletal Trauma: A Guide to Assessment and Diagnosis.* Edinburgh: Churchill Livingstone; 2011.

5. McQuillan KA, Makic MB, Whalen E. *Trauma Nursing: From Resuscitation Through Rehabilitation.* St. Louis, MO: Saunders/Elsevier; 2009.

6. Sanders MJ, Lewis LM, Quick G, McKenna K. *Mosby's Paramedic Textbook.* St. Louis, MO: Elsevier/Mosby Jems; 2012.

7. Mattox KL, Moore EE, Feliciano DV. *Trauma.* New York: McGraw-Hill Medical; 2013.

8. Marx JA, Hockberger RS, Walls RM, et al. *Rosen's Emergency Medicine: Concepts and Clinical Practice.* Philadelphia, PA: Mosby/Elsevier; 2010.

9. Campbell J, ed. *International Trauma Life Support For Prehospital Care Providers.* 6th ed. Upper Saddle River, NJ: Pearson Prentice Hall; 2008.

10. American College of Surgeons. *Advanced Trauma Life Support: Student Course Manual.* Chicago, IL: American College of Surgeons; 2012.

11. Bracey A. *Guidelines for Massive Transfusion.* Bethesda, MD: American Association of Blood Banks; 2005.

12. Andrew NP, ed. *Critical Care Transport.* Sudbury, MA: Jones and Bartlett; 2011.

13. Proehl J, ed. *Emergency Nursing Procedures.* 4th ed. Philadelphia, PA: Saunders/Elsevier; 2009.

14. Lustenberger T et al. The reliability of the pre-hospital physical examination of the pelvis: a retrospective, multicenter study. *World J Surg.* 2016;40(12):3073-3079.

18

Burn Trauma

HEATHER MCLELLAN

COMPETENCIES

1. Identify the pathophysiology of burn wounds.
2. Describe the initial assessment of the patient with burns.
3. Describe the management of the patient with burns during transport.

Etiology and Epidemiology

A *burn wound* is an injury caused by the interaction of an energy form (thermal, chemical, electrical, or radiation) and biologic matter. Most burns are *thermal:* flame burns, scalds, or contacts with hot substances (Fig. 18.1). Frostbite is often included in this category; however, no current statistics are available regarding its incidence rate.

Chemical injuries occur when the source of energy contacted is capable of causing tissue necrosis. Examples of necrosis-causing chemicals include strong acids, which cause coagulation necrosis from protein precipitation, and alkalis, which cause liquefaction necrosis.

Electrical burns occur when contact is made with a high-voltage current. The current itself is not considered to have any thermal properties while traveling through material of low resistance; however, the potential energy of the current is transferred into thermal energy when it meets resistance with biologic tissue and is dispersed throughout that tissue. This action is accomplished primarily by conduction.

Radiation injuries can be caused by both ionizing and nonionizing radiation. Radiation injuries make up a very small percentage of burn injuries.

Nearly 500,000 individuals receive medical treatment for thermal burn injuries in the United States each year.[1] Of these, 40,000 need hospitalization, and 6600 die.[1] The World Health Organization estimates that 265,000 fire-related deaths occurred worldwide in 2014, with most of these in developing countries.[2] The survival rate from major burns has increased significantly and is now up to 96.8%.[1]

Electrical injuries are largely accidental in nature with a minor number of self-inflicted or suspected child abuse circumstances.[1] There are an estimated 3000 admissions for burn-related electrical injuries with a mortality rate of approximately 40%. All ages are affected, and the most common victims are those who work with electricity professionally. The 20- to 50-year-old age group has the greatest electrical injury rate.[1] Injuries occur predominantly in the male population and are caused by work and industrial accidents. There are approximately 300 injuries and an estimated 100 people are killed by lightning each year in the United States.[3] Most lightning injuries occur in the daytime hours of the summer and fall months. The outdoors enthusiast, athlete, camper, farmer, or golfer is more prone to lightning injury because of more frequent exposure to the elements.[3] Newer forms of electrical injuries are those incurred from electrical weapons such as stun guns and Tasers. They deliver a burst of high-voltage energy direct current (DC). Injuries can include cardiac dysrhythmias and electrolyte abnormalities, but such incidence is rare.[3] This incidence increases with coexisting intoxication or preexisting cardiovascular disease.

Pathophysiology of Burn Wounds

The causes of burns may vary, but the local and systemic responses are generally similar. The extent of the injury is influenced by three factors: (1) the intensity of the energy source, (2) the duration of exposure to the energy source, and (3) the conductance of the tissue exposed. The relationship between the duration of exposure to and intensity of the energy source is significant in determining the magnitude of the injury. Increased intensity with increased exposure causes increased amounts of tissue damage. Conductance can be affected by the presence of hair, water content of the tissues, and thickness and pigmentation of the skin. Significant factors that determine severity of electrical injury are (1) voltage and amperage, (2) resistance of internal body structure and tissue, (3) type and pathway of current, and (4) duration and intensity of contact.[4-6]

For a better understanding of the pathophysiology of burn wounds, one must know the anatomy and functions of the skin. Skin is composed of two layers: the epidermis and the dermis. The *epidermis,* the outer layer, consists of the basement layer of cells that migrate upward to become surface keratin. The inner layer, the *dermis,* consists of collagen and elastic fibers and contains hair follicles, sweat and sebaceous glands, nerve endings, and blood vessels. Beneath

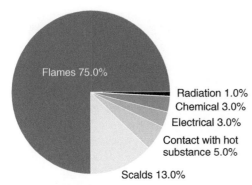

• **Fig. 18.1** Causes of burn injuries.

the cutaneous layers is a layer of subcutaneous tissue that consists primarily of connective tissue and fat deposits; this layer overlies muscle and bone.

The primary functions of skin include (1) the regulation of body temperature through dilation and constriction of the dermal and subcuticular vessels in response to environmental temperature, (2) protection against injury and bacterial invasion, (3) prevention of body fluid loss, and (4) sensory contact with the environment. A burn injury interrupts and compromises these functions.

Thermal Burn Injury

Responses of the body to thermal injury consist of varying degrees of tissue damage, cellular impairment, and fluid shifts. Locally, a brief initial decrease in blood flow to the area occurs, followed by a marked increase in arteriolar vasodilation. Release of toxic mediators of inflammation is activated with the burn, creating a complex circulatory dysfunction. These mediators include histamine, serotonin, kinins, oxygen free radicals, prostaglandins, thromboxanes, and interleukins. Although inflammatory activity is a necessary part of the healing process, excess production of mediators, especially oxidants and proteases, causes more capillary endothelial and skin cell damage.[4-6] This increases capillary permeability, particularly once the burned area reaches a size that is approximately 30% of the body surface area (BSA), which causes intravascular fluid loss and wound edema.

Hypoproteinemia that results from the increase in capillary permeability aggravates edema in the nonburned tissue. Myocardial contractility is thought to be decreased because of a release of tumor necrosis factor-α. Insensible fluid loss from the burn wound increases the basal metabolic rate and, along with fluid shift, leads to hypovolemia, hypotension, and inadequate end organ perfusion.[4-7]

The decrease in circulating plasma causes hemoconcentration of hematocrit, which in turn can cause hemoglobinuria when the hemoglobin is filtered through the kidneys and can contribute to renal failure. Increased peripheral vascular resistance leads to a decrease in venous return to the heart, decreased cardiac output, impaired tissue perfusion, and a decrease in renal perfusion, which can also contribute to renal failure.[4-6]

A decrease in splanchnic blood flow occurs, which increases the occurrence of mucosal hemorrhages in the stomach and duodenum. An increased risk of sepsis from bacterial translocation may also be seen as a result of diminished mucosal barrier function in the intestine. Patients with burns on more than 20% of the BSA can also have a dynamic ileus, which can be of special concern for the patient transported by air at high altitudes.

Decreased immune response in both cell-mediated and humoral pathways increases the patient's susceptibility to infection.[6,8] Thus the transport team must take precautions to prevent further injury to the burn victim through exposure to contaminated environments.

Thermal burns and pregnancy should be considered in any female of reproductive age. The outcome of the pregnancy is determined by the extent of the mother's burn injury. Spontaneous abortions can be anticipated with burns greater than or equal to 60% percent of BSA. The incidence rate of preterm labor or spontaneous abortion is reduced with adequate oxygenation, fluid resuscitation, and electrolyte imbalance correction.[1,2]

Electrical Injury

Electrons flowing through the body produce injury by depolarizing muscles and nerves. They can also disrupt electrical rhythms in the brain and heart. Electrical energy is also converted to thermal energy when it meets resistance from tissues. Resistance is described as the degree of hindrance to electron flow. Those tissues that contain the most electrolyte media, nerves, blood vessels, and muscles transmit current most easily because they have the least resistance. Tissues, tendons, and fat are most resistant and do not allow conduction, which causes burning and surrounding deep muscle damage. The intensity of the electrical current that passes through victims shows a direct correlation to the tissue damage produced.[3,9]

Voltage is defined as the force with which the electrical movement occurs. High-voltage injuries (>1000 V) and low-voltage injuries (<1000 V) are both common, and either type can cause death. Large amounts of electrical high voltage cause more significant injury to the patient and result in tissue charring and extensive blistering. The type of current, alternating or direct, can also determine the significance of injury.[4,9] Alternating current (AC) produces a tetanic contraction of muscles that "freezes" the victim to the source. This reaction is not seen with DC; therefore low-voltage AC exposure, such as to a household current of 110 V, can be more dangerous than a low-voltage DC. AC also has a greater potential to cause ventricular fibrillation from tetanic chest muscle contractions (Table 18.1).

The current pathway is critical because it may determine the severity of injury. Current passing through the head and thorax involves the respiratory center or heart and is likely to produce instant death. Current passing from hand to foot may not affect the respiratory center but may damage the heart. From the entry point, the electrical current follows the path of least resistance, causing one or more tracks of

TABLE 18.1	Effects of Amperage by Household Currents (60-Hz Alternating Current)	
mAmps	**Effect**	
1–2	Tingling of skin	
15–20	Muscle tetany: the "let go" current	
50–90	Respiratory arrest (if directed through the medulla)	
90–250	Ventricular fibrillation (if the myocardium is transversed)	

damage. The energy collects at the grounding point, causing significant tissue necrosis, subsequently causing an explosive exit through the skin.[3,10] The mortality rate of hand-to-hand current passage is reported to be 60%, hand-to-foot current passage is 20%, and foot-to-foot current passage is 5%. DC has been noted to leave a discrete exit wound (Fig. 18.2), whereas AC tends to be more explosive (Fig. 18.3).

With electrical injury, flame burns occur as the result of the ignition of clothing or other items by the current. These wounds could be severe when the victim is unconscious and has a long exposure to the flame. The ignition of clothing usually occurs with high-voltage injuries that are greater than 350 to 1000 V. Frequently, high-voltage injuries cause combinations of all types of electrical burns, and determination of the proper course of therapy may become difficult.[3,10]

As electrical current passes through the body, severe dysrhythmia may occur. Ventricular fibrillation is frequently

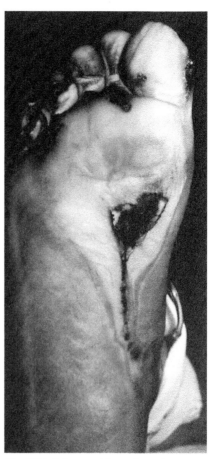

• **Fig. 18.3** Exit wound from alternating current.

induced as a 60-cycle AC passes through the ventricles. DC injuries predominantly result in asystole by depolarizing the entire myocardium. In addition to those fatal rhythms, other dysrhythmias may occur, such as atrial fibrillation, sinus bradycardia, ventricular and atrial ectopy, supraventricular tachycardia, bundle branch block, and first- and second-degree block. Coronary artery spasm, coronary endarteritis, and direct myocardial injury are thought to be the cause of these dysrhythmias. Damage to the myocardium, including myocardial rupture, is also a result of an electrical injury. These injuries are believed to be caused by the heat generated by the current. Myocardial damage manifests itself in the same manner as injury induced by ischemia.[3]

The skull is a common entry point of electrical current; thus the brainstem is often affected, which can lead to respiratory arrest and potential cerebral hemorrhage or edema.[3] Nervous system tissue is an excellent conductor of electrical current, so central nervous system damage is not uncommon. Effects of electrical injury to the central nervous system are manifested by unconsciousness, seizures, disorientation, or amnesia. Other neurologic complications that have been identified are spinal cord injuries, particularly those associated with electrical current traversing a hand-to-hand or head-to-foot course, and local nerve damage with peripheral neuropathies.[3,9] Incomplete spinal cord transection is a common delayed lesion caused by damage

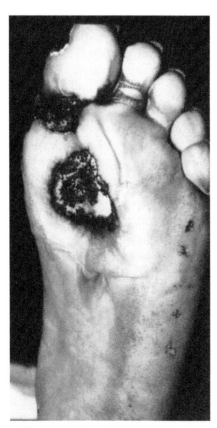

• **Fig. 18.2** Exit wound from direct current.

to the spinal cord by the heat of the electrical current or by blunt trauma from falls or severe tetanic contractions of the muscles surrounding the cord. Headaches, cerebellar dysfunction, optic atrophy, ascending paralysis, and transverse myelitis are neurologic sequelae that are delayed.[3]

Extensive necrosis over vessels resulting from electrical injury may precipitate delayed hemorrhage from large blood vessels. Arterial thrombosis, deep vein thrombosis, and abdominal aortic aneurysms may also result. A major vessel that has been only partially damaged may cause difficulty with homeostasis in open or newly closed wounds. Injuries to the abdominal cavity commonly identified after electrocution are submucosal hemorrhages in the bowel, liver failure, pancreatitis, nausea and vomiting, paralytic ileus, and various forms and degrees of ulcerative disease.[3,9]

Long bone fractures and dislocations and vertebral fractures are caused by the rigorous tetanic muscle contractions that occur. Bilateral scapular fractures have been reported from exposure to a 440-V, 60-cycle current passing briefly through a person's upper extremities. Amputations have also been the result of severe muscle contractions caused by high-voltage electrical injuries.[3,10]

Immediate burns to the eyes, optic atrophy, and the development of cataracts are not uncommon, particularly if the entrance or exit wounds appear on or around the head. Cataracts may develop unilaterally or bilaterally and occur as soon as 4 months or as late as 3 years after the injury.[3]

For the pregnant patient, the hand-to-foot pathway of current invariably passes through the fetus. The amniotic fluid and abundant uteroplacental vascularity have a low resistance to current flow, and the fetus becomes an easy victim of electrical injuries. Regardless of how slight the injury may appear, the mother must be transported to a hospital in which extensive fetal monitoring can be done.

Acute renal failure is a complication that results from direct damage to the kidney by the electrical current or blunt trauma to the kidney or from myoglobinuria. Myoglobin is released as a result of extensive muscle necrosis, and myoglobinuria is proportionate to the amount of muscle damage incurred.[3]

Assessment

The assessment of the patient with burn injuries begins with the ABCDEs of the primary assessment. Burn wounds are often dramatic in appearance and can lure the transport team's attention away from more immediate life-threatening problems.

The subjective assessment includes as thorough a history as circumstances permit. The history should include the mechanism and time of the injury and a description of the surrounding environment, such as injuries incurred in an enclosed space, the presence of noxious chemicals, the possibility of smoke inhalation, and any related trauma. The time of the injury is especially important in the calculation of fluid resuscitation. Information regarding tetanus immunization status should also be obtained with the history.[4]

Thermal Burns

Assessment of a thermal burn includes estimating the burn size and depth, associated inhalation injuries, and calculation of fluid resuscitation needs. The size of a burn wound is most frequently estimated with the rule of nines[3-6] method, which divides the body into multiples of 9% (Fig. 18.4). A more accurate assessment can be made of the burn injury, especially for pediatric patients, with a Lund and Browder chart,[3-6] which takes into account growth changes (Fig. 18.5). For estimating scatter burns, a fairly accurate approximation can be made with the patient's entire palm size to represent 1% of the total BSA and visualization of that palm over the burned area. Use of electronic assessment tools is becoming popular because these tools not only increase the accuracy of assessment but also enhance continuity of care because they are easily transmitted to each level of caregiver.[3,4,5,11]

Primarily, the temperature of the burning agent, the duration of exposure, and the conductance of the tissue involved determine the depth of a thermal burn wound. Initially, the estimation of injury depth is difficult.

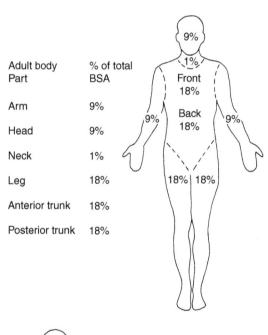

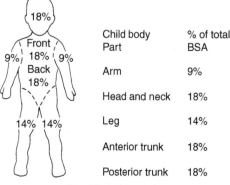

Fig. 18.4 Rule of nines.

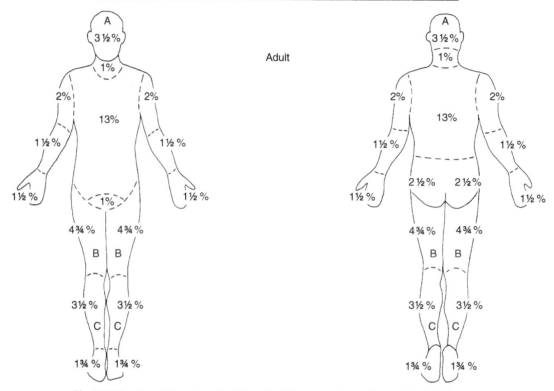

Age	0-1	1-4	5-9	1-14	15
A — ½ of head	9½%	8½%	6½%	5½%	4½%
B — ½ of one thigh	2¾%	3¼%	4%	4¼%	4½%
C — ½ of one thigh	2½%	2½%	2¾%	3%	3¼%

• **Fig. 18.5** Lund and Browder method for calculating percentage of burned body surface area.

Burn wounds typically present in a bull's-eye pattern, with each ring representing a different zone of intensity. A *superficial partial-thickness* injury, formerly known as a first-degree burn, involves the epidermis and is represented by the outermost ring, the zone of hyperemia. This type of injury is usually red in appearance, is painful, and heals in 7 to 21 days.[3-5]

A *deep partial-thickness* injury, formerly known as a second-degree burn, involves both the epidermis and dermis. This burn is seen as the middle ring and is called the zone of stasis, which is potentially viable tissue, despite the heat injury. This wound is characterized by reddened skin that is wet or blistered, is painful, and generally heals in 14 to 21 days. However, these diagnostic signs can be misleading because a full-thickness burn is possible under a blister.[3-5]

Full-thickness injuries are the center ring, called the zone of coagulation. These injuries, formerly known as third-degree injuries, encompass wounds that consist of both dermal layers and extend into the subcutaneous tissue. Subdermal burns destroy both layers of tissue and extend into fat, tendon, muscle, and bone. Full-thickness injuries are charred and leathery in appearance or white and waxy, with thrombosed vessels that are easily visible under the surface.[3-5] They

are painless because of destruction of sensory nerves, with no epithelial growth for healing. These wounds necessitate grafting and scarring frequently produces contractures.

Inhalation Injuries With Thermal Burns

The three types of identifiable inhalation injuries are (1) asphyxiation from carbon monoxide poisoning; (2) supraglottic injury, which is primarily thermal in nature; and (3) infraglottic injury, which is primarily chemical in nature. Inhalation injuries are the primary cause of death at the scene of a burn injury, and they contribute significantly to the overall morbidity and mortality rates of burn patients.[4,6,8,12]

Carbon monoxide intoxication occurs because the affinity for carbon monoxide to hemoglobin is markedly greater than that of oxygen (approximately 12 times greater); therefore the carbon monoxide displaces the oxygen and binds with the available hemoglobin to form carboxyhemoglobin, with resultant hypoxia. The signs and symptoms of carbon monoxide poisoning include pink to cherry-red skin, tachycardia, tachypnea, headache, dizziness, and nausea. Carboxyhemoglobin levels are helpful in determining the management approach for these patients. Levels of 0% to 15% rarely cause symptoms and may be normal, especially for a heavy smoker. Levels of 15% to 40% cause varying amounts of central nervous system disturbances, such as confusion and headache. Levels greater than 40% can cause mental depression and coma. Any patient with suspected carbon monoxide injury should be given 100% oxygen.[4,6,8,12] The treatment of carbon monoxide poisoning is discussed in Chapter 27.

Supraglottic injury should be suspected when facial burns, singed facial hair, or carbonaceous sputum are present. Other signs and symptoms of upper airway injury include the presence of redness or blistering in the posterior pharynx, stridor, wheezing, bronchorrhea, or any other sign of respiratory difficulty. Absence of these signs and symptoms initially does not exclude the possibility of inhalation injury because upper airway edema may not be present until after the onset of fluid resuscitation.

Infraglottic injury is often more difficult to ascertain because the injury is progressive in nature. With the exception of steam, it is caused by the inhalation of the particulate by-products of combustion. It is manifested by an increase in both pulmonary vascular resistance and pulmonary capillary permeability, which causes pulmonary edema. The primary symptom is hypoxemia that is resistant to oxygen therapy. Inhalation injuries are unpredictable in onset. Any patient with suspected inhalation injuries should be closely observed for 24 hours for onset of respiratory complications. Some experts advocate fiber-optic bronchoscopy or xenon ventilation-perfusion scanning to identify inhalation injury early.[4,6,8,12]

Electrical Injuries

If the patient actually becomes part of the circuit, they may incur direct-contact burns. These wounds may appear devastating, and they frequently resemble a crush injury rather than a burn (Fig. 18.6). The most common point of entry is the hand or skull, and the most common exit site is the feet. The sizes of these entrance and exit wounds are no real indicator of the amount of damage done to internal tissue. When the current leaves the body on its course to the ground, arc burns occur.[3,4,9] The arcing current produces extremely high energies, ranging from 3000°C to 20,000°C. Wounds are deeper because the heat intensity is closer to the body. Deep partial-thickness and full-thickness thermal burns may be indistinguishable when the heat source is more distant from the body.

Cutaneous injuries from electrical contact are frequently apparent because the skin is the first point of contact with the electrical current. Dry skin has a greater resistance than wet skin, producing greater generation of heat and subsequently a larger burn. AC produces tetanic contractions of the flexor muscle of the upper extremities, causing the skin layers at the flexed joint to be more closely apposed. As the current path passes through the apposed skin layers, typical arc burns are produced at the wrist, elbow, and antecubital fossa.[3,4,9]

Oral commissure burns are commonly seen in children under the age of 2 years. These burns are typically caused by a child chewing or sucking on a low-tension (110-V) electrical cord. This type of burn is frequently localized but can cause associated injuries to the tongue, palate, and face (Fig. 18.7).

Lightning Injuries

Lightning injuries are dissimilar to those caused by high-voltage contact; therefore the effects and injuries differ. A lightning bolt may have a voltage of up to 1 billion volts and induce currents greater than 200,000 A. Although the intensity of lightning is much greater than high-voltage electricity, the duration of exposure is much shorter, ranging from 1/10 to 1/100 of a second. Because of this lesser duration, skin burns are less severe than those burns seen

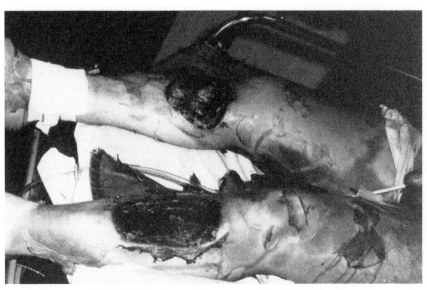

• **Fig. 18.6** Direct-contact burns resembling crush injuries.

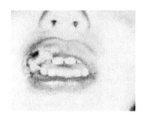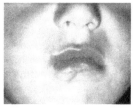

• **Fig. 18.7** Oral commissure burns in a child less than 2 years of age.

with high-voltage injuries.[3] Linear and punctate burns are frequently seen with lightning injuries, and feathering burns are pathognomonic to lightning injuries. With a lightning strike, the electrical current turns moisture on the skin to steam and frequently blows off or shreds clothing or shoes (Fig. 18.8). Blunt trauma is frequently associated with lightning injuries and is caused when the victims are hurled to the ground by the current.[3] A victim may suffer a direct strike from a lightning bolt or may experience a splash

injury. The splash injury occurs when lightning strikes an object and the stroke jumps to another object that acts as a better conductor. This mechanism causes multiple lightning strikes in people standing in close proximity to an object or to another individual who has been struck.

Patients with minor injuries usually are conscious; however, they may have lost consciousness transiently and are frequently confused and amnesic. Patients with moderate lightning injuries show more obvious altered mentation and may be combative or comatose. They may fall or be thrown down forcibly from the current, which may cause fractures and dislocations. Superficial and deep partial-thickness burns may be apparent with a moderate lightning strike injury as well as tympanic membrane rupture caused by the explosive force of the lightning strike. Difficulty in palpating peripheral pulses and a mottled appearance of the patient's lower extremities is caused by arteriospasm and is frequently characteristic with a moderate injury. The condition usually clears in a few hours. Severe lightning injuries can be more dramatic. If the lightning current passes through the brain, the DC or blast effect caused by the strike may damage the brain. The patient is comatose and may possibly be undergoing a seizure. A closed head injury caused by a fall must also be considered in these cases.[3]

Cardiac arrest with ventricular fibrillation should be anticipated. The most common cause of death in lightning injuries is cardiopulmonary arrest. Lightning may cause paralysis to the medullary respiratory center, first causing respiratory arrest and then cardiac arrest. If immediate ventilation does not occur, a subsequent cardiac arrest follows, and brain death occurs from anoxia. Multiple arrhythmias are associated with lightning strikes, including ventricular tachycardia, premature ventricular contractions, and atrial fibrillation. ST changes associated with ischemia are also common. Many ocular injuries have been reported, including detached retina, hyphema, direct thermal burn, corneal lesion, and cataract. As with electrical injuries, cataracts may appear as late as 2 years after the strike, but they are most commonly present in the first few days after the injury. Patients must be assessed for other signs of trauma caused by the impact of the strike and for life-threatening injuries.[3]

For the pregnant victim of a lightning strike, the fetus must be assessed with immediate use of fetal heart tones to determine viability. The prognosis of the unborn child is difficult to determine. Half of such pregnancies go on to normal delivery and produce no recognizable abnormality to the child, whereas the other half results in stillbirths.

Chemical Burn Injuries

Chemical burns differ from thermal burns in that the burning process continues until the agent is inactivated by reaction with the tissues, is neutralized, or is diluted with water. The degree of damage by a chemical agent depends on the concentration and quantity of the agent, its mechanism of action, and the duration of contact. Alkalis cause deeper and more significant wounds than acids.[4,13]

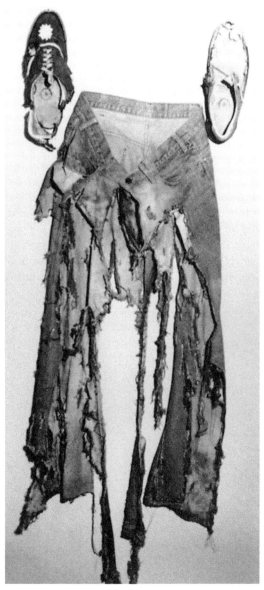

• **Fig. 18.8** Clothing of a patient struck by lightning.

Radiation Burn Injuries

Dealing with radiation burns caused by ionizing radiation is a rare occurrence. Transport after a radiation accident is probably for more critical injuries than for radiation exposure itself.[5]

Management of Burn Injury

Transport of a burn patient requires an orderly prioritized approach. Equipment and supplies should be organized in advance when possible to expedite assessment and stabilization of the burn patient. Although supplies and equipment vary among transport programs, depending on protocols and primary service populations, little is needed beyond the standard emergency medical supplies to provide quality burn care. Sheets and blankets should be carried even in the summertime to prevent hypothermia during transport.

Scene Safety

If transport of the burn patient involves scene response, the safety of all responders must be ensured. Safety precautions may include vigilance for toxic substances with the victim of a chemical burn, extinguishing sources of flame for the thermal burn, or use of special personnel and equipment for removal of electrical lines. Communication with ground personnel regarding the type of scene and landing zone is mandatory before approaching.

Removing the victim from any source of electrical current may place rescuers at risk. Wooden poles, rubber gloves, and ropes are not without risk and should be used only by those trained to work with electricity. The transport team must not assume that a downed wire is not dangerous because it is not producing sparks and because the surrounding areas are dark. Extrication is safe only when the power is turned off. If victims must be removed immediately because of injury, only trained individuals should attempt to do so. Management of the burn patient begins with the ABCDEs of the primary survey, including airway, breathing, and circulation, with a brief baseline neurologic examination. During assessments and interventions for life-threatening problems in the primary survey, the transport team should take precautions to maintain cervical spine immobilization if trauma is suspected. The transport team must be sure that the burning process has been stopped, which may require copious irrigation of the burn wound, as in the case of chemical burns, or simple removal of clothing and jewelry from the patient. The patient must be protected from further injury, and the safety of the transport team members must be ensured. The primary survey should then be performed.

Airway/Breathing/Inhalation Injury Management

Intubation may need to be accomplished early because it could become impossible later with the onset of edema after the initiation of fluid replacement to manage the burned patient's airway. Assessment for dyspnea is more difficult during transport because of the noise and vibration, so the transport team should learn to rely on other parameters for assessment of respiratory status.[4,6,8] Securing an endotracheal tube (ETT) may be difficult because tape, which is most often used, does not adhere to burned skin. Several alternatives are available, such as the use of cotton twill ties or suturing or stapling the tube to the nose or lip. Commercial ETT holders that go around the head may be considered, but caution must be taken to avoid dislodging the tube during transfers.

Inhalation injury is considered one of the most frequent causes of death in burn patients.[6] Management includes careful assessment of the airway and rapid early intervention for signs of obstruction. Early intubation, before massive edema formation, is key for the patient with airway damage. Administration of humidified oxygen helps minimize inspissation of secretions, and frequent suctioning helps remove accumulated secretions. Use of bronchodilators is helpful for minimizing bronchospasm and encouraging mucociliary clearance.[6] Other medications that may be used include N-acetylcysteine alone as a mucolytic agent or in combination with heparin as scavengers for oxygen free radicals that are produced by activation of alveolar macrophages or nitric oxide to decrease pulmonary vasoconstriction.[6] Mechanical ventilation during transport should begin with low tidal volumes and low airway pressures to minimize ventilator-associated lung trauma.[6]

Circulation/Fluid Resuscitation

Two intravenous (IV) lines should be initiated peripherally with large-bore catheters. The fluid of choice for initial resuscitation is variable, but crystalloid is the most common. Ideally, lines should be placed in nonburned areas, but they may be placed through the burn if they are the only veins available for cannulation. IV lines should be sutured in place if any danger of dislodgment exists because venous access may not be available peripherally after the onset of generalized edema. Blood should be obtained for initial laboratory studies when IV lines are initiated if that has not already been done. Intraosseous access can be used for fluid resuscitation when IV access cannot be obtained.

The goal of initial fluid resuscitation is to restore and maintain adequate tissue perfusion and vital organ function, in addition to preserving heat-injured but viable tissue in the zone of stasis.[3-5,7,8,11,14-16] Fluid needs are based on the size of the patient and the extent of the burn. Research on the use of formulas to calculate fluid requirements is varied and should be used as a guideline rather than an end goal.[14]

The two most commonly used formulae for estimating fluid needs are the Parkland formula, which is 4 mL/kg/% total BSA (TBSA) burned and the Modified Brooke, which is 2 mL/kg/% TBSA burned. One-half of the total amount of fluids should be given over the first 8 hours from the time of the injury, with the second half to be given over the following 16 hours.[14,16] Both over- and underresuscitation have negative outcomes for the patient. The current theory of "fluid creep" (fluid administered in excess of predicted amounts) would suggest that patients are frequently being overresuscitated by more than 1.5 times the highest recommended amount of fluid. Use of alternative end points for resuscitation offer more appropriate markers, such as urine output of 0.5 to 1.0 mL/kg/h in adults and 1.0 to 1.5 mL/kg/h in children.[6,14,16]

Some controversy exists over the most appropriate fluid to be used in burn resuscitation. There are proponents of various combinations of hypertonic and isotonic solutions, crystalloid, and colloid. Choice of fluid largely is a matter of local opinion and current research. The transport team must consult with the physician or burn center that is accepting the patient to obtain orders for fluids and fluid resuscitation guidelines.

Emphasis in pediatric fluid resuscitation is shifting to the minimum amount necessary to maintain vital organ function. Estimation of burn size for children has found to be greater by referring hospitals then at burn centers. This has contributed to administration of more fluid at the referring facility.[7] Current research also suggests that children tolerate rapid initial volume infusion, with half the calculated volume given over 4 hours and the remainder given over 20 hours, a formula that differs somewhat from the adult regimen. The goal with pediatric fluid resuscitation is a urine output of 1 to 1.5 mL/kg/h.[14]

Burn Wound Management

Care of the burn wound includes covering the burned area with a dry, clean dressing and, in the case of a large burn wound, placing the patient on one dry, clean sheet and covering with blankets added over the sheets as needed. Wet dressings should not be used because they provide an open pathway for bacteria, cause additional tissue injury, and leave the patient at risk of hypothermia because of loss of skin integrity from the burn injury.[4,6,8,16]

With the exception of escharotomies, open chest wounds, and actively bleeding wounds, wound management in transport consists of simply placing the patient on and covering the patient with clean, dry linen. Wet dressings are contraindicated because of the decreased thermoregulatory capacity of patients with large burns and the possibility of hypothermia. The burn patient should be covered with blankets to avoid hypothermia, and IV fluids should ideally be warmed. Some commercial wound care products are available. These should not be used without consulting a burn center.

Circumferential burns to the chest or extremities represent the more easily recognizable complications in burn care. Circumferential burns to the chest wall decrease chest wall compliance, creating respiratory insufficiency and hypoxia, especially in the pediatric population in which chest walls are more pliable. This problem can be further aggravated by generalized edema.

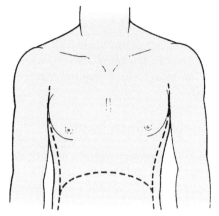

• **Fig. 18.9** Chest escharotomy sites.

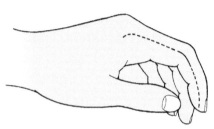

• **Fig. 18.10** Escharotomy site on the finger.

Circumferential burns to the extremities or digits can be equally threatening to the circulatory stability of the affected limb, producing the "5 Ps" that represent the signs and symptoms of an arterial injury: pain, pallor, pulselessness, paresthesia, and paralysis. An ultrasonic Doppler scan device may be helpful in locating pulses in a particularly edematous area.

Escharotomies are the traditional way to deal with compression from circumferential burns (Figs. 18.9 and 18.10). However, because this skill is difficult to teach and maintain, some recommendations are that a decompression technique should be used until a skilled provider is available. Whichever method is used to relieve the compression, it should be performed before transport and should be performed only under the direction of the receiving physician. When bleeding does occur, the appropriate treatment is direct pressure to the wound. The incisions should extend slightly beyond the constricted area for maximal effect. (See Box 18.1 for possible escharotomy sites.) Major vessels, nerves, tendons, ligaments, and joints should be avoided because future range of motion can be adversely affected. Results of the escharotomy should be carefully monitored. In most cases, relief of the constriction should be immediate.

Decompression is a more continual process with use of the least invasive methodology appropriate for the situation, including positioning, fluid management, ongoing clinical assessment, and incisions through eschar and superficial fascia only.[6]

For those burn patients who may not be transported until later in the disease process or those who may need long-distance transport to receive care, some debriding and

• BOX 18.1   Possible Escharotomy Sites

Chest

Anterior axillary incisions bilaterally joined with a transverse incision along the costal margin (Fig. 18.9).

Extremities

Axially on medial or lateral aspect; if a single incision is insufficient to relieve the constriction, then an incision on both sides should be performed.

Elbow

Medial aspect anterior to the medial epicondyle.

Hand

Axially on the dorsum, between the tendons rather than across them.

Fingers

Midlateral axial (Fig. 18.10).

Ankle

Medial aspect anterior to medial malleolus.

Foot

Axially on the dorsum between the tendons rather than across them.

---

dressings may be necessary. Mild soap and water may be used to clean simple burns. Blisters should be managed according to the burn center's wound care protocols.

When cleaning burns that are the result of contact with tar or asphalt, mixtures of cool water and mineral oil have been reported to be useful. The removal of these substances stops the burning process and helps decrease the patient's pain.[4]

Pain Management

Burn pain varies depending on burn injury type and size. Factors that can affect burn pain include actual stimulation of nociceptors, fear of procedures, and anxiety regarding change in body image. Regardless of what types of medications are administered, they should all be given IV. The generalized edema during this time allows for only sporadic absorption of the medication if given intramuscularly. As fluid shifts reverse, a "dumping" and potential overdose of any medications that were given intramuscularly can occur.[14] The exception to this is a tetanus booster, which can be given intramuscularly.

For acute burn injury pain, opioids such as morphine are the analgesic of choice, particularly in conjunction with anxiolytic sedatives, such as benzodiazepines.[14,17] Nonopiod analgesics that have proven effective include medications such as ketamine and dexmedetomidine for short periods for procedures. Adjunctive activity, such as diversion, guided imagery, and relaxation therapy, although of limited use during transport because of the distractions in transport vehicles, may be helpful during patient preparation.[17] For

longer transport times, such as international repatriation, use of virtual reality such as computer games might prove effective in diverting attention.[17]

Antibiotics should be given only at the direction of the receiving burn center.

Other Transport Considerations

Electrocardiographic monitoring should be instituted on any patient with a large burn, an electrical injury, or preexisting heart disease.[4,14] Electrode patches may be a problem to place because the adhesive does not stick to burned skin. If alternate sites for placement cannot be found, an option for monitoring is to insert skin staples such as those used for wound closure and attach the monitor leads to them with alligator clips.

A urinary catheter with a urimeter should be placed to accurately monitor urinary output. As with intubation, the catheter should be inserted early, especially for the patient with perineal burns, because edema may make insertion impossible at a later time.

To combat the problem of adynamic ileus, the transport team should insert a gastric tube in all burn patients with significant burns to decompress the stomach. This process is especially important for the patient being transported at high altitudes. Initial diagnostic studies should include hematocrit and electrolyte levels, urinalysis, chest radiograph, arterial blood gases with carboxyhemoglobin levels as indicated, and electrocardiography.[6,8,16]

Accurate documentation of all treatment provided before and during transport of the burn patient is essential. This information provides the necessary history of the incident and its initial treatment to allow for consistent and quality planning of patient care at the receiving facility.

Electrical Injury Management

As soon as the scene is secured and the patient is away from the current, primary and secondary assessment can proceed. Dysrhythmia should be treated with advanced cardiac life support algorithms or the transport program's individual protocols. Evaluation for cardiac injury is important because of the high incidence of dysrhythmias and autonomic dysfunction with electrical exposure.[3]

Cervical spine injury is of special concern for victims of electrical injury because of possible blunt trauma and because of severe tetanic contractions caused by the electrical current; therefore the cervical and thoracic spine must be immobilized.[3,4]

Initially, a minimum of two large-bore IVs with normal saline or lactated Ringer's solution should be started. Assessment of the area of surface burns is difficult because of the deep injury produced. Adequate volume replacement, treatment of acidosis, and management of myoglobinuria must also be initiated. Fluid volume replacement formulas are not helpful with electrical injuries because of the deep tissue damage seen with the apparently mild cutaneous burns.

Higher rates of urinary output are essential to maintain because hemoglobinuria and myoglobinuria are common with electrical injuries.[3,4] The fluid resuscitation must be based on actual urine flow. A minimum urine output of 100 mL/h should be maintained for adults and 1.5 to 2.0 mL/kg/h for children.[3]

Lactic acidosis is common because of the significant muscle damage caused by electrical injury. Sodium bicarbonate may be used to alkalinize the urine. Mannitol should be considered in the resuscitative phase to increase urinary output and to minimize acute tubular necrosis.[3]

Lightning Injury Management

Primary survey does not differ with the victim of a lightning strike. The patient's cardiopulmonary status must be assessed immediately, and cardiopulmonary resuscitation should be initiated on finding the patient in cardiac arrest. As with any unknown injury, the cervical spine must be immobilized before intubation and transport. The patient's cardiac status must be monitored continuously.

Burns seen with lightning injuries are not as extensive as those seen with high-voltage injuries; therefore massive amounts of fluids are not necessary unless the patient is in hypovolemic shock. Two IV lines should be established: one as a "keep open" line and one as a medication route. Observation and history taking must be performed with care to treat and transport these victims rapidly.[3]

Chemical Injury Management

Treatment of chemical injuries necessitates removal of all saturated clothing and a copious irrigation of the burn wound. In the patient with an otherwise stable condition, wound irrigation takes priority over transportation unless the irrigation can continue en route.[4,14,13] The transport team needs to ensure their safety and avoid placing a contaminated patient in a transport vehicle.

Dry chemicals such as lime should be brushed off before irrigation. Water with low pressure can be used for wound irrigation.[4] The time spent searching for a specific neutralizing agent may be more harmful than simply irrigating with water. The exogenous heat production by neutralization reaction can cause further tissue destruction. In the treatment of chemical burns, the transport team must be aware of the possibility of exposure to the noxious agents and don appropriate protective gear before coming into contact with the patient or the patient's clothing.[4,14,13]

Radiation Injury Management

Radiation burns are treated like other kinds of burns as the initial injuries occur from the heat of the explosion. Victims of radiation injury should initially be treated by those trained in managing hazardous materials. The focus beyond the lifesaving measures is to avoid contaminating the transport team and the transport vehicle and limiting further damage.[18]

Evaluation

Evaluation of the burn patient consists primarily of assessment of the effectiveness of problem intervention and the recognition of future potential complications. Not all complications are, however, predictable or correctable.

Vital signs are not the most accurate method of monitoring a patient with a large burn because of the pathophysiologic changes that accompany such an injury. Blood pressure may be difficult to ascertain because of increasing generalized edema. An invasive monitoring device may not be accurate because of the peripheral vasoconstriction caused by release of vasoactive mediators such as catecholamines. Pulse may be somewhat more helpful in monitoring the appropriateness of fluid resuscitation, as is urine output.[4,6,14,15,19] The presence of more than a mild tachycardia or a persistent tachycardia may be evidence of hypovolemia. However, even this can be confusing because tachycardia may be the result of pain and the stress response. The transport team should be careful not to overlook young, otherwise healthy adults whose normal resting heart rate may be in the 40- to 60-beats/min range or the elderly patient who may be taking medications, such as β-blockers, which interfere with the normal physiologic responses. A heart rate of greater than 70 beats/min may not indicate the underlying volume deficit for this type of patient.

A decrease in level of consciousness not associated with trauma may also be indicative of hypoxia or hypovolemia. This problem should be alleviated with appropriate adjustments in ventilatory and circulatory support. If the level of consciousness does not improve with increased hydration and oxygenation, other problem sources such as carbon monoxide poisoning or electrolyte imbalance should be suspected and investigated.[4,6,14,15,19]

The urinary output in children should be maintained at 1 to 1.5 mL/kg/h for children less than 30 kg. Oliguria is an indication of inadequate fluid volume and should be easily corrected by increasing the rate of fluid administration. When this method is ineffective and fluid volume needs have been accurately assessed and administered, an osmotic diuretic such as mannitol can be given to avoid acute renal failure.

Myoglobinuria that occurs from the release of myoglobin after deep muscle damage can precipitate in the renal tubules and cause acute renal failure. This problem is especially common after electrical burns, and urine should be monitored in such cases for color changes (dark tea color) that indicate the presence of myoglobin. Alkalinization of the urine through the addition of bicarbonate to the IV fluids is done to prevent the myoglobin from progressing to its nephrotoxic metabolites. Diuresis through mannitol or loop diuretics also helps dilute the urine and flush the renal tubules.[4,6]

Pulmonary edema can occur from either overzealous fluid resuscitation or smoke inhalation, and the transport team should be careful to monitor respiratory function as fluid administration progresses. This problem is especially apparent when the transport of the burn patient has been delayed.[6,12]

Acidosis from the increased lactic acid production can occur and be treated with sodium bicarbonate if increased fluid administration is ineffective.[4] Hyperkalemia from potassium released from the heat-damaged tissues can be reversed in several ways, including administration of sodium bicarbonate, glucose and insulin, or ion exchange resins. Hypoglycemia is a complication that frequently occurs with infants and young children because of their inability to maintain adequate glycogen stores. Blood glucose should be assessed frequently for pediatric patients. IV fluids may be changed to lactated Ringer's solution with 5% dextrose if hypoglycemia becomes a problem.[16]

Impact of Transport

For burn patients, two phases of transport usually occur. The first is the entry of the burn patient into the emergency medical services system with transport from the scene of the incident to the initial care facility. The second phase is the interfacility transport of the stabilized patient from the initial care facility to a burn center or tertiary care center.

The increasing use of critical care ground and air medical services has had an impact on both phases of burn transport. In early transport, it has made a higher level of medical expertise more rapidly available to a larger service area, which has decreased the amount of time before assessment and resuscitation begins and enabled the critically injured patient to reach a definitive care facility quickly. In the second phase of transport, it has markedly decreased the amount of time spent out of a stable environment during transfer to a burn center.[2,18] A shift in the admission patterns for burn patients has been seen; increasingly, significant burn injuries are being transported to specialized burn care centers. These changes have had the combined effect of decreasing the morbidity and mortality rates of burn patients.[1,2]

The decision to transport to a burn center is made on the basis of the condition of the patient; the size of the burn; and, in the case of scene response, the distance to the burn center. Patients with concurrent traumatic injuries should first be evaluated at a trauma center if the traumatic injuries present the greatest immediate risk. If the burn injury is the greater risk to the patient and initial burn care can be facilitated en route, then transfer to a burn center may be appropriate. The American Burn Association has identified criteria for the transfer of burn patients to a burn center (Box 18.2).

• BOX 18.2 Burn Unit Referral Criteria

1. Partial-thickness burns greater than 10% of the total body surface area.
2. Burns that involve the face, hands, feet, genitalia, perineum, or major joints.
3. Third-degree burns in any age group.
4. Electrical burns, including lightning injury.
5. Chemical burns.
6. Inhalation injury.
7. Burn injury in patients with preexisting medical disorders that could complicate management, prolong recovery, or affect mortality.
8. Any patients with burns and concomitant trauma (such as fractures) in which the burn injury poses the greatest risk of morbidity or mortality. In such cases, if trauma poses the greater immediate risk, the patient may be stabilized initially in a trauma center before being transferred to a burn unit. Physician judgment is necessary in such situations and should be in concert with the regional medical control plan and triage protocols.
9. Burned children in hospitals without qualified personnel or equipment for the care of children.
10. Burn injury in patients who need special social, emotional, or long-term rehabilitative intervention.

From *American Burn Association: Advanced Burn Life Support Referral Criteria.* Excerpted from Guidelines for the Operation of Burn Centers (pp. 79–86), Resources for Optimal Care of the Injured Patient 2006, Committee on Trauma, American College of Surgeons. <http://www.ameriburn.org/BurnCenterReferral Criteria.pdf>; 2006.

Summary

Burn and electrical injuries can present a major challenge to transport team members, but an orderly, prioritized approach can greatly simplify management. Patients may exhibit a wide spectrum of injuries from minor flesh burns to multiple traumas. Special burns such as chemical and electrical injuries have unique consequences that must be observed early in management. The quality of treatment that the patient initially receives may determine the ultimate level of rehabilitation. A clear understanding of the pathophysiology of burn injuries is essential in providing quality burn care. Assessment and also underlying principles of intervention and resuscitation rely on this knowledge base. Transportation of these patients to an appropriate hospital and early involvement of a burn care specialist are invaluable.

CASE STUDY

The transport team is called to the scene for a 21-year-old male who sustained a burn injury while trying to protect his property from a northern wildfire. He was found by firefighters while they were battling the blaze. He is transported by ground EMS to rendezvous with the flight team for transport to the burn center. Report from EMS is that he has sustained deep partial-thickness burns to approximately 40% of his body. They have initiated one IV and have a liter of NS running wide open. His weight is estimated at 70 kg.

On arrival of the flight team the patient is quickly assessed and found to have supraglottic airway involvement with red, shiny mucous membranes with sooty deposits. Preparations are made for immediate airway management. The patient is orally intubated and the tube secured.

Head-to-toe assessment reveals deep partial-thickness burns to his face, both arms, anterior torso, and right thigh. Their estimate of the burn injury was increased to 54%. He has received 1500 mL of NS. The time of injury is estimated

Continued

at 3 hours prior. A second IV is initiated and fluid is calculated using the Modified Brooke formula: 70 kg × 2 mL × 54% = 7560 mL. The IV rates are adjusted to run at approximately 460 mL/h until urine output can be measured for more accurate monitoring.

No other trauma or injuries are assessed. Cardiac monitoring is initiated, placing the electrodes on nonburned skin. The patient is placed on clean sheets and covered with a thermal blanket and secured to the stretcher. The patient is placed on mechanical ventilation for the transport.

During transport vital signs including oxygen saturation and end-tidal CO_2 are monitored. Report is called to the burn center and he is transported directly to the burn unit for assessment of the burn injury.

Key learning points:
- Burn injuries should not distract from higher priorities for intervention such as airway management.
- Assessment of burn injury should be carefully documented for follow-up on resuscitation decisions, and the use of a nomogram or assessment tool can aid in consistency.
- In the prehospital environment isolated burn care management is relatively straightforward, focusing on maintaining respiratory and circulatory status and preventing further injury.

EMS, Emergency medical services; *IV,* intravenous; *NS,* normal saline.

References

1. National Burn Repository. *Report of Data from 2006–2015.* Chicago, IL: American Burn Association; 2016.

2. World Health Organization. *Burns Fact Sheet No 365.* Retrieved from http://www.who.int/mediacentre/factsheets/fs365/en/; 2014.

3. Pinto DS, Clardy PF. Environmental and weapon-related electrical injuries. In: Grayzel J, ed. *UpToDate.* Waltham, Mass.: UpToDate; 2016. Retrieved from www.uptodate.com.

4. Emergency Nurses Association. *Trauma Nursing Core Course (TNCC): Provider Manual.* 7th ed. Des Plaines, IL: Emergency Nurses Association; 2014.

5. Rice PL, Orgill DP. Classification of burns. In: Collins K, ed. *UpToDate.* Waltham, Mass.: UpToDate; 2016. Retrieved from www.uptodate.com.

6. Rice PL, Orgill DP. Emergency care of moderate and severe thermal burns in adults. In: Grayzel J, ed. *UpToDate.* Waltham, Mass.: UpToDate; 2016. Retrieved from www.uptodate.com.

7. Goverman J, Bittner E, Friedstat J, et al. Discrepancy in initial pediatric burn estimates and its impact on fluid resuscitation. *Journal of Burn Care & Research.* 2015;36(5):574-579.

8. Jeschke Marc G, Kamolz LP, Sjoberg F, et al. *Handbook of Burns Volume 1: Acute Burn Care.* 1st ed. Vienna: Springer Verlag; 2012.

9. Marques EG, Júnior GAP, Neto BFM, et al. Visceral injury in electrical shock trauma: proposed guideline for the management of abdominal electrocution and literature review. *International Journal of Burns and Trauma.* 2014;4(1):1.

10. Coughlin MJ, Saltzman CL, Anderson RB. *Mann's Surgery of the Foot and Ankle.* 9th ed. 2v. Beaverton, OR: Ringgold Inc; 2013:730.

11. Malic CC, Karoo ROS, Austin O, Phipps A. Resuscitation burn card—A useful tool for burn injury assessment. *Burns.* 2007;33(2):195-199.

12. Micak RP. Inhalation injury from heat, smoke, or chemical irritants. In: Collins K, Finlay G, eds. *UpToDate.* Waltham, Mass.: UpToDate; 2016. Retrieved from www.uptodate.com.

13. Kaushik S, Bird S. Topical chemical burns. In: Grayzel J, ed. *UpToDate.* Waltham, Mass.: UpToDate; 2015. Retrieved from www.uptodate.com.

14. Pham TN, Cancio LC, Gibran NS, American Burn Association. American burn association practice guidelines burn shock resuscitation. *Journal of Burn Care and Research.* 2008;29(1):257-266.

15. Endorf FW, Dries DJ. Burn resuscitation. *Scandinavian Journal of Trauma, Resuscitation and Emergency Medicine.* 2011;19(1):69.

16. Gauglitz FF, Williams FN. Overview of the management of the severely burned patient. In: Collins K, ed. *UpToDate.* Waltham, Mass.: UpToDate; 2016. Retrieved from www.uptodate.com.

17. Wiechman S, Sharar SR. Burn pain: Principles of pharmacologic and nonpharmacologic management. In: Collins K, ed. *UpToDate.* Waltham, Mass.: UpToDate; 2015. Retrieved from www.uptodate.com.

18. Wingard JR, Dainiak N. Treatment of radiation injury in the adult. In: Tirnauer J, ed. *UpToDate.* Waltham, Mass.: UpToDate; 2016. Retrieved from www.uptodate.com.

19. Luo Q, Li W, Zou X, et al. Modeling fluid resuscitation by formulating infusion rate and urine output in severe thermal burn adult patients: A retrospective cohort study. *BioMed Research International.* 2015;2015:508043.

19

Neurologic Emergencies

CATHLEEN VANDENBRAAK

COMPETENCIES

1. Identify neurologic pathophysiology in terms of pressure-volume relationships and the components of the cerebral vault and its effect on patients who require air or surface transport.
2. Integrate the components of neurologic anatomy and physiology to perform a focused neurologic examination.
3. Implement the evaluation and management of the patient with a stroke and seizure before and during transport.

Introduction

Neurologic illness or injury is a common reason for air medical transport because of its potentially disabling or fatal consequences. The transport team is instrumental in assessing and determining the need for intervention on the basis of expert knowledge of the physiology of neurologic pathologies and how they relate to air medical transport. The two priorities of the air medical crew are effective management of those secondary injuries and rapid transport to an acute care facility.[1-3]

Neurologic Pathophysiology

A basic understanding of neuropathophysiology assists with the ability to critically think through management of patients with neurologic insults. This chapter examines pressure-volume relationships and the volumetric components (cerebrospinal fluid [CSF], blood, and brain) of the neurologic system to gain an understanding of how changes in each of these components affect intracranial pressure (ICP), maintenance of ICP, alterations in ICP, and management of ICP changes.[4-7]

Pressure-Volume Relationships

The main components of volume in the skull are the brain, blood, and CSF. The latter two drain into the dural sinuses.

In healthy individuals, venous pressure is the main determinant of ICP. However, any increase in the volume of one of these components without a corresponding decrease in the volume of the other two results in raised ICP. Alteration in ICP is the prime concern in the care of patients with neurologic emergencies.[1,2,8]

Monro-Kellie Doctrine[2,4,5,7]

The Monro-Kellie doctrine was discovered by Alexander Monro, a Scottish anatomist, and his student George Kellie. This principle states that cerebral blood flow is constant; there is a constant outflow of venous blood flow to make room for new incoming arterial blood, and the brain is enclosed in a rigid box. Under normal conditions the volume of the brain is 80%, blood 10%, and CSF is 10%. When a condition changes a volume in one of the three areas, the other areas are affected. These changes in volume of one area and decrease in another area results in increased ICP (Fig. 19.1).

Cerebrospinal Fluid [2,4,5,7]

CSF is actively secreted by the choroid plexus in the lateral, third, and fourth ventricles. CSF leaves the ventricular system, circulates throughout the subarachnoid space, and finally reaches the subarachnoid space overlying the cerebral convexities. Here, the CSF is absorbed passively by way of the arachnoid granulations located parasagittally along the sagittal sinus. The fluid passes through the structures of the granulation into the cerebral venous system and is carried away with venous blood.[2,4,5,7]

Absorption is pressure driven. The rate of CSF absorption is proportional to the ICP. CSF volume can be pathologically increased by an interference with absorption. This increase can be caused by a mass or stricture in the ventricular system that prevents the CSF from exiting into the subarachnoid space. This accumulation of CSF is termed obstructive or noncommunicating hydrocephalus.[2,4,5,7]

Alternatively, after the CSF leaves the ventricular system, its circulation may be disturbed so that the fluid cannot reach the arachnoid granulation, resulting in communicating or

$$K \sim V_{CSF} + V_{Blood} + V_{Brain}$$

• **Fig. 19.1** Modified Monro-Kellie hypothesis.

nonobstructive hydrocephalus. Given that the subarachnoid space is so large, a focal lesion such as a tumor ordinarily does not produce this type of obstruction. Instead, a widespread disorder such as inflammation of the meninges or increased CSF protein results from such an obstruction.[2,4,5,7]

Volume-Pressure Relationship[2,4,5,7]

There is a reciprocal compensatory mechanism in the Monro-Kellie doctrine to maintain a constant intracranial volume in the following areas: displacement of venous blood through jugular and scalp veins, displacement of intracranial CSF through the foramen magnum and to the spinal subarachnoid space, and decreased production of CSF. This displacement is limited. Once the limitations are exceeded, ICP rises. If left untreated, then the result is intracranial hypertension.

Compliance[2,4,5,7]

Compliance is the adaptability of the capacity of the intracranial contents. Compliance is affected by any increase in volume over a specific time period. One area that can affect compliance is edema that alters brain volume. Brain volume, except for a relatively insignificant alteration in interstitial water, does not change under ordinary circumstances. However, with injury, cerebral brain water may accumulate in the form of cerebral edema. An accumulation of water can be found in the intracellular space, extracellular space, or both. The three types of cerebral edema are vasogenic, cytotoxic, and interstitial.

Vasogenic edema is an extracellular edema of the white matter that results from increased capillary permeability as a result of the breakdown of the tight endothelial junctions and increases in pinocytotic vesicles at the level blood-brain barrier. Vasogenic edema is seen locally around brain tumors, although it can develop around a cerebral infarct or a cerebral abscess as well. Generalized vasogenic edema occurs with cerebral trauma or meningitis. Cytotoxic edema is an increase in fluid in the neurons, glia, and endothelial cells as a result of ATP-dependent sodium-potassium pump failure so that fluid and sodium accumulate within the cell, leading to diffuse brain swelling. Development of cytotoxic edema is associated with a severe hypoxic or anoxic episode, such as a cardiac arrest or asphyxiation. It is also seen with hypoosmolarity conditions, such as water intoxication, hyponatremia, and the syndrome of inappropriate secretion of antidiuretic hormone.

Interstitial edema occurs with hydrocephalus. The edema is found in the periventricular white matter when the intraventricular pressure is greater than the ability of the ependymal cells to contain the CSF within the ventricle.

Cerebral Blood Volume and Flow[2,4,5,7]

Cerebral blood volume comprises two relatively independent components: the arterial blood volume and the venous blood volume. Arterial blood volume accounts for approximately 25% of the total cerebral blood volume, and venous blood volume accounts for the other 75%. Arterial cerebral blood flow (and volume) under normal circumstances remains relatively independent of systemic mean arterial blood volume and pressure through a process called autoregulation. Autoregulation is influenced by pressure and biochemical parameters. As mean systemic arterial pressure increases, cerebral arterial blood vessels constrict, preventing the increase in blood volume and flow that normally occurs. If the mean systemic arterial blood pressure decreases, then the cerebral arteries dilate, increasing cerebral blood flow. Alternatively stated, the blood flow is directly proportional to the perfusion pressure and inversely proportional to the total resistance of the system. Cerebral blood flow is maintained in a constant state between a mean systemic arterial pressure of approximately 60 and 140 mm Hg. Normal blood flow to the cerebral cortex averages 50 mL of blood flow/100 g of brain tissue (expressed as mL/100 g/min). At perfusion less than 20 mL/100 g/min, neuronal cell membranes become impaired, which results in neurologic dysfunction. Despite this impairment, if the blood flow is restored, this damage is reversible. At perfusion flow less than 10 mL/100 g/min, the neuronal tissue rapidly becomes irreversibly damaged. In a no-flow state, cell death may occur within minutes.[2,4,5,7] Arterial blood volume is also influenced by complex biochemical or metabolic action that can be summarized by the association of PaO_2, $PaCO_2$, and cerebral blood flow. Increased $PaCO_2$ or decreased PaO_2 results in dilation of the blood vessel, presumably in response to greater cerebral metabolic needs. Thus this component of autoregulation may be influenced by respiratory control, with hyperventilation resulting in decreased cerebral blood flow and hypoventilation resulting in increased cerebral blood flow. Venous blood volume is passively influenced by the delivery of blood from the arterial side and the ability of the cerebral venous system to drain from the head. This drainage depends on two influences: hydrostatic pressure and central venous pressure. Elevation of the head increases hydrostatic pressure on the venous side, permitting more rapid drainage from the cerebral venous system, mainly through the internal jugular veins bilaterally. Increased central venous pressure, whether caused by increased intrathoracic pressure or by right heart failure, decreases cerebral venous return.[2,4,5,7] Respiratory management can greatly influence the volume of cerebral venous blood. If intrathoracic pressure is increasing because, for example, then the patient is straining on an endotracheal tube that is blocked, a decrease in cerebral venous drainage (and thus an increase in cerebral venous blood volume) occurs.

All of the earlier concepts are important in understanding the cerebral hemodynamic portion of this chapter.

The most common areas that a critical care transport nurse would apply these principles in the critically ill neurologic patient is the cerebral perfusion pressure (CPP) and ICP. There are two calculations to apply:

$$CPP = MAP - ICP$$

$$MAP = DBP + (SBP - DBP)/3$$

where MAP = mean arterial pressure, DBP = diastolic blood pressure, and SBP = systolic blood pressure.

Application of Neurologic Pathophysiology to Cerebral Perfusion Pressure and Mean Arterial Pressure[1,4,5,7,9]

The native autoregulatory system refers to the brain's ability to keep the cerebral blood flow at a relatively constant level over a wide range of CPPs, which is accomplished by varying the resistance in the precapillary arterioles. A CPP greater than or equal to 70 mm Hg ensures adequate cerebral perfusion; ICP is normally 5 to 20 cm H_2O or 3 to 15 mm Hg. Constant cerebral blood flow is obtained with MAPs ranging from 50 to 150 mm Hg, but these values may be higher in patients with chronic hypertension. At the low end of this curve (Figs. 19.2 and 19.3), CPP drops and cerebral hypoperfusion ensues; however, at the high end of the curve, cerebral hyperperfusion with cerebral edema occurs. In disease states, the curve becomes linear and the CPP approximates the cerebral blood flow because of the loss of vessel autoregulation. Elevation of ICP or decrease in MAP results in cerebral hypoperfusion.

To understand the ability of the intracranial components to compensate for the development of a mass (thinking of the combined volume of cerebral edema as mass is helpful), a look at the pressure-volume curve is useful (see Fig. 19.2). As a change in volume of mass occurs, at first, no change in

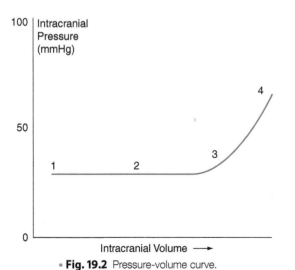

• **Fig. 19.2** Pressure-volume curve.

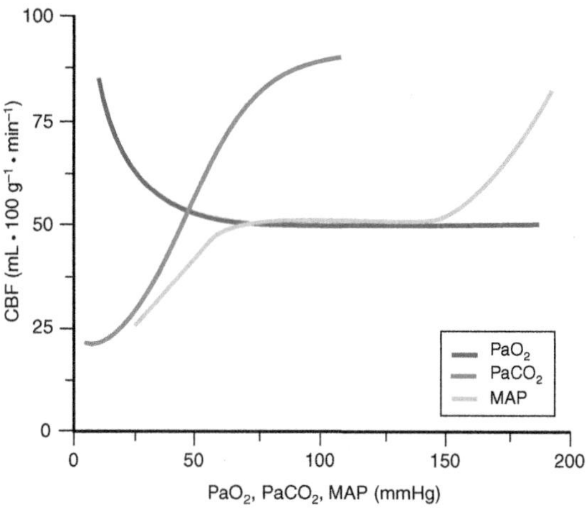

• **Fig. 19.3** Changes in cerebral blood flow (CBF) caused by independent alterations in $PaCO_2$, PaO_2, and mean arterial pressure (MAP). (From Piyush M, Patel PM, Drummond JC. Cerebral physiology and the effects of anesthetics and techniques. In: Miller RD, ed. *Miller's Anesthesia*. 6th ed. Philadelphia, PA: Churchill Livingstone; 2005.)

ICP occurs. This phenomenon is the result of compliance and is accomplished by the reduction in volume of CSF and blood. At some point, however, compliance is lost, and additional changes in volume result in great increases in ICP. In the acute state of cerebral edema, or rapidly developing ICP, the total shifts in volume amount to approximately 50 to 75 mL.[2,4,5,7]

Neurologic Examination[2,7]

A comprehensive neurologic assessment of the patient to be transported is important. After completion of a primary assessment, chief symptoms, history of present illness (including but not limited to onset, duration, and sequence of symptoms), and medical history should be obtained. If the patient has an altered mental state, then ruling out causes of mentation changes is important (Box 19.1). The examination should be conducted in a systematic, stepwise approach that proceeds from the highest level of function (cerebral cortex) to the lowest level of function (reflexes). The cranial nerves (CNs), motor system, and reflexes should be assessed as well. In many cases, serial focused neurologic examinations are necessary for appropriate and timely interventions.

A rapid assessment of the patient's mental status should be made. Is the patient awake? Can the patient talk? Can the patient answer questions appropriately? Can the patient protect the airway? Life-threatening concerns are addressed immediately. A complete mental status examination focuses on the following areas: awareness and mental function as well as reception and interpretation of sensory stimuli, including an awareness and responsiveness to self, to the environment, and to the impressions made by the senses, and of cognitive function.

There are 12 pairs of CNs (a pair consists of a right and left nerve). Each nerve (right and left) must be evaluated

---

• BOX 19.1   Mnemonic for the Differential Diagnosis of Coma

U: Units of insulin
N: Narcotics
C: Convulsions
O: Oxygen
N: Nonorganic
S: Stroke
C: Cocktail
I: ICP
O: Organism
U: Urea
S: Shock

---

separately to completely identify the extent of dysfunction that may be unilateral (Fig. 19.4). Findings are compared for symmetry. As a brief review, CN I is the olfactory nerve. Testing of this nerve is oftentimes deferred, unless an anterior fossa mass is suspected. CN II is the only nerve that can be examined directly. Testing encompasses an evaluation of visual acuity, visual fields, and an ophthalmoscope examination. An ophthalmoscope examination is rarely completed in the transport environment because of the need to balance a comprehensive examination with a rapid transport and

relatively short bedside time. CNs III, IV, and VI are all tested together because all three supply the extraocular eye muscles. CN V is composed of both sensory and motor components. Sensation on the face is tested here along with masseter and temporal muscle strength (clench/open jaw). CN VII is the facial nerve. This nerve also has both sensory and motor components. The sensory component includes the sense of taste on the anterior two-thirds of the tongue. The motor component is tested by observing symmetry of the face at rest and during deliberate facial movements. CN VIII, also called the acoustic nerve, is a pure sensory nerve. Testing of this nerve involves the use of a tuning fork to test air and bone conduction. CNs IV and X are tested together because of their intimate association with function in the pharynx. Having the patient open the mouth and say "ah" allows visualization of the uvula for midline location and voice quality analysis and also allows for the testing for the presence of a gag reflex. CN XI is the spinal accessory nerve and is tested by having the patient shrug the shoulders against resistance and by having the patient turn the head to the side against resistance. Finally, CN XII is the hypoglossal nerve. Testing this nerve involves having the patient protrude the tongue and move it from side to side. Clinical judgment must be used when deciding whether or not a judicious use of time involves performing a complete or

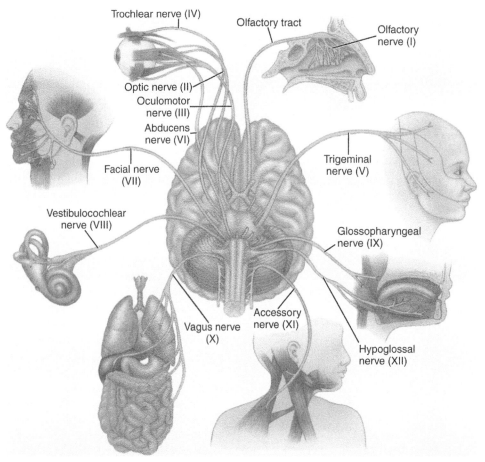

• **Fig. 19.4** Ventral surface of the brain showing attachment of the cranial nerves. (From Patton KT, Thibodeau GA. *Anatomy and Physiology.* 8th ed. St. Louis, MO: Elsevier, 2013.

partial CN assessment. This decision is based on the type of patient being transported and the agency's standing medical orders.

The next part of the neurologic examination is the motor system examination. The neck; upper limbs; trunk; and finally, the lower extremities should be examined (in that order). Generally speaking, muscle size, tone, and strength are examined.

The sensory system is examined next and is done with the patient's eyes closed. This portion of the examination is not generally included in a standard neurologic examination unless numbness, pain, trophic changes, or other sensory abnormalities are present.[2] Superficial, deep, and discriminative sensations are tested.

The cerebellar system is tested by beginning with a finger-to-nose test. If this test is completed successfully, then a further examination of upper extremity coordination is not necessary. Lower extremity tests are generally not done in the transport environment.

The final portion of the neurologic assessment involves the testing of reflexes. Knowledge of how to test reflexes in both the upper and the lower extremities is useful because many transport vehicles limit patient access to the lower extremities. Reflex testing involves muscle-stretch reflexes, superficial reflexes, and pathologic reflexes. Testing of reflexes is a routine part of the examination of a patient with acute spinal cord injury.

Overview of Neurologic Emergency Treatment

In treatment of a patient with a neurologic emergency, maintaining a blood pressure adequate enough to perfuse the brain tissue, while ensuring that the pressure is not high enough to cause injury to the vascular beds in the brain, is imperative. Factors that must be considered when determining the target blood pressure include the type of neurovascular emergency, the level of hypertension that exists, the patient's blood pressure history, and the perceived condition of the patient's native autoregulatory system. If the CPP is allowed to drop below the limits of autoregulation, then ischemic damage may result. If the CPP is above the upper limit, then autoregulatory breakthrough occurs, leading to increased intracranial blood volume, increased ICP, and vasogenic edema. In addition, each type of neurologic emergency can have a significant impact on cerebral blood flow in its own unique way.[2,4,7,9,10]

Stroke: Epidemiology, Types, and Initial Treatment

The American Heart Association (AHA) has increased public awareness for the need to recognize that a stroke is an emergency. Additional education provided to prehospital and transport personnel since 2013 from the AHA has

focused on rapid assessment and transport to the nearest primary stroke center. In 2015 the AHA and the American Stroke Association (ASA) updated these guidelines for rapid assessment, treatment, and intervention for this population. Because of a lack of primary stroke centers in certain areas of the United States, air medical resources are often used for the rapid transport to decrease out-of-hospital time.[3,6,11-13]

In 2015 the AHA reported that close to 800,000 people will suffer a stroke in the United States. Stroke is the fourth leading cause of death. Health care and indirect stroke-related costs are known to be billions of dollars annually in the United States. With the increased use of intravenous (IV) thrombolytics (currently tissue plasminogen activator [tPA]) and endovascular stroke treatment, there is a more positive prognosis for the patient who has suffered a stroke.[3,6,11-13]

Strokes are characterized as ischemic or hemorrhagic. Over 80% of strokes are classified as ischemic stroke, which is characterized by a sudden loss of blood circulation of the brain. Ischemic stroke is caused by a thrombus or a clot that occludes a cerebral artery. The location of the cerebral perfusion loss dictates what neurologic functions are impaired.[3,6,11-13]

Another type of stroke is called hemorrhagic stroke, which is caused from bleeding directly into the parenchyma of the brain. The term intracerebral hemorrhage may also be used to describe this type of stroke.[3,4,6,9,11-13]

Prehospital assessment of a suspected stroke requires the assessment of symptoms in any patient with acute change in mental status. Patients may present with an abrupt loss of movement and sensation and present with deficits. Visual loss, diplopia, dysarthria, aphasia, and facial droop also may present.[14]

Differentiation of ischemic versus hemorrhagic stroke is difficult in the field. Historically a patient with acute loss of consciousness, headache, and nausea and vomiting may be more likely to have a hemorrhagic stroke.

Rapid transport of these patients by air medical services from the field versus interfacility makes a keen assessment important for the critical care transport nurse. Ruling out a stroke mimic, most commonly hypoglycemia, is imperative. Any patients presenting with a Glasgow Coma Score of 14 or less need to have their glucose levels evaluated. The Cincinnati Prehospital Stroke Score examines three areas for the presence or absence of facial droop, arm drift, and abnormal speech.[3,6,11-14]

Pathophysiology of Stroke

The brain receives its blood from two sets of vessels. Two common carotid arteries in the anterior neck bifurcate, each into an external carotid artery that supplies primarily facial tissue and the internal carotid arteries that provide most of the blood supply to the brain through its major subdivisions (the anterior cerebral and the middle cerebral arteries). In the posterior aspect of the neck on either side lie the vertebral arteries. These combine shortly after they pass through the foramen magnum into the single basilar artery, which mainly supplies the brainstem. The posterior cerebral arteries from the vertebral basilar system communicate through two posterior communicating arteries with the internal carotid arteries. A small anterior artery permits communication between the two anterior cerebral arteries. Thus at the base of the brain, a significant collateral circulation called the circle of Willis is formed in which blood can flow as needed from one internal carotid system to the opposite internal carotid system, or to the vertebral basilar system, or to any combination of connections between the internal carotid systems and the vertebral basilar system.[2,7,12,13]

In addition, extensive collateral vessels may develop between the external carotid system and the internal carotid system. These collaterals are supplied mainly through facial anastomoses by way of the ophthalmic artery and through anastomoses between scalp vessels and vessels of the dura and arachnoid, which is called leptomeningeal collateral circulation. Beyond this, however, in the depths of the brain, no collaterals assist deficient circulation. Therefore occlusion of smaller vessels from the surface of the brain inward results in ischemia and infarction.[2,7,12,13]

The most common cause of vascular occlusion, resulting in the classic appearance of a stroke, is an embolus from some other part of the vascular system. Approximately one-third of these emboli (especially in older persons) come from disease in the heart. Previous myocardial infarctions or valvular heart disease may result in the development of mural thrombi, which are the source of emboli. In the great vessels a common location for thrombi formation is the bifurcation of the common carotid into the internal and external carotid. Disease at this location can often be detected with the auscultation of a bruit over the carotid bifurcation at the border of the involved sternocleidomastoid muscle just at the level of the angle of the mandible. Auscultation must be performed carefully to prevent the dislodging of thrombi in the underlying vessel.[2,7,12,13]

The next most common cause of cerebral ischemia is spontaneous intracerebral hemorrhage from cerebral aneurysms or arteriovenous malformations; that of accompanying hypertension is the most prevalent. As a result of this hemorrhage, the first vascular response is to contract and constrict to control hemorrhage in the region of the vascular injury. Second, as the hematoma develops in the brain tissue, the mass effect can place significant pressure on the distal arterioles, and capillary blood pressure becomes relatively low. Approximately 85% of hemorrhagic cases involve the cerebral hemispheres, and only a relatively small number of cases occur in the cerebellum and brainstem as a result of involvement of the vertebral basilar system. In the case of hemorrhage in the cerebellum, the fourth ventricle may be acutely obstructed by the hematoma, resulting in a sudden increase in ICP caused by impeded CSF flow. This increase is managed by the neurosurgeon with ventriculostomy drainage.[2,7,12,13]

A small subset of hemorrhagic cases involves the rupture of intracranial aneurysms into the subarachnoid space. This subarachnoid hemorrhage, along with causing primary brain injury, may result in cerebral ischemia caused by cerebral vasospasm. Little is found to distinguish this condition from other strokes except the symptom of severe, often focal, headache just before the hemorrhage.[2,7,12,13]

Assessment of the Stroke Patient

When a critical care transport team is requested to transport a patient with stroke, time is of the essence. A thorough history from the referring facility is important. Time of onset of symptoms (or time last seen normal), associated symptoms, computed tomographic (CT) scan interpretation, and treatment should be ascertained. The National Institutes of Health Stroke Scale (NIHSS) is an assessment tool used to evaluate neurologic status in acute stroke patients (http://www.ninds.nih.gov/doctors/nih_stroke_scale.pdf). Reassessment of stroke patients with the NIHSS provides a standard way for critical care nurses and doctors to evaluate the patient who has had a stroke as well as to evaluate the effectiveness of selected treatments that may be initiated for the management of the stroke.[2-4,6,7,12-14]

Planning Care of the Stroke Patient

The AHA and ASA guidelines are the standard for stroke care from prehospital care to discharge home. The critical care transport team should be familiar with all levels of care because the referring staff may require assistance with them. Prehospital recommendations for the stroke patient include the following[2-4,6,7,12-14]:

- Use of prehospital screening tolls such as Los Angeles Prehospital Stroke Screen or Cincinnati Prehospital Stroke Scale
- Rapid transport to closest available comprehensive stroke center with prehospital notification
- Management of the primary survey
- Administration of oxygen if pulse oximetry is less than 94%
- Maintaining nothing by mouth status
- Evaluating other causes of stroke symptoms such as hypoglycemia

Emergency department recommendations for the management of a stroke patient include the following[2-4,6,7,12-14]:

- Adherence to time goals, which includes door to physician time of 10 minutes; door-to-CT scan of less than 25 minutes, and door-to-drug of less than 1 hour.
- Use of stroke rating scale; preferred scale is NIHSS.
- Limitation of hematological and coagulation blood studies. Only blood glucose is required. Troponin is preferred.
- Treatment of hypoglycemia or hyperglycemia aggressively to reduce poor outcomes.

- Treatment of hypovolemia with IV normal saline.
- Baseline 12-lead electrocardiogram.
- Continuous cardiac monitoring is recommended to screen for atrial fibrillation.
- Blood pressure should be carefully lowered with a goal of SBP of less than 185 mm Hg and DBP of less than 110 mm Hg.[10]
- Blood pressure needs to be lowered and stabilized before tPA is administered.[10,12]
- Blood pressure should be maintained at or below 185/105 mm Hg for a minimum of 24 hours post-tPA.[10,12]
- For patients eligible for tPA but their blood pressure is greater than 185/110 mm Hg, AHA recommends labetalol 10 to 20 mg IV over 1 to 2 minutes and repeat once, or nicardipine infusion at 5 mg/h; titrate at 2.5 mg increments every 5 to 15 minutes with a maximum infusion of 15 mg/h. Hydralazine and captopril may be considered appropriate.[10,12]
- If blood pressure is not maintained below 185/110 mm Hg, do not administer tPA.[8,10,12]
- Post-tPA management blood pressure goal is 185/105 mm Hg.[10,12]
- If patient presents with SBP greater than 180 to 230 mm Hg or DBP greater than 105 to 120 mm Hg, then consider labetalol 10 mg IV followed by continuous infusion of 2 to 8 mg/min or nicardipine, as mentioned previously.[10,12]
- Sodium nitroprusside IV is considered if blood pressure is not controlled or DBP is greater than 140 mm Hg.[10,12]

IV fibrinolysis for acute stroke is widely accepted. Indication and contraindications for use need to be carefully assessed before medication is given. Consent for medication from the physician in charge of the case is required. Outcomes are increased the sooner the drug is initiated; the goal is within 3 hours of onset. However, multiple National Institute of Neurologic Disorders and Stroke clinical trials have shown decreased disability in those who received the drug greater than 3 hours post onset of symptoms.[8]

When called to transport a patient with an ischemic stroke, the transport team should have a protocol that addresses all of the components of the care of the stroke patient. Continuing tPA is important (tPA dose is 0.9 mg/kg with 10% as an IV push and the remainder over 1 hour via infusion pump) and flushing it through the IV site with normal sterile saline at 50 mL/h is widely accepted practice to ensure that all of the drug is infused. Continued monitoring and vital signs every 15 minutes are recorded. Any changes in patient status may require additional treatment.[2-4,7,6,12-14]

Other important components included in the transport include obtaining a full medical record, with attention to initial neurologic examination and NIHSS. CT scan, magnetic resonance imaging (MRI), or magnetic resonance angiogram (MRA) availability, online or on disk, is imperative

to continue the best practice of treatment for this population of patients.[2-4,7,6,12-14]

Critical care transport teams may transfer the patient directly to an interventional radiology recovery area (INR Suite). The receiving team may elect multiple procedures, with or without tPA given.[2-4,7,6,12-14]

Endovascular therapy with stent-retriever thrombectomy is one of the newest Class 1 recommendations from the AHA/ASA. There are multiple types of stent retrievers and trials associated with favorable outcomes to decrease disability. Many have had patients completely recover from their stroke.[2-4,7,6,12-14]

Intracerebral Hemorrhage Events

Intracerebral hemorrhage occurs when there is bleeding within brain parenchyma. Oftentimes this is caused by trauma or is spontaneous in nature. Approximately 20% of suspected strokes are diagnosed with a hemorrhage and not eligible for fibrinolytic treatment. Intracerebral hemorrhage may result from hypertension, and vascular malformation rupture can be caused by drug abuse.[2,7]

Assessment, treatment, and initial interventions for the stroke patient have been previously discussed. Further testing such as CT angiography, MRI, MRA, and cerebral angiogram may reveal further data to help determine the course of treatment. Surgical decompression of hemorrhage may be indicated in some cases.

Patients with an intracerebral hemorrhage may have an ICP monitor placed to continually measure the pressure exerted by intracranial content (blood, brain, and CSF). Types of monitoring devices and the location placed within the neurologic system will influence the accuracy and incidence of complications. Some ICP monitors will also allow for drainage of CSF and blood. The transducer should be level at the external auditory meatus, which approximates the level of the foramen of Monro.[2,7]

During a critical care transport of a patient with ICP monitoring in place it is important to understand your agency's limitations for monitoring in transport. Patient position during transport, vehicle movement, and the outside environment will all influence the accuracy of the monitor. Will the device function within the transport environment? Do the team members have the knowledge and education to continue to use the equipment and interpret and manage the data that may be obtained from the device?

The alternative to monitoring an increasing ICP is to closely monitor for external signs of increased ICP, such as deterioration of the level of consciousness, pupillary change, or report of change in CT scan interpretations. Remember, these are late and often irreversible signs.

Seizures

Seizures result from abnormal electrical activity in the brain. Seizures may be the result of epilepsy or other underlying causes such as traumatic brain injury, electrolyte abnormalities, fever, or a stroke. It is important to note that in patients with an underlying seizure disorder, an illness or injury may precipitate a seizure.[1,2,7,9]

The onset of epileptic seizures is associated with several types of generalized and focal brain lesions. The underlying neuropathophysiology, however, is poorly understood. Although the belief is reasonable that an alteration exists in the neuronal pool or in the extracellular environment (both general theories have their advocates), neither laboratory investigations nor clinical experience with specific antiepileptic drugs have yielded a common therapy.[1,2,7,9]

Similar epileptic syndromes, however, are known to occur and are caused by focal lesions such as brain tumors, arteriovenous malformations, stroke, and generalized states such as head trauma and viral or metabolic encephalopathies. In addition, in some idiopathic epilepsy syndromes, no obvious underlying cause is apparent. With more sophisticated recording techniques, several idiopathic epileptic syndromes are being associated with the presence of focal lesions, such as occult infarcts or sclerosis after birth trauma.[1,2,7,9]

Some patients present with status epilepticus. Traditionally, status epilepticus is defined as 30 minutes of continuous seizure activity or a series of seizures without return to full consciousness between the seizures. Many believe that a shorter period of seizure activity causes neuronal injury and that seizure self-termination is unlikely after 5 minutes, whereas some suggest times as brief as 5 minutes define status epilepticus. In any case, these patients are considered to have true neurologic emergencies because of the neuronal injury that results.[1,2,7,9]

Neuronal ischemic changes were once thought to be caused by decreased respiratory effort. They are theorized to occur in combination with ictal events and include a marked increase in metabolic rate and membrane changes that affect the transport of small ions at the neuronal level.[1,2,7,9]

Assessment

Several classification schemes for epilepsy have been used. These include the following:

1. Focal (partial) seizures: These begin in small localized areas of the brain and may or may not spread generally.
2. Generalized seizures: These are diffuse and uncontrolled, with neuronal changes that begin bilaterally and are symmetric; generalized tonic-clonic seizures are also known as grand mal seizures.
3. Absence or petit mal seizures: These generally involve the thalamocortical activating system in the brain.
4. Continuous seizure activity or status epilepticus.[1]

The same assessment criteria should be used regardless of the classification of seizure activity exhibited. The assessment criteria should include a thorough history, physical examination, and neurologic evaluation. The onset, type,

and duration of seizure activity should be determined from the history. Additional pertinent information includes allergies, medications, medical history, family history, recent illness, or injury.

Patient and transport team safety must always be a priority when providing care for the patient with a seizure. The airway is always of primary importance. The transport team must be alert to signs of trauma that may have occurred before or concurrent with the seizure activity. The physical assessment should then include motor, sensory, and psychomotor evaluation. The degree of involvement of these areas depends on the individual patient presentation. Involvement may range from isolated focal activity to generalized status involvement.

Regardless of the level of involvement, motor activity during epileptic seizures is involuntary. Motor activity varies greatly depending on the type and neural focus of the seizure. In generalized tonic-clonic seizures, movement begins with the tonic phase, which is a continuous tense muscular state. This phase is followed by a hypertonic phase with hypertension and muscle rigidity. The clonic phase is characterized by rapidly alternating muscle rigidity and relaxation. During the clonic phase, sphincter control can be lost and the patient may be incontinent. Tachycardia, hyperventilation, and salivation result from autonomic discharge during seizure activity. Sensory assessment is subjective because the patient's symptoms may include visual, auditory, or proprioceptive phenomena. Psychomotor assessment is the determination of the level of consciousness, which may vary widely depending on the type of seizure activity and the time of evaluation. Other psychomotor observations include amnesia and repetitive behavioral patterns.[1,2,7,9]

The transport team should be watchful for additional examples of seizure presentation including staring spells, a loss of motor control, blinking, lip smacking, and cycling extremity movements.

Planning of Care of Seizure Patient

A plan of care for the patient with seizure who needs transport includes a rapid thorough assessment, appropriate interventions, and safe transfer to tertiary care.

Implementation of the plan involves management of the airway for prevention of hypoxia with simultaneous protection of the patient from physical injuries and additional complications. Ongoing support of the cardiovascular system and treatment of the seizure activity is important. Management of the underlying illness or injury that predisposed the patient to seizures may also be necessary. Initial management includes completion of a glucose level to rule out hypoglycemic seizure.[1,2,7,9]

Seizure management in the transport setting generally involves the use of a benzodiazepine (lorazepam or midazolam) and a longer-acting anticonvulsant, such as phenytoin or levetiracetam.[1,2,7,9]

All patients with a generalized presentation of seizures characterized by bilateral tonic-clonic activity, altered level of consciousness, and possibly urinary or fecal incontinence should undergo aggressive treatment. Conditions can quickly become relatively hypoxic as a result of the seizure activity. Hypoxia tends to aggravate the seizure disorder and make treatment more difficult. The hypoxia occurs at two levels: generalized tissue hypoxia and cellular hypoxia. General tissue hypoxia occurs because the intense motor activity of the seizure interferes with adequate respiration. This aspect of the seizure disorder can be managed with the use of neuromuscular blocking agents in association with proper airway management. However, the intense neuronal activity characterized by sustained or rapidly intermittent bursts of neuronal discharge produces additional hypoxia at the cellular level. This hypoxia can result in a more long-term neuronal injury and is the reason for the aggressive use of an antiepileptic drug. The patient with a focal seizure (or partial seizure) characterized, for example, by facial twitching or motor activity limited to one extremity with no alteration of consciousness need not undergo aggressive management for short periods of time if attention must be paid to a more serious medical problem. However, a focal epileptic syndrome could become generalized fairly rapidly, so such a progression should be anticipated. Status epilepticus is a dangerous syndrome. It is the most refractory to treatment, and the stress of the intense motor activity can cause not only respiratory insufficiency but also, in the elderly, myocardial strain that leads to myocardial injury. Severe hypertension may also occur during status seizures, resulting in expected complications such as intracerebral hemorrhage.[1,2,7,9]

Practically speaking, the acute management of a generalized seizure syndrome is simple and straightforward. Accessible IV lines should be placed for medication administration. Intraosseous placement should be considered immediately if traditional peripheral lines cannot be placed. Alternative medication routes including rectal administration may need to be considered in the transport environment.[1,2,7,9]

Attention to the airway is most important, and intubation should be considered for any patient whose ability to control the airway is compromised. Rapid-sequence induction should precede any intubation attempts because of the neuroprotective benefits achieved with adequate sedation of the patient before intubation. Continued sedation is recommended. As mentioned previously, sedation with benzodiazepines is used to treat any additional seizure activity that might occur. The use of ongoing neuromuscular blockade is controversial in the transport environment because of the inability of the critical care team to assess the presence of seizure activity. The safety of the patient (including maintenance of an airway) is the primary concern in the transport setting.

Generalized epilepsy leading to status epilepticus is most often seen in the acute state in one of two situations: (1) with generalized encephalopathy, including that immediately following trauma; and (2) in patients who are known epileptics, who have reduced drug intake, and whose blood levels have fallen below therapeutic concentrations.[1,2,7,9]

Status epilepticus is treated with IV medications including: benzodiazepines as initial treatment and urgent control antiepileptic drug therapy (IV fosphenytoin/phenytoin, valproate sodium, or levetiracetam). All of these medications place the patient at risk for potential side effects such as respiratory depression and cardiac arrhythmias. For these reasons, the patient must be carefully monitored during transport. Every transport program must have well-developed, updated medical guidelines for seizure management during transport or have immediate access to medical direction.[1,2,7,9]

Evaluation

Patient outcome depends not only on the intervention but also on precipitating factors and any complications the patient might experience. The optimal goal in caring for the patient with seizures is prompt control of the seizure activity to minimize cerebral insult and prevent complications.

Evaluation data might include arterial blood gas values, chest radiographs, and laboratory results, including medication blood levels, and possibly CT scan or MRI to rule out cerebral pathology on the patient's admission to the receiving facility. In the trauma patient with seizure activity, radiographs of the skull and cervical spine are also evaluated. Copies of all radiologic studies performed from an outside hospital should be copied or transmitted and made available for transport with the patient.

Patients who present with seizure activity pose special problems. The most obvious is the safety of the uncontrolled seizure patient during transport. The patient, crew, and transport vehicle must be protected from the danger associated with the unpredictable motor responses of the seizure patient. Extra care should be taken in the application of protective patient restraints, and aggressive pharmacologic therapy should be instituted for all seizure patients.

Of particular note are visually induced seizures. The photosensitivity type is most prevalent. These seizures are induced by light flashes; patients prone to these seizures may experience them in flight as a result of the strobe effect of aircraft lights. Pattern-induced seizures may occur in response to the light–dark pattern caused by a slowly rotating main rotor during start-up and shutdown.

Summary

Patients experiencing a neurologic emergency are frequently transported by air and ground. Research has demonstrated that rapid transport to a designated stroke center can positively impact patient outcomes and quality of life. Competent and safe transport of the patient with a neurologic emergency does make a difference in patient care.

CASE STUDY

HISTORY

The transport team is dispatched for an interfacility transport from a 12-bed emergency department of a local community hospital to a comprehensive stroke center. The patient is a 72-year-old female weighing approximately 90 kilograms with a diagnosis of an acute ischemic cerebral vascular accident (CVA).

The patient has a past medical history of a TIA (transient ischemic attack) less than a month ago. She has a history of hypertension, hypothyroidism, and anxiety. Medications include lisinopril, an 81-mg aspirin, levothyroxine, and a daily multivitamin. The patient has no history of any allergies.

The patient was last seen without complaints at "bedtime" per her husband. He awoke early in morning to hear a "thump" and found her lying on the floor. The patient was awake with dysarthria; and complete right-sided weakness. A local emergency medical service (EMS) was called to transport her to the community hospital.

The EMS transport team established cardiac monitoring, which showed a normal sinus rhythm at a rate of 88 beats per minute, blood pressure 190/110, and respiratory rate of 18 breaths per minute. SpO_2 reading was 96% on room air. Blood glucose reading was 127 mg/dL. A heparin lock was placed and transport was uneventful.

Assessment

In the emergency department, a 12-lead ECG was performed and no acute changes were found. Routine labs were drawn including electrolytes, a complete blood count, PT/INR, and a urinalysis. Computerized axial tomography (CT) of her head showed no hemorrhage. Initial National Institutes of Health (NIH) Stroke scale was 11.

Based on the findings of CT of the head, initial assessment, and NIH Stroke scale, the emergency department doctor consulted with a comprehensive stroke center located 90 minutes from the hospital. Using telemedicine to repeat the assessment and review findings, it was agreed, due to unknown time last seen normal, tissue-type plasminogen activator (tPA) was not to be given, and the patient would be flown directly to the interventional suite at the stroke center.

The transport team arrived and received the bedside hand-off communication from the referring staff. The transport team received a copy of the chart and a CD of the imaging that was done. The purpose of the transport was explained to the patient's husband and other family members. Directions to the receiving facility were provided to the family.

The patient's blood pressure remained elevated with a MAP greater than 130 mm Hg. A nicardipine infusion was started at 5 mg/hr. The transport team, using an evidenced-based protocol, titrated the nicardipine for a goal of 10% to 15% reduction of her MAP.

Transport

The patient was secured to a stretcher and the head of bed was placed at 45 degrees to assist with maintaining her airway and decreasing the risk of increasing her intracranial pressure. The environment in the aircraft was managed so that the patient remained normothermic.

Approximately 10 minutes into the transport, the patient began drooling and became nonverbal and completely flaccid on the right side. She was unable to protect her airway and had snoring respirations. The transport team elected to perform rapid-sequence intubation utilizing etomidate and rocorurium based on their advanced airway management protocols. The patient was successfully intubated on the first pass with 8.0 mm endotracheal tube secured at 23 mm at teeth. An oral gastric tube was placed without difficulty. She was placed on a portable ventilator with AC 14, tidal volume 550 FiO_2 60%, and PEEP of 5 cm H_2O.

The transport team notified their dispatch center in order to provide an update that was relayed to the awaiting interventional team. The patient's blood pressure decreased to MAP 108 mm Hg and her Glasgow Coma Score was now 3. No further interventions were initiated.

The interventional radiology team took the patient directly to the CT scanner upon arrival. A hemorrhagic CVA was found in the left parietal to the left temporal lobes. No interventions were performed.

Outcome

The patient was admitted to the neuro ICU for care. After 24 hours, a repeated scan demonstrated worsening hemorrhaging. Honoring the patient's advanced directives, the family withdrew care, and the patient expired peacefully with her family at her bedside.

References

1. Hall J. States of brain activity-sleep, brain waves, epilepsy, psychosis, and dementia. In: Hall J. ed. *Guyton and Hall Medical Physiology.* 13th ed. Philadelphia, PA: Elsevier; 2016:763-772.
2. Hickey JV. *The Clinical Practice of Neurological and Neurosurgical Nursing.* 7th ed. Philadelphia, PA: Lippincott Williams & Wilkins; 2014.
3. Lukovits T, Von Iderstine S, Brozen R, et al. Interhospital helicopter transport for stroke. *Air Medical Journal.* 2013;32(1):36-39.
4. Boss B, Huether S. Alterations in cognitive systems, cerebral hemodynamics, and motor function. In: McCance K, Huether S, eds. *Pathophysiology: The Biologic Basis for Disease in Adults and Children.* 7th ed. St. Louis, MO: Elsevier; 2014:527-580.
5. Hall J. Cerebral blood flow, cerebrospinal fluid, and brain metabolism. In: Hall J, ed. *Guyton and Hall Medical Physiology.* 13th ed. Philadelphia, PA: Elsevier; 2016:787-794.
6. Hawk A, Marco C, Huang M, Chow B. Helicopter scene response for stroke patients: A five-year experience. *Air Medical Journal.* 2016;35(6):352-354.
7. McQuillan K, Belden J. Neurologic system. In: Alspach JG, ed. *Core Curriculum for Critical Care Nurses.* 6th ed. Philadelphia, PA: Saunders Elsevier; 2006:381-524.
8. Lyerly MJ, Albright KC, Boehme AK, et al. Safety protocol violations in acute stroke tPA administration. *Journal of Stroke and Cerebrovascular Diseases.* 2015;23(5):855-860.
9. Boss B, Huether SD. Disorders of the central and peripheral nervous systems and the neuromuscular junction. In: McCance K,

Huether S, eds. *Pathophysiology: The Biologic Basis for Disease in Adults and Children*. 7th ed. St. Louis, MO: Elsevier; 2014: 581-640.

10. Kim A, Johnston SC. Neurologic complications of hypertension. In: Aminoff M, Josephson SA, eds. *Aminoff's Neurology and General Medicine*. 5th ed. London: Academic Press Elsevier; 2014: 119-145.

11. Hutton CF, Fleming J, Youngquist S, et al. Stroke and helicopter emergency medical service transports: An analysis of 25, 332 patients. *Air Medical Journal*. 2015;34(6):348-356.

12. Jauch EC, Saver JL, Adams HP, et al. Guidelines for the early management of patients with acute ischemic stroke: A guideline for healthcare professionals from the American Heart Association/American Stroke Association. *Stroke*. 2013;44:870-947.

13. Latimer A, Bell J, Powell E, Tilney P. A 77-year-old man with acute ischemic stroke. *Air Medical Journal*. 2015;34(5): 230-234.

14. Kummer BR, Gialdini G, Sevush JL, et al. External validation of the Cincinnati Prehospital Stroke Severity Scale. *Journal of Stroke and Cerebrovascular Diseasese*. 2016;25(5):1270-1274.

20

Cardiovascular Emergencies

CINDY GOODRICH

COMPETENCIES

1. Perform a detailed cardiovascular assessment before, during, and after transport.
2. Identify patients with acute cardiac events and provide appropriate treatment.
3. Recognize the potential for lethal events and initiate appropriate interventions.
4. Utilize invasive monitoring during transport.
5. Provide treatment for patients with acute cardiac events and hemodynamic abnormalities.

Cardiovascular emergencies will challenge even the most experienced transport team. Critical care transport of patients with acute cardiovascular events requires rapid assessment and critical thinking skills to provide life-saving treatment. The demand for medical transport of patients who are dependent on invasive devices and new sophisticated technology has continued to increase over time.[1] This chapter describes advances in clinical care for patients with acute coronary syndromes (ACSs) including acute myocardial infarction (AMI), cardiogenic shock, heart failure (HF), aortic dissection, and other manifestations of cardiovascular disease, with a focus on assessment and management relative to the medical transport environment.

Individuals experiencing acute cardiac events, decompensated HF, or an aortic dissection in a small, isolated, resource-limited, community-based hospital often require rapid critical care transfer to a tertiary care facility for further evaluation and emergent intervention. Transport of these critically ill patients involves a number of issues unique to the transport environment, which include the potential effects of altitude and the difficulty associated with initiation of resuscitative interventions in a limited space and uncontrolled environment, such as in an aircraft or in the back of a transport vehicle.

Alterations of Cardiovascular Physiology at High Altitudes

One of the greatest threats to patients with cardiovascular disease is hypoxia. Decompensation of patients with acute cardiovascular disease during transport at high altitudes is generally caused by hypoxic hypoxia, which is defined as an oxygen deficiency in the body tissues, sufficient enough to cause impaired function.[1,2] Individual patient tolerances vary, but patients with cardiac disease are usually at risk for compromise when the cabin pressure exceeds 6000 feet. Physiologic changes occur as barometric pressure decreases, resulting in a lower partial pressure of oxygen. This reduction in the amount of oxygen in the blood decreases oxygen availability to the tissues. As altitude increases, the availability of oxygen for gas exchange decreases, causing a reduction in oxygen saturation. Compensatory mechanisms are activated in an effort to maintain adequate oxygen delivery to the tissues. These include increases in heart rate (HR), respiratory rate, and cardiac output (CO). The increased workload on the heart increases myocardial oxygen consumption and necessitates the need for increased blood flow to the heart muscle.

In healthy individuals, cardiac reserve allows the body to compensate for reduced blood flow to the tissues by altering HR and stroke volume (SV). Blood flow to the heart muscle is also increased by dilating the coronary artery microvasculature. Cardiovascular disease may limit a patient's ability to maximize CO in response to increasing oxygen demand. Patients with coronary artery disease (CAD) who are unable to compensate for the increased workload imposed on the heart because of decreased oxygen tension at high altitude may experience chest pain, cardiac dysrhythmias, HF, pulmonary edema, or even cardiac arrest.[2-4]

Supplemental oxygen should be given to patients during transport when indicated. The current 2015 American Heart Association (AHA) Guidelines Update for Cardiopulmonary Resuscitation and Emergency Cardiovascular Care continue to recommend arterial oxygen saturation (SaO_2) of greater than 93%.[5] The potential detrimental effects of altitude can be minimized by administering supplemental oxygen and aircraft pressurization at higher altitudes. In fixed-wing transport, limiting cabin altitude to a maximum of 6000 feet has been shown to eliminate problems for patients with cardiovascular disease. Cabin pressure is not a fixed variable and may need to be adjusted to accommodate patient condition. Cabin pressure can be adjusted to as low as sea level; however, a decrease in cabin pressure may come at the expense of travel time at a lower altitude. Flights at lower altitude may result in decreased speeds and therefore longer flights with an increased need for refueling stops during the trip. This will lengthen the time a patient is out of a controlled environment.

Decisions regarding altitude restrictions or limitations must be based on patient history, current clinical condition, and pilot-in-command expertise and judgment. These decisions need to be evaluated throughout the mission and may need to be adjusted as a result of continued in-flight patient surveillance.[3,6]

Special Considerations for Cardiopulmonary Resuscitation in the Transport Environment

Cardiac arrest is of special concern to those involved in the transport of critically ill patients. Cardiopulmonary resuscitation (CPR) in the confined space of an aircraft cabin or ground transport vehicle is both difficult and challenging. Advanced cardiac life support (ACLS) guidelines are used as the standard of practice for resuscitation of the patient in cardiac arrest by most transport programs.[7] Team members are expected to have current verification of ACLS skills through the AHA to participate in patient care within the transport environment.[6,8] Detailed pretransport assessment, planning, and intervention along with prompt correction of dysrhythmias, repletion of electrolytes, and continuous maintenance of adequate oxygenation and ventilation may help to prevent the need for resuscitation during transport.

Transport teams must maintain a state of perpetual readiness for emergencies such as cardiac arrest. Preparation includes ensuring proper functioning of resuscitation equipment and that an adequate oxygen supply is readily available. ACLS drugs should be well labeled, not expired, and ready for quick administration. Generally, the number of crew members available to perform basic and advanced life support resuscitation is limited to only two medically trained personnel. Resuscitation roles and responsibilities must be well defined for effective and rapid response during an emergency.

Cardiopulmonary Resuscitation and Defibrillation During Transport

High-quality CPR and defibrillation are the two interventions that have been shown to increase neurologically intact survival.[9]

Cardiopulmonary Resuscitation High-quality, uninterrupted CPR is essential for improved survival from cardiac arrest. Manual chest compressions remain the standard of care for the treatment of cardiac arrest.[9] The performance of manual CPR during out-of-hospital cardiac arrest is often less than optimal, and affects survival.[10] Providing high-quality, effective CPR in a moving ambulance or in an aircraft during flight can be challenging and often dangerous

for the providers. Transport personnel should aim to provide the best-quality CPR possible within the constraints and limitations of their operating environment. The recently published 2015 AHA Guidelines Update for Cardiopulmonary Resuscitation and Emergency Cardiovascular Care identify specific settings in which the use of mechanical CPR devices may be considered as a strategy for delivering high-quality compressions during CPR.[11] Specific settings identified include prolonged CPR, situations in which the number of rescuers is limited, during hypothermic cardiac arrest, in the angiography suite, during preparation for extracorporeal CPR, and in moving ambulances. In these guidelines they stress the importance of limiting interruptions in CPR during deployment and removal of these devices.

There are many benefits to using mechanical CPR devices in the resource-challenged, transport environment. Mechanical CPR can improve the consistency of chest compressions (rate and depth), minimize interruptions in chest compressions, reduce rescuer fatigue during prolonged resuscitation, and allow for CPR to continue during patient transfer. Use of these devices will allow providers to complete other necessary tasks and eliminate the safety concerns related to the performance of CPR by an unrestrained crew in a moving vehicle or aircraft. Use of these devices requires a commitment to training and quality review.

Special consideration should be given to transport vehicle configuration in anticipation of the potential need for CPR and resuscitation during transport. The position and height of the stretcher in relationship to the transport crew is important. It must allow the crew the ability to change positions, facilitating proper hand and arm positioning during chest compressions. A well-designed configuration minimizes the need for crew members to extend or release restraint devices during the administration of therapeutic interventions.[6]

Defibrillation During Transport

The most critical factor in the determination of the success of a resuscitative effort is time to restoration of effective spontaneous circulation.[9] Immediate defibrillation is the priority in the treatment of confirmed ventricular fibrillation (VF) and unstable ventricular tachycardia (VT).[9] The close quarters, metallic composition of transport vehicles, and proximity of vital electronic equipment, particularly in the rotor-wing environment, previously generated concern among transport personnel about the safely of defibrillation in this environment. Holleran[6] addressed the potential electrical risks of airborne defibrillation and showed that defibrillation with modern equipment in a medically equipped twin-engine helicopter is safe. Despite cramped quarters and sensitive electrical equipment, defibrillation can be performed without hesitation, whether the aircraft is on the ground or in the air, provided that standard defibrillation precautions are observed. Transport crew should use self-adhesive defibrillation pads and follow the ACLS defibrillation standards for the selection of energy levels.[7] The crew should inform the pilot before defibrillation and maintain clearance from the patient and stretcher when discharging the current.

Temporary Pacing During Transport

Temporary pacing is used when the heart's normal conduction system fails to produce myocardial contraction, resulting in hemodynamic instability. It is indicated when a patient's HR is too slow or too high to maintain adequate CO, or in those at risk for developing significant bradycardias. The purpose of pacing is to reestablish normal hemodynamics in a compromised heart that is beating either too fast or too slow. During transport, transcutaneous pacing (TCP) may be used until a transvenous pacemaker can be inserted. Ventricular pacing is used more often in emergent situations, but atrial or atrioventricular (AV) sequential may be indicated in some settings.

Transcutaneous Pacing

TCP provides immediate, temporary pacing during critical situations, without the risks associated with placing an invasive pacemaker. It is an external, rapid, noninvasive, and time-saving method to pace the heart.[12] This temporary method stimulates ventricular myocardial depolarization through the chest wall via two large electrodes that are placed on the anterior and posterior chest wall or on the anterior and left lateral positions. These are placed in addition to the standard electrodes placed for cardiac monitoring. These patches are attached by a cable to an external pulse generator. Energy (milliamps [mA]) is delivered to the myocardium via the external pulse generator based on the set rate, sensitivity, and output. TCP is a quick method for pacing, but it also requires a significant amount of energy to achieve capture and successful pacing of the heart. Patient discomfort is common and will require the use of medications for pain and sedation. The reliability of TCP is dependent on the skin-to-pad contact and the thoracic impedance that must be overcome during pacing. Because of these limitations, TCP should only be considered as a temporary method of pacing until more definitive treatment with a transvenous or permanent pacemaker can be achieved. TCP should be performed according to current ACLS protocols.

Transvenous Pacing

Transvenous pacing is indicated when more prolonged pacing is required. It is most commonly used for short-term management of symptomatic bradycardias, either as a bridge to permanent pacing or for self-limited bradycardias. Transvenous pacing is more reliable than TCP because a pacer lead is directly in contact with the myocardium. This method of pacing is much more reliable than TCP, but requires placement of pacing wires by an experienced physician. A pacing lead wire is inserted through a vein into the right atrium or right ventricle. Once inserted, the lead wires are attached to a battery-operated, external pulse generator. The transport crew should become familiar with the types of transvenous pacemakers that are used by local hospitals.

Before leaving the referring facility, the pacemaker setting should be verified. These settings include the rate, sensitivity (mV), and output (mA). Mechanical capture should be confirmed by the presence of a pulse. Problems encountered during transvenous pacing include lead disconnection from the generator and battery failure. Additional batteries should be taken on all transports. The transport crew must know how to reattach loosened lead wires and how to change the battery of the pacemaker if warranted during transport.

Complications that may be encountered during transport include sensing problems, failure to capture, myocardial penetration, and cardiac tamponade. Pacemaker malfunctions include failure to sense or failure to capture. Undersensing or failure to sense occurs when the pacemaker does not see the native cardiac activity and pacing occurs randomly in the middle of, or after, a P wave or QRS complex. It may be caused by malposition of the catheter, poor intracardiac signal quality, or generator malfunction. Undersensing is managed by turning the sensitivity setting of the pulse generator to the full-demand position.[13] Oversensing, which results in pauses in the paced rhythm, can result from sensing of atrial electrical activity if the pacing lead is positioned near the tricuspid valve, from sensing of T waves; or from sensing voltage transients that are the result of lead wire fracture, environmental influences, or signals from the generator. The problem of oversensing can be resolved by turning the sensitivity setting toward the asynchronous position until the unwanted signals are no longer sensed.[13]

Failure to capture during transvenous pacing can be related to the patient's clinical condition or to the mechanics of the pacing unit. Clinical conditions resulting in loss of capture include acidosis, hypoxia, antiarrhythmic drugs, and electrolyte imbalances. Mechanical causes of loss of capture include poor endocardial contact, lead fracture or dislodgment, or myocardial perforation. The pacer output (mA) should be increased while the underlying cause is identified and treated. Most authors suggest setting the output to three times the initial threshold to prevent later loss of capture. Failure to capture can be related to malposition of the lead, resulting in poor endocardial contact, catheter dislodgment, or fracture, or to an increase in the myocardial stimulation threshold. It is identified by a pacing spike on the electrocardiogram (ECG) without a P wave or QRS complex. To resolve this problem, the current output should be increased until consistent capture occurs. If electrolyte imbalance is the underlying problem, then it should be corrected. The position of the lead should be checked and repositioned if necessary.

Myocardial penetration or perforation into the pericardial space is usually accompanied by a pericardial friction rub and often by a squeaking systolic sound or murmur. If the pacing wire has migrated, it should be repositioned.

If cardiac tamponade occurs in association with perforation, immediate pericardiocentesis should be performed. If a pericardiocentesis is not in your scope of practice, continue aggressive fluid resuscitation.

Targeted Temperature Management

The new AHA guidelines recommend that targeted temperature management should be used in comatose, adult patients who achieve return of spontaneous circulation after cardiac arrest.[7] Comatose patients are defined as those without any meaningful response to verbal commands. A constantly maintained temperature between 32°C and 36°C is recommended for at least 24 hours.[9,14] The induction of this mild-to-moderate hypothermia in comatose patients after cardiac arrest has been shown to be beneficial with improved neurologic outcomes and reduced mortality.[15,16] Currently, the routine prehospital administration of cold intravenous (IV) fluids is not recommended because available evidence suggests there is no direct benefit and that there may be some potential harmful effects.[17-21]

Acute Coronary Syndromes

ACS is a spectrum of clinical conditions caused by varying degrees of coronary artery occlusion. The three presentations of ACS include unstable angina, acute non-ST elevation MI (NSTEMI), and acute ST elevation MI (STEMI). ACS may result from a variety of conditions in which coronary arteries are narrowed or occluded by clots, plaque (fat), or spasm. Any of these syndromes may cause sudden cardiac death.[22]

Pathophysiologic Factors

An abrupt change in the caliber of a coronary artery can occur as a result of coronary blood vessel spasm or the abrupt worsening of an atherosclerotic plaque. Atherosclerotic plaques can suddenly become more narrowed because of the formation of atheroma in the wall of the vessel or the formation of a thrombus on the surface of a damaged plaque.[23]

ACSs begin with a disruption of the endothelium overlying an atherosclerotic lesion. Lesions more likely to be involved in ACS are the mild-to-moderate lesions with thin fibrous tissue caps. The continuum of unstable angina, acute NSTEMI, and acute STEMI is, in truth, a varying degree of the same underlying problem: a mild-to-moderate lipid-laden atherosclerotic plaque that suddenly ruptures exposing the underlying cholesterol gruel to the circulating blood and setting in place multiple mechanisms that attempt to repair the damaged vessel wall. Platelets, once activated, bind to exposed areas of the vessel wall. More platelets are drawn to the area, and the activated platelets begin to bind to each other via receptors on their surface, known as glycoprotein IIb/IIIa receptors. The activation of platelets during this process causes release of regulatory substances, which cause further aggregation of platelets and vasoconstriction. Platelet activation also leads to the secretion of vasoconstriction substances, which limit

blood flow in the affected coronary artery.[24] At the same time, the clotting cascade is activated, leading to formation of thrombin. Thrombin is a potent stimulant of platelet activation and is responsible for the conversion of fibrinogen in the bloodstream to fibrin. As platelets accumulate in the area, a platelet plug forms, which itself can intermittently occlude flow in the coronary. As this mass of platelets becomes organized, fibrin interconnects, resulting in the formation of a stable blood clot, or thrombus.[25]

Once platelets have aggregated on the surface of the ruptured plaque, the competition between antithrombotic and thrombotic processes in the body becomes intense. The vessel may reocclude at any time or heal without further symptoms, or the ruptured plaque/platelet plug may be incorporated into the atherosclerotic plaque, contributing to the progressive growth of atherosclerotic CAD.

The degree to which a coronary artery is occluded and whether or not it remains occluded by this process subsequently determines in which part of the continuum of ACSs an event is classified. For example:

1. One event is unstable angina caused by an acute change in the caliber of a coronary artery as a result of plaque rupture and thrombus formation. If transient occlusion of a coronary by activated platelets at the site of a ruptured plaque occurs with subsequent recanalization of the vessel, the patient may be symptomatic at rest (while the coronary is occluded) and have symptoms that resolve spontaneously with recanalization of the vessel. Transient ECG changes may occur while the patient is symptomatic, but the episode is often too short to show either ECG changes or evidence of myocardial injury.

2. An event classified as an NSTEMI infarction begins in the same manner, but either occlusion of the coronary is prolonged (with myocardial necrosis) or distal embolization of small platelet clumps occurs, leading to occlusion of smaller distal coronary branches and therefore myocardial necrosis. Spontaneous recanalization may occur, but biochemical evidence of myocardial necrosis is found (troponin, CPK-MB). In both of these instances, a significantly narrowed coronary artery (although recanalized) remains, and therapy is aimed at keeping the activated platelets present on the artery surface from progressing into a stable thrombus.

3. Acute STEMI represents the syndrome of acute plaque rupture, which continues to its ultimate end point, which is an organized thrombus made up of activated platelets with cross-linked fibrin, resulting in a stable thrombus. These patients have continued chest pain and associated ST segment elevation because of injury caused by total occlusion of coronary blood flow. At this point, therapy must be aimed at immediate reperfusion.

Acute Coronary Syndromes: Diagnosis, Assessment, and Treatment

The diagnosis of ACS is based on patient presentation, serum markers of cardiac injury, and findings on a 12-lead ECG.

It is important to exclude other nonischemic causes of chest pain including aortic dissection, esophageal rupture, and pulmonary embolism.

The initial assessment should include evaluation of chest pain and other associated signs and symptoms. Chest pain can be evaluated by using the OPQRST mnemonic. This involves assessing onset, provocation and palliation, quality, radiation, site, and time course. A quick, focused examination should be done by transport crews to determine the presence of other conditions that may complicate the management of these patients. These include evaluation for HF, cardiogenic shock, or other causes of hemodynamic compromise. A 12-lead ECG should quickly be obtained to determine whether ECG changes consistent with ACS are present. ECG changes indicative of unstable angina or NSTEMI include ST depression and inverted T waves, without the presence of Q waves. ECG changes seen with STEMI include ST elevation greater than or equal to 1 mm in two contiguous leads or greater than or equal to 2 mm in V2 and V3. Laboratory values including electrolytes, coagulation studies, hemoglobin and hematocrit, and cardiac biomarkers including troponin and CPK-MB should be reviewed for abnormalities.

Treatment goals in ACS include quick identification of the cause of the chest discomfort and aggressive management using evidence-based interventions.[22] Initial management involves rapid assessment and treatment of any abnormalities in airway, breathing, and circulation (ABCs). Continuous cardiac monitoring, oxygen saturation, supplemental oxygen, as indicated, and IV access should always be continued during transport. The current 2015 AHA Guidelines Update for Cardiopulmonary Resuscitation and Emergency Cardiovascular Care continue to recommend an arterial oxygen saturation of SaO$_2$ of greater than 93%.[5] Cardiac dysrhythmias should be treated according to ACLS protocols. Combi-pads should be placed and available for defibrillation and pacing if needed. Resuscitation equipment and emergency medications should also be readily available.

Immediate treatment of ACS includes the administration of oxygen, aspirin, nitroglycerin (NTG), and morphine as outlined in the ACS ACLS protocol.[22,26] A major goal in the treatment of ACS is to augment the anticoagulant properties that the body possesses and to interfere with the clot formation process. ACSs begin primarily as a process mediated by activated platelets; therefore therapeutic strategies are aimed at inhibition of platelets and interference with platelet-to-platelet interactions. Initial pharmacologic treatment begins with the administration of 325 mg of nonenteric-coated aspirin (ASA). Aspirin is a potent inhibitor of thromboxane, a stimulated platelet aggregation. Aspirin has clearly been shown to decrease MI and death in patients who present to the hospital with ACS.[22]

NTG works by relaxing vascular smooth muscle, leading to both arterial and venous vasodilation. Venodilation results in decreased preload and a decrease in ventricular wall tension. Arterial vasodilation leads to a decrease in systemic blood pressure (BP). These actions work to decrease myocardial oxygen consumption and demand. Coronary vasodilation also occurs, leading to increased myocardial oxygen supply. Initially three sublingual NTG tablets (0.4 mg) or one to two sprays are given under the tongue every 3 to 5 minutes for ongoing symptoms as tolerated by the patient or until the pain is relieved. An NTG drip is usually started if the pain is not relieved by initial sublingual doses (unless contraindicated). NTG is contraindication if a phosphodiesterase inhibitor has been taken within the last 24 to 36 hours depending on the specific medication. It should be used with extreme caution in patients with an inferior wall MI with right ventricular (RV) infarction, hypotension (systolic BP [SBP] <90 mm Hg), tachycardia, and bradycardia.

Morphine, which is a narcotic analgesic agent, may also be used to treat the pain associated with ACS. Usually 2 to 4 mg IV is given with repeated doses as indicated for ongoing chest pain per individual program protocols. Morphine helps to decrease workload on the heart by reducing sympathetic stimulation caused by pain and anxiety.

Other medications that may be used for treatment of ACS include β-blockers, heparin, and glycoprotein IIb/IIIa inhibitors. β-Blockers work by decreasing myocardial oxygen demand. These agents interrupt sympathetic impulses by competing with the neurotransmitter norepinephrine at the β-sympathetic nerve endings. β-Receptor inhibition results in decreased HR, decreased myocardial contractility, and slowed impulse transmission through the cardiac conduction system. These effects lead to decreased myocardial oxygen consumption. In addition, β-blockers decrease MI size and improve survival rates because of a decreased incidence of myocardial rupture and VF.[22]

Heparin is a potent anticoagulant that augments the body's ability to reduce thrombin generation and fibrin formation. Heparin does not dissolve a clot that has already formed; however, it does halt the propagation of existing clot or any new clots. Clinical evidence supports the use of heparin in ACSs.[22] The transport team should follow individual program protocols.

The glycoprotein IIb/IIIa receptors on the surface of platelets are responsible for the attachment of platelets to one another. Drugs that inhibit this process block the common final pathway of platelet aggregation; therefore they are inhibitors of the formation of thrombus. The agents currently in use, such as abciximab, eptifibatide, and tirofiban, all have different mechanisms of actions, dosing strategies, and half-lives. A review of these drugs is not included here because it is beyond the intended scope of this chapter. These medications, which have become an important part of the treatment of patients with ACSs, should be familiar to transport personnel. Current AHA 2015 guidelines recommend the use of glycoprotein IIb/IIIa inhibitors in addition to aspirin and heparin for patients with an NSTEMI or refractory ischemia.

Acute Myocardial Infarction: Assessment and Diagnosis

An *acute myocardial infarction* occurs as a result of coronary artery occlusion from a thrombus forming on the surface of a ruptured atherosclerotic plaque. When flow no longer exists in the coronary artery, the entire distribution of that coronary artery is at risk for injury or myocardial cell death. Initially, that wall of the heart becomes stiff and then stops moving, which results in a loss of left ventricular ejection fraction, potentially leading to significant valvular dysfunction and ventricular arrhythmias. The length of interruption in coronary blood flow will determine the resultant extent of myocardial injury and damage.

The cardiac blood supply is made up of three principal coronary arteries supplying nutrients during diastole. These vessels, the first branches off the aorta, originate from the coronary ostia at the level of the aortic valve cusps. The left main coronary artery divides into the left anterior descending (LAD) and the left circumflex arteries. The LAD supplies the anterior surface of the heart, the anterior two-thirds of the septum, and part of the lateral wall. The LAD distribution is represented on the surface ECG in the V or chest leads. The circumflex coronary artery supplies branches to the lateral and posterior surfaces of the heart. The circumflex is not well represented on the standard ECG. Changes caused by ischemia or infarction in the circumflex coronary artery may be seen in the lateral (I, aVL, and V5, V6) leads or in the posterior wall by inference from changes in the V1 and V2 leads, which appear as ST segment depression that is actually elevation on the posterior surface of the heart.

In 85% of patients, the right coronary artery (RCA) supplies blood to the inferior surface of the heart and to the posterior third of the interventricular septum by way of one of its branches, the posterior descending coronary artery. These areas of the heart are represented on the ECG as the inferior leads or leads II, III, and aVF. On the way to the inferior surface of the heart, the RCA is also responsible for supplying blood flow to the right ventricle. When an inferior wall MI is seen it is import to do a right-sided 12-lead ECG to search for the concurrent presence of an RV infarct because the RV is also supplied by the RCA. If an RV infarct is present, ST elevation will be seen in V4R. The maintenance of RV preload, with the administration of fluids, is the initial therapy for support of RV infarction. Positive inotropic agents, such as dobutamine, may be indicated to augment contractility of the damaged RV. Nitrates and other drugs that decrease preload should be used with caution because they may cause decreased CO and BP.

ECG changes seen with STEMI include ST elevation greater than or equal to 1 mm in two contiguous leads (leads that represent an area of the heart that is supplied by a single coronary), or greater than or equal to 2 mm in V2 and V3. A full discussion of 12-lead interpretation is beyond the scope of this chapter. Ongoing chest pain associated with 12-lead ECG changes that show ST segment elevation in contiguous leads known as an acute injury pattern together make the diagnosis of an AMI. ST segment elevation on the ECG represents ischemia, injury, and subsequent myocardial cell necrosis in the area of the occluded coronary artery.[27]

Initial assessment of patients with suspected AMI should include a detailed history, evaluation of chest pain and other associated signs and symptoms, and assessment for other concurrent conditions that could complicate management such as HF or cardiogenic shock. Chest pain can be quickly evaluated by using the OPQRST mnemonic. Patients who present with an AMI describe chest heaviness, discomfort, or pressure, often associated with shortness of breath (SOB), diaphoresis, nausea, and vomiting. The discomfort may radiate to the neck, jaw, or arms. Excessive sympathetic stimulation may result in an elevated BP and an increased HR. The patient should be evaluated for the presence of an S3, rales, or distended neck veins, which indicate the presence of HF caused by either severe left ventricular failure from the AMI or flash pulmonary edema resulting from the acute onset of severe mitral regurgitation.[28] The patient should also be evaluated for contraindications for specific types of therapy such as fibrinolytics.

Acute Myocardial Infarction: Management

Management of AMI has dramatically changed over the last decade because of improvement in pharmacologic support, hemodynamic monitoring, mechanical and surgical support, and the development of ventricular assist devices (VADs). Once the diagnosis of an AMI is clear, it should immediately prompt the decision of reperfusion therapy with primary angioplasty and associated pharmacologic therapy.

In AMI patients, the preferred reperfusion strategy is restoration of the normal blood flow in the infarct-related artery using primary percutaneous coronary intervention (PCI). It is recommended that fibrinolytic agents be used if PCI is unavailable in patients within 120 minutes without contraindications to use of these drugs.[22]

Critical care transport is essential for the rapid transport of these patients to tertiary institutions with angioplasty facilities. Acknowledgment of the presence of an AMI in the prehospital setting or at a referring institution should prompt the receiving institution to activate their cardiac catheterization laboratory staff. This process can be facilitated by transport personnel who can take AMI patients directly to the cardiac catheterization laboratory to reduce the "door to catheter" time. Direct physician-to-physician contact and the timely fax of electrocardiographic results can avoid unnecessary delays in reperfusion therapy.

As with the other ACSs, an AMI begins as a platelet problem but evolves into a process that ends in the formation of a thrombus through the formation and infiltration of the platelet plug by fibrin cross-links. The initial treatment goals are therefore similar to those for other ACSs. The use of aspirin, heparin, and glycoprotein IIb/IIIa inhibitors in addition to a definitive reperfusion strategy, such as emergent angioplasty, are the basic concepts of AMI therapy. Fibrinolytic therapy destroys fibrin in the intracoronary thrombus. In doing so, activated platelets are released from the thrombus. These activated platelets can reassemble and reocclude the vessel if adjunctive anticoagulation and antiplatelet strategies are not used. Oral antiplatelets will also be given in addition to ASA including clopidogrel, ticagrelor, and prasugrel.

Agents such as β-blockers, NTG, and morphine sulfate for pain control are important to decrease myocardial oxygen demand. In patients with adequate BP, IV morphine sulfate (2–4 mg) and IV NTG therapy can be used for pain control. β-Blockers (metoprolol 5 mg IV q 5 minutes for three doses) can help decrease myocardial oxygen demand in the patient with no contraindication (i.e., severe congestive HF, bradycardia, or diffuse wheezing).

Emergency *coronary artery bypass grafting (CABG) surgery* is performed in the setting of an AMI for patients with severe left main disease, failed angioplasty, and multivessel CAD not amenable to percutaneous revascularization. The time needed to activate a pump team and to place patients on bypass limits CABG as an initial strategy for reperfusion. Critical care transfer of these patients via air or ground is essential, and the transport crew should be knowledgeable and skilled in the care of these challenging patients.

Dysrhythmias

Serious electrical abnormalities of the HR and rhythm are classified as *dysrhythmias.* The function of the heart's electrical system is to transmit electrical impulses from the sinoatrial node (SA) to the atria and ventricles, causing contraction and delivery of blood to the lungs and body.

Altered blood flow to the myocardium during AMI or other cardiac conditions can affect the heart's conduction system leading to dysrhythmias. Dysrhythmias can be described as being too fast *(tachycardia)* or too slow *(bradycardia);* in regularity, one or more beats occurring earlier or later than expected; or in a different pattern of activation of the cardiac muscle. Dysrhythmias can originate in any area of the heart. They are usually divided into those that start in the atrium, the AV node, or the ventricle.

Identification of the origin of the dysrhythmias is based on the following[27]:
1. Rate: Normal is 60 to 100 beats/min, slow is less than 60 beats/min, and fast is greater than 100 beats/min.
2. Rhythm: Regular or irregular.
3. P waves: Present, morphology, one P wave before every QRS complex.
4. PR interval duration: Normal, shortened, or prolonged; normal is 0.12 to 0.20 second.
5. QRS morphology and duration: Normal duration is 0.06 to 0.12 second. Does QRS follow every P wave?

Pathophysiologic Factors

Cells that conduct the electrical current through the heart are known as pacemaker or automatic cells. The normal pacemaker of the heart, the SA node, is located at the junction of the superior vena cava and the right atrium. An electric impulse is initiated at this node, and it travels through the internodal pathways to the AV node. The AV node is located in the right atrium, directly above the tricuspid valve and anterior to the coronary sinus. The electrical impulse travels through the AV node and then moves through a common bundle of His, which divides almost immediately into the right and left bundles. The left bundle divides further to form two direct pathways to the anterior and posterior papillary muscle. The electrical impulse then permeates the many small fibers of the Purkinje network, beginning at the endocardium and ending in the ventricular myocardium.[13]

The primary pacemaker of the heart is the SA node, which normally pacing the heart at a rate of 60 to 100 beats/min. Secondary pacemakers include the AV junction with an inherent rate of 40 to 60 beats/min and the ventricles with an inherent rate of 20 to 40 beats/min. Dysrhythmias are the result of an irritable focus or foci in the electrical conduction system. Several mechanisms contribute to the development of dysrhythmias. The ischemic process and postnecrotic entities and underlying cardiac disease may enhance myocardial electrical instability leading to dysrhythmias. In addition, the development and treatment of myocardial failure result in mechanical dysfunction, metabolic changes, and electrolyte shifts as well as contribute to rhythm disturbances. Invasive cardiac instrumentation or pharmacologic therapies also have the potential to provoke serious dysrhythmias.

Dysrhythmias Originating in the Sinoatrial Node

Sinus Tachycardia

Sinus tachycardia originates in the SA and is characterized by a HR greater than 100 beats/min. It is a physiologic response to the body's demand for increased oxygen caused by conditions such as anxiety, exercise, smoking, infection, anemia, hypotension, and hyperthyroidism. Treatment is directed toward correcting the underlying cause of the tachycardia, as opposed to correcting the rapid HR. CO may be reduced as a result of decreased ventricular filling with rates greater than 180 beats/min, leading to further ischemia and tissue damage during AMI. IV or oral β-blockers may be used when the tachycardia produces symptoms, as long as the underlying cause is corrected first.[27,29]

Sinus Bradycardia

Sinus bradycardia originating in the SA is defined as a HR less than 60 beats/min. Relative bradycardia involves a HR that is not sufficient enough to maintain adequate CO and may be greater than 60 beats/min.[26] Sinus bradycardia may be caused by disease of the SA node, hypoxia, normal athletic heart, vagal stimulation, AMI, or by various medications. Patients with asymptomatic bradycardia require no treatment and should be observed for decompensation. Those that become symptomatic as HR falls, usually below 50 beats/min, will require treatment because of decreased CO and coronary perfusion. They may become hypotensive, have altered mental status, complain of chest pain and SOB, or have signs and symptoms of HF.[26] It is important to distinguish between asymptomatic and symptomatic bradycardia to determine when treatment is required.

The current AHA 2015 guidelines should be used for the treatment of symptomatic bradycardia, beginning with the administration of IV atropine.[7] The first dose is usually 0.5 mg IV and it may be repeated every 3 to 5 minutes to a maximum dose of 3 mg. Atropine enhances sinus node automaticity and AV conduction. If atropine is ineffective, prepare for TCP or the initiation of a vasopressor infusion using either dopamine or epinephrine. TCP should be started immediately if IV access is not available. Ultimately these patients may require transvenous pacing. The use of lidocaine can be lethal to a patient with bradycardia when the bradycardia is a ventricular escape rhythm.[30]

Dysrhythmias Originating in Atria

Supraventricular Arrhythmias

Supraventricular arrhythmias originate above the ventricle and reflect atrial irritability. An ectopic pacemaker outside the SA node, in the atria or AV junction takes over at a rate of 150 to 250 beats/min. It is referred to as paroxysmal supraventricular tachycardia (SVT) when it starts and ends abruptly. Atrial tachycardia, atrial flutter, and atrial fibrillation (AF) are examples of these dysrhythmias.

Atrial Tachycardia

Atrial tachycardia is a regular rhythm, greater than 150 beats/min, and is usually associated with a narrow QRS. The QRS may be prolonged if a bundle branch block or aberrant conduction is present. An impulse originating outside the SA node in the atria takes over as the pacemaker of the heart. The HR is usually between 160 and 240 beats/min. P waves precede the QRS but are often obscured because of the rapid HR.

Atrial Flutter

Atrial flutter presents as a series of rapid, regular flutter waves, often described as sawtooth in appearance. An ectopic pacemaker outside the SA node in the atria takes over as the pacemaker with an atrial rate of 220 to 350 beats/min. The ventricular rhythm is usually regular if the AV conduction ratio is constant, but it may be irregular if there is variable conduction through the AV node.

Atrial Fibrillation

AF occurs when multiple atrial ectopic atrial pacemakers fire chaotically in rapid succession with a usual atrial rate of 350 to 600 beats/min.[29,31] Impulses are randomly conducted through the AV node to the ventricles, resulting in a typically irregular ventricular response. The rhythm is described as being irregularly irregular. AF results in loss of effective atrial contraction (atrial kick), which may reduce CO by as much as 25%, and also promotes mural thrombus formation.[31]

Treatment of Supraventricular Tachycardia

Treatment of supraventricular dysrhythmias begins with determining whether the patient is stable or unstable, and then to provide treatment based on clinical condition and identified rhythm. The objectives of treatment are to control the rate, convert the rhythm, and use anticoagulation therapy when appropriate. Unstable patients have signs and symptoms such as altered mental status, hypotension, or chest pain attributed to the existing tachycardia. Patients who are symptomatic must be treated immediately to reverse the consequences of increased workload on the heart and reduced CO. These patients require immediate cardioversion as outlined in ACLS guidelines. If the patient is stable, the rhythm should be evaluated, and pharmacologic treatment is indicated according to ACLS guidelines. Initial treatment of stable SVT includes vagal maneuvers and administration of IV adenosine. Adenosine will not terminate atrial flutter or AF, but will help to slow AV conduction. Slowing AV conduction will assist in the identification of flutter or fibrillation waves. β-Blockers and calcium channel blockers may also be used if indicated.

Dysrhythmias Originating in the Atrioventricular Node

First-Degree Atrioventricular Block

First-degree AV block is characterized by a constant, prolongation of the PR interval greater than 0.20 second. There is a constant delay in the conduction of an impulse through the AV node. P waves are identical and precede every QRS complex. First-degree AV block has been associated with congenital structural heart disease such as endocardial cushion defects. Other causes include ischemia, anoxia, digitalis toxicity, and AV node malfunction. It is rarely treated, but the cause should be determined and corrected.

Second-Degree Atrioventricular Block

Mobitz type I (Wenckebach AV block) is characterized by the progressive lengthening of the PR intervals until a QRS complex is completely dropped, and the cycle is repeated. Each atrial impulse takes progressively longer to travel through the AV node until conduction is completely blocked. This is a less serious form of second-degree AV block and usually does not require treatment unless the patient becomes symptomatic.

Mobitz type II is recognized when the P waves are periodically blocked from conduction to the ventricles without a progressive prolongation of the PR interval. In this type of block, the PR interval of all conducted beats is constant. The P waves are identical and precede each QRS complex when they are present. Mobitz type II is more serious than Mobitz type I and often progresses to third-degree AV block. If the patient is symptomatic, immediate treatment with pacing or β-adrenergic support (dopamine or epinephrine infusions) may be required as outlined in the current ACLS guidelines.[26] Atropine is usually ineffective in reversing type II AV blocks with widened QRS complexes.[26]

Third-Degree Atrioventricular Block or Complete Heart Block

Third-degree AV block is a potentially lethal conduction abnormality characterized by separate and independent atrial and ventricular activity. Either sinus or ectopic atrial pacemakers control the atria, and a pacemaker that is distal to the AV block controls the ventricles. The ECG shows completely dissociated P waves and QRS complexes. Immediate treatment in symptomatic third-degree AV block involves the use of TCP or a transvenous pacemaker, if available. Pharmacologic therapy can include atropine at 0.5 to 1.0 mg (although normally ineffective unless the QRS is narrow) or the initiation of a vasopressor infusion using either dopamine or epinephrine.[26] Dopamine infusions are started at a rate of 2 to 20 μg/kg per minute and epinephrine infusion of a rate of 2 to 10 μg/min, and titrated to patient response. Ultimately these patients will require transvenous pacing.

Dysrhythmias Originating in Ventricles

Ventricular Arrhythmias

Ventricular ectopic activity is a common phenomenon in AMI, and *ventricular arrhythmias* are the major cause of sudden cardiac death in the United States. The most common cause of ventricular arrhythmia is ischemic CAD. Ventricular arrhythmias arise in the ventricles beyond the bifurcation of the bundle of His.

Death from a ventricular arrhythmia occurs through its interference with the cardiac pumping function. Several conditions that occur during the ventricular arrhythmia contribute to the decrease in CO, which in turn can cause syncope and lead to cardiac arrest. The loss of the normal AV sequence is associated with a significant decrease in CO. The rate of the ventricular arrhythmia also determines hemodynamic instability. A rate below 150 beats/min does not usually cause hemodynamic compromise if the duration is short. If the VT exceeds 200 beats/min, significant symptoms are usually present and can include dyspnea, lightheadedness, loss of vision, syncope, and cardiac arrest. Patients with ventricular tachyarrhythmias should be closely monitored because they have increased risk of progression to VF, especially with a history of compromised ejection fraction.

Ventricular Tachycardia

VT originates from an ectopic pacemaker in the ventricles, usually with a rate of 150 to 250 beats/min.[29] The QRS complexes appear wide and bizarre. The rhythm may be well tolerated or associated with hemodynamic compromise. Current emphasis related to treatment methods is still placed on whether the patient's condition is deemed stable or unstable, and with or without pulses. In assessment of the patient in VT, instability is determined by symptoms displayed such as chest pain, hypotension, decreased level of

consciousness, shock, SOB, or pulmonary congestion that can be attributed to the rapid HR, usually greater than 150 beats/min. If the patient's condition is determined to be unstable, the rhythm is wide and regular (monomorphic), and pulses are detected, then immediate synchronized cardioversion is indicated. If the rhythm is wide but irregular (polymorphic) with pulses present, defibrillation instead of cardioversion should be instituted. VT without pulses should be immediately defibrillated according to current ACLS guidelines.[26] In stable patients, VT is first treated with pharmacologic agents. The current ACLS guidelines recommend the use of amiodarone, procainamide, and sotalol as the antiarrhythmics of choice at this time. Lidocaine can also be used as an alternative agent in these stable patients. Magnesium should be considered in the patient with torsades de pointes. Current ACLS guidelines for specific algorithms should be used for treatment of all dysrhythmias.

Ventricular Fibrillation

VF is chaotic depolarization from multiple ectopic pacemakers in the ventricles. No effective contraction occurs, which results in severe hemodynamic compromise caused by a lack of CO. It is characterized by rapid, abnormal, fine or coarse fibrillatory waves, and the absence of QRS complexes. VF is the most common mechanism of cardiac arrest from myocardial ischemia or infarction. The best treatment for VF is early, high-energy unsynchronized defibrillation. High-quality CPR should be performed until defibrillation is available. If defibrillation fails, start pharmacologic treatment with epinephrine 1 mg IV push every 3 to 5 minutes. Vasopressin was removed from the most current ACLS guidelines because it was found to offer no advantage over epinephrine in cardiac arrest.[7] Antiarrhythmic drugs including amiodarone and lidocaine may also be given during cardiac arrest from VF between countershocks. Again, adherence to current ACLS guidelines regarding CPR, defibrillation, and pharmacotherapy is important.

Pulseless Electrical Activity and Asystole

Pulseless electrical activity (PEA) is defined as any organized rhythm without a pulse, and there is electrical activity but no mechanical contraction of the heart. The QRS complex may be wide or narrow, fast or slow, and regular or irregular. This excludes asystole, VF, and VT without a pulse. Asystole is characterized by an absence of ventricular contraction and CO without a pulse. The ECG will show a flat line with no discernible electrical activity, and no pulse will be present. Both PEA and asystole are life-threatening conditions, resulting in death unless they are quickly treated. Treatment for both PEA and asystole begins with high-quality CPR followed by the administration of 1 mg of epinephrine IV or interosseous every 3 to 5 minutes. CPR should not be interrupted during resuscitation. If during resuscitation a shockable rhythm arises, immediate defibrillation should be instituted. The current ACLS guidelines do not recommend the use of TCP for patients in asystole. Efforts should be focused on quick identification of reversible causes using the Hs (hypovolemia, hypoxia, hypo/hyperkalemia, hydrogen ion [acidosis], and hypothermia) and Ts (tension pneumothorax, tamponade [cardiac], toxins, and thrombosis [coronary and pulmonary]), as outlined in the current ACLS guidelines. Reversible causes must be rapidly searched for and treated immediately to have a successful resuscitation.

Cardiogenic Shock

Cardiogenic shock is a clinical condition of extreme pump failure leading to an inability of the heart to perfuse the vital organs. It is pump failure that results in inadequate tissue perfusion. Classic signs of cardiogenic shock include significant systemic hypotension and evidence of end-organ hypoperfusion, such as altered mentation and low urine output.[32,33] Hemodynamic parameters are often used to define this condition. These include persistent SBP less than 80 to 90 mm Hg or a mean arterial pressure (MAP) of 30 mm Hg lower than baseline, a reduced cardiac index (CI) of less than 1.8 L/min per square meter without support or less than 2 to 2.2 L/min per square meter with support, and elevated ventricular filling pressures (pulmonary artery wedge pressure [PAWP] of >18 mm Hg).[34] Often this diagnosis is made using a pulmonary artery catheter (PAC), which allows for measurement of both CI and filling pressures (PAWP). An alternative method involves using echocardiography. The most common cause of cardiogenic shock is MI in which there is extensive ischemic damage involving greater than 40% of the left ventricle.[32,33,35,36]

During the last two decades, the primary goal of therapy for the patient with AMI has been to manage or prevent pump failure. Because the amount of ventricular failure is directly related to the extent of infarction, therapies aimed at limiting MI size and early revascularization are imperative in reducing the incidence and extent of pump failure.

There are many other causes of cardiogenic shock including severe RV infarction, acute exacerbation of severe HF, stunned myocardium as a result of cardiac arrest or hypotension, advanced septic shock, significant dysrhythmias, valvular disorders, ruptured ventricular wall aneurysm, cardiac tamponade, and tension pneumothorax.[35,36]

Pathophysiologic Factors

Cardiogenic shock results when the heart is unable to pump blood forward, resulting in a decreased SV, CO, and tissue perfusion. Oxygen delivery falls causing a reduction in the delivery of oxygen and nutrients to the tissues. Ultimately end-organ damage and multisystem organ failure occur if this process is not reversed.

Assessment and Diagnosis

Cardiogenic shock is usually diagnosed based on clinical presentation and physical findings. The classic presentation includes severe systemic hypotension, signs of tissue hypoperfusion (altered mental status, cold, clammy skin, decreased urine output, and metabolic acidosis), and respiratory distress caused by pulmonary congestion. Patients in cardiogenic shock appear acutely ill and are in acute distress. They may complain of difficulty breathing and chest pain. Physical examination often reveals profound hypotension, signs of peripheral hypoperfusion, jugular venous distention (JVD), hypoxemia, acidosis, rales, and oliguria.[37,38] They often have an ashen or cyanotic appearance, and the skin is cool and clammy with mottled extremities. Some patients have a depressed sensorium as a result of hypoxemia. Pulses may be irregular if dysrhythmias are present, and peripheral pulses are faint and rapid. JVD is usually present. A repeat 12-lead ECG should be done to look for the presence of ischemia, injury, and infarct. A PAC may be placed in patients who do not respond to initial resuscitative efforts to allow for monitoring and guidance therapy related to CO and cardiac filling pressures.

Hemodynamically, patients in cardiogenic shock manifest marked hypotension, with an SBP of 80 to 90 mm Hg, or MAP of 30 mm Hg lower than baseline; a reduced CI of less than 1.8 L/min per square meter without support or less than 2.0 to 2.2 L/min per square meter with support; abnormal mental status; cold, clammy skin; decreased urinary output (UO); elevated HRs; and a PAWP of greater than 18 mm Hg.[34] They may also exhibit pulmonary congestion, arterial hypoxemia, and evidence of metabolic acidosis (low serum bicarb and elevated serum lactate). Dysrhythmias often occur as a result of hypoxemia, and the chest x-ray (CXR) may reveal pulmonary vascular congestion.

Patients in cardiogenic shock require frequent assessment of hemodynamic parameters, including BP, HR, and pulmonary artery pressures (if a PAC is present). They should be frequently assessed for peripheral perfusion, presence of edema, color and warmth of skin, blood gases, hemoglobin, and hematocrit to assess oxygen-carrying capacity and function.

Management

Initial management of cardiogenic shock includes early identification and rapid, aggressive stabilization before the onset of hypotension. Severe hypotension and hypoperfusion are treated with both pharmacologic and nonpharmacologic methods of circulatory support. Specific issues to be addressed include correction of hypoxemia, correction of electrolyte levels and acid-base balance, maximization of volume status, treatment of sustained dysrhythmias, inotropic and vasopressor support, early revascularization, and consideration of intraaortic balloon pump (IABP) support and the use of VADs. Oxygenation and airway support are imperative, and correction of hypoxemia may include intubation and mechanical ventilation. Patients with severe pulmonary congestion will require intubation and the use of positive end-expiratory pressure (PEEP). Electrolyte imbalances, such as hypokalemia and hypomagnesemia, create vulnerability to ventricular dysrhythmias, whereas acidosis may depress myocardial contractility.

Maximization of volume status necessitates fluid resuscitation unless pulmonary edema is present. PAWP should be maintained at the lowest value that results in adequate CO. Intake and output should be monitored carefully. Patients with inferior wall myocardial infarction often have an associated RV infarction. The maintenance of RV preload, with the administration of fluids, is the initial therapy for support of RV infarction. Discreet fluid boluses such as 250 mL of isotonic saline can be used with careful evaluation after each bolus to determine whether CO and perfusion have improved. Frequent assessment of PAWP and CO is essential. Pulmonary edema may result in the setting of overzealous, unmonitored fluid administration. Antiarrhythmic drugs, cardioversion, and pacing should be used promptly as necessary to correct any dysrhythmias or heart blocks that affect CO. Inotropic agents and vasopressors should be initiated for cardiovascular support in the presence of inadequate tissue perfusion with adequate intravascular volume. Nitrates, β-blockers, and angiotensin-converting enzyme (ACE) inhibitors, normally used to improve outcomes after AMI, can worsen hypotension and should be avoided in true cardiogenic shock. Mechanical circulatory support, IABP, and VADs may be needed to stabilize patient conditions until coronary angioplasty and can be used as a bridge to surgical revascularization or heart transplantation.

Pharmacologic Therapy

It is essential to aggressively treat severe hypotension and tissue hypoperfusion in cardiogenic shock to maintain vital organ perfusion. Pharmacologic management includes the use of both inotropic and vasopressor agents. Severe hypotension leads to hypoxemia and lactic acidosis, which may decrease responsiveness to vasopressors as well as cause further myocardial depression. Vasopressors used for the initial treatment of hypotension include norepinephrine and dopamine. The effect of dopamine is dose dependent. In higher doses, usually greater than 10 μg/kg per minute, it acts as an α-agonist causing vasoconstriction. Norepinephrine has both α-agonist and some β-agonist activity resulting in potent vasoconstriction as well as some positive inotropic effects. Some evidence suggests that outcomes may be better with norepinephrine versus dopamine.[39]

Dobutamine is a positive inotropic agent that can be used in patients that have an SBP greater than 80 mm Hg when CI is low and PAWP is high. This drug improves CO by increasing myocardial contractility. An alternative to the inotropic agent is milrinone. It is both a positive inotrope agent as well as a vasodilator. It is important to remember that dobutamine and milrinone do not reverse the hypotension that is seen in post-MI shock. Generally, vasopressors are used in patients who have severe hypotension, and a

positive inotropic agent is used when severe hypotension is not present. Both of these agents are often used in patients with cardiogenic shock.

Patients who are not hypotensive but in a low CO state may also require afterload reduction with vasodilators to decrease workload on the heart. Vasodilators should be used with extreme caution because they can cause further hypotension and a decrease in coronary blood flow. Vasodilators are used to increase forward flow by reducing afterload; these drugs include sodium nitroprusside and NTG. Sodium nitroprusside reduces afterload by decreasing filling pressures and can also increase SV. NTG reduces PAWP and left ventricular filling pressure and redistributes coronary blood flow to the ischemic area. Diuretic therapy is limited to treating pulmonary congestion and decreasing intravascular volume, improving oxygenation.[30,40]

Intraaortic Balloon Pump Counterpulsation

When pharmacologic support and adjunctive therapies fail to improve low CO and poor perfusion associated with cardiogenic shock, an IABP may be used as a temporary stabilizing therapy.

In the setting of cardiogenic shock complicated by AMI, the optimal strategy involves revascularization and adjunctive IABP support. Coronary reperfusion can be achieved by PCI, emergent CABG, or by fibrinolysis. Primary PCI is the preferred method of revascularization if it can be implemented within 90 to 120 minutes of initial hospital presentation.[41,42] Ideally, it should be performed within 90 minutes of first medical contact.[22] IABP can be used effectively to stabilize patients before angiography and revascularization. Stabilization with IABP and appropriate hemodynamic management, followed by transfer to a tertiary care facility, is the treatment option for those facilities without direct angioplasty capability.[41,42] Further discussion of IABP counterpulsation is discussed in Chapter 21.

Heart Failure

Definition and Pathophysiologic Factors

Acute heart failure (AHF) is common and potentially fatal in the critically ill. It occurs when the heart is unable to pump sufficient blood to meet the metabolic needs of the body, resulting in inadequate tissue perfusion.[28,43] Any condition that decreases the heart's ability to pump will cause HF. Blood begins to back up into the pulmonary and/or systemic circulations. Signs and symptoms seen in AHF are the result of the accumulation of fluid behind the left or right ventricle or both. This results in congestion of the vascular system draining into the heart. The most common cause of AHF is left ventricular systolic (inability to pump blood forward) or diastolic dysfunction (impaired ventricular filling). Damage to the myocardium for any reason will result in failure of the heart as an effective pump. There are many causes of AHF, including prolonged myocardial ischemia or infarct, heart valve disorders, conduction defects, wall damage from cardiomyopathies, and hypertension.[28] HF is a progressive, debilitating condition that ultimately results in death unless the patient is a candidate for cardiac transplant.

Assessment and Diagnosis

A careful history usually reveals the cause of HF, such as MI, hypertension, or valvular disorders. Left ventricular dysfunction from CAD and advanced age are the primary risk factors that contribute to the development of HF. Other risk factors include diabetes, angina, hypertension, a history of cigarette smoking, obesity, an elevated high-density lipoprotein, abnormally high or low hematocrit levels, proteinuria, and a history of CAD or previous MI. The patient has SOB, which begins initially with exertion and progresses to SOB at rest. In severe HF, the patient has orthopnea and must sit upright or lean over a table to breathe.

Physical examination reveals signs and symptoms resulting from excess fluid accumulation behind the left or right ventricles. In RV failure, JVD, elevated central venous pressure (CVP), hepatomegaly, and peripheral pitting edema without venous insufficiency may be present. In left ventricular failure, dyspnea at rest, orthopnea, cough, fatigue and weakness, elevated PAWP, laterally placed point of maximal intensity, and an S3 gallop may be present.[28]

Electrocardiographic monitoring may show the development of dysrhythmias such as AF, complete heart block, and rapid tachycardia, which could exacerbate pump failure. Laboratory data are nonspecific, although arterial hypoxemia and metabolic acidosis are common, and respiratory alkalosis may be present with significant tachypnea. CXRs can reveal cardiomegaly and may show pulmonary vascular congestion and interstitial edema. Invasive monitoring reveals an elevated right atrial (RA) and PAWP, elevated systemic vascular resistance, and low CO.[28] Transport crews must remain alert to factors that can aggravate the underlying cardiac dysfunction. These factors include extension of active ischemia or infarction, uncontrolled hypertension, or heavy alcohol consumption. Viral infections and pneumonias frequently trigger the onset of symptoms and may necessitate weeks of close supervision for recovery, if recovery is even possible. AF, which can cause or result from worsening failure, warrants the restoration of sinus rhythm to improve cardiac function. Obesity is both a primary cause and an aggravating factor for HF. Orthopnea is a sensitive symptom of elevated filling pressures, and the degree of orthopnea parallels the amount of increased pressure. JVD indicates the presence of elevated resting filling pressures. Peripheral edema may be seen in those with chronic HF. Weight gain may indicate an impending episode of HF. Abdominal symptoms can result from hepatic congestion. Once the patient is determined to be in failure, they must be evaluated for manifestations of hypoperfusion. Evidence of hypoperfusion includes low BP, narrow pulse pressure, cool extremities, and altered mentation.

Management

Knowledge of precipitating factors, physical findings, and past management of HF will assist in the treatment of these complex and challenging patients. Management of AHF focuses on the reduction of preload for relief of pulmonary edema, reduction of afterload with vasodilators to enhance SV, and use of positive inotropic agents to enhance contractile function. IV diuretics and nitrates are used for preload reduction. Afterload reducing agents and ACE inhibitors are used in the chronic, as opposed to acute, setting. Inotropic agents are rarely used to enhance contractility because of the increase in myocardial oxygen demand, unless shock is present.[28,30] Currently, β-blockers are used to improve LV performance and improve survival.[44]

Airway and oxygenation are the first priorities in management of AHF patients. The airway should be rapidly assessed and stabilized in patients presenting with acute dyspnea. Supplemental oxygen and assisted ventilation should be provided when indicated. Routine use of oxygen is not recommended unless hypoxemia (an Sao_2 of <94%) is present.[5] Noninvasive ventilation (NIV) is gaining more popularity as a way to reduce the need for intubation.[45,46] Patients with respiratory failure who fail NIV or have contraindications to its use should be intubated. Use of PEEP is often used to improve oxygenation when patients are mechanically ventilated. Pulse oximetry and waveform capnography measuring end-tidal CO_2 should be used to monitor ventilation and oxygenation during transport. Continuous ECG monitoring is needed to monitor for dysrhythmias that may occur as a result of electrolyte imbalances. Strict intake and output measurements must be maintained and recorded. Responses to medications should be closely evaluated and documented. All medication infusions should be maintained on IV pumps and titrated as indicated.

Acute Pericarditis

Pericarditis refers to inflammation of the pericardial sac. It is one of the most common disorders involving the pericardium, and it has many different causes. The pericardium is a closed fibrous sac that surrounds the heart. It consists of an inner serous membrane, called the visceral pericardium, which closely adheres to the superficial myocardium and coronary vessels. The fibrous outer layer that surrounds the heart is the parietal pericardium. The space between the visceral and parietal layers normally contains 10 to 20 mL of pericardial fluid that acts as a lubricant between the contracting surfaces. The exact role of the pericardium is unclear; however, it is believed to serve as a lubrication system, ensuring that cardiac motion is unimpaired by surrounding mediastinal structures. Because the pericardium resists stretching, it functions as a protective mechanism to prevent sudden dilation of the heart. The pericardium may also protect the heart from infection.

Pericarditis is often associated with AMI. It results from an extension of the infarction to the epicardial area and is associated with an inflammatory response localized to the pericardium bordering the infarction. It may also be a delayed response to a more generalized inflammatory process, such as in Dressler's syndrome. Other common conditions associated with the development of pericarditis include infection, collagen vascular diseases, uremia, malignancy, drug therapy, and trauma.[47,48]

Assessment and Diagnosis

Pericarditis may present as an isolated process or be a manifestation of another underlying condition.[47,48] The presentation of pericardial heart disease depends on the pericardium's response to injury and the subsequent effect on cardiac function. The presentation will vary depending on the underlying cause. Diagnosis and recognition of acute pericarditis in the emergent situation are largely dependent on a patient history of pleuritic chest pain and the presence of a pericardial friction rub.[47,48] Typical chest pain is described as severe, sharp, and substernal and increases with inspiration or in the reclining position. This pain may be further aggravated by coughing or movement and is reduced when the patient sits up and leans forward. Sitting up and leaning forward reduces pressure on the parietal pericardium, allowing for splinting of the diaphragm.[49] Substernal pain may radiate to the neck, shoulder, and back. It is important to distinguish chest pain caused by pericarditis from that of other life-threatening conditions such as MI, aortic dissection, and pulmonary embolism.

Physical examination reveals a pericardial friction rub that may be heard at various times and in various locations during the patient's course. This is highly specific to pericarditis. The friction rub resembles a high-pitched grating or scratching sound. It is best heard with the diaphragm of the stethoscope placed at the lower left sternal border or apex with the patient sitting up and leaning forward during expiration. Pericardial friction rubs may be distinguished from pleural rubs by having patients hold their breath during auscultation. Pleural rubs will disappear during this period because they are caused by friction between the inflamed visceral and parietal pleuras. A pericardial friction rub will continue to be heard because it is caused by friction between the two inflamed layers of the pericardium. The presence of a friction rub does not exclude the presence of a large pericardial effusion or tamponade. Associated signs and symptoms of pericarditis include fever and leukocytosis, dyspnea related to increased pain with inspiration, dysphagia related to irritation of the esophagus by the posterior pericardium, and sinus tachycardia. A normal BP should be present, without paradoxical pulse or venous distention.

ECG changes that may be seen include ST elevation and atypical T wave abnormalities caused by inflammation of the epicardium. Diffuse ST segment elevation across most leads of the 12-lead ECG in conjunction with PR segment depression is the typical ECG presentation.

Management

Careful evaluation should be done to distinguish pericarditis from other life-threatening conditions such as MI, aortic dissection, and pulmonary embolism. Most patients with pericarditis can be managed with medical therapy. Treatment is focused on relief of pain and resolution of the underlying inflammation. This is accomplished by treating with nonsteroidal antiinflammatory drugs (NSAIDs) unless they are contraindications. These include ibuprofen, indomethacin, and aspirin. Ketorolac, a parenteral NSAID, has also been found to be effective in the treatment of pericarditis.[50] It is also recommended that patients receiving aspirin or NSAIDs also receive a proton pump inhibitor for gastrointestinal protection.[48] During transport, a major priority of care is appropriate pain control and continued reduction of inflammation using the prescribed NSAID agents. Narcotic analgesia agents such as morphine or fentanyl should be considered for additional control of pain. Patients should be monitored for complications of pericarditis, such as pericardial effusion, which can rapidly accumulate resulting in cardiac tamponade.

Cardiac Effusion and Tamponade

The pericardium is a closed, fibrous sac surrounding the heart, consisting of a visceral and parietal layer. The space between the two layers normally contains between 10 and 20 mL of pericardial fluid that acts as a lubricant between the contracting surfaces. A *pericardial effusion* is present when there is an accumulation of more than the normal amount of fluid in this sac. Pericardial effusions may occur rapidly or over time. Effusions can be caused by any pericardial condition such as acute pericarditis, post-MI or cardiac surgery, infection, aortic dissection extending proximal into the pericardium, collagen vascular disease, and chest trauma.[49,51]

Cardiac tamponade occurs when the accumulation of fluid results in increased pressure and subsequent compression of all chambers of the heart to such an extent that early diastolic filling diminishes and CO is significantly compromised.[52]

Pathophysiologic Factors

The hemodynamic effects of effusion are related to the speed of accumulation of the fluid. Rapid accumulation of 150 to 200 mL may produce acute cardiac tamponade; in contrast, large pericardial effusions, which develop slowly, can be totally asymptomatic. Under normal conditions, between 10 and 20 mL of fluid may be present in the pericardial space. The development of a larger volume of fluid may result from pericardial inflammation of any cause, HF, traumatic injury to the heart, aortic dissection, or neoplasm. Accumulation of additional fluid in the pericardial sac begins to impede cardiac filling as intrapericardial pressure begins to rise. This leads to impaired CO, which ultimately results in cardiac tamponade.[52]

Assessment and Diagnosis

Mild-to-moderate pericardial effusions may not produce symptoms. If the fluid accumulates slowly, the fairly noncompliant pericardium stretches to accommodate the increasing volume with little or no rise in intrapericardial pressure until it reaches a size where it can no longer stretch. However, if the fluid accumulates rapidly, a small volume can be life-threatening. The clinical diagnosis of tamponade is usually made based on history and physical findings. Clinical symptoms of cardiac tamponade are related to systemic venous congestion, a reduction in cardiac SV, and respiratory effects of impaired ventricular filling. Early tamponade manifests as tachycardia, tachypnea, edema, and elevated venous pressure. The classic signs, described as Beck's triad, include distended neck veins resulting from elevated CVP, decreased BP, and muffled heart sounds. Pulsus paradoxus (abnormal fall in systolic pressure during inspiration caused by differential filling of the ventricles) may be present. The ECG will typically show sinus tachycardia and low voltage. Electrical alternans, a beat-to-beat alteration in the QRS complex, may also be present, reflecting movement of the heart in the pericardial fluid.[52] CXRs may show a widening cardiac silhouette with a clear lung field. Echocardiography is the recommended method for rapid and accurate diagnosis of tamponade, if available.

Cardiac tamponade from trauma is usually the result of penetrating injuries, but blunt injury may also cause the pericardium to fill with blood from either injury to the heart itself or from the surrounding great vessels. Cardiac tamponade should be suspected in any trauma patient with PEA or lack of response to volume resuscitation.[53] If early signs of cardiac tamponade are not treated, severe hypotension and RA and RV collapse occur, resulting in profound circulatory failure and shock.

Management

Emergent evacuation of the pericardial fluid is definitive therapy in the presence of acute cardiac tamponade. Hemodynamic support during preparation of the patient for pericardiocentesis includes administration of blood, plasma, normal saline solution, or lactated Ringer's solution. Pericardiocentesis is accomplished with needle aspiration of pericardial fluid via the subxiphoid method. Removal of even small amounts of fluid will result in temporary relief of symptoms. A positive pericardiocentesis caused by trauma necessitates an open thoracotomy for definitive treatment.

Nontraumatic Aortic Dissection

Aortic dissection is one of the most challenging disorders of the aorta that the transport crew will encounter. Despite advances in treatment, mortality from aortic dissection remains between 25% and 30%.[54] Survival is dependent on early recognition and rapid, aggressive treatment.

Aortic dissection occurs when an intimal tear or separation develops in the aorta, resulting in hematoma formation in the medial layer. The dissection can occur distal or proximal to the initial tear, and may involve the aortic valve or other branches of the aorta. Dissections can originate anywhere along the length of the aorta and are classified according to anatomic location.

Two commonly used anatomic classification systems are the DeBakey[55] and Stanford system.[56] The DeBakey system classifies dissections based on their site of origin. In type I, the dissection originates in the ascending aorta and extends distally; in type II, the dissection is limited to the ascending aorta; and in type III, the dissection originates in the descending aorta and extends proximally or distally. The Stanford system is more widely used and classifies dissections as type A or type B. Type A dissections involve the ascending aorta regardless of the primary intimal tear location, and type B includes all other dissections.

Conditions associated with aortic dissection include systemic hypertension, congenital abnormalities of the aortic valve, advanced age, and heritable disorders of connective tissue such as Marfan's syndrome, which is a nonatherosclerotic disorder of connective tissue that involves massive degeneration of elastic fibers in the aortic media. Complications of aortic dissection include compromised blood flow to visceral organs and the extremities and neurologic deficits because of interruption of flow in branch vessels. Patients with distal dissection are usually treated medically, unless the dissection is complicated by rupture of the aorta or compromise of blood supply to vital organs.[54] Surgery, emergent if necessary, is indicated for most patients with proximal dissection.[54]

Assessment and Diagnosis

The classic symptom seen in aortic dissection is the sudden onset of pain, described as ripping, sharp, knife-like, and tearing, that often originates in the back (interscapular) or substernal area and possibly extends down into the legs. This occurs in 90% of the patients who present with aortic dissections.[57] Anterior chest pain is seen with ascending dissections, whereas posterior chest or back pain is seen when the dissection is distal to the left subclavian artery.[58] The pain may be migratory as the dissection increases in size. Impaired or absent blood flow to peripheral vessels caused by the dissection will result in a bilateral or unilateral pulse deficit. Pulse deficit is defined as a weak or absent femoral, brachial, or carotid pulse.[58] A new diastolic heart murmur may be heard if the dissection propagates proximal to the aortic valve. Severe chest pain associated with this murmur signifies the presence of acute aortic regurgitation. Other signs result from obstruction of major vessels that originate from the aorta. Depending on the location of the dissection and the compromised vessels involved, the patient may have ischemia of various organ systems and signs and symptoms of cardiac disease. MI, cerebral insufficiency, cerebrovascular accident, hemiplegia or paraplegia, renal failure, and intestinal infarction may all result from dissections. A delay in diagnosis or misdiagnosis is common because of the diverse presentation that may occur with aortic dissections.

The patient with acute dissection is often in severe distress and appears to be in shock with pallor, sweating, peripheral cyanosis, and restlessness. Hypotension and shock-like symptoms are most commonly seen in patients with ascending aortic dissections.[59] Hypotension is usually a result of rupture of the dissection into the pericardial space and may lead to cardiac tamponade. Rupture into the pleural space or mediastinum is more common with proximal dissection.[60] However, the BP may also be elevated, often as high as 200 mm Hg systolic, with a significant difference between both arms in the presence of descending aortic dissections.[59] Differential BP and pulses may indicate compromise of blood flow to one or both subclavian arteries. Absence of femoral pulses may indicate extension of the dissection into the aortic bifurcation, with compromised circulation to one or both legs. Clinical diagnosis of aortic dissection is often made based on clinical presentation, but confirmation of the diagnosis requires imaging. Acute ascending thoracic aortic dissections are considered a surgical emergency and require immediate intervention. Descending thoracic aortic dissections in hemodynamically stable patients are managed medically unless continued bleeding or organ ischemia occurs, requiring surgical intervention.

Transport of suspected aortic dissections should not be delayed to obtain imaging studies. However, if available, they may be useful in conjunction with other diagnostic signs. Cardiovascular imaging used to demonstrate dissections includes computed tomographic angiography, magnetic resonance imaging, and transesophageal echocardiography. Radiographic findings suggestive of an acute aortic dissection include mediastinal widening, extension of the aortic shadow beyond a calcified aortic wall, a localized bulge on the aortic arch, a left apical cap, tracheal deviation, and left pleural effusion.[57]

Management

Prompt initiation of therapy and transport of patients with acute aortic dissection remains a challenge for transport crews who often care for these patients during the brief interval between the onset of symptoms and the occurrence of life-threatening complications. Acute management of dissections is aimed at controlling pain and halting the progression of the dissecting force by reducing BP and HR. Pain may be managed with IV narcotic analgesia while the transport crew constantly observes for signs of respiratory compromise. BP should be aggressively lowered to the lowest level compatible with adequate visceral, renal, and cerebral perfusion. In most cases a target BP of 100 to 120 mm Hg is used in the hypertensive patient with an aortic dissection.[61-63] Initial BP management involves the use of IV β-blockers to reduce the HR. This will minimize aortic wall stress and shearing forces on the aortic wall

before the addition of any vasodilator. IV β-blockers that are commonly used are propranolol, labetalol, and esmolol. The advantage of esmolol is that it is short-acting, cardioselective, and easy to titrate to the desired effect. Nitroprusside, a vasodilator, can then be added to the β-blockade if the systolic pressure remains elevated above the target BP. The goal of therapy in the hypertensive patient is to lower the BP as low as possible without compromising mentation or urine output.[61,63] Continuous BP monitoring with an arterial line is recommended for patients on nitroprusside drips using the arm with the highest BP.[61,63] Some programs are also using nicardipine drips as their second-line drug if β-blockade alone does not achieve the desired target BP. Nicardipine, a calcium channel blocker, has also been shown to be an effective agent for control of hypertension. In hypotensive patients, the cause should be determined and treated if possible before administering fluid.

Transport crews must be prepared to initiate intubation and assist with ventilation if the patient's condition deteriorates and he or she becomes hemodynamically unstable. At least two large-bore IV access sites should be established for transport. Fluids should be kept to a minimum unless severe hypotension or rupture of the aorta occurs in flight. Blood should be available for transfusion during transport. Cardiac rhythm, BP, and continuous waveform capnography if the patient is intubated should be monitored during transport. Inadequate pain or BP control and evidence of progressive dissection indicate an urgent need for surgical intervention. The transport team should not delay transfer to wait for laboratory results or radiograph results. Coordination of efforts among transport personnel and the referring and receiving hospitals expedites admission to the surgical department for prompt intervention.

Hypertensive Crisis

Hypertensive crisis is a potentially life-threatening complication of hypertension. It may occur in patients with or without chronic hypertension. Patients without prior hypertension may not tolerate BP levels as high as those patients with chronic hypertension.

The presence of end-organ damage determines whether the crisis is defined as urgent or emergent. Critical elevation of the BP without end-organ damage is considered a hypertensive urgency and can be treated with oral medication over the course of 24 to 48 hours.[28,30] Those with severe hypertension and manifestations of acute, ongoing end-organ injury are said to have a hypertensive emergency. Hypertensive emergency requires immediate reduction in BP to prevent end-organ damage.[28,30] The SBP often exceeds 200 mm Hg, with a diastolic BP greater than 120 mm Hg. No predetermined criteria exist for the level of BP necessary to produce a hypertensive emergency because an acute rise in BP from a normal baseline may produce symptoms of end-organ damage. This may occur in pregnant patients who develop eclampsia. The rate of rise of the BP and the difference between the patient's usual level and the level present during crisis are the more important factors. A hypertensive crisis is a rapid progressive rise in BP sufficient to cause potential irreversible damage to vital organs. The major organs at risk are the brain, heart, and kidneys. A variety of serious end-organ effects are associated with hypertension. These include CAD, ischemic and hemorrhagic stroke, aortic dissection, renal failure, and HF. A hypertensive crisis may cause aortic dissection, cerebral hemorrhage, renal failure, and left-sided HF.[28,30]

Assessment and Diagnosis

There are many risk factors for hypertension including advanced age, family history of hypertension, race, high sodium intake, excess alcohol use, excess weight, diabetes, dyslipidemia, renal disease, sleep apnea, endocrine disorders, various medications, and physical inactivity. Hypertensive emergencies are diagnosed based on the presence of severe hypertension with manifestations of end-organ damage.

The purpose of the physical examination is to identify signs of end-organ damage. Retinopathy, congestive HF, arrhythmias, or focal neurologic deficits may be present on clinical examination. Funduscopic examination findings consistent with retinopathy include retinal hemorrhages, papilledema, and exudates. Palpitations, angina, or congestive HF can present with cardiovascular decompensation. Signs and symptoms of left ventricular failure include chest pain, dyspnea, pink frothy sputum, rales, and bronchospasm. Neurologic symptoms may include altered mental status, headache, nausea, and seizures.[13,28]

Hypertensive encephalopathy is one of the most severe complications seen in hypertensive emergencies. It is characterized by the presence of progressive central nervous systems signs and symptoms, including severe headache, nausea, vomiting, and visual difficulties. Focal neurologic findings can include blindness, seizures, aphasia, and hemiparesis. If left untreated, symptoms may progress to convulsions, stupor, coma, and death. Hypertensive emergencies are often caused by mismanagement or patient nonadherence to treatment regimens.

Management

Therapy should be based on the clinical situation, critical organ involvement, and the desired time frame for lowering the BP. Identification of the specific antihypertensive agent and BP goals for optimal management varies depending on the specifics of the hypertensive emergency. Immediate, but careful reduction in BP is indicated. Rapid, uncontrolled BP reduction may result in ischemic damage to vascular beds that are accustomed to a higher BP. The majority of hypertensive emergencies can be managed by lowering mean arterial BP gradually by 10% to 20% in the first hour and by a further 5% to 15% over the next 23 hours.[64,65] The major exceptions to this include patients with ischemic strokes, acute aortic dissections, and nontraumatic hemorrhagic

stokes.[64,65] Target BP goals should be known before departing the referring facility.

Frequent, accurate BP measurement is often difficult during transport. Arterial pressure monitoring will provide the easiest and most accurate method for monitoring BP. Monitoring of cardiac rhythm, level of consciousness, and assessing for signs of impending pulmonary edema or cardiac failure will help the transport team evaluate whether the antihypertensive agents are effective. Several parenteral and oral agents are available to use in a hypertensive crisis. The choice of drug is dependent on the type of hypertensive crisis and the specific medications that are available. Examples of antihypertensive drugs that can be given IV include sodium nitroprusside, NTG, nicardipine, labetalol, esmolol, clevidipine, fenoldopam, hydralazine, and phentolamine. These are generally used in hypertensive emergencies. Oral agents are generally reserved for use in hypertensive urgencies in which there is hypertension but no signs of end-organ damage.

Sodium nitroprusside is one of the more common agents used to treat hypertensive emergencies. It acts by direct peripheral vasodilation with balanced effects on arterial and venous blood vessels. The antihypertensive effects of IV sodium nitroprusside are apparent in seconds and is dose dependent. Once the drug is discontinued, the pressure will rapidly rise to the previous level in 1 to 10 minutes. Infusion rates must be closely monitored to avoid sudden fluctuations in BP.

Hemodynamic Monitoring in Cardiovascular Assessment

Critical care transport requires specialized knowledge and skills related to hemodynamic monitoring. Use of these technologies allows for assessment of cardiopulmonary status and responses to therapy. Clinicians must be familiar with hemodynamic monitoring technologies and have the knowledge and skill to provide safe and effective care during transport. Space limitations, noise levels, and vibration in the transport environment may complicate the use of sophisticated hemodynamic monitoring equipment. Transport team members must refine their use of visual and tactile assessment skills for clinical patient evaluation. These skills should be used in conjunction with hemodynamic monitoring.

Cardiac Output

The circulatory system is responsible for maintaining adequate perfusion so that oxygen and nutrients are delivered to the tissues, meeting the metabolic needs of the body. Hemodynamic monitoring assists in the identification and timely initiation of interventions aimed at maintaining or restoring adequate tissue perfusion.

CO, defined as the amount of blood ejected from the heart into the systemic circulation per minute, is a major contributor to maintaining adequate oxygen delivery to the tissues. The normal range for CO is 4 to 8 L/min.[66] CI is determined by dividing CO by body surface area (BSA). BSA is based on height and weight. CI is a more precise measurement of cardiac performance because it allows for differences in body size. Normal CI ranges from 2.5 to 4 L/min per square meter.[66]

CO is determined by HR and SV. The SV, which is the amount of blood ejected from the heart per heartbeat, is dependent on preload, afterload, and contractility. Preload can be defined as the amount of blood in the ventricles at end diastole. Increased preload causes the cardiac muscle to stretch, resulting in an increase in the force of the following cardiac contraction. Starlings law states that an increase in preload or stretch will result in an increase in the subsequent force of contraction, improving CO.[67] Afterload is the amount of resistance the ventricles must overcome to eject their contents into the systemic or pulmonary circulations. Contractility is the force of ventricular contraction. It is determined by the amount of muscle fiber shortening that is needed to cause the force of contraction in the absence of changes in preload and afterload.

Invasive Hemodynamic Monitoring

Invasive hemodynamic monitoring is used to monitor a patient's hemodynamic state and allows for assessment of volume status and administration of fluids and medications. Invasive measurements are obtained using a fluid-filled, pressure monitoring system. The insertion of invasive lines should be done by qualified physicians or designated personnel who have validated skills and practice with these lines. Appropriate setup and maintenance of the pressure monitoring system are critical for obtaining accurate and reliable measurements. Transport crews must be familiar with hemodynamic monitoring technologies and have the knowledge and skill to provide safe and effective care during transport. These include the use of arterial lines, central venous catheters (CVCs) and PACs. Transports of these patients require careful monitoring and maintenance of the invasive lines to prevent accidental movement or dislodgement.

Basics of Pressure Monitoring

Invasive measurements are obtained using a fluid-filled, pressure monitoring system. Waveforms that are generated by the heart (mechanical signal) are detected by the pressure transducer and converted to an electrical signal that is displayed on the bedside or transport monitor.

Ensuring Accurate Measurements Setup

Appropriate setup and maintenance of the pressure monitoring system are critical for obtaining accurate and reliable measurements. This system consists of pressure tubing with a transducer and flush device, flush solution, a pressure bag, and a reusable pressure cable. Noncompliant pressure tubing should be used between the transducer and the invasive

catheter so that the physiologic signal is transmitted without distortion. Soft, compliant IV tubing should not be used because it may absorb a portion of the generated signal before it reaches the transducer leading to inaccurate pressure readings. A continuous flush system must be used to maintain patency of the system and to minimize clot formation.[68] Most often this is accomplished by placing the flush bag into a pressure bag that is inflated to 300 mm Hg. This allows the system to be flushed at a constant rate of 3cc/h. An alternative method involves placing the system on an infusion pump to maintain patency of the system. This is often done in small children and neonates. The system should be flushed to gravity including all ports before attaching to the invasive line. Gravity flushing prevents microbubble formation in the system. All stopcock ports should be flushed and any air removed from the system. Air bubbles present anywhere in the system will cause distortion of the signal, resulting in inaccurate measurements.[68] Once the system has been flushed to gravity, and all air eliminated from the system, it should be placed into the pressure bag and inflated to 300 mm Hg. Now the pressure monitoring system is ready to be attached to the invasive line once it has been placed into the patient.

Leveling and Zeroing The system must be leveled and zeroed to obtain accurate pressure measurement. The patient should be placed supine with the head of the bed flat or elevated 45 degrees.[68-70] Leveling eliminates the effects of the weight of the fluid-filled catheter tubing and fluid column.[67] This involves placing the air-fluid interface of the stopcock closet to the transducer at the phlebostatic axis (Figs. 20.1 and 20.2). The phlebostatic axis is used as the

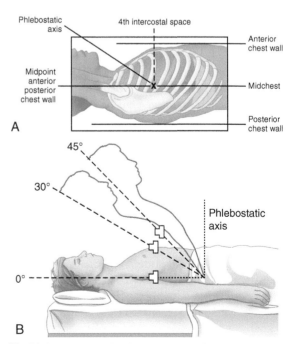

• **Fig. 20.1** Location of the phlebostatic axis. (From Lough ME. *Hemodynamic Monitoring: Evolving Technologies and Clinical Practice.* St. Louis, MO: Elsevier; 2016.)

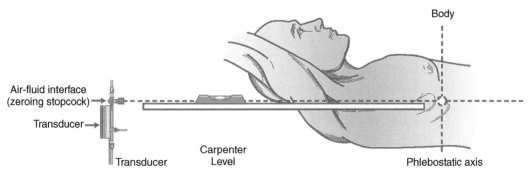

• **Fig. 20.2** Air–fluid interface. (From Preuss T, Wiegard DL. Single-pressure and multiple-pressure transducer systems. In: Wiegard DL, ed. *AACN Procedure Manual for Critical Care.* 4th ed. St. Louis, MO: Elsevier/Saunders; 2011.)

zero reference point and is considered to be at the level of the atria.[68-70] It is defined as the intersection of the fourth intercostal space and the midchest (midway between the anterior and posterior chest walls; Fig. 20.1). Marking the phlebostatic axis with an X on the chest will allow for future identification of this reference point. A carpenter level or laser level should be used to align the air–fluid interface with the phlebostatic axis. The system must be releveled with every position change to obtain accurate values. A 2-mm Hg error can result from every inch of discrepancy between the phlebostatic axis and the air–fluid interface.[67] If the air–fluid interface is above the phlebostatic axis, then erroneously low values result; if it is below the phlebostatic axis erroneously, then high values will result because of the effects of hydrostatic pressure.[71] In the transport environment, an effective strategy involves taping the transducer at the phlebostatic axis until the patient arrives at the receiving facility. This will eliminate the need to relevel with every position change. Zeroing and leveling of the system to the phlebostatic axis eliminates the effects of hydrostatic and atmospheric pressure. It assures that only heart or vessel pressures are measured. It is important to reconfirm that the appropriate pressure waveform is seen on the monitor screen after zeroing the system. Zeroing should be done once the pressure system is attached to the transport monitor and anytime questionable values are displayed. Once the invasive catheter is placed, the preprimed fluid-filled pressure monitoring system should be attached, making sure the pressure bag is inflated to 300 mm Hg.

Reading Pressure Waveforms All pressure measurements should be obtained at end expiration. End expiration is the point in the respiratory cycle in which there is the least effect of intrathoracic (pleural) pressure on intracardiac pressures.[67,72]

Dynamic Response Testing (Square Wave Test)

Dynamic response testing determines the system's ability to accurately reproduce a physiologic signal. The dynamic response should be assessed for all pressure monitoring systems using the square wave test. During a square wave test, the fluctuations that result from a fast flush are analyzed.

If an optimal square wave results, the system is assumed to be able to accurately record the patient's pressure waveform during monitoring.[67]

Selected Invasive Pressure Monitoring Technologies

Transport crews must have the knowledge and skills to safely care for patients with invasive pressure monitoring technologies including arterial lines, CVC lines, and PACs. This includes setup, zeroing, and leveling of the hemodynamic monitoring system.

Arterial Pressure Monitoring

Arterial lines are inserted when continuous BP monitoring is required or when frequent arterial blood gas analysis is indicated. Continuous monitoring of BP allows for timely titration of vasoactive and antihypertensive infusions. Common sites for insertion include the radial, femoral, brachial, and dorsalis pedis arteries. The radial artery is the most frequently used site because the hand has a secondary source of blood supply from the ulnar artery. It also runs over a bone, allowing for compression of the site in case of bleeding.[67] Complications of arterial lines include limb ischemia, infection, and bleeding.[67]

Transport crews are usually not trained and credentialed to place arterial lines but must be familiar with the setup, maintenance, and interpretation of values. The pressure monitoring system is set up and maintained as previously described earlier. Use of this pressure monitoring system allows for direct, real-time, and continuous monitoring of systolic and diastolic pressures as well as MAP. In adults, the previously described pressure bag setup with a continuous flush device should be used to maintain catheter patency to prevent clot formation.

Central Venous Pressure Monitoring

CVP monitoring allows for the assessment of right heart hemodynamics and may aid in evaluating responses to therapy. CVP is monitored using a fluid-filled pressure monitoring system that is attached to the distal port of the CVC. This allows for continuous monitoring of the CVP. Normal CVP ranges from 2 to 8 mm Hg in adults.[67] Serial measurements and trending of this value are recommended over interpreting a single static value. CVP measurements should be obtained at end expiration. The system must be set up correctly, leveled, and zeroed to obtain accurate measurements. The use of CVCs provides access to the central circulation for providing fluids, medications, venous blood sampling, and monitoring the CVP, if indicated. Common sites include right internal jugular, subclavian, and femoral veins. Complications include pneumothorax, hemothorax, infection, and bleeding.

Pulmonary Artery Monitoring

This invasive technology allows for direct measurement of RA pressure, pulmonary artery pressure, PAWP, and CO as well as the calculation of systemic and pulmonary vascular resistance. Some specialized catheters also allow for intracardiac pacing, continuous measurement of CO, and for fiberoptic measurement of continuous mixed venous oxygen saturation (SvO_2).

Transport crews must be competent in the use and clinical application of hemodynamic values and waveforms obtained from PACs. It is critical to understand the principles of proper placement and potential for migration of the catheter that can lead to life-threatening pulmonary artery infarct or rupture. This includes an understanding of its various lumens or ports and the use of pressure monitoring systems. Values obtained with a PAC provide information that may be trended to improve the care of patients with hemodynamic stability.

A PAC is a flow-directed, multilumen, balloon-tipped catheter inserted into the right side of the heart (pulmonary artery). It is used to assess volume status, administer fluids and medications, and to assess CO in the critically ill.[69] The balloon at the tip of the catheter allows blood flow to float the catheter through the vena cava into the heart, terminating in the pulmonary artery (Fig. 20.3). The standard 7.5 Fr

PAC has four lumens, is 110 cm in length, and has black markings every 10 cm starting at the distal tip of the catheter (Fig. 20.4). These markings are helpful for positioning during insertion as well as establishing the insertion depth once the catheter has been placed. Catheters that are placed from the subclavian vein should have an insertion depth of 35 to 50 cm, those placed from the internal jugular vein should have an insertion depth of 40 to 55 cm, and those placed via the femoral vein should be at 60 cm, 70 cm from the right antecubital fossa and 80 cm from the left antecubital fossa.[73] The catheter has multiple lumens or ports including the proximal injectate port, pulmonary artery distal port, balloon inflation port, and thermistor connector. Some PACs have additional infusion ports that can be used for the administration of fluids and medications. The proximal port opens up in the right atrium and is used to monitor RA pressure and for injection of a fluid bolus during intermittent CO measurement. The distal port opens up in the pulmonary artery and is used to monitor systolic, mean, and diastolic pressures in the pulmonary artery. This port also allows for sampling of mixed venous blood. Both of these ports should be transduced using a pressure monitoring system so that there is continuous display of the values and waveforms on the monitor. The balloon inflation port is used to obtain a PAWP, which is obtained by slowly inflating the balloon with air, using a preset 1.5-mL syringe until the pulmonary artery pressure converts to a PAWP waveform (Fig. 20.5). Normally it should take between 1.25 and 1.5 mL of air to convert from a pulmonary artery to a PAWP waveform.[73] The balloon should not be inflated for more than 2 to 4 respiratory cycles (8–15 seconds), and once a PAWP reading is obtained, it should be passively deflated by removing the syringe from the balloon port. Active deflation by pulling back on the syringe may result in tearing of the balloon. Pulmonary rupture resulting in life-threatening hemorrhage may result from prolonged

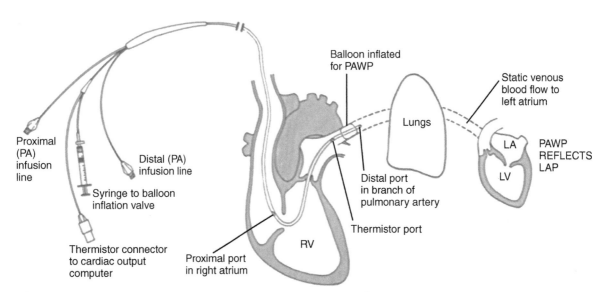

• **Fig. 20.3** Position of pulmonary artery in the heart. (From Preuss T, Wiegard DL. Single-pressure and multiple pressure transducer systems. In: Wiegard DL, ed. *AACN Procedure Manual for Critical Care.* 4th ed. St. Louis, MO: Elsevier/Saunders; 2011.)

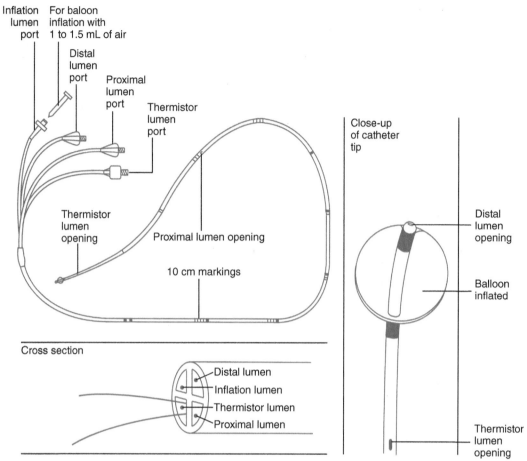

• **Fig. 20.4** Characteristics of the pulmonary artery catheter. (From Preuss T, Wiegard DL. Single-pressure and multiple pressure transducer systems. In: Wiegard DL, ed. *AACN Procedure Manual for Critical Care.* 4th ed. St. Louis, MO: Elsevier/Saunders; 2011.)

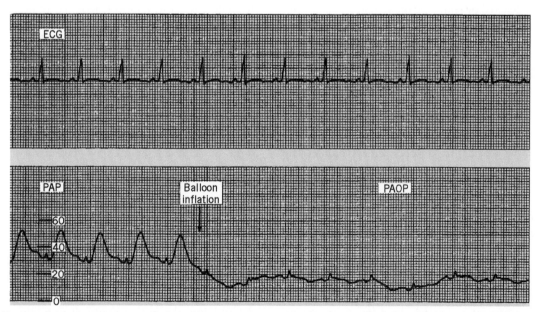

• **Fig. 20.5** Change of pulmonary artery waveform to pulmonary artery wedge pressure waveform. (From Preuss T, Wiegard DL. Single-pressure and multiple-pressure transducer systems. In: Wiegard DL, ed. *AACN Procedure Manual for Critical Care.* 4th ed. St. Louis, MO: Elsevier/Saunders; 2011.)

balloon inflation.[73] The thermistor port allows for monitoring of a temperature change during bolus CO measurement and for the monitoring of core body temperature.

Complications include dysrhythmias, pulmonary artery rupture, pulmonary infarct, embolic events, and infection. Routine use of these catheters has decreased over the years, but the transport crew may still encounter their use in select populations including patients with cardiogenic shock, complicated MI and HF, trauma, acute respiratory distress syndrome, and pulmonary hypertension.[73] Because of this, transport crews should be familiar with normal values and waveform morphology for each of the measurements obtained with a PAC.

Verification of correct PAC position is made using CXR and waveform analysis. Dysrhythmias may result if the catheter is pulled back into the right ventricle. A catheter that is positioned too distal into the pulmonary artery may become spontaneously wedged, resulting in a pulmonary infarct or rupture.[69] Steps must be taken to ensure accurate measurement of hemodynamic values including appropriate setup, leveling, zeroing, validating correct catheter position, and assessing the dynamic response of the pressure monitoring system.

Transport considerations specific to PACs include the following: (1) documentation of insertion depth to allow for identification of catheter migration; (2) always transducing the distal port using a pressure monitoring system, confirming the presence of a pulmonary artery waveform; and (3) watching for catheter migration. Catheters that migrate proximal into the RV or that become permanently wedged must be repositioned to prevent life-threatening complications including dysrhythmias and pulmonary artery rupture. This should be done following specific programs, procedures, and protocols, such as (4) verifying that the balloon is deflated by removing the syringe and allowing for passive deflation, (5) taking the original 1.5-mL syringe with the catheter, (6) never flushing the catheter in a wedged positon, and (7) never using the distal port to administer fluids or medications other than the saline flush at 1 to 3 mL/h.

General Transport Safety and Consideration (Invasive Hemodynamic Lines)

On arrival to the bedside, the transport crew should evaluate the pressure monitoring setup, hemodynamic waveforms, and values being obtained with invasive hemodynamic technologies. The catheter site and insertion depth (CVC and PACs) should be documented and the CXR reviewed for placement if available. The catheter site should be assessed and covered with an occlusive dressing. Catheters must be secured and the patency of all ports confirmed before changing over to the transport monitor. Vented caps on stopcock ports should be replaced with sterile, nonvented caps to prevent accidental blood loss or infection. Excess tubing and stopcocks should be removed from the pressure monitoring system to reduce distortion in the system. Once the invasive line is connected to the transport

monitor, it should be zeroed and leveled to the phlebostatic axis. The pressure bag should be inflated to 300 mm Hg and monitored periodically during transport to maintain patency of the system. Waveforms and hemodynamic data should be evaluated during transport. The distal port of all PACs must be transduced with a pressure monitoring system to monitor for catheter migration. Monitor alarms should be set to alert the transport crew that a change in the patient's condition has occurred or that the catheter has migrated or become dislodged. Potential complications that can occur during transport include catheter migration or dislodgement, clot formation at the catheter tip, and hemorrhage from line disconnection. Loss of distal circulation can occur with arterial lines. Direct pressure should be held to the site of any dislodged catheter until bleeding stops.

Less Invasive Hemodynamic Monitoring

Less invasive hemodynamic monitoring technologies now allow for the evaluation of flow-determined hemodynamic parameters in the critically ill. Some of these include CO, SV, pulse pressure variation, and SV variation. Most of these systems are based on arterial waveform analysis in which SV is estimated based on variation in the pulse waveform.[74] These less invasive hemodynamic technologies differ in several ways including the algorithm used to determine the values, the way the information from the arterial waveform is transformed, requirement for calibration, the required site for arterial catheter placement, and the accuracy with which the parameters such as CO are achieved.[74] Several of the currently available technologies that analyze the arterial pulse wave morphology include the FloTrac (Edwards Lifesciences Corporation, Irvine, California), PiCCO (Pulsion, Feldkirchen, Germany), and LiDCO (LiDCO Ltd., London, United Kingdom) systems.[75] An accurate arterial waveform is required to obtain valid data from these technologies. These systems use the previously described fluid-filled arterial line setup. The system should be leveled and zeroed to the phlebostatic axis. Distortion of the arterial waveform caused by technical issues, such as inaccurate leveling to the phlebostatic axis, over or under damping, or from dysrhythmias, may result in erroneous values.[76] Because these systems are based on the arterial waveform, it is imperative that an accurate arterial waveform be achieved for accurate measurement of SV and therefore CO. Currently, an additional monitor is required for these technologies.

Noninvasive Hemodynamic Monitoring

Noninvasive methods used to assess the hemodynamic status of the patient include the monitoring of the capillary refill, pulse rate and quality, BP, mentation, UO, and skin temperature. Mental status changes are important when determining the patient's overall condition. Significant changes in mentation occur in shock when flow is compromised to the vital organs. Skin temperature and color, capillary refill, and UO in the absence of renal disease reflect tissue perfusion as it relates to CO and intravascular volume. A combination of noninvasive methods such as capillary refill time, quality of the heart rate, and quality of the pulse or pulse contour should be used in conjunction with hemodynamic monitoring to assess the adequacy of CO during transport of critically ill patients.

BP measurements are frequently used to make clinical decision during transport. The gold standard for monitoring BP is direct measurement using an arterial pressure monitoring system.[77] Direct BP monitoring via an arterial line is more accurate than indirect pressures specifically in the presence of hypertension, hypothermia, and shock.[77] Unfortunately, invasive arterial pressure monitoring is not always feasible in the transport environment. Because of this, noninvasive or indirect BP monitoring is frequently relied on for measurements of BP. BP can be obtained noninvasively using mechanical Doppler augmentation, automated BP devices (NIBP), or palpation of the radial pulse with a sphygmomanometer and cuff. These noninvasive, indirect measures assess flow, whereas direct arterial pressure monitoring measures pressure. It is important to keep in mind that direct and indirect measures will not always correlate because of the differences between measuring flow versus pressure. Inaccuracies in noninvasive BP monitoring frequently occur because of inappropriate cuff size or positioning of the extremity during BP measurement. The BP cuff width should be 40% of the arm circumference or one that covers two-thirds of the extremity being used.[71,78,79] Using a cuff that is too large will result in erroneously low readings. A cuff that is too small will result in erroneously high readings. Because of this, the transport crew should carry several sizes of cuffs to accommodate for patient size and age. Accuracy is also affected by the position of the extremity in which the BP is being taken. The extremity should be positioned at the phlebostatic axis (mid chest level) for accurate BP reading. Elevation of the extremity above the phlebostatic axis will result in erroneously low values and if placed below this level will result in erroneously high vales. Although BP measuring devices can be useful for monitoring trends in the patient's hemodynamic status, the patient's hemodynamic status should be evaluated with multiple methods rather than one specific parameter such as BP.

The stresses of flight, such as the effect of vibration on biomedical equipment and electromagnetic interference, has not been defined totally.[77] Thus transport crews must use a combination of invasive and noninvasive assessment methods to evaluate patient status throughout the transport process.

Critical Care Transport of the Cardiovascular Patient

Specialized skills and knowledge are required for transport of patients with cardiovascular emergencies. Proper patient preparation, stabilization, and resuscitation should be performed during the transport of these challenging and critically ill patients. This should include assessment, planning, intervention, and evaluation.

Assessment

Assessment of the cardiovascular patient begins with the initial information elicited from the referring agency by dispatch personnel. This information can be invaluable for evaluating the best vehicle for patient transport and is helpful for air transport (especially when flying in an aircraft with limited space and weight restrictions), for anticipating in-flight emergencies, and for preparing the receiving agency for the patient. Time en route to the referring agency can be spent developing a preliminary plan of care based on initial information obtained from dispatch and the referring agency when available.

For the cardiovascular patient, assessment and preparation for transport are directed toward recognition, prevention, and correction of hypoxia and maintenance of adequate tissue perfusion and CO. The amount of time spent on assessment of the cardiovascular patient depends on the severity of the illness and the need for rapid intervention. The transport crew should obtain as much information as possible to provide safe and efficient transport to a definitive care institution and to ensure continuity of care.

A brief history of the event may be elicited from the patient, family members, or referring agency personnel. A general appraisal of the patient can be made while approaching the bedside and observing at that time the skin color, diaphoresis, activity or position of comfort, and respiratory distress. This should include observing for the presence of IV drug infusions, the amount of oxygen that is being delivered, the presence of invasive hemodynamic monitoring lines, and the cardiac rhythm displayed on the monitor. An initial perception of the situation helps to organize and direct management of the patient for efficient and safe transport.

The physical examination is often abbreviated because of time constraints and is based on the transport crew's judgment in determining what information is vital for transport. Hands-on assessment of the patient includes confirmation of vital signs and hemodynamic readings and the identification of implications for continued emergency care. Initial evaluation of airway, breathing, and circulation are of paramount importance. If the patient is not in immediate need of CPR, the overall cardiovascular status should be evaluated. Any necessary procedures should be performed at this time, such as intubation, IV or central line insertion, chest thoracostomy tube insertion, or additional therapeutic interventions as indicated.

Planning and Intervention

Adequate management and preparation of the patient for transport can greatly reduce the need for resuscitative measures en route to receiving facilities. Planning care for transport of the critical cardiovascular patient includes anticipating complications that may occur as a result of the disease process. This requires a strong critical care knowledge base and ongoing competency in the transport of the critically ill.

Evaluation

Throughout the transport process, the transport team must systematically evaluate the patient's progress, analyze data, and modify the plan of care based on the patient's response to therapy. In the transport environment, continual assessment and monitoring of the patient provide data regarding the success or failure of each intervention.

Summary

Technologic advancement is driving the medical industry, which in turn affects air and ground medical transportation programs. The critical care transportation industry must adapt to and be proficient with the ever-changing technology that patients and their families are using in their communities. Chapter 21 contains a thorough explanation of the current methods used for mechanical management of the patient with cardiovascular disease. One day these patients will inevitably need emergent transportation, and critical care transport programs must be educated and prepared to provide optimal patient care.

References

1. McBride LE. Transfer of patients receiving advanced mechanical circulatory support. *J Thoracic Cardiovasc Surg*. 2000;119(5):1015.
2. Hainsworth RD. Cardiovascular adjustments for life at high altitude. *Respir Physiol Neurobiol*. 2007;158(2-3):204-211.
3. Damergis JA. Physiological parameter changes of high altitude and their correlation with acute Mountain sickness. *Ann Emerg Med*. 2008;51(4):536.
4. Erdmann JS. Effects of exposure to altitude on men with coronary artery disease and impaired left Ventricular function. *Am J Cardiol*. 1998;81(3):266-270.
5. Callaway CW, Donnino MW, Fink EL, et al. Part 8: post-cardiac arrest care: 2015 American Heart Association Guidelines Update for Cardiopulmonary Resuscitation and Emergency Cardiovascular Care. *Circulation*. 2015;132(suppl 2):S465-S482.
6. Holleran RS. *ASTNA Patient Transport: Principles and Practice*. 4th ed. St. Louis, MO: Mosby Elsevier; 2010.
7. Link MS, Berkow LC, Kudenchuk PJ, et al. Part 7: adult advanced cardiovascular life support: 2015 American Heart Association Guidelines Update for Cardiopulmonary Resuscitation and Emergency Cardiovascular Care. *Circulation*. 2015;132(suppl 2):S444-S464.
8. Hickman BM. Stress and the effects of air transport on flight crews. *Air Med J*. 2001;20(6):6-9.
9. Kleinman ME, Brennan EE, Goldberger ZD, et al. Part 5: adult basic life support and cardiopulmonary resuscitation quality: 2015 American Heart Association Guidelines Update for Cardiopulmonary Resuscitation and Emergency Cardiovascular Care. *Circulation*. 2015;132(suppl 2):S414-S435.
10. Wik L, Kramer-Hohansen J, Myklebust H, et al. Quality of cardiopulmonary resuscitation during out-of-hospital cardiac arrest. *JAMA*. 2005;293(3):299-304.
11. Brooks SC, Anderson ML, Bruder E, et al. Part 6: alternative techniques and ancillary devices for cardiopulmonary resuscitation: 2015 American Heart Association Guidelines Update for Cardiopulmonary Resuscitation and Emergency Cardiovascular Care. *Circulation*. 2015;132(suppl 2):S436-S443.
12. Hulleman M, Mes H, Blom MT, Koster RW. Conduction disorders in bradysystolic out-of-hospital cardiac arrest. *Resuscitation*. 2016;106:113-119.
13. Woods SL. *Cardiac Nursing*. 4th ed. Baltimore, MD: Wolters Kluwer/Lippincott Williams & Wilkins; 2010.
14. Nielsen N, Wetterslev J, Cronberg T, et al. Targeted temperature management at 33(C versus 36(C after cardiac arrest. *N Engl J Med*. 2013;369(23):2197.
15. Hypothermia after Cardiac Arrest Study Group. Mild therapeutic hypothermia to improve the neurologic outcome after cardiac arrest. *N Engl J Med*. 2002;346(8):549-556.
16. Bernard SA, Gray TW, Buist MD, et al. Treatment of comatose survivors of out-of-hospital cardiac arrest with induced hypothermia. *N Engl J Med*. 2002;346(8):557-563.
17. Kim F, Olsufka M, Longstreth Jr WT, et al. Pilot randomized clinical trial of prehospital induction of mild hypothermia in out-of-hospital cardiac arrest patients with a rapid infusion of 4 degrees C normal saline. *Circulation*. 2007;115(24):3064-3070.
18. Kämäräinen A, Virkkunen I, Tenhunen J, et al. Prehospital therapeutic hypothermia for comatose survivors of cardiac arrest: a randomized controlled trial. *Acta Anaesthesiol Scand*. 2009;53 (7):900-907.
19. Bernard SA, Smith K, Cameron P, et al. Rapid Infusion of Cold Hartmanns Investigators. Induction of prehospital therapeutic hypothermia after resuscitation from nonventricular fibrillation cardiac arrest. *Crit Care Med*. 2012;40(3):747-753.
20. Kim F, Nichol G, Maynard C, et al. Effect of prehospital induction of mild hypothermia on survival and neurological status among adults with cardiac arrest: a randomized clinical trial. *JAMA*. 2014;311(1):45-52.
21. Debaty G, Maignan M, Savary D, et al. Impact of intra-arrest therapeutic hypothermia in outcomes of prehospital cardiac arrest: a randomized controlled trial. *Intensive Care Med*. 2014;40 (12):1832-1842.
22. O'Connor RE, Al Ali AS, Brady WJ, et al. Part 9: acute coronary syndromes: 2015 American Heart Association Guidelines Update for Cardiopulmonary Resuscitation and Emergency Cardiovascular Care. *Circulation*. 2015;132(suppl 2):S483-S500.
23. Corti RH. Evolving concepts in the triad of atherosclerosis, inflammation, and thromboses. *J Thrombolysis*. 2004;17(1):35-44.
24. Freedman JL. The role of platelets in coronary disease. Available at http://www.UpToDate.com; Accessed September 2016.
25. Klein L. Clinical implications and mechanisms of plaque rupture in acute coronary syndromes. *Am Heart Hosp*. 2005;33(4):249-255.
26. American Heart Association. *Advanced Cardiovascular Life Support Provider Manual*. Dallas, TX: American Heart Association; March 2016.
27. Dubin, D. *Rapid Interpretation of EKG's*. 6th ed. Tampa, FL: Cover Publishing Company; 2000.
28. Kasper DL. *Harrison's Principles of Internal Medicine*. 19th ed. New York: McGraw-Hill Medical; 2015.
29. Hammond BB, Zimmermann PG, eds. *Sheehy's Manual of Emergency Care*. 7th ed. St. Louis, MO: Emergency Nurses Association. Elsevier/Mosby; 2013.

30. Papadakis MA. *CURRENT Medical Diagnosis and Treatment 2016.* 55th ed. New York: McGraw-Hill; 2016.

31. Wesley K. In *Huszar's Basic Dysrhythmias and Acute Coronary Syndromes: Interpretation & Management.* 4th ed. St. Louis, MO: Elsevier/Mosby; 2011.

32. Reynolds HR, Hochman JS. Cardiogenic shock: current concepts and improving outcomes. *Circulation.* 2008;117(5):686.

33. Hochman JS. Cardiogenic shock complicating acute myocardial infarction: expanding the paradigm. *Circulation.* 2003;107(24): 2998.

34. Hochman JS. Clinical manifestations and diagnosis of cardiogenic shock in acute myocardial infarction. Available at http://www.UpToDate.com; Accessed September 2016.

35. Hollenberg SM, Kavinsky CJ, Parrillo JE. Cardiogenic shock. *Ann Intern Med.* 1999;131(1):47-59.

36. Hochman JS, Boland J, Sleeper LA, et al. Current spectrum of cardiogenic shock and effect of early revascularization on mortality. Results of an International Registry. SHOCK Registry Investigators. *Circulation.* 1995;91(3):873-881.

37. Menon V, Slater JN, White HD, et al. Acute myocardial infarction complicated by systemic hypoperfusion without hypotension: report of the SHOCK trial registry. *Am J Med.* 2000;108 (5):374-380.

38. Menon V, White H, LeJemtel T, et al. The clinical profile of patients with suspected cardiogenic shock due to predominant left ventricular failure: a report from the SHOCK Trial Registry. Should we emergently revascularize Occluded Coronaries in cardiogenic shock? *J Am Coll Cardiol.* 2000;36(3 suppl A):1071-1076.

39. De Backer D, Biston P, Devriendt J, et al. Comparison of dopamine and norepinephrine in the treatment of shock. *N Engl J Med.* 2010;362(9):779-789.

40. Williams SW. Management of cardiogenic shock complicating acute myocardial infarction towards evidence based practice. *Heart.* 2000;83(6):621-626.

41. O'Gara PT, Kushner FG, Ascheim DD, et al. 2013 ACCF/AHA guideline for the management of ST-elevation myocardial infarction: executive summary: a report of the American College of Cardiology Foundation/American Heart Association Task Force on Practice Guidelines. *Circulation.* 2013;127(4):529-555.

42. O'Gara PT, Kushner FG, Ascheim DD, et al. 2013 ACCF/AHA guideline for the management of ST-elevation myocardial infarction: a report of the American College of Cardiology Foundation/American Heart Association Task Force on Practice Guidelines. *Circulation.* 2013;127(4):e362-e425.

43. Wright SM. Pathophysiology of congestive heart failure. *J Cardiovasc Nurs.* 1990;4(3):1-16.

44. Capomolla S, et al. Beta blockade therapy in chronic heart failure: diastolic function and mitral regurgitation improvement by carvedilol. *Am Heart J.* 2000;193(4):596-608.

45. Heart Failure Society of America, Lindenfeld J, Albert NM, et al. Heart Failure Society of America 2010 Comprehensive Heart Failure Practice Guideline. *J Card Fail.* 2010;16(6):e1-e194.

46. Vital FM, Ladeira MT, Atallah AN. Non-invasive positive pressure ventilation (CPAP or bilevel NPPV) for cardiogenic pulmonary edema. *Cochrane Database Syst Rev.* 2013;CD005351.

47. LeWinter M. Clinical practice. Acute pericarditis. *N Engl J Med.* 2014;371(25):2410-2416.

48. Imazio M, Gaita F. Diagnosis and treatment of pericarditis. *Heart.* 2015;101(14):1159-1168.

49. Spodick DH. Acute, clinically noneffusive ("dry") pericarditis. In: Spodick DH, ed. *The Pericardium: A Comprehensive Textbook.* New York: Marcel Dekker; 1997.

50. Arunasalam S, Siegel RJ. Rapid resolution of symptomatic acute pericarditis with ketorolac tromethamine: a parenteral nonsteroidal antiinflammatory agent. *Am Heart J.* 1993;125(5 Pt 1): 1455-1458.

51. Troughton RW, Asher CR, Klein AL. Pericarditis. *Lancet.* 2004; 363(9410):717-727.

52. Spodick DH. Acute cardiac tamponade. *N Engl J Med.* 2003;346 (7):684-690.

53. Bursi FE. Heart failure and death after myocardial infarction in the community; the emerging role of mitral regurgitation. *Circulation.* 2005;111(3):295-301.

54. Hagan PG, Nienaber CA, Isselbacher EM, et al. The International Registry of Acute Aortic Dissection (IRAD): new insights into an old disease. *JAMA.* 2000;283(7):897-903.

55. DeBakey ME, Henley WS, Cooley DA, et al. Surgical management of dissecting aneurysms of the aorta. *J Thorac Cardiovasc Surg.* 1965;49:130-149.

56. Daily PO, Trueblood HW, Stinson EB, et al. Management of acute aortic dissections. *Ann Thorac Surg.* 1970;10(3):237-247.

57. Pape LA, Awais M, Woznicki EM, et al. Presentation, diagnosis, and outcomes of acute aortic dissection: 17-year trends from the international registry of acute aortic dissection. *J Am Coll Cardiol.* 2015;66(4):350-358.

58. Black JH. Management of acute aortic dissection. Available at http://www.UpToDate.com; Accessed September 2016.

59. Nallamothu BK, Mehta RH, Saint S, et al. Syncope in acute aortic dissection: diagnostic, prognostic, and clinical implications. *Am J Med.* 2002;113(6):468-471.

60. Theroux P, Willerson JT, Armstrong, PW. Progress in the treatment of acute coronary syndromes: a 50-year perspective. *Circulation.* 2000;102(20 suppl 4):IV2-IV13.

61. Erbel R, Alfonso F, Boileau C, et al. Diagnosis and management of aortic dissection. *Eur Heart J.* 2001;22(18):1642-1681.

62. Tsai TT, Nienaber CA, Eagle KA. Acute aortic syndromes. *Circulation.* 2005;112(24):3801-3813.

63. Manning WJ. Overview of acute aortic syndromes. Available at http://www.UpToDate.com; Accessed September 2016.

64. Elliott WJ. Clinical features in the management of selected hypertensive emergencies. *Prog Cardiovasc Dis.* 2006;48(5): 316-325.

65. Elliott WJ. Evaluation and treatment of hypertensive emergencies in adults. Available at http://www.UpToDate.com; Accessed September 2016.

66. Klein DG. Cardiac output measurement techniques (invasive). In: Wiegard DL, ed. *AACN Procedure Manual for Critical Care.* 4th ed. St. Louis, MO: Elsevier/Saunders; 2011.

67. Lough ME. *Hemodynamic Monitoring: Evolving Technologies and Clinical Practice.* St. Louis, MO: Elsevier; 2016.

68. Preuss T, Wiegard DL. Single-pressure and multiple pressure transducer systems. In: Wiegard DL, ed. *AACN Procedure Manual for Critical Care.* 4th ed. St. Louis, MO: Elsevier/Saunders; 2011.

69. Preuss T, Wiegard DL. Pulmonary artery catheter insertion (assist) ad pressure monitoring. In: Wiegard DL, ed. *AACN Procedure Manual for Critical Care.* 4th ed. St. Louis, MO: Elsevier/Saunders; 2011.

70. Preuss T, Wiegard DL. Pulmonary artery catheter and pressure lines, troubleshooting. In: Wiegard DL, ed. *AACN Procedure Manual for Critical Care.* 4th ed. St. Louis: Elsevier/Saunders; 2011.

71. Darovic GO. *Hemodynamic Monitoring: Invasive and Noninvasive Clinical Application.* 3rd ed. Philadelphia, PA: WB Saunders; 2002.

72. Berryhill RF, Benumoff JL, Rauscher LA. Pulmonary vascular pressure reading at the end of exhalation. *Anesthesiology.* 1978;49 (5):365-368.

73. Fleck DA. Pulmonary artery catheter insertion (Perform). In: Wiegard DL, ed. *AACN Procedure Manual for Critical Care.* 4th ed. St. Louis, MO: Elsevier/Saunders; 2011.

74. Campos ML, et al. Techniques available for hemodynamic monitoring: advantages and limitations. *Med Intensiva.* 2012;36(6): 434-444.

75. Marik PE. Noninvasive cardiac output monitors: a state-of-the-art review. *J of Cardiothoracic and Vascular Anesthesia.* 2013;27(1): 121-134.

76. Vincent JL, Pelosi P, Pearse R, et al. Perioperative cardiovascular monitoring of high-risk patients: a consensus of 12. *Critical Care.* 2015;19:224.

77. McMahon N, Hogg LA, Corfield AR, Exton AD. Comparison of non-invasive and invasive blood pressure in aeromedical care. *Anaesthesia.* 2012;67(12):1343-1347.

78. Dobbin KR. Noninvasive blood pressure monitoring. *Crit Care Nurse.* 2002;22(2):123-124.

79. McEvoy M, Handley C, Steel D. Hemodynamic Monitoring. In: Pollak AN, ed. *Critical Care Transport.* Boston, MA: American College of Emergency Physicians. Jones and Bartlett Publishers; 2011.

21

Mechanical Circulatory Support Devices in Transport

TONYA ELLIOTT, LESLIE C. SWEET, AND ALLEN C. WOLFE, JR.

COMPETENCIES

1. Identify the indications for the use of a mechanical circulatory support device.
2. Perform an assessment of the patient with a mechanical circulatory support device.
3. Manage specific mechanical circulatory support devices before, during, and after the transport process.

Mechanical circulatory support (MCS) is indicated in patients who, in spite of optimal medical therapy, remain in cardiogenic shock or refractory advanced heart failure. This chapter will review the MCS devices (MCSDs) currently implanted in this very ill population who may then need to be transported, the challenges of assessing and treating these patients, and the related transport considerations and recommendations.

The modern era of mechanical support has ushered in important changes to the technology that impacts prehospital care. There are two advancements that have enabled thousands of patients to be treated with MCS every year. The first area of improvement is the early recognition of advanced heart failure. Over the last several years, there have been tremendous strides in the diagnosis and treatment of all forms of heart disease, resulting in improved survival rates, but with more patients with advanced heart failure requiring advanced therapies such as MCS. The second area of evolution is the technological advancements in the MCSDs.

Additionally, in the 1990s, it was recognized that transporting patients in cardiogenic shock to MCS implanting centers improved outcomes. The New York City area created a referral network so that the pathway to implanting centers was well established to facilitate early treatment.[1] A large implanting center in Germany mobilized their MCS program to provide emergent circulatory support.[2] McBride et al. reviewed their results from a small cohort of patients transported into their institution. They determined

that although only 8 of 16 patients transported had long-term survival, there were no complications related to the transport.[3]

Another consideration is cardiac congenital anomalies, which can alter blood flow through the cardiopulmonary system rendering pediatric patients unable to oxygenate and/or circulate blood in a manner compatible with life. These children require extracorporeal membrane oxygenation (ECMO) until a more permanent therapy for heart failure can be provided, such as long-term left ventricular assist devices (LVADs) and heart transplantation. Transporting pediatric patients on ECMO to ventricular assist device (VAD)/heart transplant centers is paramount to survival. Coppla et al. provided a review of decades of cases in which pediatric patients in cardiogenic shock were transported on ECMO with comparable outcomes to patients supported on ECMO within their institution.[4]

All of these studies demonstrated the need to have knowledgeable transport services readily available to safely transport critically ill patients on MCSD.

Historic Perspective

In 1966 Dr. Michael DeBakey implanted the first successful cardiac assist device in a young female patient who could not be weaned from cardiopulmonary bypass (CPB). The patient was successfully supported by the device for 10 days[5] and was ultimately discharged home. This landmark success fueled the interest in further development and use of MSCDs for severe end-stage heart failure. Subsequently, researchers and physicians turned their focus to total replacement of the injured myocardium with the use of a total artificial heart (TAH). In 1969 Dr. Denton Cooley implanted a TAH (the Liotta heart) in a patient with failure to wean from CPB. The patient was supported for 64 hours before undergoing cardiac transplant. Additional modifications and clinical use continued into the 1980s with the first permanent implantation of a TAH in 1982 into an elderly dentist, Dr. Barney Clark, at the University of Utah by Dr. William Devries. The device, the

Jarvik-7 TAH, was designed by Dr. Robert Jarvik and associates for total cardiac replacement. Although Dr. Clark ultimately died of multiple complications, he was fully supported for an unprecedented 112 days,[5,6] which was a pivotal achievement for the field of artificial organs. The Jarvik-7 has undergone further modifications and enhancements since then, and is currently known as the SynCardia temporary TAH (SynCardia Systems, Inc., Tucson, Arizona). Limitations of the earlier technology, however, prompted scientists and physicians to refocus on developing technology to *assist* the failing heart versus completely replacing it.[5]

In the 1980s, while heart transplantation gained prominence in the cardiac surgery arena, many end-stage heart failure patients died awaiting transplant because of an insufficient number of donor organs compared with the profoundly increasing number of transplant candidates.[7] In light of this skewed supply/demand ratio, medical researchers and engineers were tasked with developing a device that was readily available and capable of sustaining patients until a suitable donor organ became available, or providing lifetime support to advanced heart failure patients deemed ineligible for heart transplant. The mid-1980s and early 1990s ushered in the early designs of VADs, the fill-to-empty or pulsatile pumps, which were successfully used in patients awaiting heart transplant.[8] With further enhancements, they even allowed VAD-supported patients to be discharged home into the community.[5] With the increased cost of LVAD patient management within the hospital setting, hospital discharge of VAD patients into the community had a profound impact on patient quality of life and survival with proper caregiver and community support, education, and training.

These successful applications of VAD therapy prompted clinicians to consider using VADs in patients deemed ineligible for transplant. The Randomized Evaluation of Mechanical Assistance for the Treatment of Congestive Heart Failure (REMATCH) trial, which was a randomized, multicenter clinical trial, demonstrated that the HeartMate Vented Electric Left Ventricular Assist System (HeartMate VE LVAS; Thoratec Corporation, Pleasanton, California), a pulsatile VAD, significantly improved survival and quality of life compared with optimal medical management in this very ill patient cohort. The survival benefit was limited (52% and 23% at 1 and 2 years postimplant), and device comorbidities were significant enough that the clinical community continued to look at developing improvements and alternative technologies.[5,9] Hence, the clinicians and researchers became focused on developing smaller pumps, with increased durability and hemocompatibility, decreased power demands, ideally without drivelines, and associated with minimal comorbidities and improved clinical outcomes, including quality of life.

Meanwhile, the development of the intraaortic balloon pump (IABP) support began in 1958 when Dr. Dwight Harken described a method to treat left ventricular failure (LVF) with counterpulsation. His recommendation was the removal of a certain amount of blood volume from the femoral artery during systole, with rapid replacement of this volume during diastole.[10] Complications arose because of the need for bilateral femoral arteriotomies, requiring surgical insertion and removal, and hemolysis of cells in the pumping apparatus.[10] Later in the 1960s, Dr. Spiro Moulopolous, a researcher at the Cleveland Clinic, developed a form of treatment for LVF that expanded significantly in the years that followed.[11] With the concepts of his predecessors, he made a simple, effective, and affordable circulatory assist device, what is today known as the IABP, and successfully used it to support three patients in cardiogenic shock.[12] This groundbreaking research gave rise to other great work at that time. In 1968 Dr. Adrian Kantrowitz continued to work with counterpulsation and demonstrated reversal of cardiogenic shock in 27 patients with both hemodynamic and clinical improvement.[11]

In summary, the evolution of all of these MCSDs have created a more sophisticated set of treatment strategies to offer today's complicated advanced heart failure and cardiogenic shock patient cohorts who are supported with both air and surface transport.

The Basics

MCSDs are mechanical devices or pumps designed to support the pumping function of a failing heart, whether attributable to acute cardiogenic shock or severe chronic cardiomyopathy. These devices may be separated into two major categories: TAHs and VADs. The *TAH* is a device that completely *replaces* the native heart physically and functionally. Implantation of a TAH involves removal of the native heart similar to cardiac transplantation. Typically, the TAH is attached to the atria and great vessels of the heart (pulmonary artery [PA] and aorta), with complete excision of the remaining heart muscle. The caveat of the TAH, however, is that if the device should fail, no "backup" native heart exists to compensate for device failure. In addition, because of the inherent size of a TAH, the patient must have adequate thoracic space to accommodate the pump. TAHs are most ideally suited for patients with medically refractory biventricular heart failure.

Conversely, *VADs* are designed to *assist* the native heart in pumping adequate blood to vital body organs. The native heart remains intact, and the VAD is attached to the appropriate great vessels and heart chambers, typically with inflow and outflow cannulas. The degree of circulatory support by the VAD varies depending on the design of the VAD and the capabilities of the native heart. With some devices, the native heart may serve primarily as a "funnel" or conduit through which the circulating blood is delivered to the artificial pump, which then provides complete cardiac output (CO) for that side of the heart.

VADs may be categorized by the side of the heart they support and the design of the pump itself. VADs that support the right side of the heart are *right ventricular assist devices* (RVADs), and VADs that support the left side of the heart are LVADs. When the technology is used to support both sides of the heart, it is a *biventricular assist device* (BVAD or BiVAD), and in some cases may involve two totally different devices (a hybrid configuration).[13] With full BiVAD support, a patient in sustained ventricular fibrillation could be completely coherent and the arrhythmia clinically insignificant because of adequate circulation from the BiVAD alone.

Indications for Ventricular Assist Device Therapy

The specific indications for VADs include the following: (1) bridge to recovery (BTR), (2) bridge to more definitive therapy, (3) bridge to transplant, and (4) lifetime or destination therapy (DT). BTR is indicated when there is a suspicion that, given the opportunity to "rest" on a VAD, the native heart function may be able to sufficiently recover and adequately support circulation, ultimately allowing for explantation of the device. Initially, this indication was thought to be limited to acute cardiogenic shock patients only, but clinical experience has shown in a few cases that myocardial recovery may be achieved with the longer duration of support provided by more long-term "durable" devices.[12,14]

Bridge to more definitive therapy describes the use of a short-term device to temporarily support the failing heart through an acute event. With time to stabilize the patient's condition, the cardiac function may be more thoroughly evaluated to better determine whether the insult is reversible, or whether a more definitive, long-term therapy is indicated and whether the patient is eligible for such therapy. Definitive therapy strategies may include more conventional percutaneous coronary interventions and coronary artery bypass graft surgery or may expand to cardiac transplantation or permanent MCSD.

Bridge to cardiac transplantation (BTT) is the use of a VAD to provide ongoing ventricular support to a transplant candidate whose heart becomes refractory to conventional pharmacologic support and for whom a suitable donor heart has not yet become available. The VAD is intended to provide adequate circulatory support until the donor heart becomes available. It is then removed along with the native heart during the transplant surgery. Current data from the United Network of Organ Sharing (UNOS) Registry continues to show that there are twice as many heart transplant candidates as there are recipients, reaffirming the ongoing shortage of available donor organs.[15] Historically, approximately 30% of transplant candidates die while awaiting a suitable donor heart. More recently, the mortality rate has decreased to 11%.[16,17] This reduction in pretransplant mortality is attributable to multiple factors, including the use of VADs to bridge these patients, as shown by the increase of LVAD BTT cases from 3% in 1990 to greater than 28% in 2004, to 42% in 2013.[15,18,19] Per the Organ Procurement Transplant Network/Scientific Registry of Transplant Recipients (OPTN/SRTR), the pretransplant mortality rate for patients on VAD support at the time of listing for transplant has also dropped from 68.4 per 100 waitlist years in 2003–2004 to 9.9 in 2013–2014.[15] Table 21.1 shows the breakdown of MCSD use for BTT.[19]

Lifetime or *DT* describes the use of a VAD to sustain circulatory support in patients with medically refractory end-stage heart failure who are also deemed ineligible for cardiac transplant because of other comorbidities. Historically, these patients would be sent home, if possible, with palliative or hospice care for the duration of their lives. With the advent of more durable devices, these patients may be adequately sustained on VADs and still be active members of their families and communities. Clinical trials with these durable devices show sustained improvement in quality of life and functional capacity in the majority of patients supported by VAD therapy.[20]

Further categorization of VADs includes the intended length of support and the design of the device. *Acute VADs* are those devices typically implanted for short-term use, especially in the setting of cardiogenic shock, for 7 to 10 or even up to 30 days. *Chronic* or *long-term (durable) VADs* are devices implanted for more long-term support, typically

TABLE 21.1 Adult Heart Transplants: Donor and Recipient Characteristics

Preoperative Support (Multiple Items May Be Reported)	1992–2003 (n = 48,061) (%)	2004–2008 (n = 17,366) (%)	2009–6/2014 (n = 19,770) (%)	p-Value
Mechanical circulatory support	22.2[a]	26.0	43.0	<0.0001
LVAD	13.2[a]	21.8	36.6	<0.0001
RVAD	—	4.4[b]	3.2	<0.0001
TAH	0.0[a]	0.5	1.4	<0.0001
ECMO	0.3[c]	0.9	1.2	<0.0001

ECMO, Extracorporeal membrane oxygenation; *LVAD,* left ventricular assist device; *RVAD,* right ventricular assist device; *TAH,* total artificial heart.
[a]Based on 11/1999–2003 transplants.
[b]Based on 2005–2008 transplants.
[c]Based on 5/1995–2008 transplants.
From ISHLT International Registry for Heart and Lung Transplantation 2105. *J Heart Lung Transplant.* 2015;34(10):1244-1254.

with the intent to discharge the patient into the community. Some indications exist for implanting devices from either of these categories for a duration of support between these two time lines.

Device Characteristics and Designs

Regarding the design of VADs, the technology has evolved significantly over recent years. The earliest designs of MCS included roller pumps for CPB and the IABP for cardiogenic shock. Although the use of IABPs for acute cardiogenic shock may increase the CO by 10% to 15%, a significant mortality rate remains in shock patients. Both CPB and IABPs are limited in the duration of support that they can provide. The goal of advancing VAD support is to provide even higher blood flow than the more conventional IABP, with potentially longer, more tolerable support to assist in improving both acute and long-term outcomes. The vast improvements in technology have returned the ECMO as a favorable treatment option in the acute setting of medically refractory cardiogenic shock and heart failure patients. The advent of the Impella Ventricular Support Systems (Abiomed, Inc., Danvers, Massachusetts) has provided another option for prophylactic device support for high-risk percutaneous angioplasty procedures, as well as interim support of severe left or right heart failure as a bridge to more definitive therapy.

The different devices developed in recent years may also be categorized per device design, regardless of indication for short-term or long-term use. *Pulsatile flow pumps or VADs (PF-VADs)* are devices that are considered *fill-to-empty* or *volume-displacement pumps.* These pumps typically have a blood sac or chamber in which blood collects before being ejected into the circulation, similar to the native heart's diastole and systole. The rate at which these devices pump is often dependent on filling of the blood chambers and does not necessarily correlate with the patient's native heartbeat. Unlike an IABP with electrocardiogram (ECG) tracing capabilities, any apparent synchrony of pumping rates between PF-VADs and the native heart is coincidental. These devices have inflow and outflow valves to ensure unidirectional blood flow through the pump.

Continuous flow pumps or VADs (CF-VADs), contrary to the volume-displacement pumps, draw blood continuously from the supported heart. CF-VADs do not have a blood-collecting chamber or unidirectional valves, and they do not pause for optimal filling. They do have inflow and outflow cannulas, similar to the PF-VADs, but instead of the blood chamber they contain a high-speed impeller. The impeller is likened to a turbine engine or propeller. Because CF-VADs draw blood continuously from the supported ventricle, pulsatility of the sustained circulation may be dampened significantly. If the VAD is supporting the left side of the heart, for example, then a peripheral pulse may be difficult to palpate, necessitating the use of a Doppler flow probe to auscultate and confirm blood flow. Basic assessment skills of adequate circulation (e.g., capillary bed refill, adequate

mentation, urine output) have heightened importance in these patients.

CF-VADs may be further differentiated into the axial flow and centrifugal flow pumps. The CF-VAD impeller uses rotational energy to propel blood through the pump. It may be cylindrical or disk shaped, and uses blades or vanes to direct the blood flow forward. The blood flow path of the axial flow devices is linear across the cylindrical impeller, relying on circumferential energy (Fig. 21.1). The rotational speed of an axial flow device is typically 8000 to 15,000 rotations per minute (rpm).

The blood flow path of the centrifugal flow devices involves a 90-degree turn through the disk impeller via the perpendicular inflow and outflow ports, combining both centrifugal and circumferential energy to propel the blood forward (Fig. 21.2). The rotational speed of the centrifugal pump is typically 2000 to 6000 rpm. In addition, the centrifugal blood pump impeller is magnetically and/or hydrodynamically suspended (elevated by the blood flow through the pump), which eliminates the amount of contacting

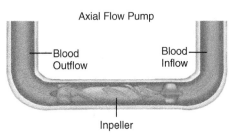

• **Fig. 21.1** Blood flow through an axial flow impeller (Thoratec Heart-Mate II LVAS). (From Mancini D, Colombo P. Left ventricular assist devices: a rapidly evolving alternative to transplant. *J Am Coll Cardiol.* 2015;65(23):2542-2555.)

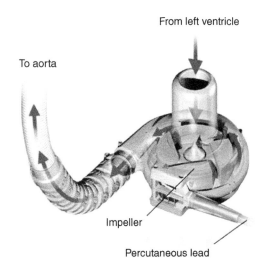

• **Fig. 21.2** Blood flow through a centrifugal flow impeller (HeartWare HVAD Pump). (From Aaronson KD, Slaughter MS, Miller, LW et al. Use of an intrapericardial, continuous-flow, centrifugal pump in patients awaiting heart transplantation. *Circulation.* 2012;125(25):3191-3200.)

mechanical surfaces that otherwise could wear with time.[2,16] Hence, centrifugal pumps are often referred to as "wearless" pumps. As the technology advances, these devices, inherent to their design, have become smaller, more energy efficient, and have fewer contacting parts. The benefits of these advances are that the pumps will likely last longer and can be implanted in a wider range of body sizes, which makes the technology more accessible to more patients.

Acute Cardiogenic Shock Devices

As previously described, VADs used for acute cardiogenic shock are those devices indicated for immediate stabilization of the patient's condition, with an average projected support time of 7 to 10 days. Common indications for these devices include acute cardiogenic shock associated with myocardial infarction (MI), postcardiotomy shock, viral myocarditis, and temporary right ventricular failure (RVF) associated with implantation of a permanent LVAD. The advantage of these short-term devices is that they allow the clinical team the opportunity to stabilize the patient's condition for a more clear understanding of the clinical pathology and etiology of the cardiogenic shock, and the most appropriate course for further therapy. Strategies at this time include the addition of maximal pharmacologic therapies to optimize the potential for recovery and removal of the VAD versus confirming that the VAD cannot be weaned. In the latter case, the next strategies to consider are patient eligibility for cardiac transplant versus lifetime VAD therapy. In extreme cases, withdrawal of pharmacologic and mechanical support may be warranted and requested by next of kin.

Typical acute cardiogenic shock devices that may necessitate medical transport are the IABP, ECMO, and the CentriMag Blood Pumping System (Thoratec Corporation, St. Jude Medical, Pleasanton, California). The major components of these blood pumps typically include cannulas and blood tubing that are attached to the native circulation (i.e., major blood vessels versus the heart) and then to the blood pump; the blood pump itself; and the console that runs the pump and provides electrical power to the system, with backup batteries for patient transportation while on support. All of these devices currently require systemic anticoagulation to minimize the potential for thrombus formation and occlusion, in balance with minimizing the potential for excessive bleeding and its associated complications, including blood transfusions and subsequent right

heart failure. Heparin is used most often, although an alternative agent such as argatroban or bivalirudin may be needed if the patient has tested positive for heparin-induced thrombocytopenia (HIT).

Intraaortic Balloon Pump

An IABP is a device whose primary purpose is to increase coronary perfusion and CO, while decreasing cardiac workload through counterpulsation. As the native heart begins systole, the IABP balloon deflates, augmenting the overall CO by as much as 40%. As diastole begins, the balloon inflates, increasing blood flow to the coronary arteries. Secondary effects of IABP are outlined in Table 21.2.[21] This device is ideal for patients with poor CO, chest pain unrelieved with medical therapy, and failed pharmacologic therapy associated with poor perfusion related to cardiogenic shock.

Placement of the IABP typically involves inserting a flexible catheter into the femoral artery and advancing it into the descending thoracic aorta (Fig. 21.3). The placement of the catheter is confirmed with fluoroscopy or chest x-ray. As illustrated in Fig. 21.3, proper location of the catheter is essential for ideal functioning. Poor placement of the IABP catheter can create other complications that are discussed later in this section.

The fiber-optic IABP offers operator flexibility, which allows the flight crew members the capability to care for a broad range of patients. These pumps are designed to work in conditions unique to the operating room, to the cardiac catheterization laboratory, to the Intensive Care Unit, and to air and surface transport. The technology uses speed and quick algorithms, supplying support to patients with arrhythmias.[22] The balloon pumps have colorful display panels combined with pneumatic and electronic innovations. These balloon pumps possess cardiosynchronization capabilities, with autoselect trigger selection and timing. The IABP adapts its deflation automatically while supporting ventricular ectopy or other arrhythmias.[13] If the timing is not correct, then a number of physiologic changes can occur, as outlined in Table 21.3.

The automatic mode of the IABP uses the ECG trigger, but if the ECG trigger is lost, then the pump searches for the next best trigger source and resets the timing accordingly. A manual mode allows the transport team members to select and control all of the triggers and their timing even during changes in rhythm. This technology allows the flight

TABLE 21.2	Secondary Effects of Intraaortic Balloon Pump Support							
Clinical Parameter	CO	SV	LVEF	CPP	Systemic Perfusion	HR	PCWP	SVR
Secondary effect	↑	↑	↑	↑	↑	↓	↓	↓

CO, Cardiac output; *CPP,* coronary perfusion pressure; *HR,* heart rate; *LVEF,* left ventricular ejection fraction; *PCWP,* pulmonary capillary wedge pressure; *SV,* stroke volume; *SVR,* systemic vascular resistance.

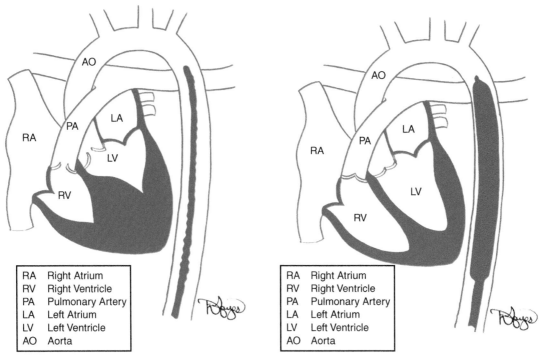

The IABP is deflated during systole, as the heart contracts.

The IABP is inflated during diastole as it improves coronary circulation.

RA	Right Atrium
RV	Right Ventricle
PA	Pulmonary Artery
LA	Left Atrium
LV	Left Ventricle
AO	Aorta

• **Fig. 21.3** Placement of intraaortic balloon pump balloon-tipped catheter. The goal of inflation is to produce a rapid rise in aortic pressure, which optimizes diastolic augmentation and increases oxygen supply to the coronaries. During deflation, the reduction in end aortic diastolic pressure (afterload) causes improved cardiac performance. (Courtesy David Hayes.)

team members to focus more on the patient and aviation safety rather than the pump.

Because of the large amount of background noise in air medical transport, the IABP console supports a large visual alarm display. The balloon is filled with a predetermined amount of helium. In the manual mode, the pump needs manual filling of the balloon catheter to compensate for the changes in balloon volume during air transport. This is done by the transport teams every 2000 feet on ascent and every 1000 feet on descent.[22] The newest generation IABP automatically refills the helium based on volume sensors, which detect changes in the volume of helium, prompting auto refill. This refilling also occurs every 2 hours automatically in manual or auto modes. In situations of very

TABLE 21.3	**Intraaortic Balloon Pump Timing Errors**

Timing Error	Effect
Early inflation 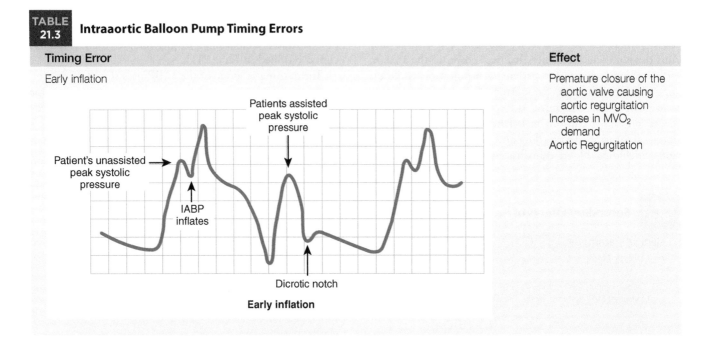	Premature closure of the aortic valve causing aortic regurgitation Increase in MVO$_2$ demand Aortic Regurgitation

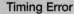

TABLE 21.3	Intraaortic Balloon Pump Timing Errors—cont'd

Timing Error	Effect
Late inflation 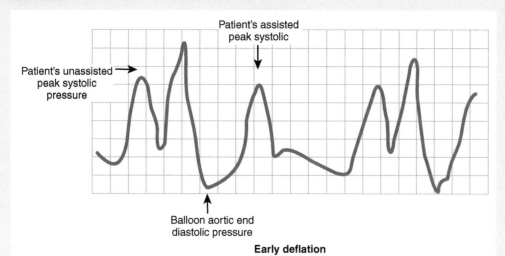 **Early deflation**	Suboptimal coronary perfusion
Early deflation 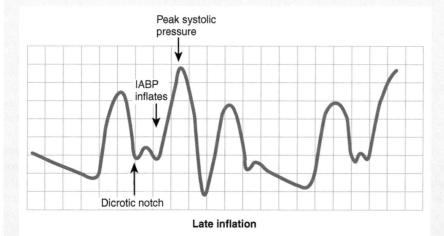 **Late inflation**	Retrograde coronary blood flow Suboptimal coronary perfusion and cause angina Suboptimal afterload reduction Increase in MVO$_2$
Late deflation 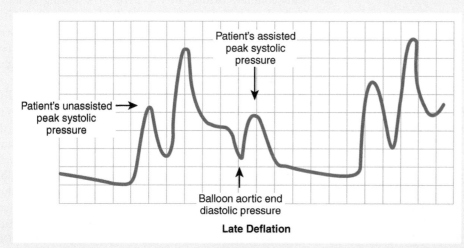 **Late Deflation**	Impedes ejection of left ventricle, therefore increasing the resistance the balloon pumps against (afterload) Increase MVO$_2$

MVO$_2$, Mixed venous oxygen saturation.

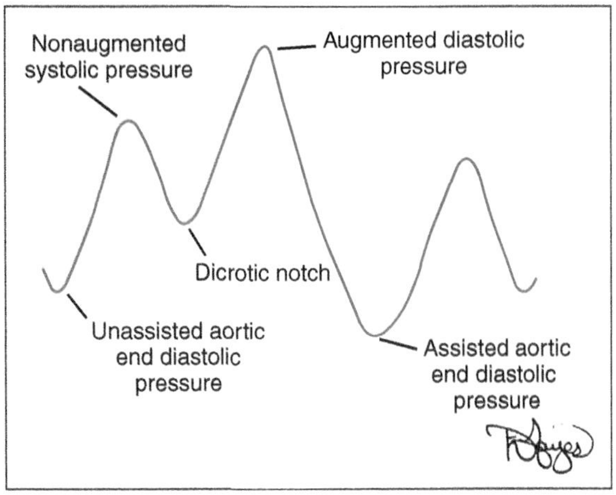

• **Fig. 21.4** Intraaortic balloon pump counterpulsation waveform. (Courtesy David Hayes.)

rapid descent, the pump refills many times, quickly causing a helium loss alarm.

The frequency of IABP counterpulsation is ordered by the physician. In most cases, it is 1:1; thus for each contraction of the native ventricles and opening of the aortic valve, the IABP catheter is triggered to inflate during the subsequent diastolic phase timed to the dicrotic notch (Fig. 21.4). The computerized system allows the IABP to manage the patients at more rapid heart rates than previous generations using 1:1 counterpulsation. The counterpulsation can be set for other frequency modes, such as 1:2 and 1:3, for which inflation of the balloon occurs on the dicrotic notch on every second or third beat, respectively. The balloon then deflates again at the onset of native ventricular systole. These types of balloon pumps have undergone significant changes in the last decade. The pumps are more operator friendly, and their computerized monitoring systems allow for automatic timing of the inflation and deflation of the balloon catheter. The pumps also have transport designs that are more lightweight and safety conscious for air surface transport personnel.

Patient Assessment

A complete assessment of the patient's hemodynamic status is vitally important before the transport of a patient with an IABP; however, the assessment should start with the primary survey. After the primary survey assessment and any interventions, a baseline neurologic examination is warranted. This examination is important because a highly placed IABP catheter can block blood flow to the subclavian and carotid artery.

The hemodynamic assessment should consist of evaluation of the patient's CO, cardiac index, LV stroke work index, systemic vascular resistance, pulmonary vascular resistance, and other pulmonary catheter data, if available. Assessment of heart sounds should be done with the IABP on standby so that the sounds are clearly heard, with the baseline assessment monitoring for the possible accumulation of an excessive amount of fluid around the pericardium (cardiac tamponade). In air transport, hearing capabilities are impaired; therefore all the important sound-assessed information should be obtained before leaving the referring facility. The assessment of the IABP includes diastolic augmentation, pump timing, and any alarms.

Although the use of PA catheters has decreased significantly in the last several years, standard practice in critical care transport of these devices is the continuous monitoring of the PA catheter waveforms. Hence, transport teams should be properly trained in the management of PA catheters and waveform analysis. If the catheter migrates into the PA, then a wedge waveform is visualized on the monitor. This displacement can result in occlusion or perforation of the PA, which can cause pulmonary infarct and possibly death. In this situation, the caregiver needs to ensure that the balloon is deflated before pulling the catheter back until the PA waveform is visualized on the monitor. In instances in which the PA catheter slips into the right ventricle, the catheter should be withdrawn to the right atrium (RA).

Physical assessment of the patient is important because it will also ensure proper anatomic positioning of the IABP. The patient may have specific clinical assessment deficits if the device is malpositioned. If the patient's left brachial pulse is absent, for example, then the catheter may be positioned too high, causing occlusion of the subclavian artery and ultimately affecting blood flow to the left arm. A radiograph or fluoroscopy is best for identification of this misplacement. If the catheter is too low, then the patient may have oliguria or anuria as a result of the catheter blocking the renal arteries, decreasing renal blood flow. The patient's distal pulses may also no longer be palpable.

Important laboratory values to review before transport include the most recent complete blood count (CBC), prothrombin time, partial thromboplastin time, platelet counts, and basic metabolic panel. If oozing at the insertion site is present or occurs, then careful placement of a liter bag of intravenous (IV) fluids over the exit site may be helpful. This placement applies light pressure without interfering with counterpulsation of the IABP. The oozing is most likely the result of the decrease in platelets caused by IABP counterpulsation or anticoagulation effects from other medications. The head of the bed or stretcher should be less than 30 degrees to prevent occlusion of the catheter. Light restraints or sedation may be helpful in securing the leg in which the catheter is inserted to prevent accidental IABP dislodgement or interference with balloon pump functioning. The diameter of the catheter varies from patient to patient; therefore assessment for distal pulses is important to ensure perfusion of both extremities. An occlusion can cause ischemia of the affected extremity and result in clot formation, decreased circulation, and total arterial occlusion with possible amputation if the IABP is not adjusted or removed. The transport personnel must perform a thorough assessment and relay any complications from IABP therapy to the accepting physician with complete documentation in the flight chart.

Transport Considerations of the Patient With an Intraaortic Balloon Pump

1. In any vehicle, whether ground, or fixed or rotor wing, verify that the inverter can supply power to the IABP.
2. The two main manufacturers of IABPs (Arrow International, Tampa, Florida, and Maquet, Rastatt, Germany) both have adapters specifically for transport personnel in the event the transport team's pump is different from the one at the referring facility. These adapters allow interfacing between the two different pumps.
3. A transport bag should accompany all IABP transports with auxiliary supplies for IABPs.
4. Ensure that sufficient helium and a backup helium tank are provided.
5. The changes in altitude affect the amount of helium in the tank because of autofilling. The transport provider should calculate the number of autofills to prevent running out.
6. All blood pressure readings should be taken from the IABP console and not the noninvasive blood pressure cuff (NIBP) or manually. The highest pressure sensed or heard is the diastolic augmentation, not systolic. Therefore documentation of the NIBP or manual pressures provides inaccurate information.
7. Positioning the patient with the head toward the front of the fixed aircraft decreases the patient's preload. The opposite occurs if the patient is positioned with the feet toward the front.
8. Ensure that the IABP console is plugged in to alternating current (AC) power whenever possible (e.g., in the transport vehicle and immediately on arrival at the bedside of the sending facility).
9. Ensure that the fiber-optic catheters are properly zeroed and calibrated to the specifications of the manufacturer. Of note, at altitudes greater than 10,000 feet in an unpressurized cabin, the fiber-optic catheters may be altered and inoperable. They are more accurate below 10,000 feet.[22]

Management of Common Intraaortic Balloon Pump Emergency Procedures

In the transport environment, preparation for the worst-case scenario in patient care and safety is a fact of life. Table 21.4 lists some emergencies that can occur with IABP therapy and their management.

Extracorporeal Membrane Oxygenation

Heart transplant remains the gold standard for treating end-stage, advanced heart failure in eligible candidates. OPTN and UNOS set national policies to ensure fair organ allocation. In 2006 the policies were modified to promote transplanting the sickest patients on the list to reduce mortality during the waiting period. At the time of this writing in 2016, the policies will be enhanced to further favor transplanting the sickest patients (https://optn.transplant.hrsa.gov/governance/public-comment/adult-heart-allocation-changes-2016). Under these guidelines, patients supported on ECMO will be given priority listing status. Hence, more transplant-listed patients who decompensate quickly may be put on ECMO, and may then require transport to the transplanting center for urgent upgrade to the sickest status.

ECMO is used in patients in emergently decompensating cardiac, cardiopulmonary, or pulmonary failure. Candidates for ECMO support include patients who experience cardiac and or pulmonary collapse, for example, patients with severe flu or acute respiratory distress syndrome (ARDS); lung transplant patients who cannot oxygenate; or severe cardiomyopathies resulting in rapid, catastrophic circulatory shock. The ECMO system is designed to remove carbon dioxide and oxygenate the blood. ECMO support may allow for changes in the ventilator settings to reduce inhaled oxygen and positive end-expiratory pressure, reducing the risk of barotrauma injury.

The inflow cannula for ECMO drains blood from the venous circulation into the circuit. Blood is pumped

TABLE 21.4	Intraaortic Balloon Pump Emergency Interventions
Problem	**Intervention**
Ventricular fibrillation or pulseless ventricular tachycardia arrest	1. Follow ACLS guidelines 2. Stopping the pump is not necessary 3. Pump is grounded and can accommodate electrical shocks
Cardiopulmonary arrest: asystole or pulseless electrical activity	1. Begin ACLS guidelines, and place pump on pressure mode during compressions 2. IABP pump will continue to pump with compressions as pressure is sensed
Power failure	1. Attach 60-mL syringe to proximal stopcock 2. Inflate IABP catheter once every 3–5 min to prevent clot formation on catheter
Diastolic hypertension	1. Provide afterload reduction or decrease augmentation volume in IABP if possible
Rapid heart rate <200	2. Leave the IABP in 1:1 counterpulsation
Balloon rupture (evidenced by blood in the sheath, loss gas alarm, and rust-colored flacks)	3. Stop the pump immediately; clamp the catheter 4. Position patient in the left lateral position 5. IABP needs to be removed as soon as possible

ACLS, Advanced cardiac life support; *IABP,* intraaortic balloon pump.

through the system by a centrifugal pump head, then into the oxygenator, and back to the patient's body. Cannula placement is based on the patient's need for support. For cardiac and cardiopulmonary failure, the cannulas drain from the venous system (e.g., inferior vena cava or RA via the femoral or jugular veins) into the circuit then into the arterial system (e.g., ascending aorta for central ECMO or femoral artery). This approach is known as venoarterial ECMO. In patients with pulmonary or ventilatory failure, the cannulas drain from the venous system (e.g., femoral and/or jugular vein) into the circuit and back into the venous system. This is known as venous-venous ECMO. The ECMO system is heparinized to prevent clot formation.

The Extracorporeal Life Support Organization (ELSO) has developed guidelines for transporting patients on ECMO. The guidelines are available at www.elso.org. Patients may need to be emergently transported to a center that has the capacity to implant ECMO, or if already supported on ECMO, may need to go to a center with access to transplant or durable VADs. The distance between centers and weather conditions impacts which mode of transport is appropriate, so careful planning is required. The team who accompanies the ECMO patient usually includes a perfusionist who will attend to the ECMO circuit during the transport. Other equipment considerations must include the ability to provide power to the circuit and to have a redundant system in the event of device malfunction. Because many ECMO patients have coagulopathies, for long transports it may be necessary to have additional blood products to ensure adequate blood volume. Specific check lists can be accessed on the ELSO website.

Impella Ventricular Support Systems

The Impella Ventricular Support Systems are catheter-based devices that are indicated for temporary support in the setting of refractory cardiogenic shock following cardiac surgery and acute MI. The device is intended to support circulation for hours to days, allowing the ventricle to rest and recover, if possible. The system may also be used to support circulation during high-risk cardiac catheterization procedures. The Impella 2.5, Impella CP, and Impella 5.0 (Fig. 21.5) are microaxial catheters that are placed percutaneously in the femoral or axillary artery and threaded up to the heart to provide LV support. The Impella LD is surgically placed directly into the ascending aorta and advanced into the left ventricle. The Impella 2.5 and Impella CP devices deliver up to 2.5 and 3.3 L/min blood flow, respectively, and have a pigtail catheter at the distal tip, which is intended to keep the Impella stable within the ventricle and decrease the incidence of ectopy. The Impella 5.0 and Impella LD both deliver up to 5.0 L/min blood flow. All of these devices directly unload blood from the left side of the heart, resulting in a decrease in LV end-diastolic volume and end-diastolic pressure, and increasing aortic pressure and flow.

The Impella RP is a right ventricular support system and is inserted percutaneously into the femoral vein and threaded up to the PA. The Impella RP is indicated for

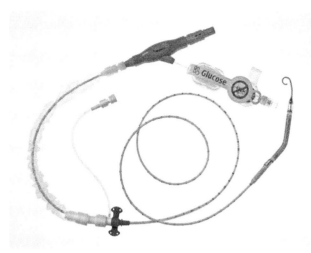

• **Fig. 21.5** Impella 5.0 catheter. The Impella family of heart pumps have the unique ability to unload the heart and enable native heart recovery, potentially allowing patients to return home with their own hearts. As the world's smallest heart pump, the Impella platform has supported more than 50,000 patients in the United States alone, and is the only Food and Drug Administration (FDA)-approved percutaneous ventricular assist device (pVAD) indicated as safe and effective for PCI in high-risk patients and patients with acute myocardial infarction complicated by cardiogenic shock (AMICS). (Courtesy Abiomed, Inc, Danvers, Massachusetts.)

patients who develop right heart failure following LVAD implant, cardiac transplant, cardiac surgery, and an MI, and delivers up to 4 L/min blood flow.

The Impella catheter has an inlet port, through which blood flows into the catheter, to the impeller. The impeller spins thousands of times a minute to accelerate blood flow through the catheter, ejecting it out the outlet port into the great vessel. For LV support, the inlet port is located within the LV, whereas the Impella RP has the inlet port within the inferior vena cava. The outlet ports are in the aorta and PA, respectively (Fig. 21.6).

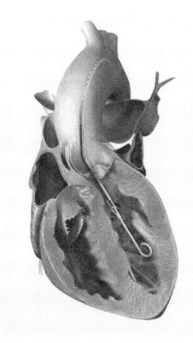

• **Fig. 21.6** Impella catheter placement. (By Skire913 (Own work) [CC BY-SA 4.0 (http://creativecommons.org/licenses/by-sa/4.0)], via Wikimedia Commons.)

These catheters are inserted under fluoroscopy to ensure proper positioning of the catheter and the inlet and outlet ports, and are anchored to the groin with sutures.

The motor housing sits just above the outlet area on the cannula. Proximal to the motor housing is a pressure sensor that monitors pressure seen in the aorta and ventricle relative to the placement of the catheter across the valve. The sensor readings create a waveform that is displayed on the controller and indicates proper placement of the catheter. There is a repositioning sheath on the catheter to limit the incidence of limb ischemia and catheter migration. The red plug on the back end of the Impella houses a memory chip and pressure transducer, which remembers the setting when transferring consoles.

The Impella catheter is connected to the purge system. The purge system is comprised of a bag of IV fluid (typically heparinized dextrose solution) attached to the purge cassette, which is then loaded into the controller, and attached to the catheter on the other side. The purge cassette flushes the catheter with the viscous IV fluid to reduce the risk of clot formation and prevent blood from entering the motor housing.

The catheter is attached externally to the controller (Fig. 21.7), which performs three functions: it facilitates user interface to monitor and control the device, it delivers the purge fluid to the catheter, and it has a backup power supply. The controller allows for the speed of the impeller rotation to be adjusted to control the intensity of ventricular emptying. The system displays the speed with "P levels": zero (P-0 = no rotation) is the lowest, ranging from P-1 at 10,000 rpm to P-9 at 33,000 rpm. Other information

obtained from the monitor includes the placement signal derived from the pressure gradient detected by the pressure sensor in the catheter. This confirms the inlet and outlet positions on opposite sides of the pulmonary or aortic valve, for right or left support. The motor current waveform is also displayed, along with the flow rate in liters per minute, purge system flow (mL/h), power status (AC or battery), and any active alarms.

Patient Management

The implanting center will set the P level, which should not be adjusted during transport except in two situations. Suction events are the most common clinical issues causing alarms. A suction event indicates that the impeller is offloading more blood than the amount filling the ventricle. This can result in collapse of the ventricle/vessel or the catheter tip sucking up against the inside of the heart. Reducing the P level and the rotations per minute will allow better filling. If a patient's condition deteriorates during transport requiring cardiopulmonary resuscitation, then the P level should be reduced to P-2.

Patients on these systems are anticoagulated to prevent thromboembolic events. The manufacturer recommends an activated clotting time (ACT) of 160 to 180 seconds.

Transport Considerations

Motor current is monitored to determine whether the pump is placed correctly across the valve. Any alarms indicative of loss of motor current or malpositioning of the catheter should be considered a high priority or critical alarm and be addressed promptly per the device manual. If this occurs, then the patient should be treated medically because he or she is not being treated by the device.

Patients may be transported via ground or air, including fixed-wing aircraft and helicopters. Do not raise the head of the bed above 30 degrees, and consider a knee immobilizer to stabilize the catheter placement. Do not reposition the catheter in the aircraft; this should occur in the accepting facility under fluoroscopy. Monitor the exit site for bleeding and hematoma formation and assess the distal pulses.

The Impella Controller can operate the system on a battery for 60 minutes and will beep intermittently as a reminder. The internal battery must be charged for 5 hours for the system to run for 1 hour. The device should be attached to AC power when in the vehicle or at the referring facility. When loading the device into the transport vehicle, make sure the engine is running and the inverter is operational before attaching to AC power. This will prevent a significant drain on the transport vehicle battery and affect its ability to start. The controller is on a cart that has to be secured to prevent rolling and possible catheter dislodgement. The method will vary by transport provider.

According to the 2016 guidelines for transport by Abiomed, before leaving with the patient, ensure the following:
1. The catheter placement should be verified by echocardiography.

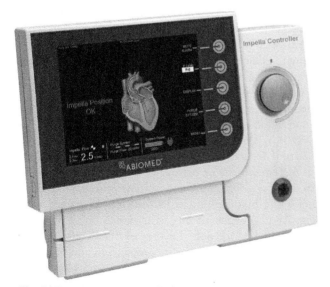

• **Fig. 21.7** Automated Impella Controller with Impella catheter. The Impella family of heart pumps have the unique ability to unload the heart and enable native heart recovery, potentially allowing patients to return home with their own hearts. As the world's smallest heart pump, the Impella platform has supported more than 50,000 patients in the United States alone, and is the only Food and Drug Administration (FDA)-approved percutaneous ventricular assist device (pVAD) indicated as safe and effective for PCI in high-risk patients and patients with acute myocardial infarction complicated by cardiogenic shock (AMICS). (Courtesy Abiomed, Inc, Danvers, Massachusetts.)

2. Tighten proper connections on the Impella Catheter to prevent catheter migration.
3. The connection cables should be free of stress.
4. Assess purge pressures during changes in altitude.
5. Place the red plug of the Impella at the level of the heart.
6. Heparinized dextrose IV fluid is the purge solution.
7. In the event of chest compressions, decrease the flow to P-2.

Maintaining optimal patient hemodynamic status and correct Impella position are two key factors in managing patients supported with the Impella System during transport.

CentriMag Blood Pumping System

The CentriMag Blood Pumping System is a short-term, extracorporeal, magnetically levitated centrifugal blood pump capable of providing RVAD, LVAD, or BiVAD support (Fig. 21.8). The blood pump typically provides 4 to 5 L/min blood flow, with normal pump speeds of 3000 to 4000 rpm. The CentriMag System is approved for 6 hours of circulatory support, and for up to 30 days when used as an RVAD in patients with cardiogenic shock attributable to acute RVF. The components of the CentriMag System include the blood pump itself, which contains the magnetically suspended impeller; the motor, which houses and drives the pump; the blood tubing, which is connected from the patient to the blood pump; an ultrasonic flow probe, which provides a direct measurement of the pump flows; and the console and backup console, which are capable of supporting one blood pump per console.

With the ultrasonic flow probe placed directly onto the outflow blood tubing, the CentriMag System has the unique ability to provide a direct measure of pump output, unlike the other acute devices in which flows are calculated. The flow probe can also detect retrograde flow and alarm accordingly. A minimum of 1000 rpm is suggested to ensure forward blood flow through the pump. The location of the flow probe should be changed regularly by approximately 1 cm to avoid creating a cinched area in the tubing, in which blood flow could slow and become susceptible to thrombus formation. The CentriMag Blood Pump uses one of two consoles: the primary console or the backup console (Fig. 21.9). The display screen of the primary console

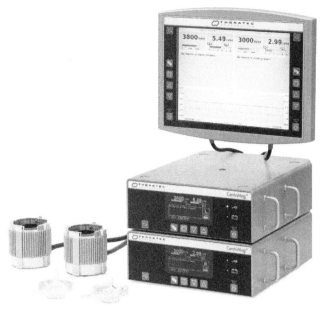

• **Fig. 21.9** CentriMag second-generation console with monitor and motors. (CentriMag, HeartMate 3, and St. Jude Medical are trademarks of St. Jude Medical, LLC, or its related companies. Reproduced with permission of St. Jude Medical, ©2017. All rights reserved.)

provides the pump speed, pump flow, power source and status, and alarm messages. Console adjustments include the ability to adjust the speed ranges from 500 to 5000 rpm, along with low- and high-flow alarm triggers. The backup console is designed to temporarily replace a failed primary console by providing support to the blood pump until a functioning primary console is available. The display screen of the backup console provides limited information (pump speed, remaining battery time, and alarm messages), although it delivers the same speed and flow capabilities as the primary console.

Implantation of the CentriMag Blood Pump is most often performed intraoperatively via a sternotomy, with venous and arterial cannulation of the RA and PA, respectively, for RVAD support and similarly, the left atrium (LA) and aorta for LVAD support (Fig. 21.10). Percutaneous placement may be performed with femoral venous and arterial access for inflow and outflow cannulation, respectively. The blood pump is locked into the pump motor (Fig. 21.11), which in turn is mounted on a bracket attached to a bedside pole. Locking of the blood pump into the motor is critical to ensure proper function of the system. A motor cable attaches the motor and blood pump to the console, which is secured on a bedside stand. If a BiVAD is implanted, then two consoles and two pump motors are needed for the two blood pumps, with backup consoles available for emergency support.

Assessment of the CentriMag Blood Pump includes monitoring patient hemodynamics; recognizing that the continuous flow pump may dampen arterial waveforms and minimize palpable pulses in the patient with LVAD

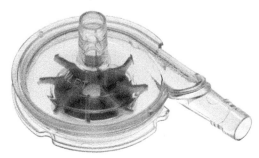

• **Fig. 21.8** CentriMag Blood Pump. (CentriMag, HeartMate 3, and St. Jude Medical are trademarks of St. Jude Medical, LLC, or its related companies. Reproduced with permission of St. Jude Medical, ©2017. All rights reserved.)

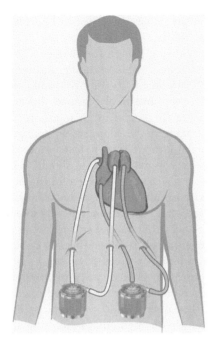

• **Fig. 21.10** CentriMag BiVAD cannulation. (CentriMag, HeartMate 3, and St. Jude Medical are trademarks of St. Jude Medical, LLC, or its related companies. Reproduced with permission of St. Jude Medical, ©2017. All rights reserved.)

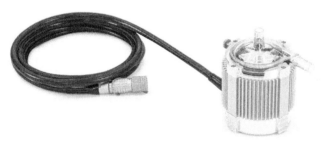

• **Fig. 21.11** CentriMag motor with CentriMag blood pump inserted. (CentriMag, HeartMate 3, and St. Jude Medical are trademarks of St. Jude Medical, LLC, or its related companies. Reproduced with permission of St. Jude Medical, ©2017. All rights reserved.)

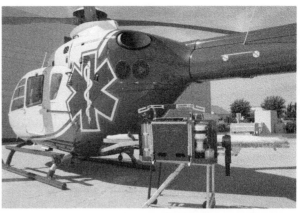

• **Fig. 21.12** Second-generation CentriMag System on CMS Transporter. (CentriMag, HeartMate 3, and St. Jude Medical are trademarks of St. Jude Medical, LLC, or its related companies. Reproduced with permission of St. Jude Medical, ©2017. All rights reserved.)

support; and monitoring for suction events as demonstrated by blood tubing chattering, presence of air in the tubing, and drops in pump flows. The blood tubing must be free of kinking and obstruction at all times, specifically on the inflow side, to help prevent air from entering the arterial tubing. Prevention of suction is achieved with improving blood volume and decreasing pump speed. Full anticoagulation is required for the CentriMag System, with systemic IV agents (e.g., heparin or argatroban if patient is HIT positive). Monitoring for thrombus formation or fibrin layering includes a focus on the tubing connections, which are frequently secured with tie-bands, and the blood pump. If the pump must be stopped at any time, then a tubing clamp must be applied to the outflow graft before turning off the pump. An extra motor, console, and flow probe should be available at all times for the patient with CentriMag Blood Pump support (Fig. 21.12).

Table 21.5 provides a brief overview of all of these acute cardiogenic shock devices.

TABLE 21.5	Acute Cardiogenic Shock Devices: Characteristics and Features		
Device name	**ECMO**	**Impella Recover**	**CentriMag**
Type	Centrifugal	Centrifugal	Centrifugal
Ventricle support	BiVAD	LVAD, RVAD, BiVAD	LVAD, RVAD, BiVAD
Rate/speed	1000–4000 rpm	10,000–33,000 rpm	1000–5500 rpm
Flow (L/min)	3–4	1.7–3.5	4–5, maximum 9.9
Flow probe	Yes	No	Yes
Internal backup console	No	No	No
Console backup battery (mins)	90	60	Primary 60; backup: 120
Manual pump	Yes	No	No
Defibrillation/cardioversion	—	Yes	Yes, without disconnect
CPR	Per doctor only	Per doctor	Per doctor
Anticoagulation	Heparin	Heparin	Heparin

BiVAD, Biventricular assist device; *CPR,* cardiopulmonary resuscitation; *ECMO,* extracorporeal membrane oxygenation; *LVAD,* left ventricular assist device; *rpm,* rotations per minute; *RVAD,* right ventricular assist device.

Transport Consideration and Assessment of Acute Ventricular Assist Devices for Interfacility Transports

The transport of acute VADs requires a competent staff. The transport staff should have critical care experience and be trained on the management of VADs or plan to transport a third rider who is considered the expert during the transport. Patient conditions are often unstable from recent surgery. As more community hospitals implant VADs, the need for transport to more definitive centers for heart transplantation or more permanent devices is warranted. Before any transport on any device, an assessment for a properly working inverter is crucial. Consult the operational manual for specific information, which may vary with each device, and have clamps and heparin available for the transport. Of note, the weight and space issues are also important for rotor-wing and fixed-wing transports.

The physical assessment of the patient includes the primary and secondary survey with a review and analysis of laboratory values, advanced hemodynamics, adequate perfusion indicators, and adequate ventilation. In addition, auscultation of native heart sounds are recommended because peripheral pulses may be difficult to palpate if a centrifugal device is used. An assessment of device alarms and battery status should also be included, with review of the device display screen to obtain more specific information about device performance, including pump flow, rate, and speed. These data should be reviewed with a physician to ensure that specific device parameters are maintained.

Regardless of whether a patient has a stable (closed) or unstable (open) sternum, the sternum is weakened and a plan should be discussed on how to perform external compressions in the event of an emergency. The patients are typically sedated with IV medications. Therefore it is important to ascertain the preimplant Glasgow Coma Score to compare it with newer findings should the patient awaken during transport. Vasoactive medications, a PA catheter, intubation, a possible IABP, and systemic anticoagulation are common in all patients with acute devices. The higher-than-normal clotting time may be related to the earlier operating room procedure (VAD implantation). The ACT should be greater than 200 seconds. All patients have some type of chest tube and should be watched carefully for increased bleeding. Epicardial pacing wires are available if temporary pacing is needed. If a patient has an automatic implantable cardioverter defibrillator, then the transport crews should assess whether it is activated or disabled. If the patient has a CF-RVAD, then extreme caution should be used when disconnecting any central vascular access device and exchanging IV bags. The continuous VADs could potentially pull air into the circulatory system if the lines are left uncapped. The most common postoperative issues facing acute patients with VADs are bleeding, arrhythmias, cardiac tamponade, hemodynamic instability, and sepsis. Other potential complications include ARDS, pulmonary embolism, and hypothermia related to heat loss from the external pump tubing.

When transporting patients on devices with externally exposed cannulas and/or blood tubing, additional precautions must be considered. The external cannulas should be visible at all times, and never covered. Ensure that the straps that secure the patient to the transport stretcher do not kink or compress the cannulas. In emergency situations in which pump function is considered compromised, only the outflow cannula should be clamped. Clamping the inflow cannula can result in air entrainment within the system. Additionally, inherent in the acute indication design, these devices are typically intended to be temporary and may therefore be susceptible to movement and/or dislodgement. It is imperative that stable positioning of the cannulas and catheters are a high priority throughout transport. Consideration of immobilization of the blood tubing as well as the affected patient limb, if appropriate, should be included in the planning phases of transport, along with methods for securing the console near the patient.

Durable Devices for Refractory Advanced Heart Failure

When a patient develops severely decompensated acute or chronic heart failure refractory to conventional pharmacologic and mechanical therapies such that hospital discharge is not feasible, or frequent rehospitalizations are needed to stabilize the patient's symptoms, the clinical team may consider more definitive therapeutic options. Cardiac transplant is the current gold standard for treating patients with end-stage heart failure who are deemed eligible, and it offers a 50% survival rate at 10 years posttransplant.[17] VAD technology can offer comparable clinical outcomes and quality of life, without the delay for treatment (e.g., waiting for a suitable donor organ) and without the side effects of immunosuppressive therapy. The quest is to design mechanical support devices that are durable, applicable to multiple body sizes, easy to implant, easy to manage technically and clinically, with minimal concurrent medication requirements including anticoagulation therapy, and suitable for all refractory heart failure indications. There is an overview of both TAHs and VADs that are currently being implanted in the following section.

Pulsatile Flow Devices

In review, the pulsatile devices, whether a TAH or a VAD, are those devices that contain a blood sac or chamber that allows for blood to collect before being ejected into the native circulation, either pneumatically or mechanically. Inflow and outflow valves, whether tissue or mechanical, ensure unidirectional, forward blood flow. Patients will typically have a palpable pulse with these devices.

Total Artificial Hearts

The *SynCardia temporary TAH* (SynCardia Systems, Inc., Tucson, AZ), an artificial heart (Fig. 21.13) currently available in the United States, received approval from the Food and Drug Administration (FDA) in October 2004 as a bridge to transplant in eligible patients at risk for imminent death, and is undergoing FDA evaluation for Human Device Exemption for DT. The device consists of blood pumps with one percutaneous pneumatic cable per pump and the external hospital-based (Companion 2 Hospital Driver) and portable (Freedom Portable Driver) consoles. The 70-mL blood pump is currently approved for commercial use, but there is a smaller 50-mL blood pump undergoing clinical trial evaluation at this time for applicability to the smaller patient cohort (e.g., women and adolescents).

As previously described, the SynCardia temporary TAH completely replaces native heart function and is surgically implanted, following removal of the native ventricles, by connecting to the native atria, PA, and aorta. The pump has unidirectional mechanical valves to replace the native heart valves, which are also removed at implant. The blood sacs will partially fill with the assist of vacuum pressure from the driver and then completely eject with a specific amount of pulsed air delivered back through the pneumatic cable. The SynCardia temporary TAH is capable of improving CO and end-organ perfusion, with pump flows up to 9.5 L/min. The pump rate is fixed, but the blood sacs can accommodate an increased blood volume return, as with exercise, allowing for an increased CO. Patients supported by the TAH no longer need inotrope, pacemaker, and/or defibrillator support. To optimize pump performance, the Companion 2 Hospital Driver allows the clinicians to adjust the pump parameters while in the hospital, including pump rate, left and right pump and vacuum pressures, and a percentage of time in systole.

The Freedom Portable Driver (Fig. 21.14) is the portable pneumatic driver for the SynCardia TAH, which allows patients to be discharged home on support. It can be carried in a backpack or shoulder bag, and runs on electricity, batteries, or a car battery. The system needs two batteries to function, each with a 2-hour capacity. The driver's display screen provides the pump rate in beats per minute, fill volume (FV), and CO when the display button is pushed. The pump rate is a fixed setting adjusted by the implanting center with special equipment and cannot be altered in the field. The default beats per minute is 125 and is the common setting to help fill and empty the TAH. The FV maximum is 70 mL, but it is usually maintained at approximately 60 mL.[23] CO should be sufficient to restore stable outputs and is usually more than 4 L/min. The driver also contains an internal backup system, which is activated automatically if the primary system fails, triggering an alarm until the console is replaced by the backup console; otherwise, no lights or sounds are active on the driver unless there is an alarm.

Patient Assessment

The TAH creates pulsatile blood flow so that patients have a systolic and diastolic pressure. The chest should be auscultated to ensure pump function, which can be heard without a stethoscope. Because the TAH replaces the native ventricles, patients do not have an ECG tracing; hence, there is no need to monitor the ECG or place electrodes. Clinical assessment, then, is focused on the blood pressure and the TAH parameters on the Freedom Portable Driver console, with the target parameters outlined in Table 21.6.

Fluid balance is delicate with the SynCardia TAH because the pump ventricles are stiff; therefore the system can only move a fixed amount of blood. Judicious use of fluids to treat patients is paramount to ensuring that patients are not flooded into volume overload.

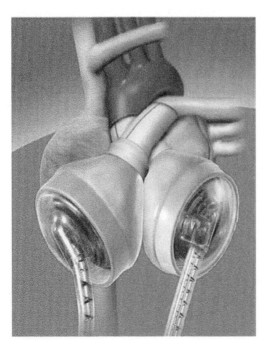

• **Fig. 21.13** SynCardia temporary Total Artificial Heart. (Courtesy SynCardia Systems, Inc., Tucson, Arizona.)

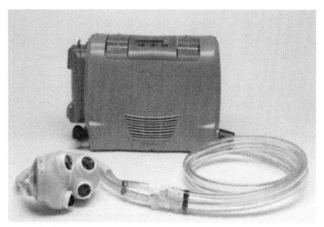

• **Fig. 21.14** Freedom Portable Driver with the SynCardia Temporary Total Artificial Heart. (Courtesy SynCardia Systems, Inc., Tucson, Arizona.)

TABLE 21.6	Clinical Targets for the SynCardia Temporary Total Artificial Heart		
Blood Pressure	TAH Bpm	TAH FV	TAH CO
<140 mm Hg	~120 bpm	>50 mL	>3.5 L/min

bpm, Beats per minute; *CO,* cardiac output; *FV,* fill volume; *TAH,* total artificial heart.

Ensure that backup batteries are present during transport. It is also essential to bring the backup Freedom Portable Driver in the event of emergent need to switch drivers, and 12V vehicle power is needed for proper operation.

Emergency Management

There are three alarms on the Freedom Portable Driver: battery status, temperature, and fault. The only way to silence these alarms is to resolve the issue. Transport teams should reference the Freedom Driver System Operator Manual or emergency medical services (EMS) VAD field guides to troubleshoot these alarms.[24]

Parameters

1. A systolic blood pressure greater than 140 mm Hg will result in an inability of the system to empty efficiently and requires immediate treatment. Contact the implanting center for orders for appropriate medications.
2. An FV less than 50 mL may indicate a problem with the diaphragm within the pump and necessitate a switch to the implant console. The patient should be transported to the implant center as soon as possible.
3. CO less than 3.5 L/min is an emergency.
4. Vasopressor agents are *not* to be given.
5. Chest compressions are contraindicated.
6. Defibrillation is not effective because there are no native ventricles.
7. Contact the implanting center for instructions while the patient is emergently transported to that center.

For an emergent transport, transport teams unfamiliar with the device should transport the patient's significant other to assist in management of the device. Assess if the significant other has been trained on the device at the implantation center and if he or she is able to assist with management of the device. Another option is to ask the conscious patient questions about the operation and emergency management of the device, such as how to change the batteries or exchange the Freedom Portable Driver if necessary. This will provide a quick review of the basics to transport the patient "emergently" from point A to point B.

Continuous Flow Devices

As previously described, VADs, unlike TAHs, are designed to support the native heart without removing it. Initially, the FDA approval of these technologies required specification of the intended indication for commercialization as BTT or DT. Over time, clinical application and use of the approved devices has evolved to a more general indication of medically refractory, advanced heart failure. As described by Felker and Rogers,[25] the ultimate treatment goal of the therapy is driven by the patient's outcome following implant.

Although the original predecessors were pulsatile VADs, the currently available long-term VADs are CF-VADs intended for LVAD support only. Although some of these devices are being evaluated in preclinical work for RVAD and BiVAD support,[26] the current approved strategy is LVAD only. The major components of these devices are the blood pump, with an inflow cannula and an outflow graft; the controller, which runs the pump and provides device status and alarm indicators; and the power source. Not all of these devices use a bedside console, but they do provide interchangeable access to electricity and battery power. As LVADs, these devices cannulate the LV apex for the inflow access, with outflow anastomosis primarily to the ascending aorta, although some clinicians have limited experience with alternative anastomotic sites such as the descending thoracic aorta.[27] It is possible to anastomose the outflow cannula in the descending aorta if it is determined that the aortic arch is calcified, avoiding the increased risk of stroke or difficulty sewing to a friable arch.

Blood flow dynamics through the pumps are impacted by the differential pressures at the inflow (LV) and outflow (aorta) cannulas, with sensitivity to preload and afterload. The higher differential pressure (higher aortic pressure relative to ventricular pressure) results in a lower pump outflow. Conversely, the lower differential pressure (increased ventricular pressure relative to aortic pressure) results in a higher pump outflow. Hence, systemic hypertension, for example, will diminish the pump output. Anticoagulation of these devices currently includes at least one antiplatelet (usually aspirin) and antithrombin therapy (warfarin).

In contrast to the PF-VADs, CF-VADs have the advantage of finer control of LV unloading with manual impeller speed control, which helps to minimize the risk of RVF. Alternatively, they do not have the capability for manual drive (e.g., hand pumping) should the device fail. The physiologic and subsequent geometric changes that occur with LV support may perpetuate otherwise benign RVF, prompting the need for additional inotropic support if not temporary mechanical support for the RV. If necessary, it is possible to support the RV with a temporary device and the LV with a durable device. The temporary RVAD may then be weaned and explanted after several days of RV myocardial rest.

Another feature of the CF-VADs is that they are valveless. Because these devices draw blood continuously through the pump, valvular assurance of unidirectional blood flow is not needed. However, without valves and no mechanism for manually running the pump, pump failure and subsequent stoppage may potentially result in a significant retrograde blood flow (approximately 1–2 L/min) from the aorta back through the pump into the LV. Hence, efforts to prevent device failure have a heightened importance.

Axial Flow Ventricular Assist Devices

The *axial flow VADs* are continuous flow blood pumps with a linear blood path across the impeller. Two axial flow long-term blood pumps currently available in the United States are the HeartMate II LVAS (Thoratec Corporation, St. Jude Medical, Pleasanton, California) and the Jarvik 2000 Ventricular Assist Device (Jarvik Heart, Inc., New York). The HeartMate II LVAS received FDA approval for BTT and DT in April 2008 and January 2010, respectively. The Jarvik 2000 is currently involved in FDA investigational trials for BTT and DT.

HeartMate II Left Ventricular Assist System

The *HeartMate II LVAS* is an axial flow VAD, with its inflow cannula and outflow graft attached to the LV apex and ascending aorta, respectively, with placement of the blood pump itself in a subdiaphragmatic, preperitoneal pocket (Fig. 21.15). The inflow cannula has a textured surface intended to stimulate the development of a biological (pseudointimal) layering to help reduce the risk for thrombus formation on the cannula. The driveline is tunneled across the abdomen and exits through the skin, connecting the implanted pump to the external components of the system. The HMII System Controller essentially runs the pump, monitors the system and provides alarm and power statuses, and transmits power from the power source to the pump. The display button on the controller screen will allow the user to toggle through pump parameters, including speed, flow, and pulsatility index (PI), as well as power indicators. This allows the provider to assess the VAD performance.

Alarms and lamps along with messages in the display alert providers to pump issues and instruct the providers on actions to be taken.

The controller has two power cables that connect to either the electrical power module or to portable batteries with battery clips. The green light on the controller confirms that both power connections are good. The batteries can provide up to 10 to 12 hours of power, depending on the patient activity. The controller and power source are kept close to the patient, along with the backup controller. In the event of a primary controller malfunction, the controllers must be exchanged. Although the controller icons include the pump running symbol, confirmation should also be made by auscultating the chest.

Jarvik 2000 Ventricular Assist Device

The Jarvik 2000 axial flow pump has a number of nuances that differentiate it from the other axial flow pumps. The inflow cannula contains the impeller, which is placed directly into the LV apex (Fig. 21.16). The potential advantage of this intraventricular placement is that the pump pocket used by the other devices is obviated, as is the potential for pump pocket infections. The outflow graft is anastomosed to the aorta. Another nuance of the Jarvik 2000 is tunneling of the driveline. As a part of the current US clinical trial, the driveline may be tunneled through the abdomen, as with other CF-VADs, or it may be tunneled under the skin to a pedestal located behind the ear. The postauricular position is being studied in the DT trial.

Similar to other LVAD controllers, the Jarvik 2000 controller runs the pump, provides power to the pump, and monitors and triggers alarm statuses (Fig. 21.16). In addition to these standard features, the Jarvik 2000 controller uniquely allows the patient the ability to adjust the speed of

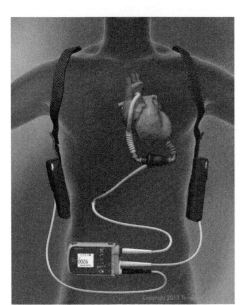

• **Fig. 21.15** Implantation approach of the Thoratec HeartMate II Left Ventricular Assist System. (Courtesy Thoratec Corporation, Pleasonton, California.)

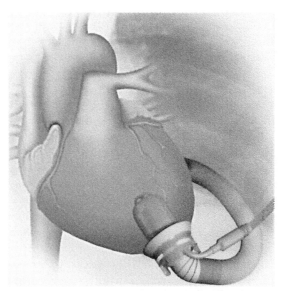

• **Fig. 21.16** Implantation approach for the Jarvik 2000 Left Ventricular Assist Device. (Courtesy of Robert Jarvik, MD.)

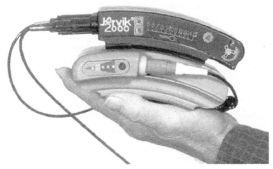

• **Fig. 21.17** Jarvik 2000 controller and battery. (Courtesy of Robert Jarvik, MD.)

the pump to accommodate the body's physiologic demands (e.g., lower speeds for rest, intermediate speeds for everyday activity, higher speeds for strenuous activity). The speed-adjustment knob is located on the side of the controller next to the speed settings indicator. The speed settings are numbered 1 to 5, with 1000-rpm incremental speed rates per speed setting, ranging from 8000 to 12,000 rpm. The speed rates correlate with a volume of augmented blood flow, which is not necessarily actual blood flow. Adequate filling of the blood pump affects the pump flow, as with any of the other devices. A setting of 1 provides an estimated augmented blood volume of 1 to 2 L/min, whereas a setting of 5 provides an estimated augmented blood volume of 5 to 7 L/min. The watts used to drive the pump are indicated on the controller and range from 3 to 13. The cables that connect the pump to the external components include an extension cable with a retractable coil that allows up to an additional 6 feet from the patient to the controller.

The Jarvik 2000 is designed to be powered by battery sources only and not electricity. The pump may be attached to the battery recharger for battery support, but it does not draw electricity even though the battery charger is plugged into a wall socket. The two types of battery sources for the Jarvik pump are the portable batteries that provide up to 7 to 12 hours of support per battery and the reserve batteries that provide up to 24 hours of support. All of the batteries recharge by being plugged into electricity.

Centrifugal Flow Rotary Pumps

The centrifugal blood pumps are continuous flow pumps with disk impellers that are magnetically and/or hydrodynamically suspended. These pump designs suggest a "wearless" system with maximal durability because there are no contacting mechanical parts to wear down over time. The disk impeller uses both centrifugal and circumferential energy to propel the blood through the blood path, which includes a perpendicular turn as the blood enters and exits the impeller. These centrifugal pumps boast smaller drivelines to help minimize the driveline infection issues of their predecessors. They are also more energy efficient to allow for the possibility of smaller and lighter batteries for longer periods of time, pending technologic advancement. Centrifugal flow

pumps currently available are the HeartWare Ventricular Assist System (HeartWare, Inc., Framingham, Massachusetts), and the HeartMate 3 LVAD (Thoratec Corporation, St. Jude Medical, Pleasanton, California). Both pumps have received commercial approval (CE Mark) in Europe. The HeartWare System has BTT approval in the United States and has completed enrollment in the DT trial, whereas the HeartMate 3 LVAD is undergoing a clinical trial in the United States. Primary components of these pumps, as with their axial flow pump predecessors, include the blood pump, the external controller, and the power source. Similarly, the pump flow dynamics of the centrifugal LVAD are sensitive to the differential pressure relationships of the inflow and outflow cannulas, and to preload and afterload. Additionally, these devices currently require both antithrombin and antiplatelet therapy.

HeartWare Ventricular Assist System

The *HeartWare Ventricular Assist System* received FDA approval for BTT in 2012, and is finalizing the data for DT submission. Unlike the other centrifugal pumps, the HeartWare pump is implanted within the pericardial space (Fig. 21.18), with outflow graft anastomosis to the ascending aorta and subcutaneous driveline tunneling to either the right or left upper quadrant of the abdomen. The driveline is significantly smaller than in its predecessors and is connected to the external controller (Fig. 21.19), which is then connected to the appropriate power source. The controller provides the pump speed, flow, and watts parameters; alarm messages and interventions to correct them; and power source and status. A unique characteristic of this pump is that the patient's hematocrit (Hct) value is entered into the controller at the implanting center and is combined with pump speed and watts to provide a highly accurate calculated pump flow. As such, an incorrect entry of the patient's Hct or an outdated value may affect the flow estimate and

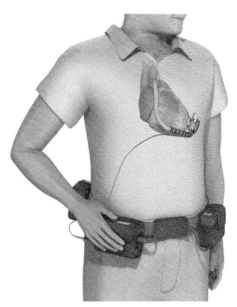

• **Fig. 21.18** HVAD system. (Courtesy of HeartWare, Framingham, Massachusetts.)

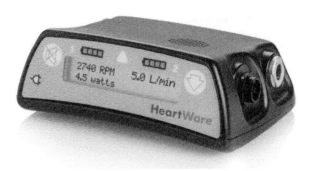

• **Fig. 21.19** HeartWare Controller. (Courtesy of HeartWare, Framingham, Massachusetts.)

trigger an inappropriate low- or high-flow alarm. Power sources include external batteries, AC adaptor to an electrical outlet, and a direct current adaptor to a car outlet. One battery provides 4 to 6 hours of support and will automatically switch over to the fully charged battery when necessary. External batteries are recharged by a portable battery charger.

HeartMate 3 Left Ventricular Assist System

At the time of this writing, the HeartMate 3 LVAS (Fig. 21.20) is an investigational LVAD in the United States with design modifications that may theoretically reduce complications common in VAD patients. The pump has a centrifugal design with an impeller that is completely magnetically suspended in the middle within the pump housing. The speed of the impeller rotation is set by the clinicians at the implanting center and is usually approximately 4800 to 5600 rpm. An additional design feature is that the speed of the impeller pulses up and down 30 times a minute or every 2 seconds, disrupting the blood movement inside the pump and potentially reducing thrombus formation. Because of this small variation in speed, there is a different characteristic to the sound of the pump on auscultation. This pulsation, however, cannot be felt with palpation, and happens so quickly that it is not captured by the setting that displays the speed on the controller.

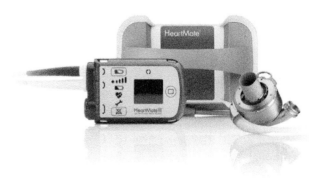

• **Fig. 21.20** HeartMate 3 Left Ventricular Assist System and Controller. (CentriMag, HeartMate 3, and St. Jude Medical are trademarks of St. Jude Medical, LLC, or its related companies. Reproduced with permission of St. Jude Medical, ©2017. All rights reserved.)

Another design modification is the modular driveline. A known device complication is damage to the external driveline, resulting in pump stoppage. The modular driveline allows clinicians to replace the external portion of the driveline by unlocking the connection and attaching a new driveline. This connection point needs to be protected from accidental stress and disconnection. The connection is a heavy, metal two-piece section on the driveline. It should be inspected to ensure that a yellow ring between the two metal pieces cannot be seen. If the yellow ring is visualized, then stabilize the connection and contact the implanting center for instructions on ensuring that the two metal halves are screwed together.

The interface on the controller for the HeartMate 3 LVAS is very similar to the HeartMate II. The controllers for the two systems can be distinguished by the color scheme of the body of the controller. The back of the HeartMate 3 pocket controller is black, which allows the care team to quickly identify that the patient has a HeartMate 3 simply by looking at the controller. The back of the HeartMate II controller is white. All external components are similar in appearance and operation as with the HeartMate II.

Table 21.7 provides a brief overview of all of these chronic heart failure devices.

Interfacility or Scene Transport Consideration of Long-Term Ventricular Assist Devices

The number of patients discharged in the community with VADs has increased in recent years. Because heart failure can be treated with VADs and the improved durability of the devices means longer support times, transport crews are likely to encounter this patient population. Most of these patients have long-term devices with more stable conditions, unlike their acute VAD counterparts who are more likely being transported in the immediate postoperative period. Some of the more stable patients have had their devices for weeks or months, and others for years. With the increased number of VAD options, transport crews are challenged to remain competent on all of them. Therefore the educational leadership of these programs must ascertain which devices are in their area and develop training programs accordingly.

Patient Assessment

As many patients attempt to normalize their appearance when managing the equipment, identifying that a supported patient actually has a CF-VAD may be the first assessment challenge. If any of the external components are seen, quickly confirm if the patient has a VAD because this will dramatically change your assessment.

Once it is determined that the patient has a CF-VAD, next confirm if the patient has a palpable pulse, because the patient assessment will need to be modified due to pulseless

TABLE 21.7 Chronic or Refractory Heart Failure Devices: Characteristics and Features

Device name	SynCardia	HeartMate II	Jarvik	HeartWare	HeartMate3
Type	Vol. disp.	Axial	Axial	Centrifugal	Centrifugal
Ventricle support	TAH	LVAD	LVAD	LVAD	LVAD
Typical rate/speed	120–135 beats/min	8000–12,000 rpm	8000–12,000 rpm	2400–3000 rpm	4000–9000 rpm
Flow (L/min)	4.9–9.5	4–10	Up to 8	2–10	4–10
Motor current (watts)	Not displayed	6–8	3–10	3.5–5.0	4–8
Built-in backup controller	Backup motor	Yes	No	No	Yes
Battery support (hours/battery set)	2	10–12	7–12	8–12	8–12
Manual pump	No	No	No	No	No
Defibrillation/ cardioversion	No	Yes	Yes	Yes	Yes
CPR	No	Per doctor	Per doctor	Per doctor	Per doctor
Antithrombin	Yes	Yes	Yes	Yes	Yes
Antiplatelet	Yes	Yes	Yes	Yes	Yes

CPR, Cardiopulmonary resuscitation; *LVAD*, left ventricular assist device; *rpm*, rotations per minute; *TAH*, total artificial heart; *Vol disp.*, volume displacement.

blood flow. Auscultate the chest to listen for native heart sounds and the pump. Because a pulse oximeter uses the surge in blood flow during systole to calculate an accurate saturation, it may not be accurate in these patients, so clinical decisions should not be based on this number. Peripheral blood pressures must be measured using a sphygmomanometer, a Doppler flow probe, and gel. Automated blood pressure machines rely on pulsatility, which is dependent on the native heart function and filling. Assessing the patient's level of consciousness, skin color and temperature, heart rhythm using a monitor, and signs of dehydration versus volume overload are important first steps.

It is important to know the model of the device, whether it is axial or centrifugal flow, and whether backup equipment is readily available. Having the contact information from the implanting center will be especially helpful. If the site can be contacted, then the clinicians may be able to provide patient-specific information to help with the clinical assessment and management. The controller will provide VAD parameters, which are important to monitor and trend throughout the transport. The controller can also be helpful during alarm conditions, because it may provide information about troubleshooting the alarm and specific actions to take. Controller alarms need to be reported immediately to the implanting center.

Low-flow alarms occur with poor filling of the pump or obstruction to emptying. The Mechanical Circulatory Assist Guidelines from the International Society of Heart Lung Transplant state several etiologies that result in poor pump filling. These patient-pump interface issues can be summarized in an acronym SHAB DORC:

S: Sepsis or sedation: Assess the patient for signs and symptoms of infection, and/or use of sedatives that can cause vasodilatation.

H: Hypertension: Mean arterial pressure (MAP) greater than 90 mm Hg may create too much resistance, limiting forward blood flow through the pump; typical MAP target is 65 to 85 mm Hg.

A: Arrhythmias: Obtain rhythm strip.

B: Bleeding: Approximately 25% of all patients with VADs experience gastrointestinal bleeding.[28]

D: Dehydration: This may be the result of aggressive diuretic regimen or poor oral intake.

O: Overdrive: The speed is too fast for the patient's current volume status, or there is an obstruction, especially seen in the immediate postoperative period caused by tamponade.

R: Right heart failure.

C: Clot: Clot formation inside the pump is a possible complication and can change the blood flow dynamics through the pump.

Patient monitoring and management should include establishing IV access, monitoring heart rhythm, and obtaining results of the most recent blood tests to include CBC, blood chemistries, and international normalized ratio.

Assessment of the Equipment

Assessment of the device function involves reviewing the VAD parameters displayed on the controller. The VAD parameters should be monitored frequently and routinely for the duration of the transport, and include the pump flow, speed, and power. The pump flow is the amount of blood flow through the pump, which is calculated by the system in liters per minute. The Jarvik 2000 LVAD, as previously described, does not provide a calculated measure of flow; rather, it provides a dial setting providing an estimate of augmented flow volume. The pump speed is how fast the impeller inside the pump is spinning and is measured in rotations per minute. The pump speed is set at the implanting center and is a fixed speed. Only the Jarvik 2000 LVAD has the ability to adjust the speed outside of the hospital setting. The power is how much energy in watts the pump uses to rotate the impeller to move the blood flow at the set speed. The HeartMate devices have an additional parameter, the PI. It is a unit of measure unique to those devices that provide the end user with a number that represents the filling of the pump. A number above 3.5 is adequate.

In addition to the pump parameters, the controllers or consoles for each VAD are designed to provide information to clinicians on their display screens regarding urgent or emergent conditions that require interventions. Alarms are announced through audible alerts and/or illuminated lamps on the controllers/consoles. Each system has a way to differentiate noncritical versus hazard alarms based on the warning signals. The battery status is typically monitored by the controller or console and should be checked frequently to avoid power interruption. Issues with connections or component functionality will trigger alarms. Contact the implanting center to obtain instructions on how to intervene.

The alarm guides for each device may be accessed by referring to the device-specific manufacturer website, which is the most reliable source of current information. Additionally, the MCS guidelines published in 2013[29] reference the use of the EMS VAD field guides as a resource for providers interfacing with VAD equipment. The VAD coordinator professional organization, the International Consortium of Circulatory Assist Clinicians, has endorsed the use of the field guides as best practice. The most current versions of the field guides are available electronically on www.MyLVAD.com.

The patients are instructed to always carry a travel bag with all of the equipment needed to manage the device in an emergency. This bag should contain extra batteries, backup controllers, and other specific equipment for the device. Also inside the travel kit is a reference card for the alarms and contact information for patient management. This equipment should always be transported with the patient. The patient is also instructed to be in the company of another person who is trained in emergency management of the device. If an emergency arises that renders the patient unconscious, then the secondary caregiver should take over management of the pump. The secondary caregiver must also be transported if weight and space allow.

The patients who return for readmission to the local hospital return for a number of reasons. Along with device-related failure alarms unresolved by the patient, they may also return for non–device-specific issues, including altered mental status, falls, peripheral venous thrombosis (deep vein thrombosis), stroke or transient ischemic attacks, chest pain, sepsis, and nutritional and psychosocial issues.

Summary

The use of VADs will only increase as the technology continues to evolve and improve. The next frontier of MCSD projects to be smaller, more energy efficient, and possibly less invasively implanted. The potential for easier technology with easier implantation approaches allows smaller hospitals the opportunity to implant these devices and potentially transport these patients to larger facilities. This progress will have a significant impact on the volume of critical care air and surface transports. As this occurs, transport teams must remain competent in transport and develop specific policies and guidelines related to the management and transport of this special patient population. Because the number of devices in this country is expanding, most prehospital personnel and transport personnel cannot remain comfortable and competent. Box 21.1 outlines a series of questions each transport team member can ask the patient, secondary caregiver, or knowledgeable physician to ensure safe and swift transport by the teams. These questions provide the information needed to safely transport patients with MCSD during an interfacility or scene flight if a situation occurs in which a patient presents with an unfamiliar device.

• **BOX 21.1** **Checklist Review for Mechanical Circulatory Support Device Transport**

1. Can I do external cardiopulmonary resuscitation?
2. If not, is a hand pump or external device available for use?
3. If the device slows down (low flow state), what alarms are triggered?
4. How can I speed up the rate of the device?
5. Do I need to use heparinization for the patient if the device slows down?
6. Can the patient undergo defibrillation while connected to the device?
7. If the patient can undergo defibrillation, does anything need to be disconnected before defibrillation?
8. Does the patient have a pulse with this device?
9. What are acceptable vital sign parameters?
10. Can this patient be externally paced?

References

1. Helman D, Morales D, Edwards N, et al. Left ventricular assist device bridge-to-transplant network improves survival after failed cardiotomy. *Ann Thorac Surg.* 1999;68(4):1187-1194.
2. Reiss N, El-Banayosy A, Posival H, et al. Transport of hemodynamically unstable patients by a mobile mechanical circulatory support team. *Artif Organs.* 1996;20(8):959-963.
3. McBride LR, Lowdermilk GA, Fiore AC, et al. Transfer of patients receiving advanced mechanical circulatory support. *J Thoracic Cardiovasc Surg.* 2000;119(5):1015-1020.
4. Coppola AP, Tyree M, Larry K, DiGeronimo R. A 22-year experience in global transport extracorporeal membrane oxygenation. *J Ped Surg.* 2008;43(1):46-52.
5. Kirklin JK, Frazier OH. Developmental history of mechanical circulatory support. In: Frazier OH, Kirklin JK, eds. *ISHLT Monograph Series Mechanical Circulatory Support.* Vol 1. Philadelphia, PA: Elsevier, Inc; 2006.
6. Devries W. The permanent artificial heart: four case reports. *JAMA.* 1988;259(6):849–859.

7. American Heart Association. *Heart Disease and Stroke Statistics: 2005 Update.* Dallas, TX: American Heart Association; 2005.

8. Portner P, Oyer P, McGregor C. First human use of an electrically powered implantable ventricular assist system. *Artif Organs.* 1985;9(a):36.

9. Rose EC, Gelijns AC, Maskowitz AJ, et al. For the REMATCH Study Group: Long-term use of a left ventricular assist device for end-stage heart failure. *N Engl J Med.* 2001;345(20):1435-1443.

10. Overwalder PJ. Intra-aortic balloon pump (IABP) counterpulsation. *Internet J Thoracic Cardovasc Surg.* 1999;2(2).

11. Bolooki H. *Clinical Application of the Intraaortic Balloon Pump.* Armonk, NY: Futura Publishing Company, Inc; 1998.

12. Farrar DJ, Holman WR, McBride LR, et al. Long-term follow-up of Thoratec ventricular assist device bridge-to-recovery patients successfully removed from support after recovery of ventricular function. *J Heart Lung Transplant.* 2002;21(5):516-521.

13. Samuels LE, Shemanski KA, Casanova-Ghosh E, et al. Hybrid ventricular assist device: HeartMate XVE LVAD and Abiomed AB5000 RVAD. *ASAIO J.* 2008;54(3):332-334.

14. Wood C, Maiorana A, Larbalestier R, et al. First successful bridge to myocardial recovery with a HeartWare HVAD. *J Heart Lung Transplant.* 2008;27(6):695-700.

15. Organ Procurement and Transplantation Network and the Scientific Registry of Transplant Recipients. *OPTN/SRTR 2014 Annual Data Report Heart; Special Issue: OPTN/SRTR Annual Data Report 2014.* 2016;16(S2):4-7. (OPTN/SRTR Annual Data Report 2014: Preface. American Journal of Transplantation, 2016; 16: 4–7. doi: 10.1111/ajt.13664)

16. Colvin M, Smith JM, Skeans MA, et al. OPTN/SRTR Annual Data Report 2014: Heart. *Am J of Transplant.* 2016;16(S2):115-140.

17. Taylor DO, Edwards LB, Boucek MM, et al. Registry of the International Society for Heart and Lung Transplantation: twenty-fourth official adult heart transplant report. *J Heart Lung Transplant.* 2007;26(8):769-781.

18. Kirklin JK, Holman WL. Mechanical circulatory support therapy as a bridge to transplant or recovery (new advances). *Curr Opin Cardiol.* 2006;21(2):120-126.

19. Lund LH, Edwards LB, Kucheryavaya AY, et al. ISHLT International Registry for Heart and Lung Transplantation 2015. *J Heart Lung Transplant.* 2015;34(10):1244-1254.

20. Slaughter MS, Rogers JG, Milano CA, et al. Advanced heart failure treated with continuous-flow left ventricular assist device. *N Engl J Med.* 2009;361(23):2241-2251.

21. Gravelee GP, Davis RF, Stammers AH, et al. *Cardiopulmonary Bypass: Principles and Practice.* 3rd ed. New York: Lippincott, Williams & Wilkins; 2008.

22. Arrow International. *Counterpulsation Applied: an Introduction to Intra Aortic Balloon Pumping.* Reading, PA: Educational Materials Cardiac Assist; 2012.

23. Slepian MJ, Smith RG, and Copeland JG. The SynCardia CardioWest Total Artificial Heart. In: Baughman KL, Baumgartner WA, eds. *Treatment of Advanced Heart Disease.* Boca Raton, FL: Taylor and Francis; 2006.

24. SynCardia. *TAH Manual.* Tucson, AZ: SynCardia Systems, Inc; 2014.

25. Felker GM, Rogers JG. Same bridge, new destination. *J Am Coll Cardiol.* 2006;47(5):930-932.

26. Yoshioka D, Toda K, Yoshikawa Y, Sawa Y. Over 1200-day support with dual Jarvik 2000 biventricular assist device. *Interact Cardiovasc Thorac Surg.* 2014;19(6):1083-1084.

27. Sorensen EN, Pierson RN, Feller ED, Griffith BP. University of Maryland surgical experience with the Jarvik 2000 axial flow ventricular assist device. *Ann Thorac Surg.* 2012;93(1):133-140.

28. Harvey L, Holley CT, John R. Gastrointestinal bleed after left ventricular assist device implantation: incidence, management, and prevention. *Ann Cardiothorac Surg.* 2014;3(5):475-479.

29. Feldmen D, Pamboukian SV, Teuteberg JJ, et al. The 2013 international society of heart and lung transplantation guidelines for mechanical circulatory support. *J Heart Lung Transplant.* 2013;32(2):121-146.

Reference Manuals

Abiomed. *Impella Ventricular Support Systems for use during Cardiogenic Shock.* Danvers, MA: Abiomed, Inc; 2011.

Abiomed. *Impella RP with the Automated Impella Controller.* Danvers, MA: Abiomed, Inc; 2015.

Abiomed. *Patient Transport with the Automated Impella Controller.* Danvers, MA: Abiomed, Inc; 2011.

Abiomed. *Transport Guidelines for the Patient with the Impella System.* Danvers, MA: Abiomed, Inc; 2016.

HeartWare. *HeartWare Ventricular Assist System instructions for use.* Rev 21. Miami Lakes, FL: HeartWare, Inc; 2015.

Jarvik. *Jarvik 2000 Operator Manual.* New York: Jarvik Heart, Inc; 2009.

Jarvik. *Jarvik 2000 Patient Handbook.* New York: Jarvik Heart, Inc; 2009.

Maquet CS 100 Educational Materials: IABP Counterpulsation. Mahwah, NJ: Datascope Corporation; 2012.

Maquet Cardiosave Operators Manual. Mahwah, NJ: Datascope Corporation; 2013.

SynCardia. *SynCardia Temporary Total Artificial Heart (TAH-t) with the Freedom Driver System Operator Manual.* Tucson, AZ: SynCardia Systems, Inc; 2005.

Thoratec. *HeartMate II Left Ventricular Assist System instructions for use.* Pleasanton, CA: Thoratec Corporation; 2016.

Thoratec. *HeartMate II LVAS Operating Manual.* Pleasanton, CA: Thoratec Corporation; 2013.

Thoratec. *CentriMag Blood Pump Instructions for use.* Pleasanton, CA: Thoratec Corporation; 2013.

Thoratec. *2nd Generation CentriMag System Operating Manual.* Pleasanton, CA: Thoratec Corporation; 2013.

www.Thoratec.com, Accessed 17.06.16.

22

Pulmonary Emergencies

LUKE GASOWSKI AND CHAD POGGEMEYER

Anatomy and Physiology Overview

Anatomy

Airway

The human airway can be divided into two sections, the upper and lower airway. The upper airway consists of the nose, mouth, and pharynx, and the lower airway includes the trachea and the multiple generations of the tracheobronchial tree. The responsibilities of the upper airway include an entranceway for air, a filter and humidification system, a sense of smell, phonation, and protection for the lower airway. The pharynx is subdivided into the nasopharynx, oropharynx, and the laryngopharynx. Air enters the nares and is filtered by nasal hair, which traps external particles. Turbulent flow is created as air passes over the bony prominences of the conchae. This assists in the collection of foreign matter on the posterior mucous-lined surfaces. Because the nasal cavity is highly vascularized, the incoming air is warmed and humidified as it continues its transit of the airway. Olfactory nerve fibers located around the cribriform plate provide the sense of smell as air passes through. The epiglottis is the leaf-shaped flexible cartilage that covers the larynx during swallowing. Its primary function is to prevent food and liquids from entering the trachea and is a primary landmark structure for intubation. The larynx is an extension of the airway involved in the continuation of protective mechanisms and the generation of sound. Palpated outward landmarks of the larynx include the thyroid and cricoid cartilage. These structures can also be used to externally manipulate the laryngeal anatomy to optimize visualization of the vocal cords during endotracheal intubation. The cricoid area is often the site for emergency surgical access when conventional methods of definitive airway placement have failed or are implausible.[1,2]

The lower airway consists of the trachea, the right and left mainstem bronchi, and extended structures of further bronchi, bronchioles, alveolar ducts, and alveolar sacs. These structures can be physiologically divided into various categories such as conducting versus respiratory zones and cartilaginous versus noncartilaginous formation with sites of actual gas exchange. The cartilaginous airways consist of the trachea, mainstem bronchi, lobar bronchi, and segmental and subsegmental bronchi. The noncartilaginous airways include the bronchioles and terminal bronchioles and extend to the respiratory bronchioles, alveolar ducts, and alveolar sacs. There are approximately 270 to 300 million alveoli in the average-size adult, with the total surface area equivalent to a tennis court.[1,2]

The trachea starts at the distal portion of the cricoid cartilage and is approximately 10 to 12 cm long. It is made up of 16 to 20 C-shaped cartilaginous rings that provide stability. The mucosal surface of the trachea is made up of columnar epithelium and mucous-secreting cells. The trachea continues distally to the bifurcation, called the carina, which is at the angle of Louis at the level of the second rib. The right mainstem bronchus bifurcates off the trachea at an angle of around 20 to 30 degrees in comparison to the left, which is about 45 to 55 degrees. This makes the incidence of foreign body aspiration or endotracheal intubation at higher risk on the right side than left.

The right and left mainstem bronchi branch into further distal bronchi and bronchioles. The lobar bronchi divide into segmental bronchi, which are excellent anatomic identification markers for sites of infections or lung masses. The next two divisions after the subsegmental bronchi include the bronchioles and terminal bronchioles, which are the beginning of the noncartilaginous airways and decrease to less than 1 and 0.5 mm, respectively. Distal to the terminal bronchioles the cross-sectional area increases considerably, and these respiratory zones are the working entity in which gas exchange takes place and alveolar budding begins. These next three regions, the respiratory bronchioles, alveolar ducts, and alveolar sacs, are also referred to as the acinis. At this point in the tracheobronchial tree, the size of the respiratory bronchioles is only about 0.4 mm in diameter and continues to bifurcate further into three to four generations. The alveolar ducts and alveolar sacs are where the major transaction of oxygen and carbon dioxide takes place, with the latter being the largest site of gas exchange. The alveolar sacs are made up of Type I and Type II cells. Type I cells are squamous epithelial cells and Type II cells are granular pneumocytes. The alveolar wall is lined by thin, flat Type I cells. They contain a large amount of capillaries because they are the site of gas exchange. Type I cells cannot replicate like Type II cells can. Type II cells exhibit a number of functions, including the production of surfactant and surfactant-associated proteins, division and differentiation into Type I cells that may have been damaged, and transport of sodium and water toward the endothelial cells and blood to help minimize fluid accumulation in the alveolar space.[3] Surfactant produced by these Type II cells decreases the surface tension and helps prevent alveolar collapse.[1,2,4]

Thoracic Cage

The thoracic cavity encompasses and protects the cardiopulmonary structures and other organs. The skeletal framework includes the ribs, sternum, costal cartilages, and the posterior thoracic vertebrae. There are two layers that line the surface of the lung: the visceral pleura, which covers the outermost lining of the lung, and the parietal pleura, which lines the thoracic wall. Between the two pleura linings is a potential space that contains a small amount of serous fluid, approximately 20 mLs, which acts as a lubricant. This allows the two linings to glide over each other during inspiration and exhalation. These intact structures of the thorax are vital to create pressure gradients needed to facilitate the process of ventilation. Other organs found in the thorax include the esophagus, thymus gland, lymphatic vessels, and nerves.

Muscles of Ventilation

The process of ventilation has two phases: inspiration and expiration. Inspiration is an active process. Contraction of the diaphragm causes it to descend, and the external intercostal muscles increase the anterior posterior diameter of the thorax by raising the ribs and lowering the diaphragm. As chest cavity size increases, a negative pressure gradient is created, and air is inspired. As the diaphragm relaxes it ascends by natural elastic recoil and causes an increase in the intrapleural and intraalveolar pressure, and air flows out of the lungs.

The accessory muscles are a group of muscles used in the acute stages of respiratory distress or in the presence of chronic lung disease. Normally, the diaphragm and intercostal muscles are able to provide adequate ventilation without recruiting other muscles to aid in the process. Observation of which muscles are used in your assessment is key to the evaluation of the pulmonary patient. On inspiration the major muscles used are the scalene, sternocleidomastoid, trapezius, pectoralis, and external intercostal muscle. The majority of these muscles increase the anteroposterior diameter of the chest, which assists in creating a larger pressure gradient between the intrapleural pressure and outside environment. The muscles of expiration are enlisted when airway resistance is heightened and the muscles are used to push up on the diaphragm or decrease the lateral and anteroposterior

diameter of the chest. These include the abdominal muscles and internal intercostal muscles.[1,2,4]

Volumes and Capacities

Volumes and capacities have several individualized factors that contribute the average numerical value. These include age, height, gender, and ethnicity. For the purpose of this book the average amount will be given with the volumes and capacities approximately 20% to 25% smaller in women compared with men. When taking into account the volume of air in the lung, four distinct sections can be derived. These sections can then be divided in another four capacities. When these values are known, they provide cardinal information for the diagnosis and understanding of specific pulmonary diseases and management (Table 22.1).[3]

Physiology

Effective ventilation depends on an intact thoracic cage, patent airway, integrity of the alveolar-capillary membrane, normal compliance, normal airway resistance, and adequate nutrition.

Oxygen Delivery and Consumption

Oxygen is carried in the blood in two forms: dissolved in blood plasma and bound to hemoglobin. At physiologic PO_2, only a small amount of oxygen is dissolved in plasma because oxygen has such a low solubility.[5] To express O_2 content in its proper units, the amount of O_2 that dissolves in 100 mL of plasma for each millimeter of mercury (mm Hg) of PO_2 is 0.003 mL/dL.[6] The second carried form of oxygen is bound to the hemoglobin inside the erythrocyte. This is where the majority of oxygen is transported in the blood. Each molecule can contain four heme groups to which oxygen can combine. Through cooperative binding almost all the hemoglobin becomes saturated with oxygen after it passes through the lungs. The body is dependent on the oxyhemoglobin transport during increased metabolic demands.[6]

Oxygen delivery is the product of cardiac output and total arterial oxygen content ($DO_2 = CO \times CaO_2$). Cardiac output is based on stroke volume and heart rate, whereas CaO_2 is derived from the amount of dissolved oxygen plus the total hemoglobin content, oxygen binding capacity of hemoglobin, and the hemoglobin's oxygen saturation. With normal values placed for PaO_2 100 mm Hg, hemoglobin concentration 15 g/dL, and hemoglobin saturation with oxygen 97%, approximate normal CaO_2 is 20 mL O_2 per deciliter or 200 mL O_2 per liter. With a cardiac output of 5 L/min, this would give 1000 mL O_2 per minute. Under normal physiologic conditions, the tissues use 250 to 300 mL O_2 per minute; this leaves the remaining three-fourths in available reserve for increased metabolic demands.[6]

TABLE 22-1 Volumes and Capacities

Lung Volume Measurements	Male (mL)	Female (mL)
TV: Volume of gas that normally moves into and out of the lungs in one quiet breath	500	400–500
IRV: Volume of air that can be forcefully inspired after a normal tidal volume	3100	1900
ERV: Volume of air that can be forcefully exhaled after a normal tidal volume exhalation	1200	800
RV: Amount of air remaining in the lungs after a forced exhalation	1200	1000
Lung Capacity Measurements		
VC: VC = IRV + TV + ERV; volume of air that can be exhaled after a maximal inspiration	4800	3200
IC: IC = TV + IRV; volume of air that can be inhaled after a normal exhalation	3600	2400
FRC: FRC = ERV + RV; lung volume at rest after a normal tidal volume exhalation	2400	1800
TLC: TLC = IC + ERV + RV; maximal amount of air that the lungs can accommodate	6000	4200
Residual RV/TLC ratio (RV/TLC × 100): Percentage of TLC occupied by the RV	$600\overline{)1200} = 20\%$ (approximately)	$4200\overline{)1000} = 25\%$ (approximately)

ERV, Expiratory reserve volume; *FRC*, functional residual capacity; *IC*, inspiratory capacity; *IRV*, inspiratory reserve volume; *RV*, residual volume; *TLC*, total lung capacity; *TV*, tidal volume; *VC*, vital capacity.
From Jardins TDR, Burton GG. (2015). *Clinical Manifestations and Assessment of Respiratory Disease.* St. Louis: Mosby; 2015, Table 3.2.

Alveolar-Capillary Membrane and Diffusion of Pulmonary Gases

The process of a gas molecule moving from an area of higher concentration to an area of lower concentration is called diffusion. There are several barriers that need to be overcome for gas exchange to occur. In the lungs, a gas molecule must diffuse through the alveolar-capillary membrane, which is composed of (1) the liquid lining of the intraalveolar membrane, (2) the alveolar epithelial cell, (3) the basement membrane of the alveolar epithelial cell, (4) loose connective tissue (the interstitial space), (5) the basement membrane of the capillary endothelium, (6) the capillary endothelium, (7) the plasma in the capillary blood, (8) the erythrocyte membrane, and (9) the intracellular fluid in the erythrocyte until a hemoglobin molecule is encountered.[4] The amount of time for this to take place is approximately 0.25 second. Diffusion is affected by the alveolar surface area, driving pressure, and the thickness of the alveolar capillary.[2]

Ventilation-Perfusion

Alveolar ventilation is the volume per minute that reaches the alveoli and physiologically takes part in the process of gas exchange. The variables that make up the total in this equation are tidal volume, respiratory rate, and dead space. This is approximately 4 L/min.[1]

Perfusion is the amount of blood flow to the respiratory capillaries. Normally, the amount of blood that perfuses the alveoli is 5 L/min (i.e., cardiac output). In a perfect physiologic state, the ventilation of every alveolus is matched by an equivalent of perfusion, resulting in an average ventilation-perfusion ($\dot{V}/\dot{Q}$) ratio of 4:5 or 0.8.

There are a multitude of physiologic conditions that alter the $\dot{V}/\dot{Q}$ relationship. When inadequate ventilation occurs relative to a normal state of perfusion, as occurs in pneumonia, the $\dot{V}/\dot{Q}$ ratio is said to be low and is referred to as a shunt. Pulmonary shunting can be subdivided into relative and absolute shunts, and the latter can be further divided into anatomic and capillary shunting. These can essentially affect oxygen uptake, which results in hypoxia. The severity of the shunt depends on whether oxygen therapy is effective. As the $\dot{V}/\dot{Q}$ ratio lowers, the less responsive it will be and it will be completely unresponsive to oxygen in the presence of an absolute shunt. An anatomic shunt exists when blood travels from the right side of the heart to the left side without undergoing gas exchange.[1,2,4,6]

When there is normal ventilation or an increase in ventilation and perfusion is compromised, a $\dot{V}/\dot{Q}$ mismatch occurs. The classic example would be a pulmonary embolus, which causes an increase in the $\dot{V}/\dot{Q}$ ratio. This has also been referred to as dead space ventilation. As the name implies, dead space is the volume of air that does not come in contact with the pulmonary capillary blood and is essentially wasted. Anatomic dead space consists of the volume of air that does not partake in gas exchange and is approximated by 2 mL/kg or 1 mL/lb.[2,6]

In the setting of poorly ventilated arterioles, constriction occurs, diverting the blood to better ventilated areas.

Similarly, poorly perfused alveoli collapse, causing atelectasis or alveolar consolidation, which results in the diversion of airflow to more effectively perfused areas. This is termed a silent unit and helps to compensate for imbalanced $\dot{V}/\dot{Q}$ ratios.

Distribution of the ventilation and perfusion is heavily weighted by gravity. It can, however, be used to maximize the $\dot{V}/\dot{Q}$ ratio in the compromised lung. By placing the patient where the functional alveoli are in the dependent position and the affected units are elevated, the parallel of ventilation and blood flow can be maximized, improving gas exchange (Fig. 22.1).

Oxygen-Hemoglobin Dissociation Curve

The oxygen-hemoglobin dissociation curve illustrates the relationship between hemoglobin saturation of oxygen and PaO_2. This sigmoid-shaped curve depicts the ability of hemoglobin to bind and release oxygen into the tissues and is affected under certain physiologic conditions. The relationship between oxygen content and the pressure of oxygen in the blood is not linear. The upper portion of the curve is relatively flat and shows that small changes in PaO_2 have little effect on the percentage saturation in hemoglobin. However, when looking at the PaO_2 as it drops below 60 mm Hg, there is a drastic drop in the saturation of hemoglobin. This emphasizes the importance of maintaining a PaO_2 greater than 60 mm Hg in clinical practice. There are many factors that influence the oxyhemoglobin dissociation curve and affect the loading and unloading of oxygen. These include the pH, temperature, 2,3-diphosphoglycerate (2,3-DPG), abnormal hemoglobin, and carbon dioxide (Fig. 22.2).[1,2,4,7]

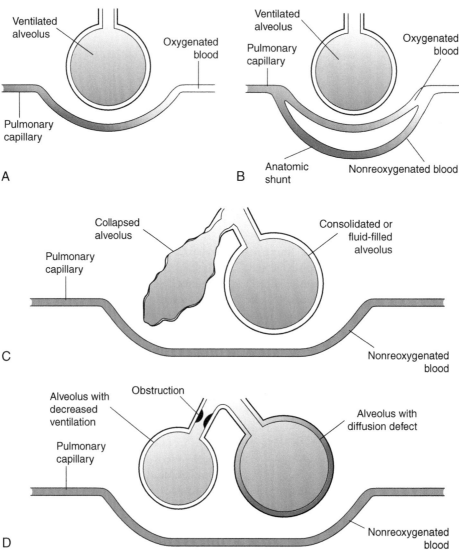

• **Fig. 22.1** Pulmonary shunting. (A) Pulmonary embolism (PE). (B) Bronchial smooth muscle constriction; (C) atelectasis; and (D) alveolar consolidation are common secondary anatomic alterations of the lungs. (Modified from Des Jardins T. *Cardiopulmonary Anatomy and Physiology: Essentials for Respiratory Care.* 2nd ed. Albany, NY: Delmar; 1993.)

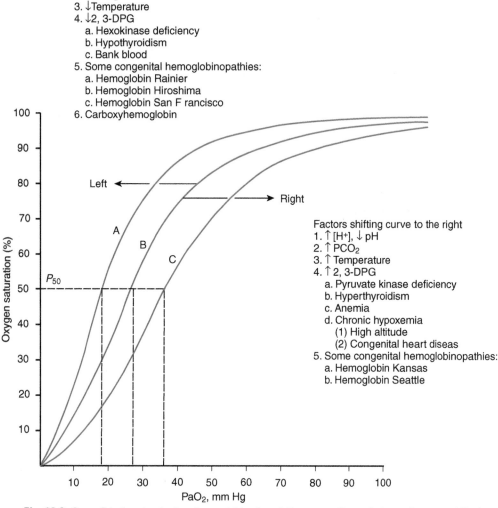

Factors shifting curve to the left
1. ↓ [H+], ↑ pH
2. ↓PCO$_2$
3. ↓Temperature
4. ↓2, 3-DPG
   a. Hexokinase deficiency
   b. Hypothyroidism
   c. Bank blood
5. Some congenital hemoglobinopathies:
   a. Hemoglobin Rainier
   b. Hemoglobin Hiroshima
   c. Hemoglobin San F rancisco
6. Carboxyhemoglobin

Factors shifting curve to the right
1. ↑ [H+], ↓ pH
2. ↑ PCO$_2$
3. ↑ Temperature
4. ↑ 2, 3-DPG
   a. Pyruvate kinase deficiency
   b. Hyperthyroidism
   c. Anemia
   d. Chronic hypoxemia
      (1) High altitude
      (2) Congenital heart diseas
5. Some congenital hemoglobinopathies:
   a. Hemoglobin Kansas
   b. Hemoglobin Seattle

• **Fig. 22.2** *Curve B* is the standard oxyhemoglobin dissociation curve. *Curve A* shows the curve shifted to the left because of hemoglobin's increased affinity for oxygen. *Curve C* shows the curve shifted to the right because of hemoglobin's decreased affinity for oxygen. Factors responsible for shifting the curve are listed adjacent to Curves A and C. (From Kinney MR, et al. *AACN's Clinical Reference for Critical Care Nursing.* St. Louis: Mosby; 1988.)

pH

The pH of blood is a measurement of the hydrogen ion concentration of blood. It is used to express a state of acidity or alkalinity. As the hydrogen ion concentration increases, there is a decrease in the pH, a state of acidity, and a subsequent decrease in the affinity for oxygen, which leads to the hemoglobin giving up oxygen to the tissues. This is represented by a right-sided shift in the oxygen-hemoglobin dissociation curve. Conversely, because there is a decrease in hydrogen ions, the pH increases, and physiologically there is an increased affinity of hemoglobin for oxygen augmenting its uptake from the alveoli.

Temperature

As body temperature rises, such as during exercise or an increase in metabolic production, there is a shift to the right

in the curve and oxygen is released to the tissues. A shift to the left because of a drop in temperature, as in a state of hypothermia, would not allow oxygen to be released to the tissues as readily.

2,3-Diphosphoglycerate

2,3-DPG is a phosphate found in large quantities in the red blood cells. An increase in 2,3-DPG will shift the curve to the right, and low levels will result in a left-sided shift. Its presence is oftentimes referred to as a chisel aiding in the drop-off of oxygen to the tissues. It should be noted that factors such as hypoxia and the presence of anemia lead to an increase in 2,3-DPG levels, whereas blood being stored as little as 1 week has been shown to have low concentrations of the intermediate metabolite.

• BOX 22.1 **Oxygen Content Components**

Oxygen content = (Oxygen capacity × oxygen saturation) + (0.0031 × PaO_2)

Oxygen capacity = Maximal amount O_2 blood can carry	Stated as milliliters of O_2 per 100 mL of blood (vol%)	Multiply hemoglobin by 1.34
Oxygen saturation = % of hemoglobin saturated with oxygen	Stated as percentage	SpO_2 or SvO_2

Systemic oxygen transport (mL/min) = Arterial oxygen content (mL/100 mL) × cardiac output × 10 (conversion factor) = 1000 to 1200 mL/min.

Abnormal Hemoglobin

Abnormalities in the hemoglobin molecule can also affect oxygen loading and unloading. Structural abnormalities occur when the amino acid sequence alters the shape of the molecule's polypeptide chains, varying it from normal.[8] By altering the shape of the molecule, there is a tendency for changes in oxygen affinity. Carboxyhemoglobin, methemoglobin, and fetal hemoglobin all cause a left-sided shift and an increased oxygen affinity.[1]

Carbon Dioxide

As there is an increase in carbon dioxide, the blood becomes more acidotic, which causes a right-sided shift. This acidity is caused by the reaction of carbon dioxide with water to form carbonic acid, with the end result being a drop in pH. This inverse ratio of pH and PCO_2 is termed the Bohr effect. A decreasing PCO_2 leads to an alkalotic state, increased O_2 affinity, and a left-sided shift. The understanding of this relationship is significant for clinical applications (Box 22.1).

Respiratory System Support

Oxygen Therapy

Many critically ill and injured patients need oxygen therapy to support adequate tissue oxygenation. In addition to concurrent identification of a physiologic cause, oxygen therapy is a common means for hypoxia support.

Oxygen delivery systems are classified into two categories: high-flow systems and low-flow systems. *Low-flow systems* are devices that deliver at or below the patient's physiologic minute ventilation. These low-flow systems allow the patient to draw a supplemental amount of oxygen from the apparatus, with part of the inspired tidal volume from the room air within or around the apparatus. Therefore the amount of oxygen that is inspired varies depending on the patient. The flow of oxygen depends on the device and is constant to the set flow. The concentration of inspired oxygen is variable and depends on the patient's minute ventilation.[9-11] For example, a patient with a high minute ventilation above 20 L/min inspires less oxygen than a patient with a lower minute ventilation at 10 L/min using an oxygen device set at 15 L/min because the patient with high minute ventilation uses a greater amount of room air per minute.[11,12]

High-flow oxygen systems are devices that deliver above the patient's physiologic minute ventilation. These devices result in the patient inspiring the total present fraction of inspired oxygen (FiO_2). The high flow makes the concentration of inspired oxygen less dependent on the patient's ventilatory pattern and volume because the flow exceeds that of the patient's demand.

Ventilatory Support

Many patients with pulmonary emergencies, ventilatory failure ($PaCO_2$ >50 mm Hg), and respiratory failure (PaO_2 <60 mm Hg) need mechanical ventilation during transport. See Chapter 12 for an extensive discussion about the use of ventilators during transport, including management of the machine and the patient.

Respiratory Monitoring Methods

Measurement of respiratory function during transport assists the team in the assessment of acute changes in pulmonary function. Respiratory system monitoring is important to diagnose and anticipate potential deterioration and compromise to ventilation or oxygenation. Pressure monitoring of the airway and vascular system are a few invasive means to help monitor ventilation. Electrocardiograms (ECGs), blood laboratory, blood gases, pulse oximetry, end-tidal capnography, and pulmonary function testing are other means to investigate and monitor the status of the respiratory system. Capnography may also be used to monitor gas exchange and pulmonary ventilation. Fig. 22.3 illustrates a normal capnogram. Both pulse oximetry and capnography assist in patient evaluation and management during transport.[10,13]

Chapter 12 contains an in-depth discussion of current methods that can be used to monitor a patient's pulmonary status during transport.

Respiratory Support Tools

In addition to maintaining oxygenation and ventilation, there are other considerations to help support the respiratory

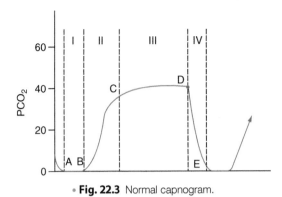

• **Fig. 22.3** Normal capnogram.

care. Humidity can be helpful. Dry cool gases delivered to the patient can cause narrowing and constriction to the airways. Asthmatics may have a greater effect with potential bronchospasm. Dry air can prevent mucous mobility and create more viscous secretions and potentiate mucous plugging. Lung humidity is important to maintain for the lung environment to be most compliant.

Aerosol therapy is a mode for medication delivery. The type of device used to deliver an aerosol will make a difference to the delivery of the medication. Each device is able to nebulize a medication to a certain particle size. The particle size will allow medication to travel to the targeted lung area. The smaller the particle size, the farther the medication will go in the lung airways. An aerosol device should be selected for the specific medication and desired particle size based on the target area of the lung. Refer to manufacturer specifications for targeted particle size.

Lung hygiene is the clearance of mucus and secretions. Moisture and mucolytics can help to decrease secretion viscosity. Other therapies and equipment that can also help to improve secretion mobility to facilitate clearance include chest physical therapy, vibratory devices, cough assist, positional drainage, and pressure resistance, which are all used to support lung hygiene.

These tools are used to enhance pulmonary therapy by a combination of mobilizing secretions, decreasing viscosity, and fragmenting mucous plugs to allow pulmonary toileting of secretions. With good therapies, deep breathing, and coughing, these tools can help to achieve improved lung clearance.

Respiratory Gases

Compressed gases are used to allow access and availability of necessary support and treatment. A few commonly used gases are medical air consisting of room air (21% oxygen, 78% nitrogen, and 1% other gases), oxygen, heliox, and nitrous oxide. Oxygen and room air are the most common and most supportive gases, with heliox and nitrous oxide as specialty gases used to support specific physiologies.

Acute Respiratory Failure

Acute respiratory failure can occur when chronic pulmonary disease or other factors affect the patient's ability to maintain adequate oxygenation. Acute respiratory failure is defined as a PO_2 less than 60 mm Hg and commonly includes ventilatory failure defined as inadequate gas exchange with a carbon dioxide pressure ($PcCO_2$) greater than 50 mm Hg.[1] The transport team's initial concern is for adequate oxygenation then ventilation, followed by management of the underlying process that led to acute respiratory failure.

Acute Respiratory Distress Syndrome

Etiology

Acute respiratory distress syndrome (ARDS) is a lung injury that has many causes (Fig. 22.4). It may be a complication of other diseases or injuries, with the most common being severe sepsis with a pulmonary source of infection.[14] ARDS is an inflammatory lung condition that can complicate any physiology and can manifest from severe pneumonia, trauma, sepsis, inhalation injuries, aspiration of gastric contents, and prolonged volutrauma, as well as many other conditions. ARDS leads to further injury of the lung, with edema to the lung tissue causing poor gas diffusion across the alveolar capillary membrane resulting in low oxygen levels in the blood. The poor oxygenation is usually due to $\dot{V}/\dot{Q}$ and intrapulmonary shunting.

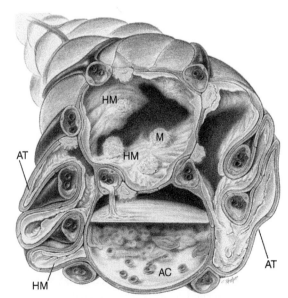

• **Fig. 22.4** Cross-sectional view of alveoli in adult respiratory distress syndrome. *HM,* Hyaline membrane; *AT,* atelectasis; *AC,* alveolar consolidation; *M,* macrophage. (From Des Jardins T, Burton GG. *Clinical Manifestations and Assessment of Respiratory Disease.* 4th ed. St. Louis: Mosby; 2002.)

Pathophysiologic Factors

ARDS results from a severe alteration in pulmonary vascular permeability, which leads to a change in lung structure and function. It is divided into two phases. The first phase is the disease process that initiates an exudative state with an overwhelming expression of a proinflammatory response. This response results in damage to pulmonary endothelium and epithelium and in accumulation of fluid in the alveoli.[13] The second phase causes extensive pulmonary fibrosis and loss of normal alveolar structure.[10,13] The outstanding characteristic of ARDS is hypoxemia refractory to oxygen therapy. Because ARDS is a complication of other illnesses or injuries, the transport team must also consider the pathophysiology of the underlying problem. ARDS has a very high mortality rate of about 50%.

Assessment

Assessment of the patient with ARDS includes the history of the present illness to determine the predisposing factors that led up to the diagnosis. Patients with ARDS report sudden onset of dyspnea; cyanosis occurs, and intubation with mechanical ventilation often becomes necessary. The patient appears in obvious acute distress. If the transport team is using mechanical ventilatory support for the underlying illness or injury, pulmonary compliance may decrease.[10,13]

Chest radiographs reveal widespread pulmonary infiltrates. Hypoxemia is present and may be severe. As the process worsens, accumulation of fluid in the alveoli significantly reduces pulmonary compliance. The patient's condition may progress to hypercapnia respiratory failure as the ability to maintain an effective minute ventilation is lost.[13] A decreased PaO_2/FiO_2 ratio indicates reduced arterial oxygenation with adequate or increased available alveolar oxygen. ARDS is defined by mild ARDS, 201 to 300 mm Hg; moderate ARDS, 101 to 200 mm Hg; and severe ARDS, less than or equal to 100 mm Hg.

Intervention

Management of the patient with ARDS is a challenge. Positive end-expiratory pressure (PEEP) is added to mechanical ventilation in an attempt to improve arterial oxygenation. In addition, PEEP increases functional residual capacity, reduces closing volume, improves overall lung compliance, reduces $\dot{V}/\dot{Q}$ mismatching, mitigates end-expiratory alveolar collapse, maintains alveolar recruitment, and reduces ventilator-associated lung injury. Reducing atelectasis with PEEP may also more evenly distribute inflation stresses produced by repetitive opening/closing of alveolar structures during ventilation. As lung compliance decreases, higher levels of PEEP may be needed to maintain oxygenation levels. The management of the ventilated patient with ARDS is oxygenation support with high PEEP and low lung protective volumes to prevent higher-than-desired peak inspiratory pressures.[1,10,13,15]

Supplemental oxygen is necessary because hypoxemia is significant. The oxygen delivery system and FiO_2 used depends on the patient's condition. Advanced ventilation strategies including inverse ratio ventilation, adaptive pressure release ventilation, and high-frequency oscillation are other considerations for improving oxygenation in the ARDS patient. Because of the difficulty oxygenating and ventilating these patients, priority to oxygenation over ventilation may be needed, and permissive hypercapnia is accepted.

Fluids should be restricted unless shock is present. The impaired pulmonary capillary membrane allows fluids to leak into the alveoli. In the presence of shock, fluids must not be withheld. The main pulmonary system goal of air medical transport is to maintain adequate oxygenation and ventilation.

Chronic Obstructive Pulmonary Disease

Chronic obstructive pulmonary disease (COPD) can be considered as a single disease state or in combination with verifying degrees of asthma, chronic bronchitis, and/or emphysema.[15] Emphysema and chronic bronchitis coexisting in varying degrees is not unusual. Although each entity is discussed separately, remember that each can be present in the same patient.

One should not discount the effect of altitude on the patient with COPD because the ability to increase ventilation and cardiac output in response to stress is limited.[1]

Asthma

Etiology

Asthma is a reversible obstructive pulmonary disorder caused by airway inflammation that results in the restriction of airflow secondary to inflammation. The characteristics of asthma include airway inflammation, increased airway responsiveness to various stimuli, airway bronchoconstriction, and increased mucous production.[16] Acute management of asthma is directed at management of inflammation and reversal of bronchoconstriction.

Pathophysiologic Factors

Various stimuli can trigger increased airway responsiveness. Once stimulation takes place, an inflammatory response occurs. Cellular infiltration and mucosal edema are seen (Fig. 22.5). Airway hyperreactivity with smooth muscle contraction and additional mucous production and diminished secretion clearance also occurs and results in $\dot{V}/\dot{Q}$ abnormalities, increased airway resistance, and hyperinflation of the lungs with an increase in residual volume. Status asthmaticus is a severe attack that is refractory to bronchodilator therapy.[10]

Assessment

The transport team should elicit a careful history to identify precipitating factors. For example, a viral illness or other environmental exposure may precede the acute exacerbation of asthma. The patient may report a cough and dyspnea.

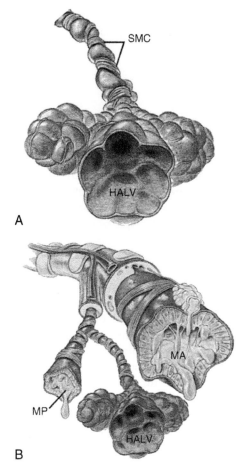

SMC

HALV

A

MA

MP

HALV

B

• **Fig. 22.5** Obstructive lung disorders. (A) Bronchial smooth muscle constriction *(SMC)* accompanied by air trapping. (B) Tracheobronchial inflammation accompanied by mucous accumulation *(MA),* partial airway obstruction, and air trapping. *MP,* Mucous plug. (From Des Jardins T, Burton GG. *Clinical Manifestations and Assessment of Respiratory Disease.* 3rd ed. St Louis: Mosby; 1995.)

A patient with a long history of asthma can usually rank the relative severity of the illness. A thorough medication history regarding timing and dosage is helpful. (Other useful questions should include: Any previous intensive care unit admissions? and Any admissions that required intubation? These can be useful in determining how sick the patient might become.

The physical examination reveals different degrees of respiratory distress based on the severity of the current episode. Tachypnea, wheezing, and a prolonged expiratory phase are not uncommon. If no wheezing is heard and the patient has difficulty talking, the transport team should consider the situation as emergent. Absence of wheezing may indicate that the patient is not able to ventilate sufficiently to produce breath sounds. Inspiratory retractions may be seen, as may the use of accessory muscles. The blood pressure is variable, and pulsus paradoxus may be present. Cyanosis and lethargy are late signs, and the presence of cyanosis or lethargy necessitates immediate attention.[10]

Diagnostic studies help determine the severity of the asthma. Resistance to airflow is measured with spirometry or a peak flow meter. Spirometric measurement of forced expiratory volume in 1 second (FEV_1) is done before and after treatment to ascertain treatment success. Peak expiratory flow rate can be accomplished with a handheld meter and has been used to determine whether arterial blood gas (ABG) measurement is necessary.[16,17] Pulmonary function testing is helpful with management and monitoring; however, clinical presentation is key for identification in the acute case.

In addition to measurement of resistance to airflow, a chest radiograph may be done if other parameters are abnormal. ABG measurement may be helpful in patients with severe asthma. Table 22.2 illustrates the stages of asthma with corresponding ABG results.

Intervention

Ensuring an adequate airway and providing supplemental oxygen are initial interventions. Asthma medications are divided into controller and rescue medications. Controller medications include orally inhaled corticosteroids, leukotriene modifiers, mast cell stabilizers, theophylline, omalizumab, and systemic corticosteroids. Rescue medications include short-acting β_2-agonists and, in some cases, inhaled anticholinergics and short-acting theophylline. Intubation and mechanical ventilation are used only in severe cases. The indications for intubation and mechanical ventilation are listed in Box 22.2. Mortality rate increases for asthma patients who need intubation.[16] This reactive airway disease can be challenging because management is very

---

TABLE 22-2   Stages of Asthma

Stage	pH	PO$_2$	PCO$_2$	Interpretation
I	↑	Normal	↓	Hyperventilation: ED treatment
II	↑	↓	↓	Hyperventilation; ED treatment consists of correcting hypoxemia
III	Normal	↓	Normal	Obstruction prevents hyperventilation; patient may need hospitalization
IV	↓	—	↑	Severe; ICU admission; may necessitate mechanical support of respirations
V	↓	↓↓↓	↑↑	"Crossed" gases: PaCO$_2$ > PaO$_2$; hospitalization and mechanical support of respirations after intubation necessary

ED, Emergency department; *ICU,* intensive care unit.
From Hammond BB, Lee G. *Quick Reference to Emergency Nursing.* Philadelphia: Lippincott; 1984.

• **BOX 22.2** **Seven Indications for Intubation and Mechanical Ventilation in the Patient With Asthma**

1. Decreased level of consciousness.
2. Progressive exhaustion.
3. Absent breath sounds or severe wheezing despite therapy.
4. pH 7.2.
5. PCO_2 >55 mm Hg.
6. PO_2 <60 mm Hg despite high-flow oxygen.
7. Vital capacity decreases to level of tidal volume.

pharmacologically involved. In addition to bronchodilators and antiinflammatory medications (corticosteroids), systemic β-adrenergics and smooth muscle relaxants are used to manage reversal. Heliox is also a consideration to help facilitate oxygenation in the severely constricted lung.

Evaluation

The transport team should evaluate the patient's condition at regular intervals to ensure success of therapy. A decrease in dyspnea or in the degree of tachycardia and absence of accessory muscle use are parameters for evaluating the success of treatment. Improvement is evaluated by exhaled capnography waveform and patient presentation. The patient should also be able to verbalize a subjective improvement in respiratory effort.

Chronic Bronchitis

Etiology

Chronic bronchitis is defined as having a productive cough for a least three consecutive months for two successive years, in which the cough cannot be attributed to any other cause. Several contributing factors are known to be instrumental in the etiology of chronic bronchitis. Smoking and inhaled pollutants contain irritants that aid in the pathologic changes that contribute to exacerbations, recurrent infections, and hospitalizations. Secondhand smoking and work-related environments can also be influential and directly related to the origin of the disease process.[3]

Pathophysiologic Factors

Pathologic changes are common to the large- and medium-size airways, which have direct implications to the distal airways. Because of the chronic inflammation and bronchospasms caused by external irritants, there is a reduction in the cross-sectional diameter in the airways. This chronic inflammatory state leads to a hypersecretion of copious amounts of sputum in which the body's normal protective mechanisms become easily overwhelmed and ineffective from impairment of the mucociliary blanket. This can progress to partial or complete airway blockage. These manifestations can occur with or without measurable airflow

obstruction. The progressive result of these combinations of factors can lead to hypercapnia and hypoxia.

Emphysema

Etiology

Emphysema is defined pathologically as the presence of permanent enlargement of the airspaces distal to the terminal bronchioles, accompanied by destruction of their walls and without obvious fibrosis.[1] Factors that contribute to the diseased state include smoking, inhaled pollutants, occupational hazards, gender, socioeconomic factors, and α_1-antitrypsin deficiency.

Pathophysiologic Factors

Pathologic changes begin to occur years before the onset of symptoms. The alveoli are damaged or destroyed and the airspaces beyond the terminal bronchioles are enlarged. This leads to an increase in the ratio of air to lung tissue in the alveoli. Once the alveolar capillary interface becomes anatomically altered, the gas exchange is impaired. As the proximal structures to the alveolus fail to keep the airways open, the expiratory phase becomes essential to CO_2 elimination, as the resistance to airflow increases. This allows air to be trapped in the alveoli increasing residual volumes. Typically, the patient's vital capacity is close to normal until the disease has advanced to a severe stage.[1,3] Fig. 22.6 illustrates the pathophysiology of COPD.

Assessment of Chronic Bronchitis and Emphysema

The history is important in determining the primary etiology of the disease. Exacerbations may occur with minor pulmonary infections, stress, changes in weather, or continued exposure to environmental pollutants (including smoking). The patient's subjective assessment of the condition is important for determining the usual status of the disease, and the historical hospitalization course will aid in the severity of the current pulmonary state. The patient may report increased dyspnea, change in sputum production, or an increase in the malaise that may accompany the disease.[18]

The clinical presentation of chronic bronchitis and emphysema each have individual characteristics that may overlap each other, with patients having a combination of the two diseases. Physical examination may reveal rhonchi, expiratory wheezes, or diminished breath sounds. Rales may be present during a state of pulmonary infections. Accessory muscles for inspiration and expiration are actively used due to the increased work of breathing. Tachycardia and the presence of dysrhythmias are not uncommon in either condition. With the emphysema patient the thorax is hyperresonant to percussion because of hyperinflation of the alveoli, and the anterior

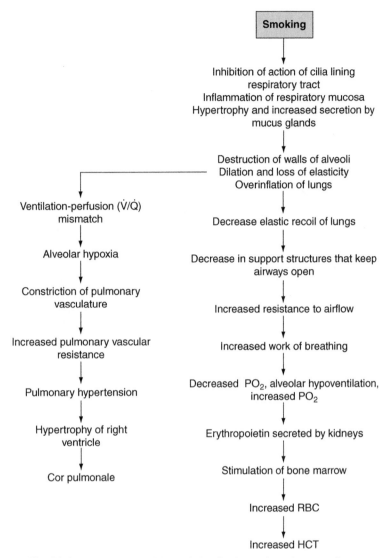

Smoking

Inhibition of action of cilia lining
respiratory tract
Inflammation of respiratory mucosa
Hypertrophy and increased secretion by
mucus glands

Destruction of walls of alveoli
Dilation and loss of elasticity
Overinflation of lungs

Ventilation-perfusion ($\dot{V}/\dot{Q}$)
mismatch

Decrease elastic recoil of lungs

Alveolar hypoxia

Decrease in support structures that keep
airways open

Constriction of pulmonary
vasculature

Increased resistance to airflow

Increased pulmonary vascular
resistance

Increased work of breathing

Pulmonary hypertension

Decreased PO_2, alveolar hypoventilation,
increased PO_2

Hypertrophy of right
ventricle

Erythropoietin secreted by kidneys

Cor pulmonale

Stimulation of bone marrow

Increased RBC

Increased HCT

• **Fig. 22.6** Basic pathophysiology of chronic obstructive pulmonary disease.

posterior diameter of the chest is increased, which can also lead to muffled heart sounds. Observation of the patient's respiratory pattern reveals pursed lips with a prolonged expiratory phase. The patient frequently wants to sit and lean forward, with hands on knees in a tripod position, which aids in the stability of the accessory muscles. Emphysema patients are often referred to as "pink puffers" because they are markedly dyspneic and can maintain a relatively normal arterial oxygenation level in less severe stages. Conversely, patients with chronic bronchitis are frequently referred to as "blue bloaters" because they appear edematous and cyanotic. They tend to have a larger physical build and can tend to be overweight. A chronic, loose productive cough is a classic presentation.[1,3,4]

Mental status is an important component of the transport team's objective assessment of the patient. Retention of CO_2 occurs in the later stages of the disease process, and once the CO_2 level in the arterial circulation increases beyond the baseline level, one of the first signs is behavioral

and emotional changes. These may vary from confusion, irritability, and a decrease in intellectual performance caused by obtundation. Any alterations should be aggressively investigated and treated.[19]

If available, ABG results contain valuable information to the extent of distress or failure but should also be matched with the patient's clinical condition. Other worthy common laboratory findings may include polycythemia, hypochloremia (as HCO_3- rises), and hypernatremia.[8]

Radiologic findings for patients with chronic bronchitis may include translucent lung fields, fibrotic-appearing lung markings caused by bronchial wall thickening, depressed or flattened diaphragms, and right atrial enlargement (cor pulmonale). The patient with emphysema may also show similar manifestations, such as translucency, flattened diaphragms, and occasional atrial and ventricular enlargement, along with a narrowed heart silhouette.[3]

ECG findings in advanced stages may show low-voltage complexes, right axis deviation, and flattened or inverted P waves in I and aVL. These common diagnostic tools may be available during interfacility transfers and benefit in the continuance of care when combined with a thorough patient assessment.

Intervention

Supplemental oxygen is given in an attempt to correct the patient's hypoxia to his or her baseline level. It should be noted that the peripheral chemoreceptors are located at the bifurcations of the aortic arteries and the aortic arch. These chemoreceptors are responsive to low levels of oxygen in the arterial blood and become active only when the PaO_2 is less than approximately 60 mm Hg. However, the major influence of stimulation, received by the medulla, is excessive levels of hydrogen ions from the cerebrospinal fluid by the central chemoreceptors. This hypoxic response is far slower than signals sent by the central chemoreceptors.[5]

Other approaches to the care of the COPD patient should be based on clinical presentation and assessment. In acute management, short-acting β_2-agonists are commonly used for bronchial smooth muscle relaxation in addition to anticholinergics such as ipratropium bromide. Systemic glucocorticosteroids can also be implemented because of the inflammatory process; however, the onset of action is usually within 1 to 2 hours. This population of patients oftentimes is already on combination long-acting β_2-agonist/glucocorticosteroids, long-acting anticholinergics, and uncommonly methylxanthines. The patient may need assistance with removal of secretions via nasotracheal suctioning or endotracheal suctioning if intubated. Intravenous (IV) fluids for rehydration may be necessary, and these should be administered cautiously in the presence of heart failure. Antibiotic therapy and expectorants are generally prevalent because of recurrent infections. Cardiac monitoring is necessary, and life-threatening dysrhythmias should be treated according to standard advanced cardiac life support protocols. During acute exacerbations, delineations between distress and failure need to be identified immediately, with appropriate action taken. When indications exist, bilevel noninvasive ventilation has been used with extreme success in curbing the progression of distress into deterioration. If intubation and mechanical ventilation are necessary because of hypoxia refractory to other interventions or respiratory failure, aggressive pulmonary toilet measures should be undertaken and evaluated for results.

With advances in invasive and noninvasive ventilation, the transport team will be exposed to various brands of equipment. Instances may occur in which the team may not be familiar with the facilities equipment, modes of ventilation, or they may not have the equivalent device. Diligence in continuation and familiarization with such equipment and advances are a must in the transport setting.

Spontaneous Pneumothorax

Etiology

A pneumothorax is defined as the accumulation of air in the pleural space. Spontaneous pneumothoraces can be categorized as primary and secondary types. A primary spontaneous pneumothorax occurs in the absence of an underlying lung disease process, and a secondary process occurs in the presence of a condition. Various risk factors include age, gender, genetics, lung disease, smoking, and a history of previous pneumothoraces. There are three ways in which air or gas can enter the pleural space: from an opening in the chest wall, gas-forming bacteria in an empyema in the pleural space, or perforation of the visceral pleura.[20]

Pathophysiologic Factors

The pathophysiology is similar to that of a pneumothorax caused by thoracic trauma (Fig. 22.7). The lung collapses in varying degrees, and hypoxemia may occur. If the pneumothorax is significant, a tension pneumothorax may occur when the air is trapped in the pleural space under pressure. This may lead to pressure being placed on the great veins; decreased venous return; and, consequently, hemodynamic compromise.[3]

With a primary spontaneous pneumothorax, the patients are typically tall, thin, and adolescent males. One possible reason putting the patient at an increased risk could be the expeditious growth of the chest during adolescent years, resulting in a thinner pleural wall and airspace enlargement. This results in the formation of small subpleural airspaces known as blebs. These blebs can rupture in conditions that may cause an increase in intrapulmonary pressure, such as coughing. When this occurs air will travel into the pleural space and cause the pneumothorax.[1,4,21]

A secondary spontaneous pneumothorax occurs in the presence of an underlying lung disease. Some of these diseases include, but are not limited to, asthma, emphysema, tuberculosis, and a collection of interstitial lung diseases. Because of the pathologic or structural changes that each of these conditions places on the pulmonary system, any increased resistance, decreased compliance, or loss of integrity of the pleural wall, especially during exacerbated states, predisposes the patient for an increased risk of a spontaneous pneumothorax to occur.

Assessment

In most cases the hallmark complaint is an acute onset of severe stabbing chest pain and dyspnea, which occurs primarily on inspiration. Frequently there is associated pain present in the tip of the shoulder on the affected side. The degree of pain and dyspnea are usually directly related to the size of the pneumothorax. Breath sounds are decreased or absent on the affected side and can be difficult to auscultate in the presence of an obstructive lung disease. Acute

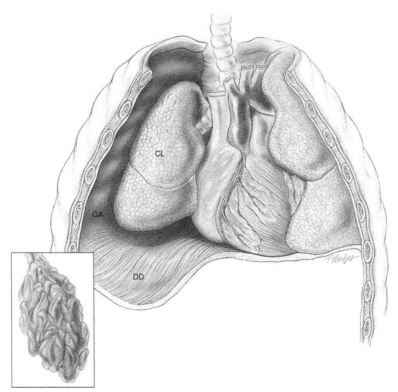

• **Fig. 22.7** Pneumothorax. A right tension pneumothorax. *CL,* Collapsed lung; *DD,* depressed diaphragm; *GA,* gas accumulation in the pleura cavity; *Inset,* atelectasis, a common secondary anatomic alteration of the lungs. (From Jardins TDR, Burton GG. *Clinical Manifestations and Assessment of Respiratory Disease.* St. Louis: Mosby; 2015.)

signs also include tachypnea, tachycardia, anxiety, and acute alveolar hyperventilation with hypoxia. If the pneumothorax progresses to more advanced stages, then the patient's hypoxia will worsen, with ventilator failure and accompanying changes in mental status. The prehospital use of ultrasonography in the air transport environment can provide quick, early diagnostic detection to facilitate decisions for treatment or reevaluation before or during transport.

Intervention

In some patients who are asymptomatic or have mild signs and symptoms of a small lung collapse, diagnosis can oftentimes go undetected. When identified, hospitalization for observation may be all that is necessary; however, even in these circumstances it may take weeks for a full recovery. Treatment is driven by symptoms rather than size of the pneumothorax. With involvement of less than 20% of the affected lung, no invasive treatment is usually needed. Simple bed rest and oxygen may be all that is necessary in most conservative approaches. Symptomatic patients are usually treated with an evacuation by needle decompression with a one-way valve device placed or tube thoracostomy, with both including supportive care. A needle decompression is performed at the second intercostal space on the affected side, two fingerbreadths lateral to the sternal border. The fourth intercostal anterior axillary is also acceptable for

needle decompression, and it may be the location of choice in the obese patient. Definitive care involves chest tube placement in the fourth intercostal space, with the anterior axillary line on the affected side. If recurrence continues chemical pleurodesis is often considered.

The implications for transfer, particularly air transport, are significant and should involve careful forethought. The transport team should not transfer a patient with a pneumothorax, even in a helicopter at low altitudes, without considering whether a chest tube should be inserted. The transport providers should always be diligent, and if the decisions are made not to insert a chest tube before transfer, constant reassessment and readied equipment should be available for emergent needle thoracostomy if needed. In transporting a patient with any preexisting pulmonary disease directly affecting intrapulmonary pressure, baseline parameters should be closely assessed before transport. Reevaluation of symptoms, vitals, mental status, observation of accessory muscle use, changes in SpO_2, and ensuring patency of the chest tube (if present) should all be monitored. Sudden deterioration should lead to an evaluation of signs of a tension pneumothorax (tracheal deviation, jugular venous distention, absent breath sounds, or chest movement on the affected side). In the intubated patient, consideration of peak inspiratory and plateau pressures along with end-tidal CO_2 monitoring is beneficial in the detection of patient changes. Any interventions taken during transport should be constantly reassessed.

Pulmonary Embolism

Etiology

Acute pulmonary embolism (PE) is a common and sometimes fatal disease with a highly variable clinical presentation.[21] The incidence of a PE is estimated to be approximately 60 to 70 per 100,000, and that of venous thrombosis approximately 124 per 100,000 of the general population. After coronary artery disease and stroke, acute PE ranks third among the most common types of cardiovascular diseases.[22] PE refers to obstruction of the pulmonary artery or one of its branches by material (thrombus, tumor, air, or fat) that originated elsewhere in the body.[23] In dealing with thrombus formation, risk factors involve conditions of stasis, such as prolonged sitting, local pressure, and immobilization. Other forms of status are congestive heart failure, shock, and varicose veins. Recent surgeries, trauma, cancer, hypercoagulation disorders, and inherited factors enhance the occurrence for a PE.

Pathophysiology

Once the pulmonary artery becomes partially or completely obstructed, the luminal area becomes compromised and leads to respiratory and hemodynamic alterations (Fig. 22.8). This impacts the patient's well-being parallel to the degree of cross-sectional area involvement. Effects include an initial high $\dot{V}/\dot{Q}$ ratio (distal the embolism, measurably infinite, if the presence of no perfusion), a decrease in pulmonary surfactant, bronchoconstriction, and hemodynamic collapse. The $\dot{V}/\dot{Q}$ mismatch occurs because of a normal-to-high ventilation rate compared with poor perfusion, creating an area of physiologic dead space. Bronchoconstriction is a result of histamine, prostaglandin, and serotonin release. Collectively, alveolar atelectasis, consolidation, tissue necrosis, and bronchial constriction lead to decreased alveolar ventilation relative to the alveolar perfusion (decreased $\dot{V}/\dot{Q}$ ratio).[24] Right ventricular failure often is caused by an increase in workload to maintain adequate cardiac output and oxygen delivery.

Assessment

Physical assessment alone is not always a reliable indicator because signs and symptoms can mimic other conditions, and the onset can be variable. These signs and symptoms may include tachycardia, tachypnea, dyspnea, pleuritic pain, cough, wheezes, hemoptysis, lightheadedness, jugular venous distention, orthopnea, dependent edema, and an accentuated S2 heart sound or an S3 noted. A history could show evidence of prolonged travel or immobilization, recent surgeries, oral contraceptive use, congestive heart failure, neoplasms, or family heritable or prothrombotic tendencies. Laboratory tests aiding in the clinical suspicion include ABGs, D-dimer, and biochemical markers of right ventricular dysfunction such as brain natriuretic peptide (BNP), N-terminal pro-brain natriuretic peptide, and troponin I and T. These all have limited diagnostic value, but may be used in conjunction with, history, assessment, and further testing. ECG abnormalities can show nonspecific ST segment and T wave changes, SI QIII TIII pattern, and right axis deviation. A chest radiograph is typically performed in most patients suspected of a pulmonary embolism to look for an alternative cause of the patient's sysmptoms.[24] Pleural effusions, atelectasis, an elevated hemidiaphragm, and cardiomegaly are common. Definitive imaging includes computed tomographic pulmonary angiography and less commonly, $\dot{V}/\dot{Q}$ scanning or other imaging modalities.[14] Bedside echocardiography may be performed in the presence of hemodynamic instability caused by a high index of suspicion and urgency of intervention.

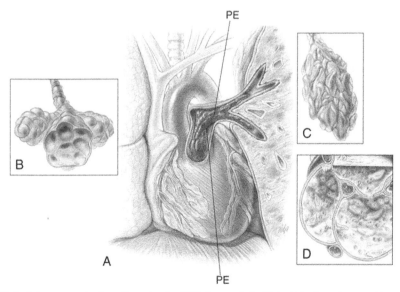

• **Fig. 22.8** Pulmonary embolism. (From Jardins TDR, Burton G.G. *Clinical Manifestations and Assessment of Respiratory Disease.* St. Louis: Mosby; 2015.)

Intervention

Most patients are hemodynamically stable on presentation, and attention should be targeted to supportive measures such as oxygen therapy, IV access, and cardiac monitoring. Initiating anticoagulation versus thrombolytic therapy is based on patient stability, index of clinical suspicion, and diagnostic evaluation. The continuum of therapy and constant reevaluation during transport is essential and open to redirection. Respiratory failure, hypoxia, or hemodynamic instability should encourage the provider to consider intubation and mechanical ventilation. IV fluids should be given as first-line therapy for hypotension; however, care should be taken in patients with right ventricular dysfunction, because excessive amounts could be detrimental. Norepinephrine is the most frequently used agent in this population because of its effectiveness, and it is less likely to cause tachycardia.[21] Familiarization with validation tools, scores, and criteria used by local sending facilities to assist in treatment options are beneficial to the transport provider.

Pulmonary Hypertension

Etiology

Pulmonary hypertension (PH) is defined by a mean pulmonary arterial pressure (mPAP) greater than or equal to 25 mm Hg at rest and is usually confirmed by a right heart catheterization. Normal pulmonary arterial systolic pressure ranges from 15 to 30 mm Hg, diastolic pressure from 4 to 12 mm Hg, and normal mPAP is less than or equal to 20 mm Hg. Many clinicians consider an mPAP of 21 to 24 mm Hg as borderline elevated and of uncertain clinical significance.[25] PH has been formerly classified into two separate categories, primary and secondary, according to the existence of causes and risk factors. Since then, a clinical classification was established by the World Health Organization (WHO) to individualize different categories of PH sharing similar pathologic findings, similar hemodynamic characteristics, and similar management.[26] This classification has been adopted worldwide. The five groups include pulmonary artery hypertension and the following four groups, which classify PH according to its subsidiary mechanisms and similarities. In each group the pulmonary pressure is listed, as previously noted. Early recognition and identification is essential because of the added complication of other cardiovascular and respiratory diseases and the less responsive it is to therapy in the advanced stages.

Pathophysiology

Pulmonary artery hypertension (Group 1) is the narrowing of the vessels to the lungs, adding stress to the right side of the heart. Over time, this leads to right-sided heart failure and eventual compromise to the left side of the heart. Group 1 consists of heritable, drug- and toxin-induced, and connective tissue disorders to name a few. In Groups 2 to 5,

the WHO classification system can be used to understand the pathophysiology and associated similarities and treatment options of the PH. In Group 2, pulmonary hypertension is characterized by left ventricular involvement and valvular disease. This leads to left-sided heart failure and a back pressure of fluid into the lungs. Group 3 consists of chronic lung disease and hypoxia, which is generally considered the origin for the narrowing of the pulmonary arteries. Group 4 consists of chronic thromboembolism, which causes the vessels to become narrowed and vasoconstrict because of blood clots. Group 5 is PH caused by unspecified multifactorial mechanisms, including hematologic, systemic, and metabolic disorders.[25,26]

Assessment

Signs and symptoms are generalized and may include, but are not limited to, shortness of breath, chest pain, tachycardia, fatigue, hemoptysis, peripheral dependent edema, lightheadedness, and cyanosis. because of the general line of complaints, time from symptom onset to diagnosis can be an extensive period of time. This causes the diagnosis not to be made until further progression or advanced stages are present. A detailed past medical history involving associated ailments such as drug and toxin exposure or use, HIV infection, connective tissue disorders, COPD, chronic kidney disease, or thyroid disorders may be considered significant when combined with other clinical data. After physical examination and history, tests that would contribute to the assessment and suspicion of a PH diagnosis involves a systematic progression of steps. These would include chest radiograph, ECG, echocardiogram, $\dot{V}/\dot{Q}$ scan, Pulmonary function tests (PFTs), overnight oximetry, HIV, antinuclear antibody test, liver function tests, and right-sided heart catheterization for the gold standard of diagnosis.[27] These are chiefly done on an outpatient basis or when an acute exacerbation would lead to suspicion of such a diagnosis.

Interventions

Treatment is guided toward the underlining cause with the goal to prevent further escalation of symptoms and to reduce them. A large share of the patients transferred would already have a diagnosis, and the prehospital provider would possibly see these medications or interventions already implemented and group therapy could overlap. Of all groups the following lists of recommendation are general and may not be feasible or available in the prehospital environment. Group 1 interventions are aimed at relaxing the blood vessels in the lungs using calcium channel blockers, prostanoids, phosphodiesterase-5 inhibitors, and endothelin receptor antagonists. These are commonly prescribed after a vasoreactivity test. Because Group 2 consists of left ventricular involvement and valvular disease, acute care should be toward management of preload, afterload, and contractility, keeping in mind the left ventricular function. For Group 3, managing the root of hypoxia is the primary goal. Group 4 may include blood-thinning medication, and Group 5 as a heterogeneous group should again be treated by the cause.[26-28]

Neurologic Disorders

Etiology

The respiratory system can be separated into two areas, which are both essential to the normal operation of the pulmonary system: the lungs and its network of gas exchange and the respiratory muscles, which are associated with the neuroanatomical structures of the brainstem and nerves. Neurologic disorders influencing respiratory function can also be subdivided into the location of the interaction. These include the cerebral cortex, brainstem, myopathies, the neuromuscular junction, and peripheral nerves. Even though there are a variety of causes and sequel of action, these diseases oftentimes follow a similar course of events. It is essential to identify these patients at risk of respiratory complications early, whether it is an emergent state or in the evolution of their disease process. Either of these requires appropriate intervention for their current situation.

Pathophysiology

Injury to the brain, whether due to trauma, hemorrhage, or infection, can lead to a depressed level of consciousness and inability to protect the airway. Mechanisms of disruption involving the pons, medulla, and other automatic ventilation controls can induce abnormal respiratory patterns or inefficiencies such as hypoventilation. These direct disturbances in the acute setting are often managed with airway protection and mechanical ventilation oftentimes before an actual diagnosis can be made, but they are treated with a high index of suspicion from precipitating factors and presentations.[29]

The respiratory manifestations of spinal cord injury depend on the level of injury and extent of damage.[30] Partially affected areas can lead to added improvement of function compared with a complete discontinuance of activity. High cervical injury above the origin of the phrenic nerve (C1-C3) leads to paralysis of all the major respiratory muscles except the accessory and bulbar muscles.[9] These insults require chronic respiratory support. Injury at the level of the phrenic nerve roots (C3-C5) results in weakness or total paralysis of the diaphragm.[4] Lower cervical injuries (C5-C6) involve intercostal and abdominal muscle involvement and commonly lead to ineffective vital capacities, cough, and subsequent mucus withholding. Depending on the severity, without aggressive support, these lower cervical injuries can lead to the necessity for airway and ventilator management.

Myopathies such as Duchenne muscular dystrophy and myotonic dystrophy refer to an assortment of progressive hereditary diseases that involve muscle fibers.

Complications associated with these neurologic diseases result in the direct effect of muscle weakness to the respiratory system. It is often accompanied by other deficits, such as an abnormal respiratory drive, sleep-related breathing disorders, and an ineffective cough. A single or multifactorial inadequacy leads to respiratory insufficiency and many times respiratory failure.

Myasthenia gravis is a chronic disorder of the neuromuscular junction that interferes with the chemical transmission of acetylcholine between the axonal terminal and the receptor sites of voluntary muscles.[3] The common presentation is weakness of voluntary muscles and improvement with rest and/or the dosing of an anticholinesterase medication such as Tensilon. Acute respiratory failure can occur on initial presentation; an increase, decrease, or discontinuation of anticholinergics; administration of neuromuscular blocking medication; and surgery (thymectomy). Other than the acute setting of airway and ventilator management, treatment includes anticholinesterase medication, corticosteroids, thymectomy, and plasmapheresis.

Guillain-Barré is a peripheral nerve syndrome that usually presents with hyporeflexia with or without sensory symptoms, pain, and numbness, which can last days to weeks. In extreme cases this can lead to eventual ascending symmetric paralysis. The exact cause is not known; however, it usually follows a respiratory or gastrointestinal bacterial or viral infection, recent surgeries, and lymphomas. Treatment involves immunoglobulin therapy, corticosteroids, and plasmapheresis.

Assessment

The primary focus is to assess for signs of respiratory distress and failure along with neurologic investigation. Physical examination should reveal evidence of any spinal abnormalities causing a restrictive lung pattern. The transport team should be diligent in a careful history, which can lead to a high index of suspicion rather than a definite acute diagnosis in some cases. This information may contain valuable evidence showing a progression of a known ailment versus an acute onset of impending respiratory dysfunction. In the advancing disease, signs of hypoventilation, decreased muscle strength, and an altered level of consciousness may be present. With interfacility transfers, information such as ABGs, chest radiograph, and PFTs is beneficial in trending muscle strength and pulmonary status. Effort-dependent spirometry may be diminished because of weakening muscles, such as serial measurements of a forced vital capacity. Specific symptoms and tests associated with an illness and interventions should also be sought out.

Interventions

Immediate priority in patients presenting with respiratory failure caused by neurologic disorders are airway management, oxygenation, and prompt treatment of precipitating factors, such as pneumonia, in addition to assessment for more specialized therapies. Noninvasive ventilation may be appropriate to support ventilator effort when the patient is able to maintain his or her own airway without the risk of vomiting or diminished respiratory effort, is hemodynamically stable, is able to maintain an adequate mask seal, and is neurologically intact. Intubation with mechanical ventilation may be needed in the presence of the patient's inability to maintain his or her own airway and respiratory failure associated with hypoventilation, hypoxia, and mucus accumulation.[3,29,31]

Drowning

According to the WHO, in 2012 an estimated 372,000 people died from drowning, making drowning a major public health problem worldwide. Injuries account for over 9% of total global mortality. Drowning is the third leading cause of unintentional injury death, accounting for 7% of all injury-related deaths.[32]

In the past there has been debate in definitions and nomenclature of drowning, creating degrees of confusion and the subsequent need for a more consistent approach in studying this group of incidents. Although there may be dry, wet, or near-drowning, depending on whether water is inhaled into the lungs, there is no clinical difference in how the victim is treated or whether the final outcome is good or bad.[33] However, some authors have argued that because pulmonary complications may follow the aspiration of water without the loss of consciousness, nonfatal drowning should be defined as survival, at least temporarily, after aspiration of fluid into the lungs ("wet nonfatal drowning") or after a period of asphyxia secondary to laryngospasm ("dry nonfatal drowning").[34]

In its 2010 resuscitation guidelines, the American Heart Association recommended that the Utstein definitions and methods of data reporting for drowning and related events should be used to improve consistency in reporting and research. According to the Utstein guidelines, drowning refers to "a process resulting in primary respiratory impairment from submersion or immersion in a liquid medium." The Utstein guidelines further suggest that ambiguous or confusing terms such as "near drowning," "secondary drowning," and "wet drowning" should not be used.[9] The most influential factors that determine outcomes are duration and severity of the hypoxia. Therefore definitions now used include drowning, which is the process of experiencing respiratory impairment from submersion or immersion in a liquid; submersion, which is when the airway is below the surface of the liquid; and immersion, which is when the airway is above the surface of the liquid.[35]

Etiology

The instigation of drowning is usually accidental and preventable. One of the major risk factors is age, with the highest rates among children 1 to 4 years of age.[32] Other elements that increase the incidence is gender, especially males; accessibility and traveling on water; medical emergencies including heart attacks, seizures, hypoglycemia, or diabetic coma; and stroke.

Alcohol and substance abuse also increases the incidence of drowning. Unfortunately, submersion injury also can be an indication of child maltreatment and abuse.

Pathophysiology

Persons who are submersed in a substance, most often water, panic and hold their breath. They may also hyperventilate, which can lead to aspiration and the swallowing of water. Swallowed water may cause vomiting and further aspiration of fluid in the lungs, resulting in direct pulmonary injury and hypoxia. A small percentage of drowning patients have laryngospasms, which is the natural protective reflex that prevents foreign material from entering the lungs; however, they can still suffer from obstructive asphyxia. Approximately 90% aspirate. In small amounts the fluid is usually quickly absorbed; however, even small amounts can lead to catastrophic results. This aspiration of fluids leads to bronchospasms, atelectasis, alveolar consolidation caused by contaminated materials, alveolar-capillary damage, and an increase in surface tension caused by a decrease in pulmonary surfactant, all of which contribute to hypoxia. These manifestations show why most of the morbidity from drowning is the consequence of cerebral hypoxia.[35]

It should be noted that a rapid change in body temperature, as seen in ice-cold water engagement, can ignite the mammalian dive reflex phenomenon, which acts as a protective mechanism. The body is cooled so quickly that the body's metabolic rate is slowed and residual oxygen levels are enough to maintain basic organ viability. Some reported cases have found a return of spontaneous circulation even after approximately 1 hour of downtime.

Assessment

The assessment of the near-drowning victim begins with evaluation and management of the patient's airway, breathing, and circulation. The evaluation should include consideration of whether the patient may have sustained a cervical spine injury from falling or jumping into the water, and cervical spinal precautions should be taken.

Interventions

Because most drowning patients involve some degree of hypoxia, hypercapnia, and acidosis, rapid evaluation and intervention with mechanical ventilation should be a high priority. Lung protective strategies should be used because of an increased incidence of barotrauma and ARDS, and high levels of PEEP are often needed. Establishment of IV access and correction of hypovolemia is necessary because drowning victims may become hypovolemic following prolonged

• BOX 22-3 **Drowning Prevention**

When children are around water (swimming, bathing), they must be watched by an adult at all times.
Never swim alone.
Never drink alcohol or use drugs when swimming or boating.
People with backyard pools or ponds or who live near bodies of water should learn cardiopulmonary resuscitation.
Never use air-filled swimming devices (water wings) in place of life jackets or approved life preservers.
Know the local weather conditions to prevent being caught out on the water in a storm.
Follow beach warnings about dangerous tides, rip currents, or presence of danger in the water.

Modified from Carden DL, Smith JK Pneumonias. *Emerg Med Clin North Am.* 1989;7(2):255-278.

immersion caused by the hydrostatic effects of water.[35] Thermoregulation is also a continuant whether for rewarming or neurologic cooling strategies (Box 22.3).

Pneumonias

Etiology

Pneumonia is an inflammation of the lung parenchyma caused by either a bacterium or a virus (Fig. 22.9). Box 22.4 lists the different types of pneumonia with their causative organisms. The severity can be dependent on the specific pathogen and any underlying risk factors the patient may have. Pneumonias can be classified as community acquired, hospital acquired (including ventilator acquired), or from aspiration. Identification of the classification can be helpful with the start of treatment and focusing on the common pathogens from each type of pneumonia.

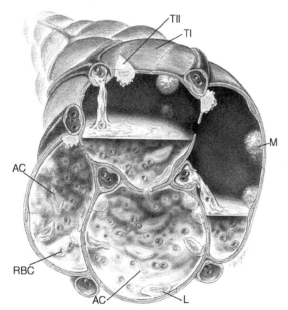

• **Fig. 22.9** Cross-sectional view of alveolar consolidation in pneumonia. *TI,* Type I cell; *TII,* Type II cell; *M,* macrophage; *AC,* alveolar consolidation; *L,* leukocyte; *RBC,* red blood cell. (From Des Jardins T, Burton GG: *Clinical Manifestations and Assessment of Respiratory Disease.* 4th ed. St. Louis: Mosby; 1995.)

Pathophysiologic Factors

Pneumonia is an inflammatory process in which the affected alveoli are diffusely involved. Bacteria, neutrophils, and protein pass from one alveolus to another and produce compact infiltrates. The dense alveolar consolidations prohibit volume loss and produce air bronchograms on chest radiography.

Bronchopneumonias occur with areas of normal lung parenchyma interspersed with affected lung parenchyma. The condition is multilobar and bilateral, with areas of atelectasis. *Staphylococcus aureus* is the most common organism. *Interstitial pneumonia* is the result of an inflammatory process that affects the support structures of the lung.

Assessment

The history of the patient with suspected pneumonia includes fever and purulent sputum production. The specific signs and symptoms for different types of pneumonia are listed in Box 22.3. In addition to a careful history, a physical examination should include not only a thorough pulmonary assessment but also an assessment of the patient's overall health. Testing includes chest radiograph, sputum cultures, Gram stains, and possibly a bronchoscopy.

Intervention

Interventions include oxygenation and ventilation support, identification of the type, antibiotics, and prevention of spreading. The type-specific interventions are summarized in Box 22.3.

Pleural Effusion

Pleural effusion is a collection of fluid in the pleura space. The fluid is mobile and will gravitate to the most dependent area of the pleural cavity. The more significant the volume of accumulated fluid, the more the lung is compressed, creating less space for lung expansion and a decreased area for oxygenation. Treatment includes identification using auscultation and chest radiograph with intervention being evacuation or drainage of the effusion. Ongoing care may include identification of the fluid and management of the cause.

• BOX 22-4 Pneumonias

Streptococcus Pneumoniae (Pneumococcal)

Organism
S. pneumoniae: Gram-positive, lancet-shaped Diplococcus; aerobe

Risk Factors
Young, elderly, immunosuppression, alcoholism, COPD, cardio-vascular disease, diabetes mellitus, hyposplenia; highest risk in winter months

Pathophysiology
Bacteria is normal inhabitant of upper respiratory tract; aspiration, inhalation, or hematogenous seeding are routes of entry; damage occurs from overwhelming growth, which impairs gas exchange

Clinical Manifestations
Malaise, sore throat, rhinorrhea, chills, fever, rust-colored sputum, pleuritic chest pain, nausea, vomiting, abdominal pain, tachycardia, tachypnea, dyspnea, decreased breath sounds, dullness, rales, pleural friction rub; in elderly patients, change in mental status or congestive heart failure is a possible presentation

Diagnostic Findings
Leukocytes up to 40,000 mL with left shift
Leukopenia
Liver function tests abnormal
CXR: Homogeneous lobar or sublobar infiltrates

Treatment
Antibiotics
Fluids
Oxygen

Staphylococcus Aureus

Organism
S. aureus pneumonia: Gram-positive nonmotile spherical organism

Risk Factors
IV drug abuse, immunocompromised, and complication of influenza epidemic

Pathophysiology
Aspiration from upper respiratory tract leads to infections; growth occurs rapidly in the debilitated host; hematogenous seeding occurs with dialysis or IV drug use

Clinical Manifestations
Abrupt onset of fever, chills, cough, dyspnea, pleuritic chest pain; purulent sputum ranging from yellow to pink; frank hemoptysis common; toxic appearance; tachypnea, tachycardia, rales, rhonchi

Diagnostic Findings
White blood cell >150,000/mL
Positive blood cultures in 20% of cases
CXR: Bilateral lower lobe bronchopneumonia, early abscess formation or pleural effusion possible

Treatment
Antibiotics
Fluids
Oxygen

Klebsiella Pneumoniae

Organism
K. pneumoniae: Gram-negative, nonmotile, encapsulated rods

Risk Factors
Men, over 50 years of age, alcoholism, heart disease, diabetes mellitus, COPD, aspiration

Pathophysiology
Results in necrosis of alveolar walls, multiple abscesses, loss of lung volume, friable blood vessels

Clinical Manifestations
Fever, rigors, dyspnea, productive cough, hemoptysis, copious purulent sputum that is green or blood streaked

Diagnostic Findings
Leukopenia or leukocytosis
CXR: Lobar consolidation, typically of right upper lobe; rapid appearance of lung abscesses; pleural effusion common; bronchopneumonia in lower lobes

Treatment
Antibiotics
Fluids
Oxygen

Pseudomonas Aeruginosa

Organism
P. aeruginosa: Gram-negative motile rod, not encapsulated

Risk Factor
Second most common nosocomial, decreased host defenses or antimicrobial therapy, alcoholism, diabetes mellitus

Pathophysiology
Aspiration, necrosis of alveolar walls, multiple abscesses, loss of lung volume, friable blood vessels

Clinical Manifestations
Same as those for Klebsiella infection

Diagnostic Findings
Leukocytosis with left shift
Arterial hypoxemia
Hypocapnia
Positive blood cultures in 33% to 50% of cases
CXR: Patchy infiltrates in lower lobes; cavitation, empyema

Treatment
Antibiotics
Fluids
Oxygen

Haemophilus Influenzae

Organism
H. influenzae: Gram-negative, pleomorphic motile rod; encapsulated and nonencapsulated strains

Risk Factors
50 years of age; >50% have alcoholism, COPD; upper respiratory infection, 2 to 6 weeks previously
Encapsulated strain: Alcoholism, diabetes mellitus, COPD, impaired immune system
Nonencapsulated strain: Exacerbation of bronchitis, nonbacteremic pneumonia

Pathophysiology
Bacterial infection that produces inflammation

Clinical Manifestations
Minimal elevations in temperature, pulse, and respiration; dyspnea; rales; rhonchi; pleuritic chest pain; nausea; vomiting

Diagnostic Findings
Leukocytosis
CXR: Bronchopneumonia, lower lobe and multilobular pleural effusions

Treatment
Antibiotics
Fluids
Oxygen

COPD, Chronic obstructive pulmonary disease; CXR, chest x-ray; IV, intravenous.

CASE STUDY

Pulmonary System

History

The transport team was called to the scene of a near-drowning. A 15-year-old boy was playing ice hockey with his friends on a farm pond. He suddenly fell through weak ice. He was pulled out by his friends, and cardiopulmonary resuscitation was begun.

On arrival of the transport team, the patient was found with a palpable pulse and a Glasgow Coma Scale of 5 (E–1), (V–1), (M–5); pupils were 4 mm, and both were reacting equally. The patient's airway was secured with endotracheal intubation and rapid-sequence intubation after an IV access was obtained. His wet clothing was removed, and he was wrapped in a warm blanket. A cervical collar was applied, and the patient was placed on a backboard and prepared for transport to the trauma center.

During transport, lorazepam and fentanyl were administered for agitation. His vital signs were blood pressure 110/50 mm Hg, pulse rate 130, and assisted ventilations at 16. A pulse oximetry reading could not be obtained because of his cold extremities. His CO_2 level was measured at 30 on the end-tidal monitor.

Outcome

The patient was admitted to the critical care unit, where his level of consciousness continued to improve. However, pneumonia and sepsis developed, which were believed to be the result of aspiration of the water in the farm pond. *Pseudomonas* was cultured from his sputum. He needed a tracheostomy for ventilatory support. However, after several weeks, he was able to have the tracheostomy tube removed and eventually made a full recovery.

Discussion

One important point this case makes is the success of basic life support at the scene by this patient's friends. Mouth-to-mouth ventilation was started immediately once his friends pulled him out of the water, resulting in a limited amount of time that the patient was without ventilation. Some experts also believe that the water temperature may increase the chances of survivability.

References

1. Kacmarek RM, Stoller JK, Heuer AH. *Egan's Fundamentals of Respiratory Care*. 10th ed. St. Louis: Elsevier Health Sciences; 2012.
2. Jardins TDR. *Cardiopulmonary Anatomy & Physiology: Essentials of Respiratory Care*. 6th ed. Clinton Park, NY: Delmar Cengage Learning; 2012.
3. Jardins TDR, Burton GG. *Clinical Manifestations and Assessment of Respiratory Disease*. St. Louis: Mosby; 2015.
4. Hess DR, MacIntyre NR, Mishoe SC, Galvin WF. *Respiratory Care: Principles and Practice*. 2nd ed. Sudbury, MA: Jones and Bartlett Publishers; 2011.
5. Pittman RN. *Regulation of Tissue Oxygenation*. San Rafael, CA: Morgan & Claypool Life Sciences; 2011. Chapter 4, Oxygen Transport. Available from http://www.ncbi.nlm.nih.gov/books/NBK54103.
6. Beachey W. *Respiratory Care Anatomy and Physiology: Foundations for Clinical Practice*. 3rd ed. Edinburgh, UK: Elsevier Health Sciences; 2013.
7. Collins J-A, Rudenski A, Gibson J, et al. Relating oxygen partial pressure, saturation and content: The haemoglobin–oxygen dissociation curve. *Breathe*. 2015;11(3):194-201. Retrieved from http://www.ncbi.nlm.nih.gov/pmc/articles/PMC4666443/.
8. American College of Surgeons. *Advanced Trauma Life Support-Skills Procedure*, Chest Trauma Management, Needle Thoracentesis (Student Manual). 7th ed. Chicago, IL: American College of Surgeons; 2004.
9. Brashers V. Structure and function of pulmonary system. In: McCance KL, Huether SE, eds. *Pathophysiology: the Biologic Basis for Disease in Adults and Children*. 5th ed. St. Louis: Mosby Elsevier; 2006.
10. Ellstrom K. The pulmonary system. In: Alspach G, ed. *Core Curriculum for Critical Care Nursing*. 6th ed. Philadelphia, PA: Saunders Elsevier; 2006.
11. Randhawa R, Bellingan G. Acute lung injury. *Anaesth Intens Care Med*. 2007;8(11):477-480.
12. Rozet I, Domino KB. Respiratory care. *Best Pract Res Clin Anaesthesiol*. 2007;21(4):465-482.
13. Deal EN, Hollands JM, Schramm GE, et al. Role of corticosteroids in the management of acute respiratory distress syndrome. *Clin Therapeutics*. 2008;30(5):787-799.
14. Cottrell JJ. Altitude exposures during aircraft flight. *Chest*. 1988; 93(1):81-84.
15. Selfridge-Thomas J, Hoyt S. Respiratory emergencies. In: Hoyt S, Selfridge-Thomas J, eds. *Emergency Nursing Core Curriculum*. 6th ed. Philadelphia, PA: Saunders Elsevier; 2007.
16. Krouse JH, Krouse HJ. Asthma: guidelines-based control and management. *Otolaryngol Clin North Am*. 2008;41(2):397-409.
17. Spahn JD, Covar R. Clinical assessment of asthma progression in children. *J Allergy Clin Immunol*. 2008;121(3):548-557.
18. Kanellakis NI, Jacinto T, Psallidas I. European respiratory society. Retrieved June 4, 2016, from http://breathe.ersjournals.com/; 2015, September 1.
19. American Thoracic society-assessment. http://www.thoracic.org/copd-guidelines/for-health-professionals/exacerbation/definition-evaluation-and-treatment/assessment.php; 2015, February.
20. Huang T-W, Lee S-C, Cheng Y-L, et al. Contralateral recurrence of primary spontaneous Pneumothorax. *Chest Journal*. 2007;132 (4):1146-1150.
21. Tapson VF. Treatment, prognosis, and follow-up of acute pulmonary embolism in adults. Retrieved April 19, 2016, from http://www.uptodate.com/contents/overview-of-the-treatment-prognosis-and-follow-up-of-acute-pulmonary-embolism-in-adults; 2016, April 7.
22. Bělohlávek J, Dytrych V, Linhart A. Pulmonary embolism, part I: Epidemiology, risk factors and risk stratification, pathophysiology, clinical presentation, diagnosis and nonthrombotic pulmonary embolism. *Experimental and Clinical Cardiology*. 2013;18(2). Retrieved from http://www.ncbi.nlm.nih.gov/pmc/articles/PMC3718593/.
23. Thompson BT, Kabrhel C. 2016. Overview of acute pulmonary embolism in adults. Retrieved April 19, 2016, from http://www.uptodate.com/contents/overview-of-acute-pulmonary-embolism-in-adults.

24. Thompson BT, Kabrhel C. Clinical presentation, evaluation, and diagnosis of the adult with suspected acute pulmonary embolism; 2016. Retrieved 19, 2016, from http://www.uptodate.com/contents/clinical-presentation-evaluation-and-diagnosis-of-the-adult-with-susptected-acute-pulmonary-embolism.

25. Rubin LJ, Diego S, Medicine. Overview of pulmonary hypertension in adults. Available at http://www.uptodate.com/contents/overview-of-pulmonary-hypertension-in-adults; 2016, March Accessed 19.04.16.

26. Simonneau G, Gatzoulis MA, Adatia I, et al. Updated Clinical Classification of Pulmonary Hypertension. *J Am Coll Cardiol.* 2013;62(suppl 25):D34-D41.

27. Gibbons GH. Related director's message. How is pulmonary hypertension treated. Available at http://www.nhlbi.nih.gov/health/health-topics/topics/pah/treatment; 2015 Accessed 22.04.16.

28. Hoeper MM, Granton J. Intensive care unit management of patients with severe pulmonary hypertension and right heart failure. *Am J Respir Crit Care Med.* 2011;184(10):1114-1124.

29. Critical Care Research and Practice. Volume 2012 (2012), Article ID 207247; 2016. From http://dx.doi.org/10.1155/2012/207247. Retrieved April 19, 2016, from http://1http://www.hindawi.com/journals/ccrp/2012/207247/.

30. Anderson FA, Wheeler HB. Venous thromboembolism risk factors and prophylaxis. *Clin Chest Med.* 1995;16(2):235.

31. Mangera Z, Panesar G, Makker H. Practical approach to management of respiratory complications in neurological disorders. *International journal of general medicine.* 2012;5:255-263. Retrieved from http://www.ncbi.nlm.nih.gov/pubmed/22505823.

32. WHO. "Drowning." World Health Organization. http://www.who.int/mediacentre/factsheets/fs347/en/; Feb 3. 2016. Web. Apr 19. 2016.

33. Wedro B. "Drowning: Facts about wet and dry drowning." eMedicineHealth; 2016. WebMD. Apr 19, 2016. http://www.emedicinehealth.com/drowning/article_em.htm.

34. Chandy D, Weinhouse GL, et al. "Drowning (submersion injuries)." n.d. Web. Apr 19. 2016. http://www.uptodate.com/contents/drowning-submersion-injuries.

35. Immersion submersion and drowning. Retrieved April 19, 2016, from http://www.derangedphysiology.com/main/required-reading/trauma-burns-and-drowning/Chapter%204.0.7/immersion-submersion-and-drowning; 2016, January 23.

23

Abdominal Emergencies

KYLE MADIGAN

COMPETENCIES

1. Perform a comprehensive assessment of the patient with an abdominal emergency.
2. Initiate the critical interventions for the management of an abdominal emergency during transport.
3. Identify the management of specific abdominal emergencies during transport.

Disorders encountered by transport teams may include esophageal obstruction and esophageal varices with rupture; stomach disorders, such as gastric or duodenal hemorrhage, ulceration, perforation, or pyloric obstruction; gallbladder and biliary tract disorders; liver disease; pancreatic disorders; and intestinal obstruction or rupture, ruptured diverticula, acute appendicitis, and abdominal compartment syndrome.

Transport via air may cause specific problems for the patient with an abdominal emergency.[1] The aerodynamics and biophysics that govern air medical care are especially important in relation to the gastrointestinal (GI) system, which encompasses 26 feet of liquid-producing and gas-producing viscous matter. Careful patient history, assessment, and pretransport planning are imperative for the patient transported via air or ground.[2]

Selected Abdominal Emergencies

Esophagus

The esophagus is a hollow tube of striated and smooth muscle that is approximately 10 inches long in an adult. It lies posteriorly to the trachea, closely aligns the left main stem bronchus, and exits the thoracic cavity at the diaphragmatic hiatus, or approximately at the T11 level. The esophagus provides the primary functions of peristaltic movement of food bolus, prevention of reflux with lower esophageal sphincter activity, and venting for gastric pressure changes.[2,3]

Vascular supply to the esophagus is through branches of the descending thoracic aorta. Venous return from the esophagus is through the superior vena cava, azygos system, and portal vein system.

Neurologic intervention is initiated in the medulla and performed by the vagus nerve. Because the esophagus lies in the thoracic cavity, in normal atmospheric conditions, it maintains a subatmospheric pressure of -5 to -10 mm Hg, whereas the stomach, which is in the abdominal cavity, rests at an atmospheric pressure of $+5$ to $+10$ mm Hg. Acute esophageal occurrences are esophageal obstruction, esophageal varices, and esophageal rupture.

Esophageal Obstruction

Three areas in the esophagus are narrow and may be potential sites for obstruction and injury. These areas include the cricoid cartilage, the arch of the aorta, and the point at which the esophagus passes through the diaphragm.[1,3]

Esophageal obstruction is fairly common. Strictures, webs, tumors, diverticula, foreign bodies, achalasia, and lower esophageal rings can all reduce or eliminate the venting property of the esophagus for the upper GI system. When air medical transport of a patient with obstruction is undertaken, intermittent exposure to variations in altitude is of great importance. Esophageal obstruction and an expanding gastrum can pose a serious threat if rapid decompression occurs at 35,000 feet. The venting property needs to be established before flight and depends on whether rotor-wing or fixed-wing transport is to be used.[4]

Assessment

The transport team will need to carefully correlate physical assessment with interpretation of radiologic and laboratory data to anticipate any potential problems that may occur during the transport process.

The transport team should ascertain the patient's chief symptom and medical history. Included in these subjective data should be the patient's clinical course since the incident occurred. Medical history helps the transport team identify and anticipate any other additional problems that may arise during transport.

The transport team performs a physical examination that includes assessment of the following:
- The patient's ability to protect the airway.
- The patient's ability to clear secretions by swallowing.
- The presence and location of pain.

Diagnostic Tests

Radiographic studies of the obstruction should accompany the patient. If an esophagoscopy has been performed, a report should be provided to the transport team so they can prepare for any potential problems that may occur during transport.

Plan and Implementation

If the patient is being transported via air, the plan of care depends on the anticipated transport altitude. The transport team should carefully evaluate the patient's ability to maintain the airway. Even with aircraft pressurization, adequate gastric venting is extremely important if high altitude will be maintained. Pretransport medications and antiemetic therapy are often helpful not only for the antiemetic effect, but some agents can also provide sedation, especially in patients at risk for motion sickness.[5]

When not contraindicated, a gastric tube should be placed and gastric contents emptied before and during transport. If the gastric tube is hooked to suction, its flow and contents should be closely monitored during transport. Continuous monitoring of respiratory status is also necessary.

Intervention

Caution must be exercised when a patient is placed on suction devices during transport. Intermittent disconnection of suction from the gastric tube allows the pressures to equalize and prevents extreme suction against the gastric wall.

Children with a potential esophageal obstruction may benefit from an accompanying parent or other caregiver to decrease anxiety and prevent crying or other movement that may increase the risk of airway compromise.

Esophageal Varices

The most common cause of *esophageal varices* is hepatic congestion, and they are present in as much as 50% of patients with cirrhosis. Torturous, fragile, and dilated esophageal veins can bleed from spontaneous rupture caused by increased portal hypertension or physical or chemical trauma. Esophageal varices are usually associated with hepatic dysfunction as related to cirrhosis, renal failure, coagulopathies, and sepsis.[5,6] Varices occur frequently at the distal esophagus and hemorrhoidal plexus, and hemorrhagic shock from an esophageal bleed can occur rapidly. Bleeding occurs in 30% to 40% of patients who have esophageal varices.[5-7]

Assessment

Sequential history of the patient with esophageal varices helps the transport team anticipate probable needs during transport. Patients with a preexisting history of coronary artery disease, congestive heart failure, and hepatic disease have a higher rate of mortality and may require advanced intervention in anticipation of transport.[5-7]

The transport team should obtain a history related to the cause of the esophageal varices, which can also provide information about other potential problems that could develop during transport. For example, the patient with severe liver disease also has bleeding and clotting problems. Patients with a history of alcoholism may experience withdrawal, which could put them at risk for seizures.

Careful consideration of the patient's most recent pretransport laboratory data (hematocrit and hemoglobin levels, prothrombin time [PT]/partial thromboplastin time [PTT] or international normalized ratio [INR], and electrolyte profile) helps the transport team anticipate the patient's needs during transport.

For patients who have undergone angiography, the transport team must secure the cannulization site before any patient movement and monitor the site frequently throughout transport for bleeding and potential for an expanding hematoma.

Plan and Implementation

The transport team's primary priority is to ensure adequacy of the airway before transport. The transport team must consider what supplies are needed should an acute hemorrhagic episode occur during transport. Continuous gastric suction can produce large volumes of secretions, and a system to adequately dispose of secretions during transport needs to be ready, such as a supply of sealable bags or containers with tight seals.

An experienced transport member must maintain adequate care of any esophageal balloon tamponade device, such as the Sengstaken-Blakemore, Linton, or Minnesota tubes. Although infrequently used, traction-dependent or specialized esophageal tubes can pose a problem for transport. Traction maintained with a football helmet can be used during transport (Fig. 23.1).[7]

Airway loss from these particular types of tubes can be from either physiologic deterioration or tracheal obstruction. Endotracheal intubation is accomplished before placement of a balloon tamponade device in most situations.[8] Pressure changes associated with altitude should be considered by the

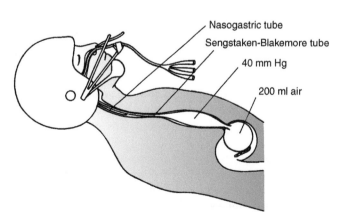

Nasogastric tube
Sengstaken-Blakemore tube
40 mm Hg
200 ml air

• **Fig. 23.1** Traction maintained with football helmet for Sengstaken-Blakemore tube.

flight team; saline solution, rather than air, can be used to inflate the cuffs to prevent further expansion during flight.

Intervention If an acute hemorrhagic episode occurs, maintenance of airway and circulating volume is the first priority. Blood and blood products may be needed during transport. In patients experiencing acute gastroesophageal bleeding, transfusion resuscitation should be initiated promptly to maintain hemodynamic stability.[9] Caution must be taken with blood volume resuscitation, because over resuscitation may increase portal vascular pressures leading to rebleeding.[8,9]

Effective pretransport planning to prevent vomiting and ensure adequate venous access and volume resuscitation is crucial. Management of medications such as octreotide and less commonly used, vasopressin, should be anticipated during transport.

Esophageal Rupture

Esophageal rupture commonly results from penetrating trauma but may also result from a blunt insult to the thorax. Rupture from invading lesions, tumors, or caustic exposure also occurs, but to a lesser extent. If esophageal rupture has occurred, the venting properties and pathways have been altered. During transport, and with possible altitude changes, the distribution and displacement of gases are no longer circumvented by the appropriate course. Complications of gastric pneumonitis, hemopneumothorax, and alteration in gas exchange may all occur.

Assessment

The transport team evaluates the history of preceding incidents leading to the current episode. Drugs known to have corrosive effects on the esophagus are doxycycline, tetracycline, acetylsalicylic acid, clindamycin, potassium chloride, quinidine, and ferrous sulfate. Caustic substances can quickly lead to burning or complete erosion of the tissue. Estimation of the degree and size of burns is extremely difficult and can quickly compromise respiratory status. If the rupture is caused by an extravasating tumor, hemorrhage and airway control can become quite difficult to manage.

Plan and Implementation Priorities

The transport teams' priorities are as follows:
1. Ascertain adequacy of airway, ventilation, and oxygenation.
2. Maintain adequate venous access and volume support.
3. Placement of gastric tube with adequate suctioning, if not contraindicated.

Stomach

The stomach lies beneath the diaphragm and is secured in the peritoneum by the lesser omentum. The stomach is subject to alterations in intraabdominal pressure (IAP), unlike the esophagus, which has negative atmospheric

pressure. The cardiac sphincter separates the esophagus from the stomach. Vascular supply is from the celiac artery branches, and venous return is through the superior mesenteric, splenic, and portal veins.

The stomach functions as a receptacle of ingested substances and attempts to provide chemical and mechanical breakdown. As the stomach expands, peristaltic action increases. The average time of gastric emptying is 1 to 8 hours. Chyme is then propelled through the pyloric sphincter into the duodenum. Decreased gastric motility and alterations in altitude can lead to complications.

Acute Gastric Occurrences

Acute gastric occurrences can take the form of gastric duodenal hemorrhage, gastric perforation from both mechanical and chemical means, pyloric obstruction, and gastric and duodenal ulceration (Fig. 23.2).[6]

Bleeding from peptic or duodenal ulceration occurs more frequently than esophageal variceal bleeding, representing up to 50% of all such cases. Several methods may be used to manage the bleeding, including insertion of gastric tubes, such as Linton or Minnesota tubes (rarely used anymore for the management of bleeding esophageal varices); pharmacologic management; endoscopy; thermal therapy; injection therapy, and if bleeding is massive and cannot be controlled, surgery. Anticipatory planning and thorough preparation can ensure a safe patient transport.[10-12]

Ulcerative lesions of the stomach or duodenum that lead to bleeding or perforation are in part caused by mucosal membrane erosion. The tissue beneath the mucosa is then subjected to general tissue corrosion. Ulcerations can lead to hemorrhage, perforation, or obstruction and may occur after an attempted repair.

Intervention

In the event of an acute hemorrhagic episode during transport, a transport team member should perform volume resuscitation, including administration of blood, blood products, and medications to manage the bleeding.[4,8,9,11,12] Complications may arise if the gastric tube becomes obstructed.[12] Gastric dilation and excessive hydrochloric acid can cause nausea and vomiting, which may mechanically induce hemorrhage. Maintenance of adequate gastric venting is imperative throughout any altitude changes when the patient is transported via air.

Movement can cause nausea whether via air or ground. The transport team should consider administration of an antiemetic to decrease the risk of vomiting, which may precipitate bleeding and potential airway compromise during transport.

Gallbladder and Biliary Tract

The primary function of the gallbladder and biliary tract is to receive approximately 2 L of bile a day from the liver. Bile, which is stimulated not only by food ingestion but also by

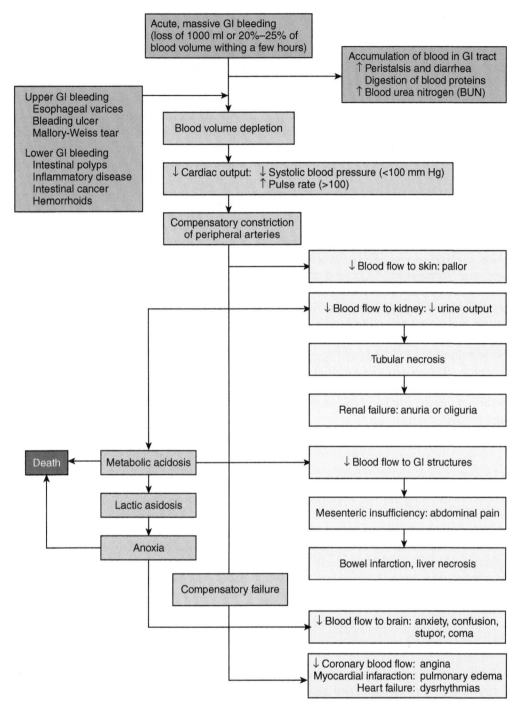

• **Fig. 23.2** Pathophysiology of gastrointestinal bleeding. (From McCance K, Huether S, eds. *The Biologic Basis for Disease in Adults and Children.* 7th ed. St. Louis, MO: Elsevier/Mosby; 2014.)

stress and acute illness, flows into the duodenum through the common bile duct. Fluid and electrolyte reabsorption takes place in the gallbladder before the bile enters the duodenum; therefore, with generalized volume deficit, an even more concentrated efficacious bile enters the duodenum.

Bile, which is composed of fatty acids, bile salts, phospholipid, cholesterol, conjugated bilirubin, and water, mixes with the chyme to aid digestion.

The ampulla of Vater and sphincter of Oddi are common sites of disease or injury that dramatically affect the entire tract. The gallbladder and biliary tracts are stimulated sympathetically by the splanchnic nerve and parasympathetically by the vagus. Vascular supply is provided by the hepatic artery and cystic vein.

Gallbladder and biliary disorders that necessitate acute medical transport are infrequent. However, necrotic gangrenous cholecystitis can progress to septicemia, acute pancreatitis, or gallbladder rupture, hepatic failure, or both, because of obstruction of bile flow and production.

Plan and Implementation

Transport of patients with gallbladder and biliary tract disorders includes pretransport evaluation and determination of adequate drainage of gastric or cholecystotomy tubes or both. Careful observation during transport is imperative for prevention of flow obstruction. As with any major abdominal disease or trauma, careful monitoring of oxygen tension and saturation should occur during transport.

Liver

The incidence of liver disease and its associated illnesses is relatively frequent. Because of its varied synthetic and metabolic functions, the liver may be affected by a host of disorders, trauma, and ingestions.[5] Acute and chronic hepatic diseases are common in the general public.

An adult liver weighs approximately 3 lb and is supplied by the hepatic artery and portal vein. The liver is a very vascular organ and receives as much as 30% of the cardiac output via the portal vein and hepatic artery.[5]

The most commonly encountered diseases of the liver encountered by transport personnel are cirrhosis, liver failure, or associated biliary atresia; also common are patients who are candidates for liver transplantation.

Assessment

Hepatic encephalopathy is a common presentation in the patient with decompensating chronic liver disease.[13] Hepatic encephalopathy can cause confusion, somnolence, asterixis, hyperreflexia, cognitive deficits, and progression to coma. A confused and irritable patient could potentially become a safety threat in the transport environment. Other causes of altered mental status, such as electrolyte imbalances, hypoglycemia, and ingestion, should be considered and treated pretransport.

Plan and Implementation

Hepatic encephalopathy, acid base imbalance, and electrolyte imbalances may make the patient confused and combative and can contribute to the challenge of transport, especially during transport.

When transporting a patient with liver disease, knowledge of which medications may be affected by liver dysfunction is important. For example, benzodiazepines may have extended half-lives because of the metabolism pathway of the liver. The prolonged sedative effects may be misinterpreted as progressing encephalopathy.

Hepatic encephalopathy is often treated with medications such as aminoglycoside antibiotics and lactulose in an effort to reduce and absorb ammonia production. A side effect of lactulose administration is excessive diarrhea, which may result in fluid and electrolyte imbalances.[12] The transport team needs to ensure that the patient is appropriately "padded" to prevent skin damage from the rectal output and possible contamination of equipment.[9]

Hepatitis

The transport team is very likely to encounter patients with hepatitis and must use appropriate personal protection equipment to protect themselves. Hepatitis is most commonly caused by a virus, although it may also be induced as a side effect to medications.

Assessment

The most common strains of viral hepatitis include type A, type B, type C, and delta viruses. These strains are responsible for the most severe cases of viral hepatitis. Hepatitis A is transmitted primarily enterally, where both hepatitis B and C are contracted through exposure to blood and body fluids.

The transport team will want to elicit a thorough history related to both prescribed and recreational drug use because this may be the cause of the hepatitis.[13]

The transport team should evaluate the patient's laboratory data before transport, with particular focus on signs of infections, anemia, and elevated liver enzymes and bilirubin. As synthetic production becomes inhibited, evaluation of coagulation studies is indicated.

The patient with hepatitis generally describes flulike signs and symptoms including general malaise, body aches, and fever. Without the presence of jaundice, the presentation may be misleading.

Scleral icterus becomes present as bilirubin levels elevate in the presence of hepatitis. On physical examination, abdominal tenderness, palpated hepatomegaly, and increased temperature are common findings the transport team will encounter. As bilirubin levels continue to rise, cutaneous jaundice may be appreciated on physical examination.

Diagnostic Tests

Laboratory tests are the primary diagnostic tool for establishing a diagnosis of hepatitis. Hyperbilirubinemia, elevated liver function tests including serum aspartate aminotransferase and alanine aminotransferase are indicative of the presence of hepatitis. Elevated PT and INR are indicative of a worsening clinical picture.

Plan and Implementation

Anticipated treatment during patient transport is aimed at supportive therapy. Correction of fluid and electrolyte imbalances may be required by the transport team. Administration of an antiemetic should be anticipated because continued vomiting may induce upper GI bleeding. Avoidance of hepatotoxic medications should be a prime consideration of the transport team.

It is important for the transport team to always practice standard precautions before, during, and after the transport of a patient with suspected or diagnosed hepatitis. Equipment should be inspected and cleaned to reduce the risk of transmission of blood-borne pathogens.

Pancreas[6]

The pancreas is positioned horizontally across the abdomen and is located retroperitoneal and posterior to the spleen. The pancreas receives its vascular supply through the celiac and mesenteric arteries. The pancreas consists of endocrine, alpha, beta, and delta cells, and is responsible for the production of insulin and glucagon. Pancreatic disorders include pancreatitis, hemorrhagic pancreatitis, cancer, and damage caused by trauma. Devastation of this organ leads to difficult care management of fluid and electrolyte balance, hemodynamic stability, and pain control (Fig. 23.3).[4]

Assessment

A thorough history is helpful in determining the cause of the pancreatic disease process. A history of alcohol abuse

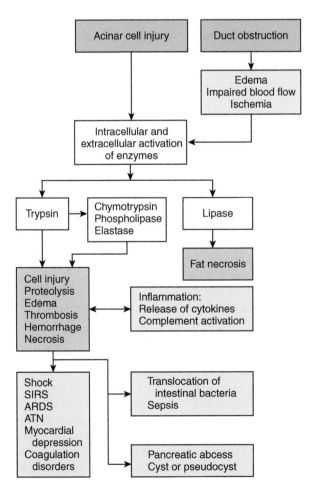

• **Fig. 23.3** Pathophysiology of acute pancreatitis. (From McCance K, Huether S, eds. *The Biologic Basis for Disease in Adults and Children.* 7th ed. St. Louis, MO: Elsevier/Mosby; 2014.)

and dependence is present in up to 35% of all cases of pancreatitis.[5] Careful evaluation of electrolyte balance may help the transport team determine additional treatment. A gastric tube must be in place before transport. If the patient has already undergone surgery and drains have been placed, the transport team must ensure proper venting for collection bulbs and surgical dressings. Pain management is an important transport intervention in the care of the patient with pancreatitis.

Patients presenting with both acute and chronic pancreatitis often describe constant, severe abdominal pain localized to the epigastrium or left upper quadrant.[9] The pain is often described as positional, with recumbent positions causing an increase in symptoms.

Elevated vital signs may be indicative of pain and an indication of hypovolemia in the patient with pancreatitis. Patients may sequester as much as 6 L of fluid in their retroperitoneum secondary to leaky capillary syndrome and vasodilatation.

Evaluation of the white blood cell count, hemoglobin, metabolic panels, and arterial blood gases may assist in determining the severity.[9]

Diagnostic Tests

Evaluation of the patient's laboratory tests for elevated levels of amylase and lipase, along with visualization via computerized tomography, can be helpful in determining the presence of pancreatitis. Hypocalcemia may also present through cardiac dysfunction and compromise.[9]

Intervention

Because of the potential for multiorgan involvement, priorities for the patient with pancreatitis include oxygenation and restoration of hemodynamic stability. Early and aggressive volume resuscitation is very important in the management of pancreatitis. Pain management is a concern for these patients and should be evaluated and treated by the transport team before and during transport.

Intestines

The small intestine (duodenum, jejunum, and ileum) is approximately 23 feet long. The primary functions of the intestines are absorption and digestion. The large intestine is composed of the cecum, ascending colon, transverse colon, descending colon, and sigmoid colon. This extensive, enclosed, and gas-producing system can pose many difficulties for transport of a patient who has either direct intestinal disease or general acute illness.

The intestinal problems most frequently encountered by transport teams are obstructions, ruptures, ruptured diverticula, acute appendicitis, ischemic bowel, and mesenteric infarct.[1,14] Many of these patients have sepsis and septic shock.

Assessment

A careful history is necessary to determine whether the intestinal disease is a primary or secondary illness. A physical examination by the transport nurse should check specifically for abdominal distention, hyperactive high-pitched bowel sounds, and rectal blood. Also, the transport team should assess the patient for signs and symptoms of peritonitis or sepsis.

Plan and Implementation

The transport team should evaluate venous access and volume needs before transport. The patient in shock may require fluid resuscitation and vasopressors to support hemodynamics. During transport, the team must ensure an adequate airway and provide oxygen, consider aircraft altitude or pressurization to reduce gas expansion, and ensure gastric tube patency. Continuous gastric tube suctioning is imperative throughout transport for a patient with an intestinal obstruction. Patients with stomas need adequate collection-bag capacity and venting.

If the patient has sepsis or septic shock, the transport team should direct care toward early goal-directed therapy. See Chapter 13 for the management of sepsis.

Abdominal Compartment Syndrome

Abdominal compartment syndrome contributes to organ dysfunction and occurs in concert with many injury and disease processes.[2,14] It may be linked to primary disease processes, such as pancreatitis, or secondarily to the treatment interventions of other diseases. Increased intraabdominal pressure results in hypoperfusion to the abdominal organs, increased intrathoracic pressure causing respiratory compromise, and ultimately multisystem dysfunction.

Assessment

Patients at risk for abdominal compartment syndrome include those with both traumatic and medical diagnoses. Abdominal surgical patients, and those suffering major trauma or thermal burns, are at risk because of aggressive volume resuscitation, along with leaky capillary syndrome. Medical diagnoses with abdominal compartment syndrome include, but are not limited to, pancreatitis, sepsis, liver dysfunction and cirrhosis, and intraabdominal and retroperitoneal tumors.

The presence of an open abdomen post damage control surgery does not preclude a patient from developing abdominal compartment syndrome. The transport team should always consider abdominal compartment syndrome in patients exhibiting early signs of shock including altered mental status and poor perfusion.

As with all gas-filled cavities, the transport team must take into consideration altitude changes. Gastric decompression with a gastric tube should be considered before transport.

An expanding abdomen, along with diminished abdominal wall compliance, is a common sign of developing abdominal compartment syndrome. Other symptoms include decreased urinary output, hypoxia, and hypercarbia.[13] Increased pressure in other parts of the body including an increased intracranial pressure without a head injury and an increased peak airway pressure without the presence of a thoracic injury may occur.

Diagnostic Tests

Abdominal compartment syndrome is present when IAP exceeds 20 mm Hg. IAP is routinely measured via transducing a urinary catheter in the bladder, in which normal pressures approximate the central venous pressure.[13]

Plan and Implementation

Nonsurgical approaches to reducing the effects of IAP include gastric decompression, sedation, and chemical paralysis to reduce ventilator asynchrony and subsequent decrease in intrathoracic pressure. Achieving fluid volume balance is important because volume boluses and aggressive resuscitation may be detrimental. The transport team may encounter patients who have undergone abdominal laparotomy in an effort to acutely reduce IAP.

Abdominal Aortic Emergencies

Patients with abdominal aortic injuries may require transport to definitive, specialized care.[7] The mortality rate from ruptured abdominal aortic aneurysms (RAAAs) exceeds 80%.[12] Risk factors for abdominal aortic aneurysms (AAAs) include increasing age, male gender, family history of abdominal aortic aneurysm, and smoking. New data suggest that one-half of all AAAs occur in woman under 65 years of age and nonsmokers.[11] Once the AAA has ruptured, operative intervention is emergently indicated.

Assessment

Most patients with AAA or RAAA come from a referral center and have been diagnosed. Many are also in hemorrhagic shock. Because time is one of the most important factors for potential survival, the transport team's assessment should be focused on critical problems such as hypoxia, hypotension, and bleeding.

Plan and Implementation

Rapid transport to an appropriate care facility is one of the most important interventions that can be provided by the team. Decreased time to the operating room has shown decreased mortality rates. A focused rapid assessment should be performed by the transport team. Blood and blood products are needed if a rupture has occurred and the patient is in hemorrhagic shock. However, the transport should not be delayed for diagnostic or laboratory data. A coordinated effort to decrease time to surgical intervention should be the goal. The transport team needs to be prepared for cardiac arrest during transport and consider when possible allowing the family to see the patient before transfer or even accompany the patient because of the high mortality rate associated with RAAA.

Volume resuscitation should be administered with caution. Over resuscitation can lead to increased bleeding from clot dislodgement and dilutional coagulopathy. Correction of hypotension should be goal directed at maintaining adequate cerebral and myocardial perfusion.[12]

Summary

Careful planning by the transport team before transport of the patient with an abdominal emergency, especially via air, helps anticipate potential decompensation, while providing effective, safe care.

Because patient problems are difficult to predict, the transport team should plan for equipment and treatment methods that can be applied easily to all patients before transport. Gases that expand with altitude are ever present in the GI system; proper venting mechanisms should be placed before flight, and backup devices should be available on the aircraft. Calculation of flight time, ground time, and unanticipated diversions helps the transport team estimate the amount of volume, battery time, capacities, and therapeutic support needed for the entire transport time.

CASE STUDY

Gastrointestinal Medical Emergencies

The helicopter was called to transport an 82-year-old man with an upper GI bleed from a community hospital to a tertiary care center. Refractory massive hemorrhage had occurred during the previous 12 hours, and simple endoscopy by the local community hospital revealed what they believed to be a mass, greater than 13 cm, in the gastric pouch. Because of the size of the mass, clear visualization of the probable hemorrhagic sites was obstructed. This patient had a history of hospital admission 1 week before this occurrence for mild upper GI bleed brought on by food ingestion. A diagnosis of thrombocytopenia and hypertension was made at that time.

Transport Team Examination

The patient was a mildly obese man who was pale and diaphoretic, in semi-Fowler's position on an emergency department stretcher. He was actively bleeding from a gastric tube and periodically vomiting large amounts of bright red blood and clots. The patient was visibly anxious and expressed fear of dying.
Cardiovascular: Skin was pale, cool, and diaphoretic, with petechiae over chest, abdomen, and thighs anteriorly.
Electrocardiogram: Global ischemia with occasional multifocal PVCs was noted. Two large-bore IV catheters were in the upper extremities.
Respiratory: Nasal cannula delivered 4 L/min. Breath sounds revealed faint rales at bilateral bases. The chest radiograph revealed bilateral lower lobe infiltrates and a markedly distended gastrum elevating the left diaphragm. An approximately 13-cm mass with varying densities was seen.
GI-GU: Normoactive bowel sounds were auscultated, and a large mass was palpated in the left upper quadrant. A urinary catheter was in place and draining clear yellow urine. A #18 Salem sump was in place and lying posteriorly to the gastric mass draining bright red blood. The emergency department staff was performing saline solution lavage.
Medications given before the transport team's arrival were as follows:
Furosemide 40 mg IVP
Lorazepam 2 mg IVP

5 units of packed red blood cells
3200 mL of crystalloid
Laboratory data were as follows: Hct 27, PT 12.9, PTT 22.5; platelets 73,000; ABG on 4 L/min nasal cannula O_2 shows pH 7.38, PO_2 68, PCO_2 32; vital signs are blood pressure 110/68 mm Hg, AP 108, respiration 30; temperature 96°F, patient shivering.

Interventions

The transport team prepared the patient for transport and took iced saline solution in a cooler and four additional units of packed red blood cells. The stretcher was prepared with dry warmed linen and a space blanket. The oxygen was changed to 100% nonrebreather mask, and the patient was given safety orientation before flight.

The flight time to the tertiary facility was 20 minutes. Vital signs remained stable, and the saline solution lavage was continued throughout the flight, with noted clearing on landing. Units no.14 and 7 of red packed blood cells were infusing. Patency of the gastric tube during air medical transport was crucial for this patient, and frequent manipulation of the tube was necessary to prevent occlusion.

Workup of this patient revealed that the gastric mass was a product of small bones, Styrofoam, hair, and paper products. The patient was taken to the operating room for removal of the foreign-body mass. It was noted at that time that the patient had no body hair.

Discussion

Pretransport planning for the needs of the patient for the initial admission time and during the flight to the receiving facility is imperative. This patient continued to receive colloid replacement during type-matching and cross-matching at the receiving facility.

The gastric bleeding was caused by mechanical lacerations from small bones. The patient underwent surgical repair and psychiatric evaluation after admission. In this extremely complicated case, a diagnosis of bezoar was made, and further psychological evaluations were to follow.

ABG, Arterial blood gas; *AP,* apical pulse; *GI,* gastrointestinal; *GU,* genitourinary; *Hct,* hematocrit; *IV,* intravenous; *IVP,* intravenous push; *PT,* prothrombin time; *PTT,* partial thromboplastin time.

References

1. Emergency Nurses Association. *Emergency Nursing Core Curriculum.* 6th ed. ENA: Des Plaines, IL; 2008.
2. Thibeault D. ed. *Transport Professional Advanced Trauma Course Manual.* 6th ed. Aurora, CO: Air & Surface Transport Nurses Association; 2014.
3. Doig A, Huether S. Structure and function of the digestive system. In: McCance K, Huether S, eds. *The Biologic Basis for Disease in Adults and Children.* 7th ed. St. Louis, MO: Elsevier/Mosby; 2014:1393-1422.
4. York-Clark D, Johnson J, Stocking J, et al, eds. *Critical Care Transport Core Curriculum.* Aurora, CO: Air & Surface Transport Nurses Association; 2017.
5. Barros A, Haffner F, Duchateau F, et al. Air travel of patients with abdominal aortic aneurysm: urgent evacuation and nonurgent commercial air repatriation. *Air Medical Journal.* 2014;33:109-111.
6. Doig A, Huether S. Alterations of digestive function. In: McCance K, Huether S, eds. *The Biologic Basis for Disease in Adults and Children.* 7th ed. St. Louis, MO: Elsevier/Mosby; 2014:1423-1485.
7. Treger R. Sengstaken-Blakemore tube placement. *Medscape.* http://emedicine.medscape.com/article/81020-overview#a6; 2015 Accessed 31.07.16.
8. Wolfson A. (Ed in chief). *Harwood-Nuss' Clinical Practice of Emergency Medicine.* 6th ed. Philadelphia, PA: Wolters Kluwer; 2015.
9. Villanueva C, Escorsell A. Optimizing general management of acute variceal bleeding in cirrhosis. *Current Hepatology Reports.* 2014;13(3):198-207.
10. Barnet J, Messmann H. Management of lower gastrointestinal tract bleeding. *Best Pract Res Clin Gastroenterology.* 2008;22(2):295-312.
11. Goralnick E, Meguerdichian D. Gastrointestinal bleeding. In: Marx J, Hockberger R, Walls R, eds. *Rosen's Emergency Medicine.* 8th ed. Philadelphia, PA: Elsevier Saunders; 2014:248-253.
12. Hearnshaw S, Travis S, Murphy M. The role of blood transfusion in the management of upper and lower intestinal tract bleeding. *Best Pract Res Clin Gastroenterology.* 2008;22(2):355-371.
13. Murphy N. Diagnosis and management of liver failure in the adult. In: Parillo J, 7 R.P, eds. *Critical Care Medicine: Principles of Diagnosis and Management in the Adult.* 4th ed. Philadelphia, PA: Elsevier Saunders; 2014:1309-1333.
14. De Waele J, De laet I, Malbrain M. Understanding abdominal compartment syndrome. *Intensive Care Medicine.* October 2015; 42(6):1068-1070.

24

Metabolic, Endocrine, and Electrolyte Disturbances

MOLLY BONDURANT AND RENEÉ SEMONIN HOLLERAN

COMPETENCIES

1. Perform a comprehensive assessment of the patient, including past medical and current illness history, detailed physical examination, and laboratory and pertinent radiographic data.
2. Identify key clinical points related to metabolic, endocrine, and electrolyte disturbances that may arise during transport.
3. Describe appropriate interventions, and treatment considerations, for patients with specific metabolic/endocrine imbalances and select electrolyte disorders.

Metabolic, endocrine, and electrolyte disturbances are commonly encountered in the transport environment. Recognition of abnormalities and potential adverse effects is essential for effective holistic treatment and prevention of complications. Because of the variety of hormones, electrolytes, and their effects, these emergencies can affect all body systems. Whether one of these abnormalities is the primary reason for their transport-related illness or a secondary concern, the transport team should be vigilant in the identification of precipitating events and detection of potential complications.

As is the hallmark of quality patient care delivery by the transport team, thorough and frequent reassessment is vital to the survival of these patients.

Endocrine System Physiology

The endocrine system is composed of a collection of glands: the hypothalamus, pituitary, parathyroid, thyroid, adrenals, pancreas, ovaries, and testes. The hormones each of these glands produces have distinct functions.[1,2]

Hormone levels that are too high or too low indicate a problem with the endocrine system. When circulating hormones are at a high level, hormone release is inhibited. Conversely, when circulating hormone levels are low, hormone release increases. Hormone diseases also occur if one's body does not respond to hormones in the appropriate ways. Stress, infection, renal and liver function, and changes in the blood's fluid and electrolyte balance may also influence hormone levels.

Hypothalamus

The hypothalamus releases or inhibits hormones relating to endocrine functions and emotions. One of the most significant roles of the hypothalamus is to link the nervous system to the endocrine system via the pituitary gland. It is linked to the posterior pituitary both by function and proximity. The synthesis of posterior pituitary hormones occurs in the hypothalamus but is then transferred along axons and stored in the posterior pituitary. Anterior pituitary action is regulated in the hypothalamus by inhibiting or releasing certain hormones.

Pituitary

The pea-sized pituitary gland is located at the base of the brain, within the sella turcica of the middle cranial fossa. It produces many hormones and also causes other organs to produce hormones. The anterior of the pituitary gland produces the following hormones: prolactin, growth hormone, adrenocorticotropin, thyroid-stimulating hormone (TSH), luteinizing hormone, and follicle-stimulating hormone. The posterior of the pituitary gland stores and secretes antidiuretic hormone (ADH) and oxytocin (Fig. 24.1).[1]

Parathyroid

On the posterior side of the thyroid gland are four small glands known as the parathyroid. These glands produce parathyroid hormone (PTH), which balances calcium levels in the body, allowing the muscular and nervous systems to function effectively. Calcium-sensing receptors release PTH when serum calcium levels decrease. PTH causes osteoclasts to release calcium, increasing blood calcium levels. PTH also facilitates calcium reabsorption by the kidneys.

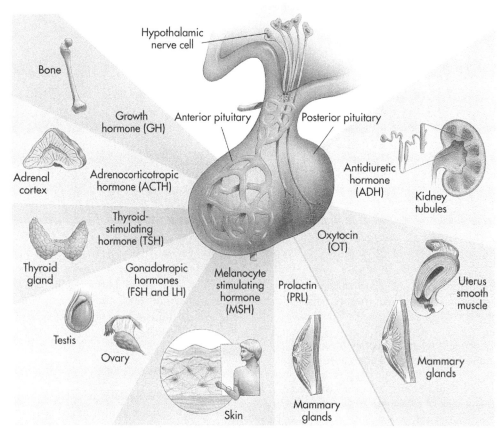

• **Fig. 24.1** Pituitary hormones and their target hormones. (From Brushers V, Jones R, Huether S. Mechanism of hormonal regulation. In: McCance K, Huether S, eds. *The Biologic Basis for Disease in Adults and Children.* 7th ed. St. Louis, MO: Elsevier/Mosby; 2014.)

Thyroid

The thyroid, a butterfly-shaped gland, sits in the anterior neck below the cricoid cartilage. It partially surrounds the trachea and consists of two lobes connected together in the middle by an isthmus. The thyroid cells secrete thyroxine (T4) and triiodothyronine (T3) when stimulated by the pituitary. The parafollicular cells in the thyroid produce calcitonin, which affects calcium metabolism.

Adrenals

The adrenal gland consists of two layers, an outer cortical layer and an inner medullary layer. They are located above the kidneys in the retroperitoneal area. Mineralocorticoids (e.g., aldosterone), glucocorticoids (e.g., cortisol), and androgens are produced by the adrenal cortex. Glucocorticoids allow the body to resist stress, and aldosterone helps to maintain internal fluid balance. The catecholamines, epinephrine and norepinephrine, are released from the adrenal medulla in response to sympathetic stimulation.

Pancreas

The pancreas lies in the left upper abdomen behind the stomach and between the spleen and duodenum. It functions as both an exocrine and endocrine gland. As an exocrine gland, it produces enzymes and bicarbonate that promote digestion. As an endocrine gland, the pancreas secretes hormones directly into the bloodstream, carried to different cells, aiding in glucose balance.

Endocrine and Metabolic Emergencies

There is a wide array of endocrine and metabolic disorders that could potentially present in the transport environment. Because of ongoing treatment and response, metabolic/endocrine patients can be some of the most likely to experience a change in clinical status during transport. The importance of continuous monitoring and careful reassessment cannot be overstated. This section focuses on some of the most frequent endocrine and metabolic emergencies encountered in the transport environment.

Hyperglycemia

Hyperglycemia or an elevated blood sugar may be precipitated by multiple factors. These may include infections such as urinary tract infections, pneumonia, and skin infections. Medications such as atypical antipsychotics and corticosteroids may cause hyperglycemia. Abuse of alcohol and cocaine also has the potential to cause hyperglycemia. The most life-threatening causes of hyperglycemia are diabetic ketoacidosis (DKA) and hyperosmolar hyperglycemic state (HHS).[3]

Diabetic Ketoacidosis[4,5]

DKA can occur in both diagnosed and undiagnosed diabetes mellitus. It can often prompt an initial diagnosis of diabetes. DKA can be initiated by stress, substance abuse, illness, infection, or pregnancy in previously undiagnosed patients, as well as failure to maintain a proper insulin regimen in diagnosed patients. The resulting gluconeogenesis creates an insulin deficiency.

Four acute problems can result from prolonged insulin deficiency: hyperglycemia, dehydration, electrolyte depletion, and metabolic acidosis. Osmotic diuresis, caused by severe hyperglycemia, leads to urinary losses of water, sodium, potassium, magnesium, calcium, and phosphorus. In DKA, profound volume depletion can occur, and an adult patient typically loses 6 L of body water.

Hyperosmolarity promotes insulin resistance, and without insulin glucose cannot be used. Serum blood glucose levels, urine glucose concentrations, and osmotic diuresis are increased. Energy is derived from fats and muscle proteins. Lipolysis then occurs causing a buildup of fatty acids leading to ketoacidosis.

Onset of the disease process occurs over a short period of time, usually 2 or 3 days. Patient history may include polydipsia, polyuria, weakness, fatigue, and weight loss. Nausea, vomiting, decreased appetite, and abdominal cramping may be noted as the condition worsens. Other findings may include focal or global neurologic signs and symptoms, especially confusion and loss of consciousness. The patient may have a fruity odor on the breath and rapid, deep Kussmaul respirations, which are caused by respiratory compensation for a metabolic acidosis. A decreased PCO_2 level will be notable in the patient's blood gas values caused by forced physiologic increased respiration. Skin examination will reveal dry, hot skin and dry-appearing mucous membranes. Severe dehydration may lead to hypotension. Sinus tachycardia is most often seen, but dysrhythmias related to electrolyte disturbances might also be notable.

The focus of the management of the patient with DKA is correction of fluid loss with intravenous (IV) fluids; correction of hyperglycemia with insulin; correction of electrolyte disturbances; correction of acid-base balance; and treatment of the potential cause, such as an infection. Transport teams must use evidence-based medical protocols to safely manage these patients before and during transport. These protocols should be reviewed on a frequent basis so that team members feel comfortable managing these patients.

Patients with DKA are profoundly volume depleted, and fluid replacement is of primary importance in DKA care. Fluid replacement alone will result in a drop of whole blood glucose 20 to 50 mg/dL per hour. Correction of blood glucose that occurs too fast can cause a rebound effect related to improved insulin sensitivity.[6] Use 0.9% normal saline for initial resuscitation per patient care protocols.

Serum potassium will fall markedly as patients are rehydrated and as acidosis corrects. Insulin administration can exacerbate serum hypokalemia. Insulin therapy is generally held until a potassium greater than 3.5 mEq/L can be obtained. If the potassium is less than 5.2 mEq/L but greater than 3.5 mEq/L, it is safe to start potassium repletion along with insulin.[6] Potassium replacement should be based on evidence-based protocols.

After an initial fluid bolus, patients with DKA should receive an insulin infusion per transport patient care protocols. Glucose should be monitored frequently, particularly after any rate change. Only short-acting insulin should be used when treating DKA, and IV infusion is the preferred route.

In patients with DKA, literature suggests a detrimental effect from sodium bicarbonate therapy. Administer bicarbonate to DKA patients only in conjunction with specific medical direction in cases in which there is cardiac dysfunction caused by profound acidosis (pH <6.9).[7]

Hyperosmolar Hyperglycemic State

HHS occurs most often in patients who are over the age of 50 years, have type 2 diabetes managed by oral medication and diet, or have undiagnosed diabetes. Many of them are taking other medications, such as diuretics, which exacerbate the problem. Many older patients have comorbidities contributing to the onset of this condition. Illness, surgery, or injury to the body can create an increase in glucose levels. Type 2 diabetic patients may not produce enough insulin to prevent hyperglycemia from occurring.

Severe dehydration is caused by an increase in serum glucose levels. These patients have a fluid deficit that can approach 10 L. Patients worsen when they are not able to replace lost fluids. The body begins to metabolize fat and muscle tissue, and this increases fatty acid and amino acid levels. The existing hyperglycemia is then worsened by hepatic gluconeogenesis. Intravascular volume depletion or underlying renal disease will decrease the glomerular filtration rate and glucose levels will rise. When more water than sodium is lost, the result is hyperosmolality. There is an insufficient level of insulin available to reduce blood glucose levels, especially with insulin resistance.

HHS can be precipitated by a number of causes such as acute myocardial infarction, stroke, or underlying infections. Medications and treatment of noncompliance, undiagnosed diabetes, substance abuse, certain medications, and the presence of other diseases can also be igniting factors.

Symptoms of HHS can develop over days or even weeks and may be so subtle that the patient does not seek treatment readily. Initial symptoms include mild abdominal pain, a decrease in appetite, polydipsia, and polyuria. Headaches, blurred vision, and confusion develop as the condition progresses. Hypotension, tachycardia, and dysrhythmias may also be present, and seizures or coma can occur.

The fruity smell of DKA is not present in patients with HHS, although respirations may be increased. A change in the patient's mental status is usually described as the presenting concern and reason for hospital or transport encounter.

Treatment includes establishing and maintaining fluid and electrolyte balance by initiating IV fluids with normal saline solution, monitoring intake and output, and managing blood sugar based on transport medical protocols. Profound volume deficit is present in HHS patients and resuscitation should be managed closely. After an initial fluid bolus, patients with HHS should receive an insulin infusion per departmental patient care protocols. Rapid reduction in serum glucose is dangerous and without benefit. Glucose should be monitored frequently and particularly after any rate change. For HHS patients, insulin infusion is typically discontinued when glucose falls to 250 to 300 mg/dL or declines by more than 100 mg/dL per hour.[2,7] If seizures have occurred, ensure that safe patient positioning and padding is used to protect the patient in transport.[2,7]

Hypoglycemia

Hypoglycemia affects patients with type 1 diabetes and is present when glucose drops below 50 mg/dL in adult or pediatric patients or 40 mg/dL in neonatal patients. The age of the patient, a description of the symptoms, and the method of measurement all determine the degree of hypoglycemia and what medical treatments are warranted. A patient can become symptomatic if the glucose level in the body drops too precipitously. Because glucose is the brain's most important source of energy, the effects of hypoglycemia are primarily neurologic. The brain must have a continuous flow of glucose from the circulatory system because it cannot synthesize or store glucose for more than a few minutes. Any patient presenting with a neurologically altered profile or any unresponsive patient should be evaluated for hypoglycemia.[8]

Iatrogenic insulin effects in patients with type 1 diabetes are often the typical cause of hypoglycemia, but it can also be caused by adrenal insufficiencies, sepsis, pancreatic tumors, and congenital metabolic disorders. Some diabetes medications such as sulfonureas and meglitinides can also cause hypoglycemia. Other medications, such as α-glucosidase inhibitors, biguanides, and thiazolidinediones combined with other diabetes medications may also precipitate hypoglycemia. Increased physical stress, liver disease, lack of food intake, changes in insulin or oral agents, pregnancy, alcohol consumption, nonsteroidal antiinflammatory drugs, phenytoin, thyroid hormones, and β-blockers can also contribute.

Many diabetic patients can recognize the symptoms of hypoglycemia and are able to remedy the condition independently. These symptoms include anxiety, diaphoresis, dry mouth, shakiness, pallor, palpitations, pupil dilation, and hunger. Some patients, however, may not notice the onset because the sympathetic response is masked by α-blocker therapy.

Symptoms such as irritability, confusion, difficulty speaking, headaches, ataxia, paresthesia, abnormal mentation, and stupor occur when the brain is not receiving glucose. These symptoms can make it difficult for a patient to seek treatment, and without treatment neuroglycopenia can cause seizures, coma, or possibly death.[1]

Treatment should be based on evidence-based medical transport protocols, which include establishing and maintaining fluid and electrolyte balance by initiating IV fluids with rapidly available glucose, D_{10}, D_{50}, or oral glucose solution. Glucagon may be considered in patients with adequate hepatic reserves (e.g., nonalcoholic). Patients who overdose on sulfonylureas may require octreotide. Resolution of symptoms should be rapid with appropriate therapy.[8]

Thyroid Storm[9]

Thyroid storm (thyrotoxicosis) is caused by a release of excessive thyroid hormones resulting in exaggerated adrenergic activity. Excessive release of thyroid hormones can be increased by thyroid tumors and nodules. Iodine and iodine-containing drugs such as amiodarone and lithium can also precipitate hyperthyroidism. The autoimmune disorder, Graves disease, in which thyroid-stimulating immunoglobulins increase thyroid activity, accounts for 60% to 80% of all cases of hyperthyroidism.[9]

When hyperthyroidism or thyrotoxicosis (symptomatic hyperthyroidism) is not properly managed, a thyroid storm can occur. Clinical findings include hyperthermia, agitation, tremors, tachydysrhythmias, and signs of heart failure. Delirium, syncope, or coma may be notable neurologic symptoms. Care must be taken to not confuse the symptoms with mania or psychosis. Management of acute agitation must be considered to ensure a safe transport.

Other symptoms may include abdominal discomfort, shortened attention span, tremors, and manic behavior. Older patients may exhibit new-onset atrial fibrillation. Tachycardia may be appreciated and pulmonary crackles auscultated. In severe cases, the patient's mental status can progress to coma.

Signs of dehydration, such as changes in the skin from warm and diaphoretic to hot and dry, will occur as dehydration worsens. Increased gastric motility may cause diarrhea, nausea, and vomiting. Thinning of the hair, jaundice, and hepatic tenderness may be present, and goiter (an enlarged thyroid gland) can develop. The patient may exhibit a staring gaze with heavy eyelids, and periorbital edema can develop.

Without swift and proper intervention, cardiac failure and death can occur, and mortality rates can be as high as 25%. Hormone levels can elevate as a result of surgery, infection, hospitalization, trauma, emotional stress, childbirth, or a sudden discontinuation of antithyroid medications.[9]

The patient's history plays an important role in identifying thyroid storm including recent illnesses and medications. It is important to ascertain if there has been any recent discontinuation in a prescribed medication, particularly a thyroid medication. A history of recent loss is significant.

Rapid, aggressive steps need to be taken if thyroid storm is suspected. Hormone levels must be reduced and hemodynamic integrity must be protected. β-Adrenergic blockade is the mainstay of thyroid storm therapy. Goals of treatment include identifying and managing the condition precipitating the thyroid storm. Management of life-threatening airway, breathing, and circulatory problems will take priority. Cooling measures may be required to manage hyperthermia. Antipyretics may be effective in treating fever. Avoid salicylates because there is an association with thyroid hormone displacement.

β-Adrenergic blockers are administered to manage cardia arrhythmia. Medications that may be administered to reduce thyroid hormone levels include propylthiouracil or methimazole. Glucocorticoids are used to reduce peripheral thyroid hormone deiodination and prevent adrenal insufficiency. A saturated solution of potassium iodide may be administered an hour after the other medications to reduce and stabilize the production of thyroid hormones. When standard management does not work, lithium may be used.

Hyperglycemia and hypercalcemia are frequently present and should improve with fluid therapy. The patient's hemodynamic status and electrolyte levels determine the fluid of choice.

The recognition and management of the patient in a thyroid storm is complicated. It is important that evidence-based medical transport programs or the medical director is consulted to assist with the safe management of these patients.

Myxedema Coma[10]

Untreated hypothyroidism can progress over time to myxedema coma. All patients who develop myxedema coma have hypothyroidism, and most are 60 years or older. Many cases occur during the winter months.

Myxedema coma can occur as a result of autoimmune thyroiditis (e.g., Hashimoto's disease), iodine deficiency, tumor activity, ablation therapy, or drug therapy. Pituitary dysfunction causes secondary hypothyroidism. Thyroid hormone secretion is lowered by alterations in pituitary function, which decreases TSH release. When the hypothalamus secretes inadequate amounts of thyrotropin-releasing hormone (TRH) or TRH does not reach the pituitary gland, tertiary hypothyroidism occurs.

Medications can also cause myxedema coma. These include amiodarone, lithium, β-blockers, anesthesia, and several anticonvulsants. Gastrointestinal hemorrhage (GI bleed), hypoglycemia, hypothermia, burns, infection DKA, and trauma can also precipitate the condition.

Symptoms include shortness of breath, weight gain, doughy edema, characteristic deep tendon reflex delays, fatigue, decreased activity tolerance, and tongue swelling. Patients may appear confused and be slow to respond to questions. Hallucinations, paranoia, depression, decreased concern for personal appearance, and combativeness may also be present. These symptoms are termed *myxedema madness*. This could present as both a patient safety and transport team safety risk during transport.[10]

Proper intervention is essential for patients with myxedema coma. In patients who are unconscious or have a depressed level of consciousness, their tongue may be partially or fully obstructing their airway. Pulmonary infection can occur with alveolar hypoventilation caused by weak respiration and decreased respiratory drive. Hypercarbia can follow alveolar hypoventilation, which can further complicate the patient's mental status. The respiratory system can be further impaired by obesity-related sleep apnea. Death is usually caused by respiratory failure.

Decreased heart rate, decreased cardiac volume, and decreased stroke volume are notable cardiac changes. Body temperature is usually less than 96°F (35.5°C), and skin is pale and cool. Glomerular filtration rates, renal blood flow, and sodium reabsorption decrease. The patient's normal volume of excreted fluid is lessened, and generalized non-pitting edema may be noticeable. Increased insulin sensitivity and decreased oral intake may cause hypoglycemia to develop, and constipation also can occur as a result of system metabolic slowing.

Decreased white blood cell count, decreased hemoglobin and hematocrit, and decreased thyroid levels are observable on diagnostic tests. Radiographs, scans, and other diagnostic tests may be performed as the patient becomes stabilized.

Treatment based on evidence-based medical transport protocols may include the administration of thyroxine. Hypotension is addressed with volume resuscitation, glucocorticoid support, and thyroid replacement. Vasopressor administration may increase the risk of arrhythmias and/or angina, and they do not work as effectively in the absence of thyroid hormone. Thus vasopressor therapy should be considered only in cases of severe hypotension unresponsive to other therapies. Associated adrenal insufficiency can be seen in primary or secondary hypothyroidism. Stress doses of glucocorticoids should be considered until the possibility of adrenal insufficiency is excluded.

Mechanical ventilation should be considered to facilitate management of respiratory acidosis, compromised respiratory musculature, and increased oxygen demand. Measures should be initiated to decrease the potential risk for hypothermia. Passive or slow warming is preferred because increased oxygen demands related to warming can overtax an already overstressed system. Gastric decompression should be performed before transport to prevent/treat paralytic ileus.

Acute Adrenal Insufficiency[11]

Acute adrenal insufficiency is a rare but serious condition. It is also known as adrenal crisis, or addisonian crisis. It is characterized by depletion of adrenal glucocorticoids and mineralocorticoids. It can occur as a result of destruction of the pituitary gland, injury to or removal of the adrenal glands, sudden ending of long-term steroid therapy, or in a person who has Addison disease. In a person with Addison disease, trauma, surgery, stress, or infection can be strong risk factors. Severe physiologic stressors such as myocardial infarction, complicated pregnancy, or septic shock can cause massive bilateral adrenal hemorrhage. Sodium and water loss from the kidneys and GI tract occur as a result of a failing adrenal system. This can be followed by water loss, leading to hypovolemia, which presents as refractory hypotension. This can further progress to cardiovascular collapse, coma, and death. Serum potassium increases as sodium decreases. This leads to hyperkalemia and sometimes fatal dysrhythmias. Without enough cortisol gluconeogenesis fails. Activities of the adrenal medulla are also compromised by decreased cortisol levels.

Symptoms of adrenal insufficiency are nonspecific, making diagnosis difficult. Obtaining a patient's recent medical history is vital. Complaints may include fatigue, weight loss, palpitations, headache, weakness, nausea, abdominal pain, anorexia, and diarrhea. Patients may experience sudden pain in the legs, lower back, or abdomen; high fever; dehydration; and hypotension. These symptoms may result in an altered mental status or loss of consciousness.

Physical findings may include orthostatic changes/hypotension, dry mucous membranes, poor skin turgor, lethargy, tachycardia, and delayed capillary refill. Hyperpigmentation of the skin and mucous membranes may also be noted on examination. Patients usually have hypoglycemia, and hyponatremia, hyperkalemia, and hypercalcemia may also be present.

Treatment includes establishing and maintaining fluid and electrolyte balance by initiating IV fluids with normal saline solution or 5% dextrose in normal saline, administration of IV hydrocortisone and plasma as a volume expander per protocol or as ordered, and monitoring intake and output. The possibility of adrenal hemorrhage should be considered in anticoagulated patients with ongoing hypotension. Potassium levels should be checked to guard against hyperkalemia. Vasopressors are appropriate after adequate volume placement is achieved. Measures should be taken to provide as quiet and as relaxed an environment as possible, with sedatives administered as needed for transport.[11]

Pituitary Disorders

Other states including pituitary disorders may be seen in the critical care transport environment. These conditions and other less commonly seen states may also cause characteristic electrolyte abnormalities. When transporting metabolic/endocrine cases in which the diagnosis and therapy are not familiar, the transport team should discuss appropriate care with the treating physicians and/or medical control before and during transport, as indicated by the patient's condition.

Diabetes Insipidus[10]

Diabetes insipidus (DI) is caused by inadequate or impaired secretion of ADH or impaired or insufficient renal response to ADH. Treatment is dependent on proper determination of the disturbance. Central DI occurs when the secretion and release of ADH is impaired. This can happen as a result of a tumor, surgery, and head trauma or can also be genetically induced.

There are four types of DI: nephrogenic, neurogenic, dipsogenic, and gestagenic.

Nephrogenic DI is caused when urine is not properly concentrated by the kidneys; it can be caused by genetics or it also can be acquired. Alterations in the kidneys account for acquired forms of the condition. This is most often a result of disease, drugs, or other conditions such as hypokalemia, hypercalcemia, pregnancy, and sickle cell anemia.

Neurogenic DI is most often caused by decreased secretion of ADH from the posterior pituitary gland. Causes include neoplasm of the hypothalamus or anterior pituitary gland, infection (e.g., bacterial meningitis, viral encephalitis), head trauma (e.g., basilar, sphenoidal, facial skull fractures), or surgery, granulomas (e.g., sarcoidosis, histiocytosis), vascular anomalies (e.g., ischemia, aneurysms, hematoma, inflammation), chemical toxins, use of ADH-inhibiting medications (e.g., phenytoin [Dilantin] ethanol, glucocorticoids, adrenergic agents, narcotic antagonists), autoimmune disease, and/or a genetic link.

Dipsogenic DI, also known as primary or psychogenic polydipsia, is caused by excessive fluid intake secondary to an abnormal thirst mechanism. Primary polydipsia is caused by granuloma (e.g., neurosarcoid), infection (e.g., tuberculous, meningitis), autoimmune disease (e.g., multiple sclerosis), and use of certain medications (lithium [carbamazepine]). Psychogenic polydipsia is the result of psychological disorders such as schizophrenia, mania, and neurosis.

Gestagenic DI is caused by a transient increase in the breakdown of ADH and can develop in pregnant women with eclampsia, preeclampsia, multiple gestation, or abnormal liver function. This form of DI is characterized by decreased circulating ADH and a massive increase in the activity of vasopressinase (i.e., an enzyme produced in the placenta and broken down in the liver). These women do not respond to replacement vasopressin. The condition typically resolves with delivery of the placenta.[9]

Diagnosis is made through laboratory tests that measure urine osmolality. Urine osmolality less than 200 mOsm/kg in the presence of polyuria indicates DI. To differentiate between central and nephrogenic DI, the water deprivation test can be used.

Managing a patient with DI requires monitoring of fluid status, neurologic status, electrolyte levels, and resulting electrocardiographic (ECG) rhythm. Distinguishing between central and nephrogenic DI and the monitoring of fluid intake, output, and urine osmolality are essential to the treatment of DI. Hormone replacement therapy may be required. Desmopressin acetate or vasopressin may be administered per physician order or protocol. Isotonic maintenance fluid should be provided at a rate that at least matches hourly urine output.

Syndrome of Inappropriate Antidiuretic Hormone Secretion[1,10]

The syndrome of inappropriate antidiuretic hormone (SIADH) occurs when the pituitary gland releases excessive amounts of ADH, which originates in the hypothalamus and is stored in the pituitary gland. When the hypothalamic secretion osmoreceptors or hypothalamic-pituitary-adrenal axis is changed by disease, SIADH can occur. It can also be caused by tricyclic antidepressants, narcotics, thyroid or pituitary lesions, oral hypoglycemic medication, and carbamazepine. The patient might present with related disorders such as pneumonia, tuberculosis, abscesses, porphyria, hypothyroid disorders, or a traumatic brain injury.

Urine volume is decreased resulting from increased distal renal tubular permeability to water. ADH is typically determined by serum osmolality and circulatory blood volume. Release of ADH is stimulated by an increase in serum concentration. The kidneys respond by increasing water absorption, and serum concentration decreases. Urinary output slows as circulating volume expands. This creates a fluid overload and hyponatremia by association.

Patients may describe symptoms such as nausea, vomiting, diarrhea, weakness, abdominal and/or muscle cramps, weight gain, fatigue, headache, and decreased urinary output. They may appear disoriented or confused, and seizures may occur as hyponatremia worsens. Cerebral edema and hyponatremic encephalopathy can occur when severe hyponatremia leads to changes in fluid levels.[9]

Laboratory results may show serum sodium levels less than 125 mEq/L and low serum osmolality less than 280 mOsm/kg.

Management of SIADH depends on the severity of hyponatremia. In many cases, water restrictions starting at 800 to 1000 mL/day is sufficient. Some cases may require a restriction to 500 mL/day, however. Close monitoring is essential, because acute hyponatremia can cause seizures and create a risk for cerebral edema and hyponatremic encephalopathy.

Select Electrolyte Disturbances[2,11-13]

Electrolytes are crucial for nearly all cellular reactions and functions. They direct acid-base balance, regulate water distribution, transmit nerve impulses, and contribute to blood clotting. Electrolyte abnormalities can manifest in a variety of ways. Electrolyte balance is influenced by normal cell function, fluid intake and output, acid-base balance, and hormone secretion. Normal levels are maintained within very narrow ranges through complex processes within the renal and endocrine systems.

Sodium

Sodium is the body's most abundant solute in extracellular fluid. It helps in the regulation of normal extracellular fluid osmolality, maintenance of acid-base balance, activation of nerve and muscle cells, and influences water distribution (with chloride).

Hyponatremia

Hyponatremia is defined as a state in which there is a relative deficiency of sodium concentration in relation to the amount of water in the plasma (extracellular compartment). A sodium level of less than 135 mEq/L indicates hyponatremia; a level less than 120 mEq/L is considered a critical value. Causes can be dilutional (i.e., blood becoming too dilute) or the result of direct or indirect sodium loss.

Conditions associated with hyponatremia include the following: congestive heart failure, excessive water intake, cirrhosis, SIADH, acute renal failure with oliguria, renal injury or sepsis, diarrhea, vomiting, excessive sweating, adrenal insufficiency, and renal lesions.

In patients with hyperglycemia, factitious hyponatremia can develop because of intracellular to extracellular fluid shifts. This condition usually corrects itself as the glucose levels are corrected.

Symptoms of hyponatremia vary from patient to patient. They are also variable depending on how precipitous the patient's sodium level has dropped. If the level drops quickly, the patient is more likely to be symptomatic.

The initial symptoms are primarily neurologic including headache or disorientation. Progression to muscle twitching, tremors, weakness, and changes in level of consciousness may ensue. When sodium levels fall below 110 mEq/L, symptoms may become severe usually because of brain edema leading to delirium, ataxia, psychosis, seizures, or coma.

There are multiple medications associated with hyponatremia, e.g., anticoagulants, anticonvulsants, antidiabetics, diuretics, and sedatives. Medications can cause hyponatremia by potentiating the action of ADH or by causing SIADH. Diuretics may also cause hyponatremia by inhibiting sodium reabsorption in the kidneys.

Hypernatremia

Hypernatremia is caused by dehydration and is defined as a sodium level of greater than 145 mEq/L. Causes may include gastric fluid losses; osmotic diuresis; hypothalamic disorders, such as a lesion-impairing thirst; exercise; seizures; and intake or administration of hypertonic saline solutions.

Neurologic signs are the most critical signs of hypernatremia because fluid shifts have a significant effect on brain cells. Early signs to look for include agitation or restlessness, anorexia, weakness, low-grade fever, flushed skin, and nausea and/or vomiting. Severe hypernatremia can lead to seizures, coma, and permanent neurologic damage.

Medications associated with hypernatremia include antacids with sodium bicarbonate, certain antibiotics, salt tablets, IV sodium chloride preparations, sodium polystyrene sulfonate, and corticosteroids.

Identification and management of the cause as well as controlled fluid replacement generally will correct this electrolyte imbalance. Volume depletion should be carefully reversed with normal saline/lactated Ringer's infusion with attention to avoidance of a too-rapid decrease in sodium. The goal for sodium reduction is no more than 0.5 mEq/L per hour.

Potassium

Potassium plays a crucial role in many metabolic cell functions and is subject to multiple influences within the body; it is the body's major intracellular ion. An important contributor to potassium balance is acid-base balance. ECG changes are frequently associated with potassium abnormalities, which may or may not correlate with severity.

Hypokalemia

A potassium level of less than 3.5 mEq/L indicates hypokalemia. Excessive diarrhea and vomiting, excessive diuresis, intestinal obstruction, GI suctioning, renal insufficiency, overuse of laxatives or steroids, severe trauma, and excessive sweating are all associated with hypokalemia. It also can be a result of intracellular shifting of potassium caused by alkalosis.

Hypokalemia may be associated with cardiac conduction abnormalities, which are refractory to therapy until K levels are corrected. Ventricular ectopy is the most common dysrhythmia. IV potassium replacement should never exceed 40 mEq/h, and typically half that rate is a reasonable target. Oral potassium is well absorbed and safe, although nausea and/or vomiting may occur.

Hyperkalemia

A potassium level of greater than 5.5 mEq/L indicates hyperkalemia. Causes include oliguria, tissue breakdown (i.e., released potassium from lysed or damaged cells), or excessive potassium intake. Various ECG changes correlate well with severity in hyperkalemia. Elevated T waves occur when serum potassium reaches 5.5 to 6.6 mEq/L, and prolonged PR interval and widened QRS complexes are evident when levels reach 6.5 to 8.0 mEq/L. Hyperkalemia is also observed frequently in patients with chronic renal disease and renal failure.

Hyperkalemia primary risks are cardiac, and include refractory ventricular arrhythmias. Treatments as outlined in ACLS (advanced cardiac life support protocols) include measures to protect the myocardium (calcium chloride/calcium gluconate) and shift potassium into the intracellular space (bicarbonate, insulin/glucose, albuterol), whereas longer-acting agents (sodium polystyrene sulfonate, furosemide) or dialysis are instituted to reduce total body potassium.

Calcium

Calcium is stored primarily in the skeleton, but approximately 2% of the total body calcium is located in the extracellular fluid. Calcium is an essential electrolyte for cardiac and neuromuscular function. Abnormalities in calcium levels are often associated with magnesium and phosphorus abnormalities.

Hypocalcemia

A calcium level of less than 8.5 mEq/L indicates hypocalcemia. Causes of hypocalcemia include hypoparathyroidism, malabsorption syndrome, osteomalacia, acute pancreatitis, chronic renal failure, vitamin D or magnesium deficiency, hyperphosphatemia, and increased calcitonin.

Clinical findings are significant for positive Chvostek sign (light facial tap eliciting abnormal facial spasms) and positive Trousseau sign (carpal spasms induced by the inflation of a blood pressure cuff on the upper arm). As a result of increased excitability of brain tissue, seizures are also occasionally seen. Patients may display other symptoms such as numbness or tingling of the fingers, toes, nose, lips, or earlobes; facial grimacing; muscle twitching hyperactive deep tendon reflexes; and abdominal pain. Critical symptoms include laryngospasms, seizures, bronchospasms, and cardiac collapse. ECG signs include potential for prolonged QT interval.

Hypomagnesemia should be excluded before treatment for hypocalcemia because patients with low serum magnesium levels respond poorly to calcium replacement. Hypocalcemia can be easily managed with the administration of IV calcium. During administration the patient should be carefully observed to include hemodynamic monitoring, cardiac rhythm, and repeat calcium levels.

Ionized calcium levels may be low in patients receiving blood transfusions despite normal total calcium because of the citrate in banked blood that binds ionized calcium. Consequently, providers may be advised to administer 1 g of calcium chloride IV for every 3 to 4 units of transfused blood in patients with shock who are receiving multiple rapid transfusions. Providers should follow departmental patient care protocols.

Hypercalcemia

A calcium level of greater than 10.5 mEq/L indicates hypercalcemia. Causes include increased mobilization of calcium from bones as seen in hyperparathyroidism, immobilization, thyrotoxicosis, excessive calcium intake, renal tubular acidosis, and chronic thiazide therapy. Chronic hypercalcemia is associated with renal lithiasis, peptic ulcer, and pancreatitis. Patients taking digitalis will have enhanced calcium effects.

Symptoms of hypercalcemia can be vague, including irritability, fatigue, general malaise, nausea, vomiting, constipation, headache, or difficulty concentrating. Primary symptoms are often neurologic. Patients may be confused or have a depressed level of consciousness. They may also express polyuria, polydipsia, or have an ileus. ECG changes include QT interval shortening.

Treatment of the underlying cause and increasing renal excretion of calcium with IV hydration and loop or osmotic diuretics is the priority in correction of hypercalcemia. Although rare, serum calcium levels of higher than 13.5 mg/dL require urgent attention.

Patient Handoff and Preparation for Transport[13]

History

Obtain a complete past medical and current illness or injury history through subjective and objective review with patient, family, and referring facility/agency providers. A reliable and complete history in patients with metabolic, endocrine, or electrolyte problems can help with identifying the cause of the metabolic or endocrine problem.

1. In some cases, aspects of the history are critical to the diagnosis; for example, previous thyroid surgery, steroid-dependent reactive airway disease, and hemodynamic instability after receiving iodinated contrast.
2. Obtain and record patients' past medical history, any surgical history, medications, and any precipitating factors in their current illness. When possible, data should be gathered about patients' social history, alcohol use, use of illicit substances, and family history.

Physical Examination

1. Perform a primary and secondary survey.
2. General inspection of the patient may provide useful clues (e.g., thyroidectomy scars, fruity breath in DKA, presence of insulin pump, etc.). Assess the patient's hydration status (e.g., skin and mucous membranes, volume status, intake and output).
3. Although the transport team may be time limited in some of the very detailed examinations, some findings specific to the clinical circumstance can be quickly performed (e.g., Kussmaul respirations in DKA, abnormally delayed deep tendon reflexes in hypothyroidism, Trousseau sign in hypocalcemia). Consider the lengthier examinations in transport if time and patient access allows.
4. Initial intervention focuses on maintaining airway, breathing (specifically oxygen administration to maintain an oxygen saturation of at least 90%) and circulation, initiating IV access, and assessing pain. Continuous vital sign monitoring should be initiated before and during transport.

Monitoring

1. Ensure that all cardiac and hemodynamic monitors and equipment are functioning including noninvasive blood pressure equipment, pulse oximetry monitor, cardiac telemetry, defibrillator, and transcutaneous cardiac pacemaker.
2. Ensure that all medications for emergent administration as recommended by the American Heart Association

guidelines for advanced cardiac and advanced life support are available.

3. Ensure that airway management equipment is available in the event that the patient's condition deteriorates. If necessary, use positive-pressure ventilation devices such as noninvasive positive-pressure ventilation, bag-mask device, or positive end-expiratory pressure to maximize oxygen-carbon dioxide exchange.
4. Identify and manage the underlying cause of the condition.
5. Establish and maintain fluid and electrolyte balance by initiating IV fluids with isotonic or other solution, as ordered; insert a urinary catheter as indicated by the patient's condition; and monitor intake and output.

Vascular Access

1. Ensure adequate peripheral or central vascular access for crystalloid and medication administration.

Radiography

1. Radiography (e.g., chest imaging revealing lung mass in SIADH) and ECG (e.g., peaked T waves with hyperkalemia) are infrequently diagnostic but can provide useful clues to the presence and/or explanation of metabolic/endocrine disorders.

Laboratory Data

Laboratory data are of paramount importance in diagnosing and in guiding therapy of metabolic/endocrine/electrolyte disorders.

1. Basic labs (electrolytes, blood urea nitrogen [BUN]/creatinine, glucose, complete blood count, urinalysis) should be assessed in all cases.
2. Arterial blood gases can assist in determining acid-base balance, which is helpful in many patients with significant metabolic/endocrine disorders. Use point-of-care testing (e.g., an i-STAT System if available), particularly during long transports.
3. Specialized testing (e.g., thyroid panel, hemoglobin A1C) may be performed as clinically indicated; however, it should generally not delay critical care transport.
4. The osmolarity (number of dissolved particles per liter of solution) is frequently important in metabolic/endocrine cases.
   a. Calculated osmolarity: $(2 \times Na) + BUN/2.8 + glucose/18$.
   b. Normal range for osmolarity is 275 to 295 mOsm/L.
   c. The osmolarity may also be directly measured by the laboratory at most hospitals.
   d. The osmolar gap may be helpful in the differential diagnosis of various conditions. The difference between the calculated and measured osmolarity is called the osmolar gap. The normal osmolar gap is 10 to 15 mOsm/L; a greater gap suggests the presence of another solute (e.g., lactate, ethanol, methanol, ethylene glycol, isopropyl alcohol).
5. In some instances, "abnormal" laboratory data are factitiously elevated. To prevent inappropriate treatment,

transport teams should be familiar with corrections for at least two common factitious entities.

   a. Pseudohyponatremia is usually caused by hyperglycemia, hyperlipidemia, or hyperproteinemia. Correction of Na levels for hyperglycemia should be calculated.

   b. Apparent hyperkalemia may be caused by hemolysis, leukocytosis, or thrombocytosis.

Medication Administration

1. Medication administration will be guided by clinical circumstances, with physician orders or using evidence-based medical transport protocols.
2. IV fluid therapy choices are more important in metabolic/endocrine conditions than in most other critical care transports. The specific fluid being administered, the rate of administration, and the rationale for fluid selection should be clear to the transport team.

Pretransport Stabilization/Planning and Intratransport Care

Pretransport stabilization and planning for intratransport care should include specific interventions as dictated by the patient's disease process.

1. Ensure optimal patient positioning. Stressors of transport can exacerbate symptoms in response to pain and changes in vital signs.
2. Continue monitoring the patient during treatment and transport for changes in vital signs, signs of deterioration, development of hypoxia, and evidence of pain and/or discomfort. If seizures have occurred, ensure padding is used to protect the patient during transport.
3. Metabolic/endocrine patients are among those most likely to have a change in status during transport because of ongoing treatment and response. Examples in which transport providers should closely follow patients include ECG rhythm in hyperkalemia, glucose in patients on insulin infusions, and potassium (when possible) in patients being treated for DKA.
4. Explain all aspects of critical care transport to the patient, including plans, interventions, and expectations, both during transport and on arrival at the receiving facility.
5. Ensure that all laboratory results, imaging studies, and the patient care record accompany the patient for interfacility transport.
6. If the patient becomes combative or difficult to control physically, advise the pilot of a need to land immediately or the driver to pull over until the patient can be safely managed in transport.

7. Continual assessment of volume/perfusion status includes monitoring of hemodynamics and urine output, with adjustment of IV infusions (and consideration of medications such as hydrocortisone), as indicated by the clinical circumstances.
8. Other intratransport care should follow the disease-specific guidelines as outlined in departmental patient care protocols.

References

1. Brashers V, Jones R, Huether S. Mechanism of hormonal regulation. In: McCance K, Huether S, eds. *The Biologic Basis for Disease in Adults and Children*. 7th ed. St. Louis, MO: Elsevier/Mosby; 2014:689-716.
2. Tucci V, Sokari T. The clinical manifestations, diagnosis, and treatment of adrenal emergencies. *Emergency Medicine Clinics of North America*. 2014;32(2):465-484.
3. Corwell B, Knight B, Olivieri L, Willis G. Current diagnosis and treatment of hyperglycemic emergencies. *Emergency Medicine Clinics of North America*. 2014;32(2):437-452.
4. Hamdy O. Diabetic ketoacidosis treatment and management. *Medscape Reference Drugs, Diseases & Procedures*. http://emedicine.medscape.com/article/118361-treatment; 2016 Accessed 27.07.16.
5. Howard PK, Steinmann RA. *Sheehy's Emergency Nursing Principles and Practice*. 6th ed. St. Louis, MO: Elsevier; 2010.
6. Nyenwe E, Kitabchi A. The evolution of diabetic ketoacidosis: An update of its etiology, pathogenesis and management. *Metabolism*. 2016;65(4):507-521.
7. Kitabchi A, Umpierrez G, Miles J, Fisher J. Hyperglycemic crisis in adults with diabetes. *Diabetes Care*. 2009;32(7):1335-1343.
8. Llamado R, Czaja A, Stence N, Davidson J. Continuous octreotide for sulfonylurea-induced hypoglycemia in a toddler. *Journal of Emergency Medicine*. 2013;45(6):e209-e213.
9. Robertson G. Diabetes insipidus: Differential diagnosis and management. *Best Practices & Research Clinical Endocrinology & Metabolism*. 2016;30(2):205-218.
10. Brashers V, Jones R, Huether S. Alterations of hormone regulation. In: McCance K, Huether S, eds. *The Biologic Basis for Disease in Adults and Children*. 7th ed. St. Louis, MO: Elsevier/Mosby; 2014:717-767.
11. Sharp C, Wilson M, Nordstrom K. Psychiatric emergencies for clinicians: The emergency department management of thyroid storm. *Journal of Emergency Medicine*. 2016;51(2):155-158.
12. Doig A, Huether S. The cellular environment: Fluids and electrolytes, acids and bases. In: McCance K, Huether S, eds. *The Biologic Basis for Disease in Adults and Children*. 7th ed. St. Louis, MO: Elsevier/Mosby; 2014:103-134.
13. York-Clark D, Johnson J, Stocking J, et al, eds. *Critical Care Transport Core Curriculum*. Aurora, CO: Air & Surface Transport Nurses Association; 2017.

25

Infectious and Communicable Diseases

JASON COHEN

Infectious diseases are routinely encountered by transport personnel. Patients suffering with the ill effects of such disease, and those that are asymptomatic carriers of infection, present challenges to daily practice. In time-critical emergencies, many of the precautions that exist to prevent transmission of infectious agents can become a hindrance to efficient care. Additionally, transporting patients from the scene of motor vehicle collisions or an emergency department may limit the available background information, such as culture results or sensitivities. Given the greater than 1400 known human pathogens that are continuing to evolve and adapt, an understanding of infectious diseases, and their associated risks, is critical to providing efficient and appropriate care.[1] Additionally, this knowledge allows transport professionals to protect themselves, their loved ones, and their future patients.

As recently as the 1970s, there was a general impression that infectious diseases would soon be an affliction of the past. Antibiotics, vaccines, and knowledge of hygiene led to what appeared to be a victory over the war on infection. The global pandemic of HIV quashed this optimism in 1992 with a publication from the Institutes of Medicine titled "Emerging Infections: Microbial Threats to Health in the United States."[2] Since then the increasing threats of developing pathogens have been recognized. These threats range from increasing microbial resistance, the rise of pathogenic viruses spread widely by travel that used to be locally limited, deliberate terroristic releases of infectious pathogens, and the increasing evolution of pathogens capable of transmission from human to human.

In 2003, severe acute respiratory syndrome (SARS) was initially described in Asia as a new infectious disease leading to high mortality. Eventually traced to a coronavirus, high risk of transmission to health care workers became a major concern as spread in medical personnel defined the outbreaks in Taipei and Toronto.[3] During the outbreak, the disease not only affected the actual provider, but had a large impact on the daily operations of emergency and health care personnel because of illness, quarantine, and concerned personnel absenteeism.

Perhaps one of the most high-profile microbial threats of the past few years was the Ebola virus outbreak of 2014. The evolution of that outbreak caught the public's attention because of its dramatic clinical presentation and high mortality associated with infection. The fear associated with infection and the risk of transmission brought medical transport of these patients to the forefront of the general population (along with the medical community). The infection of medical providers, and the death of some within medically advanced countries, led to intense public scrutiny of transport preparations.

Because of the impact of these and countless other life-threatening communicable disease outbreaks on the medical transport professional, the Air & Surface Transport Nurses Association developed a position statement on the transport of patients with serious communicable diseases.[4] Highlights of this statement are noted in Box 25.1.

This chapter starts with an overview of communicable disease transmission and prevention with an emphasis on the "all-hazards" approach to maintaining responder, crew, and community safety. It is followed by a review of specific high-risk pathogens, their treatment, and perhaps most importantly the precautions necessary to safely care for these patients in the unique transport environment.

Infection Control Policies

Our world is dependent on microorganisms for innumerable processes. The vast majority of these microorganisms present no pathogenic threat to humans as they coexist in a symbiotic relationship with their environment. These organisms are so commonplace that world is, at times, forgetful of the potential threat they present to human and population health. We become complacent and perhaps, naive, regarding the need to protect ourselves and our patients from their transmission whenever possible.

• BOX 25.1 **Air & Surface Transport Nurses Association Position Statement**

Transport of Patients with Serious Communicable Diseases

"The transport team is likely to be at added risk of exposure due to factors such as environmental conditions and interventions performed, and thus must be aware of the most current information available from infectious disease specialists to make informed practice decisions."

Precautions

- *Standard precautions* should be used in caring for all patients. Gloves, surgical masks, and eye protection must be worn whenever potentially splashing or creating droplets of potentially infectious fluids. Gloves must be changed between patients, with hand hygiene performed before applying and after removing gloves. Care providers must not eat or purposefully touch their mucous membranes or nonintact skin in areas with likely exposure to infectious microorganisms. All surfaces in patient care areas should be disinfected between patient encounters.
- *Airborne precautions* should be used when caring for patients with known or suspected infections spread by airborne droplets. Airborne precautions include use of N95 masks, and should be utilized by all members of the transport team, and if possible, a surgical mask should be worn by the patient. When possible, maximize fresh air ventilation and air exchange in the transport vehicle.
- *Droplet precautions* should be used when caring for patients with known suspected infections spread by large particle droplets. Droplet precautions require use of surgical masks by all members of the transport team, and if possible, a surgical mask should be worn by the patient. When possible, maximize fresh air ventilation and air exchange in the transport vehicle.
- *Contact precautions* should be used when caring for patients with known or suspected infections spread by direct or indirect patient contact. Contact precautions require use of gloves and gown or coveralls during direct patient contact

and procedures. Hand washing and/or waterless hand sanitizers should be used after each patient contact and after contact with items or equipment that have been in contact with the patient even after wearing gloves. Attention must be paid to the cleaning of all surfaces and equipment upon completion of transport.

Education

- Medical teams transporting patients with potential infectious illnesses should follow infection control procedures outlined by the World Health Organization (WHO), the Occupational Safety and Health Administration (OHSA), Center for Disease Control and Prevention (CDC), and the Commission on Accreditation of Emergency Transport Services (CAMTS).

Cleaning and Disinfection

- Transport vehicles should be terminally cleaned and decontaminated after transport of patients with highly infectious diseases. Ability to decontaminate the vehicle may factor into choice of transport vehicle.
- Appropriate Personnel Protective Equipment (PPE) should be donned prior to entering area to decontaminate.
- Cleaners should be EPA registered with labeling specific for the suspected pathogens.
- Emphasis should be on cleaning patient care areas surfaces. Stretchers and litters, including wheels, brackets, and other areas likely to become contaminated, should receive special attention. Railing, medical equipment and control panels, flooring, walls, and work surfaces in the vehicle also should be cleaned and disinfected.
- Only mattresses and pillows with plastic or impermeable covers should be used.
- All soiled supplies and patient-generated waste should be disposed of in accordance with CDC and local guidelines.

Adapted from ASTNA. <https://c.ymcdn.com/sites/astna.org/resource/collection/4392B20B-D0DB-4E76-959C-6989214920E9/ASTNA_Position_Statement_Transport_Pt_Serious_Commuicable_Disease_FINAL_(002).pdf>.

Prearrival preparation begins before the initial communication with a dispatch or call communication center. Basic screening information should be acquired using standardized questions to assess for the potential of communicable diseases (both active and nonpathogenic). For prehospital environments, standardized prompting from Emergency Medical Dispatch cards, such as those from the International Academies of Emergency Dispatch or similar organizations, can screen for potential infectious disease risks. These questions are important because they screen for some of the previously mentioned highly contagious/high-impact emerging infectious diseases by asking about recent travel to an area with active disease. These answers can inform the responding crew as to the level of precautions to take. Similarly, for interfacility transports, querying for and recognizing a potentially infectious diagnosis and using precautions in the sending facility are critical to the transporting personnel.

Historically the precautions taken to prevent the spread of "commonplace" microbes have been called *universal precautions*. Perhaps more appropriate terminology would be *routine practices* and then *additional precautions*. This would imply that a baseline level of precautions is practiced for all patient encounters, with additional protection when clinically indicated. This approach is necessary because the risks of communicable diseases may not be apparent on initial or prearrival assessment. This is especially the case when the presenting medical condition is not caused by the infectious agent and is a complicating or sometimes colonizing condition instead. Many factors go into the ability of a microorganism to cause an infection. This is defined as the invasion and multiplication of microorganisms in or on body tissues that causes cellular damage through the production of toxins, multiplication, or competition with host metabolism.[5] Recognizing that not all infectious agents are immediately apparent on prearrival or on first contact necessitates a preventative strategy using routine precautions to maintain the safety of the transportation team.

By far, the most effective preventive medical measure to combat the spread of infectious disease has been the development of safe and effective vaccinations associated with large-scale population-based immunization programs. This should be considered the baseline of "routine precautions." Based on some estimates, routine childhood vaccination in the United States prevents approximately 20 million illnesses with savings approaching $70 billion in direct and indirect community costs for each birth group vaccinated.[6] The Commission on Accreditation of Medical Transport Systems, the primary and most widely recognized medical transport accreditation organization, includes specific preventive health measures for employees in its accreditation standards. In addition to routine health care, vaccinations specific to the transport population of the individual program must be included in personnel policies. These vaccinations include, at a minimum, routine prophylaxis against tetanus, measles, mumps, rubella, and hepatitis B, along with specific international immunizations, based on the Centers for Disease Control and Prevention (CDC) recommendations.[7]

As we build on these basic interventions to prevent the spread of infectious disease, the next step would be hand hygiene. Compliance of medical providers with hand hygiene has repeatedly been shown to be very poor.[8] Frequently cited within the hospital staff setting, the consistency of hand hygiene by prehospital providers has not been shown to be any better.[9] Importantly, because this intervention should occur before and after patient contact, time pressures typically associated with the transport of emergent or critically ill or injured patients should theoretically not play a role in preventing this as routine practice. As a direct intervention, hand hygiene is probably one of the most important measures one can take to prevent both self-contamination and cross-contamination with pathogenic microorganism. Additionally, routine hand hygiene can theoretically help reduce nosocomial transmission through reduced contamination of patient care equipment and environment. As a specific intervention in the health care setting, implementation of dedicated hand-hygiene education and resource allocation significantly reduced overall infections by drug-resistant organisms in health care systems.[10]

Transmission of pathogenic microorganisms from health care workers requires several sequential steps. The organism must be present on a patient or surrounding surface (fomite), the organism must be transferred to a medical provider's skin, the organism must be able to survive on the skin of the provider for several minutes, and the provider must touch another patient or fomite. Breaking this chain anywhere in its progression greatly limits the spread of nosocomial infections. Assessing for contamination is not a reliable predictor of organism transfer on the skin as multiple studies have shown significant transfer of microorganisms onto medical providers even after "clean procedures," such as touching intact skin.[11,12] Hand hygiene prevents the survival of microorganisms on the skin when performed correctly, and it should be performed frequently and regularly throughout the course of patient care, even if gloves are used (Box 25-2).

Hand washing with soap and water and alcohol-based applications are effective for decreasing the volume and viability

---

BOX 25.2 Indications to Perform Hand Hygiene

- At beginning and end of shift
- Before and after each patient contact
- If moving from contaminated body site to clean body site during patient care
- After handling potentially contaminated materials including medical or transport equipment, clothing, and so forth
- After decontaminating equipment
- Before eating, drinking, applying cosmetics, or smoking
- Before and after using the bathroom

---

of pathogens on the hands. The alcohol-based rubs have been shown to increase compliance with hand hygiene significantly and decrease the spread of multidrug-resistant organisms.[10] With the slightly greater complexity involved in the transport environment, this may be the preferred option. However, it is important to recognize situations in which alcohol-based applications are less appropriate than hand washing. Indications specifically for washing with soap and water (and not waterless sanitizers) include the following:

- Hands become visibly soiled
- Contamination with greasy substances
- Potential exposure to specific pathogens including norovirus, *Cryptosporidium*, *Clostridium difficile*, and other spore-forming organisms

Personal Protective Equipment

Transport personnel should use barrier precautions to prevent potentially infectious substances from contacting skin or mucous membranes. This personal protective equipment (PPE) should be routinely provided by the transport agency and ensure they are accessible to the crew members throughout the different phases of patient contact. These barrier devices must include gloves, which must be worn whenever potentially coming into contact with bodily fluids, mucous membranes, or the nonintact skin of patients. Additionally, masks, eye shields, and clothing coverage should be available and used in situations that droplet formation or aerosolization of bodily fluids is possible, such as during intubation, suctioning of an airway, or wound irrigation.

Many respiratory contagious diseases are transmitted via exhaled or expelled airborne droplets from an infected person. Routine surgical masks may not adequately protect against these respiratory pathogens, and specialized masks or respirators may be necessary. Knowledge of the specific etiology of a respiratory infection is not always possible before transport personnel exposure; thus preparation must assume potential exposure risks. Using properly fitted N95 masks can protect against most of the airborne droplet diseases. These masks, when properly used, have the ability to filter submicron particles at a 95% efficiency. There are multiple models of these masks available, although selection should be limited to those certified by the National Institute of Occupational Safety and Health (NIOSH). They are, by design, disposable and should not be used when caring for more than one patient. It is important to consider policies to address these airborne droplet exposures in all transport personnel, including pilots and drivers, as appropriate. N95 masks should at least be used whenever there is potential exposure to the following pathogens[13,14]:

- Measles
- Tuberculosis (TB)
- SARS
- Middle East Respiratory Syndrome (MERS)
- Varicella
- Avian and pandemic influenza

Clean, disposable gloves of appropriate size and material must be made available and used before initiation of patient care. Care should be taken to avoid tears or disruptions of the gloves during patient care, and, if a tear is found, hand hygiene should be performed and new gloves used. In some situations it may be appropriate to double or triple gloves to ensure redundancy in case of disruption to the first layer of gloves. To prevent transmission to other transport personnel, it is critical to remove gloves before entering the driver/pilot compartment of the vehicle.

During the "in-hospital" portion of patient care delivery, impermeable gowns are standard PPE whenever large volumes of potentially infectious material are encountered (severe hemorrhage, child birth, massive emesis, etc.) or during patient care that may "splash" potentially infectious material. This is clearly the ideal scenario, but the unique conditions in the air medical environment prompted the Occupational Safety and Health Administration (OSHA) to render an opinion that allows employers to choose "appropriate" PPE considering both the risks of exposure and the performances of the employee. Thus jumpsuits or Nomex flight suits are suitable PPE if they prevent potentially infective material from passing through to the caregivers under normal use in a nominal period of time. In case of soilage, the garment should be removed for cleaning or repair as soon as feasible and at the cost of the employer.[15] This practice, however, does not decrease risks of nosocomial infection if it is not possible, due to mission tempo, to launder or change the jumpsuit between patients. Thus it is still recommended to use an impermeable gown whenever possible when treating patients potentially infected with communicable diseases known to be transmitted through contact. These diseases include the following[4]:

- Gastrointestinal, respiratory, skin, or wound infections
- Known colonization with drug-resistant bacteria
- Enteric infections with organisms with known prolonged survival on environmental surfaces
- Hepatitis A
- Rotavirus
- Respiratory syncytial virus
- Parainfluenza virus or enterovirus infection
- Contagious skin infections
- Viral or hemorrhagic conjunctivitis

Injury to crew members or assistants by potentially infected sharps is another area of significant concern. NIOSH reported that needle-stick type injuries are the most common source of infection by blood-borne pathogens in the health care setting.[16] Engineering safeguards, such as needleless systems, are the most effective way to reduce the opportunity for these types of injuries. Needles should never be recapped and should not be bent or broken before disposal. Sharps must be disposed of in a puncture-resistant container meeting OSHA requirements with clear labeling. Additionally, education and training on safe sharps management and hazard mitigation should be routine for new employees in the transport environment and should include immediate reporting of exposure and ensuring appropriate medical follow-up as indicated.

Decontamination

Transport vehicles are difficult environments to thoroughly decontaminate and require attention to detail to prevent nosocomial transmission between patients and to the transport crew. During cleaning, crew members should wear appropriate PPE. Physical cleaning with the appropriate Environmental Protection Agency (EPA)-registered cleaner is necessary for all equipment and surfaces, with special attention to any areas potentially contaminated with bodily fluids. Knowledge and understanding of the potential pathogens can help direct the appropriate cleaning product. All agencies should have dedicated and explicit infection control policies including decontamination protocols. There are varying levels of cleaning and decontaminating both vehicle and medical equipment and supplies. Ideally, one would provide the fullest level of decontamination between each patient; however, operational realities may preclude this in practice. At the least, medical equipment and vehicle surfaces should be cleaned after every patient contact. The highest level of decontamination and cleaning should be performed on a regularly scheduled basis and after transport of patients with highly pathogenic conditions.

Following each patient, all equipment should be removed from vehicle storage locations before cleaning. All surfaces should be wiped or sprayed with an approved disinfecting agent and wiped clean. Any visible contamination should be washed with soap and water or a disinfecting wipe as well. Following this cleaning, it is necessary to let the vehicle air dry. Medical equipment and transport devices should be likewise inspected and individually decontaminated. Following completion of the decontamination, the team member should remove his or her PPE and dispose of it appropriately. Multiuse cleaning supplies such as mops should be allowed to soak in a bleach and water or disinfecting solution for greater than 30 minutes. Following transport of patients with highly contagious or pathogenic conditions, such as *C. difficile,* specific cleaning protocols should be used because routine disinfection may not be sufficient. Recommendations for specific pathogens can be found in Table 25.1.

TABLE 25.1	Infectious Diseases and Recommended Precautions
Disease	**Precaution**
HIV	Standard
Anthrax	Standard
Bronchiolitis	Contact
Clostridium difficile	Contact
Epiglottitis	Droplet
Epstein-Barr/mononucleosis	Standard
Cholera	Standard
Gangrene	Standard
Gastroenteritis	Standard
Rotavirus	Contact
Hepatitis A	Contact
Hepatitis B/C	Standard
Herpes-zoster virus	Airborne/contact
Influenza	Airborne/droplet
Impetigo	Contact
Measles	Airborne/droplet
Bacterial meningitis	Droplet
Pertussis	Droplet
Scabies	Contact
Severe acute respiratory syndrome	Airborne/droplet/contact
Pulmonary tuberculosis	Airborne/droplet
Viral hemorrhagic fevers	Airborne/droplet/contact

Adapted from *Healthcare Infection Control Practices Advisory Committee (HICPAC).* 2007 Guideline for Isolation Precautions: Preventing Transmission of Infectious Agents in Healthcare Settings. https://www.cdc.gov/hicpac/2007IP/2007ip_appendA.html; 2007.

Transport of Patients With Specific Conditions

Respiratory Presentations

Acute respiratory infections are one of the largest areas of infectious disease growth in the world, including many new and reemerging infections. Respiratory infections include both the upper and lower airways and are inclusive of pharyngitis, epiglottitis, bronchitis, pneumonia, influenza, empyema, and so forth. Upper airway infections are defined as those above the epiglottis, and lower airway infections are defined as below the epiglottis. The majority of deaths related to infectious diseases in the United States are caused by lower airway infection, especially pneumonia.[17] They are a leading cause of overall mortality in both developed and developing countries. The impact of these infections is highest among children globally with over 40% of lower respiratory tract deaths in children under the age of 5.[18]

Respiratory infections should be suspected whenever the patient has a fever with dyspnea, chest pain, or cough. This presentation may be significantly altered in those patients with altered immune systems, including the very young and very old.

Pneumonia

Pneumonia, an infection of the lower respiratory tract, is usually caused by the inhalation of aerosols containing pathogenic microorganisms or by aspiration of oropharyngeal flora. It may also be caused by hematogenous spread from a distant focus of infection. The most typical causative agents are *Staphylococcus aureus, Haemophilus influenza, Moraxella catarrhalis, Mycoplasma pneumonia, Legionella pneumoniae, Chlamydia pneumonia,* and *Streptococcus pneumoniae. S. pneumoniae* is the most common etiology identified in community-acquired pneumonia when an identification is obtained. The incidences of the other organisms vary throughout different regions of the country and vary significantly when nosocomial infections are considered. Classic pneumonia presents with abrupt onset of fever, chills, cough, dyspnea, and physical examination findings of fever, tachycardia, and rales. The atypical causes of pneumonia may present with more indolent findings along with other associated nonrespiratory complaints. Again, those at the extremes of age or who are immunocompromised may present with nonrespiratory complaints including diarrhea, headaches, and abdominal pain. Diagnosis can be suspected clinically, and it is confirmed or excluded by radiographic findings while in the hospital. Treatment is supportive with prompt administration of *appropriate* antimicrobial therapy based on the most likely pathogen. Many studies have demonstrated increases in mortality when appropriate antibiotics are delayed in administration for hospitalized patients beyond 8 hours from identification. Ensuring adequate coverage of potential pathogens while weighing the risks of increasing microbial resistance to antibiotics is crucial. Knowledge of local microbiological prevalence and their susceptibility to particular antibiotics is crucial for effectively selecting antimicrobial therapy.

Pertussis

Vaccinations against pertussis have been available since the 1940s. Despite this, pertussis is the least well-controlled vaccine-preventable diseases in the United States.[19] The highest mortality rates with pertussis are for children younger than 1 year of age, in which death is usually caused by a complicating pneumonia. Pertussis should be considered in all patients with chronic cough; however, diagnosis can be challenging because of its three poorly defined stages and symptomatic overlap with most other upper respiratory infection syndromes. Pertussis, or "whooping cough," is caused by infection with *Bordetella pertussis* and is easily transmitted by airborne droplets; thus airborne and droplet precautions are necessary to decrease the risk of nosocomial infection. Antibiotics are effective in the early, first part of the illness to decrease the overall length of infection as well as the duration of infectivity.

Influenza

Influenza is arguably one of the most talked about infectious diseases, especially when considering its pandemic possibilities. One of the most dramatic examples of the power and impact of infectious diseases is the Spanish Influenza pandemic of 1918. The virus swept across the globe in waves, with more than 50 million fatalities worldwide and an estimated 675,000 killed in the United States.[20]

There are three predominant types of influenza: A, B, and C. Type C is not known to cause significant clinical symptoms or outbreaks. Type A influenza is further broken down into subtypes based on their expressed surface proteins (H and N). The Type A viruses are found in humans, ducks, chickens, pigs, whales, and seals. Type B virus is only found in humans. Because the virus slowly changes its genome in the host animals (called antigenic drift), the flu vaccine may only be partially effective in raising antibodies in an immunized person. Thus it is critical to apply appropriate respiratory PPE when caring for these patients.[1]

Individuals infected with influenza potentially present with fever, cough, myalgias, headaches, and sore throat. However, variations on this presentation are the norm. Transmission occurs primarily via airborne droplets from an infected individuals cough or sneeze, or direct contact with surfaces contaminated with respiratory secretions. Airborne precautions and strict hand hygiene are necessary to prevent self-infection. The mortality of influenza often presents as complicating coinfections, and usually impacts those at the extremes of age and the immunocompromised patient. Most commonly the complicating infection is a pneumonia, although myocarditis and encephalitis also occur. In modern, developed countries, mortality rates approach 1 in 1000 cases.

Treatment for influenza is primarily supportive. There are several antiviral medications currently approved for treatment in the United States. Generally, only the neuraminidase inhibitors are recommended for treatment of those at high risk for complications from the disease. The efficacies of these medications are such that they only shorten the length of illness by 1 day and possibly attenuate the severity of illness. They are not recommended for otherwise healthy people unless they are in a high-risk occupation, such as health care, and only when it can be started within the first 48 hours of illness. Because of the limitations in therapy, many health care organizations are requiring masks be worn by all nonimmunized health care workers.

Avian Influenza

Avian influenza is a subtype of influenza Type A (H5N1). First described in an infected 3-year-old in Hong Kong in 1997, it has now been reported in at least 15 countries. Surprisingly, Avian flu seemed to have a higher attack rate and mortality rate among young adults, with less than 10% of the cases being greater than 40 years of age. The mortality rate was a striking 62% of those known to be infected, making it highly pathogenic. It is primarily found in birds but can be transmitted to humans via virus shedding in animal saliva, nasal secretions, and feces. Transmission seems to be limited to humans in direct contact with infected poultry and surfaces, although aerosolization of viruses in droplets may also spread the disease. Precautions and disinfection strategies should therefore reflect these potentials.

Tuberculosis

Mycobacterium TB can cause infection anywhere in the body, although predominantly active TB is found in the lung. The bacterium is transmitted by aerosolized respiratory droplets from sneezing, coughing, or during airway interventions (such as intubation or bronchoscopy). Those patients without active pulmonary TB are generally not considered infective. Active pulmonary TB is characterized, by those with competent immune systems, by fever, weight loss, night sweats, malaise, and a minimally productive cough. This presentation may not be different than other respiratory diseases; thus it is imperative for the caregivers to keep TB in their working diagnosis with most respiratory complaints. Certain demographic and historical factors increase the risk for active TB, including emigration from an endemic area, prison exposure, homelessness, exposure to others with active TB, active HIV, transplantation, or other immunocompromised state.

Given the airborne droplet transmissibility of TB, limiting exposure to high concentrations of potentially aerosolized droplets is an important part of personal protection. During transport of infected patients, all members of the crew should wear submicron, N95 disposable masks during all phases of patient care. Transport vehicles should maximize fresh air exchange. Aircraft with one-direction airflow capabilities should use this during transport to minimize recirculation. Nonintubated patients with active pulmonary TB should be asked to wear a surgical mask, whereas intubated patients should use a high-efficiency particulate arresting (HEPA) filter on the exhalation limb of the vent circuit.

TB is predominantly a treatable condition. Potential exposures should be reported to the transport organization or public health system as soon as possible. Reporting facilitates close follow up of the caregiver and definitive diagnostic testing of the potential patient. Most infections remain inactive or "latent" throughout a person's lifetime; however, 10% of people with latent infections will progress to active infection. Treatment for latent TB may range from 6 to 9 months using isoniazid (INH). Those individuals that progress to active infection require therapy with a four-drug regimen including INH, rifampin, pyrazinamide, and ethambutol. Multidrug-resistant TB is increasingly prevalent and is resistant to standard therapy with INH and rifampin. Extensively drug-resistant (XDR) TB is a very rare disease with resistance to INH, rifampin, quinolones, and at least one of the second-line agents. Patients with XDR TB may be forcibly quarantined in the United States because of its limited treatability and high risk of death for those with compromised immune systems who acquire the disease.[21]

Severe Acute Respiratory Syndrome

SARS presents similarly to other respiratory infections with a higher prevalence of extrapulmonary symptoms being the norm including vomiting and diarrhea. It was only first described in February 2003 with the last known case reported in July of the same year. An explosive outbreak of adult respiratory distress syndrome seeming to have an epicenter in a hotel in Hong Kong during a single weekend quickly spread across multiple continents including the Americas and Europe. Later determined to be from a coronavirus (similar to those that cause the common cold), it appears to have been carried to that hotel from a physician in an adjacent Chinese province.[22] Most patients diagnosed with SARS were young adults in their twenties, with very few cases in children less than 15 years old. Strikingly, over 20% of those infected were health care workers who were most linked to "superspreader" events.[23] These events caused the aerosolization of infective droplets during inpatient medical care (i.e., bronchoscopy, intubation, etc.) Symptoms included fever, chills, and myalgias followed 3 to 7 days later by nonproductive cough and dyspnea. At least 20% of affected patients went on to require intubation because of progressive hypoxemia.

Because of the high attack rate of health care providers and the explosive nature of the outbreak, many regional, national, and international precautions were put in place to regulate the transport of potentially infected patients. Within the United States, transportation requires coordination with the CDC Quarantine Station and other federal and state authorities. Specific guidance from the CDC for air travel of potential SARS patients is summarized in Box 25.3. Given the risks associated with the enclosed transport environment, several companies offer portable isolation units that may facilitate safer transfer of SARS patients in vehicles that do not have separate isolated cockpit or driver compartments.

Following transport, maximal aeration should be performed to allow at least one entire cabin air exchange, if not more, before cleaning. Limit the potential for reaerosolization of droplets by avoiding blowers and fans. All surfaces and medical equipment involved in the transfer should be cleaned with hospital-grade, EPA-registered disinfectant.[24]

Middle East Respiratory Syndrome

Similar to SARS, MERS is a newly discovered coronavirus that seems to have originated on the Arabian Peninsula. The first reported case was in July 2012 in a man from Saudi Arabia. Since that index case, it has been found to be the causative organism in over 80 subsequent infections, with only two in the United States. All cases were in the Arabian Peninsula or

---

> ● **BOX 25.3** Air Medical Transport of Severe Acute Respiratory Syndrome Patients

- Patients should be on dedicated air medical transport with the minimum number of crew.
- A single primary caregiver should be assigned to the patient.
- Consider PPE breaks during extended transports that must be secured "upwind" of the patient.
- Coordinate with the Centers for Disease Control and Prevention and other state/federal authorities before initiating transport.
- International transports require coordination with over flown, en route, and destination localities and facilities.
- Fixed-wing aircraft with forward-to-aft air flow with a separate cockpit cabin are strongly preferred.
- Aircraft that recirculate air without a HEPA filter should not transport a SARS patient.
- Aircraft ventilation should remain on at all times during transport including ground delays.
- In rotor-wing and small unpressurized aircraft, all crew should wear disposable and properly fitted N95 or higher level respirators.
- Nonintubated patients should wear surgical masks, and intubated patients should use HEPA filter on the ventilator circuit.
- Patients should be positioned as far "downwind" in regard to ventilation as possible.
- A minimum distance of 6 feet from the patient should be designated a dirty "zone" with full PPE required.
- Following transport and before cleaning, the vehicle should be thoroughly aired out.
- At the conclusion of transport, personnel should self-monitor and report at least daily on the development of fever or respiratory symptoms.

HEPA, High-efficiency particulate arresting; *PPE,* personal protective equipment; *SARS,* severe acute respiratory syndrome.
Adapted from *Centers for Disease Control and Prevention.* Guidance on air medical transport for SARS patients. <https://www.cdc.gov/sars/travel/airtransport.html>; 2005.

---

in people having recently returned from travel there. It appears the virus originally came from animal reservoirs in the dromedary camel and perhaps bats, as well. Similar precautions used for SARS should be followed for MERS.

Dermatologic Presentations

Measles

Childhood vaccination against infection with measles has significantly decreased the spread of the disease in the United States. With an efficacy of 95% in preventing the disease in exposed persons, vaccination is an effective method for potentially eliminating it from our population completely. Unfortunately, increasing rates of intentional avoidance of vaccination within the United States has led to increasing size and frequency of local and regional outbreaks compared with only a few years ago. This was emphasized in 2014 following an outbreak related to a California theme park that led to more than 140 cases of measles.[25] Young infants and elderly people, who cannot be immunized, are most at risk for contracting serious forms of the disease and are also most dependent on herd immunity for protection. Annually, over 100,000 deaths occur from complications of the disease, predominantly in developing and resource-poor countries.

Clinical manifestations of infection with the measles virus are initially nonspecific upper respiratory illness symptoms typified by fever, cough, runny nose, and conjunctivitis. Following this stage, a rash develops centrally on the body and progresses outward to the face, hands, and feet over the subsequent 3 days. Initially blanchable, the rash develops into nonblanchable spots over the subsequent 4 days. In severe cases, the lesions may become hemorrhagic. The extent of the rash correlates with the severity of disease. Characteristic of measles infection are Koplik spots described as small blue-white lesions on the buccal mucosa. Upward of 30% of measles cases develop complications, some of which may be severe.[26] Most commonly, a secondary infection complicates measles because of the immunosuppressive effect of the virus. Pulmonary involvement is the leading cause of childhood mortality from measles, followed by diarrhea and central nervous system involvement.

Measles virus is transmitted by respiratory droplets, and aerosolization and precautions against exposure are necessary for at least the first 4 days after onset of rash. Measles virus has been found to be suspended in the air up to 2 hours after patient departure. At least a full cabin air exchange should occur before reuse.

Varicella

Varicella-zoster virus (VZV) causes two distinct clinical diseases: varicella (chickenpox) and herpes zoster (shingles). Primary infection with VZV causes chickenpox and reactivation of the virus later in life causes shingles. Varicella is usually a mild disease when presenting in childhood, although it can progress to life-threatening when initial presentation is in adults or in immunocompromised patients. Since the introduction of the varicella vaccine in 1995, rates of infection and subsequent morbidity and mortality have significantly dropped.[27]

Following infection with varicella, a prodrome similar to other viral illnesses occurs including fever and malaise, which is quickly followed by a general vesicular rash within 24 hours. The rash starts as macules and papules that progress to characteristic vesicles, which are extremely pruritic. The vesicles then crust over and form crusted papules. Characteristic of varicella are "crops" of these lesions in different stages of development across the body. New lesions stop appearing usually within 4 days.

Complications of varicella, similar to measles, include primarily superinfection. Central nervous system involvement may occur leading to meningitis or encephalitis. Reye syndrome is a rare complication that is unique in its association with salicylate exposure. This syndrome includes nausea, vomiting, headache, delirium, combativeness, and even coma. Since advising parents against using aspirin in febrile children, this has essentially disappeared from clinical practice. In adults, development of varicella pneumonia

is more common than in children, and it carries a mortality rate of 10% to 30%. Those that require mechanical ventilation for pneumonia have mortality rates approaching 50%.[28] Pregnant patients are at risk for maternal varicella, leading to possible transmission to the neonate with significant mortality. Additionally, primary varicella infection before 20 weeks' gestation puts the fetus at risk for congenital varicella.

VZV is transmitted primarily via aerosolization of nasopharyngeal droplets or by direct contact with fluid found within the vesicles. Patients are contagious until all of the vesicles have crusted over and dried. If possible, nonimmune crew members who may be pregnant should not be involved with the care of a potentially infected patient or in handling articles potentially contaminated with nasopharyngeal or vesicular discharge. During patient care, crew members should use an N95-level respirator and PPE for droplet precautions. This is important even for those crew members who believe they are immune to protect against incomplete immunity and to model behavior for other members of the crew.

Scabies

Scabies is a mite infestation of the skin by *Sarcoptes scabiei* that leads to an intensely pruritic reaction. The itching is a type of hypersensitivity reaction to the mite, its feces, and eggs. The mite itself is barely visible with the unaided eye, and its burrowing habits make it usually unobservable to the patient. Typically, the distribution of the infestation aids in the clinical diagnosis because it usually affects the web spaces of the digits, wrists, elbows, the area immediately around the nipples in women, the posterior aspect of the feet, and the lower buttocks. Scabies in and of itself is an unlikely reason for emergent or critical care transport. However, patients may harbor an infestation during transport for an unrelated condition. Because transmission is from direct contact or contact with heavily infested clothing/linens, knowledge of the infestation can prevent spreading of this unwanted guest. Strict barrier precautions, including gown and head cover, is essential to prevent spread to health care workers. If possible, removal of equipment and linen from use for 3 days after exposure will prevent cross-contamination because the mite cannot survive long away from its human host. If this is not possible, linens and clothing should be washed in hot water and placed in a hot dryer or dry cleaned to kill the mites. Cabins should be vacuumed and cleaned thoroughly, and pesticides are not indicated.[29]

Neurologic
Meningitis

Bacterial, viral, parasitic, and fungal infections of the central nervous system or its surrounding structures cause inflammation of the meninges that cover the brain and spinal cord. Infection may occur from spread of an adjacent infective source, from contamination during trauma, or from hematogenous spread from a distant foci. Typical presentations include fever; headache, neck stiffness, and, frequently, altered mental status. Presentations may vary based on the patient's immune status and preexisting diseases.

Viral meningitis is the most frequent cause of meningitis and generally requires only supportive care with an excellent prognosis in those with normal immune function. Parasitic or amoebic meningitis is relatively rare and can have devastating consequences. *Naegleria fowleri,* an amoeba found naturally in warm water and soil, is an example of a particularly aggressive infection that often affects young otherwise healthy patients. Fungal meningitis, usually caused by inhaling spores of these organisms, typically affects those with HIV or poorly controlled diabetes. Bacterial meningitis requires rapid identification and treatment to impact its high mortality rate, and it is the focus of this section.

Most commonly caused by *Neisseria meningitidis* or *Streptococcus pneumoniae,* bacterial meningitis accounts for over 135,000 deaths worldwide per year with a large portion of the survivors carrying significant chronic neurologic sequelae. Previously, *Haemophilus influenzae* type B was a common etiology, although after vaccine development, these cases have been greatly reduced in the United States. The epidemiology of health care–acquired meningitis is very different and depends on previous neurologic surgery or antibiotic exposure. It is most commonly caused by staphylococci or bacilli species.[30] Patients with community-acquired bacterial meningitis are typically quite ill and present quickly (typically less than 1 day) after developing symptoms. Aggressive resuscitation with appropriate antibiotics in addition to supportive care is usually necessary. Ideally, a definitive diagnosis should be attempted before initiation of antibiotics; however, if lumbar puncture will be delayed for any reason, blood cultures should at least be gathered because most cases of bacterial meningitis also involve bacteremia. Before antibiotic administration, a dose of dexamethasone should be given because it has been shown to decrease mortality and neurologic complications when given before antibiotics and has no benefit shown after antibiotics.

Commonly, meningitis and meningococcemia are confused entities and much of the precautions center around meningitis. *N. meningitides,* also known as meningococcus, can cause both meningitis and bacteremia. This is termed meningococcemia. Meningococcemia is a particularly feared entity because of its rapid progression to multisystem organ failure and death along with its relatively nonspecific initial presentation. In addition to the fever, malaise, and headache typical of meningitis, meningococcemia often includes leg pain, pale or mottling of skin, and cool extremities (manifestations of early shock). The rash of meningococcemia is present in approximately 50% of cases and is described as nonblanching petechial hemorrhages most frequently on the limbs and lower trunk.[31] These petechiae can coalesce into large areas of purpura or bruising. The degree of apparent petechiae can correlate with severity of disease as microvascular coagulopathy progresses along a spectrum to disseminated intravascular coagulation.

As the infectious etiology of meningitis is not always known before patient transport, it is important to proceed with precautions such that infection may be from meningococcemia or other virulent pathogens. As transmission is primarily from oropharyngeal droplets and aerosolization, airborne and droplet precautions are necessary including gloves, gowns, and masks. Generally, close contact (i.e., those providing bedside care during transport) should receive antibiotic prophylaxis if the pathogen was meningococcus or *H. influenzae* type B. Prophylaxis usually entails a single dose or short course of antibiotics including ciprofloxacin or rifampin. The vehicle and equipment should undergo standard cleaning and disinfection. Close follow up with the health care facility is necessary to ensure that diagnostic culture data are forwarded to the crew members and transport agency.

Gastrointestinal

Diarrhea

Diarrhea is usually defined by the passage of loose or watery stools with a frequency of at least three times in 24 hours. Its presence implies impaired gastrointestinal function such that there is impaired water absorption or active excretion of water. When the diarrhea includes blood or mucus, the diagnosis leans toward invasive diarrhea (dysentery). Acute diarrhea lasts less than 14 days, whereas chronic diarrhea is defined as lasting more than 30 days. Persistent diarrhea falls in between the two time lines. There are an estimated 2 to 4 billion cases of diarrhea per year with a predominance of infectious causes.[32] Infectious diarrhea is one of the top five killers worldwide, with mortality concentrated in resource-poor areas. Mortality is usually from dehydration and malnutrition and typically can be prevented in developed and resource-rich areas. However, even when not life-threatening, infectious diarrhea can have profound effects on personal productivity as well as impacts on the health care system, especially when outbreaks occur among health care workers.

Infection is the leading cause of acute diarrheal illness. The majority of such infections are self-limited and require little medical intervention or support. Infectious diarrhea can be caused by virus, bacteria, and protozoa. For those patients who had cultures of their stool for diagnosis, the most common causes were presumed to be viral because no bacteria were identified from the culture medium. Travelers (i.e., transient) who develop diarrhea tend to have a bacterial etiology. Severe cases of diarrhea also are usually caused by bacteria. Transmission is predominantly person to person and hand to mouth; however, contaminated food and water are also sources of sporadic outbreaks of infective diarrhea. Norovirus can also be spread via airborne droplets.

As noted, infective diarrhea is usually self-limited and responds well to supportive therapy and attention to hydration. This hydration may be oral or intravenous if not tolerated by mouth. Traditionally, antibiotic therapy is not indicated because of the self-limited nature of the illness.

The marginal benefits of antibiotics in most cases of acute diarrhea do not seem to outweigh the real risks of potential side effects, bacterial resistance, and risk for *C. difficile* infection that unnecessary antibiotics pose. However, some specific pathogens do warrant antimicrobial therapy, and at times clinical and historical information may indicate empiric therapy before laboratory diagnosis. Specific indications for antimicrobial therapy are beyond the scope of this chapter; however, clinical benefit has been demonstrated when treating *Vibrio cholera, Shigella, Salmonella, Campylobacter, Yersinia, C. difficile, Cyclospora, Entamoeba,* and *Giardia lamblia.* Additionally, those that are immunosuppressed or have evidence of severe or invasive disease (bloody stool, fever) may benefit from early antimicrobial therapy.[33]

Clostridium Difficile

C. difficile is the most common health care–related infectious diarrhea and has significant potential morbidity and mortality associated with it. It is a spore-forming, toxin-producing anaerobic bacteria that proliferates in the human intestinal tract when the normal flora has been altered by antibiotics. It is also a common form of diarrhea in patients with poorly controlled HIV infection. Clinical manifestations of *C. difficile* infection may range from asymptomatic carriage to severe colitis and megacolon with subsequent perforation and peritonitis. Symptoms of infection include watery diarrhea and abdominal cramping, often with low-grade fever.[34] Leukocytosis is common and may be the only presenting problem, especially when the patient is not interactive for the examination. Often treatment must be initiated before definitive diagnosis and a low threshold for empiric therapy is necessary. Standard therapy includes prompt recognition and intravenous metronidazole and enteric vancomycin. In severe cases, colectomy is necessary to provide source control and remove ischemic complications.

Strict contact precautions are necessary to prevent nosocomial spread of *C. difficile* bacteria and spores. Because of the presence of asymptomatic carriers, it is reasonable to maintain these precautions beyond the duration of diarrhea. It is unclear how long after diagnosis these precautions are necessary and it is an area of active research.[35] The spores can survive on surfaces for several months, so careful attention to decontamination is critical after patient transfer. Given the difficulty in decontaminating some multiuse equipment, such as blood pressure cuffs, the use of disposable supplies may be appropriate. Environmental cleaning should be performed with products specifically labeled as EPA approved as sporicidal for *C. difficile* or bleach based, because most products that do not carry this label are not sporicidal and are not effective. Frequent hand hygiene is a critical step in decreasing transmission as well. Alcohol-based products are *not* sufficient to clean after exposure to *C. difficile*. Vigorous hand washing with soap and water is necessary to remove the spores; however, alcohol-based products are better at killing the actual bacteria. Thus it is reasonable to adopt an approach to hand hygiene of washing with soap and water followed by an alcohol-based product.

Blood-Borne Infections

Hepatitis B

It is estimated that there are over 245 million carriers of hepatitis B in the world. After the implementation of vaccination programs, the incidence has decreased significantly, but still over 600,000 people die per year because of related liver disease.[36] Infections with hepatitis B virus can range from asymptomatic carriage through fulminant hepatitis and chronic disease. Acute infection is similar to most other viral infections with nonspecific fatigue and malaise, often accompanied by a low-grade fever. Subsequently, right upper quadrant abdominal pain may develop, associated with mild nausea and vomiting. Jaundice may develop (70% of cases) and be evidenced by darkening of urine or off-colored stool. Diagnosis of hepatitis would be suspected by hepatic enzyme elevations (aspartate transaminase and alanine transaminase) and confirmed with serologic testing. Most patients recover uneventfully from acute hepatitis B infection, although a very small percentage (<0.5%) will develop fulminant hepatitis with consequent hepatic failure and significant fatality rate.[37] Acute hepatitis B progresses to a chronic state and varies by age and ranges from 50% in young children to 5% of adults. Chronic infection may be asymptomatic or progress to cirrhosis and liver failure. Additionally, chronic hepatitis B infection significantly increases the risk of developing hepatocellular carcinoma. There are multiple treatment regimens now for hepatitis B, but they all carry significant side effect profiles and significant costs.

Hepatitis B is transmitted by percutaneous or mucous membrane exposure to bodily fluids that contain the virus. For health care workers, percutaneous exposure by needle stick is the most common method. With successful completion of the hepatitis B vaccine series, however, this route of transmission is rare. If the exposed individual does not have these vaccinations or is found to have incomplete immunity, hepatitis B immunoglobulin may be administered following exposure.

Hepatitis C

Slightly less prominent on a global level than hepatitis B, it is estimated that over 185 million people carry or have carried hepatitis C. The acute presentation is similar to hepatitis B and nonspecific as well. Diagnosis can be made using serologic testing. A major difference, however, is that a high percentage of patients infected with hepatitis C convert to chronic infection, reaching 85% in some reports. Up to 30% of individuals with chronic infection develop cirrhotic liver disease and the complications associated with that ailment. Although progression is variable, it seems 20 to 30 years of chronic disease is usually necessary to form the fibrosis necessary for cirrhosis.[38]

Similar to hepatitis B, percutaneous and mucous membrane exposure is the greatest risk for health care workers. The CDC estimates approximately 385,000 sharps-related injuries per year among hospital workers, and that does not include the moving, rarely stable, transport environment.[39] The risk of seroconversion after a needle stick from a patient infected with hepatitis C is approximately 1.8%.[40] There is no vaccine prophylaxis against hepatitis C, and no postexposure prophylaxis has yet been shown to be effective in preventing infection. Thus strict droplet precautions should be followed when performing any bedside care that may spread potentially infected fluids (venipuncture, intubation, etc.).

Human Immunodeficiency Virus

HIV was first described in a group of 12 men in 1981. During the subsequent decades, over 35 million fatalities related to HIV have been documented worldwide, making its impact similar to the influenza pandemics of the early 20th century. Although the mortality rate from HIV-related diseases has decreased significantly, the incidence of HIV-infected patients has continued to rise. It is estimated that over 36 million people are living with HIV infection, with the majority in Sub-Saharan Africa. Similar to hepatitis, the initial acute phase of HIV infection is nonspecific and may be attributed to an upper respiratory infection. Although some infected patients will have no symptoms, many will develop fever, malaise, nonspecific lymphadenopathy, headache, and a sore throat. Following the onset of this acute phase, most patients recover over the subsequent 1 to 2 weeks and are asymptomatic. During this subsequent chronic phase, the virus replicates and the patients' immune system is slowly weakened to the point that opportunistic infections occur.[41]

Like other blood-borne pathogens, transmission to health care workers is possible from splashing of infected fluid onto open skin (i.e., open wounds or mucous membranes) and from sharp needle-stick type events. There are many factors that go into the potential transmissibility of HIV after these exposures, including the patient's viral load and host immune system. The overall risk of developing HIV from infected needle sticks is approximately 1 in 435 exposures; and from mucous membrane exposure is 1 in 1000. Exposure characteristics that impact the potential for transmission are visible contamination with infected body fluids, deep injury to the health care worker, injury with an object that was in the patient's vein or artery, and terminal illness in the patient.[42]

Viral Hemorrhagic Fevers

Viral hemorrhagic fevers (VHFs) are a class of diseases characterized by acute febrile illness with bleeding diathesis. There are several distinct classes of viruses that cause VHF, but they are common in their ability to cause severe multisystem organ dysfunction including significant damage to the microvascular system of the body. These illnesses cause bleeding, although it is rare for the hemorrhage itself to be life-threatening. All of the viruses are dependent on animal or insect hosts as reservoirs to propagate infection; however, humans are not the natural host. Although there are several known VHFs, this section will concentrate on the Ebola virus because clinical management and personal protection applies to all VHFs.

Ebola infections are severe and often life-threatening in their presentations. A recent significant outbreak from 2014 to 2016 in West Africa affected thousands of people in the region. During the outbreak, residents from around the world traveled to the region to aid those afflicted by the disease, and residents of those areas traveled out of the area. This movement of people in and out of the affected area developed into a situation in which Ebola was being diagnosed and treated outside of the outbreak region. It illustrated the ability for such diseases to be spread easily throughout the world by rapid air travel and ease of transportation. Unfortunately, some of the aid workers who responded to the West African area of need became infected with the Ebola virus, demonstrating the need for coordinated and thoughtful planning to prevent further spread of the infection.

Symptoms of Ebola (and all VHFs) include the complex of fever, headaches, and myalgias/arthralgias, followed by vomiting and diarrhea with abdominal pain. A few days after symptom onset, maculopapular rashes develop followed by bleeding from ruptured capillaries and microvascular structures. Clinically this bleeding may be from the gastrointestinal tract, ocular mucosa, respiratory tract, and skin. Severe shock and multisystem organ failure than ensue. Treatment is purely supportive.[17] Experimental vaccines and therapy with antiviral medications is ongoing without clear clinical benefit yet.

Transmission of the virus occurs during contact with an infected animal or (in the case of other VHFs) from bites from infected mosquitoes or ticks. Once a human is infected, transmission can be passed directly through contact or by contact with contaminated objects. There is some concern that Ebola has the ability to be transmitted by airborne droplets during events that may splash bodily fluids such as intubation, venous catheterization, and so forth. Infection control practices are incredibly important during transport of these patients and take significant coordination to prevent further nosocomial spread. Unplanned events can alter transport plans and destinations because of security concerns, accidents, and patient clinical events. Having dedicated equipment and specifically trained personnel handle these high-risk transports is crucial to handling these unforeseen events.

Specific instructions in preparing a transport vehicle are beyond the scope of this chapter but are available in several places. Communication and planning with local, regional, and federal health authorities is crucial to a safe transfer and can assist with pretransport planning. Crew members should be well trained and regularly refreshed on the use of appropriate PPE and contingency plans. Box 25.4 lists the CDC recommendations for PPE in caring for potentially

● **BOX 25.4** **Recommended Personal Protective Equipment for Ebola Patients**

- Single-use impermeable gown (to calf) or coverall
- Powered air-purifying respirator
- N95 is allowed with full face mask and hair covering
- Double-gloved with extended cuffs
- Single-use disposable boots
- Single-use disposable apron

Adapted from *Centers for Disease Control and Prevention*. Ebola virus. <https://www.cdc.gov/vhf/ebola/healthcare-us/ppe/guidance.html>.

infected patients. During patient care, regular and repeated cleansing of gloved hands should be performed using alcohol-based cleanser. A dedicated monitor should observe and ensure compliance with appropriate donning and doffing of PPE. Following transport (even with appropriate PPE) of patients with Ebola, personnel should be monitored for fever at least twice daily for 3 weeks postexposure. If the crew member develops fever greater than 38.3°C, immediate hospitalization and isolation are mandatory.

Summary

Despite the predictions of a few decades ago, infectious and communicable diseases are far from becoming "an affliction of the past." Recent lessons from pandemic and epidemic infections with SARS and Ebola demonstrate just how relevant these diseases are. Given the number of affected health care workers and the nosocomial transmission of these microbes, attention to and planning for these types of infective events are crucial. Transport agencies must devote adequate resources in planning, oversight, and supplies to safely care for and transport these patients. Education toward proper PPE, its utility and function, and its limitations, is crucial to keep crew members safe and ready for the next patient.

References

1. van Doorn H. Emerging infectious diseases. *Medicine*. 2014;42(1):60-63.
2. Institute of Medicine. *Emerging Infections: Microbial Threats to Health in the United States*. Washington, DC: National Academy Press; 1992.
3. Varia M, et al. Investigaton of nosocomial outbreak of severe acute respiratory distress syndrome (SARS) in Toronto, Canada. *CMAJ*. 2003;169(4):285-292.
4. Air & Surface Transport Nurses Association. *Transport of Patients with Serious Communicable Diseases*. Retrieved from http://c.ymcdn.com/sites/astna.org/resource/collection/4392B20B-D0DB-4E76-959C-6989214920E9/ASTNA_Position_Statement_Transport_Pt_Serious_Commuicable_Disease_FINAL_(002).pdf; 2015.
5. Association for Professionals in Infection Control and Epidemiology. *APIC Text of Infection Control and Epidemiology*. Washington, DC: APIC; 2002.
6. Zhou F, et al. Economic evaluation of the routine childhood immunization program in the United States, 2009. *Pediatrics*. 2004;133(4):1-9.
7. Commission on Accreditation of Medical Transport Systems. *Accreditation Standards*. Retrieved from http://www.camts.org/Accreditation-Standards.html; 2015.
8. Garus-Pakowska A, Sobala W, Szatko F. Observance of hand washing procedures performed by the medical personnel before patient contact. Part I. *Int J Occup Med Environ Health*. 2013;26(1):113-121.
9. Bucher J, et al. Hand washing practices among emergency medical services providers. *Western Journal of Emergency Medicine*. 2015;16(5):727-735.
10. World Health Organization. *Evidence of Hand Hygiene to Reduce Transmission and Infections by Multidrug Drug Resistant Organisms in Health-Care Settings*. Retrieved Oct 22, 2016, from http://www.who.int/gpsc/5may/MDRO_literature-review.pdf?ua=1; 2009.
11. Grabsch EA, et al. Risk of environmental and healthcare workers contamination with vancomycin-resistant enterococci during outpatient procedures and hemodialysis. *Infection Control and Hospital Epidemiology*. 2006;27(3):287-293.
12. Pessoa-Silva CL, et al. Dynamics of bacterial hand contamination during routine neonatal care. *Infection Control and Hospital Epidemiology*. 2004;25(3):192-197.
13. National Institute for Occupational Safety and Health. *Respirators*. Retrieved June 12, 2016, from http://www.cdc.gov/niosh/topics/respirators/default.html; 2016.
14. Doyle TJ. Infection Control in Air and Ground Medical Transport. In: Blumen IJ, ed. *Principles and Direction of Air Medial Transport*. Salt Lake City, UT: Air Medical Physician Association; 2015.
15. United States Department of Labor. *Bloodborne Pathogens (Regulation 29 CFR 1910.1030)*. Retrieved Nov 30, 2016, from Occupational Safety and Health Administration: https://www.osha.gov/pls/oshaweb/owadisp.show_document?p_table=STANDARDS&p_id=10051; n.d.
16. National Institute of Occupational Health and Safety. *Preventing Needlestick Injuries in the Health Care Setting*. Retrieved from https://www.cdc.gov/niosh/docs/2000-108/; 2014.
17. Khabbaz RBB. Emerging and Reemerging infectious disease threats. In: Bennett JE, et al, eds. *Bennett's Principles and Practice of Infectious Diseases*, Updated Edition. 8th ed. Philadelphia, PA: Elsevier/Saunders; 2014.
18. World Health Organization. *The Global Burden of Disease: 2004 Update*. Retrieved from http://www.who.int/healthinfo/global_burden_disease/GBD_report_2004update_full.pdf?ua=1; 2008.
19. Berger JT, et al. Critical pertussis illness in children: a multicenter prospectie cohort study. *Pediatr Crit Care Med*. 2013;14(4):356-365.
20. Moresn D, et al. The 1918 influenza pandemic: lesssons for 2009 and the future. *Crit Care Med*. 2010;38(S4):e10-e20.
21. Centers for Disease Control and Prevention. *Multdrug-Resistant Tuberculosis*. Retrieved from Tuberculosis: http://www.cdc.gov/tb/publications/factsheet/drtb/mdrtb.htm; 2016.
22. Hui DS, Chan PK. Severe acute respiratory distress syndrome and coronavirus. *Infect Dis Clin North Am*. 2010;24(3):619-638.
23. Dye C, Gay N. Modeling the SARS epidemic. *Science*. 2003;300(5627):1884-1885.
24. Centers for Disease Control and Prevention. *Guidance on Air Medical Transport for SARS Patients*. Retrieved Sept 12, 2016. https://www.cdc.gov/sars/travel/airtransport.html; 2005.

25. Zipprich J, et al. Measles outbreak-California, December 2014–February 2015. *MMWR Morb Mortal Wkly Rpt*. 2015;64(6):153-154.

26. Gans H, et al. *Measles: Clinical Manifestations, Diagnosis, Treatment, and Prevention*. Retrieved from UpToDate: http://www.uptodate.com/; 2016.

27. Centers for Disease Control and Prevention. Decline in annual incidence of varicella—selected states, 1990–2001. *MMWR Morb Mortal Wkly Rpt*. 2003;52(37):884-885.

28. Albrecht M. *Clinical Features of Varicella-Zoster Infection: Chickenpox*. Retrieved from UpToDate: http://www.uptodate.com; 2016.

29. Centers for Disease Control and Prevention. *Parasites—Scabies*. Retrieved Oct 2, 2016, from https://www.cdc.gov/parasites/scabies/index.html; 2010.

30. Tunkell A. *Clinical Features and Diagnosis of Acute Bacterial Meningitis in Adults*. Retrieved from UpToDate: http://www.uptodate.com; 2016.

31. Takada S, et al. Meningococcemia in adults: A review of the literature. *Intern Med*. 2016;55(6):567-572.

32. Hodges K, Gill R. Infectious diarrhea. *Gut Microbes*. 2010;1(1):4-21.

33. Casburn-Jones A, Farthing MJ. Management of infectious diarrhea. *Gut*. 2004;53(2):296-305.

34. Wanahita A, et al. Clostridium difficile infection in patients with unexplained leukocytosis. *Am J Med*. 2003;115(7):543-545.

35. Bobulsky G, et al. Clostridium difficile skin contamination in patients with C. difficile-associated disease. *Clin Infect Dis*. 2008;46(3):447-453.

36. Ott J, et al. Global epidemiology of hepatitis B virus infection: new estimates of age-specific HBsAg seroprevalence and endemicity. *Vaccine*. 2012;30(12):2212-2219.

37. Lok A. *Clinical Manifestations and Natural History of Hepatitis B Virus Infection*. Retrieved Dec 8, 2016, from UpToDate: http://www.uptodate.com; 2015.

38. Cacoub P, et al. Extrahepatic manifestations associated with hepatitis C virus infection. A prospective multicenter study of 321 patients. *Medicine (Baltimore)*. 2000;79(1):47-54.

39. The National Institute for Occupational Safety and Health. *Stop Sticks Campaign*. Retrieved Dec 7, 2016, from https://www.cdc.gov/niosh/stopsticks/sharpsinjuries.html; 2011.

40. Strasser M, et al. Risk of hepatitis C virus transmission from patients to healthcare workers: a prospective observa. *Infect Control Hosp Epidemiol*. 2013;34(7):759-761.

41. Sterling T, et al. General clinical manifestations of human immunodeficiency virus infection. In: Mandell GJ, et al, eds. *Principles and Practice of Infectious Diseases*. 7th ed. Philadelphia, PA: Churchill Livingstone/Elsevier; 2010.

42. Baggaley R, et al. Risk of HIV-1 transmission for parenteral exposure and blood transfusion: a systematic review and meta-analysis. *AIDS*. 2005;20(6):805-807.

26

Heat- and Cold-Related Emergencies

VAHÉ ENDER AND RENEÉ SEMONIN HOLLERAN

COMPETENCIES

1. Describe thermoregulation and mechanisms of heat loss.
2. Define mild, moderate, and severe hypothermia.
3. Identify methods to prevent heat loss during patient transport.
4. Identify risk factors that contribute to heat-related illnesses.
5. Identify the different types of heat-related illnesses, including heat exhaustion and heatstroke.
6. Initiate the appropriate management of a heat-related illness in the transport environment.

Regardless of the climate prevalent in their region of clinical practice, transport professionals must be familiar with heat- and cold-related emergencies. Emergency responders working in some of the warmest climates will encounter hypothermia in their clinical practice, just as heat-related illness can be found in patients living in the most frigid of climates. Additionally, the resulting loss of thermoregulation seen in critical illness and injury can have a life-changing impact on the outcomes of patients. As such, it is essential to be aware of these syndromes to maximize the chance of survival of the critically ill patient.

The true toll of heat- and cold-related illness is unclear, yet a look back in history shows evidence of its impact on mankind. Extreme heat and cold has been linked to wars lost, as seen during the crusades in the Middle East. During the Battle of Hattin, the crusaders led by King Guy fell to the Muslim armies under Sultan Saladin. Heat exhaustion and dehydration pushed the invading forces to failure so that heavily armored knights of the crusade forces deserted their posts and sought for mercy at the hand of Saladin's armies. With every great narrative of human exploration and exploit is a story of the battle against temperature extremes, as with the bitter cold encountered by the men with Sir Earnest Shackleton. Cold has shaped history, as is seen in Hitler's failed advance on the Russian front during the Second World War, during which the technologically superior German forces (ill prepared for the winter) were defeated by the ill-equipped but veteran winter warriors of the Russian army.

Yet the toll of temperature extremes is not solely something of the past. As recently as 2003, 52,000 Europeans, predominantly the elderly, were killed by a heat wave. During the peak of this heat, almost 2000 Europeans were dying daily.[1]

Epidemiology

It is the most vulnerable patient populations who are at the highest risk of environmental injury. With age comes the progressive onset of cardiovascular and neurologic disorders, which affect one's ability to sense changes in temperature. Although the human nervous system is highly sensitive to small changes in temperature, with age comes a loss of sensory acuity. As such, an older person will not sense rising or falling core body temperatures as quickly. Additionally, underlying disease or prescribed medications can suppress intrinsic thermoregulatory mechanisms at a cutaneous and vascular level. People 75 years and older are estimated to have a five times greater chance of death from hypothermia than those younger than 75 years.[2]

One of the primary sources of body heat originates from skeletal muscle. Sarcopenia, the loss of muscle mass that comes with age, leads to a fundamental disadvantage in responding to dropping core body temperatures because of impaired shivering. Complicating the matter further is the significant effects of medications routinely prescribed to the elderly, including the subsequent interactions seen with polypharmacy. Table 26.1 lists some medicines that can affect thermoregulation and accentuate the risk of heat-related illness during hot weather. Finally, financial difficulties increasingly faced by the elderly who are no longer able to work leads to a heightened risk of exposure to temperature extremes within their homes. It is common for emergency medical services (EMS) to respond to the homes of the elderly to find near frigid temperatures inside during the winter months.

TABLE 26.1   Medications Affecting Thermoregulation

Drug Type	Example
Tricyclic antidepressants	Amitriptyline, doxepin
Selective serotonin reuptake inhibitors	Citalopram, fluoxetine, sertraline
Serotonin and noradrenaline reuptake inhibitors	Venlafaxine
Anticonvulsants	Gabapentin, pregabalin
Antipsychotics: typical and atypical	Haloperidol, risperidone
Antihypertensives: β-blockers and angiotensin-converting enzyme inhibitors	Atenolol, amlodipine, HCTZ, valsartan
Diuretics	Lasix, HCTZ
Benzodiazepines	Clonazepam, lorazepam, diazepam
Opioids	Morphine, oxycodone, hydromorphone
Medicines with anticholinergic effects	Diphenhydramine, benztropine

HCTZ, Hydrochlorothiazide.

From Westaway K. et al. Medicines can affect thermoregulation and accentuate the risk of dehydration and heat-related illness during hot weather. *J Clin Pharm Ther.* 2015;40(4):363-367.

Adipose tissue acts as an effective insulator from the cold; unfortunately, the lack of vascularity found in adipose causes it to counter attempts by the human body to cool through vasodilation. As such, the obese population is at a higher risk for heat-related injury. The additional weight of adipose tissue against the thorax and diaphragm leads to an impaired ability for the obese patient to match the increased respiratory workload associated with high metabolic rates during exposure to hot environments.

Infants and neonates are particularly vulnerable to heat- and cold-related illnesses. Because of a large head-to-body proportion and less tissue insulation compared with adults, a child's body temperature increases three to five times faster than an adult's. Additionally, poor motor development leads to infants and newborns being unable to sense and respond to temperature changes and more importantly, seek protection.

This same challenge is encountered in populations in which substance use or socioeconomic factors create limited access to water, shelter, and temperature-controlled environments, making them vulnerable during temperature extremes.

Boaters, campers, sailors, hikers, anglers, mountaineers, and other outdoor people are at risk for environmental injury. Generally, such people are healthy but become victims of the environment, physical exhaustion, or their own carelessness. Outdoor hypothermia is categorized into two groups: immersion and nonimmersion. Examples of nonimmersion hypothermia include exposure to wind, rain, snow, and freezing temperatures. Immersion hypothermia occurs more rapidly than nonimmersion hypothermia; heat loss is 35% higher if the patient swims or treads water rather than stays still.[3,4] A person with immersion hypothermia may drown sooner because the level of consciousness decreases at 30°C.

Methods of Thermal Exchange and Loss

Under normal conditions, 90% of the heat produced by the body is lost to the environment via the skin surface by conduction, radiation, convection, and evaporation. Conduction together with convection each account for 15% of heat loss.[5] *Conduction* occurs when the body comes into direct contact with a thermal conductor. Examples of good conductors are water, snow, metal, and damp ground. Normally, conduction plays a minor role in heat transfer, but it is an important factor when the patient has been immersed in cold water, is lying in a snowbank, or is lying on hot asphalt. Heat loss in water is approximately 24 times faster than heat loss in air of the same temperature.[3,4] Immersion in water in temperatures less than 10°C causes hypothermia in only a few minutes,[6] in contrast to more than an hour in air.[7]

Environmental temperature has a direct effect on the patient. The higher the temperature is, the more external heat is present. When the environmental temperature is equal to or greater than the body's temperature, passive heat loss through conduction and radiation is decreased. *Radiant heat loss,* which makes up 45% of total heat loss, occurs when the ambient temperature is lower than the body's temperature; conversely, the body readily absorbs radiant heat from the environment.

When air or water moves across the body surface, heat is lost via *convection.* An increase in the amount of air moving over the skin (forced convection) increases the amount of heat loss. The drier the air, the better the skin surface-to-air gradient, and the more heat that is lost.

The primary mechanism for heat dissipation is the *evaporation* of sweat, which makes up 25% of heat loss. Through vaporization from the body surface, a loss of 1 mL of sweat reduces body heat load by 1.7 kcal.[1,8-14] Under conditions of high ambient temperature and high ambient humidity, the skin is unable to provide effective cooling as the evaporation gradient is lost. At 75% humidity, evaporation decreases; at 90% to 95% humidity, evaporation ceases.[8]

It is in cases in which the ability of the human body to cool or warm is inhibited by illness and/or overwhelmed by the environment that injury occurs.

Heat-Related Illness

Pathophysiology of Heat-Related Illness

The human body is in a constant state of strict thermoregulation, tightly maintaining a core body temperature of 36°C to 38°C, all while being exposed to temperatures ranging from the bitter cold of the winter to the scorching heat of summer. The hub of thermoregulation is the hypothalamus. Deeply nestled within the brain, this almond-sized structure serves as a control center for the most essential parts of the human body, including body core temperature. Input from cutaneous, gastric, and neuronal sensors send stimulus through neurotransmitters and hormones to keep the body within a tight temperature range of $\pm 0.6°C$.

Heat Production

Intrinsic heat production is a by-product of the most fundamental metabolic process in the human body—glycolysis. The muscles of the skeletal system along with major organs such as the liver generate significant amounts of the total body heat during their basic cellular functions. In an average-sized adult male, approximately 1700 kcal are produced daily, although this can increase significantly to nearly twice that with even light to moderate physical activity.[8-10] This generation of heat can also be increased through intrinsic pathways, such as a response to infection or injury.

Fever is an endogenous source of heat caused by an elevation in our thermal "set point" most often as a response to bacteria or viruses that release pyrogens. These stimulate prostaglandin synthesis within the anterior hypothalamus. Fever can also be seen frequently as a response to major illness and injury such as postcardiac arrest syndrome or traumatic head injury, in which fundamental thermoregulatory mechanisms are disrupted. The mechanism for hyperthermia in heat injury differs from fever, because the human thermal set point remains normal in cases of exposure, which is why antipyretics are not an effective means of decreasing core body temperature in heat-injury victims.

This intrinsic heat production can be increased by agents such as illicit drugs, particularly stimulants acting as sympathomimetics including cocaine, amphetamines, and MDMA. Additionally, with the rising use of novel drugs such as synthetic cathinones and K2/Spice, EMS are increasingly encountering patients with drug-induced hyperthermia. In 2011 Coffee County EMS cared for close to 1500 victims of heat-illness while at the Bonnaroo Music and Arts Festival in Tennessee. Some of these cases, complicated by drug and alcohol use, required aeromedical evacuation.[15]

Finally, many over-the-counter medications and prescription drugs affect the body's ability to regulate temperature. Drugs with even mild anticholinergic properties inhibit the activation of sweat glands by sympathetic inhibition, impairing one of the primary mechanisms for thermal regulation. Of particular concern are drugs that cause primary hyperthermic syndromes, as seen with psychiatric drugs such as lithium, tricyclic antidepressants, and drugs associated with serotonin syndrome.

The human body is a veritable power plant. If unchecked by environmental heat loss, at rest, the core body temperature would rise by $1°C/h$ until it would hit the maximal temperature compatible with human life ($43°C$). Under maximal exertion, core body temperature would rise by an astonishing $5°C/h$ if there were no compensatory mechanisms to cool the human body.

Heat Loss

Thermal loss caused by the environment provides the human body with a fundamental means of offsetting its intrinsic heat generation. Heat loss primarily occurs through the conduction of heat from the warm body to the cooler ambient environment. Thick clothing acts as a barrier for the essential evaporative processes needed for cooling because of retained humidity and heat. High environmental humidity also acts as a virtual barrier for this because it decreases the skin surface-to-air gradient.

On exposure to a warm environment, the body will attempt to shift blood toward the periphery to maximize heat exchange, promoting heat loss. This change in hemodynamics results in a decrease in systemic vascular resistance and a correlated increase in cardiac output. This increases myocardial workload and oxygen demand. Although this hyperdynamic state can be well tolerated in the young, patients with underlying cardiovascular disease are placed at increased risk for myocardial injury. It is not uncommon to see rises in cardiac biomarkers in the elderly heatstroke victim as a result of this. Twelve-lead electrocardiograms (ECGs) can reveal nonspecific ST segment changes that resolve following supportive care and cooling measures.

With an increase in cooling through evaporation, predictable decreases are seen in available circulating blood volume. In severe heat stress, the body loses as much as 1.5 L/h, and even 3 L/h in extreme cases.[16,17] This leads to a progressive state of hypovolemia, which if left uncorrected, leads to a progressive cascade of injury. Hypotension is usually a sign of severe or premorbid heat illness.[16,17]

The respiratory system adapts to this hyperdynamic state by increasing respiratory rates, which leads to an increase in insensible losses of volume through the exhalation of warm, humid gases into the hot air. Metabolically, a respiratory alkalosis is caused by hypocarbia.

Ataxia, dysmetria, and dysarthria may be seen early in the onset of heatstroke because the Purkinje cells of the cerebellum are particularly sensitive to the toxic effects of high temperatures. Because these changes are seen in other neurologic events, such as stroke, heatstroke may not be recognized initially. Cerebral edema combined with associated diffuse petechial hemorrhage is often found in fatal cases.

When the hyperthermic insult is associated with status epilepticus and profound hypotension the energy requirements of the brain increase. This in turn contributes to the spiraling core temperature, increasing up to four times the metabolic rate of the brain. The cerebral vessels dilate maximally; thus the blood flow is dependent on mean arterial pressure. The added effects of dehydration (hypovolemic source) produce a pathophysiologic state conducive to brain death and damage.

Kidney function is altered from the loss of sodium and water in sweat. The kidneys retain sodium causing water retention and the excretion of potassium. Renal dysfunction occurs because of hypovolemia and hypoperfusion. Urinary output drops, and acute renal tubular necrosis may ensue. If sodium losses are of sufficient severity, signs of hyponatremia may appear. A risk of hypokalemia may develop because of the excretion of potassium in the urine.

The liver, which is particularly sensitive to temperature damage, is affected in nearly every case.[18,19] This decrease in function theoretically should aid in heat reduction because the liver is one of the major heat-producing organs. Prothrombin times (PTs) become prolonged.[20,14] Reduced hepatic perfusion caused by shunting of blood to the periphery leads to hypoglycemia in 20% of patients with exertional heatstroke, although its clinical significance is unclear.[21,22] Interestingly, the pancreas is the only organ not damaged by the toxic effects of heat stress.[16]

During heat stress, the gastrointestinal (GI) tract undergoes direct thermotoxicity and relative hypoperfusion because of the shunt of blood to the periphery. Ischemic intestinal ulceration can also occur, which may lead to frank GI bleeding.[16]

Muscle damage is evidenced by rhabdomyolysis. Muscle degeneration and necrosis occur as a direct result of extremely elevated temperatures. Elevated creatine phosphokinase (CPK) values are a diagnostic hallmark of heatstroke because of this rhabdomyolytic process. The release of destructive lysosomal enzymes occurs as a result of extensive skeletal muscle damage. The release of lysosomal enzymes into the circulation may cause widespread capillary injury and lead to disseminated intravascular coagulation (DIC), acute respiratory distress syndrome, and acute renal tubular necrosis.[22]

Stages of Heat-Related Illness

The most common forms of heat illness, from least to most severe, are heat cramps, heat exhaustion, and heatstroke.

Heat Cramps

Heat cramps of heavily exercised muscle occur during and after exercise in a hot environment and are an extreme inconvenience to the patient. These cramps usually occur in trained athletes and in physically fit, acclimatized persons. These persons sweat profusely and characteristically replace sweat losses with water and inadequate amounts of salt. Hyponatremia ensues, which hinders muscle relaxation mechanisms. Usually, the muscles show the fasciculations of fatigue. A slight or moderate rise in CPK enzymes in serum is often observed. This rhabdomyolysis has not been shown to constitute an important clinical problem.[11,17,21] No permanent effects have been shown from heat cramps.

Heat cramps involve exquisitely painful sustained muscular contractions, most commonly involving the muscles of the lower extremity; however, any muscle group in the body can be affected. The patient usually reports heavy exercise in a hot environment, with onset of cramping after rest.

Heat Exhaustion

Heat exhaustion is an ill-defined syndrome that can affect anyone. The brain cannot tolerate core temperatures greater than 40.5°C (104.9°F).[11] The typical victim of heat exhaustion is usually not acclimatized to the environment and has worked in the heat for several days. Both infants and elderly bedridden patients are at higher risk of heat exhaustion because of their impaired ability to dissipate heat and communicate thirst.

Heat exhaustion, if allowed to proceed, results in heatstroke. An essential distinction between the two entities is that cerebral function is unimpaired in persons with heat exhaustion, aside from minor irritability and poor judgment. Body temperatures are lower, and the symptoms are less severe in persons with heat exhaustion.

This syndrome results from loss of water, loss of salt, or both. Pure forms of single loss of either water or sodium are rare. Water-depletion heat exhaustion, which results from inadequate fluid replacement, is more serious and develops in a few hours. Salt-depletion heat exhaustion develops over the course of several days.

Heat exhaustion is largely a manifestation of the strain placed on the cardiovascular system because it attempts to maintain normothermia. With sodium and water loss, the patient becomes dehydrated, tachycardic, and syncopal, with orthostatic hypotension. The patient's temperature is usually less than 38°C to 39°C (100.4°F–102.2°F) and is often normal. The patient retains the ability to sweat, which gives rise to cool clammy skin. Headache and euphoria commonly occur because of dehydration and hypoperfusion. Mental status remains intact, although minor aberrations may be manifested. Flulike symptoms of nausea, vomiting, and diarrhea with muscle cramps may be present. Subjective symptoms include intense thirst, vague malaise, myalgia, and dizziness.

Laboratory values show classic signs of dehydration (elevated hematocrit, blood urea nitrogen [BUN], serum protein, and concentrated urine levels) with hyponatremia and hypokalemia. Liver function enzymes may be elevated. However, these signs may not occur until 24 to 48 hours after the heat injury.[8,11,17]

Heatstroke

Heatstroke is a life-threatening medical emergency in which the body's physiologic heat-dissipating mechanisms fail and body temperature rises rapidly and uncontrollably. The central core temperature exceeds 42°C. At 42°C and above, cellular oxygen demands surpass the oxygen supply, and oxidative phosphorylation is disrupted, which causes cell and organ damage throughout the body. The duration of the hyperthermic episode and the temperature reached may be the single most important factors in patient survival and prognosis.

The resultant damage of such severe hyperthermia has many causes. Central nervous system (CNS) disruption with altered mental status is a key diagnostic criterion in heatstroke. Early in the course of heatstroke, some persons appear confused and show irrational behavior, or even frank psychosis, whereas others become comatose or have seizures. The patient may have hot flushed skin, with or without sweating, vomiting, and diarrhea. Hyperventilation at respiratory rates up to 60 is universally seen. Respiratory alkalosis is often present with tetany and hypokalemia. Pulmonary edema is not uncommon.

The cardiovascular system responds by reaching maximal stroke volume. Because of the shunt through the dilated periphery, tachycardia is the only way to increase cardiac output. Heatstroke results in high output failure, with cardiac output of 20 L or more. Central venous pressure readings are elevated despite hypotension caused by decreased ventricular contractility at temperatures over 40°C. The hyperdynamic state persists even after cooling. The ECG results generally show nonspecific ST-T changes with various atrial and ventricular arrhythmias.[18,23,24]

Blood studies should include arterial blood gas, complete blood cell count, platelets, PT/partial thromboplastin time (PTT), electrolytes, BUN, creatinine, glucose, liver function tests, CPK and lactate dehydrogenase, and a urinalysis. White blood counts of 30,000 to 50,000 are not uncommon. The platelet count and PT/PTT are monitored for onset of hypocoagulability. Hypofibrinogenemia and fibrinolysis may occur and progress to frank DIC.

The muscle enzymes in heatstroke are elevated in the tens of thousands, which is a diagnostic hallmark of heatstroke. Muscle breakdown occurs from direct thermal injury, clonic muscle activity, or tissue ischemia. In exertional heatstroke, CPK levels up to 1,500,000 IU/L have been reported. CPK levels greater than 20,000 IU/L are ominous and indicative of later DIC, acute kidney failure, and potentially dangerous hyperkalemia.[13,16,18,25]

Reduced renal blood flow from shock and dehydration leads to ischemic kidneys. Acute renal failure is seen in 30% of exertional heatstroke cases and up to 53% of exposure cases resulting in heatstroke, and such renal function must be closely observed and treated. Concentration of the urine may lead to accumulation of uric acid and myoglobin, which have the capacity to crystallize in renal tubules. Crystallization may lead to obstructive uropathy and the development of acute tubular necrosis. BUN levels are frequently elevated. Low serum osmolarity, moderate proteinuria, and machine oil appearance of the urine occurs in patients with exertional heatstroke.[13,16,26]

The liver is frequently damaged, and frank jaundice is noted. The development of early jaundice, less than 24 hours after onset, has a worse prognosis than delayed jaundice. The engorged vessels of the GI tract may become ulcerated and hemorrhage massively.

Patterns of Heatstroke Presentation

Heatstroke is manifested in three distinct patterns: classic, exertional, and drug induced. The three essential elements in the diagnosis of heatstroke are exposure to heat stress, internal or external; CNS dysfunction; and increased body temperature greater than 40°C.

Classic heatstroke, which tends to occur in the elderly, the ill, and infants, develops over a period of several days. It often occurs during heat waves and affects persons who do not have access to a cooler environment and fluids. Often, the patient is discovered in bed and is unresponsive. In these cases, the patient has hot, red, or flushed skin; has usually ceased sweating; and is significantly dehydrated.

Initial symptoms of classic heatstroke are similar to those of heat exhaustion: dizziness, headache, and malaise, with progression to frank confusion and coma. Fever, tachycardia, and hypotension are additional presenting signs. These patients also hyperventilate, which gives rise to respiratory alkalosis.

Exertional heatstroke usually occurs in young, fit, but unacclimatized persons who are often male athletes. Many such patients perform in hot and humid weather conditions that prevent adequate dissipation of generated heat. Of these patients, 50% still sweat profusely from the rapid onset; severe dehydration has not yet had time to occur.

Exertional heatstroke has a prodrome of chills, nausea, throbbing pressure in the head, and piloerection on the chest and upper arms. Concentration wanes; a subjective sense of physical deterioration is noticed; and the person feels increasingly hot, with decreased sweat production. Paresthesia is noted in the hands and feet.

Onset of irrational behavior then occurs. The face turns ashen gray, and the skin may feel relatively cool if sweat is still being produced. This effect is followed by seizures and collapse. Patients who have exertional heatstroke often have severe metabolic acidosis from anaerobic metabolism related to muscle exertion and volume depletion. They also have significant rhabdomyolysis.[1,27,28]

Intervention and Treatment
Priorities

The most critical goal and life-saving measure in heat illness is cooling the patient to rapidly decrease body temperature. Immediate treatment often leads to prompt recovery. The more rapid the cooling, the lower the risk of mortality. Morbidity and mortality are directly related to the duration and intensity (temperature maximum) of hyperthermia.

While the patient is cooled as rapidly as possible, maintenance of the ABCs of emergency care must not be forgotten. Because the patient may not have the ability to protect the airway, the transport team must effectively ventilate the lungs, oxygenate the blood, and maintain an adequate circulatory volume with an intact pump while performing continuous assessments.

Interventions: Mild to Invasive

Cooling can be accomplished in the prehospital setting first by removing the patient from the hot environment and especially away from hot surfaces, such as concrete and pavement, even if no shaded area is nearby. The transport team should remove the patient's clothing and wet down the patient.

Covering the patient with cool fluid and increasing the movement of air over the patient enhance heat loss by increasing the evaporative gradient. The transport team should open the windows of the ambulance or make use of the air circulation of helicopter rotors during transport to further increase air movement over the patient. In one study of three cases of heatstroke, the patients were sprayed with lukewarm water while they were exposed to the downwash of a helicopter's rotors.[9,29,30]

Heat cramps constitute a mild form of heat illness. Treatment consists of removal from the source of heat, rest, and fluid and electrolyte replacement. Oral replacement should be started by having the patient drink a balanced electrolyte solution. If oral intake is contraindicated, 1000 mL of normal saline solution is administered intravenously (IV) over a 1- to 3-hour period. Mild forms of heat exhaustion are treated in a similar manner. If the patient's body temperature is elevated, the transport team should cool the skin with fans and cool compresses.[12,22,27,30,31]

More severe cases of heat exhaustion necessitate parenteral rehydration. Laboratory values (renal electrolytes, BUN, and hematocrit) are best used to guide replacement. Fluid is titrated to cardiovascular status. Normal saline solution, half-normal saline solution, and dextrose half-normal saline solution have all been used; no evidence exists of a clear superiority of any one of these fluids.[32] In 12 hours, patients generally feel well, have normal vital signs, and can be discharged without sequelae.

Heat exhaustion must be regarded on a continuum from the mild case, treated with simple cooling measures, to the severe case, which progresses to full-blown heatstroke. The most important treatment for heat illness is recognition of the hyperthermic insult and rapid initiation of cooling.

Controversy surrounds the question of which method is ideal for cooling the patient with heatstroke. Several methods are considered to be of therapeutic benefit. Packing the patient in ice and immersing the body in cold water are historic methods of cooling. However, ice water baths may cause peripheral vasoconstriction, which will inhibit cooling of the core. Additionally, decreased cutaneous blood flow and capillary sludging promotes DIC. Furthermore, ice water may cause a shivering response, which is a heat-producing mechanism. Cold water enemas have been suggested and may help decrease core body temperature; however, they are usually not necessary.[25,33]

The primary means of cooling measures in heatstroke revolve around promoting heat loss through conductive and convective heat loss. Using room-temperature water evaporated from the victim's skin with circulating air from a fan can effectively promote heat loss. Additionally, ice packs placed in areas of maximum heat transfer (neck, axillae, and inguinal area) may also be used with caution. The patient's skin must be closely monitored for injury from the ice packs.

Cooling measures should be ceased when body core temperature reaches 39°C (102°F) to avoid overshoot. Because of altered thermoregulatory mechanisms, the core temperature will continue to fall to the normal range without further intervention.[19]

Refractory hyperthermia necessitates more aggressive invasive methods. Ice water gastric lavage has been reported to be effective both in a controlled canine model[32] and in actual victim treatment.[16,34] Gastric lavage has the advantages of rapid cooling and effective use of readily available equipment. Iced peritoneal lavage, hemodialysis, and cardiopulmonary bypass (CPB) have been used as "rescue" measures in severely refractory cases.[14,17,23] These increasingly invasive operative methods require a great commitment of resources and have higher degrees of risk and complication rates. The value of critical care teams becomes more apparent in their ability to bring these critically ill patients to appropriate centers that might be able to institute these therapies.

Transport Care

Heatstroke presents a complex patient management picture. If, when the transport team arrives, cooling measures have not been implemented or need augmentation, institution of the previously discussed interventions must be of the highest priority. Therapy is best guided by invasive thermometry because tympanic and cutaneous thermometers have wide margins of error, especially at the extremes of body temperatures. Placement of an esophageal or urinary catheter with the ability to monitor temperature is essential to the care of these patients. As in any life-threatening case, a secured airway, institution of oxygenation, ventilation, and stabilization of cardiovascular status are mandated.

Endotracheal intubation is indicated for any exposure patient who has a depressed sensorium because of the risk of emesis, aspiration, and airway obstruction. Resuscitation before rapid-sequence induction may be necessary to decrease the risk of hemodynamic collapse. The combination of volume depletion and the vasoplegic effects of anesthetics requires a cautious approach. A systolic blood pressure of 90 mm Hg may be a reasonable preanesthesia goal, as the literature suggests an associated decreased risk of postintubation cardiac arrest.[35] Induction agents used should be tailored to the patient's hemodynamic state. Following intubation, careful attention should be paid to heatstroke patients requiring mechanical ventilation. Because of their hypermetabolic state, a higher minute ventilation should be preserved to avoid worsening acidosis. Patients with heatstroke are often hypotensive because of dehydration and the physiologic compensation of extreme vasodilation. In most cases, the hypotension responds to cooling. Large amounts of fluids and inotropic agents are needed only when cooling results in no response.

In patients with normotensive conditions or in whom hypotension is readily resolved with cooling, normal saline solution is most often recommended; however, fluid choice should be made in consultation with medical expertise.[23] Vasoactive medications may need to be initiated for vascular support when fluid resuscitation is not effective. Because of complications of impaired cardiac function, pulmonary edema, congestive heart failure, adult respiratory distress syndrome, and acute kidney failure, fluid replacement should be guided by physical examination and the use of ultrasound. Field guidelines for fluid replacement recommend infusion of normal saline solution until a systolic blood pressure of 90 mm Hg is obtained.[18] Solutions that contain glucose should generally be avoided to maximize absorption.[25]

In the light of the axiom that "the best defense is a good offense," monitoring the patient for multiple organ failure and prompt intervention of clinical manifestation of such failure are of the utmost importance. Placement of a gastric tube accomplishes gastric decompression and monitors for the onset of GI bleeding. To protect the GI tract administer gastric protectants such as sucralfate in a slurry (1 g/10 mL water q 8 h) and consider antibiotics to prevent sepsis from bacterial translocation and GI mucosal damage.[25]

An indwelling urinary catheter should be inserted to monitor hourly urinary output and rhabdomyolysis. Because of the possibility of kidney impairment, the transport team must closely monitor and support kidney function. If urine output becomes more than 1 mL/kg after the patient is well hydrated, consider mannitol, dopamine, and furosemide IV bolus followed by 1 mg/kg/h infusion. After urine flow is initiated, fluid therapy should be continued at two to three times maintenance levels and titrated off.[25]

Liver failure is a frequent complication of heatstroke. When liver failure is combined with kidney failure, the choice of drugs used in treatment becomes difficult. DIC occurs in severe cases; most patients who die of heatstroke have evidence of DIC.[11] Standard treatment measures are instituted.[13] For prevention of DIC, administer heparin at 200 to 250 units/kg every 8 hours subcutaneously.[18]

Electrolyte and acid-base imbalances may be manifested. Patients with low serum glucose levels are treated with glucose administration. Hyperkalemia and hypokalemia are common. Hypokalemia with respiratory alkalosis is transient and needs no treatment; hypokalemia with acidosis necessitates replacement therapy.[1,9] Hyperkalemia reflects cellular damage and acidosis.[14] Administer potassium chloride for hypokalemia correction at a rate of no more than 0.5 mEq/kg per hour. Sodium bicarbonate may have to be given for severe metabolic acidosis (pH $\leqq 6.9$). Sodium bicarbonate (0.3 × body weight [kg] × base deficit IV) should be given at 50% calculated dose, with subsequent blood gas determinations.[25]

Monitor ECG for arrhythmias. Seizures are treated with benzodiazepines. Use of prophylactic treatment has been considered because seizures may increase heat production, metabolic acidosis, and hypoxia. The neurologic status should be reevaluated constantly. If it deteriorates, consider mannitol (1 g/kg IV) or hypertonic saline and repeat corticosteroids every hour.[25]

Summary of Heat-Related Illness

Heat illness presents as a continuum from mild to severe. Heat exhaustion, if untreated, may proceed to frank heatstroke, which is a life-threatening medical emergency. Causes of heat illness encompass endogenous, environmental, and drug-related pathologies.

Prompt recognition of the problem and rapid cooling limit the severe sequelae associated with heat toxicity. Various cooling methods are used to limit the duration of exposure to hyperthermia. Research shows the length of exposure and maximum temperature reached are two critical criteria in the survival and recovery of patients with heatstroke.

Complications of heatstroke affect every organ system and can lead to multiple organ system failure. Liver and kidney failure are common. Neurologic complications are usually rare with prompt cooling to achieve euthermia. Cerebellar effects are the residual pathologies most often seen.

The onset of DIC, coma lasting more than 8 hours, cardiac dysfunction, hypotension, and high lactate and CPK levels are ominous signs and are usually predictive of mortality.

Cold-Related Injury

On May 20, 1999, Anna Bagenholm, a Norwegian surgical resident, and a friend set out into the Norwegian mountains for a day of skiing. During a descent she lost her balance and subsequently fell through a sheet of ice head first. Her body, trapped under an 8-inch layer of ice, was exposed to the frigid glacial waters. Although she was initially able to survive by breathing in an air pocket, she went into cardiac arrest while rescue teams fought to free her from the ice. By the time she was pulled out of the cold water, she had been trapped for 80 minutes. Worse yet, she had been pulseless for 40 minutes. Resuscitation was started and she was emergently flown to Tromso University Hospital, which was a leading center in the use of CPB for hypothermia. Following cannulation and placement onto bypass, she was rewarmed until her heart beat for the first time in over 2 hours. She was stabilized over 9 subsequent hours, and survived a complex Intensive Care Unit course. Today, she works as a radiologist at the very same hospital that saved her life. Anna Bagenholm is on record as having one of the lowest body temperatures ever recorded in a survivor of hypothermia at 13.7°C.

Hypothermia, defined as a core body temperature of less than 35°C, occurs because the body can no longer generate sufficient heat to maintain body functions.[6] *Accidental hypothermia,* in contrast to iatrogenic hypothermia, is the unintentional decrease in core temperature associated with trauma or exposure to the environment.[36,37,38-40] Core body temperature can be measured in the rectum, the esophagus, the tympanic membrane, or the bloodstream. Rectal thermometers provide the least reliable measurement of core body temperature. Esophageal thermometry is the most reliable.[41]

Classification

Hypothermia can be both a clinical symptom and a disease.[42] It can be classified as *primary*, with simple environmental exposure in a healthy person, or *secondary*, with hypothermia as a part of a disease process or caused by a predisposing condition.[42] Multiple predisposing factors can place a person at risk of hypothermia. Age, diseases, medications, and type and length of exposure can all contribute to the development of hypothermia. The transport environment can especially place a patient at risk for hypothermia from loss of clothing, wet clothing, lack of protection from the environment, medications, diseases and injuries, and lack of environmental control within the transport vehicle itself.[39,43-46] See Box 26.1.

Hypothermia is classified into four stages. *Mild hypothermia* is defined as a core body temperature greater than 32°C and less than 35°C (90°F–95°F) and is associated with low morbidity and mortality rates. The patient may display symptoms of ataxia, slurred speech, apathy, and even amnesia. Thermoregulatory mechanisms continue to operate.[47] *Moderate hypothermia* occurs when the core body temperature is greater than 28°C but less than 32°C (82°F–90°F). Thermoregulatory actions such as shivering continue but begin to decrease and eventually fail. The patient's level of consciousness continues to decrease, and cardiac arrhythmia may develop. *Severe hypothermia* is defined as a core body temperature of 28°C (82°F) or less and is associated with higher morbidity and mortality rates.[37,48-50] *Profound hypothermia* occurs at a temperature of 20.0°C to 9.0°C (68.0°F–48.2°F).[46] These zones and characteristics are summarized in Table 26.2.

In circumstances where core body temperature cannot readily be measured, a simplified approach to hypothermia staging has been developed. With an emphasis on clinical symptoms rather than set temperatures, the Swiss Staging of Hypothermia provides a rapid means of approximating the extent of hypothermia in a victim. This may be helpful as an initial tool in the early stages of the management of such a patient, prior to invasive thermometry being placed. This staging criteria and their respective recommended treatments are shown in Table 26.3.

Physiologic Response to Hypothermia[6,31,38,51-56]

The hypothalamus is sensitive to temperature changes as small as 0.5°C.[5] Stimuli sent from the hypothalamus to the sympathetic nervous system increase heart rate and dilate muscle blood vessels to increase heat production. In addition, shivering generates heat by increasing muscle activity. At the same time, cutaneous vasoconstriction reduces heat loss by shunting blood from the periphery to the core.[7,57-64]

The ability to shiver is affected by hypoglycemia, hypoxia, fatigue, alcohol, and drugs. Shivering is the body's main mechanism of heat production and its strongest defense against hypothermia. However, shivering requires increased blood flow to peripheral muscles. Preshivering increases heat production by 50% to 100%. Visible shivering increases heat production by 500%. An average 70-kg person produces about 100 kcal/h of heat under basal conditions and up to 500 kcal/h when shivering.[6] This degree of heat production, however, cannot be sustained for long because the patient becomes fatigued once glycogen stores are depleted. Maximal shivering occurs at 35°C and stops below 32°C. Cessation of shivering when paired with unconsciousness is a sign that the patient has made the transition from moderate to severe hypothermia.[65]

Hypothermia results when the thermoregulation system becomes overwhelmed or damaged centrally at the hypothalamic level or systemically by a decrease in heat production or an increase in heat loss. Thermoregulation is disrupted at the hypothalamic level by head trauma, cerebral neoplasm, cerebrovascular accident, acute poisoning, acid-base imbalance, Parkinson's disease, and Wernicke's encephalopathy. Acute spinal injury can eliminate vasoconstrictive control by the hypothalamus. Heat production is decreased by malnutrition, hypothyroidism, hypopituitarism, and rheumatoid arthritis. Normally, 90% of the heat produced by the body is lost to the environment by way of conduction, convection, radiation, and evaporation.

Metabolic Derangements

Complications of hypothermia result mainly from the sequelae of *metabolic derangements*. Initially, metabolism increases to generate heat. Optimal metabolism begins to decrease at 35°C. Symptoms of mild hypothermia consequently include shivering, hypoglycemia, and increased respiratory rate, heart rate, and cardiac output. A dramatic decrease in metabolic rate occurs between 30 and 33°C as the patient makes the transition from moderate to severe hypothermia. Every 10°C decrease in temperature decreases metabolism by half.[6] At 28°C, all thermoregulation ceases. The metabolic functions of the liver also begin to falter at temperatures below 33°C. The liver no longer efficiently metabolizes fats, proteins, and carbohydrates or drugs, alcohol, and lactic acid. Symptoms of severe hypothermia

---

• BOX 26.1 Predisposing Factors for Hypothermia

Diabetes
Malnutrition
Hemorrhagic shock
Stroke
Thermal injuries
Elderly
Infants
Emergency childbirth
Environmental exposure
Immersion in cold water
Fluid resuscitation with cold infusions
Aircraft frame
Failure to remove wet clothing
Lack of environmental control in the transport vehicle

Modified from Danzl D: Accidental hypothermia. In Auerbach P, editor: *Wilderness Medicine*, 5th ed. St. Louis, MO: Mosby; 2007.

TABLE 26-2   Physiologic Changes Related to Temperature

Degrees Celsius	Degrees Fahrenheit	Characteristics
38.0	99.6	Normal rectal temperature
37.0	98.6	Normal oral temperature
Mild		
36.0	96.8	Increased basal metabolic rate in an attempt to balance heat loss, tachycardia, increased cardiac output
35.0	95.0	Shivering at the maximum, usually still responsive, but level of consciousness beginning to decrease, regulatory systems beginning to falter
34.0	93.2	Dysarthria, amnesia, blood pressure still normal, oxyhemoglobin curve begins to shift to the left
32.0	91.4	Heart rate decreases to 50 to 60 bpm, ataxia, poor coordination, apathy, lethargy
Moderate		
32.0	89.6	Vasoconstriction, level of consciousness progressively falls
31.0	87.8	Shivering stops, respirations and blood pressure may be difficult to obtain
30.0	86.0	Mental confusion, delirium, increased muscle rigidity; heart rate and cardiac output begin to decrease, arrhythmias begin to develop (atrial fibrillation)
29.0	84.2	Acidosis, hyperglycemia, metabolic rate decreased by 50%, decreased respirations, bradycardia, decreased stroke volume, decreased cardiac output, pupils dilated, paradoxical undressing
Severe		
28.0	82.4	Hypotension, loss of vasoconstrictive capabilities, ventricular fibrillation if patient handled roughly, increased myocardial irritability
27.0	80.6	Prolonged PR, QRS, and QT intervals; muscle flaccidity; no voluntary movement (appears dead); no pupillary reactions
26.0	78.8	Seldom conscious, areflexia
25.0	77.0	Stuporous, hypoventilation, ventricular fibrillation may appear spontaneously, cerebral blood flow one third of normal, cardiac output 45% of normal
24.0	75.2	Coma, pulmonary edema, respiratory arrest
23.0	73.4	No spontaneous movement, rigor mortis appearance, no corneal reflexes
22.0	71.6	Maximal risk of ventricular fibrillation, 75% decrease in oxygen consumption
21.0	69.8	Apnea
Profound		
20.0	68.0	Pulse is 20% of normal
18.0	64.4	Asystole
10.0	50.0	92% decrease in oxygen consumption

TABLE 26-3   Swiss Staging of Hypothermia

Stage	Clinical Presentation	Typical Core Temperature	Treatment
HT I	Conscious, shivering	32°C–35°C	Warm environment and clothing. Active movement if possible.
HT II	Impaired consciousness, not shivering	28°C–32°C	Cardiac monitoring, minimal and cautious movements, horizontal position and immobilization, full body insulation, active external and minimally invasive rewarming techniques.
HT III	Unconscious, not shivering, vital signs present	24°C–28°C	HT II management PLUS airway management as required; ECMO or cardiopulmonary bypass in cases with refractory cardiac instability.
HT IV	No vital signs	< 24°C	HT II and HT III management plus CPR and guideline-directed cardiac arrest management.

Adapted from Brown DJ et al. Accidental hypothermia. *New Engl J Med*. 2012;*367*;20.

include absence of shivering, hyperglycemia, and decreased respiratory rate, heart rate, and cardiac output. Bowel sounds are decreased, if not absent, as a result of decreased gastric motility and gastric dilation.[50]

Hypoglycemia is associated with chronic mild hypothermia, whereas hyperglycemia is associated with acute severe hypothermia. Long-term shivering depletes glucose and glucose stored in the form of glycogen. Shivering can stop at temperatures greater than 33°C if glucose or glycogen stores are depleted or if insulin is no longer available. Shivering begins again when the core body temperature increases to 32°C if depleted glucose is replaced. Hyperglycemia occurs at temperatures below 30°C because insulin no longer promotes glucose transport into cells once metabolism significantly decreases.[10,11] Hyperglycemia does not occur if glucose and glycogen stores have been previously depleted but not replaced.

Oxygenation and Acid-Base Disorders

The respiratory rate initially increases after sudden exposure to cold but then decreases as body temperature and metabolism decrease.[42] At temperatures above 32°C, ventilation is usually adequate. At 30°C respirations are shallow and difficult to observe. Apnea and respiratory arrest commonly occur at temperatures between 21°C and 24°C. Although carbon dioxide production also decreases to about half the basal level with each 8°C drop in temperature,[46] the decreased respiratory rate is inadequate to effectively excrete CO_2 at a temperature below 33°C. Consequently, respiratory acidosis develops in the hypothermia victim.

Cellular respiration is impaired by the decrease in metabolism, drop in cardiac output, and left shift on the oxyhemoglobin dissociation curve. Hypothermia decreases cardiac output by decreasing heart rate and circulating blood volume and by increasing blood viscosity and peripheral vascular resistance. Blood shifting to the core results in a perceived overhydration, and the body responds by removing the extra volume through diuresis. Prolonged hypothermia also causes plasma to leak from the capillaries, increasing blood viscosity by 2% for every 1°C decline.[42,46]

Hypothermia begins to shift the oxyhemoglobin dissociation curve to the left at 34°C. Oxygen then binds tenaciously with hemoglobin, which results in reduced tissue oxygen delivery. In addition, oxygen consumption is half of normal at 27°C and, at 17°C, falls to one-quarter the normal value.[42,66] Anaerobic metabolism and lactic acid production increase from the combination of decreased cardiac output, oxygen delivery, and oxygen consumption. The increase in lactic acid leads to cardiac arrhythmia and death.

The cardiovascular system is more sensitive to the effects of acid-base disturbances than any other body system. Acidosis is commonly associated with asystole, and alkalosis is associated with ventricular fibrillation.[42,67-69] Hypoventilation and lactic acid production lead to respiratory and metabolic acidosis. Acidosis usually corrects itself once the patient is rewarmed. Hyperkalemia is associated with metabolic acidosis and with muscle damage and kidney failure, which may all be present in the rewarmed hypothermic patient. Iatrogenic respiratory and metabolic alkalosis is difficult to treat and should be avoided.

Central Nervous System

The CNS displays some of the most impressive sequelae in the patient with hypothermia. Complete recovery is possible even after prolonged cardiac arrest. Hypothermia protects CNS integrity and may allow the brain to withstand long periods of anoxia. Cerebral blood flow decreases 6% to 7% for every 1°C decline until 25°C is reached.[42,66] Cerebral oxygen requirements decrease to 50% of normal at 28°C, to 25% of normal at 22°C,[38,68] and to 12.5% of normal at 16°C.[59] Caroline[70] noted that the brain can survive without perfusion for about 10 minutes at 30°C, whereas it can survive for up to 25 to 30 minutes at 20°C.[59] Remarkably, Steinmann[61] noted that at 16°C the brain can survive without oxygen for up to 32 to 48 minutes.[61,62]

Patients with mild hypothermia are clumsy, apathetic, withdrawn, and irritable. Reflexes are hyperactive at temperatures above 32°C. Level of consciousness begins to decrease markedly at 32°C, and patients become lethargic or disoriented and begin to hallucinate. Hypothermia victims even remove jackets, gloves, shoes, and other protective clothing. This reaction is known as *paradoxical undressing* and is often one of the first signs that patients are becoming severely hypothermic. Patients can no longer ascertain whether they are cold.

The cough reflex is absent at decreased temperatures, and aspiration of stomach contents can occur. Coma develops between 28°C and 30°C. At temperatures below 30°C, the pupils dilate and become nonreactive. In addition, corneal and deep tendon reflexes may be absent. The patient with hypothermia must be carefully examined to rule out rigor mortis or death. At temperatures below 20°C, the electroencephalographic results, if they were available, would be flat.[61,62]

Cardiac Arrhythmia

The effects of hypothermia on heart rhythm were noted as early as 1912. Hypothermia was found to produce bradycardia that progressed to asystole.[42,66,71] In 1923, subjects reportedly showed T wave changes on ECGs after drinking 600 mL of ice water.[72,73] Up to 90% of all patients with hypothermia are believed to have some ECG abnormality, including atrial fibrillation, sinus bradycardia, and junctional rhythms.[7,47,74-78]

The heart initially responds to mild hypothermia with an increase in heart rate as a result of sympathetic stimulation; this response is short-lived. Heart rate then decreases to 50 to 60 beats/min at 33°C and to 20 beats/min at lower temperatures.[6,47] Atrial fibrillation with a slow ventricular rate is common at temperatures below 29°C. Okada et al.[79] recently noted that atrial fibrillation was unusual in mild hypothermia (temperature greater than 32°C) and was often observed in moderate (32°C–26°C) and moderately deep (less than 26°C) hypothermia. About half of the cases studied in moderately deep hypothermia remained in sinus, atrial, or junctional rhythm. Atrial fibrillation usually spontaneously converts to sinus rhythm after return to normothermia.[68,79]

Changes in the conduction system begin at 27°C and may be observed as a widened QRS interval and prolonged PR and QT intervals. The Osborne, or J, wave is seen clearly at 25°C. The J wave is described as an extra deflection at the junction of the QRS and ST segments

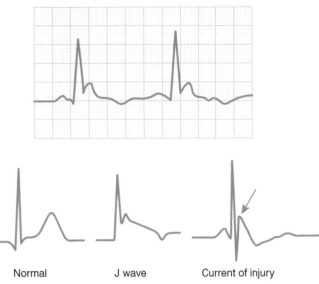

• **Fig. 26.1** Electrocardiographic tracing showing the characteristic J, or Osbourne, wave of hypothermia.

(Fig. 26.1). The origin of the J wave is unknown. According to Okada et al.,[79] the prolongation of the Q-T interval and the presence of J waves are directly related to the severity of the hypothermia. Large J waves are seen at temperatures of less than 30°C, whereas small J waves are seen at higher temperatures.

Several theories have been offered for the presence of J waves in hypothermia. The J wave may represent hypothermia-induced ion fluxes that cause delayed depolarization or early repolarization of the left ventricle. The J wave may also be a hypothalamic or neurogenic factor. J waves may also be seen in patients with CNS lesions or cardiac ischemia, in patients who are septic, or even in young healthy people.[80]

Ventricular irritability, which occurs at temperatures less than 30°C, is commonly associated with alkalosis and is the most lethal cardiovascular response to hypothermia. At 28°C, rough handling, careless intubation, or cardiac compressions can irritate the heart. Ventricular fibrillation can occur spontaneously at 25°C. Unfortunately, arrhythmia at temperatures below 30°C becomes increasingly refractory to drugs and defibrillation because of decreased perfusion and metabolic rate.

Asystole occurs at 20°C but has a surprisingly good prognosis if the patient is rewarmed quickly. Asystole is associated with acidosis and appears to be the primary arrhythmia in accidental hypothermia. Rankin and Rae[81] found that asystole was the terminal rhythm in all 22 patients they studied. Graham et al.[80] found in their study of 73 ECGs that atrial fibrillation and junctional bradycardia were associated with poor outcomes.

Circum-Rescue Collapse

Some years ago, physiologists postulated that the collapse that often occurred after victims were removed from hypothermic situations to warm environments was caused by an afterdrop in core temperature. However, research has shown this belief to be incorrect; the main problem appears to be sudden circulatory changes. This condition is now referred to as *circum-rescue collapse;* it most commonly occurs after rescue from immersion in water.[82]

In the water, an increased hydrostatic pressure around the victim's legs and trunk results in an increase in venous return and an increase in cardiac output. This increase in central volume is sensed as hypervolemia by the body; thus a diuresis and salt loss (natriuresis) occurs. Peripheral vasoconstriction occurs because of the relative cold temperate of the water, even in temperate climates, which results in a further increase in venous return and exacerbation of this response. In this way, the victim's intravascular volume becomes depleted.[4]

One suggested mechanism that leads to circulatory collapse is the stress on the myocardium from increased venous and arterial pressures that result in increased catecholamine release. Coupled with hypoxia, the increase in circulating catecholamines may provoke cardiac dysrhythmias. A second part to the theory is that vertical removal from the water causes both a sudden release in the hydrostatic pressure around the abdomen and legs and a consequent positional venous pooling in the lower limbs and reduced venous return to the heart. The resultant acute decrease in coronary perfusion may provoke ventricular fibrillation or acute myocardial ischemia, causing death.[3,4,82]

Frostnip and Frostbite[75,83]

Frostnip, a superficial form of frostbite usually found on the face, nose, and ears, is manifested by numbness and pallor of the exposed skin. Management consists of warming the area with a warm hand or wrapping or covering the area for protection.

Frostbite results from the cooling of body tissue to the point of ice crystal formation[84] and most often involves the distal extremities. Destruction of the skin produces a more severe injury than frostnip. Although frostbite is commonly associated with below-freezing temperatures, it can be produced at above-freezing temperatures by wind, altitude, humidity, and prolonged exposure and can be exacerbated by impaired vascular integrity and decreased cardiac output.[74,58]

The injury caused by frostbite has been divided into four phases: the prefreeze phase, the freeze-thaw phase, the vascular stasis phase, and the late ischemic phase. This pathophysiology results in cell dehydration and shrinkage, abnormal intracellular electrolyte imbalances, thermal shock, and denaturation of the lipid-protein complexes.[75]

Blood cells "sludge" in the vessels and eventually circulation to the tissue ceases.[75] Frostbite is classified as first, second, or third degree. First-degree injury, superficial freezing without blistering or peeling, is characterized by hyperemia and edema. The tissue becomes mottled, cyanotic, and painful after rewarming. Second-degree frostbite produces blistering or peeling of the skin and is characterized by hyperemia and vesicle or bleb formation. When rewarmed, the

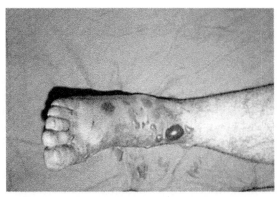

• **Fig. 26.2** Frostbite. (From Sanders MJ. *Mosby's Paramedic Textbook.* 3rd ed. St. Louis: Mosby/JEMS; 2007.)

skin is deep red, hot, and dry to touch. Third-degree frostbite is characterized by death of the dermis and even deeper tissue such as muscle and bone (Fig. 26.2).[83]

Prehospital care focuses on protecting the affected area from trauma and partial thawing. Superficial skin injury can be treated by removing any wet clothing and placing warm dry clothing on the injured area. The affected area should be kept frozen if any possibility of refreezing exists. The area must never be massaged. The patient should not be allowed to walk if the legs are involved unless it is a matter of survival.

Patients should be given ibuprofen and fluids and pain management provided with an appropriate narcotic.[37,75,85] The affected part needs to be carefully immobilized and protected from additional injury. Patients should be transported to a center familiar with the care of frostbite.

Rewarming Techniques[84,86-89]

Expert consensus is that the patient should be rewarmed as quickly as possible because the myocardium is refractory to therapy below 30°C. The three techniques for rewarming are passive external, active external, and active internal. Only passive external, active external, and limited forms of active internal rewarming can be initiated in the air medical setting. Consequently, rapid transportation to a facility that can provide more extensive rewarming techniques is imperative. Transport personnel must be aware of the existence of these facilities in their service areas.

Passive External Rewarming

Passive external rewarming is simple, inexpensive, and easily instituted. It is used only in mild hypothermia and when the patient can generate heat with shivering and vasoconstriction. The patient is placed in a warm environment, covered with blankets, and allowed to rewarm naturally. Careful attention should be paid to removing wet clothing and linens from the patient because it can significantly undermine attempts at rewarming. Passive external rewarming is available in any transport vehicle with the use of a blanket, including foil layers to promote radiant warmth, and a heater. Patients with long-term alcoholism have a lower

mortality rate when passive external rewarming is used. Passive external rewarming increases core body temperature by 1°C/h.[66]

Active External Rewarming

Active external rewarming involves placement of heat on the external surface of the body. Heated blankets, chemical warming pads, and forced air devices such as the Bair Hugger are examples of active rewarming. Devices are also available that circulate warm water around the patient's body. Large electric or chemical heating pads should be placed to come in contact with the axilla, chest, and back, which is where the highest amount of conductive heat transfer takes place.[65,90] It is imperative that precautions be taken when using active rewarming tools to avoid thermal burns; all heating pads should be wrapped in some barrier material such as towels or sheets.

Afterdrop is a phenomenon that can occur in the initial stages of passive and active external rewarming. *Afterdrop* is defined as a decline of 1°C to 2°C in the core body temperature when cool blood from the extremities moves to the core.[7,53,64] Any action that moves blood rapidly from the extremities to the heart, including moving the patient or injudiciously applying heat to the periphery, can cause this phenomenon. As such, active rewarming of the extremities should be avoided especially considering its lack of efficacy. The danger of afterdrop is likely overstated because there is only limited evidence to suggest that afterdrop is clinically significant. Savard et al.[91] suggested a possible explanation for the afterdrop phenomenon: the myocardial irritability of afterdrop is caused by a blood chemical shift and not necessarily from a blood temperature shift.

Active Internal Rewarming

Active internal rewarming delivers heat directly to the body core, avoiding the risk of afterdrop. The heart, lungs, and brain are warmed first and in turn rewarm the rest of the body. Heated oxygen, IV fluids, hemodialysis and peritoneal dialysis, gastric lavage, mediastinal lavage (after thoracotomy), and CPB are all examples of active internal rewarming. The least invasive method of active internal rewarming is used when the patient has severe hypothermia but a stable cardiovascular condition. On the other hand, the most rapid active internal rewarming methods, such as CPB, are recommended if the patient has severe hypothermia and an unstable condition with cardiovascular collapse unresponsive to drugs and defibrillation. The *continuous arteriovenous rewarming* (CAVR) method, developed at the University of Washington, uses a modified bypass technique for rapid blood rewarming with a level one fluid warmer normally used for trauma resuscitation. The treatment is preferred for patients with profound hypothermia. A spontaneous pulse is necessary because the patient's intrinsic blood pressure drives flow through the countercurrent module. (In true cardiothoracic bypass, an external pump is built into the machine.) The catheters are placed into a femoral artery and venous cordis, and the blood is warmed as it flows through the countercurrent module. The CAVR method has rewarmed patients with profound hypothermia five times more rapidly (39 minutes versus 199 minutes) than standard methods and was shown to decrease mortality rate.

Management During Transport

Management of hypothermia has been controversial since Napoleon's chief surgeon, Baron Larrey, noted that hypothermic soldiers closest to the fire were the ones who died.[10] Hypothermia experiments in human subjects can be safely performed only to 35°C, and those in animals are not equivalent because the physiologic response of animals to hypothermia is different from that of humans. Consequently, current medical management of the patient with hypothermia is based mainly on anecdotal reports in the literature.

All patients with hypothermia should be transported, regardless of cardiopulmonary status. Using the old adage "A patient is not dead until warm and dead,"[16,47,48] *warm* is defined as 32°C. Severe hypothermia takes priority over any other problem except obstructed airway or major trauma with rapid exsanguination.

Danzl[67] recommended that preparation for the transport of a patient who is hypothermic includes the following:
1. Gentle removal of all wet clothing and application of dry clothing or insulation system.
2. Keeping the patient supine and avoiding massaging of extremities.
3. Stabilization of all injuries, including application of splints and covering of any open wounds.
4. Initiation of IV fluids and administration of a fluid challenge.
5. Active rewarming during transport, which should include heated oxygen and truncal heat. Any heating pack used should be properly insulated to avoid causing burns to the patient. Covering the head with a hat or towels may help rewarming efforts.
6. Wrapping the patient in layers with access available to the airway, breathing, and monitoring equipment. The outermost layer ideally should be windproof to decrease exposure to winds encountered during aeromedical evacuation.

Management of the patient with mild hypothermia is relatively uncomplicated; covering the patient with blankets and allowing the patient to warm naturally prevents further heat loss. Management of the patient with severe hypothermia is more complicated and tests the expertise and knowledge of transport personnel.

Gentle Handling

The patient must be handled gently during transport, and stimulation should be minimized. Any movement, particularly vertical lifting, has been shown to precipitate ventricular fibrillation. As such, patients should be kept supine. Rubbing or massaging the patient is contraindicated. Medical personnel should always cut clothing rather than pull it

off. A patient with mild hypothermia must be kept quiet and not be allowed to assist with rescue.

Prevention of Further Heat Loss

Prevention of further heat loss is paramount in the management of the patient with hypothermia. Limited exposure during assessment prevents heat loss during examination. The patient's wet clothing should be removed immediately to prevent conductive and evaporative heat loss. The patient should be removed or protected from any wind source, including helicopter turbulence, which can produce wind up to 100 mph. Insulated and windproofed blankets should be placed under and over the patient, with the face left exposed and the patient's head protected with a wool hat. The cold railings of the stretcher conduct heat and should not be allowed to touch the patient during transport. The interior of transport vehicles should be warmed, ideally to 24°C. Warm oral fluids should be considered for the conscious patient only after assessment for an active gag reflex. Aspiration can be a problem, especially if the size of the transport vehicle does not permit the patient to sit upright or at least at a 45-degree angle. Beverages containing alcohol are contraindicated.

Active Internal Rewarming

The respiratory tract is a major area of heat exchange and evaporative loss. Administration of warm humidified oxygen effectively rewarms the heart, lungs, and brain by way of the bronchial circulation. In addition, the cilia become more active during rewarming and humidification and can assist in decreasing and mobilizing secretions. Warm humidified oxygen is easy to administer; is safe, relatively effective, and noninvasive; and is available in the air medical setting. Mask or bag-valve apparatus at 42°C to 46°C should administer 100% warm humidified oxygen. The rate of rewarming varies from 0.5°C/h to 2.0°C/h[9] to 3.5°C in 20 minutes.[46] A high flow rate is essential for this method to be effective. Core temperature increases an additional 0.3°C/h by increasing the ventilatory rate by 10 L/min. There are commercial products available.[57,67]

Rehydration of the patient with hypothermia with warm IV fluids increases blood flow to the heart and decreases blood viscosity, vasoconstriction, potential of afterdrop, and the likelihood of cardiac arrhythmias.[66] Patients with hypothermia appear to have a better chance of survival when a bolus of warm IV normal saline solution is given before the patient is moved or externally rewarmed.[66] The transport team should establish an IV line in the largest vein available. If needed, a small amount of heat may be applied to the area to facilitate venous access. The fluid of choice is normal saline, because lactated Ringer's solution is not fully metabolized by the liver in severe hypothermia.[66] An adult patient may be infused with at least 200 mL/h, and the pediatric patient with at least 4 mL/kg/h, with adjustment if the patient needs additional fluid resuscitation. Pulmonary edema, jugular vein distention, and other problems associated with fluid overload are monitored. IV fluids are administered at a temperature of 40°C. Fluids can be warmed en route by wrapping them in an electric blanket or other commercial warming devices. Some transport vehicles now come with environmental drawers that keep fluids warm during transport. Fluids can additionally be warmed during administration through the use of commercially available devices, which include a heating core through which infusing fluids pass. These battery-powered portable devices provide an effective means of warming fluids to a temperature of 38°C during transport.

Monitoring Vital Signs

The patient's temperature, heart rate, and respirations should be monitored carefully and on a regular basis. A special thermometer capable of registering to 20°C is necessary for the patient with profound hypothermia. The most accurate means of thermometry is an esophageal thermometer inserted into the lower third of the esophagus, approximately 24 cm for the average adult. The placement of an esophageal probe also avoids the repeated exposure of the patient to obtain temperatures by other means. Both temporal artery and tympanic thermometers frequently used in other health care settings are unreliable for the measurement of temperature in hypothermia and should not be used. Danzl[67] noted that rectal temperature lags behind actual core temperature and is influenced by leg temperature and placement of the rectal probe. Volunteers were placed in freezing cold water for 15 minutes, and all the classic signs of hypothermia were noted. The body was able to compensate and core body temperature remained unchanged for at least 15 to 20 minutes.[36,83,87]

Inaccurate assessment of the patient's respirations can lead to improper management and can precipitate life-threatening arrhythmias. The patient must be observed carefully for at least one full minute for the presence of respirations to be determined. A spontaneous respiratory rate of 4 to 6 beats/min is adequate in hypothermia. An effective cardiac rhythm may be assumed if the patient is breathing spontaneously. Cardiac monitoring may be difficult because of muscle tremors. Baseline oscillations on the ECG may be the only sign that the patient is shivering. Blood pressure may not be obtainable or may be inaccurate because of vasoconstriction.

Cardiac Resuscitation

Cardiac resuscitation in the patient with hypothermia is a controversial topic. The main concern is that chest compressions could be initiated on a patient with a slow but viable rhythm. As such, pulse checks should be performed for a full minute. External cardiac massage on a hypothermic bradycardic heart can precipitate ventricular fibrillation. Established ventricular fibrillation or asystole on the heart monitor is the only indication for prehospital cardiopulmonary resuscitation (CPR) of the patient with severe hypothermia.[69] Maximal amplification should be used on the cardiac monitor to detect QRS complexes.

Some investigators believe that chest compressions should be withheld in any patient with a core temperature of less than 28°C. Adequate evidence supporting these deviations from advanced cardiac life support (ACLS) guidelines for CPR is lacking. Although hypothermia does protect the brain from anoxic damage, this "safe period" has not been established, and brain damage occurs after cardiac arrest unless CPR is started.[59,60] Therefore cardiac compressions should be started according to ACLS guidelines once ventricular fibrillation or asystole is established. If spontaneous respirations are present at any rate, a viable rhythm may be assumed, and CPR may be deferred. Danzl and Pozos[66] proposed that CPR be initiated in all cases except the following: (1) a do-not-resuscitate order is confirmed, (2) obvious lethal injuries are noted, (3) chest-wall compression is impossible, (4) rescuers are jeopardized during evacuation, or (5) signs of life are present. In cases of avalanche rescue, it is reasonable to withhold resuscitative measures for victims who have spent more than 35 minutes with an airway obstructed by snow.[92] Mechanical CPR devices may play a role in the transport of the hypothermic cardiac arrest because these devices offer a safer means of providing compressions in-flight while also minimizing interruptions encountered during litter carries and patient loading procedures. An ultrasound may be of use in assessing the presence of cardiac activity and guide in the resuscitation of the hypothermic patient. The use of end-tidal capnography can also be an adjunct to guide rescuers in resuscitative efforts, but guidelines lack clear evidence to guide its use beyond the monitoring of the intubated patient.

Although defibrillation may not be as effective in profound hypothermia, some studies suggested that efficacy of defibrillation is higher than previously thought. Although defibrillation is generally more successful at 30°C and above, there are case reports of successful defibrillation at temperatures as low as 26°C. It is reasonable to defibrillate ventricular tachycardia/ventricular fibrillation in hypothermia while performing rewarming measures. If core body temperature is below 30°C, deliver a single shock until rewarming has increased core body temperature. Once 30°C has been achieved, standard American Heart Association defibrillation guidelines can be followed.[65]

Pharmacologic Therapy

Little clinical evidence to confirm or rule out the effectiveness or complications of pharmacologic therapy has been noted.[66] Medications should be used with extreme caution. Decreased circulation pools medications in the extremities; a toxic reaction can occur when the patient is rewarmed and medication flows to the core. In light of this possibility, several authors have suggested withholding all medications from the patient with hypothermia.[66] Considering the limited evidence currently available to state otherwise, it is reasonable to consider vasopressors during resuscitation once core temp has reached 30°C. Overzealous resuscitation can precipitate ventricular fibrillation, so dosing intervals should be increased to twice-normal intervals.[92]

Pharmacologic manipulation of pulse, blood pressure, and respiratory rate should be avoided.[66] Medications given during hypothermia can have prolonged mechanism of action caused by decreased metabolic rates, so dosing should be adjusted accordingly. Medications given for the purpose of anesthesia including anesthetics and paralytics should have their doses decreased to the lowest reasonable dose. Medications should not be given orally or intramuscularly because of decreased absorption rates. Other medications should be deferred until the core temperature is 30°C. The administration of vasopressors and other advanced treatments should never undermine rewarming and resuscitative efforts.

Special Considerations

Transport personnel in the management of cold-related emergencies should consider the following principles:

1. Treat major trauma as the first priority and hypothermia as the second.
2. Remove all wet clothing and apply dry blankets as quickly as possible.
3. Notify the receiving facility while en route to the scene, clinic, or hospital to give the receiving facility time to activate appropriate resources.
4. Consider transport to an extracorporeal membrane oxygenation (ECMO)/CPB-capable center.
5. Monitor temperature via esophageal thermometry when feasible.
6. Avoid vasopressors. Consider them only if rewarming shock is unresponsive to fluids.
7. Follow ACLS guidelines and continue CPR until the patient is rewarmed to 32°C.

Summary

The toll of temperature extremes is most felt by the vulnerable, including children and the elderly. These patients pose a particular challenge to transport teams, but fundamentally the care of these patients is focused on correction of core body temperature through escalating levels of intervention. The transport team must have the appropriate equipment to care for the victims of environmental exposure. This includes the equipment necessary to warm or cool the patient while providing protection from the environment. Teams should anticipate multiorgan involvement and provide the appropriate supportive care. A collaborative approach to caring for these patients is paramount, and early notification to receiving hospitals to mobilize therapies such as active rewarming or ECMO can help provide victims of the extreme heat or cold with the best chance of survival.

References

1. Earth Policy Institute. *Setting the Record Straight: More than 52,000 Europeans Died from Heat in Summer 2003*. http://www.earth-policy.org; July 28, 2006.
2. McCauley RL, Killyon GW, Smith DJ, et al. Frostbite. In: Auerbach P, ed. *Wilderness Medicine*. 6th ed. St. Louis, MO: Mosby Elsevier; 2011.
3. Golden FS, Tipton MJ, Scott RC. Immersion, near-drowning and drowning. *Br J Anaesth*. 1997;79(2):214-225.
4. Golden F, Tipton M. *Essentials of Sea Survival*. Champaign, IL: Human; 2002.
5. Giesbrecht G, Steinman A. Immersion in cold water. In: Auerbach P, ed. *Wilderness Medicine*. 6th ed. St. Louis, MO: Mosby Elsevier; 2011.
6. Crawshaw LI, Wallace H, Dasgupta S. Thermoregulation. In: Auerbach P, ed. *Wilderness Medicine*. 5th ed. St. Louis, MO: Mosby; 2007.
7. United States Coast Guard Station. *Hypothermia* UCN 0075. New York: United States Coast Guard; April 5, 1982.
8. Epstein Y, Hadad E, Shapiro Y. Pathological factors underlying hyperthermia. *J Therm Biol*. 2004;29(7):487-494.
9. Hoffman JL. Heat-related illness in children. *Clin Pediatr Emerg Med*. 2001;2:203-210.
10. Holleran RS. *Prehospital Nursing: A Collaborative Approach*. St. Louis, MO: Mosby;1994.
11. Huether SE, Defriez CB. Pain, temperature regulation, sleep and sensory function. In: McCance KL, Huether SE, eds. *Pathophysiology*. 5th ed. St. Louis, MO: Elsevier Mosby; 2007.
12. O'Brien DJ. Heat illness. *J Aeromed Healthcare*. 1985;2:6.
13. Sidman RD, Gallagher EJ. Exertional heat stroke in a young woman: gender differences in response to thermal stress. *Acad Emerg Med*. 1995;2(4):315.
14. Tek D, Olshaker JS. Heat illness. *Emerg Med Clin North Am*. 1992;10(2):299-310.
15. Kavner L. *Bonnaroo Festival Report Tenth Death since 2002*. http://www.huffingtonpost.com; June 14, 2001.
16. Gaffin SL, Hubbard R. Experimental approaches to therapy and prophylaxis for heat stress and heatstroke. *Wilderness Environ Med*. 1996;7(4):312-334.
17. Platt M, Vicario S. Heat illness. In: Marx J, ed. *Rosen's Emergency Medicine Concepts and Clinical Practice*. 8th ed. Philadelphia, PA: Mosby Elsevier; 2013.
18. Gaffin SL, Moran DS. Pathophysiology of heat-related illnesses. In: Auerbach P, ed. *Wilderness Medicine: Management of Wilderness and Environmental Emergencies*. 6th ed. St. Louis, MO: Mosby Elsevier; 2011.
19. Hart LH, Dennis SL. Two hypothermias prevalent in the intensive care unit: fever and heatstroke. *Focus Crit Care*. 1988;15(4):49-55.
20. Bledsoe BE, Benner RW. *Critical Care Paramedic*. Upper Saddle River, NJ: Pearson Prentice Hall; 2006.
21. Centers for Disease Control and Prevention. Heat-related illnesses and deaths—United States, 1994-1995. *MMWR*. 1995;44(25):465-468.
22. Karrimi FA, et al. Adult respiratory distress syndrome and disseminated intravascular coagulation complicating heat stroke. *Chest*. 1986;90(4):571-574.
23. Tomarken JL, Britt BA. Malignant hyperthermia. *Ann Emerg Med*. 1987;16(11):1253-1265.
24. Wagner C, Boyd K. Pediatric heatstroke. *Air Med J*. 2008;27(3):118-122.
25. Hubbard RW, Armstrong LE. Hyperthermia: new thoughts on an old problem. *Phys Sportsmed*. 1989;17(6):97-113.
26. Huether SE, Defriez CB. Pain, temperature regulation, sleep and sensory function. In: Rodway GW, Huether SE, Belden J, eds. *Pathophysiology*. 7th ed. St. Louis, MO: Elsevier Mosby; 2016.
27. Harker J, Gibson P. Heat stroke: a review of rapid cooling techniques. *Intens Crit Care Nurs*. 1995;11(4):198-202.
28. Lee-Chiong TL, Stitt JT. Heatstroke and other heat-related illnesses: the maladies of summer. *Postgrad Med*. 1995;98(1):26-28, 31-33, 36.

29. Lim MK. Occupational heat stress. *Ann Acad Med (Singapore)*. 1994;23(5):719-724.

30. Pouton TJ, Walker RA. Helicopter cooling of heat stroke victims. *Aviat Space Environ Med*. 1987;58(4):358-361.

31. Proehl J. Environmental emergencies. In: Kitt S, ed. *Emergency Nursing*. Philadelphia, PA: Saunders; 1995.

32. Syverud SA, et al. Iced gastric lavage for treatment of heat stroke: efficacy in a canine model. *Ann Emerg Med*. 1985;14(5):424-432.

33. Walter BGB, Callahan CW, Hing M. The first enemy you meet; acclimatization and the mastery of desert heat. *Infantry Magazine*. Nov-Dec, 2004;93(6):10.

34. Moran DS, Gaffin SL. Clinical management of heat-related illnesses. In: Auerbach P, ed. *Wilderness Medicine: Management of Wilderness and Environmental Emergencies*. 5th ed. St. Louis, MO: Mosby Elsevier; 2007.

35. Kim WY, Kwak MK, Ko BS, et al. Factors associated with the occurrence of cardiac arrest after emergency tracheal intubation in the emergency department. *PLoS One*. 2015;9(11):e112779.

36. Antretter H, Muller LC, Cottogni M, et al. Successful resuscitation in severe hypothermia following near drowning. *Dtsch Med Wochenschr*. 1994;119(23):837-840.

37. Cauchy E, Chetaille E, Marchand V, et al. Retrospective study of 70 cases of severe frostbite lesions: a proposed new classification scheme. *Wilderness Environ Med*. 2001;12(4):248-255.

38. Ehrmantraut WR, Ticktin HE, Fazekras JF. Cerebral hemodynamics and metabolism in accidental hypothermia. *Arch Intern Med*. 1957;99(1):57-59.

39. Frakes M, Duquette L. Body temperature preservation in patients transported by air medical helicopter. *Air Med J*. 2008;27(1):37-39.

40. Jurkovich G, Gaser W, Luterman A. Hypothermia in trauma victims: an ominous sign. *J Trauma*. 1987;27(9):1019-1024.

41. Gordon AS. Cerebral blood flow and temperature during deep hypothermia for cardiovascular surgery. *J Cardiovasc Surg (Torino)*. 1962;3:299-307.

42. Collins KJ. *Hypothermia: the Facts*. New York: Oxford University Press; 1983.

43. Gregory J, Flanbaum I, Townsend M. Incidence and timing of hypothermia in trauma patients. *J Trauma*. 1991;31(6):795-800.

44. Gregory RT, Patton JF, Whitby JD, et al. Treatment after exposure to cold. *Lancet*. 1972;1(7746):377-378.

45. Hattfield ML, Lang AM, Han ZQ, et al. The effect of helicopter transport on adult patient's body temperature. *Air Med J*. 1999;18(3):103-106.

46. Hauty M, Esrig B, Long W. Prognostic factors in severe accidental hypothermia: experience from the Mt. Hood tragedy. *J Trauma*. 1987;27(10):1107-1112.

47. Giesbrecht G, Steinman A. Immersion in cold water. In: Auerbach P, ed. *Wilderness Medicine*. 5th ed. St. Louis, MO: Mosby Elsevier; 2007.

48. Arthurs Z, Cuadrado D, Beekley A, et al. The impact of hypothermia on trauma care at the 31st combat support hospital. *Am J Surg*. 2006;191(5):610-614.

49. International Commission of Alpine Rescue, Subcommission of Medicine. Field and base treatment of cold injuries. Presented at the Fifth International Symposium on Mountain Medicine, Innsbruck, Austria: November 13, 1976.

50. Jolly T, Ghezzi K. Accidental hypothermia. *Emerg Med Clin North Am*. 1992;10(2):311-327.

51. Purdue GF, Hunt JL. Cold injury: a collective review. *J Burn Care Rehabil*. 1986;7(4):331-342.

52. Reuler JB. Hypothermia: pathophysiology, clinical settings and management. *Ann Intern Med*. 1978;89(4):519-527.

53. Vaughn PB. Local cold injury-menace to military operations: a review. *Mil Med*. 1980;145(5):305-311.

54. Weast RC. *Handbook of Chemistry and Physics*. 55th ed. Cleveland, OH: CRC Press; 1974.

55. Wilson FN, Finch R. The effect of drinking iced water upon the form of the T deflection of the electrocardiogram. *Heart*. 1923;10:275.

56. York-Clark D, Stocking J, Johnson J. *Flight and Ground Transport Nursing Core Curriculum*. 2nd ed. Denver, CO: Air & Surface Transport Nurses Association; 2006.

57. Slovis CM, Bachvarov HL. Heated inhalation treatment of hypothermia. *Am J Emerg Med*. 1984;2(6):533-536.

58. Smith DS. Accidental hypothermia: giving "dead" victims the benefit of the doubt. *Postgrad Med*. 1987;81(3):38-43, 47.

59. Smith DS. *The Cold Water Connection*. Kingston, Jamaica: First International Hypothermia Conference; January 23-27, 1980.

60. Steinman AM. The hypothermic code: CPR controversy revisited. *JEMS*. 1983;8(10):32-35.

61. Steinmann S, Shackford S, Davis J. Implications of admission hypothermia in trauma patients. *J Trauma*. 1990;30(2):200-202.

62. Tek D, Mackey S. Non-freezing cold injury in a marine infantry battalion. *Wilderness Environ Med*. 1993;4(4):353-357.

63. Tolman KG, Cohen A. Accidental hypothermia. *Can Med Assoc J*. 1970;103(13):1357-1361.

64. Wilkerson JA, Bangs CC, Hayward JS. *Hypothermia, Frostbite and other Cold Injuries*. Seattle, WA: Mountaineers; 1986.

65. Zafren K, Giesbrecht GG, Danzl DF, et al. Wilderness Medical Society practice guidelines for the out-of-hospital evaluation and treatment of accidental hypothermia; 2014 update. *Wilderness Environ Med*. 2014;25(suppl 4):S66-S85.

66. Danzl DF, Pozos RS. Multicenter hypothermia survey. *Ann Emerg Med*. 1987;16(9):1042-1055.

67. Danzl D. Accidental hypothermia. In: Auerbach P, ed. *Wilderness Medicine*. 5th ed. St. Louis, MO: Mosby; 2007.

68. Okada M. The cardiac rhythm in accidental hypothermia. *J Electrocardiol*. 1984;17(2):123-128.

69. O'Keefe KM. Accidental hypothermia: a review of 62 cases. *JACEP*. 1977;6(11):491-496.

70. Caroline NL. *Emergency Care in the Streets*. 2nd ed. Boston, MA: Little, Brown and Company; 1983.

71. Knowlton FP, Starling EH. The influence of variations in temperatures and blood pressure on the performance of the isolated mammalian heart. *J Physiol*. 1912;44(3):206-219.

72. Rango N. Exposure-related hypothermia mortality in the United States, 1970–1979. *Am J Public Health*. 1984;74(10):1159-1160.

73. Rango N. Old and cold: hypothermia in the elderly. *Geriatrics*. 1980;35(11):93-96.

74. Lunardi N. Case review: ED management of hypothermia in an elderly woman. *Austral Emerg Nurs J*. 2006;8(4):165-171.

75. McAniff JJ. *The Incidence of Hypothermia in Scuba-Diving Fatalities*. Kingston, Jamaica: First International Hypothermia Conference; January 23-27, 1980.

76. McCauley RL, Killyon GW, Smith DJ, et al. Frostbite. In: Auerbach P, ed. *Wilderness Medicine*. 5th ed. St. Louis, MO: Mosby Elsevier; 2007.

77. Miller JW, Danzl DF, Thomas DM. Urban accidental hypothermia: 135 cases. *Ann Emerg Med*. 1980;9(9):456-461.

78. White JD. Hypothermia: the Bellevue experience. *Ann Emerg Med.* 1982;11(8):417-424.

79. Okada M, Nishimura F, Yoshiro H. The J-wave in accidental hypothermia. *J Electrocardiol.* 1983;16(1):23-28.

80. Graham CA, McNaughton GW, Wyatt J. The electrocardiogram in hypothermia. *Wilderness Environ Med.* 2001;12(4):232-235.

81. Rankin AC, Rae AP. Cardiac arrhythmias during rewarming of patients with accidental hypothermia. *Br Med J (Clin Res Ed).* 1984;289(6449):874-877.

82. Golden FS, Hervey GR, Tipton Jr MJ. Circum-rescue collapse: collapse, sometimes fatal, associated with rescue of immersion victims. *Nav Med Serv.* 1999;77(3):139-149.

83. Mills WJ, Whaley R. Frostbite: experience with rapid rewarming and ultrasonic therapy. reprinted in Lessons from History. *Wilderness Environ Med.* 1998;9(4):226-247.

84. Lloyd EL. Accidental hypothermia treated by central rewarming through the airway. *Br J Anaesth.* 1973;45(1):41-48.

85. Butler FK, Zafren K. Tactical management of wilderness casualties in special operations. *Wilderness Environ Med.* 1998;9(2):64-66.

86. Davies DM, Miller EJ, Miller IA. Accidental hypothermia treated by extracorporeal blood-warming. *Lancet.* 1967;1(7498):1036-1037.

87. Dobson JAR, Burgess JJ. Resuscitation of severe hypothermia by extracorporeal rewarming in a child. *J Trauma.* 1996;40(3):483-485.

88. Lloyd EL, Frankland JC. Accidental hypothermia: central rewarming in the field (correspondence). *Br Med J.* 1974;4(5946):717.

89. Morrison JB, Conn ML, Hayward JS. Thermal increment provided by inhalation rewarming from hypothermia. *J Appl Physiol Respir Environ Exerc Physiol.* 1979;46(6):1061-1065.

90. Hayward JS, Collis M, Eckerson JD. Thermographic evaluation of relative heat loss areas of man during cold water immersion. *Aerosp Med.* 1973;44(7):708-711.

91. Savard GK, Copper KE, Veale WL, Malkinson TJ. Peripheral blood flow during rewarming from mild hypothermia in humans. *J Appl Physiol.* 1985;58(1):4-13.

92. Brugger H, Durrer B, Elsensohn F, et al. Resuscitation of avalanche victims: evidence-based guidelines of the International Commission for Mountain Emergency Medicine: intended for physicians and other advanced life support personnel. *Resuscitation.* 2012;84(5):539-546.

27

Toxicologic Emergencies

MICHAEL D. GOOCH

COMPETENCIES

1. Identify the common sources of poisoning.
2. Describe the care of the poisoned patient during transport.
3. Name three antidotes for specific poisons.

The human environment contains natural and manu-factured toxins from plants, animals, chemicals, drugs, and chemotherapeutic agents. A phenome-non that has been increasing over the last few decades is the abuse of prescriptive medications, which has led to an in-crease in poisonings from medications that include seda-tives, opioids, and stimulants.[1]

Each year, more than two million human poison expo-sures are reported to the American Association of Poison Control Centers, which compiles the Toxic Exposure Sur-veillance System, the largest database of information about toxic exposures in the United States. Over half of these exposures involve medications, and more than 90% of all exposures occur in the victim's home. Others occur in loca-tions such as the workplace, schools, public areas, and numerous other locations. Half of the poisonings occur in children less than 6 years of age. Almost 80% of poisonings continue to be unintentional. Sources of unintentional ex-posure include therapeutic error (too much medication taken/given), bites and stings, environmental exposures, and food poisoning. Intentional poison exposures usually result from suicide attempts, abuse, and intentional misuse of medications.[2]

Safety must be the number one concern when transport-ing a potentially poisoned patient. Some toxins can cause injury to caregivers, so appropriate decontamination must be accomplished before transport. Decontamination is ad-dressed in the Scene Operations and Operational Safety sections of this text. Additionally, the team must consider the risks from a patient's current or potential future aggres-sive behavior related to the poisoning. Clinically, the vast majority of care for a poisoned patient is supportive.[3,4]

The purpose of this chapter is to discuss the general man-agement of the poisoned patient, identify the pathophysiology of selected substances, and describe the care of the poisoned patient during transport.

General Management of the Poisoned Patient

Once team safety is ensured, the initial approach to patient management for a poisoned patient is the same as for any other patient: primary assessment and stabilization, history and physical examination, and laboratory and other clinical studies. Clinical care is always directed at ensuring physio-logic safety (patients with inadequate oxygenation or venti-lation are supported as described in the Airway Manage-ment, Pulmonary Emergencies, and Mechanical Ventilation chapters). Patients with shock are managed as described in that section of this text. It is on this standard clinical foun-dation that considerations for specific antidotes and thera-pies are overlaid.[4-6] Box 27.1 summarizes the care for the poisoned patient.

A patient's medical history and any known history of the events around a toxic exposure provide important in-formation that can help identify a toxin. It is important to have a high index of suspicion; a poisoning should be sus-pected in any patient whose history suggests the possibility or in any patient whose clinical symptoms are not well explained by other sources. Poisoning or an overdose should be suspected in patients with mental status changes, seizures, altered body temperatures, metabolic and electro-lyte derangements, and cardiac arrhythmias. The converse is also true. Pathologic causes of body system alterations must be excluded before attributing them to a toxicologic cause. Any patient rescued from a fire, particularly from a fire in an enclosed space, should be considered as a possible poisoning.[4-6]

The patient may be exposed to a toxin by absorption, inhalation, ingestion, or injection. In the case of a known poisoning, the history should include the type of sub-stance or suspected substance that was taken, the exposure route, the time of the exposure, and the size or dosage of the exposure.[4-6]

If a thorough history cannot be obtained, the environ-ment in which the patient was found should be explored for

1. Provide basic and advanced life support after ensuring that the environment is safe for the transport team.
2. Remove the patient from the toxic environment.
3. When indicated, decontaminate the patient by removing clothing and washing off toxin.
4. Administer appropriate antidote when indicated.
5. Assess respiratory, neurologic, and cardiovascular status frequently.
6. Document or obtain baseline data.
7. Ensure the patient and transport team's safety in transport with the use of chemical or physical restraints. With use of chemical restraints, provide adequate analgesia and sedation.
8. Explain to the patient and family the plan of care, along with the patient's destination.
9. Transfer appropriate records and specimens.
10. Consult an expert when patient management questions arise.

TABLE 27.1 Odors Associated with Poisonings

Odor	Possible Poison
Bitter almond	Cyanide
Freshly mowed grass/hay	Phosgene
Fruity or sweet	Isopropyl alcohol ingestion, acetone
Garlic	Arsenic, organophosphates
Wintergreen	Methyl salicylate

Adapted from Erickson TB, et al. The approach to the patient with an unknown overdose. *Emerg Med Clin North Am.* 2007;25(2), 249-281.

clues to the cause of the poisoning; however, this should not delay treatment. Prescription medications, even those prescribed for someone other than the patient; nonprescription medications; and substances in the environment can suggest the etiology of a poisoning. This may be particularly true for pediatric patients. Bottles, containers, or other items may provide additional information about a suspected or unknown toxic substance. These items should be transported with the patient as long as there is no risk of harm to the transport team. Identification of witnesses to the event can add more information concerning what may have caused the poisoning or toxic exposure.[4-6]

Medical history, including allergies, previous surgeries, and past hospitalizations, should be noted. When possible, assessment of whether the patient has attempted suicide in the past is important.

In the care of the pediatric or elderly patient, the possibility of abuse or neglect must be kept in mind. A referral may be necessary to outside agencies, including law enforcement, so that the patient's environment may be evaluated to see whether it is appropriate and safe.[4,6]

The physical examination of a poisoned patient should be as orderly and complete as the physical examination of any patient with illness or injury. As always, baseline assessment data are particularly important to illuminate changes in the patient's condition during transport.

Some elements of the physical examination can be particularly helpful in identifying a poisoned patient or the nature of a poisoning[4-6]:

- *Neurologic*: Seizure-like activity and abnormal motor movements, mental status, pupil size, shape, reactivity, and eye movements, hallucinations, or psychotic symptoms.
- *Respiratory*: Rate, depth, breathing pattern, and adventitious lung sounds. Breath and other odors may suggest a particular poisoning or help rule out another cause. For example, the smell of oil of wintergreen can indicate salicylate poisoning. Table 27.1 lists odors associated with certain poisonings.[5]

- *Cardiovascular*: A full 12-lead electrocardiogram (ECG), ECG rhythm abnormalities, and conduction intervals, especially the QRS duration and corrected QT interval (QTc).
- *Cutaneous*: Skin color, temperature, moisture, and the presence of abnormal rashes, erythema, cutaneous bullae, petechiae, or the presence of injection or burn marks.

Assessment findings rather than laboratory results alone should guide the management. The single most important laboratory study is a rapid glucose assessment in any patient with a mental status change or presumed poisoning. Other baseline studies, such as the metabolic panels, complete blood count, coagulation studies, and a blood gas, can be helpful. Evaluation of the anion gap can be helpful in developing differentials in patients who are acidotic and suspected of a toxic poisoning. The anion gap can be calculated by using this formula: $(Na^+ \pm K^+) - (Cl^- + HCO_3^-)$. A normal serum gap is often considered to be 12 ± 4 mEq/L. Transport providers should be concerned about toxic exposures in any patient with a metabolic acidosis and an elevated anion gap.[4-6] Table 27.2 lists common causes of a gap acidosis.

TABLE 27.2 Causes of Anion Gap Metabolic Acidosis

M	Methanol
U	Uremia (renal failure)
D	Diabetic ketoacidosis
P	Propylene glycol (preservative in some intravenous medications)
I	Ingestion, iron, isoniazid
L	Lactic acidosis
E	Ethylene glycol
S	Salicylates (aspirin)

Adapted from Erickson TB, et al. The approach to the patient with an unknown overdose. *Emerg Med Clin North Am.* 2007;25(2), 249-281; Murray L, et al. *Toxicology Handook.* 2nd ed. Syndey, Australia: Churchhill Livingstone; 2011.

Serum levels of therapeutic drugs and "tox screens" can be difficult to interpret because the level of specific toxins may be incongruous with clinical manifestations. Most drug screens evaluate for the metabolites of commonly abused drugs; if the patient has not been exposed to those substances, or has received them as part of a treatment regimen, then these screens are not helpful. The timing is also important. If the specimen is collected too late or early, it may affect the results. Some substances or screens may yield false-positive and false-negative results.[4-6] Some regular screening, however, is important. Any patient with a presumed or possible ingestion should have aspirin and acetaminophen levels tested. In particular, the history does not suggest ingestion in up to 2.2% of patients with toxic acetaminophen levels. Female patients with any possibility of fertility should have a pregnancy test.[5,7-9]

Although multiple substances and various sources of toxins and poisons exist, only a limited number of specific antidotes are available. Again, supportive, standard critical care is the foundation of toxicologic management. Table 27.3 lists most of the available antidotes that may be useful in the management of a poisoned patient.

Drug removal can also be helpful. The most common method of gastrointestinal (GI) decontamination is accomplished with the administration of activated charcoal. Charcoal is effective in limiting the absorption of some ingested substances but must be given within the first few hours, or less, of the ingestion to have a significant benefit.[4-6] Enhanced elimination can also be accomplished with the alkalinization of the poisoned patient's urine, which causes an ion-trapping diuresis. For alkalinization of urine, sodium bicarbonate is added to intravenous (IV) fluids, which are

TABLE 27.3 Toxin Antidote Table

Toxic Agent	Antidote-Reversal Agents
Acetaminophen	*N*-Acetylcysteine (Mucomyst, Acedote)
Acetylcholinesterase inhibitors (cholinergic agents, e.g., organophosphates, nerves agents, carbamates)	Atropine and pralidoxime (2-PAM)
Anticholinergics (e.g., antihistamines, antispasmodics, some antiparkinsonism, antipsychotics, some antidepressants, phenothiazines)	Physostigmine, rarely used
Benzodiazepines	Flumazenil (Romazicon), rarely used
β-Blockers and calcium channel blockers	Glucagon, calcium, high-dose insulin therapy, intravenous lipid emulsion therapy
Carbon monoxide	High-flow oxygen
Cyanide	Hydroxocobalamin (Cyanokit)
Digoxin	Digoxin Fab antibodies
Heavy metals (e.g., lead, mercury, arsenic)	Edetate calcium disodium (EDTA), dimercaprol (BAL), Succimer, or D-penicillamine
Heparin	Protamine
Iron	Deferoxamine
Methemoglobinemic agents (e.g., nitrates, topical anesthetics)	Methylene blue
R: Reserpine	Naloxone (Narcan)
O: Opioids	
C: Clonidine	Opioids: 0.4 mg and titrate to effect
L: Lomotil	
A: Aldomet	All others: 10 mg
V: Valproate	
A: Angiotensin-converting enzyme inhibitors and angiotensin-receptor blockers	
X: Zanaflex	
Selective serotonin reuptake inhibitors (serotonin syndrome)	Cyproheptadine, benzodiazepines
Sympathomimetics (e.g., cocaine, amphetamines, 3,4-methylenedioxymethamphetamine [MDMA] and phencyclidine [PCP])	Benzodiazepines
Toxic alcohols (e.g., ethylene glycol, methanol)	Fomepizole (Antizol) or ethanol
Tricyclic antidepressants and aspirin	Bicarbonate infusion therapy
Warfarin (Coumadin)	Vitamin K ± fresh frozen plasma or prothrombin complex concentrate

Adapted from Murray L, et al. *Toxicology Handook*. 2nd ed. Syndey, Australia: Churchhill Livingstone; 2011; Mazor SS. Poisoning antidotes. In: Schaider JL, et al., eds. *Rosen & Barkin's 5-Minute Emergency Medicine Consult*. 5th ed. Philadelphia, PA: Wolters Kluwer; 2015.

administered to yield a urine pH of 7.5. The patient must be monitored closely for complications from fluid and electrolyte imbalances.[4-6] Some poisons are amenable to removal by dialysis.

Pharmacologic Properties of Drugs

Therapeutic dose responses are affected by multiple variables including the rate of absorption, distribution, binding or localization in tissues, inactivation, and excretion. The *rate of absorption* is defined as the time needed for ingested substances to cross the enterovascular barriers and circulate in the cardiovascular system. Agents dissolved in solution are absorbed more rapidly than those in solid forms. Timed-release or enteric-coated products are engineered to greatly decrease the absorption rate. Medications given in higher concentrations are absorbed more rapidly.

Most drugs are administered orally. Sites of absorption include the oral mucous membranes, stomach, and small intestine. Sublingual or buccal administration usually promotes quick absorption and rapid distribution. Absorption in the stomach is a passive process mediated by dissolution and diffusion. The nonionized form of a dissolved medication passes the mucosal barriers and enters the vascular compartment. Most drugs are either weak bases or weak acids. Gastric pH and contents affect both dissolution and diffusion. Weak acids, such as salicylates and barbiturates, are predominantly nonionized in a strongly acidic environment; therefore they are readily absorbed. Weak bases are in an ionized form in the stomach and are poorly absorbed. The intestinal pH is approximately 6.0 and much less acidic than the stomach pH of 1.5 to 3.0. Weak bases are readily absorbed, but weak acids cross the mucosal barrier less readily. In addition, the gastric mucosa is a lipid membrane, which absorbs lipid-soluble substances, such as alcohol, rapidly. Factors that change gastric emptying time also alter the rate of absorption of a drug. IV injection achieves the most immediate and is the most immediate and consistent blood concentration for any drug. After injection, a redistribution phase may significantly decrease the blood level of the drug. Absorption of medications given subcutaneously or intramuscularly depends on the site of injection, the solubility of the drug, and the vascularity of the injection area.

Once the drug is absorbed into the cardiovascular compartment, distribution occurs throughout the body. Agents enter or pass through the various body-fluid compartments (plasma, interstitial, and cellular fluids). Medications are restricted in distribution by their ability to pass through cellular membranes and the blood-brain barrier.

Drugs may accumulate in storage depots because of protein binding, fat accumulation, and active transport. Medications are stored in equilibrium and released as plasma concentrations are reduced. Storage depots permit maintenance of plasma levels for long periods, prolonging pharmacologic effects. Anatomic components that act as storage depots include plasma proteins, connective tissue, adipose tissue, and transcellular fluids.

The mechanism responsible for drug transport across cell membranes may be an active or passive process. Passive transfer is diffusion driven by concentration gradients. Active transport is mediated by a carrier and requires expenditure of energy. The ultimate fate of a drug is metabolism and excretion. Biotransformation involves chemical reactions, classified as either nonsynthetic or synthetic. The nonsynthetic class involves oxidation, reduction, and hydrolysis. The parent drug is changed to a more active, a less active, or an inactive metabolite. However, there are some medications that undergo little or no hepatic biotransformation. Hepatocytic enzymes mediate most nonsynthetic reactions. Exceptions include nonenzymatic hydrolysis in the plasma, plasma cholinesterase and pseudocholinesterase, and synaptic metabolism of neurotransmitter analogs.

Synthetic reactions or conjugation occur in the liver or kidney. The process couples the parent drug or its metabolites to endogenous substrates (usually carbohydrates, amino acids, or inorganic sulfates). Conjugated drugs form inactive, highly ionized, and water-soluble substances that are excreted in the urine. Conjugation is an active process that requires energy expenditure.

Active parent drugs and metabolites are excreted in the urine as a primary route of disposal. Drugs are also eliminated through excretion of feces. Metabolites are dissolved in bile, secreted into the alimentary tract, and passed through the GI tract. In addition, the unabsorbed parent drug is removed with fecal passage.

This discussion has focused on the incidence of poisoning; general considerations in the care of the poisoned patient; general management of the poisoned patient; signs and symptoms of toxicity; physical examination of the poisoned patient; useful laboratory studies; removal, elimination, or disruption of the poison; supportive and emotional care of the poisoned patient; transport nursing care of the poisoned patient; and the pharmacologic properties of drugs. The next part of this chapter focuses on the toxicity and treatment of toxicity of specific substances. Information about each of these drugs is presented for quick reference.

Toxicity and Treatment of Poisoning by Specific Substances

Acetylsalicylic Acid

Aspirin is one of the oldest nonprescription pharmaceutical agents. Its therapeutic popularity is mainly a result of its antipyretic, antiinflammatory, antiplatelet, and analgesic effects. Aspirin can be taken orally, topically, or rectally. The most common route of toxicity is via ingestion. Many over-the-counter medications contain aspirin, and multiple sources of poisoning may be involved.

An ingestion of greater than 150 mg/kg is considered toxic. Salicylate toxicity ultimately can lead to a severe aniongap metabolic acidosis. The absence of acidosis should not be falsely reassuring: salicylates directly stimulate the respiratory center, so the first acid-base abnormality is a respiratory alkalosis. Clinical manifestations of mild intoxication include headache, vertigo, tinnitus, mental confusion, sweating, thirst, hyperventilation, nausea, vomiting, and drowsiness. Severe intoxication produces similar symptoms combined with acid-base and electrolyte imbalances. Patients are agitated, restless, and uncommunicative and may have seizures or become comatose. Noncardiac pulmonary edema and hyperthermia are observed in severe poisoning, whereas bleeding diatheses are less common.[6,10]

Initial treatment of salicylate poisoning may involve administration of activated charcoal, if given within the first few hours of the ingestion, and alkaline diuresis. Alkaline diuresis is performed to increase the pH of the patient's urine to improve salicylate excretion. Supportive care and maintenance of vital functions are mainstays of treatment in this type of poisoning. If intubation is required, it is important to maintain a controlled hyperventilation to maintain the patient's respiratory alkalosis during initial management.[6,10,11]

The patient with severe poisoning may need hemodialysis. Hemodialysis not only enhances the removal of the toxic levels of the salicylate, but it can also correct the fluid, electrolyte, and acid-base imbalances that occur with salicylate toxicity.[6,10,11]

Acetaminophen

Acetaminophen, similar to aspirin, has antipyretic and analgesic properties. It is not chemically related to the salicylates. Acetaminophen has become a useful alternative to aspirin because it does not cause the GI and bleeding complications that can occur with aspirin use. Like aspirin, acetaminophen is contained in many over-the-counter drugs and may be administered orally, IV, or rectally. The main site of absorption is the small intestine, and the drug is uniformly distributed throughout most body fluids.[6,12,13]

Acetaminophen toxicity is increased by the liver because of metabolites that attach to the hepatic cell membrane and injure the lipid bilayer if they are not neutralized by the antioxidant glutathione. When hepatic glutathione stores are depleted because of an overdose of acetaminophen, the metabolites are not neutralized and cause injury and death of the hepatic cells.[6,12,13]

The classic clinical course of an acute acetaminophen poisoning occurs in four stages. The initial stage of toxicity occurs within the first 24 hours after ingestion and produces anorexia, nausea, vomiting, malaise, pallor, and diaphoresis.

The second stage begins 24 to 72 hours after ingestion. Right upper quadrant pain and tenderness may result from liver enlargement. The levels of liver enzymes, serum bilirubin, and prothrombin time begin to increase 36 hours after ingestion. Oliguria may result from acute tubular necrosis.

The third stage begins 72 to 96 hours after ingestion and is the time of peak liver function abnormalities. Anorexia, nausea, vomiting, and malaise return and jaundice become apparent. Fatalities from acetaminophen poisoning usually occur during this stage and result from fulminant hepatic necrosis.

The fourth stage, or resolution period, occurs 4 days to 2 weeks after poisoning. Patients are asymptomatic, and liver function parameters return to baseline values.[4,6,13]

Ingestions of more than 150 mg/kg are considered toxic. Activated charcoal may be helpful but must be administered within a few hours of the ingestion. The serum level of acetaminophen should be measured 4 hours after ingestion in any person who has ingested a potentially toxic dose of acetaminophen. If the acetaminophen level is still toxic at 4 hours after ingestion or if the level cannot be assayed after 8 hours have passed since ingestion and the history or evaluation of the hepatic transaminases suggests a toxic ingestion, N-acetylcysteine (NAC) should be administered. NAC replaces glutathione and is administered IV or orally at an initial dose of 150 mg/kg or 140 mg/kg, respectively. Administration is continued over a prescribed period of time. To have the most benefit administration should occur within 8 hours of ingestion; there is little benefit after 24 hours post ingestion.[6,11-13]

Anticholinergics

There are several medications (e.g., antihistamines, antipsychotics, antispasmodics, tricyclic antidepressants [TCAs]) and natural substances (e.g., jimson weed, mushrooms, deadly nightshade) that have anticholinergic properties.[14-16] These substances block the action of acetylcholine at central and peripheral muscarinic receptors. Inhibition leads to mydriasis, dry mouth, urinary retention, hyperthermia, tachycardia, altered mental status, agitation, and seizures. This is sometimes summarized by the mnemonic blind as a bat, red as a beet, dry as a bone, mad as a hatter, hotter than hades, and sick like a seizure.[14,16] Anticholinergic toxicity should be considered in any patient who presents with unexplained tachycardia, hyperthermia, and altered mental status.

Management is supportive, hypotension should initially be managed with IV normal saline solution, and a norepinephrine infusion may be needed in some patients. Agitation and seizures are best managed with benzodiazepines. If the patient is hyperthermic, cooling measures are warranted. If QRS widening is encountered, IV sodium bicarbonate therapy is preferred, as described in a later section. The use of cholinergic agents for reversal is not commonly indicated.[14-16]

Benzodiazepines

Benzodiazepines became available in the United States in 1960 for control of anxiety. These drugs are now used to decrease anxiety and as sedative-hypnotics, muscle relaxants, and anticonvulsants. Generally, a toxic level of benzodiazepines must be quite high; however, benzodiazepines are often taken in combination with other poisons, such as alcohol, which can cause death.[6,17,18]

The syndrome of benzodiazepine toxicity is nonspecific. The clinical picture is usually mild compared with those of other sedative-hypnotic poisonings. Most oral poisonings result in drowsiness and coma.

Transport team members must keep in mind that other medications and alcohol can place the patient at risk of toxicity with the administration of medications such as midazolam or lorazepam to manage a patient during transport.

The treatment of benzodiazepine poisoning begins with management of the patient's ABCDEs. Flumazenil can be administered to reverse the sedative, anxiolytic, and muscle-relaxant effects of toxic benzodiazepine ingestion. However, this drug must be administered in small doses with caution because many patients with overdoses take a combination of drugs, some of which may cause seizures at toxic levels, such as TCAs. Flumazenil reverses the anticonvulsant effects of benzodiazepines and may lead to withdrawal seizures, which also leaves patients with polyoverdoses at risk for lack of effective seizure management. Therefore its use is generally not recommended.[6,17,18] Patients with rapidly reversed overdoses may also present with aggressive behavior as their mental status suddenly improves.

Carbon Monoxide

Carbon monoxide (CO) is a colorless, odorless, tasteless gas yielded by the incomplete combustion of carbonaceous material. Sources include automobile or machine exhaust; flame-type heaters, furnaces, and ovens; defective fireplace flues; poorly ventilated charcoal and gas grills; and fires of all types. There is an increased incidence of accidental exposures during prolonged power outages caused by weather events when people attempt to stay warm from nonconventional sources and obtain electrical power from portable generators without proper ventilation.[6,19,20]

CO poisoning should be suspected in any patients with unexplained or vague symptoms, such as a headache or confusion, who may have been exposed to machinery running in an enclosed poorly ventilated space; exposed to a furnace that is new or run for the first time when the weather changes; or exposed to smoke in an enclosed space. It should be suspected with unexplained symptoms in multiple people in the same living or work space. Animals are more sensitive than humans to CO poisoning and may have been ill long before their human owners.

CO combines with the hemoglobin molecule in the red blood cell. The affinity of hemoglobin for CO is greater than 200 times that for oxygen. Not only does CO compete with oxygen for hemoglobin, but the presence of carboxyhemoglobin also greatly impedes the dissociation of oxygen from hemoglobin. This leads to a decreased partial pressure of oxygen in the blood and diminished gradient for oxygen diffusion from the red blood cell to the tissues, which results in tissue hypoxia. Arterial hypoxia results from any of the following conditions: pulmonary venous admixture from an uneven ventilation/perfusion relationship; marked inhibition of the circulatory system; direct

TABLE 27.4	Signs and Symptoms of Various Blood Levels of Carboxyhemoglobin (COHb)
Correlation of COHb and Clinical Presentations	
Level (%)	Clinical manifestations
<10	Typical smoker
10	Maybe asymptomatic to slight headache
20	Dizziness, nausea, worsening headache
30	Vertigo, ataxia, visual disturbances
40	Confusion, coma, seizures
50	Cardiovascular and respiratory failure, seizures, death

Adapted from Murray L, et al. *Toxicology Handook*. 2nd ed. Sydney, Australia: Churchhill Livingstone; 2011.

effect of CO on the pulmonary tissue, which results in increased capillary permeability and decreased production of surfactant; and shifting of the oxyhemoglobin dissociation curve to the left. Patients can develop lactic acidosis, cardiac dysrhythmias and ischemia, and seizures as the cellular hypoxia worsens.[6,19,20]

The concentration of CO in the blood has been found to relate poorly to the clinical features observed in the person who has been exposed. Table 27-4 describes the symptomatology of CO poisoning related to CO saturation in the blood.[6]

The treatment of acute CO exposure is high-flow oxygen delivery, including intubation if warranted, despite pulse oximetry readings. An important aspect of management is recalling that pulse oximetry is not reliable because it cannot differentiate between carboxyhemoglobin and oxyhemoglobin. Noninvasive CO oximetry devices exist and perform reliably within their published specifications. The available literature still does not fully support broad use of such devices to replace clinical judgment, a high index of suspicion, and blood testing in at-risk patients.[21] Carboxyhemoglobin dissociates and converts to oxyhemoglobin if high concentrations of oxygen are provided. Hyperbaric oxygen therapy has also been found to be effective in some patients, especially those who are pregnant or have levels greater than 25%.[6,19,20]

Cardiotoxic Medications

Beta and Calcium Channel Blockers

β-Blockers and calcium channel blockers have numerous benefits in managing patients with cardiovascular disease. They exert negative chronotropic, dromotropic, and inotropic effects on the heart. Calcium channel blockers also cause vasodilation. However, in an overdose scenario, these effects are exaggerated and can be lethal. Patients may experience bradycardia, atrioventricular heart blocks, and hypotension, which lead to poor tissue perfusion, and impaired glucose utilization is also common. β-Blockers may cause respiratory distress caused by the blockade of $β_2$-receptors in the lungs.

First-line treatments include the administration of IV fluids and the use of norepinephrine and epinephrine to support heart rate, blood pressure, and contractility. The administration of IV calcium can also be beneficial in β-blocker overdoses as well as with calcium channel blocker overdoses. High-dose insulin (HDI) therapy has been shown to be effective in overcoming the cardiotoxic effects of β-blockers and calcium channel blockers, as well, and is considered a first-line therapy. Sometimes referred to as hyperinsulinemia/euglycemia, this therapy increases glucose uptake in the cardiac cells and has positive inotropic effects, similar to glucagon. Careful monitoring of the patient's glucose and potassium are critically important.[6,11,22-27]

If the patient does not improve with the previously mentioned therapies, pacing, incremental increases in the HDI, and IV lipid emulsion (ILE) therapy may be beneficial. Lipids are a great source of energy for the myocardial cells, and this therapy is also theorized to create a "lipid sink," which pulls lipophilic medications out of the cardiac cells, removing the blockade and allowing for more effective contractility and conduction. With the administration of HDI and ILE therapy, vasoactive and inotropic agents may need to be adjusted to prevent overcorrection of the toxic effects. Both HDI and ILE therapies are new and consultation with toxicology may be helpful in managing these patients.[6,22,23,25,27,28]

IV glucagon can also be administered as a 3- to 5-mg bolus, followed by an infusion. Glucagon exerts positive inotropic and chronotropic effects despite blockade of the β-receptors or calcium channels. To avoid the common side effect of vomiting, glucagon should be administered slowly; premedicating with an antiemetic is sometimes helpful. Glucagon's benefit is dependent on adequate calcium stores, in the setting of hypocalcemia or a calcium channel blocker overdose, and the administration of IV calcium may improve the effect.[6,11,22-26] In some guidelines, glucagon is now considered a second-line therapy because of inconsistent clinical responses, the occurrence of side effects, and the availability of more effective therapies.[27]

Digitalis

The term cardiac glycoside is used to describe a group of drugs prescribed to treat heart failure and atrial arrhythmias. These drugs have been used throughout history, with early mention of the compound found in ancient writings in the year 1500 BC. *Digitalis* has become the most familiar of the group. It is derived from the dried leaf of the foxglove plant *Digitalis purpurea*. Several factors contribute to digitalis poisoning, including patient age; heart and renal disease; electrolyte imbalances (especially hypokalemia); and drug therapy, such as the use of diuretics.[29,30]

Clinical manifestations of digitalis toxicity are classified as cardiac and noncardiac. Cardiac manifestations including bradydysrhythmias are the result of depression through the sinoatrial and atrioventricular nodes and alteration of impulse formation and the development of

hyperkalemia. Noncardiac signs and symptoms include fatigue, anorexia, nausea, vomiting, diarrhea, confusion, restlessness, insomnia, drowsiness, hallucinations, frank psychosis, blurred vision, photophobia, and yellow-halo visual effects.[6,29,30]

Treatment of digitalis toxicity includes support of vital functions and correction of the hyperkalemia. Dysrhythmias and hyperkalemia are managed with standard care; however, the use of calcium is controversial and should be used cautiously in patients with digoxin-induced hyperkalemia. Digoxin-specific antibody fragments (Fab) are indicated if conventional supportive care to life-threatening dysrhythmias and hyperkalemia fails to correct the toxicity. Fab fragments bind to digoxin, and the Fab-digoxin complex is excreted in the urine.[6,29,30]

Tricyclic Antidepressants and Other Sodium-Channel Blocking Agents

TCAs are indicated in the treatment of refractory depression, chronic pain syndromes, and insomnia. Overdose statistics show that TCAs are one of the deadliest types of poisoning, with a high degree of morbidity and mortality in significant overdoses. Many TCAs are available in the United States.[6,31,32]

TCAs are well absorbed in the GI tract. The parent compound and active metabolites are quickly bound to plasma proteins. They exert their effects by inhibiting the amine pump mechanism responsible for the reuptake of norepinephrine and serotonin in adrenergic and serotonergic neurons. These antidepressants also block cholinergic receptors in the parasympathetic nervous system and have anticholinergic properties.[6,31,32]

The TCA agents, along with other sodium-channel blocking drugs, block the fast sodium channels responsible for the rapid depolarization (phase 0) of the cardiac action potential. In the management of patients with poisoning, it is important to understand that the list of medications that exert sodium-channel blocking effects is long and, in addition to the TCAs, includes the class I antiarrhythmics, cocaine, and some of the calcium- and β-blocking drugs. Accordingly, an evaluation of the ECG and consideration of the potential for sodium-channel poisoning is important in the management of any patient with possible ingestion.

The clinical manifestations of sodium-channel blocker poisoning include anticholinergic symptoms such as mydriasis, tachycardia, dry mucous membranes, urinary retention, and decreased peristalsis. Central nervous system (CNS) signs include confusion, agitation, hallucinations, seizures, and coma. Twitching, jerking, and myoclonic movements have also been reported. Generalized tonic clonic seizures are reported in 1% to 20% of TCA poisoning cases and are associated with the amount of QRS widening. Respiratory depression is common.

Cardiac conduction toxicity comes from conduction system poisoning and enhanced adrenergic stimulation of the myocardium. Sinus tachycardia and mild hypertension occur early in poisoning, coupled with a quinidine-like cardiac action that depresses conduction velocity, widens the QRS interval, and produces a rightward axis deviation and right bundle branch block as well as wide complex tachyarrhythmias. A terminal R wave over 3 mm in height in lead aVR is also consistent with sodium channel poisoning. Acidosis occurs because of cardiac and respiratory depression.[6,31,32]

In TCA and other sodium-channel blocker poisonings, support of vital functions is essential. Hypotension is initially managed with an IV infusion of saline solution. Vasopressor support with norepinephrine may be indicated if IV fluids are ineffective in correcting hypotension. Sodium bicarbonate therapy is indicated in any toxicologic patient with a widened QRS over 100 ms and should be given until the QRS duration normalizes. If sodium bicarbonate is not available or there is concern for the pH effect of a tremendous amount of sodium bicarbonate, hypertonic saline can be used. Seizures should be managed with benzodiazepines.[6,31,32]

Cyanide

Cyanide poisoning is rare but often fatal if not quickly identified and managed. Poisoning may result from inhalation of toxic gases from a fire involving wool, plastics, or rubber; exposure to agents used in metal refining; or prolonged infusions of high-dose nitroprusside.[33,34] Cyanide is often associated with the smell of bitter almonds, but this is not always the case. Cyanide inhibits oxygen transport, oxidative phosphorylation, and the production of adenosine triphosphate. This leads to severe tissue hypoxia, anaerobic metabolism, and a severe anion gap metabolic acidosis. The patient often displays symptoms of otherwise inexplicable metabolic acidosis and hypoxia including altered mental status, headache, GI upset, tachypnea and tachycardia, and eventually bradycardia and hypotension. Cyanide interferes with oxygen extraction, so oxygen saturation measurements are not clinically reliable in patients with cyanide poisoning.[33,34]

Management starts with the airway and administration of 100% oxygen. If available, hydroxocobalamin (Cyanokit) should be quickly administered.[33,34] Hydroxocobalamin binds with cyanide to form cyanocobalamin, which is then excreted in the urine. This reaction may cause a reddish discoloration to the patient's skin and urine.

Ethanol

Ethanol is the most widely used and abused drug in America. It is often involved in poison emergencies because it is frequently used with other drugs. Ethanol alcohol is rapidly absorbed from the GI tract. Food reduces the rate of absorption by 2 to 6 hours. Once ethanol is ingested, equilibration is rapid, and distribution uniformly occurs throughout all bodily tissues and fluids. Passage across the placenta has been documented.[6,35,36]

Ethanol metabolism occurs mainly in the liver. Acute intoxication produces psychomotor retardation; reflex

TABLE 27.5	Assessment of the Severity of Alcohol Intoxication by Blood Alcohol Level	
Serum Ethanol Concentration		Clinical Features (Dependent on Use History and Tolerance)
mg/dL	%	
50	0.05	Disinhibition and euphoria
100	0.1	Mild CNS depression, slurred speech
200	0.2	Increased CNS depression: nausea and vomiting, possible coma
400	0.4	Severe CNS depression: coma, respiratory depression, hypotension

CNS, Central nervous system.
Adapted from Murray L, et al. *Toxicology Handook.* 2nd ed. Syndey, Australia: Churchhill Livingstone; 2011.

slowing; lethargy; sleep; and ultimately, coma and death. Initially, respirations are stimulated as a result of the production of carbon dioxide. However, with increasing concentrations of alcohol, respirations can be dangerously depressed. Ethanol enhances cutaneous blood flow, which causes heat loss through vasodilation. Excessive amounts depress the central thermoregulatory mechanism, adding to the hypothermia effects. Ethanol stimulates gastric secretions, which causes an irritation of the gastric mucosa. In addition, ethanol causes diuresis mediated through inhibition of antidiuretic hormone (ADH), which decreases renal tubular reabsorption of water.[6,35,36]

Patients respond differently to alcohol poisoning. Table 27.5 correlates signs and symptoms of alcohol intoxication with blood alcohol levels.[6]

Care of the alcohol-poisoned patient consists of supportive care. Such patients may become combative, and precautions should be taken for appropriate restraint before transport.

Hallucinogens

In addition to toxic exposures to anticholinergics, two drugs that cause hallucinations are phencyclidine (PCP) and lysergic acid diethylamide (LSD). The use of both has declined over the last few decades. Marijuana is sometimes laced with PCP and is known as "whacko tobacco." Both can have effects that last hours after use. PCP was initially developed as a general anesthetic in 1958 and has similar properties to ketamine. However, because of the postanesthetic reactions that occurred with its use, it has not been used legally since 1965.[37]

PCP is often smoked, but can also be snorted or ingested and is distributed to all tissue compartments, metabolized by the liver, and excreted through the kidneys. The drug can produce bizarre and dangerous behavioral manifestations, as well as tachycardia, hypertension, and hyperthermia. In larger doses, it can cause psychosis, hostility, seizures, and coma. A common neurologic sign of PCP intoxication is nystagmus.[31,37-40]

LSD is one of the most potent hallucinogens known. Psychiatrists initially used the drug in the 1950s as an aid in clinical psychotherapy. Abuse became popular in the 1960s during the "psychedelic movement," and was listed as a schedule I controlled substance in 1966. LSD is usually taken orally. Doses as low as 25 mcg will produce clinical effects, and the intensity of its effect is dose dependent. Doses greater than 100 mcg are often needed for the full effect but also cause sympathomimetic effects similar to PCP and other stimulants. Absorption of the drug is rapid, and LSD is distributed to all tissues, including the brain. Initial effects occur in 30 to 45 minutes and may last for 10 to 12 hours. LSD is metabolized in the liver, and small amounts are excreted unchanged in urine.[41]

Psychological effects are generally pleasurable, and may include euphoria, dreams, and pseudohallucinations. The user may have enhanced color perception and experience transforming visual imagery of their surroundings and their body. Occasionally, a person may have an intense panic reaction ("bad trip") that includes frightening hallucinations and mood swings or a "flashback." Such a person may become confused, aggressive, suicidal, or violent.[38,41]

Treatment consists of supportive care. During air medical transport, patients who have taken any hallucinogen demand close observation. Patients may become hostile, belligerent, and destructive. Be observant for signs of sympathetic stimulation including hypertension, tachycardia, and hyperthermia induced rhabdomyolysis. Use of ear protection, sedation, and prophylactic chemical and/or physical restraints may be necessary before transport.[31,38,40,41]

Organophosphates

Insecticides, pesticides, and nerve agents (e.g., soman, sarin, VX) are examples of organophosphates (OPs). This toxicity may be seen in purposeful ingestions, accidental occupational exposures, and chemical exposures during a terroristic event. Some may report the associated smell of garlic with these toxins. These chemicals cause a cholinergic crisis by inhibiting acetylcholinesterase and preventing the breakdown of acetylcholine, which leads to the buildup of acetylcholine and prolonged stimulation of muscarinic and nicotinic receptors in both the central and peripheral nervous system.[42] Overstimulation of muscarinic receptors leads to the classic SLUDGE presentation: salivation, lacrimation, urination, defecation, GI, and expectoration and emesis. This also includes bronchorrhea, bradycardia, and hypotension. Nicotinic stimulation leads to tachycardia; hypertension; mydriasis; muscle fasciculations; seizures; and eventually paralysis, including the diaphragm.[42]

Safety is of the upmost priority with OPs, and the patient must be decontaminated before transport. Providers should don proper protective equipment to ensure they do not come in contact with the substance because it is easily inhaled or absorbed through the skin.[42,43] Once the patient is safe for transport personnel, the head of the bed should be elevated because of the massive amounts of airway secretions. Atropine is administered to block the overstimulation of muscarinic receptors with the goal of drying up pulmonary secretions and stabilizing the airway. The patient may require multiple large doses because there is no maximum dose for these patients.[42,43] If the patient requires intubation, then succinylcholine should be avoided because OPs prevent its breakdown and prolonged paralysis may occur. Once available, pralidoxime (2-PAM) is administered to stop the overstimulation of the receptors and reverse paralysis. 2-PAM binds to and inactivates the OPs, freeing up acetylcholinesterase. Some OPs irreversibly bind to acetylcholinesterase over time, often referred to as aging, which results in prolonged receptor stimulation. The sooner 2-PAM can be administered, the less likely this aging will occur. Patients will benefit from an initial bolus and continuous infusion. Benzodiazepines remain the agent of choice for managing seizures.[42,43]

Sympathomimetics

Cocaine, amphetamines, methamphetamines, 3,4-methylenedioxymethamphetamine (MDMA) or ecstasy (E or X), and the newer street drugs including synthetic cannabinoids, bath salts, and Molly's plant food, are commonly abused substances with sympathomimetic properties. These substances may be insufflated, smoked, ingested, injected, and now vaped. Most of these substances are metabolized by the liver and excreted by the kidney. They stimulate both the peripheral and central sympathetic nervous systems, and both α- and β-receptors. They can produce mild-to-moderate CNS stimulation manifested by euphoria; decreased fatigue; and excitement, which can progress to anxiety, paranoia, hostility, hyperthermia, and seizures. They can have significant cardiovascular effects including tachycardia, arrhythmias, hypertension, and vasospasms, which can lead to a myocardial infarction, stroke, and even death.[6,11,31,44,45]

Synthetic cannabinoids, bath salts, and Molly's plant food are newer illicit substances, which are often encountered because of their popularity. They can be obtained illegally online and at retail shops. Most are labeled "not for human consumption" and contain various chemicals. They are highly addictive and users often experience a rapid tolerance requiring more with each use to achieve the desired effect. Because these substances are synthetic, they are not detectable in the routine urine drug screen, hence, their popularity.[11,46-49]

Synthetic cannabinoids (e.g., K2 and Spice) are herbal incenses that have been treated with psychoactive chemicals, which stimulate cannabinoid receptors similar to delta-9-tetrahydrocannabinol (THC). These chemicals are more potent than THC and lead to a stronger effect including euphoria and activation of the sympathetic nervous system and inhibition of the parasympathetic system. Some patients may experience tachycardia, hypertension, paranoia, agitation, and GI distress. Bath salts (e.g., Bliss, Ivory Wave, Vanilla Sky) and second-generation bath salts (e.g., "gravel" or "flakka") are synthetic amphetamines that mimic cathinone, a naturally occurring psychostimulant found in the khat plant. These substances alter the reuptake of norepinephrine, dopamine, and serotonin, which leads to an overstimulation of the sympathetic nervous system. Bath salts have been associated with suicidal and homicidal ideations and actions.[11,46-51]

Molly's plant food or Molly, which is short for molecule, is "marketed" as pure MDMA and is usually in a powder form, unlike MDMA, which is usually a pill. Molly may or may not contain MDMA, as well as many other chemicals. However, both increase serotonin levels more than the other neurotransmitters and increase the release of oxytocin and ADH. Serotonin and oxytocin have empathogenic effects and have earned MDMA the nicknames of the "hug drug" and the "love drug." The increased release of ADH can suppress the thirst response, and users often increase their water intake knowing this effect along with the concern for overheating. This may cause some users to develop hyponatremia that leads to seizures. Both have been associated with risky sexual behaviors, disease transmission, and sexual assaults.[6,11,52,53]

The main objectives in the treatment of acute sympathomimetic exposures are to control the hyperactivity and hypertension, suppress malignant cardiac arrhythmias, correct metabolic acidosis, reduce hyperthermia, and minimize seizure activity. Benzodiazepines, such as midazolam (Versed), are the first-line intervention for patients experiencing hyperactivity, tachyarrhythmias, hypertension, hyperthermia, and seizures associated with these substances. A continuous infusion may be warranted in some patients. If the hypertension is not controlled with benzodiazepines, then vasodilators (e.g., nitroglycerin) or α-/β-blockade (e.g., labetalol) may be needed. However, pure β-blockers should not be used alone because this would leave α-receptors unopposed and could worsen the patient's condition. Sympathomimetic substances may cause sodium channel blockade, which can cause QRS widening and wide complex dysrhythmias. These rhythm changes should be managed with sodium bicarbonate and/or lidocaine if not resolved with initial therapy. Cooling measures will be needed when there is severe hyperthermia with a core temperature greater than 40°C (104°F). Patients with prolonged hyperthermia are at an increased risk for rhabdomyolysis and acute renal failure.[6,11,31,45-48,50]

Toxic Alcohols

Ethylene glycol is an odorless water-soluble solvent most commonly used in antifreeze and coolants. Ingestion usually occurs in the inquisitive toddler, as an ethanol substitute, or suicide attempt. Ethylene glycol is rapidly absorbed and reaches peak blood levels in 1 to 4 hours after ingestion. Large doses result in an inebriated patient without the odor of alcohol. Ethylene glycol approximates ethanol in CNS toxicity; however, its metabolites produce profound systemic effects, especially cardiac and renal.[6,11,54,55]

Ingestion of greater than 1 mL/kg of ethylene glycol is often lethal. It is hepatically metabolized to several metabolites including glycolic and oxalic acid. Calcium oxalate crystals are formed and deposited systemically especially in the heart

and kidneys and often lead to acute renal failure. Ethylene glycol ingestion leads to intoxication similar to ethanol ingestion. A profound anion gap metabolic acidosis is a hallmark of this poisoning, but it only occurs after metabolism has begun. Severe hypocalcemia from chelation of calcium may produce tetany and cardiac compromise.[6,11,54-56]

Methanol, a wood alcohol, is found in some fuels, windshield washing fluids, and solvents. Ingestion of greater than 0.5 mL/kg is often lethal in most patients. Initial presentation is also similar to an acute ethanol ingestion. Methanol is metabolized to formaldehyde and then formic acid. A severe gap metabolic acidosis and blindness will develop and eventually death if not treated.[6,11,54-56]

Serum levels can guide treatment for toxic alcohol ingestions; however, treatment should not be delayed while awaiting results if there is a concern for or known toxic ingestion. Fomepizole (Antizol) should be administered to inhibit the enzyme, which metabolizes alcohols. Inhibition prevents the buildup of the toxic metabolites and may prevent or limit the development of acidosis and renal failure. If fomepizole is not available, an IV ethanol drip can be initiated. (Ethanol drip is not FDA approved.) Ethanol blocks the conversion of ethylene glycol and methanol to their toxic metabolites and can slow the development of acidosis and toxicity. Dialysis may be needed to remove the toxins and stabilize any imbalances. If fomepizole is administered early enough, dialysis may not be needed in some patients.[6,11,54-56]

Snakebites

Responding to the needs of a victim of a snakebite may not be one of the most common flights encountered by the transport nurse; however, knowledge of how to care for such patients can decrease complications and save lives. Many thousands of snakebites are reported in the United States each year. Venomous snakes inflict about 4000 to 6000 of those bites. Death does occur but is rare.[57,59]

Venom is a special category of poison that must be injected by one organism into another to produce a harmful effect. It is secreted by special epithelial cells in certain organisms and is stored in the lumina or exocrine glands. The venom is comprised of multiple chemicals and enzymes, and some of them toxic. The toxins may affect particular body systems such as the neurologic, hematologic, and cardiovascular systems.[57,59]

The effects of venom are dependent on the pharmacologic complexity of the venom and the action that the venom exerts on the tissues. The location of the venom injection also affects the spread of the venom. The closer the bite is to the trunk, the higher the risk for systemic effects. However, any bite in the area of a blood vessel could potentially spread the venom more quickly.[56-60]

The most prevalent venomous snakes in the United States are the pit vipers, which include rattlesnakes, copperheads, and water moccasins (cottonmouths). These snakes produce a hemotoxin and are native to all states except Maine, Alaska, and Hawaii. Coral snakes only account for 5% of envenomations and can be found in the southwestern states, gulf coastal states, and the Carolinas. In addition to the venomous snakes native to the United States, poisonous snakes have been collected from all over the world. A bite from any one of these snakes may be fraught with complications or may even be instantly fatal.[57-60]

The following subsections describe the indigenous venomous snakes, the initial treatment of snakebites, transport nursing care of patients with snake bites, and the role of the transport team in the care of these victims.

Recognition of Venomous Bites

Fig. 27.1 compares pit viper and non-pit viper snakes. Pit vipers belong to the Crotalidae family (as shown in Fig. 27.1) and have a pit midway between the eye and nostril on each side of the head. This pit is a heat-sensing organ that helps the snake locate its prey. This particular characteristic, unlike others in Fig. 27.1, is a 100% consistent characteristic in the identification of pit vipers. Envenomation by a pit viper usually results in one or two

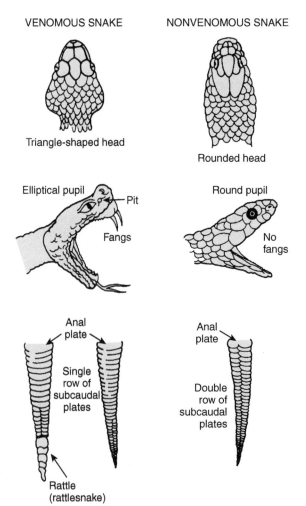

• Fig. 27.1 Comparison of pit viper (venomous) and non-pit viper (nonvenomous) snakes. (From Otten M. Venomous animal injuries. In: Marx JA, et al., eds. *Rosen's Emergency Medicine: Concepts and Clinical Practice*. 6th ed. St. Louis, MO: Mosby; 2006.)

distinct puncture wounds with symptoms of localized pain, swelling, and edema in the bitten area. Other symptoms include diaphoresis and chills, paresthesias, nausea, hypotension, faintness, weakness, muscle fasciculations, local ecchymosis, and coagulopathies.[57-60]

The second largest family of snakes in the world is the Elapidae, which contains some deadly species including cobras, mambas, sea snakes, and coral snakes. One of the distinguishing characteristics of the coral snakes found in the United States is their color pattern, which is often summarized with the mnemonic 'Red on Yellow Kills a Fellow, Red on Black Venom Lack." Envenomation by a coral snake may result in a neurotoxic course. Systemic manifestations include drowsiness, euphoria, weakness, nausea, vomiting, fasciculations, dysphagia, salivation, extraocular muscle paresis, hypotension, and cardiopulmonary failure.[57-59]

Initial Management of Snakebites

Envenomation does not always occur with a snake bite. Estimates are that 20% to 30% of crotalid bites and 50% of elapid bites do not result in envenomation; such bites are called dry bites.[57-60] In the following discussion of the general management of patients with snakebite, it is important to emphasize that experts should be consulted when questions arise about the care of patients with a snakebite. Identification of the snake is important so that appropriate treatment can be initiated and limit unnecessary care.

If the snake has not been secured, the patient should be moved to a safe environment. The patient must be kept calm and the affected part immobilized. These two interventions decrease the circulation of venom throughout the patient's system. The wound should be cleansed, any constrictive clothing removed, the extremity immobilized, and the patient transported. With coral snake bites, the application of a compression dressing to the affected area may slow systemic absorption; however, this is controversial and should never be performed with pit viper bites.[6,57,58,60]

The airway, ventilatory, and circulatory status of the patient should be constantly evaluated. Two large-bore IV lines should be started, preferably in an area away from the bite. The patient must be observed closely for progression of symptoms from a localized reaction at the wound site to a systemic reaction and development of a compartment syndrome in the affected extremity.

When possible, blood samples for baseline laboratory work should be drawn before transport. These tests may include a complete blood count, coagulation studies, a metabolic panel, creatine kinase, and urinalysis. Included in the coagulation studies should be fibrin split products and fibrinogen levels.[57,59,60]

If the patient shows signs of severe envenomation, such as worsening edema, shock, renal failure, coagulopathy, or paralysis, administration of antivenin should be started. Antivenin facilitates removal of the venom from the body but does not reverse any tissue damage. The size of the patient needs to be considered in relation to the amount of venom that the person may be able to tolerate. A child or small adult may be more severely affected.[6,57-60]

Snake antivenin is prepared from the serum of animals that were hyperimmunized against a specific venom or venoms. Unlike other drugs, the dosage of antivenin should be based on clinical findings rather than on the age and weight of the patient. Crotalidae Polyvalent Immune Fab (Crofab) is the only pit viper antivenin available in the United States. Unlike the older antivenin made from equine serum, this antivenin is ovine in nature and has less risk of allergic reactions. Skin testing and pretreatment before administration is no longer recommended, although clinicians should be prepared in case there is a reaction. Eastern coral snake antivenin is no longer manufactured but is available in those previously mentioned geographic areas of the country. Given the shortage of this antivenin, the Food and Drug Administration has extended its printed expiration date and reevaluates this on a yearly basis. There is a new antivenin currently in clinical trials. Skin testing to observe for a reaction and pretreatment is recommended before administration of coral snake antivenin. When any antivenin is given, the package instructions should be followed and resuscitation equipment kept in close range.[6,57-60]

Serum sickness may develop after antivenin administration. The incidence rate of serum sickness varies from 10% to 80% of all patients given antivenin therapy. The symptoms of serum sickness have occurred up to 3 weeks after antivenin administration. They include fever, joint pain, rash, nausea, vomiting, and neurologic symptoms. Treatment of serum sickness includes antihistamines and steroids.[57,60]

Transport Care of Patients with Snakebite

The transport team may become involved in the care of the patient with a snakebite by directly responding to the scene of the injury or by transporting the patient to more definitive care. Experts in the care of snakebites note that rapid transport of these patients to a facility that can manage the injury is imperative in saving lives and preventing complications.[57] Box 27.2 summarizes care to be provided for the patient bitten by a snake.

• BOX 27.2 Transport Care of the Patient Bitten by a Snake

1. Provide a safe environment for the transport team and patient.
2. Provide basic and advanced life support.
3. Obtain as much information as possible about the type of snake that may have envenomated the patient including a digital photograph of the snake and bite area if allowed by policy and can be done safely.
4. Immobilize the affected part.
5. Keep the patient calm.
6. Notify the appropriate receiving facility.
7. Consult an expert when patient management questions arise.
8. Establishes two large-bore intravenous lines.
9. Watch for local and systemic effects from the snakebite.
10. Administer analgesia for pain.

Summary

The transport of the poisoned patient generally involves support of the patient's airway, breathing, and circulation. Few antidotes are available for the poisoned patient, and generally the transport team may have limited resources to determine the cause of the poisoning. However, the patient management can be interesting in the detective work used to uncover cues to ingestion and, when indicated, novel therapies for specific poisonings. The transport team should always ensure safety before transport begins so they do not become victims of the poison or the patient's behavior, as well.

References

1. McCabe SE, Cranford JA, West BT. Trends in prescription drug abuse and dependence, co-occurrence with other substance use disorders, and treatment utilization: Results from two national surveys. *Addict Behav.* 2008;33(10):1297-1305.
2. Mowry JB, Spyker DA, Brooks DE, et al. 2014 Annual report of the American Association of Poison Control Centers' national poison data system (NPDS): 32nd annual report. *Clin Toxicol.* 2015;53(10):962-1147.
3. Air & Surface Transport Nurses Association. *Positon Statement: Transport Nurse Safety in the Transport Environment.* Retrieved from https://c.ymcdn.com/sites/astna.org/resource/collection/4392B20B-D0DB-4E76-959C-6989214920E9/Transport_Nurse_Safety_in_the_Transport_Environment.pdf; 2011.
4. Mycyk MB. Poisoning. In: Schaider JL, Barkin AZ, Barkin RM, Wolfe RE, Shayne PS, Hayden R, Rosen P, eds. *Rosen & Barkin's 5-Minute Emergency Medicine Consult.* 5th ed. Philadelphia, PA: Wolters Kluwer; 2015c:884-885.
5. Erickson TB, Thompson TM, Lu JJ. The approach to the patient with an unknown overdose. *Emerg Med Clin North Am.* 2007;25 (2):249-281.
6. Murray L, Daly F, Little M, Cadogan M. *Toxicology Handook.* 2nd ed. Syndey, Australia: Churchhill Livingstone; 2011.
7. Ashbourne JF, et al. Value of rapid screening for acetaminophen in all patients with intentional drug overdose. *Ann Emerg Med.* 1989;18(10):1035-1038.
8. Lucanie R, Chiang WK, Reilly R. Utility of acetaminophen screening in unsuspected suicidal ingestions. *Vet Hum Toxicol.* 2002;44(3):171-173.
9. Sporer KA, et al. Acetaminophen and salicylate serum levels in patients with suicidal ingestion or altered mental status. *Emerg Med Am J.* 1996;14(5):443-446.
10. Zell-Kanter M. Salicylate antidotes. In: Schaider JL, Barkin AZ, Barkin RM, Wolfe RE, Shayne P, Hayden SR, Rosen P, eds. *Rosen & Barkin's 5-Minute Emergency Medicine Consult.* 5th ed. Philadelphia, PA: Wolters Kluwer; 2015:998-999.
11. Roberts E, Gooch MD. Pharmacologic strategies for treatment of poisonings. *Nurs Clin North Am.* 2016;51(1):57-68.
12. Mycyk MB. Acetaminophen poisoning. In: Schaider JL, Barkin AZ, Barkin RM, Barkin, Wolfe RE, Shayne P, Hayden SR, Rosen P, eds. *Rosen & Barkin's 5-Minute Emergency Medicine Consult.* 5th ed. Philadelphia, PA: Wolters Kluwer; 2015a:20-21.
13. Olson KR. Acetaminophen. In: Olson KR, ed. *Poisoning & Drug Overdose.* 6th ed. 2012. Retrieved from http://accessmedicine.mhmedical.com/content.aspx?bookid=391&Sectionid=42069818.

14. Garlich, FM. Anticholinergic agents. In: Wolfson AB, et al, eds. *Harwood-Nuss' Clinical Practice of Emergency Medicine*. 6th ed. Philadelphia, PA: Wolters Kluwer; 2015:1463-1465.

15. Manning BH. Anticholinergics. In: Olson KR, ed. *Poisoning & Drug Overdose*. 6th ed. 2012. Retrieved from http://accessmedicine. mhmedical.com/content.aspx?bookid=391&sectionid= 42069827.

16. Whiteley PM. Anticholinergic poisoning. In: Schaider JL, Barkin AZ, Barkin RM, Wolfe RE, Shayne P, Hayden SR, Rosen P, eds. *Rosen & Barkin's 5-Minute Emergency Medicine Consult*. 5th ed. Philadelphia, PA: Wolters Kluwer; 2015:74-75.

17. Nelson ME. Benzodiazepine poisoning. In: Schaider JL, Barkin AZ, Barkin RM, Wolfe RE, Shayne P, Hayden SR, Rosen P, eds. *Rosen & Barkin's 5-Minute Emergency Medicine Consult*. 5th ed. Philadelphia, PA: Wolters Kluwer; 2015:136-137.

18. Tsutaoka B. Benzodiazepines. In: Olson KR, ed. *Poisoning & Drug Overdose*. 6th ed. 2012. Retrieved from http://accessmedicine. mhmedical.com/content.aspx?bookid=391&Sectionid= 42069845.

19. Hampson NB, Piantadosi CA, Thom SR, Weaver LK. Practice recommendations in the diagnosis, management, and prevention of carbon monoxide poisoning. *Am J Respir Crit Care Med*. 2012; 186(11):1095-1101.

20. Thompson TN. Carbon monoxide poisoning. In: Schaider JL, Barkin AZ, Barkin RM, Wolfe RE, Shayne P, Hayden SR, Rosen P, eds. *Rosen & Barkin's 5-Minute Emergency Medicine Consult*. 5th ed. Philadelphia, PA: Wolters Kluwer; 2015:178-179.

21. Wilcox SR, Richards JB. Noninvasive carbon monoxide detection: insufficient evidence for broad clinical use. *Respir Care*. 2013;58(2):376-379.

22. Barton CA, Johnson NB, Mah ND, et al. Successful treatment of a massive metoprol overdose using intravenous lipid emulsion and hyperinsulinemia/euglycemia therapy. *Pharmacotherapy*. 2015; 35(5):e56-e60.

23. Doepker B, Healy W, Cortez E, Adkins E. High-dose insulin and intravenous lipid emulsion therapy for cardiogenic shock induced by intentional calcium-channel blocker and beta-blocker overdose: A case series. *J Emerg Med*. 2014;46(4):486-490.

24. Engebretsen KM, Kaczmarek KM, Morgan J, Holger JS. High-dose insulin therapy in beta-blocker and calcium channel-blocker poisoning. *Clin Toxicol*. 2011;49(4):277-283.

25. Lim CS, Aks SE. Beta-blocker poisoning. In: Schaider JL, Barkin AZ, Barkin RM, Wolfe RE, Shayne P, Hayden SR, Rosen P, eds. *Rosen & Barkin's 5-Minute Emergency Medicine Consult*. 5th ed. Philadelphia, PA: Wolters Kluwer; 2015a:138-139.

26. Lim CS, Aks SE. Calcium channel blocker poisoning. In: Schaider JL, Barkin AZ, Barkin RM, Wolfe RE, Shayne P, Hayden SR, Rosen P, eds. *Rosen & Barkin's 5-Minute Emergency Medicine Consult*. 5th ed. Philadelphia, PA: Wolters Kluwer; 2015b:172-173.

27. St-Onge M, Anseeuw K, Cantrell FL, et al. Experts consensus recommendations for the management of calcium channel blocker poisoning in adults. *Crit Care Med*. 2017;45(3): e306-e315.

28. Schultz AE, Lewis T, Reed BS, et al. That's a phat antidote: Intravenous fat emulsions and toxicological emergencies. *Adv Emerg Nurs J*. 2015;37(3):162-175.

29. Benowitz NL. Digoxin and other cardiac glycosides. In: Olson KR, ed. *Poisoning & Drug Overdose*. 6th ed. 2012b. Retrieved from http://accessmedicine.mhmedical.com/content.aspx?bookid =391&Sectionid=42069875.

30. Troendle MM, Cumpston KL. Digoxin poisoning. In: Schaider JL, Barkin AZ, Barkin RM, Wolfe RE, Shayne P, Hayden SR,

Rosen P, eds. *Rosen & Barkin's 5-Minute Emergency Medicine Consult*. 5th ed. Philadelphia, PA: Wolters Kluwer; 2015a:322-323.

31. Aks SE. Tricyclic poisoning. In: Schaider JL, Barkin AZ, Barkin RM, Wolfe RE, Shayne P, Hayden SR, Rosen P, eds. *Rosen & Barkin's 5-Minute Emergency Medicine Consult*. 5th ed. Philadelphia, PA: Wolters Kluwer; 2015c:1164-1165.

32. Benowitz NL. Antidepressants, tricyclic. In: Olson KR, ed. *Poisoning & Drug Overdose*. 6th ed. 2012a. Retrieved from http:// accessmedicine.mhmedical.com/content.aspx?bookid=391& Sectionid=42069830.

33. Blanc PD. Cyanide. In: Olson KR, ed. *Poisoning & Drug Overdose*. 6th ed. 2012. Retrieved from http://accessmedicine.mhmedical.com/ content.aspx?bookid=391&sectionid=42069871.

34. Long H. Cyanide. In: Wolfson, et al, eds. *Harwood-Nuss' Clinical Practice Of Emergency Medicine*. 6th ed. Philadelphia, PA: Wolters Kluwer; 2015:1419-1420.

35. Kreshak A. Ethanol. In: Olson KR, ed. *Poisoning & Drug Overdose*. 6th ed. 2012. Retrieved from http://accessmedicine.mhmedical. com/content.aspx?bookid=391&Sectionid=42069880.

36. Meehan TJ. Alcohol poisoning. In: Schaider JL, Barkin AZ, Barkin RM, Wolfe RE, Shayne P, Hayden SR, Rosen P, eds. *Rosen & Barkin's 5-Minute Emergency Medicine Consult*. 5th ed. Philadelphia, PA: Wolters Kluwer; 2015:42-43.

37. Bey T, Patel A. Phencyclidine intoxication and adverse effects: A clinical and pharmacological review of an illicit drug. *Cal J Emerg Med*. 2007;8(1):9-14.

38. Witsil JC. Hallucinogen poisoning. In: Schaider JL, Barkin AZ, Barkin RM, Wolfe RE, Shayne P, Hayden SR, Rosen P, eds. *Rosen & Barkin's 5-Minute Emergency Medicine Consult*. 5th ed. Philadelphia, PA: Wolters Kluwer; 2015:480-481.

39. Wu L. Lysergic acid diethylamide (LSD) and other hallucinogens. In: Olson KR, ed. *Poisoning & Drug Overdose*. 6th ed. 2012. Retrieved from http://accessmedicine.mhmedical.com/ content.aspx?bookid=391&sectionid=42069909.

40. Aks SE. Phencyclidine poisoning. In: Schaider JL, Barkin AZ, Barkin RM, Wolfe RE, Shayne P, Hayden SR, Rosen P, eds. *Rosen & Barkin's 5-Minute Emergency Medicine Consult*. 5th ed. Philadelphia, PA: Wolters Kluwer; 2015b:856-857.

41. Passie T, Halpern JH, Stichtenoth DO, et al. The pharmacology of lysergic acid diethylamide: A review. *CNS Neurosci Ther*. 2008; 14(4):295-314.

42. Holstege CP. Organophosphate and carbamate insecticides. In: Wolfson AB, et al, eds. *Harwood-Nuss' Clinical Practice of Emergency Medicine*. 6th ed. Philadelphia, PA: Wolters Kluwer; 2015:1393-1395.

43. Vohra R. Organophosphorus and carbamate insecticides. In: Olson KR, ed. *Poisoning & Drug Overdose*. 6th ed. 2012. Retrieved from http://accessmedicine.mhmedical.com/content.aspx? bookid=391&sectionid=42069934.

44. Nordt SP. Sympathomimetic poisoning. In: Schaider JL, Barkin AZ, Barkin RM, Wolfe RE, Shayne P, Hayden SR, Rosen P, eds. *Rosen & Barkin's 5-Minute Emergency Medicine Consult*. 5th ed. Philadelphia, PA: Wolters Kluwer; 2015:1096-1097.

45. Aks SE. Cocaine poisoning. In: Schaider JL, Barkin AZ, Barkin RM, Wolfe RE, Shayne P, Hayden SR, Rosen P, eds. *Rosen & Barkin's 5-Minute Emergency Medicine Consult*. 5th ed. Philadelphia, PA: Wolters Kluwer; 2015a:244-245.

46. McGraw M, McGraw L. Bath salts: Not as harmless as they sound. *J Emerg Nurs*. 2012;38(6):582-588.

47. Mills B, Yepes A, Nugent K. Synthetic cannabanoids. *Am J Med Sci*. 2015;350(1):59-62.

48. Miotto K, Striebel J, Cho AK, Wang C. Clinical and pharmacological aspects of bath salt use: A review of the literature and case reports. *Drug Alcohol Depend*. 2013;132(1-2):1-12.

49. Terry SM. Bath salt abuse: More than just hot water. *J Emerg Nurs.* 2014;40(1):88-91.

50. Hickey JL, Lu JJ. Bath salts–synthetic cathinones poisoning. In: Schaider JL, Barkin AZ, Barkin RM, Wolfe RE, Shayne P, Hayden SR, Rosen P, eds. *Rosen & Barkin's 5-Minute Emergency Medicine Consult.* 5th ed. Philadelphia, PA: Wolters Kluwer; 2015:132-133.

51. Salani DA, Zdanowicz MM. Synthetic cannabinoids: The dangers of spicing it up. *J Psychol Nurs.* 2015;53(5):36-43.

52. White CM. How MDMA's pharmacology and pharmacokinetics drive desired effects and harm. *J Clin Pharmacol.* 2014;54(3):245-252.

53. Mycyk MB. MDMA poisoning. In: Schaider JL, Barkin AZ, Barkin RM, Wolfe RE, Shayne P, Hayden SR, Rosen P, eds. *Rosen & Barkin's 5-Minute Emergency Medicine Consult.* 5th ed. Philadelphia, PA: Wolters Kluwer; 2015b:686-687.

54. McMahon DM, Winstead S, Weant KA. Toxic alcohol ingestions: Focus on ethylene glycol and methanol. *Adv Emerg Nurs J.* 2009;31(3):206-213.

55. Stromberg PE, Cumpston KL. Ethylene glycol poisoning. In: Schaider JL, Barkin AZ, Barkin RM, Wolfe RE, Shayne P, Hayden SR, Rosen P, eds. *Rosen & Barkin's 5-Minute Emergency Medicine Consult.* 5th ed. Philadelphia, PA: Wolters Kluwer; 2015:394-395.

56. Rietjens SJ, de Lange DW, Meulenbelt J. Ethylene glycol or methanol intoxication: Which antidote should be used, fomepizol or ethanol? *Neth J Med.* 2014;72(2):73-79.

57. Norris RL, Bush SP, Smith JC. Bites by venomous reptiles in Canada, the United States, and Mexico. In: Auerbach PS, ed. *Wilderness Medicine.* 6th ed. Philadelphia, PA: Elsevier; 2012:1011-1039.

58. Weinstein SA, Dart RC, Staples A, White J. Envenomations: An overview of clinical toxinlogy for the primary care physician. *Am Fam Physician.* 2009;80(8):793-802.

59. Clark RF. Snakebite. In: Olson KR, ed. *Poisoning & Drug Overdose.* 6th ed. 2012. Retrieved from http://accessmedicine.mhmedical.com/content.aspx?bookid=391&Sectionid=42069957.

60. Lank PM, Erickson TB. Snake envenomation. In: Schaider JL, Barkin AZ, Barkin RM, Wolfe RE, Shayne P, Hayden SR, Rosen P, eds. *Rosen & Barkin's 5-Minute Emergency Medicine Consult.* 5th ed. Philadelphia, PA: Wolters Kluwer; 2015:1046-1047.

28

Gynecologic and Obstetric Emergencies

KATHRYN WADE AND TERESA GREENWOOD

COMPETENCIES

1. Perform a focused assessment of the pregnant patient, which includes subjective and objective data related to the patient's pregnancy.
2. Identify normal physiologic changes that occur during pregnancy.
3. Perform a focused assessment of the fetus before and during transport.
4. Initiate and perform appropriate interventions for the patient in preterm labor.
5. Describe and discuss common indications for transport of the high-risk obstetric case.
6. Discuss common gynecologic emergencies

Complications that arise during pregnancy and place the pregnant patient at risk have many causes. Some complications may be related to the pregnancy itself, others may be related to preexisting medical conditions that may be aggravated by the pregnancy, and yet others may be related directly to the fetus.

Transport team personnel who provide care for the obstetric patient at risk must be prepared to assess obstetric factors so that stabilizing care can be provided in preparation for transport. For recognition of the pathologies associated with pregnancy, the transport clinician must understand the normal physiologic changes that occur during pregnancy.[1] The well-being of the fetus and the mother must be considered. Identification of risk factors, early detection of possible complications, and interventions by the team during the transport can ensure a more favorable outcome for both the mother and the fetus. The transport team must be prepared to perform an obstetric assessment, determine strategies for transport, perform fetal monitoring, and initiate appropriate interventions. Complications are numerous and are usually multifocal. They can include, among other things, amniotic fluid embolism (anaphylactoid syndrome of pregnancy), delivery complications, diabetes in pregnancy, hemorrhagic complications, multiple gestation, gestational hypertension and related disorders, preterm labor (PTL) and related issues, and trauma in pregnancy. The transport team must also be prepared to identify and treat common gynecologic emergencies such as ovarian torsion, ectopic pregnancy, toxic shock, and rape.

The information gained with the general obstetric assessment (Box 28.1) aids the transport team in setting priorities for care during the transport.[2-5] The old cliché in transport and emergency medical service (EMS) was that all energies should be concentrated on the mother because "if you don't save the mother, you can't save the baby." Although this adage is true in global terms, the transport team must be aware of maternal and fetal therapies that can improve survivability and decrease morbidity of the fetus as well as the mother.

The maternal fetal triage index provides another tool that can be used to gather data for the transport of the obstetric patient. It can assist the transport team in preparing, planning, and anticipating potential problems for both the mother and the fetus during transport (see Fig. 28.1 for this tool).[6]

Determination of Team Composition for Transport of the Pregnant Patient

Determination of the members of the transport team who transport the pregnant patient continues to generate controversy. Many pregnant patients are transported by teams composed of personnel who transport a variety of patients.[2-5,7-10] However, at times, the condition of the patient or fetus may warrant personnel with high-risk obstetric (HROB) or neonatal experience. Dedicated maternal transport teams may be considered ideal from a patient care standpoint but are often cost-prohibitive or unavailable for many transport programs. The challenge becomes how to provide adequate training of nonspecialty teams in competent assessment and care of the HROB patient. This controversy is not dissimilar to the training of transport teams in care for

• BOX 28.1 General Obstetric Assessment

1. Age of patient: Age (for women less than 18 or greater than 35 years of age) predisposes the obstetric patient to many complications.
2. Gravida/para: Gravid is the number of times pregnant, regardless of outcome. Parity is broken down into four sections. The first assessment is the number of term deliveries (after 36 weeks' gestation), and the next section is the number of deliveries before 36 weeks' gestation but less than 20 weeks. The next section is the number of abortions and miscarriages. The final section is the number of now living children. This more specific assessment of parity provides a tremendous amount of obstetric history. For example, a woman has been pregnant six times. She has two term deliveries, one preterm delivery, two abortions, and one baby who died of sudden infant death syndrome. Her G/P is: G6 P 2122.
3. Estimated date of confinement (EDC): The EDC can be estimated from the first day of the last menstrual period (LMP) by using Nägele's rule, which is to count back 3 months from the LMP and then add 7 days. The due date is accurate within 2 weeks. Applications for mobile devices operating programs have free versions for calculating LMP/EDC and gestational age.
4. Ultrasound scan: Has the patient had an ultrasound scan? How many? When was the first ultrasound? In the event of an uncertain or unknown LMP or irregular menses, an ultrasound scan performed between 12 and 30 weeks is reliable for dating the pregnancy within 2 weeks. An ultrasound scan can confirm the EDC estimated by the LMP. Early ultrasound scans performed before 12 weeks are accurate for dating within 1 week. An ultrasound scan is invaluable with any question about placental location, amount of amniotic fluid present, fetal presentation, expected fetal growth, or anomalies.
5. In addition to the inquiry into medical history and allergies, obstetric history is of significance. The following information may be of some predictive value for the outcome of the current pregnancy:
   a. Did the patient deliver vaginally or by cesarean section? Has she had a vaginal birth after a cesarean section? Observe for the location and extent of any abdominal scars.
   b. Did she or the baby experience any delivery complications?
   c. Did she experience any complications associated with any past pregnancies?
   d. Has she had any preterm deliveries? At what gestation did she deliver, and what was the outcome?
   e. Has she had either spontaneous or elective abortions? Was a dilation and curettage required?
   f. How many living children does she have? What were the birth weights and genders of each child?
   g. Has less than 1 year elapsed between the last delivery and commencement of the current pregnancy?
   h. What was the length of her last labor?
6. Pertaining to the current pregnancy:
   a. Is the patient having contractions? If so, when did the contractions begin? Has there been a change in the intensity or frequency of contractions? Is there accompanying backache or pelvic or rectal pressure? How strong do the contractions palpate and how do they compare with patient reporting? What are the frequency, duration, and regularity of the contractions?
   b. Is any vaginal bleeding or bloody show present? Is there active, frank bleeding? Attempt to help the patient quantify the bleeding by the number of towels, pads, or amount of clothing soaked before arrival and observe for evidence of dried blood on the perineum, legs, and soles of the feet. Was the bleeding painless or associated with contractions or abdominal pain? Was the blood bright red or dark? Was mucus combined with the blood (bloody show)? When did, the bleeding begin? Was there any previous activity that may have precipitated the bleeding?
   c. Does the patient report leaking fluid vaginally? Does the patient believe her "bag of waters" has ruptured? Was there a gush or an intermittent trickle? A small leakage of clear fluid may be confused with urinary incontinence. Leakage of amniotic fluid is uncontrollable. What time did it happen? What color was the fluid: meconium-stained, dark (presence of blood in the fluid), or clear? Was an odor present? Is the Chux pad under the patient wet or pooling with fluid?
   d. Does the patient smoke? If so, how much? Is there any evidence of alcohol or substance abuse? Attempt to ascertain from the patient the frequency and time of last usage.
   e. Has the patient had an adequate weight gain? Does she appear malnourished or obese?
   f. Has the patient had consistent prenatal care, no prenatal care, or limited prenatal care (three or fewer visits)? Obtain prenatal record if available because it provides a tremendous amount of obstetric information including history, ultrasound scan reports, laboratory reports, vital signs, and so forth.
   g. Has there been any change in fetal activity in the past several days?
   h. Is the patient currently taking any medications? If so, what is she taking and when was the last dosage?
   i. Is the patient having any current medical problems or problems with this pregnancy?
   j. Have any diagnostic tests been done?
7. Assess initial vital signs, including temperature: The blood pressure (BP), pulse, and respirations should be assessed every 15 minutes or as indicated. The obstetric patient should be positioned in the left lateral recumbent position before the BP is taken. When the patient is in the supine position, the gravid uterus may cause obstruction of the inferior vena cava, diminishing venous return to the heart, which may lead to supine hypotension. Consequently, uteroplacental blood flow is decreased, placing the fetus at risk for compromise.
8. Fetal heart tones (FHTs): If the patient is currently being monitored with electronic fetal monitoring (EFM), evaluate the baseline fetal heart rate (FHR) and baseline variability, observing for accelerations and decelerations. FHR should be assessed with Doppler if EFM is unavailable. FHR auscultation should be assessed every 15 minutes or more frequently if any irregularities are noted. For strip interpretation, refer to the discussion in this chapter on fetal monitoring.
9. Fundal height (FH): FH should be measured in centimeters from the symphysis to the fundus. The fundal height roughly correlates to the gestation of the pregnancy in weeks. In the presence of polyhydramnios, multiple gestations, a large-for-gestation fetus, or a fetus with intrauterine growth restriction, the fundal height may not correlate with the gestation, signaling the possibility of complications. If no tape measure is available or the patient is unable to provide information, such as in the case of a trauma, assess the fundus in relation to the umbilicus. If the fundus is above the umbilicus, it is estimated the pregnancy is at least 20 to 24 weeks' gestation.
10. Lightly palpate the fundus for strength, frequency, and duration of contractions: The fingertips can indent the fundus freely with mild contractions and slightly with moderate contractions; firm tension is noted with strong contractions.

• BOX 28.1 General Obstetric Assessment—cont'd

Between contractions, palpate the abdomen for localized or generalized tenderness and observe the patient's coping response to the contractions. Gestures, posture, and facial expressions in response to contractions and verbal description should be noted. If the patient is in labor, observe for indications of advancing labor such as apprehension, restlessness, increasing difficulty coping with the contractions, screaming, nausea and vomiting, bearing-down effort, increase in bloody show, or a bulging perineum.

11. Determine the fetal position with abdominal palpation: With the fingertips and palms, lightly palpate the fundus for the head or buttocks, moving down the sides to identify the fetal spine and small parts, and palpate the lower uterine segment for the presenting part. If the fetal position remains

unclear, the fetus may be in a transverse lie. The FHT is heard most clearly over the fetal spine.

12. Assess cervical status as indicated by the presence of contractions: If the amniotic membranes are intact, cervical status just before departure should be documented. If the membranes are ruptured, a sterile vaginal examination (SVE) should never be attempted unless delivery is deemed imminent. In the presence of hemorrhage, an SVE should never be attempted unless a placenta previa has been ruled out with ultrasound scan. During transport, an SVE is not indicated unless signs of advancing labor are noted.

13. Observe for the presence of other risk factors that predispose the obstetric patient to complications.

---

specialty patients who need intraaortic balloon pumps, left ventricular assist devices, and other specialized equipment. Some suggested guidelines include the following[2-5,7-12]:

- A patient who is not in labor but needs transport for complications of pregnancy, such as preeclampsia or third-trimester bleeding, can probably be transported by a team with maternal and neonatal experience or a general transport team that has had HROB training from obstetric specialists.
- A patient not in labor but with severe preeclampsia ideally should be transported by a maternal transport team.
- A patient in labor may need both a maternal and a neonatal transport team. If this is not feasible or practical, the transport team may consider delaying the maternal transport and waiting until the baby is delivered. Now, the neonate can be safely transported in a controlled environment. Individual program-directed guidelines are imperative in assisting with transport timing decisions.

If the transport team does not routinely transport HROB cases, the Commission on the Accreditation of Medical Transport Systems[5] recommends that the team members receive training in neonatal resuscitation. The transport vehicle should allow access to both the mother and the child in the case of a delivery during transport. Each transport program should have a policy and procedure in place that addresses when transport of a pregnant patient is and is not appropriate and what team members should provide care during transport. In addition, receiving facilities are recommended to offer HROB education through the receiving facility or outside educators. Education directly leads to increased competency and confidence.

If transport services do include specialty teams as a part of their service, they must ensure that these individuals receive annual training, are competent to provide care, and are equipped and dressed for transport. This training should include the following[1,5]:

- Use of restraint systems in the transport vehicle
- Safety and survival skills

- Emergency egress training
- Postaccident/incident training

Contraindications for initiation of maternal transport should be considered before leaving a referring facility. These contraindications include the following[1,3-5,7-13]:

- Inability to stabilize the mother's condition, for example, inability to control bleeding
- Fetal status and well-being
- Imminent delivery, especially in a vehicle that does not allow access to both the mother and child
- Lack of maternal and neonatal experience by the transport team or no experienced personnel available to accompany the team
- Hazardous weather conditions that may prolong the transport time

General Strategies for Transport

The primary survey and obstetric physical assessment should be completed in a very short time because of concerns with the crew and the patient being out of belts for adjustment of the external fetal monitor. The primary survey is completed as it is in every other patient. The obstetric assessment is completed in the secondary survey. Pertinent information obtained from the patient may be gathered as the situation permits during the transport. In a life-threatening situation for the mother, the fetus, or both, lifesaving measures must take precedence. During transport, or preferably before, the team should perform the following assessments and interventions[2-5,7-16]:

1. Place the patient in a left lateral or right lateral recumbent position or displace the uterus with a wedge if the patient cannot be turned. Displacing the uterus from the inferior vena cava (IVC) provides optimal return to the heart for maintenance of adequate mean arterial pressure (MAP).

2. Note the patient's temperature if possible. The American College of Obstetricians and Gynecologists (ACOG) recommends assessment of vital signs every 15 minutes for any patient in labor or at high risk.

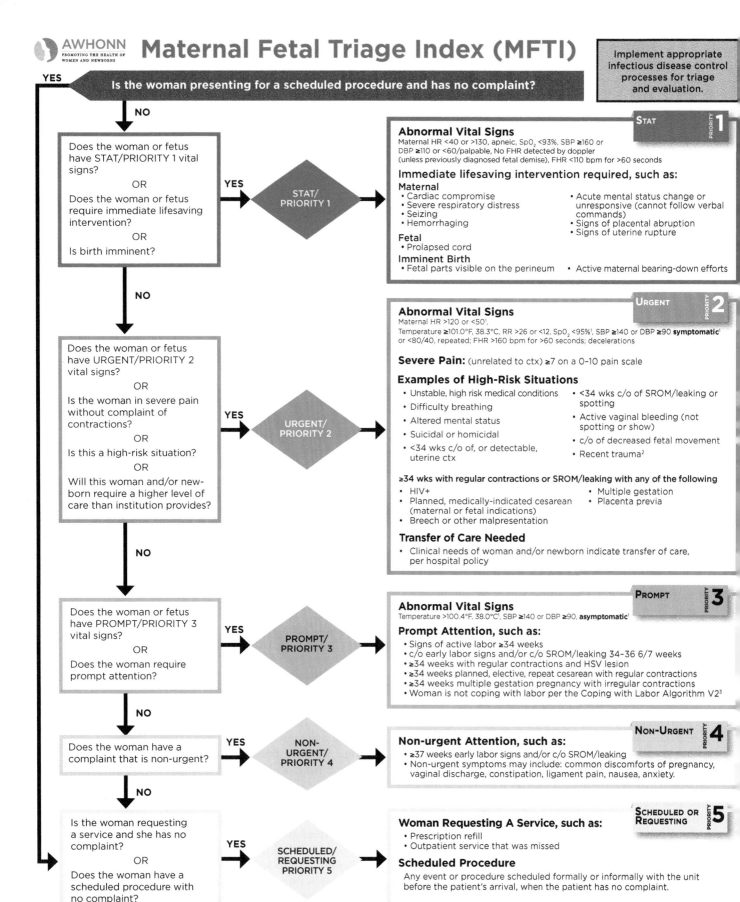

Maternal Fetal Triage Index (MFTI)

AWHONN PROMOTING THE HEALTH OF WOMEN AND NEWBORNS

Implement appropriate infectious disease control processes for triage and evaluation.

YES | Is the woman presenting for a scheduled procedure and has no complaint?

NO

Does the woman or fetus have STAT/PRIORITY 1 vital signs?
OR
Does the woman or fetus require immediate lifesaving intervention?
OR
Is birth imminent?

YES → STAT/ PRIORITY 1 →

STAT — PRIORITY 1

Abnormal Vital Signs
Maternal HR <40 or >130, apneic, SpO₂ <93%, SBP ≥160 or DBP ≥110 or <60/palpable, No FHR detected by doppler (unless previously diagnosed fetal demise), FHR <110 bpm for >60 seconds

Immediate lifesaving intervention required, such as:
Maternal
- Cardiac compromise
- Severe respiratory distress
- Seizing
- Hemorrhaging
- Acute mental status change or unresponsive (cannot follow verbal commands)
- Signs of placental abruption
- Signs of uterine rupture

Fetal
- Prolapsed cord

Imminent Birth
- Fetal parts visible on the perineum
- Active maternal bearing-down efforts

NO

Does the woman or fetus have URGENT/PRIORITY 2 vital signs?
OR
Is the woman in severe pain without complaint of contractions?
OR
Is this a high-risk situation?
OR
Will this woman and/or newborn require a higher level of care than institution provides?

YES → URGENT/ PRIORITY 2 →

URGENT — PRIORITY 2

Abnormal Vital Signs
Maternal HR >120 or <50¹, Temperature ≥101.0°F, 38.3°C, RR >26 or <12, SpO₂ <95%¹, SBP ≥140 or DBP ≥90 **symptomatic**¹ or <80/40, repeated; FHR >160 bpm for >60 seconds; decelerations

Severe Pain: (unrelated to ctx) ≥7 on a 0-10 pain scale

Examples of High-Risk Situations
- Unstable, high risk medical conditions
- Difficulty breathing
- Altered mental status
- Suicidal or homicidal
- <34 wks c/o of, or detectable, uterine ctx
- <34 wks c/o of SROM/leaking or spotting
- Active vaginal bleeding (not spotting or show)
- c/o of decreased fetal movement
- Recent trauma²

≥34 wks with regular contractions or SROM/leaking with any of the following
- HIV+
- Planned, medically-indicated cesarean (maternal or fetal indications)
- Breech or other malpresentation
- Multiple gestation
- Placenta previa

Transfer of Care Needed
- Clinical needs of woman and/or newborn indicate transfer of care, per hospital policy

NO

Does the woman or fetus have PROMPT/PRIORITY 3 vital signs?
OR
Does the woman require prompt attention?

YES → PROMPT/ PRIORITY 3 →

PROMPT — PRIORITY 3

Abnormal Vital Signs
Temperature >100.4°F, 38.0°C¹, SBP ≥140 or DBP ≥90, **asymptomatic**¹

Prompt Attention, such as:
- Signs of active labor ≥34 weeks
- c/o early labor signs and/or c/o SROM/leaking 34-36 6/7 weeks
- ≥34 weeks with regular contractions and HSV lesion
- ≥34 weeks planned, elective, repeat cesarean with regular contractions
- ≥34 weeks multiple gestation pregnancy with irregular contractions
- Woman is not coping with labor per the Coping with Labor Algorithm V2³

NO

Does the woman have a complaint that is non-urgent?

YES → NON-URGENT/ PRIORITY 4 →

NON-URGENT — PRIORITY 4

Non-urgent Attention, such as:
- ≥37 weeks early labor signs and/or c/o SROM/leaking
- Non-urgent symptoms may include: common discomforts of pregnancy, vaginal discharge, constipation, ligament pain, nausea, anxiety.

NO

Is the woman requesting a service and she has no complaint?
OR
Does the woman have a scheduled procedure with no complaint?

YES → SCHEDULED/ REQUESTING PRIORITY 5 →

SCHEDULED OR REQUESTING — PRIORITY 5

Woman Requesting A Service, such as:
- Prescription refill
- Outpatient service that was missed

Scheduled Procedure
Any event or procedure scheduled formally or informally with the unit before the patient's arrival, when the patient has no complaint.

¹High Risk and Critical Care Obstetrics, 2013
²Trauma may or may not include a direct assault on the abdomen. Examples are trauma from motor vehicle accidents, falls, and intimate partner violence.
³Coping with Labor Algorithm V2 used with permission

15003

The MFTI is exemplary and does not include all possible patient complaints or conditions. The MFTI is designed to guide clinical decision-making but does not replace clinical judgment. Vital signs in the MFTI are suggested values. Values appropriate for the population and geographic region should be determined by each clinical team, taking into account variables such as altitude.

AWHONN recommends nurses performing obstetric triage complete the online MFTI education course. Visit www.awhonn.org/mfti for more information.

©2015 AWHONN. For permission to disseminate or integrate the MFTI into the Electronic Medical Record contact permissions@awhonn.org.

Fig. 28.1 Maternal MFTI. (From Ruhl C, Scheich B, Onokpise B, Bingham D. Interrater reliability of testing of the maternal triage index. *JOAFNN.* 2015;46(6):710-716.)

3. Note fetal heart tones (FHTs). Initiate continuous electronic fetal monitoring (EFM) if available and applicable. Concerns for continuous fetal monitoring en route include vibration and movement that cause an intermittent fetal heart rate (FHR) tracing, the EFM monitoring of maternal heart rate (HR) and not the FHR, and the need for the crew members and patient to be out of belts for monitor adjustment. FHR assessment with Doppler scan should be performed at least every 15 minutes per ACOG guidelines. Document fetal movement as either present or absent. Documentation should also include current fetal movement patterns to previous fetal movement patterns. For example, is the fetus moving the same amount, more or less compared with usual movement patterns? Decreasing fetal movements may indicate progressive hypoxia and decreasing perfusion. In addition, the uterus must be palpated for contractions with assessment for frequency and duration and subjective assessment of intensity and resting tone.

4. Start an intravenous (IV) line with a large-bore 18-gauge or 16-gauge catheter and blood tubing. Use lactated Ringer's or a 0.9 normal saline solution with an infusion rate of up to 125 mL/h or titrate volume with consideration for renal, cardiac, and pulmonary status.

5. Provide supplemental oxygen with a nonrebreather mask as indicated by FHR pattern or maternal condition.

6. Monitor oxygen status with pulse oximetry, maintaining a level of 98% to 100%.

7. Have a qualified clinician assess uterine contractions and cervical status before departure. Although the assessment is subjective, a commonly used tool is palpation of the fundus during contractions. If at the peak of the contraction the fundus palpates similar to the consistency of a nose, then the contraction is considered mild. If the contraction palpates as firm as the chin, then it is considered a moderately strong contraction. If it palpates as firm as a forehead, then it is considered a strong contraction. Keep in mind that this assessment is subjective and patient perceptions should also be taken into consideration. Sterile vaginal examinations (SVEs) may be inappropriate for patients with a ruptured bag of membranes or for concerns with infection. Sterile speculum examinations are more appropriate for this patient population.

8. Note and quantify any bleeding. Blood loss should be assessed as objectively as possible. Use pad counts, weighing of blue Chux pads, or actual description on the pad (i.e., a 1 × 4-inch stain). Clots can be measured in a graduated cylinder or suction canister. Assess whether blood loss is associated with any pain or contractions.

9. Observe for leaking of fluid vaginally. Note the color and odor of the fluid and presence or absence of contractions.

Emotional and psychological support provided to the at-risk obstetric patient and her family is as vital an aspect as the emergency care provided. The team should encourage the patient to express and verbalize her anxiety, fear for the fetus, and concern regarding complications. The transport team should assess the patient's knowledge of the situation, encourage questions, and use the opportunity for patient education. The vocabulary used should be based on the education and employment background of the patient. Because most patients have never been transported via air or ground ambulance, the team should explain all medications, procedures, and equipment to allay apprehension about the unfamiliar circumstances. The team should also reassure family members about the current condition of the patient and answer any questions they may have regarding the diagnosis, treatment, or destination. This is true for *all* patients.

Inferior Vena Cava Syndrome

The IVC was once described by a cardiovascular surgeon as having the consistency of a wet paper towel roll. Use this description to imagine the weight of the fetus, amniotic fluid, placenta, and uterus compressing the IVC. Keep in mind that the IVC is responsible for transporting venous blood from the lower part of the body back to the right atrium in which it can travel through its normal cardiac flow and then be returned to the central circulation as oxygenated blood. When a gravid (pregnant) patient lies supine, she quite effectively compresses the IVC. Venous blood return is dramatically decreased, which causes a logical decrease in cardiac output (CO). If blood is not brought to the heart, the heart does not have volume to pump out. This condition is called the *inferior vena cava syndrome* (IVCS). IVCS greatly mimics hypovolemic shock. Patients present with hypotension (decreased CO), reflexive tachycardia (as a result of decreased CO), skin parameter changes (cool diaphoretic skin), and potential mental status changes (decreased cerebral blood flow leads to nausea, vomiting, and decreased level of consciousness [LOC]). Decreased blood flow to the uterus occurs secondarily. The limited amount of blood is shunted to the mother's vital organs, sacrificing the fetus. Unfortunately for the fetus, the uterus is *not* considered a vital organ. If fetal monitoring is in place, signs of fetal distress are seen as a result of hypoplacental perfusion. Luckily, for awake and alert patients, IVCS is rarely a problem because they cannot tolerate lying supine if the weight of the gravid uterus is enough to compress the IVC. The patients experience nausea and naturally flip themselves to their sides. This action increases the patency of the IVC, and the patients feel better as venous blood return increases. The greatest potential problem occurs when the pregnant patient is obtunded or unconscious, for example, a trauma patient. Appropriately, EMS puts these patients on a backboard and cervical collar. A towel roll under the backboard at the patient's hip relieves the compression of the IVC. At this time, the patient's condition should dramatically improve as blood is now able to return to the heart. If the patient is indeed in hypovolemic shock, then an objective assessment can now be made (e.g., left or right side). For years, medical personnel have all learned that the pregnant patient should be on her *left* side to increase venous and placental blood flow. The IVC lies slightly to the right midline under the uterus. In theory, if the patient is turned to the left, the IVC is the most patent. It is now known that the IVC is also patent if the patient is tilted or turned to the right. In addition, if the patient cannot be turned, the uterus can be manually displaced by gently pushing or pulling it to the left and off the IVC. Failure to treat IVCS is the most common mistake health care professionals make in the care of the pregnancy patient because they are not accustomed to "tilting" our patients, and this condition is often forgotten. Prevention is key because these patients already have compromised conditions. This is a great example of how an intervention cannot only improve the maternal condition but can also save the life of the fetus.

Fetal Monitoring Before and During Transport[17,18]

Fetal monitoring may be accomplished with intermittent Doppler auscultation, which is used most frequently for short transports, and with EFM, which is used for longer transports (approximately 30 minutes or more). An external ultrasound scan device records FHTs, and a tocodynamometer detects subjective uterine activity.[17,19] The mode of FHR assessment, be it continuous or intermittent via Doppler scan, is often program and institution dependent. One has not been clearly identified over the other as superior during transport. The ACOG does not make a statement on which method of fetal monitoring is recommended; however, they do state that FHR assessment should be done a minimum of every 15 minutes during transport.[16]

Continuous assessment of fetal well-being is best accomplished with *EFM*. FHTs are recorded simultaneously with uterine activity. The EFM works by sending ultrasound waves into the uterus; the monitor detects the fastest moving objects, which are typically the valves on the fetal heart. This information or sound is returned to the monitor in which it is converted to a number on graph paper. The monitors have a program designed to detect HRs between approximately 50 and 190 beats/min. A limitation of the EFM is that if the FHR nears the lower limits of the monitor capacities the EFM may erroneously detect the motion of one heart beat as two separate beats. This inaccuracy is called "doubling" the FHR; the monitor paper graphs the FHR at twice the actual HR. Conversely when the FHR nears the upper limits, the monitor may only recognize every other motion as a heartbeat and "halving" of the FHR occurs. So, how does one accurately assess the FHR with an EFM? The key is the audible signal on the monitor. The audible signal of the monitor remains accurate and can be compared against the printed FHR tracing to confirm accuracy. In addition, the maternal pulse should be compared with the FHR tracing to confirm that the maternal signal is not being traced. This inaccuracy has occurred in circumstances in which an intrauterine fetal demise has occurred and the EFM then monitors the maternal aorta

fluctuations and misinterprets them as a FHR. Subtle changes in the FHT are often the earliest indication of hypoxia caused by uteroplacental insufficiency or umbilical cord compression. Recognition of normal FHR tracing permits abnormalities to be realized quickly. Appropriate intervention should be aimed at correcting or alleviating the source of insult; at a minimum, actions should improve placental/uterine perfusion.

Historically, conflicting interpretations have been seen. Most of this conflict has revolved inaccuracy around nomenclature, classification, and significance of EFM patterns. Because of these inconsistent interpretations, the National Institute of Child Health and Human Development (NICHD) developed a defined terminology and classification system. This system was later adopted by the ACOG and Association of Women's Health, Obstetric and Neonatal Nurses. This chapter reflects all of the NICHD nomenclature (http://www.nccwebsite.org/resources/docs/final_ncc_monograph_web-4-29-10.pdf).

Baseline Fetal Heart Rate Assessment

The first parameter to be assessed is the FHR baseline. The baseline is the average of the FHR and typically is between 110 and 160 beats/min. The baseline is assessed over a minimum 10-minute period. In addition, it is assessed between contractions and periodic or episodic changes. Periodic changes are accelerations or decelerations, which are associated with uterine contraction. Episodic changes are accelerations/decelerations not associated with uterine contractions. The FHR baseline is the approximate mean FHR rounded to increments of 5 beats/min over a 10-minute period. In any 10-minute section, a minimum of a 2-minute period of no contractions or periodic or episodic changes is needed to determine the FHR baseline. Evaluation of the FHR baseline is a critical step in FHR interpretations. It allows interpretation of trends that occur in the baseline and can reflect subtle changes in the fetal environment.

Fetal Heart Rate Abnormalities[17,18]
Variability

Fluctuations in the FHR reflect interplay between the sympathetic and parasympathetic branches of the autonomic nervous system (ANS). A constant pull from the sympathetic nervous system increases the HR, and a push from the parasympathetic nervous system decreases the HR. These normal variations between each fetal heartbeat give the FHR tracing its "squiggly" appearance. Variability is the single most important factor in prediction of fetal well-being, based on EFM monitor interpretation. Fetal movement remains the number one nonmonitor indicator of fetal well-being. Similar to assessment of the baseline, variability can only be assessed between contractions and episodic and periodic changes (Fig. 28.2).

Absent variability occurs when the amplitude range is undetectable. Causes may include fetal metabolic acidosis,

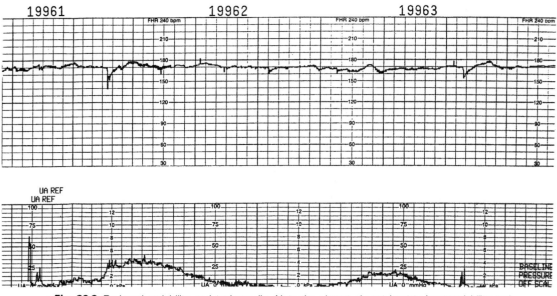

• **Fig. 28.2** Reduced variability and tachycardia. Note the almost absent beat-to-beat variability and reduced long-term variability as recorded by fetal scalp electrode; also, note the tachycardia baseline.

neurologic abnormality, marked prematurity, cardiac arrhythmia, effects of drugs, fetal sleep, or inactivity.

Moderate variability is indicative of an adequately oxygenated, normal pH, mature and intact ANS. Moderate variability is defined as fluctuations in the FHR that range between 6 and 25 beats/min. The presence of moderate variability is reassuring because it indicates that the fetus is tolerating blood flow changes within the uterus.

Minimal variability is defined as fluctuations in the FHR that are greater than undetectable but less than 5 beats/min. This variability is often associated with fetal hypoxia and acidosis. However, benign or expected minimal variability can occur in certain clinical situations including sedation, fetal sleep, and if the fetus is sick; for example, the fetal variability can decrease if the mother has received any narcotics. Narcotics are a central nervous system (CNS) depressant, and anything that decreases the maternal CNS can decrease fetal CNS as it passes through the placenta. As the maternal drug is metabolized and excreted, the effects on the fetus should also be seen to diminish. Minimal variability is not associated with maternal drug use, and other causes of decreasing variability must be assessed. Another common reason for minimal variability is immaturity in gestational age, which is associated with CNS immaturity. Fetuses that are less than 32 weeks' gestation show less variability because the ANS may not yet be fully developed. Fetal arrhythmias and cardiac or CNS anomalies may also be responsible for minimal or absent variability. These causes show variability changes from the time monitoring is initiated. The most common reason for benign minimal variability is the fetal sleep pattern. The fetus has frequent sleep periods that range from 20 to 40 minutes. A key assessment pearl is that although fetal sleep patterns are common, they are transient in nature and rarely last longer than 40 minutes.

In addition, moderate variability should be documented before and after the sleep pattern. As blood flow decreases across the placenta or umbilical cord, less oxygen is available for the fetus. If the hypoxic events are corrected, the fetus usually tolerates them well. However, if the cause of decreased perfusion is not corrected, an eventual decrease in variability is noted. Careful evaluation of the FHR tracing reflects trending of decreasing variability (minimal or absent), which is a warning sign that the fetus is losing compensatory mechanisms and fetal hypoxia and acidosis are increasing. Interestingly, the incidence rate of actual fetal acidemia in the presence of minimal or absent variability and decelerations are only 23%.[17] However, the presence of these signs remains an indicator for intervention. These interventions include measures to increase placental and uterine perfusion, such as maternal position change, IV fluid bolus to increase maternal volume/perfusion, and application of supplemental O_2.

Marked variability of more than 25 beats of fluctuation may be one of the earliest signs of hypoxia. Although it may also be an indication of increased fetal activity, constant assessment and reevaluation are necessary. If continuous EFM is used during transport, the clinician should keep in mind that a greater degree of variability may be recorded than is actually present because of vibrations from the vehicle. Variability should be assessed with NICHD terminology such as moderate, minimal, absent, or marked (Table 28.1).

Periodic Changes/Episodic Changes

Periodic changes are changes that occur in the FHR tracing related to uterine contractions. Episodic changes are changes in the FHR tracing that are not associated with uterine contractions and are often related to fetal movement. The FHR may accelerate, decelerate, or not respond.

TABLE 28.1	NICHD Terminology	
NICHD	**Fluctuations**	**Indications**
Moderate	6–25 beats/min	Well-oxygenated, nonacidotic, intact/mature CNS
Minimal	≤5 beats/min	Hypoxia, acidosis, sleep patterns, maternal drug use, cardiac or CNS insult, prematurity
Absent	Undetectable from baseline	Hypoxia, acidosis, sleep pattern, maternal drug use, cardiac or CNS insult
Marked	>25 beats/min	Fetal movement or early hypoxia

CNS, Central nervous system; *NICHD,* National Institute of Child Health and Human Development.

Acceleration Accelerations above the baseline are usually associated with fetal movement but may occur during contractions (Fig. 28.3). Because the hypoxic fetus with metabolic acidosis is unable to accelerate its HR, accelerations are viewed as a sign of fetal well-being. The true definition of acceleration is a transient increase above the baseline greater than 15 beats/min for 15 seconds or longer and typically lasting less than 2 minutes in duration. This definition is applied for fetuses that are greater than 32 weeks' gestation. The definition of acceleration for a fetus younger than 32 weeks is a transient increase over baseline of greater than 10 beats/min for at least 15 seconds and typically less than 2 minutes. Uniform accelerations are accelerations that occur with each contraction and are uniform in shape and size. This acceleration pattern may be associated with breech presentation or early and mild cord compression. In very early labor, the contractions are not strong and the fundus or top of the uterus gently compresses the breech during contractions, which causes a sympathetic response and accelerations are noted. Later, as the contractions increase in strength and the head of the fetus is pushed down into the pelvis, uniform decelerations are seen (see the section Early Decelerations).

Although the presence of accelerations and moderate variability are excellent monitor signs of fetal well-being, fetal movement remains the best nonmonitor indicator of fetal well-being. Only well-oxygenated fetuses with normal pH levels have consistent fetal movement patterns. Certainly, all fetuses have different movement patterns that are unique to themselves. During transport, the clinician should assess the current movement pattern compared with the usual movement pattern. For example, a fetus that is known to have movements of at least 15 times an hour that is now reported to have only moved once in the past 2 hours shows a significant deviation from normal patterns and further assessment and documentation are necessary. The transport team should take note of fetal movements and whether the mother has noticed a decrease, increase, or no change in fetal movement. Decreased fetal movement may be indicative of hypoxia. Although a decrease in fetal movement may be anticipated, such as in the event of maternal trauma and blood loss, the transport team is expected

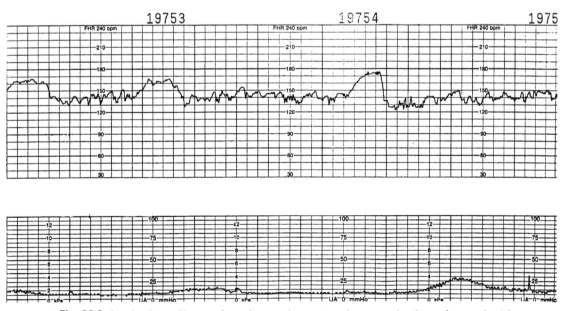

• **Fig. 28.3** Accelerations with use of an ultrasound scan transducer, accelerations of approximately 15 beats above the baseline may be noted. Long-term variability is present, and the FHR baseline range is approximately 135 to 145 beats/min.

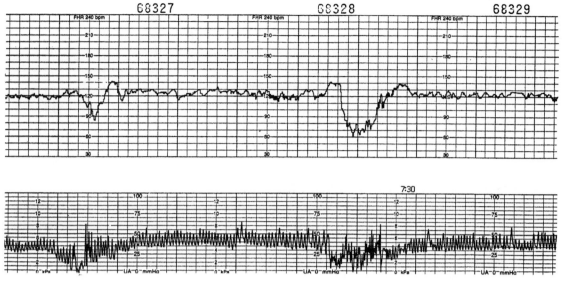

• **Fig. 28.4** Variable decelerations. Note the variable decelerations in the presence variability. The accelerations before and after the deceleration (also called shoulders) reflect adequate variability.

to inform the maternal fetal medicine physicians of this change in fetal status.

Variable Deceleration Variable decelerations can occur at any time during a contraction (Fig. 28.4). The shape may also vary and is frequently V-shaped or W-shaped. The decelerations are known as variable because of the varied shape and timing. Cord compression is typically responsible for these decelerations. However, they may also occur from head compression because of vagal stimulation in the second stage of labor (pushing). Physiologically, as the cord is compressed, blood flow through the umbilical cord is decreased. Baroreceptors cause a brief increase in the FHR to compensate. The blood flow is further impeded, and a sharp decrease occurs in the FHR. As the umbilical cord compression is relieved, the FHR responds with a quick increase above the baseline in an attempt to increase oxygenation status. After a short period of time, typically less than 5 to 10 seconds, the FHR returns to baseline with moderate variability. Initially, variables may have a characteristic appearance; frequently, a short acceleration is observed, followed by a rapid deceleration for some seconds and then a rapid rise and a short acceleration before a return to the FHR baseline. The short period of increased FHR before and after the deceleration is known as shoulders. Shoulders are associated with moderate variability and indicate that the fetus still can compensate with varying amounts of placental blood and available oxygen. Shoulders are considered a reassuring characteristic associated with variable decelerations. If the fetus continues to have variable decelerations that are progressively more consistent or deeper in nadir, then often this compensatory response is lost and only the sharp deceleration is seen without shoulders noted. The abrupt onset and sharp decline with usual rapid return to baseline makes these decelerations easily identifiable. Cord

compression may occur in a variety of circumstances. After the membranes rupture, less fluid is available to cushion the cord. Variables usually occur in response to uterine contractions but also may occur in response to fetal movement in the absence of contractions when membranes are ruptured. If a nuchal cord, short cord, or cord entanglement is present, variables usually result.

In the past, these decelerations have commonly been described as mild, moderate, or severe, depending on the drop in FHR. However, to remain consistent with NICHD nomenclature, a more conclusive method is to describe the deceleration. This description should include the depth (nadir), duration, shape, and return variability status. A better indicator of the fetal response is reflected in the baseline FHR, baseline variability, and changes in the variable decelerations. Signs that the fetus is losing its ability to tolerate the stress of repeated cord compression or that the cord compression is becoming more severe include a deeper deceleration that lasts longer, a slow return to baseline, loss of shoulders, and decreased variability. Overshoots are another type of acceleration seen with variable decelerations. These differ from shoulders in the sense that these accelerations are seen only *after* the variable deceleration as the compromised fetus attempts to improve oxygenation status. These offshoots are typically well above baseline. Offshoots are associated with minimal to absent variability and are considered nonreassuring. When interpreting the tracing, careful observations of any changes in FHT reveal more than what has just occurred during the last contraction.

Late Decelerations Late decelerations begin at or after the apex (peak) of the contraction. They gradually decelerate in a uniformed "U" shape and return to the FHR baseline well after the contraction is over (Fig. 28.5). By definition, late decelerations must be recurrent, which means they occur in

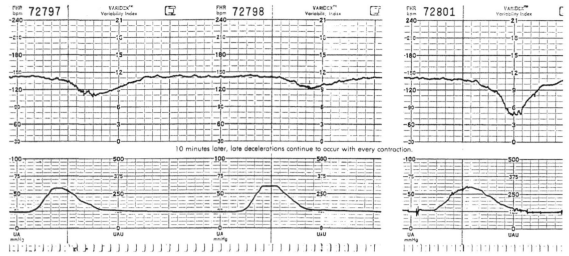

• **Fig. 28.5** Late decelerations. Note the onset of deceleration at the apex of the contraction. Also, note the minimal variability, slow recovery, and the proportional deceleration.

greater than 50% of all uterine contractions (NICHD).[3] Physiologically, during a normal contraction, a decreased amount of oxygen crosses the placenta. A healthy fetus can tolerate this decrease in oxygen via its oxygen reserves. A compromised fetus that has experienced prolonged or chronic hypoxia does not have oxygen reserves available; therefore it cannot tolerate the decrease oxygen availability found during contractions. Not until the contraction is over and the maternal–fetal exchange can resume does the FHR return to baseline. Late decelerations always mean uteroplacental insufficiency: either the placenta, the fetus, or the uterus presents with conditions that interfere with normal exchange of oxygen between the mother and fetus. One analogy is a child being dunked in a pool. The child tolerates the dunking early on, but if it continues, the child becomes fatigued, loses O_2 reserve, and ends up gasping every time he surfaces. When a contraction is stronger, the insufficiency is greater and the deceleration is proportional. However, "size does not matter." With severe hypoxia, the myocardial depression may be such that the heart is unable to decelerate in response to the stress of the contraction, and very subtle late decelerations are seen accompanied by a flat FHR baseline. Simply stated, the fetus becomes so hypoxic and acidotic that it cannot render a response to the impeded blood flow. The fetus is too sick to "wave the white flag." A FHR tracing that is tachycardia with minimal or absent variability and subtle late decelerations is considered an ominous FHR tracing and interventions must be made to improve fetal oxygenation. These interventions include measures to increase placental perfusion, such as maternal position change, supplemental O_2 via a nonrebreather mask, IV fluid (IVF) boluses, and possible delivery, if improvement is not noted.

Uteroplacental insufficiency may result from numerous maternal and fetal conditions, such as hypertensive disorders of pregnancy, diabetes mellitus (DM), cardiovascular or kidney disease, chorioamnionitis, smoking, a fetus that is past maturity, and fetal hydrops. Uteroplacental insufficiency may also result from decreased placental perfusion in placental abruption or previa, uterine hypertonus as a result of oxytocin stimulation, and hypotension. As with variable decelerations, evaluation of late decelerations with respect to FHR baseline, variability, and changes noted over time is necessary in determining the wellbeing of the fetus. Even an otherwise healthy well-oxygenated fetus can experience late decelerations in the presence of acute hypotension and hypoxia. An example of this is a mother that is obtunded and was laid flat on her back on a backboard. This position alone can cause IVCS and rapid decrease in maternal venous blood return, which then causes maternal hypotension that leads to profound fetal hypotension and results in late decelerations. Once the maternal position is tilted to the right lateral position (RLP) or left lateral position (LLP), the blood flow improves and the late decelerations resolve.

Early Decelerations Early decelerations are innocuous decelerations that begin close to the beginning of the contraction and end close to the end of the contraction. These decelerations appear to mirror the contractions. As the head is compressed, the vagus nerve is stimulated and causes a parasympathetic response that leads to a deceleration. The deceleration ends as the contraction ends because the vagus nerve (head) is no longer compressed. Early decelerations are usually associated with moderate variability and are considered benign in nature. These decelerations frequently occur in active labor when the cervix has dilated 4 to 7 cm, or they may be seen in early labor with breech presentation because, in this position, the head is compressed into the pelvic cavity with contractions. A transport consideration is that a sterile vaginal examination (SVE) or sterile speculum examination should be performed before transport to rule out advanced cervical dilation. In FHR interpretation, late decelerations should not be confused with early decelerations. Accurate placement of the tocotransducer over the fundus ensures that contractions are recorded correctly. Also, consider other reassuring attributes such as moderate variability and the presence of accelerations or fetal movement to help discern early from late decelerations.

Sinusoidal Sinusoidal is a rare FHR pattern in which a uniform sine wave pattern occurs. This FHR remains within normal baselines but has an obvious unusual appearance. It is often described as an undulating pattern that is saw-toothed in appearance. Possible causes of this pattern are fetal hypovolemia or anemia; it may occur in cases of erythroblastosis fetalis, accidental tap of the umbilical cord during amniocentesis, fetomaternal transfusion, placental abruption, or another type of accident. Neither variability nor accelerations/decelerations can be assessed. When this pattern is recognized, rapid delivery is usually recommended unless the underlying pathology can be corrected. For example, in the case of severe fetal anemia, a blood transfusion can be administered to the fetus via a percutaneous umbilical cord sampling procedure. Once the anemia is resolved, the sinusoidal pattern is resolved. However, a more commonly observed FHR pattern is a pseudosinusoidal or undulating pattern that is not pathologic (Fig. 28.6). This pattern is linked to maternal drug administration, both prescribed and illicit.

Bradycardia A baseline FHR of less than 110 beats/min for a period of 10 minutes or longer is defined as bradycardia. Bradycardia can occur as result of numerous acute or chronic conditions and can be hypoxic or nonhypoxic in nature. Many term fetuses and those past maturity may have a stable baseline between 100 and 120 beats/min, reflecting a more mature fetal neurologic system that is more parasympathetically controlled. In the absence of hypoxia, adequate variability and accelerations are also noted.

Bradycardia is a response of increased parasympathetic tone and is reflected by a decrease in fetal CO in the presence of hypoxia. The fetus can tolerate sustained bradycardia for only a short length of time before becoming acidotic. Bradycardia can be acute because of severe cord compression. It can occur minutes before delivery when the cord is drawn into the pelvis in the second stage or with a cord prolapse. Bradycardia can also occur with hypertonic or tetanic contractions as seen with placenta abruptio and any event that causes maternal hypotension. In the presence of chronic hypoxia, bradycardia is usually a late occurrence. Evaluation of variability determines how the fetus tolerates the stress.

Tachycardia A baseline FHR of more than 160 beats/min for a period of 10 minutes or longer is considered tachycardia. Tachycardia is a response of increased sympathetic tone and is reflected by a compensatory mechanism to increase CO in the presence of transient hypoxia. A decrease in variability is generally associated with tachycardia. This decreased variability and increased rate is reflective of the fetus returning to a more primitive or sympathetic response. Fetal tachycardia may be maternal or fetal in origin. Factors that contribute to tachycardia include smoking, maternal fever, use of β-sympathomimetic agents, fetal anemia, fetal hypovolemia, fetal tachydysrhythmias, chorioamnionitis, and maternal hyperthyroidism.

Assessment of FHR tracings should follow a systematic approach with these sequential steps:
1. Assessment of baseline FHR
2. Assessment of baseline variability with NICHD standards
3. Assessment of periodic/episodic changes, including accelerations or decelerations
4. Assessment for the presence of tachycardia or bradycardia

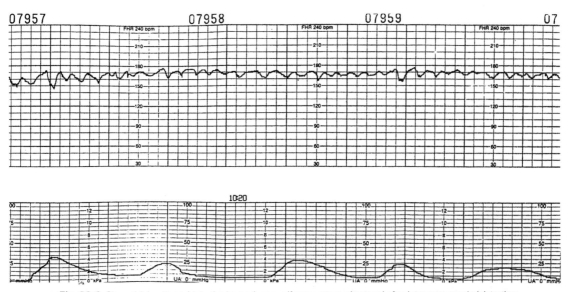

• **Fig. 28.6** Sinusoidal pattern. Note the jagged, nonuniform pattern observed after intravenous administration of butorphanol (Stadol), 1 mg, which resolved spontaneously after 20 minutes.

At any time that the transport team considers that the FHR tracing is not reassuring, medical control or receiving maternal fetal medicine physicians must be contacted for further orders. Interventions should be made to improve placental perfusion, including maternal position change, supplemental O_2 via a nonrebreather mask, and IVF boluses. If the transport team is unsure of the FHR interpretation, then the FHR strip can be faxed to the receiving facility for interpretation. If the FHR is nonreassuring en route, then medical control should be contacted (if possible) and diversion should be considered for signs of ominous fetal distress.

Nonreassuring signs of fetal well-being include a significant increase or decrease in the FHR baseline during a period of several hours, a wandering baseline, a spontaneous decrease in variability or a decrease in variability as labor progresses, bradycardia or tachycardia with reduced variability, subtle late decelerations, or any combination of these signs.

Abnormal FHR tracings are observed in situations of congenital anomalies. Frequently, variability is reduced or absent, and tachycardia or bradycardia may be noted. Table 28.2 summarizes comparative signs of acute and chronic distress. Whatever the mechanism of insult to the fetus, the plan of action for possible fetal distress is intrauterine resuscitation.

The key formula (LOCK) is as follows:

L: Place the patient in the left lateral or right lateral recumbent position.
O: Provide supplemental oxygen, via 100% nonrebreather mask.
C: Correct or improve contributing factors.
K: Keep reassessing the FHR and intervene when indicated.

Contributing Factors to Fetal Distress

Interventions that must be performed by the transport team when signs and symptoms of fetal distress are present are as follows:
1. Hypotension: Initiate a 500-mL IVF bolus, depending on the condition of the patient. If the patient has no comorbidities that promote pulmonary edema, the maternal patient can receive 2 L of crystalloids to improve maternal and placental perfusion. Correct for supine hypotension with a change to the LLP or RLP, uterine displacement, or a towel roll under the backboard.
2. Tachysystole: Consider the use of terbutaline, 0.25 mg, administered subcutaneously or via IV push. Check to ensure that the patient's HR is less than 120 beats/min before administering the medication.
3. Rule out cord prolapse. A SVE is used to confirm the presence of a cord. Lift the presenting part off the cord to relieve the cord compression and reposition the patient, following the recommendations provided in this chapter.
4. Assess for placental abruption or other complications that may affect the FHR.

TABLE 28.2	**Comparison of Signs of Chronic and Acute Distress**	
Chronic Distress (Occurs Over Time)	**Acute Distress (Occurs Suddenly)**
Mechanism of Insult	
Uteroplacental insufficiency	Umbilical cord compression or uteroplacental insufficiency
Signs of IUGR, decreased fetal movement	Initially, no indication of fetal compromise
Contributing Factors	
Gestational hypertension (preeclampsia)	Cord prolapse
Cardiac or kidney disease	Placental abruption
Severe anemia	Hypotension (vena cava compression, epidural anesthesia, hemorrhage)
Diabetes mellitus (class B-R)	Hypertonic contractions
Postdate pregnancy	Placenta previa with hemorrhage
Rh isoimmunization	
Chorioamnionitis	
Smoking	
Fetal Response (Progression Differs Depending on Circumstances)	
Tachycardia	Variable decelerations
Increased variability	Prolonged decelerations
Decreased variability	Tachycardia
Late decelerations	Increased variability
Bradycardia	Decreased variability
	Late decelerations
	Bradycardia

IUGR, Intrauterine growth restriction.

5. Change the position of the mother. If the LLP does not relieve the cord compression as indicated by continued variable decelerations, then reposition the mother to the right side; to the hands and knees; or last, to the knee-chest position. A transport consideration is the inability to restrain the maternal patient in the knee-to-chest position in some vehicles, especially small helicopters.
6. Assess for signs of maternal hemorrhage. Changes in FHR, including tachycardia and loss of variability, are often the first signs of maternal blood loss. The maternal patient has 40% to 50% more blood volume at term; therefore she can mask signs of hypovolemia. In addition, the maternal patient shunts blood to her vital organs, and the uterus is *not* considered a vital organ.

If the patient is located in an outlying area in which the transport time is expected to be lengthy, evaluation of the FHR for reassuring signs of fetal well-being aids in the decision to transport the mother or to deliver the fetus at the referring facility to increase the chance of fetal survival.

The accepting maternal fetal medicine physicians make the ultimate decision of whether or when to transport. Appropriate indications for maternal/fetal transport are if the referring facility is unable to offer specialized or HROB services or a Neonatal Intensive Care Unit. Likewise, if the transport is expected to be short and the time needed by the referring facility to prepare for a cesarean delivery is longer than the estimated transport time, maternal transport is recommended. The intent of the transport is to attain the most expedient delivery of the mother and fetus in a facility most capable of dealing with the mother and fetus at risk. Studies show improved neonatal outcomes if the fetus is delivered at a perinatal network with a level III nursery.[16]

The transport team may consider use of Doppler auscultations or EFM for transports. Advantages and disadvantages are found with both methods. Doppler auscultation is performed a minimum of every 15 minutes. This method does not allow for assessment of variability but can assess for FHR and responses to contractions if auscultation is performed during and after contractions. Continuous EFM allows for assessment of variability; however, vibration of the aircraft may artificially add artifact. Remember that this can be a problem in any transport vehicle. Because of position constraints in the aircraft, the EFM may slip and monitor maternal HR, which causes the transport team and patient to frequently be out of belts so the monitor can be adjusted. The FHR strip should clearly identify when maternal HR is monitored so that the fetal status and well-being can be documented. Trained and competent individuals must accomplish this monitoring. The age-old controversy with continuous fetal monitoring during transport is what to do with the information found. For example, if the fetal condition acutely deteriorates into fetal distress, is there adequate time to divert to another facility? Does diversion to another facility outside of the level III hospital offer services other than the referring facility? Both forms of monitoring are accepted by the ACOG as appropriate and safe. Regardless of the method chosen, if the FHR reflects acute or chronic signs of deterioration or distress, appropriate interventions must be made to alleviate the cause and to increase uterine/placental perfusion. These interventions and maternal/fetal responses need to be documented.

Normal Physiologic Changes in Pregnancy

For true appreciation and recognition of the pathologies that may be associated with pregnancy, a review of normal physiologic changes is necessary. All physiologic changes occur to prepare the body for birth, support the growing fetus, and prepare for breastfeeding. This review of systems is brief and highlights key areas[1-24]:

Airway: The failure rate with oral intubation is higher in the pregnant patient than in the nonpregnant patient. The mucosa in the pharynx of the pregnant patient is hyperemic and more edematous. The trachea of the term pregnant patient tends to be anterior, and the epiglottis is reported to be friable.

Hematologic: By term, the maternal blood volume has increased by 40% to 50%. The greater increase is in plasma then in red blood cells (RBCs), platelets, and so forth. Thus a normal dilutional anemia is often associated with pregnancy. In cases of maternal blood loss, maternal hypotension is often not noted until the patient has lost approximately 30% of the blood volume because of the extra volume created during the pregnancy. Platelets and fibrinogen slightly increase during pregnancy and cause the pregnant patient to be in a hypercoagulable state, which allows faster and more efficient clotting to prevent hemorrhage after delivery.

Respiratory: Tidal volume increases by about 40%, and respiratory rate slightly increases; thus pregnant women have compensated respiratory alkalosis. Alveolar ventilation increases by 65%.

Cardiac: CO increases by about 50% (related to the increased blood volume). HR slightly increases by about 10 beats by term. Blood pressure is normotensive (for the patient) in the first trimester, decreased in the second trimester, and returned to normotensive in the third trimester. This change is greatly related to a pregnancy hormone called relaxin. A key assessment point is that the blood pressure should never be elevated over 140/90 mm Hg during pregnancy. If it is, a pathology is always indicated.

Gastrointestinal: Slowing of peristalsis and resulting constipation occur. The stomach empties slowly, and the pregnant patient is at a high risk of aspiration with altered levels of consciousness. This effect is also related to the hormone relaxin. Because of this effect, a pregnant woman is always considered to have a full stomach no matter when her last meal was. Increased salivation is common, and frequent suctioning may be needed in the case of oral intubation. An increased incidence of cholelithiasis is found during pregnancy.

Renal: Increased renal filtration of glucose and sodium occurs during pregnancy. Blood urea nitrogen (BUN) and creatinine (CR) levels are both lower during pregnancy. Elevated levels of either renal function laboratory tests indicate pathology. Protein is a large molecule and is seen as pathologic when passed through the kidneys.

Uterus: The uterus becomes the largest intraabdominal organ. Uterine and placental perfusion increases to 600 to 800 mL of blood per minute at term. A very high risk of maternal hemorrhage is found in the presence of uterine or placental injury.

Musculoskeletal: The abdominal viscera become stretched and distended because of the growing uterus. These distorted viscera may cause abdominal pain to be referred. The effects of the hormone relaxin also cause the symphysis pubis cartilage to slightly separate, increasing pelvic instability. The gravid uterus causes the patient's center of gravity to be altered, and an increase in falls may be noted. The thoracic cavity also expands during pregnancy to allow greater lung expansion because the lungs have less distance to elongate because of the gravid uterus.

Liver: The liver is the only organ to not increase efficiency during pregnancy. Hepatic function values remain the same as nonpregnant values. However, if elevations of serum glutamate oxaloacetate transaminase (SGOT)/serum glutamate pyruvate transaminase (SGPT), or aspartate aminotransferase/alanine aminotransferase, are noted, significant pathology is implied.

Integumentary:

Elasma: This is a dark coloration or blotching of the face caused by the increase in estrogen levels which stimulates melanin production. Because of the melanin, a pregnant woman's face may develop lots of freckles. During pregnancy, higher levels of estrogen prolong the growth of hair resulting in less shedding making the hair appear fuller.

Linea nigra: This is a dark line that runs from the pubis to the umbilicus that is caused by an increase in the melanocyte-stimulating hormone produced by the placenta.

Palmer erythema: This is mottled or reddening of the palms caused by estrogen elevations.

Spider angiomas: These appear on the face, neck, chest, arms, and legs and are caused by elevated estrogen levels.

Endocrine: The follicle-stimulating hormone (FSH) ceases its activity because of increased levels of estrogen and progesterone secreted by the ovary and corpus luteum. The FSH prevents ovulation and menstruation. The corpus luteum enlarges during pregnancy and produces progesterone to help maintain the lining of the endometrium in early pregnancy. It functions until the 10th or 12th week of pregnancy when the placenta can produce progesterone and estrogen. The function of progesterone is to relax smooth muscles. Prolactin levels elevate because of maternal pituitary gland enlargement. Prolactin helps in the change of the mammary gland for lactation. Oxytocin is a hormone released by the pituitary gland and helps with production of milk and contraction. It also helps with the bonding process between mother and baby.

Metabolic: All metabolic functions increase to provide for the demands of the fetus, placenta, and uterus as well as for the mother's increased basal metabolic rate and oxygen consumption. Protein metabolism increases for maternal and fetal growth. The pancreas cannot supply the increased demand. After delivery, the mother will become hypoglycemic because insulin levels are still high. The infant's blood sugar should also be checked because there still may be a large amount of insulin in its body after delivery.

Complications of Pregnancy and Delivery

There are several complications that may occur during pregnancy and delivery. The following sections include a discussion of some of these complications and how to manage them before, during, and after transport.

Amniotic Fluid Embolism/Anaphylactic Syndrome of Pregnancy

Amniotic fluid embolism is now known as *anaphylactic syndrome of pregnancy.* Previously, it was thought that amniotic fluid gained access to the maternal circulation during labor or delivery or immediately after delivery, resulting in obstruction of the pulmonary vasculature. In addition, particulate matter in the amniotic fluid, such as meconium, lanugo hairs, fetal squamous cells, bile, fat, and mucin, was also thought to form emboli. The belief now is that the process is more likely to be an anaphylactic reaction to the amniotic fluid and the fetal cells it contains. Treatment is primarily supportive and usually necessitates immediate intubation, mechanical ventilation, pressor administration, and treatment of coagulopathy. In the United States amniotic fluid embolism causes 10% of maternal deaths. The complication is very rare and is frequently fatal, with a maternal mortality rate nearing 90%. Amniotic fluid embolism is often initially misdiagnosed as a result of the vague clinical picture of surviving patients and missed autopsy findings in fatal cases. Unfortunately, the rapid progression of this syndrome is associated with a high maternal mortality that is often not diagnosed until postmortem.[9]

Etiology and Pathophysiologic Factors

The route by which amniotic fluid enters the circulatory system of the mother is not clear. The most frequently suggested sites of entry are lacerations in the endocervical veins during cervical dilation and lacerations in the lower uterine segment, the placental site on separation and delivery of the placenta, and uterine veins at sites of uterine trauma. Under the pressure of uterine contractions, amniotic fluid gains access to the circulatory system of the mother and travels quickly to the pulmonary vasculature, where embolization and anaphylactic reaction quickly ensue.[9]

Factors that have been associated with amniotic fluid embolism include uterine rupture, cesarean section, and the use of uterine stimulants to induce labor. Other factors that place the obstetric patient at risk are a large fetus, placenta previa, placental abruption, intrauterine fetal death, meconium in the amniotic fluid, multiparity, precipitous delivery, knee-chest position, and maternal age of more than 30 years.[9]

Disseminated intravascular coagulation (DIC) is a complication that can be expected, although the pathway is unclear. Uterine atony and postpartum hemorrhage (PPH) are also frequent complications. Acute cor pulmonale, right heart failure, and pulmonary edema follow.[9]

Assessment

Of the predisposing factors that the patient may have, sudden acute dyspnea is the most characteristic symptom, followed by profound cyanosis and sudden shock. Other symptoms may include chest pain, restlessness, anxiety, coughing, vomiting, pulmonary edema with pink frothy sputum, seizures that are frequently confused with eclamptic seizures, and coma. If the patient has delivered, the transport team should watch for symptoms of PPH caused by uterine atony (and coagulation disorders, such as DIC that often follow).[9,12,15,16,21,23]

Because of the extremely rare occurrence of amniotic fluid embolism and the rapidity of onset of symptoms with deterioration, the transport team may be unsure of the clinical picture. If dyspnea appears in a patient who is in a tumultuous labor with ruptured membranes, then amniotic fluid embolism should be part of the differential diagnosis. Tachycardia, hypotension, and tachypnea indicate the severity of the embolic process. Urine output may be decreased (less than 30 mL/h), which indicates inadequate renal perfusion. Blood is shunted away from the uterus to the vital organs, and FHR changes indicative of placental insufficiency are observed. Severe fetal distress may be present. DIC can be suspected if petechiae, hematuria, bruising, or bleeding from IV sites is observed. Coagulation study results confirm DIC. Chest radiograph may show infiltrates.[9]

Strategies for Transport

If an obstetric patient with amniotic fluid embolism/anaphylactic syndrome of pregnancy is transported, supportive care should be provided. Although the clinical picture may not be clear, treatment focuses on the alleviation of presenting symptoms. The transport team should provide supplemental oxygen with a 100% nonrebreather mask if the patient is not already intubated. Positive end-expiratory pressure may be necessary because of a high association with acute respiratory distress syndrome. The transport team can provide circulatory support with additional IVFs and likely will need numerous lines or a multilumen central line. The transport team may initiate blood replacement in an attempt to correct hypovolemia, blood loss, and coagulopathy. This syndrome most commonly occurs postpartum, but if the patient is still gravid, the FHTs should be monitored for signs of severe distress.

If the fetus has been delivered, oxytocin 20 to 40 units may immediately be added to 1000 mL IV solution for uterine atony. Frequent fundal massage should be performed by supporting the lower uterine segment with one hand while massaging the fundus with the other. Morphine or fentanyl can be administered intravenously for apprehension, dyspnea, and pain. An antiemetic should be considered if the mother is nauseated or has vomited.

The transport team should expedite the transport and, if the transport will be extended because of distance, weather, or other issues, the transport team should discuss with the staff at the referring facility if delivering the baby is safer before transport. In that case, the appropriate personnel, including a neonatal team will need to be available.[9,12,15,16,21,23]

Delivery Complications

Delivery complications can be predicted in some situations and may be quite unforeseen in others. A neonatal nurse, or at a minimum, a transport nurse trained in a neonatal resuscitation program, should always be included on transports when delivery is a possibility.

The information about assessment and suggested transport care that follows makes specific reference to the complication only. General obstetric assessment and general transport principles are assumed to be considered before transport.

Breech Presentation

Breech presentation involves a fetus in a longitudinal lie with the feet or buttocks closest to the cervix. The body often can be felt through the cervix on vaginal examination. With a breech presentation, the buttocks may descend first, with the legs flexed on the fetal abdomen and the feet alongside the buttocks (complete breech); the legs may also be extended upward (frank breech), or one or both feet or knees may be present (footling or incomplete breech). At or near term, the incidence rate of breech is 3% to 4%. Because of the effects of gravity, most fetuses are cephalic or vertex. However, before 34 weeks' gestation, the incidence is considerably higher.

Etiology and Pathophysiologic Factors Breech presentation is more likely to occur in situations with uterine abnormalities, such as a septum that extends part or all of the way from the fundus to the cervix (septate uterus) or a Y-shaped uterus (bicornuate uterus). The belief is that as the pregnancy progresses, the uterine cavity provides the most room for the fetus's bulkier and more movable parts, with the extremities in the fundus of the uterus and the cephalic presenting. Before 34 weeks' gestation, the head of the fetus is disproportionately larger than the body, favoring the breech presentation. For the same reason, the hydrocephalic fetus has a high incidence of breech presentation.[6,11,16,18,22,25]

Other factors that appear to predispose to the breech presentation are grand multiparity, a previous breech delivery, multiple gestations, polyhydramnios, oligohydramnios, placenta previa, uterine tumors, and congenital anomalies.

Complications associated with breech presentation are inherent because of the position of the fetus. With the buttocks and lower extremities presenting, cord prolapse, cord entanglement around the extremities, and cord compression are more likely to occur. When delivery is managed too forcefully, birth trauma may result. Trauma to the fetal cervical spine and brachial plexus and fractures of the humerus, clavicle, skull, and neck may occur. A common concern with breech presentation is that the body of the neonate can be delivered but the head is too large to fit through the pelvis.

The fetus in breech presentation is at higher risk for birth asphyxia (hypoxia, hypercapnia, and metabolic acidosis) compared with the fetus that has a vertex presentation.

Head entrapment is a complication that occurs when the buttocks and lower extremities of the premature fetus pass through a cervix that is not completely dilated and is inadequate for the head to be delivered without trauma, asphyxiation, or both for the infant.

Assessment Although the possibility of breech presentation may be determined either through vaginal examination or ultrasound scan, this does not have any bearing on the transport of the obstetric patient unless the patient is in active labor or the membranes are ruptured. If vaginal delivery is inevitable, the transport team must be prepared to assist in a potentially difficult delivery. Vaginal delivery is imminent when the fetal buttocks are bulging the perineum and one or both legs are visible.

Strategies for Delivery Essentially, the fetus in a breech presentation should not be touched until the umbilicus has spontaneously delivered. However, the risk of hypothermia is great for these babies, and a dry warm towel should be wrapped around the torso to prevent heat loss and allow for greater control when handling a slippery baby. The team should disengage the legs if one or both have not delivered spontaneously. This maneuver can be accomplished by hooking a finger on the leg by the groin and gently reducing the leg so it is extended outside the mother's body. Caution must be taken to avoid palpating the exposed umbilical cord. At one time, it was taught to palpate the cord to assess the FHR. However, this palpation could cause venospasm and the umbilical cord could clot off. Recommendations now are that the umbilical cord should be covered with a moist gauze dressing. At this point, the arms can usually be delivered by hooking the index finger over each of the baby's shoulders in turn (Fig. 28.7). After the shoulders, have been delivered, the baby's trunk is rotated so that the back is anterior (facing up), and gentle steady downward traction is applied until the hairline is visible. The body can now rest on the palm of one hand and forearm with the index and middle fingers supporting the baby's mouth and chin to maintain flexion of the head. With the other hand supporting the back and shoulders, the body can then gently be brought upward while another member of the transport team applies gentle suprapubic pressure to facilitate the delivery of the head with a minimal amount of neck traction (Fig. 28.8).[11]

Application of suprapubic pressure can be controversial because it can lead to uterine rupture if the pressure is extreme. If gentle suprapubic pressure is not sufficient to deliver the baby, then the procedure must be stopped. Care must be taken to achieve slow and controlled delivery of the head, allowing the chin, face, and brow to sweep over the perineum. As soon as the baby's mouth has been delivered, the airway should be cleared with a bulb syringe; then, the rest of the head can be gently and slowly delivered. These deliveries can be traumatic for the neonate. Preparation for resuscitation should be initiated before delivery.

Because breech delivery is a rare occurrence for the transport team, the tendency may be to act in haste when this

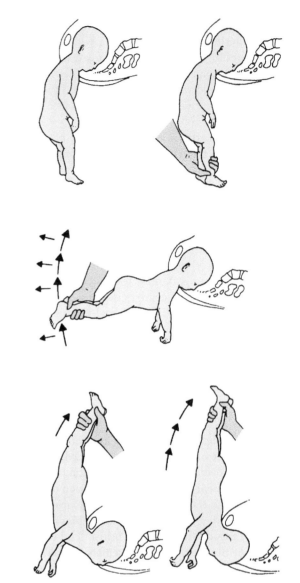

• **Fig. 28.7** Breech extraction. Upward traction to effect delivery of the posterior shoulder, followed by freeing the posterior arm. (From Hickman M. *Midwifery.* 2nd ed. Oxford, UK: Blackwell Scientific; 1985.)

situation arises. The team should guard against haste because it increases the risk for birth trauma.[1,14-17,19,20]

Hemorrhagic Delivery Complications

Once excessive bleeding occurs, quick intervention is necessary to minimize further blood loss. PPH, uterine inversion, placenta previa, placenta abruptio, gestational hypertension, and uterine rupture are delivery complications that predispose the patient to PPH and risk of hypovolemic shock. Care should be directed at correcting the cause of the hemorrhage and then managing the hypovolemic shock and associated complications such as DIC.

Postpartum Hemorrhage

There exists some controversy as to what is the exact amount of blood loss that constitutes a PPH. Some definitions state

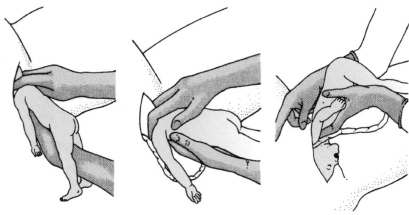

• **Fig. 28.8** Delivery of head with use of the Mauriceau maneuver. Note that as the fetal head is being delivered, flexion of the head is maintained with suprapubic pressure provided by an assistant and simultaneously with pressure on the maxilla by the operator as traction is applied. (From Hickman M. *Midwifery.* 2nd ed. Oxford, UK: Blackwell Scientific; 1985.)

that a blood loss more than 500 mL after delivery is defined as PPH. The blood loss frequently occurs in the first few hours after delivery but can occur more than 24 hours later. PPH occurs in approximately 5% of all deliveries. However, several reviews of the literature have found that a blood loss of greater than 1000 mL or more may have adverse clinical outcomes.[14]

Etiology and Pathophysiologic Factors Estimates of blood loss must be accurate. Some studies have shown that estimated blood loss was approximately half the amount actually lost. Techniques used to improve objective blood loss measurement are pad counts, weighing of Chux pads, or collection of blood clots in a graduated cylinder or suction canister. Uterine atony is the major cause of PPH. Normally, bleeding from the placental site is controlled when the interlacing muscle fibers of the uterus contract and retract in conjunction with platelet aggregation and clot formation in the vessels of the decidua. This occurs immediately after delivery of the placenta as the uterus contracts to spontaneously clamp off uterine blood vessels that once perfused the placenta. Factors that predispose to uterine atony and prevent compression of the vessels at the implantation site predispose to PPH. Uterine atony can occur after a prolonged or tumultuous labor or after general anesthetic is used. The uterus that is overdistended because of multiple gestation, uterine tumors, polyhydramnios, or a large fetus is more likely to be hypotonic after delivery. Multiparity, chorioamnionitis, previous PPH, placenta previa, and use of labor stimulants place the obstetric patient at increased risk for uterine atony and PPH.

As the uterus fills with clots, it is increasingly unable to contract and retract normally, compounding the problem of hemorrhage. In addition, when the placenta and membranes are retained, the same circumstances are created. An abnormally adherent placenta (placenta accreta) or incomplete separation may be the cause.

Another common cause of PPH is lacerations that result from delivery. Undetected lacerations of the cervix, vagina,

perineum, or lower uterine segment are all sources for hemorrhage. Hemorrhage because of lacerations is usually limited and is rarely severe. However, constant seepage over a few hours can amount to an appreciable loss. Application of forceps or use of vacuum extraction may be the reason for the hemorrhage. When a patient has had a previous cesarean section followed by a vaginal delivery, dehiscence of an old uterine scar with hemorrhage may result. Lacerations should be suspected when hemorrhaging occurs in the presence of a firmly contracted uterus. Coagulopathy associated with DIC, placental abruption, and gestational hypertension are other causes of PPH. Idiopathic thrombocytopenia or von Willebrand's disease as preexisting coagulopathies predispose to PPH.

Hemorrhage may also result from a combination of sources. Hemorrhage from uterine atony may be coupled with hemorrhage from a cervical laceration.

Assessment The transport team should determine the source of the hemorrhage. Abdominal palpation may reveal a boggy, enlarged, and soft uterus. Persistent vaginal bleeding from slight to profuse is noted with uterine atony. The team should also examine the patient for the presence of lacerations in the perineal area. Assessment for cervical, vaginal, and lower uterine segment while en route may be difficult or impossible.

Strategies for Transport A team member should palpate and vigorously massage the fundus. One hand should cup the fundus while the other provides support to the lower uterine segment just above the symphysis pubis. Often, clots are expressed, and frequent massage alone may be all the stimulation that is needed for the uterus to adequately contract and retract. Fundal massage should be performed at least every 5 to 15 minutes, and the location of the fundus in relation to the level of the umbilicus, the degree of firmness, and the vaginal flow should be noted. For example, if the fundus is at the level of the umbilicus, it is documented as U/U. If the fundus is 2 cm (fingerbreadths) above the umbilicus, it is noted as 2/U. Transport team members should use their institutional policy related to the use of abbreviations with documentation.

A full bladder is often the reason that the uterus remains boggy and cannot involute. The puffy full bladder lies directly beneath the uterus and interferes with its ability to contract. Simply having the patient void or inserting a Foley catheter for the transport tremendously decreases uterine bleeding. When the uterus is firm, it palpates like a small grapefruit and vaginal bleeding is greatly decreased. If on repeated assessment the uterus becomes boggy again, then the uterus palpates as soft and mushy and increased vaginal bleeding with clots is usually noted. Treatment is to again perform uterine massage. The awake and alert patient can be taught this treatment and can perform it herself. Also of note is that fundal massage can be painful for patients and pain relief medications should be offered and titrated to relieve pain.

Rapid infusion of 20 to 40 units of oxytocin in 1000 mL lactated Ringer's solution, or methylergonovine 0.2 mg administered intramuscularly or intravenously (rarely given IV), is recommended. Methylergonovine should be used cautiously in patients with gestational hypertension because of the pressor effects that may result in further elevated blood pressure.

The integrity of the cervix, vagina, perineum, and lower uterine segment should be documented at the referring facility. Inspection of the placenta after delivery reveals missing fragments, membranes, or both that may be retained. The team should assess blood loss and inspect the perineum; little external bleeding is observed in the presence of a pelvic hematoma. Blood from lacerations tends to be brighter red. Uterine bleeding from either a relaxed or boggy uterus or from retained parts also is bright to dark red and has numerous large clots. Maternal patients are in a hypercoagulable state. Do not pack the vagina if lacerations are seen. Instead, apply a Peri-Pad and have the patient squeeze her legs together. The pad can also be applied to the external genitalia to manage bleeding. If at any time the patient loses the ability to clot or if petechiae or bleeding from IV sites becomes apparent, the presence of DIC must be investigated (Fig. 28.9).

Uterine Inversion

Complete inversion of the uterus is extremely rare and occurs when the entire uterus turns inside out, extending out through the cervix and into the vagina in which it is visible. The uterus can partially invert with the fundus turned inside out. *Partial inversion* is not as obvious and may initially be more difficult to determine.

Etiology and Pathophysiologic Factors

Inversion may occur spontaneously after a contraction or with increased abdominal pressure caused by coughing or sneezing, and it often occurs as the result of overly aggressive

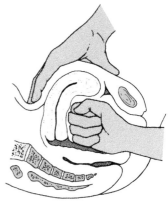

• **Fig. 28.9** This technique is very invasive; hence, the transport nurse may avoid using this procedure. As a last line of action, it is usually effective in controlling postpartum hemorrhage because of uterine atony. Note the placement of the fist in the anterior fornix. (From Hickman M. *Midwifery.* 2nd ed. Oxford, UK: Blackwell Scientific; 1985.)

management of the third stage of delivery (delivery of the placenta). Predisposing factors include excessive cord traction, fundal pressure, excessive cord traction with a placenta accreta, fundal implantation of the placenta, and uterine atony. The lesson to be learned here is do *not* pull on the umbilical cord to deliver the placenta after the baby is delivered. Within 5 to 20 minutes, the placenta spontaneously separates with a gush and lengthening of the cord. At this time, it can gently be guided out through the vagina.

Assessment

Vaginal bleeding, which may be profuse after delivery and accompanied by sudden and severe lower abdominal pain, may rarely be caused by uterine inversion. Abdominal palpation may reveal a defect in the fundus, or it may not be palpable at all, being nonglobular in shape. Signs of hypovolemic shock may develop quickly.

Strategies for Transport

If uterine inversion is recognized immediately before the uterus has had a chance to contract down and the cervix to constrict, manual replacement may be possible. Without attempting to remove the placenta, pressure should be applied with the fingertips and palm of the hand to push the fundus upward and through the cervical canal (Fig. 28.10). This procedure can be extremely painful for the patient.

While the attempt at manual replacement is being made, analgesics should be administered and the procedure and the necessity for it should be explained to the patient.[1,14-17,19,20]

Removing the placenta before attempting to replace the uterus may increase the hemorrhaging. The placenta will deliver unless some degree of placenta accreta exists, and oxytocin should be administered immediately. The best preventive measure is allowing spontaneous delivery of the placenta. If the uterus cannot be safely replaced, it should be covered with sterile moist gauze and immediate transport

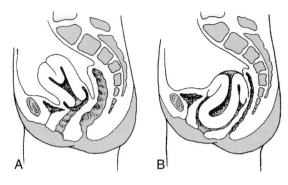

• **Fig. 28.10** Uterine inversion. (A) First degree and (B) second degree. Note the abdominal depression in which the fundus would normally be and vaginal palpation of the fundus at the cervical opening. Continued pressure with the fingertips encourages reversion of the fundus. Note the stages of inversion in the inset. (From Hickman M. *Midwifery.* 2nd ed. Oxford, UK: Blackwell Scientific; 1985.)

should ensue because surgical procedures are needed. Diversion of transport should be considered if the patient's condition is hemodynamically unstable and diversion is available and appropriate.

Uterine Rupture

A spontaneous or traumatic disruption of the uterine wall, known as *uterine rupture,* can occur. If the laceration is extensive and comes in direct contact with the peritoneal cavity, it is a complete rupture. The rupture most frequently occurs in a weak area of the myometrium, usually at the site of a previous incision. Examples of previous incisions include a previous caesarian section scar, a scar from a myomectomy, or a scar from the result of rapid deceleration forces (such as may occur with a fall or in a motor vehicle collision).

Etiology and Pathophysiologic Factors

Before further discussion of uterine rupture, differentiation between rupture and dehiscence of a scar is necessary. *Rupture* refers to the separation of an old incision and possibly an extension into previously uninvolved myometrium, with rupture of membranes. Fetal parts may extend through the rupture into the peritoneal cavity. Hemorrhage is usually present from the edges of the separation and may be massive. A *dehiscence* does not involve the fetal membranes and may not even involve the entire previous scar. Bleeding may be minimal or bloodless. Dehiscence occurs gradually, whereas rupture occurs as a sudden event. A dehiscence may become a rupture with labor or trauma.

Factors that predispose to uterine rupture include previous surgery involving the myometrium, previous cesarean section with a higher incidence of a "classic" vertical scar being involved, use of labor stimulants, trauma, previous rupture, overdistension of the uterus because of multiple gestation or polyhydramnios, and grand multiparity. Uterine rupture usually occurs during labor but can occur before the onset of labor. It can be seen with an unscarred uterus

resulting from blunt trauma. This trauma is most likely a rapid deceleration injury in which pressures inside the uterus are too high because of sudden impact and rupture occurs. Uterine rupture may also occur because of internal trauma, such as perforation with an instrument (e.g., a difficult forceps delivery); from external pressure, such as from an external version of the breech fetus; or from overly vigorous fundal pressure during delivery attempts.

In situations in which the patient has had a previous cesarean section, the probability of rupture is much greater when the scar traverses the body of the uterus vertically (classical incision) than when the scar involves the lower uterine section transversely. Dehiscence occurs more frequently without subsequent complications when the scar is low and transverse.

The degree of hemorrhage and extent of possible complications depend on the location and extent of the rupture. If the rupture does not involve the large arteries, the hemorrhage is less severe. If the rupture is complete, the mortality rate for the fetus is high. Potential complications are postpartum infection, injury to the bladder, potential for hysterectomy for uncontrolled bleeding, hypovolemic shock, kidney failure, DIC, and death.

Assessment

Signs and symptoms of uterine rupture include severe sudden continual abdominal pain and signs of hypovolemic shock. Contractions may cease or may increase in intensity and frequency. Shoulder or chest pain may result from the collection of blood under the diaphragm (Kehr's sign). Generalized tenderness with rebound pain or vaginal bleeding is likely when the rupture occurs in the lower uterine segment. However, many of these patients are obtunded from blood loss and are unable to report pain. Most bleeding is intraabdominal, and the abdomen may be distended. Frequent assessment of fundal height may be an indication that the uterus is filling with blood. Use a marker to mark the top of the fundus with ink, and frequently reassess the fundal height. Palpation of the uterus also reveals a firm or hardening uterus, which is reflective of accumulating blood. Remember the maternal patient carries 40% to 50% more blood at term and can compensate for a longer period of time before maternal vital sign changes are noted. The maternal patient can be in class III shock before any blood pressure change is noted. Another textbook description of uterine rupture is that the clinician should be able to palpate fetal parts as the uterine wall integrity is lost. Although this may or may not be true, this is a *secondary* assessment, and because of tremendous blood volume losses, it is unlikely the clinician has moved beyond the primary survey.

Strategies for Transport

Rapid recognition of the signs and symptoms of uterine rupture often mean the difference between life and death for the obstetric patient. Surgical intervention is necessary, and care is supportive. Oxytocin, 20 to 40 units in a 1000-mL solution administered IV, may incite uterine contraction with vessel constriction and reduce the bleeding after delivery of the fetus. Serial abdominal measurements can be made to further assess intraabdominal bleeding. Acute fetal distress with increasingly severe variable decelerations, late decelerations, minimal to absent variability, or absent FHT is observed.

A history of previous cesarean sections and observation of abdominal scar is of primary importance. Although the scar noted may be low and transverse, documentation is needed to determine the location of the scar on the uterus. For the patient in labor who has had a previous cesarean section, the first sign of placental abruption may actually be rupture. Tocolytics may be considered for patients with a previous classical incision that is at risk for contracting or is currently contracting. Appropriate medical staff must be contacted for direction and management.

Precipitate Delivery

Precipitate delivery occurs when the labor is abnormally rapid with strong contractions and rapid cervical dilation and descent of the presenting part. Delivery usually occurs in 2 to 3 hours from the start of contractions. The transport team's goal is to prevent an expulsive delivery and minimize trauma to both the mother and the fetus. Possible complications include uterine rupture, amniotic fluid embolism, PPH, and lacerations. Other concerns for precipitous delivery involve the neonate. This rapid and forceful delivery can lead to an increased need for resuscitation at birth and a higher incidence of birth trauma. These neonates are literally "shot out" and often need some respiratory assistance with bag-mask-valve (BVM) devices until they can acclimate to life outside the uterus. Transport professionals may not be able to control the labor, but they should have some control over the delivery. An uncontrolled delivery can cause cerebral hemorrhage in the neonate because of rapid changes in pressure. The baby's head should be guided with application of a small amount of supportive pressure.

Retained Placenta

Normally, the placenta separates spontaneously in 5 to 20 minutes after delivery of the fetus. Signs of separation include lengthening of the exposed cord and a gush of blood; the uterus appears to "ball up." Slow gentle downward traction is usually all that is needed to assist the delivery of the placenta. Do not pull on the cord with the intent of hastening the separation of the placenta from the uterine wall. This may result in the tearing of the umbilical cord and postpartum hemorrhage. When no signs of separation occur and hemorrhage is not evident, transport can be accomplished with the placenta retained. Encouraging the mother to breastfeed promotes separation of the placenta and involution of the uterus. When the placenta is partially retained, PPH results. Frequent fundal massage must be initiated until surgical services can be obtained.

Shoulder Dystocia

After delivery of the head, the anterior shoulder pushes against the symphysis, creating a situation commonly referred to as shoulder dystocia. In most circumstances, the head is the largest diameter of the fetus. Occasionally, the shoulders have a larger diameter. The obvious concern is that the head will fit through the pelvic bones and the shoulders will be unable to. The condition becomes apparent when gentle downward traction is applied to the fetal head and the anterior shoulder does not deliver. Or may be seen when the head/face deliver then "retracts back" against the perineum. This is called the turtle sign. The head extends out during a contraction but then retracts after the contraction is over because the shoulders prevent further progression. The incidence of shoulder dystocia increases significantly with birth weight.

Etiology and Pathophysiologic Factors

Several predisposing factors have been linked to shoulder dystocia. However, shoulder dystocia can occur quite unexpectedly without obvious associated factors. The complication occurs more frequently with the presence of a large fetus or with a macrosomic fetus such as those found with gestational diabetes. Other risk factors include patients with a contracted pelvis, maternal obesity, or a prolonged second stage of labor, including deliveries that require instruments for delivery.

Possible complications of shoulder dystocia include brachial plexus damage and fractured fetal clavicle. Fetal hypoxia can occur when the cord is drawn into the pelvis and compressed.

Assessment

In any situation of imminent delivery, unless the fetus is expected to weigh 2500 g or less, shoulder dystocia is a possibility. However, any fetus greater than 4000 g is at a considerably higher risk. After the head has been delivered and inspection for a nuchal cord has been performed, the delivery of the anterior shoulder should be attempted. If the anterior shoulder is unable to be delivered, consider the possibility of shoulder dystocia. Careful considerations for preparation for a difficult delivery, anticipated neonatal resuscitation, and possible diversion should be initiated.

Unnecessary haste and overly aggressive force should be avoided because of the increased possibility of birth trauma to the fetus. Excessive lateral flexion of the neck and overly vigorous traction of the head and neck increase the risk of damage to the brachial plexus.

Strategies for Delivery

Once the team member is aware of the situation, the head may be observed to retract against the perineum. Fundal pressure aggravates the shoulder impaction and should be avoided. If an episiotomy has not been made, a generous mediolateral episiotomy is recommended. The McRoberts maneuver, a simple maneuver that increases the diameter of the pelvis by stretching the pelvic joints, should be tried next. With the patient's legs flexed at the knees, the maternal nurse should help the patient draw her knees up and toward the chest (dorsal knee-chest position) and continue, with gentle downward traction of the head. Once the anterior shoulder clears the symphysis, the posterior shoulder usually delivers without resistance. The key to success in this position is to have the mother's knees as far back to her shoulders as possible. Next, gentle application of suprapubic pressure can be applied by another member of the air medical crew (the shoulder may be palpated suprapubicly). Gentle downward traction of the head should be applied concurrent with gentle suprapubic pressure. Suprapubic pressure should never be excessive because it can lead to uterine rupture and bladder trauma. The team should not persist if the shoulder does not slip under the symphysis.

Delivery of the posterior shoulder can also be attempted with rotation of the posterior shoulder downward and into the left posterior quadrant. With release of the posterior arm and shoulder, the anterior shoulder follows. Internal rotation of the fetal shoulders may also be considered. As a last resort, the infant's clavicle may be deliberately broken; however, when this is done, the chance of damage to the brachial plexus is increased. Vaginal delivery increases the risk for perinatal mortality and morbidity by 3%.[1,14-17,19,20]

Umbilical Cord Prolapse

Overt cord prolapse occurs when the cord slips down into the vagina or appears externally after the amniotic membranes have ruptured. When the cord slips down into or near the pelvis, adjacent to the presenting part, it is not palpable on vaginal examination (occult prolapse). The cord may also have slipped down to a position in which it is palpable through the cervix but in intact membranes (forelying prolapse). Varying degrees of prolapse may occur. The weight of the presenting fetal part causes compression of the umbilical cord. The amount of change in the fetal status and well-being is directly related to the degree or compression.

Etiology

Circumstances that cause maladaptation of the presenting part to the lower uterine segment or prevent descent of the presenting part into the pelvis predispose the obstetric patient to cord prolapse. These factors include breech presentation, transverse lie, premature rupture of membranes (PROM), a contracted pelvis, unengaged large fetus multiparity, polyhydramnios, multiple gestations, a long cord, and PTL. Complications include severe changes in fetal status and well-being and fetal death.

Assessment

Cord prolapse occurs suddenly and requires quick identification of the problem and quick action. Identification of the obstetric patient who is vulnerable to cord prolapse is of primary importance. Clinical signs of prolapse include sudden fetal bradycardia and recurrent variable decelerations that do not respond to a change in maternal position, administration of oxygen, or hydration. Compression of the cord between the presenting part and the pelvic tissues causes the FHR patterns that are observed.

Strategies for Transport

Actions necessary in the event of cord prolapse include elevating the presenting part off the cord with a hand in the vagina that must remain there during the entire transport to prevent further cord compression. The mother should be positioned in a Trendelenburg or knee-chest position to further reduce pressure on the cord. The cord may spontaneously retract, depending on the degree of prolapse, but should never be manually replaced because severe compression may occur. Intervention to elevate the presenting part off the cord must be maintained during the transport and through delivery. The cord should not be touched to prevent vasospasm and be gently wrapped in moist gauze and then wrapped in plastic to prevent it from drying out.

The transport team should provide supplemental oxygen via nonrebreather mask. A tocolytic agent, such as terbutaline 0.25 mg administered subcutaneously or via IV push, should be given to slow the contractions and reduce the pressure on the cord during contractions. When the cord compression is relieved, the fetus can recover from the hypoxic event in utero as long as the compression does not recur.

If cord prolapse occurs when the patient is en route, the receiving facility should be alerted to prepare for an emergency cesarean section. On occasion, the FHR pattern is normal or shows minimal abnormalities. This results from no cord compression from the presenting fetal parts. The only symptom evident is the prolapsed cord; however, the interventions are the same.

Diabetes in Pregnancy

Basically, DM is a disease in which the body is unable to produce or sufficiently use insulin to metabolize glucose. The disease is complicated by faulty metabolism of fats and proteins for energy. The course and outcome of a pregnancy complicated by diabetes depend on the severity of the disease process.

Etiology and Pathophysiologic Factors

This discussion of diabetes in pregnancy is limited primarily to how diabetes is affected by the pregnancy and how the pregnancy affects the patient with diabetes. Pregnancy is considered a diabetogenic state in which the patient has an increased need for glucose and protein and fat are metabolized to aid in the demand for higher glucose requirements. During pregnancy, the metabolism of the mother adapts to provide fuel for the growing fetus and for her own increased metabolic needs. Early in pregnancy, during the period of rapid growth of the embryo, the mother's blood glucose level decreases. The obstetric patient who has diabetes may have hypoglycemia.

At approximately 24 weeks' gestation, the diabetogenic effects of pregnancy begin. Increased hormonal activity exerts an antiinsulin effect that results in a decreased responsiveness to insulin and a rise in the level of blood glucose. Increased production of insulin by the pancreas counteracts the antiinsulin effects of the hormones, and normal blood glucose levels are maintained. If, as a result of an acquired or inherited defect in β-cell function, maternal insulin secretion fails to keep pace with the demand, a further increase in blood glucose levels occurs. At this point in the pregnancy, gestational diabetes is frequently recognized and diagnosed. For the woman who is already diabetic, an increase in insulin requirement occurs and remains increased until after delivery.

The obstetric patient with a pregnancy complicated by DM is at an increased risk compared with the remainder of the pregnant population for development of gestational hypertension and related disorders; polyhydramnios; and infections such as vaginitis, urinary tract infections, and pyelonephritis. Delivery via cesarean section and preterm delivery also occur with increased frequency because of macrosomia or changes in fetal status and well-being. As commonly found with patients with diabetes, vascular changes can affect perfusion. The placentas of women with diabetes tend to have decreased perfusion and more calcification. This in turn leads to decreased fetal perfusion and higher risks of intrauterine growth restriction (IUGR) and changes in fetal status and well-being.

The fetus of a mother with diabetes is at increased risk as well. Complications associated with the fetus include congenital anomalies, IUGR, macrosomia, delivery trauma, fetal distress, hypoglycemia, hypocalcemia, hyperbilirubinemia, respiratory distress, and intrauterine death. *Macrosomia* refers to a fetus that is large for gestational age with increased fat deposition and an enlarged spleen and liver. Macrosomia is seen more commonly when the mother has gestational DM or DM without vasculopathy. Congenital anomalies are seen more frequently when pregnant women with diabetes are in poor control of their diabetes.[1,14-17,19-21]

Assessment

Assessment of the patient with diabetes includes screening for the presence of risk factors linked to DM. All pregnant women with diabetes need to be assessed so the disease can be classified. Assessment by the transport team should include the following:

1. *Obstetric history:* Assess for the possibility that a previous pregnancy was complicated by undiagnosed diabetes. Has the patient had gestational DM with a previous pregnancy, or does she have a family history of DM? Has she delivered an infant that weighed more than 4000 g? Has she had unexplained perinatal losses, stillbirths, or traumatic deliveries? Has more than one pregnancy been complicated by gestational hypertension? Has there been gestational hypertension as a multipara? Does she have a history of polyhydramnios or preterm delivery? Is she older than 35 years?

2. *Current pregnancy:* Does the patient have signs and symptoms of DM? Is glycosuria present? Are results of a glucose challenge test abnormal? Is the patient obese? Has the patient had recurrent urinary tract infections or vaginitis? Does the patient have chronic hypertension? What are the results of ultrasound scans or other diagnostic tests? Is the diabetes controlled with diet or insulin? What is the patient's current insulin regimen? Note: If the patient has not received prenatal care with this pregnancy, most of this information is not known.

3. *History of preexisting condition:* What class is the DM, as determined by the age of onset, duration of the disease, and evidence of vasculopathy? Does the patient have cardiovascular or kidney disease? Has there been good control of the diabetes during the pregnancy? What is the patient's current insulin regimen?

Strategies for Transport

In addition to following the general guidelines for transport care, careful assessment is needed for the obstetric patient with gestational DM or diabetes because of changing metabolic demands. The transport team should obtain a diabetic history from the patient and assess for complications associated with DM in pregnancy. The time of her last meal and last insulin injection are also important to record.

If the patient is in labor, simultaneous continuous insulin and glucose infusions stabilize maternal levels and may reduce neonatal hyperglycemia or hypoglycemia. The insulin may be adjusted after delivery based on blood sugar levels, and the insulin demand decreases after delivery. The patient is given nothing by mouth. Blood glucose levels are evaluated every 1 to 2 hours and maintained at a level of 80 to 120 mg/dL (or to whatever range is desired by maternal fetal medicine physicians or endocrine physicians), with insulin as indicated by the patient's blood sugar.

The transport team should obtain a blood glucose reading just before transport. Because labor increases metabolic needs, the team should be aware of the signs and symptoms of hypoglycemia and hyperglycemia and should never administer terbutaline to a patient with insulin-dependent diabetes because of the transient hyperglycemic response seen with terbutaline. Caution is also advised with the administration of magnesium sulfate because many patients with DM have decreased renal function. Magnesium sulfate is cleared through the kidneys. In addition, many diabetic patients have the comorbidity of gestational hypertension. Use of corticosteroids to assist with maturation of fetal lungs may also influence maternal blood sugar.

Hemorrhagic Complications
Placental Abruption

Placental abruption can be defined as the premature detachment of a normally implanted placenta from the uterine wall. The separation may occur over a small area with little evidence or can separate totally with devastating results. The incidence of abruption varies widely, depending on the source. Of considerable significance is the incidence of recurrence with subsequent pregnancies.[9]

Etiology The primary cause of placental abruption is largely unknown. Hypertension, whether chronic or gestational hypertension, and previous abruption are two factors that are known to greatly increase the risk of placental abruption. Other factors that place the obstetric patient at risk include abdominal trauma, an unusually short umbilical cord, amniocentesis, multiparity, age over 35 years, uterine anomalies or tumors, and sudden uterine decompression (such as when a twin is delivered and the other twin remains in utero, or when a hypertensive crisis is acutely resolved). Other risk factors include cigarette smoking, and substance abuse, especially abuse of cocaine.

Pathophysiologic Factors Hemorrhage occurs from the arterioles that supply the decidua (lining of uterus), causing a retroplacental hematoma. Placental separation takes place at that site and may continue with the hemorrhage. As the hemorrhage continues, more vessels are disrupted, which leads to increased hemorrhage and further separation. Placental separation can be an avalanche that continues to total separation or suddenly stops for reasons unknown. Sometimes a clot blocks the hemorrhage. The decidua is rich in thromboplastin, and clotting occurs rapidly. When vaginal bleeding is observed, the blood is usually dark because of the rapid clotting and the distance it takes to reach the vagina and be seen externally. If separation occurs at the margin of the placenta (Fig. 28.11) or if the amniotic membranes are dissected from the decidua because of the hemorrhage, vaginal bleeding is observed. No vaginal bleeding is observed if the hemorrhage is completely concealed behind the placenta. Use the mental imagery of a fried egg: the yellow yolk is the abruption, and the white egg is the attached placenta. Bleeding is certainly associated with the abruption; it is just occult and cannot escape vaginally to be seen.

As the hemorrhage continues and a retroplacental clot forms, enough pressure may be exerted to force blood through the membranes, giving the amniotic fluid a port wine color, or into the myometrium, causing a condition called Couvelaire uterus. The uterine tone is increased, and irritability is noted. Contractions are frequently present. Blood is a known irritant and often leads to uterine irritability or contractions. The process is a vicious circle: as the bleeding increases, the incidence of contraction increases; as the incidence of contractions increases, so does the incidence of bleeding.

A common complication of placental abruption is DIC. Other complications include PPH, anemia, postpartum infection, hypovolemic shock, kidney failure, and fetal distress or death. As placental perfusion is altered, the risk for fetal hypoxia and acidosis is increased. The factors that predispose to placental abruption may occur preterm, predisposing to preterm delivery.

Placenta Previa

Placenta previa occurs when the placenta becomes implanted in the lower uterine segment and as a result covers or partially covers the internal cervical os. A marginal or low-lying previa extends to or close to the internal os but does not cover any part of it. Placenta previa occurs approximately once in every 200 to 400 deliveries. The incidence of placenta previa is higher preterm. As the pregnancy progresses, the fundus hypertrophies and the lower uterine segment elongates, which allows the placenta to migrate away from the internal os toward the fundus. In reality, the placenta does not move; it is merely carried up toward the fundus as the uterus grows.

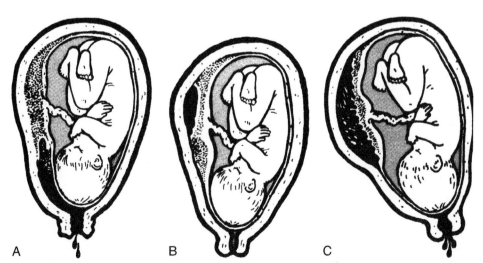

• **Fig. 28.11** Examples of placental abruption. (A) Placental separation occurs at the margin of the placenta. (B and C) Separation originates from a central area behind the placenta. (Illustrated by Vincenza Genovese, Phoenix, AZ; From Gilbert ES, Harmon JS. *High-Risk Pregnancy And Delivery.* St. Louis, MO: Mosby; 1986.)

Etiology Although the exact cause is unknown, a higher incidence of placenta previa is seen with uterine scarring. A previous cesarean section, dilation and curettage, increased parity, multiparity with short intervals, and a previous occurrence of placenta previa can scar the uterus. Other factors that place the obstetric patient at risk for placenta previa include previous chorioamnionitis, multiple gestation (for which a larger surface area is covered by the placenta), fetal erythroblastosis, maternal age over age 35 years, substance abuse, previous myomectomy, and uterine tumors.

Pathophysiologic Factors Normal placental implantation usually occurs in the fundus or body segment of the uterus. Defective perfusion of the decidua has been suggested to favor implantation of the placenta in the lower uterine segment. Because less vascularization exists in the lower uterine segment, the placenta compensates and tends to grow thinner and larger, covering a larger area and increasing perfusion.

Before the onset of labor, the cervix begins to soften, efface, and dilate. These cervical changes disrupt the placental attachment, tearing the vessels, and hemorrhage results. Bright red vaginal bleeding is observed; it is initially painless and is not initially associated with contractions. The primary episode usually involves less than 250 mL of blood and tends to cease spontaneously as clot formation rapidly occurs. Recurrence is unpredictable. Generally, the greater the extent to which the internal os is covered, the sooner the initial episode occurs. In addition, subsequent bleeds are often larger.

Potential complications of placenta previa include complications similar to those of placental abruption, such as DIC, hypovolemic shock, kidney damage (from hypoperfusion), anemia, postpartum infection, PPH, and fetal distress or death. A common complication of placenta previa and the resulting bleeds is PTL. As with other areas in the body, blood is an irritant, and as with abruptions, bleeding leads to uterine irritability and contractions, and contractions lead to more bleeding. Because hemorrhage may occur at any time without warning or precipitating events, the risk is increased with premature delivery. Furthermore, placenta accreta is a rare complication of placenta previa. With placenta accreta, the placenta (chorionic villi) attaches to the myometrium. Normal placental attachment is to the endometrium.

Assessment of Placental Abruption and Placenta Previa

Generally, the clinical findings of placental abruption vary in degree with the extent, or percentage, of the placental separation and clot formation behind the placenta. Onset of symptoms may be gradual in mild cases to sudden and without warning in severe situations. In cases of vaginal bleeding after 20 weeks' gestation, placenta previa should be considered.

Uterine Assessment (Placental Abruption) Symptoms of placental abruption may range from slight abdominal tenderness and lower back discomfort with a mild abruption to severe unceasing abdominal pain in a large abruption. Sudden severe pain without vaginal bleeding may be indicative of retroplacental hemorrhage into the myometrium. The bleeding is occult because it is behind the placenta and it is trapped. However, most presentations of placenta abruptio include vaginal bleeding. Typically, the blood is dark and clotted because of the distance it must travel from the fundus to the cervix. A key assessment point is that the color of the vaginal bleeding is related to how old the blood is not the source of the bleeding (abruptio versus previa). The intensity, frequency, and duration of contractions may vary from contractions with a slight increase in uterine tone to hypertonic (Fig. 28.12) or tetanic contractions. Tetanic contractions are very strong contractions that typically last longer than 90 seconds and have minimal resting tone in between. Assessment should include palpation of the uterus for the frequency, duration, intensity, and resting tone. The uterus is often described as boardlike, primarily because of the tetanic contractions and the accumulation of blood within the uterus. A classic presentation of placenta abruptio is profound abdominal pain that appears disproportionate to the contractions palpated. Although not a rule, often the larger the abruption, the more severe the abdominal or uterine pain. With moderate to large abruption, labor tends to progress rapidly and the risks for precipitous delivery and fetal distress are greater. Preparation must be taken for immediate vaginal delivery, or in the case of extensive hemorrhage, cesarean delivery. Radio or call ahead to the receiving facility so appropriate preparation can be made. If determination of when a contraction begins or ends is difficult and the abdomen is rigid, the patient is in profound pain and, especially with the presence of vaginal bleeding, a placental separation should be suspected.

Uterine Assessment (Placenta Previa) Contractions may or may not be present with placenta previa. The onset usually occurs during or after the hemorrhage because of increased uterine irritability. Blood is an irritant, and as a result, the uterus may become irritable or contract.

Assessment of Blood Loss (Placental Abruption) When placental abruption occurs, vaginal bleeding may vary from absent or minimal to profuse. The amount of vaginal bleeding is not an indicator of the degree of separation or of total blood loss but of the location of the separation. Assessment of a concealed hemorrhage includes any change in fundal height as an indication of continued hemorrhage. The fundus can be marked to provide a quick visual indicator of increasing uterine size. However, rising fundal height is a late sign and often requires a substantial amount of blood to accumulate in the uterus. Early signs of maternal bleeding are reflected in the FHR with an increasing baseline and loss of variability noted. Maternal tachycardia is then noted. Approximately one-third of the maternal blood volume is lost before significant changes are seen in the maternal blood pressure. The bleeding may continue until delivery of

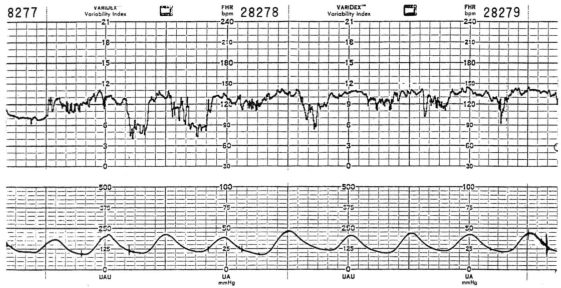

• **Fig. 28.12** Abruption pattern. Note the increased uterine tone documented with the use of an internal uterine pressure catheter (IUPC). Hypertonic contractions are occurring approximately every minute with virtually no period of relaxation between contractions. Note the distressed fetal response. An emergency cesarean section was performed with Apgar scores of 2 and 7 at 1 and 5 minutes, respectively.

the placenta, or it may stop spontaneously. The bleeding from placenta abruptio is often unpredictable. An abruption may be classified as chronic and have a constant but minimal amount of spotting or bleeding. Other abruptions may have an initial separation and bleed but then do not progress. Still other abruptions have an initial separation and then unpredictably continue to separate to varying percentages. The larger the percentage of placental separation, the more unstable the abruption.

Assessment of Blood Loss (Placenta Previa) Blood loss can be more accurately estimated with placenta previa, for which only external hemorrhage is observed. Placenta previa is characterized by repetitive and frequently more extensive bleeding episodes. Objective measurements of blood loss should always be used, such as pad counts, weighing of towel or Chux pads, and collection of blood in graduated cylinders or suction canisters.

Ultrasound Scan An ultrasound scan can confirm the location of the placenta. If an ultrasound scan is not available, a previa cannot be ruled out. An SVE may stimulate profuse bleeding by dislodging a clot and should never be done. With cervical changes that accompany active labor, occasionally an increase in bloody show is noted and may appear excessive, which may lead the transport professional to believe that a placenta previa is present. If unsure, do not attempt a vaginal examination. If the increased source of bleeding is indeed from an active bloody show, then signs of imminent delivery are also present.

Assessment of Vital Signs Signs of maternal hypovolemic shock may not be present until a blood loss of approximately

30% has occurred. However, before any change in vital signs, shunting away from the placenta to the vital organs occurs, and an FHR indicative of placental insufficiency is seen. FHR changes often include increasing or tachycardia baseline and loss of variability.

Assessment of Fetal Heart Rate Fetal distress because of placental separation or placenta previa occurs primarily from placental insufficiency (hypertonic uterus, maternal hemorrhage, or decreased placental perfusion) or fetal hemorrhage because of placental separation. The team must observe for the early signs of fetal hypoperfusion, as previously mentioned, and late decelerations and bradycardia.

Assessment of Urinary Output Urinary output of 60 to 100 mL/h suggests adequate renal perfusion and, indirectly, adequate circulating blood volume. Urinary output of less than 30 mL/h suggests decreased circulatory volume. Insertion of a urinary catheter is recommended for any circumstances in which maternal hypoperfusion or hypovolemia is suspected.

Assessment of Coagulopathy The transport team should observe for petechiae, hematuria, bruising, or bleeding from IV sites.

Assessment for Impending Shock Because of the normal physiologic changes of pregnancy, early symptoms of hypovolemia may be masked. Careful assessment of serial vital signs aids in differentiating expected blood pressure, pulse, and respirations from symptoms of impending shock. Symptoms include tachypnea, decreased blood pressure, increased pulse rate (rapid and thready), oliguria, cyanosis, pallor, and clamminess.[1,9,17] Current research suggests that trending MAPs may be more helpful in assessment of signs of shock then pure blood pressure measurement.

Strategies for Transport (Abruption and Previa)

The transport team should use the following strategies for transport of patients with abruption or previa:

1. Implement general guidelines for transport care after the primary survey and obstetric assessment are completed. Assess for contractions, the extent of hemorrhage, and estimated blood loss. Determine fundal height or mark the fundus, with frequent reassessment. Recognition of concealed bleeding is confirmed by noting an increase in the fundal height and with earlier signs of blood loss such as changes in the FHR, vital signs, and LOC.

2. Administer tocolytics as recommended. Refer to the discussion in this chapter regarding PTL for specifics about labor suppressants. Program-specific guidelines for tocolysis should be followed. Any deviation should be discussed with medical control or accepting maternal fetal medicine physicians. Maternal bleeding is a contraindication for use of β-mimetics because they cause maternal and fetal tachycardia and blur the assessment of maternal hemorrhage.

3. Assess vital signs every 15 minutes or more frequently as needed. Note any subtle changes that may indicate hypovolemia. Check capillary refill as needed to assess for peripheral perfusion. Initiate EFM, if available, to monitor FHT for changes indicative of impending fetal distress. Provide supplemental oxygen, IVFs, and maternal position change.

4. Observe for signs of DIC. Administration of fluid and blood or blood products may be necessary for the patient with active hemorrhage or shock.

5. Expedite transport if the patient's condition deteriorates. Consider diversion for active hemorrhage or fetal distress. Notify the medical director and receiving hospital to prepare for a possible emergency cesarean section delivery.

Disseminated Intravascular Coagulation

DIC is a serious and deleterious complication of pregnancy. When accelerated coagulation and activation of the fibrinolytic system occur simultaneously in pregnancy, DIC occurs as a secondary event activated by hemorrhagic complications, such as placental abruption and placenta previa, or by delivery complications, such as ruptured uterus, uterine inversion, and PPH. Other risks include traumatic labor and delivery, amniotic fluid embolism, abortions, and sepsis. DIC is also a complication of trauma in pregnancy, retained dead fetus syndrome (more than 3 weeks since intrauterine death), and hydatidiform mole.

Treatment is primarily supportive and often includes initially removing or treating the circumstance that caused the DIC, such as delivering the dead fetus. Secondarily, blood products, such as packed RBCs, fresh frozen plasma,

and cryoprecipitate, may be given to correct the coagulopathy. After the delivery of the fetus and after the patient's primary complication has been eliminated or improved, further intervention may not be needed unless the hemorrhage has been severe.[1,9,17]

Multiple Gestation

A pregnancy with more than one fetus is a multiple gestation. Twins occur in 1 in 80 to 90 births, and triplets occur in 1 in 8000 births. The use of fertility medications and in vitro fertilization has increased the occurrence of multiple gestations.

Etiology

Embryologically, twins may result from multiple ovulations, in which two distinct ova are fertilized (dizygotic, or fraternal), or from one ovum that subsequently divides into two (monozygotic, or identical). Either or both processes can also result in triplets, quadruplets, and so on. The incidence of dizygotic twins is influenced by heredity, maternal age, race, and treatment for infertility, whereas the frequency of monozygotic twins is relatively constant.

In vitro fertilization and fertility medications also contribute to the incidence of multiple fetuses.

Previous delivery of twins, maternal family history of fraternal twins, advanced maternal age, infertility treatment, and multiparity all increase the chance of multiple gestations.

Pathophysiologic Factors

Pathophysiology is related to the complications associated with multiple gestations. The large area of the uterine surface covered by the placenta is suspected in several complications. Portions are more likely to implant in the lower uterine segment where less vascularity is found, increasing the chances of IUGR, or at or near the cervical os, increasing the chances of placenta previa. The superabundance of chorionic villi appears to predispose the obstetric patient to hypertensive disorders of pregnancy, especially in a first pregnancy.

Other complications may be caused by uterine overdistension and hemodynamic and endocrinologic changes associated with multiple gestations. The mother is placed at risk for anemia, glucose intolerance, polyhydramnios, dysfunctional labor associated with uterine overdistension, and dystocia. In addition, multiple gestations predispose to PROM, PTL and delivery, placental abruption, cesarean section, uterine atony and resulting PPH, and malpresentations. The fetuses are at risk for congenital anomalies, cord prolapse or entanglement, vasa previa, twin-twin transfusion, discordant fetal growth, and intrauterine death.

The greatest threat to multiple gestations is premature labor and delivery. One theory for this is overdistension of the uterus caused by multiple fetuses. The average gestational age for onset of labor is about 36 weeks for pregnancies that have spontaneous multiple gestations. Multiple gestation pregnancies because of infertility often deliver before 36 weeks' gestation.[16] In addition, the incidence of pregnancy-induced hypertension (PIH) is significantly higher in pregnancies with multiple gestations.

Assessment

Multiple gestations are usually suspected when a discrepancy develops between the gestational age determined by the obstetric patient's last monthly period and the uterine size determined by regular fundal measurements. When the expected size of approximately 1 cm per week of gestation is exceeded, investigation may be warranted. If twinning is suspected, an ultrasound scan confirms or disproves the presence of more than one fetus. Although ACOG states that early ultrasound scans are not necessary for low-risk pregnancies, they are often considered expected by obstetric patients. Because of frequent and early ultrasound scans, multiple gestations are diagnosed commonly in the first trimester.

Strategies for Transport

The transport team must be aware that any multiple gestation is a pregnancy at risk and must assess for additional risk factors associated with a multiple gestation.

The primary survey is completed as it is for any patient with assessment of airway, breathing, circulation, disability, and exposure. The secondary assessment is the complete head-to-toe assessment with the addition of the general obstetric assessment. Assessment for the patient with multiple gestation includes a thorough assessment of PTL with palpation of the uterus for contractions and cervical examination if the patient is contracting. Other assessment priorities involve specific assessment of comorbidities such as gestational hypertension or DM. Fetal monitoring of multiple gestations during transport is extremely difficult but might be accomplished with continuous or intermittent FHR assessment via Doppler, dependent on availability and transport protocols. Of special note is that multiple gestations should be identified as A, B, C, etc., and not as 1, 2, and 3. In addition, location should also be described in relationship to the quadrants of the uterus. Numbering indicates birth order, which is not determined until the actual delivery. For example, a triplet pregnancy may have a fetus in the left lower quadrant (LLQ), the right upper quadrant (RUQ), and the right lower quadrant (RLQ). The babies are labeled as A: RLQ, B: RUQ, and C: LLQ. This distinction avoids confusion for monitoring purposes so the fetuses do not get mixed up. Caution must be taken to monitor each fetus separately.

Because of close fetal lie, a single fetus may be inadvertently monitored in more than one location. For example, triplet A may be monitored in the RUQ and may also be picked up in the LLQ. Clinicians think they are monitoring two separate fetuses, but they are actually monitoring one fetus, twice. Ultrasound scan may help to guide monitoring of separate fetuses. When the babies are actually delivered, the first fetus delivered is 1, the second is 2, and so forth.

The drug of choice in the treatment of PTL is magnesium sulfate because it has been observed that an increased incidence of pulmonary edema is associated with use of β-sympathomimetic agents in women with multiple gestations.

Hypertensive Disorders of Pregnancy

Hypertension is the most common medical problem encountered during pregnancy, complicating 2% to 3% of pregnancies. Hypertensive disorders during pregnancy are classified into four categories as recommended by the National High Blood Pressure Education Program Working Group on High Blood Pressure in Pregnancy: (1) chronic hypertension, (2) preeclampsia/eclampsia, (3) preeclampsia superimposed on chronic hypertension, and (4) gestational hypertension. This terminology is preferred over the older term PIH.[19,21,23]

Gestational hypertension refers to a group of hypertensive disorders that have their onset during pregnancy and resolve after pregnancy. Gestational hypertension, formerly known as PIH, is the new onset of hypertension after 20 weeks' gestation. The diagnosis requires that the patient have elevated blood pressure (systolic >140 or diastolic >90), previously normal blood pressure, no protein in the urine, and no manifestations of preeclampsia or eclampsia. Fifty percent of women diagnosed with gestational hypertension between 24 and 35 weeks develop preeclampsia.

Preeclampsia is a multiorgan disease process characterized by the development of hypertension and proteinuria after 20 weeks' gestation. Eclampsia is the development of convulsions in a preexisting preeclampsia or it may appear unexpectedly in a patient with minimally elevated blood pressure and no proteinuria.[19,21,23]

Persistent hypertension not associated with pregnancy that develops before 20 weeks' gestation is considered to be chronic and is called essential or primary hypertension. Chronic hypertension as a preexisting condition may be complicated during pregnancy by superimposed preeclampsia or superimposed eclampsia. HELLP syndrome (hemolysis, elevated liver enzymes, and low platelets) is considered a complication of severe preeclampsia.

Etiology

The absolute cause of gestational hypertension is unknown. Current theories point to nutritional deficiencies, immunologic deficiencies, genetic predisposition, response to chorionic villi exposure, chronic intravascular coagulation, and other factors. Certain factors are known to predispose the obstetric patient to development of gestational hypertension. Primarily, gestational hypertension is a disease of the primigravida, the teenaged primigravida, or the primigravida over 35 years of age. The patient with DM, preexisting cardiovascular or kidney disease, polyhydramnios, family history of gestational hypertension, or no prenatal care is also at risk. Other predisposing factors include pregnancy that is exposed to a superabundance of chorionic villi, such as with multiple gestation, hydatidiform mole, or fetal hydrops, or poor nutritional status, large fetus, or Rh incompatibility.

Pathophysiologic Factors

In patients with gestational hypertension, the disease process begins many weeks before the onset of any symptoms and is theorized to begin when the pregnancy is in the early weeks of gestation. A chain reaction of events is initiated as, for unknown reasons, an increased sensitivity to angiotensin II develops. As a result, vasospasm occurs, particularly arteriolar vasospasm, which initiates vasoconstriction and leads to increased peripheral resistance and eventually to hypertension. Blood perfusion to all body organs is decreased, and the function of the placenta, kidneys, liver, and brain is significantly impaired. Without forgetting the essential problem of vasospasm, the following pathophysiology is characteristic of gestational hypertension.[19,21,23]

Uteroplacental Changes

Compromised uterine and placental blood flow can lead to degeneration of the placenta and necrosis. With chronic decreased blood perfusion, IUGR can result. During labor, changes in fetal status and well-being of varying degrees can be seen, caused by uteroplacental insufficiency. As a consequence of decreased uterine blood flow, uterine activity is increased and uterine irritability and PTL are frequently seen. An old-fashioned phrase used to describe preeclampsia is *toxemia*. The belief was that the fetus was "toxic" to the mother, and the only treatment at the time was delivery.

Renal Changes

Decreased renal blood flow decreases glomerular filtration rate and in turn decreases urinary output. Cellular changes are observed in the glomerular capillary endothelial cells. The cells swell, producing narrowing of the capillary lumens, and lesions develop, causing the proteinuria (primarily albumin) seen in preeclampsia. Plasma uric acid is typically elevated because of the decreased uric acid clearance by the kidneys. In addition, CR clearance and BUN aid in the evaluation of kidney function. With decreased kidney function, sodium and water are retained. In conjunction with a decreased circulating albumin and a decrease in colloid osmotic pressure, fluid is shifted from the intravascular space to the extracellular space, which gives rise to edema that may range from slight to severe. In addition, increased sensitivity to angiotensin occurs as angiotensin I converts to angiotensin II; this conversion stimulates renin release, which causes aldosterone to be secreted. As this occurs, more salts and water are retained. This entire process is an attempt for the kidneys to improve their own renal perfusion and does initially pull more fluid into the intravascular space; however, because of osmotic changes in the blood vessels, much of the fluid leaks into the extravascular space.[14,22]

Hematologic Changes

Because of fluid shifts caused by osmotic changes, hemoconcentration is seen with a rise in hematocrit levels. An increase in the hematocrit level noted after an initial assessment may signal a deteriorating condition. The normal hypervolemia of pregnancy is decreased or nearly absent when preeclampsia is present. The pregnant patient still has a tremendous amount of volume in her body; it just is no longer in the intravascular compartment where it belongs. Also observed is intravascular platelet and fibrin deposition, which occurs in response to vessel wall damage as the disease progresses. In addition, hemolysis and coagulopathy in patients with severe gestational hypertension is more frequently associated with HELLP syndrome and the development of DIC as severe complications of preeclampsia.

Hepatic Changes

Reduction in blood flow to the liver impairs liver function. Swelling of the capsule (the fibrous sheath that completely covers the liver) and subcapsular hemorrhage may occur. Necrosis and damage to liver tissue are seen with elevated liver enzyme levels. In rare cases, subcapsular hemorrhage can be so extensive that the liver capsule can rupture with massive hemorrhage into the peritoneal cavity. Epigastric pain (right upper and mid upper quadrant pain) is associated with hepatic swelling. This epigastric pain is caused by hepatic swelling but is often misdiagnosed as heartburn, an accepted symptom associated with pregnancy. Many patients with preeclampsia have epigastric pain, but few have liver rupture. Subcapsular hemorrhage is a rare occurrence but is associated with a higher morbidity and mortality.

Cerebral Changes

Although cerebral perfusion is not initially impaired, osmotic changes and vasospasm give rise to cerebral edema, hemorrhage, and CNS irritability, evidenced by hyperreflexia, headaches, visual disturbances, clonus, nausea and vomiting, decreasing LOC, and clonic and tonic seizures.

Retinal Changes

Retinal arteriolar spasms, ischemia, and edema because of decreased perfusion are the sources of the visual disturbances seen in preeclampsia. Blurring, scotoma (blind or twinkling spots in the vision), and diplopia (double vision) may occur. Retinal detachment is a rare occurrence. Questions related to blurred vision or visual changes are key in assessment of patients with preeclampsia because they rarely offer this information. Most lay pregnant patients believe the visual changes "are just part of being pregnant"; they do not comprehend the pathology associated.

Pulmonary Changes

Changes in pulmonary capillary permeability can occur, predisposing to pulmonary edema in severe cases of gestational hypertension. A key assessment pearl is frequent assessment of lung sounds at a minimum of once an hour, which is especially true if the patient is currently on magnesium sulfate and which may also increase the risk of pulmonary edema.

Complications

Complications of gestational hypertension, some of which have already been discussed, include eclampsia, placental abruption, pulmonary edema, DIC, HELLP syndrome, hemolytic anemia, thrombocytopenia, preterm delivery and prematurity, and IUGR. Seldom-observed and grave complications include retinal detachment; kidney failure; cerebral hemorrhage; liver rupture; heart failure; intrauterine death; and rarely, maternal death.

Generally, the predisposition for the development of complications increases as the disease state deteriorates. Although prompt treatment should stabilize the condition, complications and progression to eclampsia can occur.[19,21,23]

Eclampsia

Eclampsia can occur before labor, during labor, or early in the postpartum period. It is defined as seizures that occur in patients with severe hypertensive disorders of pregnancy. Headache, visual disturbances, epigastric pain, apprehension, anxiety, and hyperreflexia with clonus in a patient with severe hypertensive disorders of pregnancy are signs of impending eclampsia. Symptoms of CNS irritability are present, and the more severe the symptoms, the more likely the patient is to have progression into eclampsia.

Seizures are characterized by clonic and tonic activity and may begin around the mouth in the form of facial twitching. The seizure may be so forceful that the patient may fall from the bed. Respirations cease during the seizure but may spontaneously resume as the seizure activity quiets. Commonly, respirations must be supported initially during the seizure and into the postictal period via BVM. Often, elective intubation is performed to further protect the patient's airway. Coma frequently ensues, and the patient remembers little of the events immediately before and after the seizure. The length of the coma varies, with the patient gradually becoming responsive. Frequently, labor spontaneously begins and progresses rapidly. As with many other severe medical states in pregnancy, the maternal host is essentially saying, "I am sick . . . get this kid out of me." Although the mechanism remains unclear, delivery of the fetus improves the maternal medical/obstetric status. With severe gestational hypertension, the risk for the mother continuing with the pregnancy and the risk of a premature delivery for the fetus are heavily weighed. Decisions regarding timing of delivery are based on these factors and responses from medications such as magnesium sulfate and steroid administration to mature fetal lungs. Pulmonary edema may develop. Massive cerebral hemorrhage and death can occur because of eclampsia, but the incidence is rare (Table 28.3). Primary treatment of the eclamptic seizure is with benzodiazepines. Drugs such as lorazepam are titrated until the seizure is eliminated. Magnesium sulfate is used to prevent the next seizure by raising the seizure threshold and is not an anticonvulsant. If the patient was on magnesium sulfate when the seizure occurred, the provider may choose to draw a magnesium sulfate level and depending on the results, rebolus the patient to raise the patient's magnesium level. Stop the seizure first, and then prevent the next one with magnesium sulfate after the patient's condition has been stabilized and the magnesium sulfate can be safely administered via bolus and maintenance dosing.

HELLP Syndrome

The HELLP syndrome was first identified and described as a serious complication of preeclampsia by Weinstein in 1982. *H* stands for hemolysis, which is confirmed with the evidence of red cell fragments and irregularly shaped red cells on peripheral blood smears. The belief is that as red cells pass through the constricted vessels that have sustained wall damage with platelet and fibrin deposition, red cell integrity is altered, and many cells are lysed. As a result,

TABLE 28.3	General Guidelines for Determining the Severity of the Disease Process[a]		
Mild	**Severe**		**Impending Eclampsia**
Blood pressure (mm Hg)	≥140/90; Diastolic increases ≥15	Diastolic, >100	Diastolic, >100
Proteinuria (dipstick)	2+/3+	3+/4+	3+/4+
Urinary output (mL/h)	>30	<20–30	<20–30
Edema	+1/+2	+3/+4	+3/+4
Pulmonary edema	Not present	May be present	Present
Headache	Not present	May be present	Present
Visual disturbances	Not present	May be present	Present
Epigastric pain	Not present	May be present	Present
Hyperreflexia and clonus	Not present	May be present	Present

[a]Some crossover of clinical findings can occur, and not all findings are absolute for each category.
Data from Magee LA. Fortnightly review: management of hypertension in pregnancy. *Br Med J.* 1999;318(7194):1332-1336.

hyperbilirubinemia is frequently seen. Hemorrhagic necrosis is a serious complication of HELLP. Hepatic infarction may occur because of gross ischemia and obstruction of blood flow from the fibrin deposits. *EL* stands for elevated liver enzyme levels. Elevated serum glutamic oxaloacetic transaminase and serum glutamic-pyruvic transaminase values are observed. *LP* stands for low platelet count. Consumptive thrombocytopenia (a platelet count lower than $100,000/mm^3$) unaccompanied by any other coagulation factor abnormalities is characteristic of the HELLP syndrome. Management of HELLP syndrome is primarily supportive and includes control of hypertension; bed rest; frequent fetal evaluation; and careful assessment of hepatic, glucose, and coagulation studies. DIC is a significant risk of HELLP.

Assessment

The "big three" in assessment of hypertensive disorders of pregnancy include hypertension, edema, and proteinuria. Easy assessment pearls start at the top and work their way down. Assessment should include the presence of a headache, blurred vision (visual changes), epigastric pain, uterine contractions, or irritability; FHR assessment for uterine perfusion; assessment of deep tendon reflexes (DTRs) on upper and lower extremities; and assessment of clonus (muscle fasciculation when the foot is sharply dorsiflexed) and generalized body edema (most commonly found in dependent areas such as the left side or sacral if the patient is lying that way). Traditional assessment also includes measurement of the blood pressure (with trending of MAP), measurement and dip of urine output, and review of laboratory tests such as complete blood cell count (CBC), platelets, liver assessment (SGOT/SGPT), glucose, and coagulation studies.

Hypertension

Hypertension is a rise in systolic pressure of 30 mm Hg or a rise in diastolic pressure of 15 mm Hg based on previously known pressures or a blood pressure of 140/90 mm Hg or higher. Current beliefs put more emphasis on the blood pressure of 140/90 mm Hg because this is the point at which destructive endothelial changes are seen. The diastolic pressure is a more reliable predictor of the disease process. The blood pressure should be taken with the patient in the left lateral recumbent position. Hypertension associated with gestational hypertension is labile and may change in the time it takes to retake the blood pressure. Careful assessment of trending MAPs may be a more reliable indicator of worsening pathology then blood pressure measurement alone.[19,21,23]

Edema

A sudden excessive weight gain of more than 2 lb in a week or 6 lb in a month is primarily attributable to fluid retention. Nondependent edema of the eyelids, face, and hands is characteristic of gestational hypertension. Pitting edema

TABLE 28.4	Assessment of Edema and Hyperreflexia	
Evaluation of Edema Score		**Score**
Minimal edema of lower extremities		+1
Marked edema of lower extremities		+2
Edema of lower extremities, face, and hands		+3
Generalized massive edema, including abdomen and sacrum		+4
Evaluation of Hyperreflexia		**Grade**
None elicited		0
Sluggish or dull		+1
Active, normal		+2
Brisk		+3
Brisk with transient clonus		+4
Brisk with sustained clonus		+5

Note: Assessment of hyperreflexia is usually accomplished with eliciting patellar deep tendon reflexes. Clonus can be assessed at the same time with swift dorsiflexion of the foot. Clonus indicates neuromuscular irritability, and each beat should be counted.
Data from Seidel HM, et al. *Mosby's Physical Examination Handbook.* St. Louis, MO: Mosby; 1999.

of the lower extremities is common. Assessment of edema is subjective, especially as clinicians do not know what patients looked like before pregnancy. For more objective assessment of overall body edema, ask a family member or the patient herself if she looks "puffy." For evaluation of edema (Table 28.4).

Proteinuria

Proteinuria usually develops after hypertension and edema. Proteins are large molecules, and proteinuria reflects significant renal deterioration.

The transport team should observe the patient for evidence of the following: (1) CNS irritability (headache, hyperreflexia evaluated with DTRs and ankle clonus [see Table 28.4], nausea, vomiting, apprehension, and anxiety); (2) impaired renal function (oliguria and proteinuria); and (3) hepatic involvement, malaise, nausea, vomiting, and in extremely rare conditions, jaundice.

Strategies for Transport

Minimization of the effects of vasospasm and hypertension and prevention of seizures and other complications are critical. Maintenance or improvement of uteroplacental blood flow minimizes the risk of insult to the fetus.

The primary survey, including assessment of airway, breathing, circulation, disability, and exposure, is done initially. The obstetric assessment is completed in the secondary survey after all the life threats identified in the primary survey. The transport team should follow general guidelines for transport care and assess for gestational hypertension and risk factors and complications associated with gestational hypertension. A history of the onset of any symptoms provides insight into the consideration of the full clinical picture.

The fetus is at increased risk for uteroplacental insufficiency. The maternal transport professional should observe the FHR tracings. Evaluation should include observation of variability, the presence or absence of acceleration or deceleration, and baseline trending. Assessment of fetal movement and trends of fetal movement reflect fetal status. However, if the patient has already received magnesium sulfate, fetal movement may be decreased.

The maternal transport professional should place a urinary catheter to monitor urinary output and proteinuria when symptoms indicate severe preeclampsia. As a result of renal deterioration, strict assessment of urine output must be made hourly. When assessing for proteinuria, avoid contamination with vaginal discharge (blood, amniotic fluid, and bacteria) to avoid inaccurate results.

Sensory stimulation is almost impossible to eliminate during transport. However, keeping lights dimmed, voices low, and sirens turned off and turning the cardiac monitor audible signal to low or off may help to decrease noxious stimuli. The transport team must be prepared to intervene in the event of an eclamptic seizure, which can be unpredictable. Magnesium sulfate, benzodiazepines, and airway supplies should be readily available.[19,21,23]

A coagulopathy is suspected if petechiae, hematuria, bruising, or bleeding from the IV sites is noted. Because these are late signs, symptoms of shock may rapidly ensue. If available, a review of laboratory values, including a CBC with platelets, prothrombin time, partial thromboplastin time, and fibrinogen, reflects progression to DIC earlier than clinical signs.

The transport nurse should evaluate pulmonary status for signs of pulmonary edema. Lung sounds and pulse oximetry (SpO$_2$) should be evaluated hourly. If acute pulmonary edema with respiratory distress occurs, morphine can be administered intravenously. Furosemide (20–40 mg administered intravenously over 2–3 minutes) can be given. Outside of acute pulmonary edema, furosemide is not commonly used in obstetrics. Furosemide crosses the placenta and can cause decreased perfusion to the placenta. The medical plan to minimize the disease includes a thorough knowledge of the action, dosage, administration, and adverse reactions of the medications that may be used in the management of gestational hypertension.

Magnesium Sulfate

Magnesium sulfate acts at the neuromuscular junction to slow transmission of impulses. By displacing calcium, it interferes with the release of acetylcholine, blocking nerve transmission to the muscle. This action, in addition to raising the seizure threshold, is thought to prevent seizures. Fifty grams of MgSO$_4$ can be added to 500 mL of lactated Ringer's solution (or 40 g added to 1000 mL) with a bolus of 4 to 6 g given slowly over 15 to 30 minutes, followed by

2 to 4 g/h infusion is highly recommended via infusion pump as the side effects of magnesium toxicity can be lethal. Therapeutic serum magnesium levels range from approximately 4 to 8 mEq/L (1.5–2.5 mEq/L is normal). When therapeutic levels are achieved, DTRs are depressed but not absent. Loss of DTRs may indicate a toxic level. Loss of lower DTRs (patella) without loss of upper (bicep) reflexes is not uncommon; it is not necessarily a sign of toxicity but does reflect higher serum magnesium levels. Changes in LOC, respiratory depression with potential for arrest, and cardiac arrest are seen with highly toxic levels (greater than 10–15 mEq/L). While a patient is receiving IV MgSO$_4$, hourly assessment of DTRs is essential. Respirations should also be closely monitored, and the infusion stopped if they reach less than 12 per minute with poor respiratory effort associated with decreasing LOC. Other respiratory concerns include the risk of pulmonary edema. Pulse oximetry should be used during transport.

The antidote for magnesium toxicity is calcium gluconate. Calcium stimulates the release of acetylcholine, stimulating nerve transmission to the muscle. Figuratively, calcium and magnesium are on a teeter totter. As serum magnesium levels increase, the serum calcium levels are driven down. Conversely, if calcium levels are increased, the magnesium levels decrease as do the associated pathologic side effects of magnesium toxicity. The recommended dosage of calcium gluconate is 1 g of a 10% solution administered intravenously over at least 3 minutes. If one ampule is not enough to reverse the side effects of hypoventilation, another ampule may be given and titrated to effect. The goal is spontaneous respiration, a return of DTRs, and a responsive LOC. If calcium is administered too rapidly, bradycardia and arrhythmias may occur.

Magnesium sulfate is not an antihypertensive agent. However, a transient drop in blood pressure after initiation of treatment is frequently seen and can be attributed to smooth muscle relaxation. Adverse reactions include flushing, sweating, nausea and vomiting, and drowsiness. A decrease in FHR variability may be observed because magnesium is a known CNS depressant. Magnesium sulfate is primarily excreted in the urine, and toxicity may develop rather rapidly in the patient with significantly impaired kidney function. The urinary output should exceed 30 mL/h while the patient is receiving the infusion. If urinary output drops below 30 mL/h, consultation with appropriate medical control or the receiving physician should be made because they may want to decrease the maintenance infusion. Magnesium should be used cautiously in patients with renal or cardiac disease.

Labetalol

Labetalol is a selective β-blocking agent that decreases systemic vascular resistance without changing CO. The standard dosage is 20 mg administered via IV push over 2 minutes; the dose may be repeated every 10 minutes until the maximum dosage of 300 mg has been given.[1] Large subsequent doses of labetalol should be avoided because profound drops in blood pressure can acutely occur. As with nonpregnant patients, labetalol can be an "unforgiving" drug in the sense that if the blood pressure drops to a hypotensive state it is slow to return to normotensive pressures. The effects of a rapid decrease in maternal blood pressure can be profound on the uterus and placenta. Neither are considered vital organs and are the first to feel the effects of hypoperfusion. The MAP should be evaluated and used to trend the decrease in maternal blood pressure. The MAP should not be dropped more than 20% to avoid causing placental hypoperfusion and increasing the risks of placental abruption.

Hydralazine

Hydralazine acts by relaxing arterioles and decreasing vasospasm. Thus it reduces blood pressure and stimulates CO. Blood perfusion to the brain, kidneys, liver, and uterus is thus improved. Hydralazine is recommended with diastolic pressure 110 mm Hg or greater for prevention of cerebrovascular accident. Transport protocol should be followed regarding titration of hydralazine. During administration, the blood pressure should be taken every couple of minutes because the onset of action is 5 to 10 minutes. If the diastolic pressure falls below 90 mm Hg, uterine blood flow may be further reduced, placing the fetus at risk. Profound decreases in maternal blood pressure not only decrease placenta perfusion but also increase the risk of placenta abruptio. The MAP should not be decreased more than 20%. Adverse reactions include reflex tachycardia, headache, palpitations, dizziness, nausea, and vomiting. Hydralazine is contraindicated in cases of lupus erythematosus and tachycardia.

Benzodiazepines

Benzodiazepines are classified as antianxiety/sedative medications but are known to prevent or arrest seizure activity, although the exact mode of action is not known. They also produce mild sedation and muscular relaxation. Benzodiazepines should be administered parentally, but in an extreme emergency when IV access is not possible, they may be given rectally. They are the first-line drug for active eclampsia. Adverse reactions include transient bradycardia, hypotension, and hypoventilation. If respirations are profoundly decreased, the antidote is flumazenil. If flumazenil is indicated, cautious and judicious administration allows for the return of spontaneous respirations without the return of seizures.

Preterm Labor and Related Issues

Regular and rhythmic contractions that produce progressive cervical changes after week 20 of gestation and before week 37 are considered to be *PTL*. Although contractions are included in this definition, note that many patients with PTL do not feel or perceive these contractions. Preterm delivery occurs in 6% to 12% of all deliveries. PTL does not always result in preterm delivery; however, the rate of preterm delivery has not decreased in recent years, and statistics have actually shown a modest increase in the incidence of PTL. With improved prenatal care, reduction of risk factors, patient education, and earlier diagnosis and treatment of PTL, it is hoped that the next decade may realize a decrease in the rate of preterm delivery.

Etiology

Although many factors predispose the obstetric patient to PTL, a few single identifiable causes exist. Infection has been recognized as a primary cause of PTL. Although the pathways frequently differ, sources of infection may include urinary tract infection, pyelonephritis, vaginitis (particularly bacterial), chorioamnionitis, and viral infection. Another identifiable cause is PROM (spontaneous rupture of membranes [SROM] before the onset of contractions and before week 37). Other factors include previous preterm delivery (the single most frequent contributing factor); uterine anomalies; poor nutritional status; poor perineal hygiene; poor weight gain; no prenatal care; less than 1 year between the last delivery and commencement of the current pregnancy; substance abuse; gestational hypertension; cigarette smoking; diabetes; chronic cardiovascular or kidney disease; previous induced or spontaneous abortion; abdominal trauma; a long commute to work; a high stress level at work or home; physical stress; overdistension of the uterus as a result of multiple gestations; polyhydramnios; uterine tumors; age (teenaged or more than 40 years); placenta previa or placental abruption; cervical incompetence; women exposed to diethylstilbestrol (DES) in utero; a retained intrauterine device (IUD); a history of pelvic inflammatory disease; and fetal anomalies, distress, or death.[15,23]

Single or multiple factors may initiate PTL. When multiple factors are present, the obstetric patient is at greater risk. Many cases have no identifiable causes. Numerous factors are theorized to lead to the progression of PTL and delivery.

Pathophysiologic Factors

In any situation in which uterine blood flow is reduced or impaired, an increase in uterine irritability can be noted and may result in the onset of labor. Viral infections with symptoms of fever, nausea, vomiting, or diarrhea may predispose to PTL primarily because of dehydration, which reduces uterine blood flow. Other similar conditions in which uteroplacental perfusion is compromised include gestational hypertension, diabetes, cardiovascular or kidney disease, overdistension of the uterus, heavy smoking, placental abruption, or placenta previa.

Hormonal influence contributes to increased uterine activity and the onset of labor. Prostaglandin release is associated with PROM, bacterial infections, abdominal trauma, and overdistension of the uterus. In at least half the patients who have PROM, labor begins in 48 hours. Meconium-stained amniotic fluid contains high levels of oxytocin, which can initiate labor. The fetus is also believed to play a role in the activation of PTL, but little is known of this contribution.

When a patient has cervical incompetence, the cervix is unable to support and maintain the growing pregnancy to term and often dilates without perceptible contractions. Cervical incompetence is characterized by premature, painless, bloodless cervical dilation in which the membranes can bulge and rupture. Obstetric history of numerous second trimester losses or "painless" PTLs and deliveries is suspect. Another concerning presentation is the patient with vaginal fullness or pressure, which is often caused by the presenting fetal part causing lower uterine segment pressure. The lower the fetus, the more pressure on the cervix and the more likely preterm delivery will occur. Even vague symptoms need to be evaluated. Advanced cervical dilation and rupture of the amniotic fluid lead to certain delivery. Congenital defects and traumatic injury to the cervix may result in cervical incompetence. Probable causes of cervical injury include trauma during a previous childbirth, cervical dilation after elective or spontaneous abortion, or gynecologic procedures. Another physiologic abnormality in which cervical anomalies and cervical incompetence are known to occur is maternal exposure to DES. For cases of known or suspected cervical incompetence, a cervical cerclage may be placed at 12 to 14 weeks' gestation. A cervical cerclage is a purse-string suture that is applied through the cervix or transabdominally and then tied off. It is intended to maintain cervical integrity so the cervix is not prematurely opened. Any patient with a cervical cerclage that has PTL is at risk of cervical dilation and tearing of the cervix. Maternal fetal medicine physicians or the receiving physician should be consulted, and decisions regarding aggressive tocolysis or removal of the cerclage and delivery by the referring facility are made before transport.

The complications associated with PTL and delivery predominantly affect the fetus. However, the side effects of tocolytic medications to maintain the pregnancy primarily affect the mother. Birth trauma and the complications associated with the transition to extrauterine life for the premature infant are primary. These complications include immature lungs, risks of infection, thermoregulating issues, intracerebral bleeding, and so forth. Neonatal sepsis can result from numerous unknown and known sources such as PROM. The intact bag of water prevents bacteria and flora from the vagina from ascending into the uterine cavity. The severity of the complications seen depend in a great measure on the gestational age of the neonate.

Maternal complications include adverse reactions to labor-suppressing agents, complications associated with cesarean section (increased incidence with PTL), endometritis, septicemia, and septic shock related to prolonged PROM and chorioamnionitis. In addition, other maternal risks include comorbidities or obstetric complications associated with the current pregnancy.

Tocolytics are used to decrease or stop contractions. Research has not shown that tocolysis has been successful in maintaining pregnancy. Thus current belief patterns are use of tocolytics not to greatly extend the pregnancy but rather to allow the administration of glucocorticoid steroid for the benefit of the fetus (Box 28.2).

Assessment

PTL should be suspected if the patient has a history of contractions 10 minutes apart or less for a period of 1 hour or longer. Another definition is more than six contractions in a 1-hour period. The transport team should assess for factors associated with PTL, remembering that the incidence of PTL increases with the number of predisposing factors. Contractions should always be palpated on the fundus or at the top of the uterus. Despite where the patient "feels" the contractions, they all initiate in the fundus and diminish as they reach the cervix. Contractions are most easily palpated in this area also. Although obstetric patients are reliable historians, they do not always perceive contractions. The smaller the uterus, related to gestational age, the less typical the contractions feel. Often, PTL patients deny they are having contractions. However, on the monitor or with palpation, contractions are evident. Further investigation reveals that the patient feels little in her uterus or abdomen but has a lower backache that comes and goes. Other common reports of preterm contractions are colicky abdominal pain similar to that with diarrhea, suprapubic cramping, pressure that comes and goes, or a feeling "like the baby is balling up." These vague symptoms are one reason that PTL is often not discovered until advanced cervical dilation has occurred. The patient is unaware of contractions until she is far progressed into labor, which also highlights the need to palpate the uterus for contractions, even when the patient denies contractions, particularly during transport. Dependent on how often the contractions occur, the uterus should be palpated every 5 minutes for a patient still contracting to every 15 to 30 minutes for patients who are acontractile. Reports of the palpation should be noted in the patient record. This palpation time allows for palpation of fetal movement, which also should be documented.

Cervical Dilation/Effacement Patterns

Cervical dilation patterns vary from primiparas to multiparas. Primiparas tend to have effacement or thinning of the cervix before dilation occurs. The multipara patient often has dilation before significant effacement occurs. For example, the PTL patient who is a primipara and is 2 cm dilated, 100% effaced, +1 station is a higher concern than the multipara who is 2 cm dilated, 10% effaced, and −2 station. Because of predictable dilation and effacement patterns, the primipara shows more signs of active labor. Of note is that cervical status is always reported in this way: dilation/effacement/fetal station (e.g., 3/90/−1). The

---

• BOX 28.2 **Common Obstetric Medications**

This brief review of common medications used in the treatment of the high-risk obstetric patient is intended to identify only key information.

Oxytocin (Pitocin): Used after delivery of placenta to promote uterine involution/prevent postpartum hemorrhage; 20 to 40 units/1000 mL wide open (or) 10 to 20 units IM.

Magnesium sulfate (MgSO₄): TX for gestational hypertension: ↓ seizure threshold to prevent eclampsia. Transient ↓ in BP. TX PTL: ↓ CA influx into cells, decreasing smooth muscle ability to contract.
- MgSO₄ level: Therapeutic: 4.8 to 8.4 mg/dL; Toxic: −10; assess patient.
- Draw level 2 hours after bolus and then q 6 h.
- Loading dose: 2 to 4 g/100 mL over 20 minutes. Patient may have systemic burning, SOB, N/V, feeling miserable. *Warn the patient.* Apply cold packs to decrease side effects.
- Maintenance dose: 20 to 40 g/1000 mL. Usually 1 to 3 g/h.
- Assessment: ABCs, lung sounds, bicep/patellar reflexes, UO, (gestational hypertension) headache, blurred vision, epigastric pain.
- Toxic: Loss of reflexes, ↓ RR, ↓ LOC, ↓ UO, ↓ BP.
- Antidote: Calcium gluconate 10%, 1 to 2 amps.

Terbutaline (Brethine): β-Sympathomimetic, relaxes smooth muscles by decreasing gap junction.
- Side effects: Maternal/fetal: tachycardia, hypotension, hyperglycemia, pulmonary edema.
- Contraindications: Maternal cardiac disease, brittle diabetic.
- Dose: 0.25 mg SQ/IV q 4 h or per protocol. 2.5 mg PO, q 4 h. Hold for HR >120.
- Laboratory tests: Check glucose, ECG for chest pain. Confirm maternal/fetal HR difference.

Indomethacin: Prostaglandin synthetase inhibitor. Prevents cytokine production thought to start labor.
- Side effects: Maternal/fetal: ↓ renal blood flow, ↓ UO, ↓ liver enzymes, ↓ AFI.

- Contraindications: Clinical suspicion of a ductal-dependent cardiac lesion; suspicion of NEC/surgical abdomen; risk of gastric perforation is increased if used concurrently with corticosteroids.
- Do not administer via umbilical arterial catheter.

Nifedipine: Ca²⁺ channel blocker. Limits influx of Ca²⁺ into cells, decreasing ability to contract. Decreases strength/effectiveness versus frequency of uterine contractions.
- Side effects: Hypotension, tachycardia, palpitations.
- Dose: Load 30 mg, then 20 mg q 4–8 h.
- Vital signs: Hold for HR >120 and BP <100/60 mm Hg.

Approved Antihypertensives in Pregnancy
- Hydralazine: Initial dose, 5 to 10 mg IV push; Labetalol: Initial dose, 20 mg slow IV; Methyldopa: Aldomet.
- Diuretics: Hydrochlorothiazide.
- Furosemide (Lasix): Rarely and cautiously used (crosses placenta barrier).

Contraindicated in Pregnancy:
- ACE inhibitors (fetal deformity, IUFD).
- Nitroprusside (Nipride), metabolizes into cyanide for the fetus.

Glucocorticoid steroids: betamethasone: Matures fetal lungs, decreases neonatal IVH, ↓ RDS.
- Side effects: Maternal, ↑ WBC, caution with PROM.
- Dose: 12 mg q 12 to 24 h times two doses. Benefits last 1 week.

ACE, Angiotensin-converting enzyme inhibitor; *AFI,* amniotic fluid index; *BP,* blood pressure; *CA,* calcium; *ECG,* electrocardiogram; *HR,* heart rate; *IM,* intramuscularly; *IUFD,* intrauterine fetal demise; *IV,* intravenously; *IVH,* intraventricular hemorrhage; *LOC,* loss of consciousness; *NEC,* necrotizing enterocolitis; *N/V,* nausea and vomiting; *PO,* orally; *PROM,* premature rupture of membranes; *RDS,* respiratory distress syndrome; *RR,* respiratory rate; *SOB,* shortness of breath; *SQ,* subcutaneously; *TX,* treatment; *UO,* urinary output; *WBC,* white blood cell count.

---

last parameter is measurement of the presenting fetal part in relation to the ischial spines, which are protruding bones on the lower pelvis. These spines can be palpated through the vaginal basement, and the presenting part is compared with the location of these protrusions. If the presenting fetal part, usually the head, is at the level of the spines, the baby is reported as a 0 station. One fingerbreadth (or 1 cm) above the spines is −1, and so forth. If the presenting part is 1 fingerbreadth below the spines, the position is reported as +1 station, and so forth. For perspective, the head begins to crown at +3 station and is delivered at +4. The transport team is not expected to be proficient in these examinations. However, they are expected to understand the implications of the examinations.

Vaginal mucus may be the first sign of cervical dilation. The mucus plug that fills the cervical canal can be dislodged by cervical changes. The cervix is considered completely dilated when it is approximately 10 cm. An important transport consideration is that with premature gestations the fetus is small and may fit though a cervix that is not completely dilated. For example, a 500-g, 23-week fetus may fit through a cervix that is only 6 to 7 cm dilated.

Spontaneous Rupture of Membranes

With any history of possible spontaneous rupture, a sterile speculum examination (SSE) is used to verify the presence of amniotic fluid leaking from the cervix and collecting in the posterior fornix of the vagina (the area underneath the cervix posteriorly). If an SSE has already been performed, the transport team should note documented results. Many transport professionals may not feel competent to perform a speculum examination. Assessment can be completed by the referring facility or fluid assessment can be obtained from fluid leaking on the external vagina. Three factors—positive pooling, positive nitrazine (which may not be accurate if obtained from fluid on the skin), and positive ferning—definitely confirms SROM. Ultrasound scan is also a useful tool when assessing amniotic fluid volumes. Pooling of fluid is seen in the vaginal vault. If none is seen, the team may encourage the patient to cough; the increased pressure usually results in the release of amniotic fluid. A sample from a site as close to the posterior fornix as possible turns nitrazine paper dark blue (alkaline) in the presence of amniotic fluid. Vaginal secretions are acidic in nature and do not affect the paper. The transport team should be aware that blood, cervical mucus, and povidone-iodine are alkaline in nature and can give a false-positive reading. Finally, a small amount of the fluid can be spread on a slide and allowed to dry completely. A frond crystallization pattern of dried amniotic fluid (with a high concentration of sodium chloride) is seen on microscopic examination; it is similar to a Boston fern in appearance. Because a microscope may not be available in small outlying areas and there may not be time to perform this procedure, the transport team must depend on the presence of pooling and a positive nitrazine test. If rupture is confirmed or suspected, an SVE should be avoided, unless delivery appears imminent, to prevent introducing microbes from the vagina into the cervical canal, which can place the patient at an increased risk for infection. If a gross rupture has occurred, if the patient has a history of a large volume loss, or if continual leaking is observed, a SSE is not necessary if it does not alter the plan for nursing care. The transport team should keep in mind that with a decreased amount of amniotic fluid, the umbilical cord is at risk for compression and variable decelerations may be seen, with or without contractions.

If a rupture has not occurred, an SVE confirms whether any cervical changes have taken place. The cervix does not have to dilate before changes can be noted. Normally, the cervix is firm, long, and closed. Any softening or effacing that may occur before dilation indicates cervical changes. If this is not the initial episode of PTL, the transport team should assess for the history of onset, current medications, other treatment such as home monitoring or bed rest, and patient compliance. Frequently, the present episode can be linked to increased activity, failure to take medication altogether, or inconsistency in following the medication regimen.

The transport team should observe the patient for any indications of the presence of infection. Symptoms of urinary tract infection, pyelonephritis, or both include dysuria, frequency of urination, fever, and flank tenderness, pain, or both. Evidence of poor perineal hygiene may be a factor not only in the development of a urinary tract infection but in vaginal infections and chorioamnionitis as well.

The transport team may assess the patient for possible chorioamnionitis; symptoms include maternal fever, maternal tachycardia, fetal tachycardia, uterine tenderness not associated with contractions, purulent vaginal discharge, and an elevated white blood cell (WBC) count. If results of laboratory tests from the referring facility are available, the laboratory tests indicated are a CBC with differential and cervical cultures for β-hemolytic streptococcus and *Neisseria gonorrhoeae*. However, most are initially asymptomatic. Commonly, the infected uterus is tender to palpation, and this is often an early clinical sign. The most common route for infection is the ascending route from the vagina to the cervix. For this reason, sterile vaginal examinations are avoided in the presence of PROM. Evidence indicates that the presence of bacteria in the vagina may locally dissolve the membrane; the bacteria then gain access to the fluid and cause a chorioamnionitis that dissolves the membrane,

resulting in SROM. With no evidence of prior infection, the incidence of infection after SROM greatly increases if the membranes have been ruptured longer than 24 hours.

Strategies for Transport

Primary goals for transport include minimization or prevention of complications, treatment of current pathologies, and improvement in or maintenance of uterine perfusion.

The primary survey and secondary survey, including the general obstetric assessment, should be done first. The transport team should then follow these general guidelines for transport care:

1. *Assess fetal well-being.* This assessment includes review of the FHR tracing for baseline rate, baseline variability, and presence or absence of accelerations or decelerations. This also includes the assessment of the presence or absence of fetal movement and comparison with usual movement patterns.

2. *Determine the contraction pattern.* Determine the phase of labor and assess whether transport can safely be attempted or whether delivery should be accomplished at the referring facility. In the event of an imminent delivery, call for the neonate team (unless *you* are the neonate team also), notify the medical director, and help the referring facility prepare for delivery.

3. *Determine the status of the amniotic membranes.* With a questionable history of fluid leakage and contractions that have slowed or stopped altogether, absolute determination of rupture is not needed before transport if it does not alter the plan for nursing care.

4. *Determine cervical status.* Determine the number of SSEs done at the referring facility, especially if an SSE was done in the presence of ruptured membranes. Assess the amount of cervical change accomplished since admission to the referring facility. Remember that once labor is established, the multiparous woman frequently has progression at a faster rate than a primipara and may need rapid transport. SSEs may be more appropriate for patients with PROM to prevent ascending infections.

5. *Maintain the patient in the LLP or RLP.* Not only do these positions improve uterine perfusion, thus decreasing uterine irritability, but they also decrease pressure on the cervix from the presenting part and may protect against further cervical changes. Having the patient stand, sit, or bend can place pressure against the cervix and should be avoided during transport. Load the patient so she is facing you in your vehicle.

6. *Assess for infection.* Observe for symptoms of urinary tract infection, pyelonephritis, vaginitis, chorioamnionitis, or signs of viral infection. These signs may include uterine tenderness, vaginal discharge, an elevated white count, uterine contractions, fetal tachycardia, maternal fever, and maternal tachycardia.

7. *Assess for cervical incompetence.* An incompetent cervix can be suspected if the patient has vague symptoms accompanied by disproportionate cervical changes. Obstetric

history in these cases is of particular importance. Placing these patients in the LLP with hips slightly elevated may further reduce any pressure on the cervix.

8. *Administer or continue tocolytic agents as prescribed.* Following transport protocols, tocolytics may be titrated to effect if they are within accepted parameters and are tolerated by the mother and fetus. Suppression of labor is always attempted to "buy time" for the transport. Current goals of buying time are 48 hours. The belief is that tocolytics do a poor job at maintaining the pregnancy and that the primary goal is to delay delivery until steroids can be given to aid in the maturation of the fetal lungs. Optimal neonatal outcome can be anticipated when the delivery occurs in a hospital that is prepared for the intensive care of premature infants. If hydration and positioning to the LLP have not slowed or arrested labor, tocolytic agents can be administered. The medications used most frequently in suppressing labor are magnesium sulfate and terbutaline.

Trauma in Pregnancy

Minor accidental injuries are common during pregnancy. The gravid uterus, loosened joints, altered center of gravity, shortness of breath, dizziness, increased fatigue, and edema all contribute to minor accidents, including falls.[8,22,26]

Serious accidental injuries during pregnancy place not only the obstetric patient but also the fetus at risk. Serious injuries during pregnancy are fortunately less common. The most common etiologies of serious obstetric trauma are motor vehicle crashes, falls, stabbings, burns, and domestic violence. The fetus is well protected in the confines of the uterus because it is surrounded by amniotic fluid, which serves as an excellent shock absorber. Physical trauma to a fetus is extremely rare, except from direct penetrating wounds or extensive blunt trauma. The fetus is at greatest risk for fetal distress and intrauterine death because of hypoperfusion from maternal trauma and death. The obstetric patient is more vulnerable to hemorrhage because of the increased vascularity surrounding the gravid uterus. Early signs and symptoms of hypovolemia may be masked by the normal physiologic changes of pregnancy. Thus blood is shunted away from nonvital organs, including the uterus, which threatens the well-being of the fetus. In dealing with a trauma patient who is pregnant, the best interest of the fetus is served by prompt assessment and interventions on behalf of the mother. Although the fetus does not survive if the mother does not survive, measures can be taken to improve fetal viability. Some of these measures include preventing IVCS by tilting the patient to the left or right and increasing uterine/placental perfusion by increasing IVFs, correcting blood or volume losses, and applying 100% O_2. Pregnant patients are sensitive to volume, and particularly in the occurrence of trauma, active volume replacement must be initiated early.[8,22,24-26]

The pregnant trauma patient needs to be appropriately immobilized for transport. Placing a small roll under the right side of the backboard and tipping the backboard 30 degrees displaces the uterus to the left or right side. Stretcher straps should be placed low and tight over the pelvis. The pregnant trauma patient is at high risk of aspiration because of the hormones of pregnancy. Early intubation should be considered. No contraindications for rapid sequence intubation (RSI) exist during pregnancy; however, be aware that the baby is also paralyzed until neuromuscular blocking agents wear off. This is not a concern if the fetus remains in the uterus because it is oxygenated via the placenta and umbilical cord. The concern for paralytics in the neonate is in the event of an immediate cesarean delivery.[8,13,24-26]

Perimortem Cesarean Section

Controversy exists over whether a perimortem cesarean section is of any value in the transport environment. Some anecdotal reports are found of these types of deliveries, but with limited survival of either the infant or the mother. Indications for this procedure may include the following[10,12,15,23]:

- Gestational age of the fetus (24–26 weeks at the youngest gestation, extending to term).
- Limited amount of time since maternal arrest. Some investigators suggest within 5 minutes of maternal arrest as ideal timing to improve fetal outcomes, but anecdotal reviews have reported fetal survival up to 20 to 30 minutes after maternal arrest. However, fetal/neonatal neurologic outcomes diminish with longer arrest to delivery time.

Experienced personnel should perform the procedure, and they must be prepared to perform neonatal resuscitation. An important transport note is to call ahead. The receiving perinatal hospital needs to be alerted to the possibility of a perimortem section so they are prepared to perform it or prepared to receive a likely compromised neonate. Another transport pearl is to perform perfect cardiopulmonary resuscitation (CPR). In the best-case scenario, CPR provides only 25% of circulating blood volume. CPR of poor quality provides less than this. Current American Heart Association guidelines advocate "push hard, push fast." To aid with adequate chest compressions, the backboard should be elevated approximately 30% from behind the area of the head and chest with manual displacement of the uterus. The advanced cardiac life support (ACLS) obstetric course recommends keeping the patient supine to increase cardiac compression and having another clinician manually displace the uterus to minimize IVCS, which may be ideal over the lateral displacement of the mother and uterus (alone) because it allows for better compression of the heart.[27] This positioning prevents IVCS and still allows adequate compressions of the heart against the spine. In the event of maternal ventricle fibrillation or ventricular tachycardia, no contraindications exist for defibrillation or cardioversion. Current ACLS algorithms should be followed during the arrest of adult pregnant patients. However, the ACLS obstetric course recommends that amiodarone be held until the baby is delivered because the fetus has delayed metabolism of amiodarone and resulting maternal hypotension.

Gynecologic Emergencies

Ovarian Torsion

Ovarian torsion is a condition associated with reduced venous return from the ovary as a result of edema, internal hemorrhage, hyperstimulation, or a mass. An ovary and fallopian tube are typically involved.

Pathophysiology[7]

Women with pathologically enlarged ovaries can develop unilateral ovarian torsion. The irregularity of the ovary likely creates a fulcrum around which the oviduct revolves. The process affects both the ovary and the oviduct (adnexal torsion). Approximately 60% of torsions occur on the right side.

Ovarian torsion can frequently arise from many anatomic changes. Torsion of a normal ovary is most common among young girls with excessively long fallopian tubes or absent mesosalpinx. Few ovarian torsion cases in pediatric patients have involved cysts, teratomas, or other masses.

During the physiologic changes in early pregnancy, which causes the presence of an enlarged corpus luteum, a cyst likely predisposes the ovary to torsion. Physiologic changes may also affect the weight and the size of the ovary, which could alter the position of the fallopian tube and allow twisting to occur. Approximately 20% of cases occur during pregnancy. Women receiving infertility treatment carry an even greater risk, in that numerous theca lutein cysts significantly expand the ovarian volume. Patients with a history of tubal ligation are at increased risk for torsion, probably because of adhesions that provide a site around which the ovarian pedicle may twist. Fifty percent to 60% of ovarian cases of torsion are associated with ovarian tumors. Ovarian torsion is the fifth most common gynecologic surgical emergency, accounting for 2.7% of cases of acute abdominal pain in the female patient. With early diagnosis and treatment, the prognosis of ovarian torsion is good.

Clinical Presentation

The classic presentation of adnexal torsion is sudden onset of unilateral lower abdominal pain, which is initially vague in character and may be accompanied by nausea and vomiting. It may radiate to the groin or flank. Patients may describe several episodes of pain over the course of hours, days, or even weeks, if the ovary has been experiencing intermittent torsion.[7]

Complications

Common complications associated with an ovarian torsion included infection, peritonitis, sepsis, adhesions, chronic pain, and rarely infertility. Early recognition of this emergency can help decrease the risk of or limit the impact of these complications.[7]

Strategies for Transport

The patient should be closely monitored for signs of shock and appropriate management for shock should be initiated (see Chapter 13). The patient should be placed in a safe position of comfort for transport. Pain should be managed using medications per transport protocols. Surgical intervention is critical and the patient should be transported to an appropriate facility as quickly and safely as possible.[7]

Toxic Shock Syndrome

Toxic shock syndrome (TSS) is a rare life-threatening complication of bacterial infection caused by *Staphylococcus aureus* and *Streptococcus pyogenes*.

Etiology and Pathophysiologic Factors[6,9]

TSS is a serious and potentially fatal disease with a mortality rate of 10%, which was discovered in the late 1980s. It presents acutely and if not aggressively treated can rapidly deteriorate to a hypotensive shock. Approximately 50% of cases are associated with menstruating women using long absorbing tampons. Most case has been associated with women, but approximately 25% have been identified in men. TSS is caused by an infectious disease affecting multiple body systems. The disease is precipitated by toxin-producing strains of *S. aureus*. Most women have antibodies to *S. aureus*, although only a small number ever develop TSS. The organism is present in normal vaginal flora in 9% of women and in urethral cultures of 5% of men without the disease. In those infected, the toxin gains entry to the bloodstream through microulcerations in the vaginal or cervical mucosa usually caused by tampons or reflux of menstrual blood from the uterus and out through the fallopian tubes onto the peritoneum caused by the obstruction of menstrual blood flow by tampons. Other cases have been associated with septic abortions, surgical and postpartum wound infections, chorioamnionitis, skin lesions, osteomyelitis, arthritis, periodontal abscess, and burns.

The organism invades tissues and produces an endotoxin that triggers an acute systemic inflammatory response. Altered capillary membrane permeability leads to extravasation of fluid. Venous blood volume is reduced with subsequent reduction in cardiac preload and impaired tissue perfusion.

Laboratory tests may demonstrate elevated SGOT, SGPT, BUN, CR, WBC, and bilirubin, with decreased platelets. Care should be taken to differentiate TSS from other diseases with similar rashes including Rocky Mountain spotted fever, measles, and scarlet fever. Blood, throat, and cerebrospinal fluid cultures as well as serology should be evaluated to rule out other diseases.

Clinical Presentation

The clinical presentation of TSS includes fever, red rash, hypotension, diarrhea, hypotension, and myalgia. As discussed previously, it can be confused with other disease processes, so a careful history of onset of symptoms and any associated causes need to be obtained.

Consequences of TSS for the pregnant patient include still births; low birth weight; conjunctivitis; pneumonia; neonatal sepsis; and congenital abnormalities including blindness, deafness, and organ damage.

Treatment

Early recognition based on history and aggressive management of sepsis and septic shock are imperative to prevent morbidity and mortality to the patient and, if the patient is pregnant, to the fetus (see Chapter 13).

Strategies for Transport

Transport considerations should be based on the condition of the patient. If the patient is septic or suffering from septic shock, management of the shock state is of utmost importance (see Chapter 13).

Ectopic Pregnancy

An ectopic pregnancy is a complication of pregnancy in which the embryo attaches outside the uterus. Ninety-five to 98% of tubal pregnancies implant in the fallopian tube. Nontubal ectopic pregnancies are rare and may occur in the ovaries, broad ligaments, and abdominal cavity. Heterotopic pregnancy, which is a rare case of an ectopic pregnancy, is one in which there may be two fertilized eggs: one embryo inside the uterus and one outside the uterus.

Pathophysiology

This can occur in the fallopian tubes, in the interstitial portion of the tube, in the horn of the uterus, in the cervix, in the abdomen, or in the ovary. One of every 100 to 200 pregnancies are ectopic and of those 95% occur somewhere within the fallopian tubes. In the United States 1 of 826 women will die of complications from an ectopic pregnancy, such as a rupture.

In most ectopic pregnancies, there exists some abnormality or constriction in the fallopian tube resulting in the delay or prevention of the fertilized ovum from reaching the uterus. The fertilized ovum then implants itself within the fallopian tube. Causes of fallopian tube narrowing or constriction can include previous pelvic inflammatory disease (causing scarring), previous inflammatory processes (from infections), endometriosis, developmental abnormalities, adhesions from previous abdominal or tubal surgeries, tubal sterilization, and use of low-dose progesterone oral contraceptives. Other causes include smoking and IUD use. If the fetus dies at an early gestation, there is no harm to the fallopian tube. However, if the fetus continues to grow within the fallopian tube, it can rupture the wall of the fallopian tube, causing significant bleeding. Slow blood loss will cause pain and lower abdominal pressure. Rapid bleeding will cause a sudden drop in blood pressure and may lead to severe hemorrhage, shock, and even death.[6,9]

Clinical Presentation

There is a clinical triad of symptoms referred to as the 3 As: amenorrhea, abdominal pain, and abnormal vaginal bleeding. The abdominal pain is usually in the lower abdomen and described as sharp. It may only occur on one side of the body. The patient may also have a positive Kehr's sign, which is acute pain in the shoulder on the side of the rupture due to blood in the peritoneal cavity. Because of bleeding, the patient may present in hemorrhagic shock.

Strategies for Transport

If the patient is suffering from hemorrhagic shock, the shock should be managed before, during, and after transport (see Chapter 13). If the patient does not present in shock, she should be monitored closely for signs of shock. The patient should be safely transported in a position of comfort. Pain management should be started and continued during transport. The patient should be transported as quickly as possible to an appropriate facility for evaluation and surgical management, if indicated.

Sexual Assault

Sexual violence is a critical global issue that affects millions of people worldwide. EMS personnel are certain to encounter sexual assault victims. Sexual violence has been defined as any form of sexual activity with another person without their express consent. After securing the scene and ensuring provider safety, lifesaving care is the top priority. Physical injuries should be detailed in the notes. Unless there is severe hemorrhage or other evidence of life-threatening genital injury, this area should not be examined. Assessment of these areas should be left to a trained sexual assault examiner. Every effort should be made to preserve evidence. Any areas on the patient that may have been exposed to body fluids or substances must be protected. Do not remove clothing unless it is necessary for medical assistance for injuries.[24]

Transport team members should be familiar with sexual assault protocols, even though the primary focus is on the safety and care of the alleged victim. Careful evaluation of a sexual assault victim will play an important role in recovery.[20]

Summary

The transport of the patient with an obstetric or gynecologic emergency requires experience and skills so that both the mother, fetus, and patient may benefit. If the mother does not receive appropriate care, the fetus suffers; but at times, the condition of the patient or fetus may warrant personnel with specific abilities not generally obtained by a general transport service. Each transport service must ensure that they are competent and capable of providing care for both the mother and fetus as well as for a patient with a gynecologic emergency.

CASE STUDY

Pregnant Patient Transport

A 22-year-old gravida 6 para 0 4 1 4 is at 28 4/7 weeks' gestation. She presents to the emergency department with symptoms of a backache and "pressure on her bottom." The patient is rapidly transferred to the labor and delivery department) in which she is placed on a monitor. Fetal heart rate (FHR) baseline is 155 beats/min with minimal variability. No accelerations or decelerations are noted now. Cervical examination reveals the cervix is 4/80%/+1. Contractions are noted via tocotransducer to be every 4 to 5 minutes, lasting 40 to 60 seconds. The patient does not feel contractions but states her back hurts every 4 to 5 minutes. Per palpation, the contractions are assessed to be moderately strong. What information does her gravidity and parity reveal? What are your transport priorities? Are you concerned that the FHR variability is minimal? What other assessment can be made to assess fetal well-being? What does the cervical examination reveal? What medications, if any, would you consider initiating?

Her gravidity reveals that she has had numerous pregnancies in a short period of time (she is only 22 years old) and that all of her deliveries have been preterm. The best indicator of preterm delivery is a strong history of previous preterm deliveries. Your transport priorities should be to start with a primary and secondary survey that includes an obstetric assessment. After this is done, and contraindications are ruled out, aggressive tocolysis and administration of steroids should be considered. That a fetus of such early gestation would have minimal to moderate variability, may be the result of central nervous system immaturity, and may not be unusual. However, continued assessment of the FHR pattern, including observation for accelerations or decelerations, should be noted. In addition, assessment of fetal movement is the number one, non-monitor method of assessing fetal well-being. The cervical examination reveals that she had advanced dilation and that successful tocolysis with extended duration of the pregnancy is unlikely. The pressure she is feeling in her "bottom" is most likely related to the low fetal position (+1 station) and pressures felt into the lower uterine segment and the vaginal vault. The goal of tocolysis is primarily to extend the pregnancy another 48 hours so tocolytics can be given to benefit the fetus. The most common tocolytic chosen is magnesium sulfate. Most likely a bolus of 2 to 4 g will be given over 20 to 30 minutes and then followed by a maintenance dose of 2 to 4 g/h. The magnesium can be titrated until tocolysis is achieved, if it is within medication parameters and the mother does not have loss of deep tendon reflexes or hypoventilation.

References

1. Jones AE, Summers RL, Deschamp C. A national survey of the air medical transport of the high-risk obstetric patients. *Air Med J.* 2001;20(2):17-20.

2. American Academy of Pediatrics. *Air and Ground Transport of Neonatal and Pediatric Patients.* Elk Gove, IL: American Academy of Pediatrics; 2007.

3. American Academy of Pediatrics and American College of Obstetricians and Gynecologists. *Guidelines for Perinatal Care.* 7th ed. Elk Grove, IL: American Academy of Pediatrics/American College of Obstetricians and Gynecologists; 2012.

4. Bickley LS. *Bate's Guide to Physical Examination and History Taking.* 10th ed. Philadelphia, PA: Walters Kluwer/Lippincott Williams & Wilkins; 2009.

5. Commission on Accreditation of Medical Transport Systems. *Standards.* 10th ed. Andersonville, SC: CAMTS; 2015.

6. Ruhl C, Scheich B, Onokpise B, Bingham D. Interrater reliability of testing of the maternal triage index. *JOAFNN.* 2015;46(6):710-716.

7. Acmi S. Acute ovarian torsion in young girls. *J Acute Dis.* 2016; 5(1):59-61.

8. Campbell J. *International Trauma Life support for Prehospital Care Providers.* 8th ed. Boston: Pearson; 2016.

9. Conde-Agudelo A, Romero R. Amniotic fluid embolism: An evidence-based review. *Am J Obstet Gynecol.* 2009;201(5):445.e1-e13.

10. Eldridge AJ, Ford R. Perimortem caesarean deliveries. *Int J Obstet Anesth.* 2016;27:46-54.

11. Fischer R. Breech presentation. *Medscape.* 2016. Accessed from *Breech Presentation.*

12. Gilbert E. *The Manual of High Risk Pregnancy and Delivery.* 5th ed. St. Louis, MO: Mosby Elsevier; 2011.

13. Hill CC, Pickinpaugh J. Trauma and surgical emergencies in the obstetric patient. *Surg Clin North Am.* 2008;88(2):421-440.

14. Kerr R, et al. Postpartum haemorrhage: Cased definition and guidelines for data collection, analysis, and presentation of immunization safety data. *Vaccine.* 2016;34(49):6102-6109.

15. Lam K. Gynecological and obstetric emergencies. In: Salyer S, ed. *Emergency Medicine for the Healthcare Provider.* Philadelphia, PA: Saunders; 2007:183-260.

16. Lohrenz LL, Metz TD. Maternal air medical transport. In: Blumen I, ed. *Principles and Direction of Air Medical Transport.* Salt Lake City, UT: Medical Physicians Association; 2015.

17. Menihan CA, Kopel E. *Electronic Fetal Monitoring: Concepts and Applications.* Philadelphia, PA: Wolters Kluwer/Lippincott Williams and Wilkins; 2008.

18. Simpson KR, Creehan PA. *Perinatal Nursing.* 4th ed. Philadelphia, PA: Wolters Kluwer Lippincott Williams and Wilkins; 2011.

19. Mammaro A, Carrara S, et al. Hypertensive disorders in pregnancy. *J Prenat Med.* 2009;3(1):1-5.

20. Norris P. Sexual assault. In: Cone D, ed. *Emergency Medical Services: Clinical Practice and Systems Oversight.* 2nd ed. Hoboken, NJ: Wiley; 2015:430-434.

21. Pettit F, Mangos G, Davis G, Henry A. Pre-eclampsia causes adverse maternal outcomes across the gestational spectrum. *Pregnancy Hypertens.* 2015;5(2):198-204.

22. Petrone P, Marini C. Trauma in pregnant patients. *Curr Probl Surg.* 2015;52(8):330-351.

23. Scott J. Obstetric transport. *Obstet Gynecol Clin North Am.* 2016;43(4):821-840.

24. Smith LG. The pregnant trauma patient. In: Makic MF, Whalen E, ed. *Trauma Nursing: From Resuscitation through Rehabilitation.* 4th ed. Philadelphia, PA: Saunders Elsevier; 2009.

25. York-Clark D, Johnson J, Stocking J, Treadwell D, Corbett P, eds. *Critical Care Transport Core Curriculum.* Aurora, CO: Air & Surface Transport Nurses Association; 2017.

26. Thibeault S. *Transport Professional Advanced Trauma Course Manual.* 6th ed. Aurora CO: Air & Surface Transport Nurses Association; 2015.

27. St. Luke's Health System. *ACLS OB: Advanced Cardiac Life Support with an OB Focus.* 4th ed. Boise, ID: St. Luke's Health System; 2016.

29

Care and Transport of the Newborn

TAMMY BLEAK AND MICHAEL A. FRAKES

The neonatal patient is an infant less than 28 chronologic days of age or under 28 days beyond the due date, for preterm infants. A term pregnancy is 38 to 42 weeks. Premature infants are defined as infants born before 37 weeks' gestation, with very preterm being 28 to less than 32 weeks, and extremely preterm if under 28 weeks' gestation. Even late preterm babies, those between 34 and 36 weeks' gestational age, have a threefold higher infant mortality rate compared with term babies.[1] Postterm infants are born later than 42 weeks' gestation. Further subgrouping is defined by birth weight: low birth weight (LBW) is less than 2500 g, very low birth weight (VLBW) is less than 1500 g, and extremely low birth weight (ELBW) is less than 1000 g.

Neonates have a unique anatomy, physiology, and pathophysiology that requires advanced knowledge and understanding to deliver appropriate care. Interfacility transport of neonates requires an emphasis on maintaining an equal or higher level of care during stabilization and transport to the receiving hospital. Teams that transport neonatal patients are expected to be specialists that can provide critical care interventions with progressive and goal-directed therapies. Specialized teams have been associated with improved outcomes compared with nonspecialized teams.[2]

The American Academy of Pediatrics (AAP) offers specific criteria for the composition, education, and operations of a neonatal transport team, and the Commission on Accreditation of Medical Transport Systems publishes industry-established standards for medical transport that can also be helpful.[3,4]

Fetal Circulation and Transition

In utero, the placenta and fetus are nourished by an umbilical vein that carries highly oxygenated blood to the right atrium via the ductus venosus and the inferior vena cava.[5] Most of this blood is directed across the foramen ovale to the left atrium, then the left ventricle, and into the ascending aorta to perfuse the coronary arteries and the brain with the most highly oxygenated blood in fetal circulation. Some of the blood from the umbilical vein, along with blood returning from the superior vena cava,

flows through the tricuspid valve to the right ventricle and out through the pulmonary valve. Most of the blood flow from the right ventricle shunts from the pulmonary artery through the ductus arteriosus and into the descending aorta as a result of the high pressure of the pulmonary vascular system. The shunted blood mixes with the remainder of the blood coming from the left side of the heart (Fig. 29.1).

The transition to extrauterine life begins the moment the neonate takes its first breath. The expansion of the lungs and exposure to oxygen at birth causes the PVR to fall and allows a rapid increase in pulmonary blood flow and a consequent decrease in flow across the ductus arteriosus. Simultaneously, as the umbilical cord is clamped, the low-resistance placental circuit is removed and an increase in systemic resistance occurs. This increase in afterload, and the increased return to the left atrium from the pulmonary circuit, helps to close the flap-like foramen ovale.

In the normal infant, once the transition to extrauterine life is complete, the ductus venosus, foramen ovale, and ductus arteriosus close, and there is not a communication between the systemic and pulmonary systems. However, if there is an abnormal connection between these two systems, shunting can take place at atrial, ventricular, or arterial levels. Blood will shunt from a higher to a lower resistance circulation, and the clinical presentation will vary by the size and location of the shunt. Shunts that occur left to right, or systemic to pulmonary, tend to be acyanotic because oxygen-rich blood is mixing with the oxygen-poor side of the heart. Abnormalities that cause blood to shunt from the right to the left side of the heart, or pulmonary to systemic, will cause the infant to appear cyanotic. Some defects require a shunt for the infant to maintain either pulmonary or systemic circulation.

Careful ongoing assessment and early intervention are critical during this time period. Neonatal hypoxia, hypoglycemia, hypothermia, sepsis, stress, and acidosis can all interfere with the normal progression of this transition, and the baby may exhibit abnormal findings such as intermittent grunting, mild retracting, tachypnea, and poor feeding.[5]

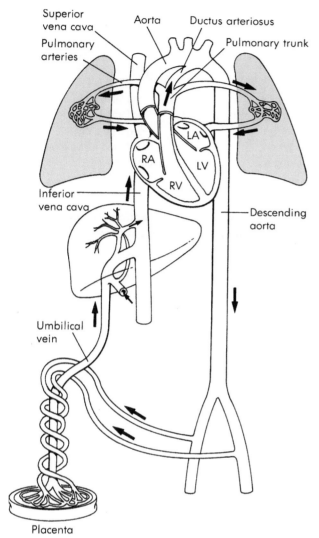

• **Fig. 29.1** Normal fetal circulation and major fetal flow patterns. (From Heymann MA. Biophysical evaluation of fetal status: fetal cardiovascular physiology. In: Creasy RK, Resnik R, eds. *Maternal Fetal Medicine.* Philadelphia, PA: Saunders; 1984.)

The infant must be observed and monitored closely until all these symptoms have been addressed or resolved. Subtle, persistent abnormalities can indicate undiagnosed congenital cardiac diseases.

Initial Priorities: Peripartum Management

Preparation for Delivery

Preparation is the key to a successful neonatal resuscitation. Approximately 4% to 10% of term and late term newborns will require some form of resuscitation.[5] In the transport setting and when available, the information to consider when preparing for delivery includes antepartum risk factors such as preeclampsia and multiple gestations, and intrapartum risk factors including maternal

anesthesia and placental abruption. The clinician will want to know the gestational age, whether the amniotic fluid is clear, the number of births anticipated, and if there are any other risk factors.[5] Transport teams attending the delivery of an infant in an uncontrolled, austere environment will want to make sure they have the ability to provide the following:
• Warmth
  • Increase ambulance temperature
  • Use a radiant warmer or provide a thermal mattress
  • Remove wet garments, dry the baby, and apply fresh, warm linens
  • Provide skin-to-skin contact with mother, or wrap body in plastic wrap to prevent heat loss
• Suction, with both bulb syringe and catheter
• Positive pressure ventilation (PPV) with various size masks and airways
• Supplies for endotracheal intubation
• Supplemental oxygen with a blender
• Emergency medications, especially epinephrine for intravenous (IV) push and infusion
• IV supplies
  • For standard IV access
  • Umbilical catheterization, if trained to do so
  • Intraosseous (IO) access equipment

Assessment

The initial assessment should be brief and focused on identification and treatment of life-threatening issues related to airway, breathing, or circulation. Evaluation of color, respiratory effort, heart rate (HR), body tone, and responsiveness to stimuli all provide an immediate snapshot of how the transition to extrauterine life is progressing at that particular moment in time and guides resuscitation.[6] The Apgar score, presented to the public in 1953 by Dr. Virginia Apgar, is a basic, rapid evaluation of the infant's overall status regarding adaptation to extrauterine life. It is not used to make real-time resuscitation decisions (Table 29.1).[7]

Provide Warmth

The temperature of the newly delivered neonate without asphyxia should be maintained between 36.5°C and 37.5°C.[8,9] If possible, provide prewarmed towels or blankets for the resuscitation. As soon as possible after delivery, the infant should be dried, wet linens removed, and an external heat source provided, such as radiant warmers. Adjuncts to the radiant warmers include plastic wrap, thermal mattresses, and heated and humidified gases. If an external heat source is not immediately available, particular attention must be paid to ambient temperature. Unintended neonatal hypothermia increases the risk of intraventricular hemorrhage (IVH), respiratory problems, hypoglycemia, and late-onset sepsis.[9]

TABLE 29-1	Apgar Score			
		Sign		
Score	**0**	**1**	**2**
Appearance, color	Blue, pale	Centrally pink	Completely pink
Pulse, heart rate	None	Less than 100 beats/min	Greater than 100 beats/min
Grimace, reflex	No response	Grimace	Cough, gag, cry
Activity/attitude	Flaccid/limp muscle tone	Some flexion	Well-flexed/active motion
Respiratory, effort	None, irritability	Weak/irregular	Good, crying

Clearing the Airway

The infant should be positioned with the neck in a neutral position, which allows for proper positioning of the airway in a sniffing position. If the airway needs to be cleared, this can be done by wiping the nose and mouth or using a bulb syringe or suction catheter with mechanical suction. The oropharynx should normally be cleared before suctioning of the nares because stimulation may cause the infant to gasp and aspirate secretions present in the oropharynx. Stimulation of the vagus nerve from suctioning too vigorously and too deeply may result in severe bradycardia; therefore suctioning after the initial clearing of the airway should be done on an as-needed basis. The Neonatal Resuscitation Program (NRP) recommends that no greater than 100 mm Hg of negative pressure should be used to avoid injury to the neonate.[5]

Aspiration of meconium-stained fluid into distal airways may significantly contribute to morbidity and mortality. It has been common practice to routinely intubate nonvigorous meconium-stained infants presenting with inadequate respirations, poor tone, or an HR less than 100 beats/min before there are many respirations. This practice is no longer supported by the American Heart Association or AAP because of insufficient evidence of benefit.[10] If an infant delivered through meconium is nonvigorous, initiate the initial steps of neonatal resuscitation as described previously.[9]

Initiation of Breathing

Most neonates initiate spontaneous breathing without intervention. Neonates that do not initiate breathing on their own may require simple interventions such as opening and positioning the airway, drying, and suctioning to stimulate breathing. If the neonate still does not have adequate respirations, appropriate tactile stimulation consists of flicking the feet or rubbing the infants back.

Neonates with spontaneous respirations but persistent central cyanosis should have pulse oximetry monitoring initiated on the right hand. Skin color is not always a reliable indicator for the need for supplemental oxygen.[5] Babies transitioning at birth take up to 10 minutes to increase their blood oxygen levels to normal extrauterine values (Table 29.2). If oximeter readings are low and not increasing, supplemental oxygen is indicated and may be delivered by oxygen mask, flow-inflating bag and mask, T-piece resuscitator, or oxygen tubing held close

TABLE 29-2	Normal Neonatal Preductal Oxygen (Right Hand) Oxygen Saturation
Minutes of Life	**SpO$_2$ Range**
1	60% – 65%
2	65% – 70%
3	70% – 75%
4	75% – 80%
5	80% – 85%
10	85% – 95%

Data from Weiner, GM, Zaichkin JG. *Textbook of Neonatal Resuscitation.* Elk Grove Village, IL: American Academy of Pediatrics; 2016.

to the baby's mouth and nose. If the neonate has labored breathing and cannot maintain target oxygen saturations with 100% free-flow oxygen, early initiation of continuous positive airway pressure (CPAP) may avoid the need for intubation and mechanical ventilation.[5,11,12]

Positive Pressure Ventilation and Intubation

If the neonate does not begin spontaneous effective respirations, if the HR remains below 100 beats/min, or if appropriate oxygen saturations cannot be maintained with 100% free-flow oxygen, PPV should be initiated at a rate of 40 to 60 breaths/min with the minimal amount of oxygen to support oxygenation. Effective ventilation should be evaluated by auscultation of breath sounds and observation of chest excursion and HR. The infant should respond to effective ventilation with an improvement in HR, oxygen saturations, and spontaneous respiratory effort.[5,13]

Neonates are at high risk for pulmonary air leaks such as a pneumothorax or pneumomediastinum, so ventilating pressures should always be monitored with a manometer. Although pressures up to 30 to 40 cm H_2O may be initially necessary to open the lungs, the lowest pressures possible to maintain adequate chest rise and oxygenation should be used. Once the infant has established spontaneous respirations and an HR of 100 beats/min, the team should reevaluate the amount of support needed.

If there is no clinical improvement with effective PPV or if PPV is required for more than a few minutes, consider intubation.[5]

TABLE 29-3	Endotracheal Tube Size and Depth for Neonatal Patients		
Gestational Age (Weeks)	Weight (g)	ETT Size	Maximum ETT Depth
<28	<750	2.5	6.75
<28	750–1000	2.5	7
28–34	1000–2000	3	8
34–38	2000–3000	3.5	9
>38	>3000	3.5–4.0	10

ETT, Endotracheal tube.
Data from Karlson K. The S.T.A.B.L.E. Program postresuscitation/pretransport stabilization care of sick infants guidelines for neonatal healthcare providers. *Learner manual*. 6th ed. Park City, UT; 2013.

An accurate gestational age can help guide the proper depth of endotracheal tube (ETT) insertion and ETT size selection (Table 29.3). For ETT depth, the nasal-tragus length method is validated: the ETT marking at the baby's lip should correspond to the calculated depth of (distance from the baby's nasal septum to the ear tragus) +1.[5] Another easy calculation for the depth of the ETT in patients greater than 750 g is 6 + weight in kilograms = ETT depth. In patients less than 750 g, this calculation could cause the ETT to be secured too deeply.[14]

Careful and immediate evaluation for right or left mainstem or esophageal intubation should be done and effectiveness of ventilation should be assessed. Clinical signs of increasing HR, symmetric chest rise, and equal, bilateral breath sounds suggest successful intubation. End-tidal carbon dioxide detection should also be done with either a colorimetric or waveform device.[5,15,16]

The laryngeal mask airway (LMA) may be a beneficial airway adjunct in patients when PPV with a face mask is unable to achieve effective ventilation or when intubation is unsuccessful or not possible.[9] This may occur when the neonate presents with facial congenital anomalies such as Pierre Robin syndrome. Placement does not require instruments, and the LMA is blindly passed using the clinician's finger to guide it into place. Limitations of the LMA include size constraints, inability to deliver high ventilation pressures, and insufficient evidence that it can be used for intratracheal medications or prolonged assisted ventilation in neonates.[5] The smallest LMA for use in neonates is for those greater than 2 kg.

Chest Compressions

Chest compressions should be initiated if the HR is less than 60 beats/min after 30 seconds of effective PPV.[5] Resuscitation for neonates should be performed at a rate of 120 "events" (compressions or breaths) per minute. Ninety compressions plus 30 breaths on 100% oxygen should occur at a ratio of 3:1. The status of the infant should be reassessed after 60 seconds of resuscitation. If the child's HR is greater than 60 beats/min, compressions can be stopped. If the HR remains below 60 beats/min, epinephrine should be given.

The recommended technique for chest compressions in neonates is the thumb-encircling-hands technique, preferred over the previously recommended two-finger technique because of the ability to have more control over the depth of compression and delivery of a more consistent pressure.[17] This method appears to provide better peak systolic and coronary artery perfusion pressure. The baby should be placed on a firm surface for delivery of effective compressions, with the caregiver encircling the infant's chest with both thumbs used to depress the infant's sternum. The infant's chest should be depressed to a depth of approximately one-third of the anteroposterior diameter of the chest, and the chest should be allowed to recoil completely by releasing pressure so that the heart can refill.[5]

Drug Support

Less than 1% of neonates will require drug intervention when effective ventilation has been established. If the HR continues below 60 beats/min with effective ventilation and chest compressions for a minimum of 30 seconds or in the absence of an HR, epinephrine should be given. The recommended IV dose is 0.1 to 0.3 mL/kg or 0.01 to 0.03 mg/kg of 0.1 mg/mL epinephrine solution followed by 0.5 to 1 mL flush of normal saline. ETT administration may be more readily accessible, but studies have shown larger doses are required and absorption is unreliable and not as effective as IV administration.[18] If the ETT route is used, administer 0.5 to 1 mL/kg or 0.05 to 0.1 mg/kg of 0.1 mg/mL epinephrine. Administration of ETT epinephrine should be followed by PPV to facilitate absorption by distribution throughout the lungs. If the first dose is given via the ETT and does not elicit an effective response, subsequent doses should be given by IV as soon as vascular access is established.[9] If the HR remains below 60 beats/min, subsequent doses of epinephrine may be given every 3 to 5 minutes.

Consider hypovolemia in patients with a history of bleeding or if the infant has poor response to resuscitation, pallor, decreased capillary refill, and/or weak pulses that persist even with adequate ventilation, chest compressions, and administration of epinephrine. If hypovolemia is suspected, normal saline should be given in 10 mL/kg aliquots over 5 to 10 minutes. Type O Rh-negative blood should be considered when severe fetal anemia is documented.

If peripheral vascular access cannot be rapidly achieved, current NRP guidelines for resuscitation in the delivery room recommend emergent line placement into the umbilical vein as the most accessible parenteral route (Fig. 29.2). IO is another vascular access route for those trained in the technique. This approach is a reasonable alternative, especially in the outpatient setting when cannulation of the umbilical vessel may not be possible. All medications and fluids that can be given in an umbilical vein catheter can be given via IO in term and preterm neonates.[5]

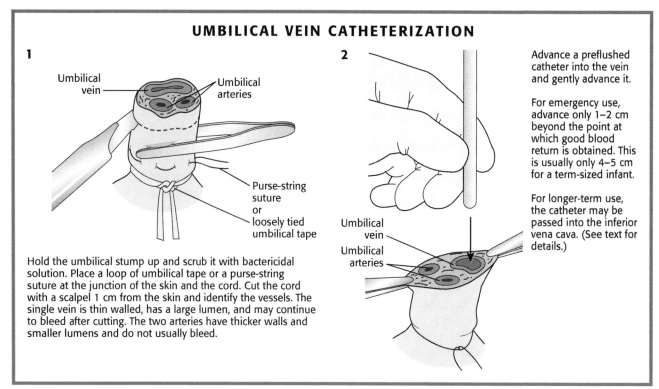

UMBILICAL VEIN CATHETERIZATION

1

Umbilical vein

Umbilical arteries

Purse-string suture or loosely tied umbilical tape

Hold the umbilical stump up and scrub it with bactericidal solution. Place a loop of umbilical tape or a purse-string suture at the junction of the skin and the cord. Cut the cord with a scalpel 1 cm from the skin and identify the vessels. The single vein is thin walled, has a large lumen, and may continue to bleed after cutting. The two arteries have thicker walls and smaller lumens and do not usually bleed.

2

Umbilical vein

Umbilical arteries

Advance a preflushed catheter into the vein and gently advance it.

For emergency use, advance only 1–2 cm beyond the point at which good blood return is obtained. This is usually only 4–5 cm for a term-sized infant.

For longer-term use, the catheter may be passed into the inferior vena cava. (See text for details.)

• **Fig. 29.2** Umbilical vein catheterization. (From Zaoutis L, Chiang V. *Comprehensive Pediatric Hospital Medicine.* Philadelphia, PA: Elsevier; 2007.)

Apgar Scoring

The AAP and American Congress of Obstetricians and Gynecologists encourage the use of an expanded Apgar score for up to 20 minutes for infants who are depressed (score less than 7) at 5 minutes of life (see Table 29.1). The Apgar score is not an accurate indicator of neonatal asphyxia and should not be used to predict mortality or neurologic outcomes.[19-21] Low scores at 5 and 10 minutes can be associated with acute peripartum or intrapartum events.[22] An infant with an Apgar score of 0 at 10 minutes of age can have resuscitative efforts discontinued because of the high probability of poor neurologic outcome if there is confirmation that there has not been a detectable HR.[21]

Special Considerations for Preterm/LBW Babies

Preterm and LBW infants are at great risk for cold stress because of their thin skin, large surface area relative to body mass, and decreased fat stores that allow for increased heat loss. In the transport setting, thermal mattresses and plastic wrap can be used to maintain body heat. Monitor temperatures frequently to avoid overheating or underheating and to maintain a goal temperature of 36.5°C.[5]

Preterm infants are at increased risk of neurologic injury because of the delicate capillaries in the germinal matrix. Transport has been associated with an increased risk for IVH in VLBW infants.[23] Evidence supports the practice of neutral head positioning to decrease the risk of IVH.[24] If possible in the transport environment, keep the head in a midline position for the first 72 hours of life along with the head of the bed elevated at 30 degrees.[25]

In the stress of the transport environment, attention should be given to careful handling of the infant. This includes avoiding a head-down position; avoiding overinflation of the lungs, which could result in a pneumothorax; assuring gradual changes in oxygenation and ventilation; and avoiding rapid volume infusions.

Evaluation of Prolonged Resuscitation

If the neonate has not responded to the initial priorities of delivery room management, the transport team must re-evaluate the clinical assessment and management of the infant. Common reasons for an inadequate response to resuscitation include the following:
1. Pulmonary sources
   a. Dislodged ETT
   b. Obstructed airway
      i. Obstructed ETT
      ii. Congenital malformation
   c. Pneumothorax
   d. Failure of oxygen supply or ventilation device
   e. Pulmonary hypoplasia
   f. Congenital diaphragmatic hernia (CDH)
2. Cardiac sources
3. Shock
4. Inborn error of metabolism

5. Hypothermia
6. Hypoglycemia
7. Blood glucose

Noninitiation and Discontinuation of Resuscitation

According to the NRP, when circumstances at birth predict "almost certain early death and when unacceptably high morbidity is likely among survivors, resuscitation is not indicated although exceptions may be appropriate." Situations that may call for noninitiation of resuscitation include:

- Birth weight less than 400 g
- Confirmed trisomy 13
- Anencephaly
- Gestational age less than or equal to 22 weeks
- No response after 10 minutes of ongoing adequate resuscitative efforts
- Severe fetal growth retardation[5,18,26]

Postdelivery Management

History and Assessment

Assessment of the newborn should include history, clinical examination, and laboratory data. The maternal history is a key part of the neonatal history. Obstetric information obtained should include the estimated day of confinement (EDC) or due date based on the mother's last menstrual period and clinical data; maternal age; gravity; parity; abortions; fetal demise; neonatal deaths; number of living children; time since rupture of membranes; and complications of the pregnancy, labor, or delivery. Maternal medications (both during pregnancy and during the perinatal period) should be assessed, along with group B streptococcus (GBS) status and associated treatment, and other maternal infections such as herpes simplex virus, chlamydia, gonorrhea, hepatitis B, syphilis, or HIV. Any maternal illicit drug use should also be obtained.

Neonatal history should include gestational age, postdelivery age, the delivery type and course, time or membrane rupture and nature of fluids, Apgar scores, resuscitation efforts, initial physical examination, and subsequent clinical course. Laboratory data and radiographic studies should also be reviewed.

A considerable amount of baseline information can be obtained strictly through simple observation before disturbing the infant. This observation should include:

- Heart
  - Rate, rhythm, heart sounds, murmurs, extra sounds
- Chest
  - Symmetry and adequacy of air entry, rales, rhonchi, wheezes
- Abdomen
  - Bowel sounds, organomegaly, masses
- Pulses
  - Quality
  - Comparison between upper and lower extremities
- Signs and symptoms of distress
  - Color, respiratory effort, posture, tone
- Obvious morphology.

Once the baseline examination has been established, the rest of the examination should proceed with an organized, systematic approach. For example, the transport team might examine the infant beginning from the head and working downward. The essential components of a detailed examination are outlined in Table 29.4. The potential value of each part of the examination must be weighed against any stress it may cause to an already compromised infant and current physiologic stability.

Glucose and Maintenance Fluids

Before birth, the fetus stores glucose in the form of glycogen to use after birth.[27] The ability of the neonate to maintain glucose stability after birth can be adversely impacted by three factors: glycogen levels, hyperinsulinemia, and glucose utilization. Glycogen storage generally occurs in the latter portion of the third trimester, which puts the preterm infant at risk for hypoglycemia. Small-for-gestational-age (SGA) infants (those in the lowest 10% of the growth curve) stressed in utero use the glucose transferred from the mother via the placenta for growth and survival. This restricts the infant's ability to make or store glycogen.

TABLE 29-4	Key Components of Neonatal Physical Exam
	Assess
Head	Symmetry, shape caput succedaneum, cephalhematoma
Fontanels/sutures	Fontanel number, fullness, depression, size, suture mobility
Symmetry of face	Development, shape, movement
Ears	Shape, position of face, presence of skin tags
Eyes	Shape, position, size, pupils, hemorrhages
Mouth	Cleft palate, teeth, abnormalities, presence of micrognathia
Neck	Webbing, length
Nose	Symmetry, septum, patency
Clavicles	Masses, intactness
Chest	Size, symmetry, shape
Umbilical cord	Number of vessels
Genitals	Development, testes, urethral and vaginal openings
Anus	Patency, meconium
Spine	Masses, symmetry, dimples
Extremities	Symmetry, development, movement, pulses
Hips	Range of motion
Reflexes	Root, suck, Moro, grasp
Tone	Flaccid, normal, jitteriness, flexion

A second factor is hyperinsulinemia, which occurs in infants of diabetic mothers (IDM) and which should be considered in infants who are large for gestational age (those in the top 10% of the growth curve). Abnormal elevation of maternal glucose concentrations will be seen in the fetus; however, maternal insulin does not cross the placenta. The fetus will increase insulin secretion in response to the increased glucose concentration. At delivery, the maternal glucose stops but the infant's insulin remains elevated and can take several days to regulate. IDM babies are also at increased risk for hypocalcemia and hypomagnesemia.

Finally, increased glucose utilization occurs in infants that are stressed or sick because increased energy needs can rapidly deplete their glycogen stores. Some maternal medications can also increase the risk of neonatal hypoglycemia such as terbutaline, β-blockers, tricyclic antidepressants, sulfonylureas, and thiazide diuretics.[27]

The healthy term infant normally reaches the nadir of the serum glucose level at approximately 2 hours after birth.[28] Glucose screening is therefore recommended for all healthy term infants between 1 and 2 hours of age. Infants identified as high risk should have screening glucose levels as soon as possible after delivery. A widely used neonatal education program for sick infants called STABLE recommends that a glucose less than 50 mg/dL should be corrected with IV therapy and monitored until the glucose stabilizes between 50 and 110 mg/dL on two consecutive measures 15 to 30 minutes apart.[27]

Hypoglycemia that is symptomatic in the neonate is associated with increased neurodevelopmental impairment. Symptoms of neonatal hypoglycemia include hypotonia, lethargy, poor feeding, jitteriness/tremors, seizures, apnea, tachypnea, and cyanosis. When hypoglycemia is suspected, a screening test should be done while a plasma glucose is sent to the laboratory. Treatment should be initiated before confirmation from the laboratory is received. Not all infants with hypoglycemia are symptomatic, and there is not currently clear evidence that asymptomatic neonatal hypoglycemia impacts neurodevelopmental outcomes. Nevertheless, infants that are asymptomatically hypoglycemic and are sick should be kept in the normoglycemic range.[27]

In the otherwise healthy infant, oral reestablishment of serum glucose is the preferred method; however, critically ill neonates cannot tolerate oral intake. Symptomatic patients will require an IV established and a glucose infusion rate of 4 to 6 mg/kg per minute. A usual starting dose is 80 mL/kg per day (5.5 mg/kg/min) followed by a bolus of 2 mL/kg (200 mg/kg) of D10W slowly over 5 minutes.[27] Do not bolus with dextrose concentrations over D10. A recheck of the blood glucose should be repeated within 15 to 30 minutes after a glucose bolus or IV rate increase. When there is continued hypoglycemia, a decision to bolus or increase fluid rates or dextrose concentration must be made on the basis of the fluid requirements and tolerance of the individual baby.

A peripheral vein may be used to administer solutions that contain glucose concentrations up to 12.5% dextrose. At concentrations over 12.5% dextrose, a central venous line should be considered. Treatment of extremely resistant hypoglycemia may include the use of glucagon, glucocorticoids, and diazoxide. Administration of these drugs, however, is beyond the scope of this chapter.

Hyperglycemia (blood glucose levels greater than 125 mg/dL) can be seen in infants less than 32 weeks' gestation or infants that are SGA because of their immature endocrine system. Generally hyperglycemia is managed by individual program protocol or medical direction.

Glucose monitoring should be conducted frequently during transport to ensure that glucose homeostasis is maintained. A point-of-care glucose check should be assessed within 15 to 30 minutes after changing IV fluids containing dextrose or increasing or decreasing infusion rates. All abnormal results should be monitored and reported as per protocol or medical direction.

Fluid Management

Maintenance of fluid and electrolyte balance in the newborn requires careful, precise calculations. The transport team should precisely calculate the infant's fluid requirement, including any abnormal losses; too much or too little fluid can be detrimental to the progress of the infant.

Generally sick infants typically need approximately 80 mL/kg per day on the first day of life. This requirement increases by approximately 10 mL/kg per day on the first subsequent day of life. Premature infants, particularly those weighing less than 1500 g, should be given special consideration of potentially increased fluid needs. Insensible water losses, immature skin surfaces, and prolonged exposure to radiant warmers can increase fluid requirements by as much as 50%.

The main sources of neonatal fluid loss are insensible water loss (skin and respiratory fluid losses) and urinary output (UO). Insensible water loss increases significantly in the extremely premature or ELBW infant. Radiant warmers, elevated environmental temperature, and respiratory distress increase insensible water loss. The use of heat shields and warm, humidified air delivered through the ventilator can significantly minimize these losses. In the sick neonate, UO should be measured as accurately as possible with urine bags, diaper weights, or catheterization. With appropriate fluid intake, UO should be 1 to 2 mL/kg per hour. During the first week of life, the infant averages a 5% to 7% loss of birth weight.[29] Subsequent changes in the baby's fluid intake are based on evaluation of these criteria.

The need for electrolyte evaluation before transport is determined based on the age of the newborn, the length of the transport, and the presence of risk factors for electrolyte imbalance. The addition of electrolytes to IV fluids is usually not necessary in the first 12 to 24 hours. Serum electrolyte levels should be checked before any additional electrolytes are added.

Thermoregulation

It is well documented that unintended hypothermia in neonatal patients adversely impacts morbidity and mortality.[27,30]

The neonate is at high risk for hypothermia because of a large skin surface area to body mass ratio and poor thermal insulation. If not corrected, hypothermia can increase metabolism and cause peripheral vasoconstriction. This decreases peripheral perfusion and can lead to metabolic acidosis. Other adverse effects of cold stress include increased oxygen consumption, pulmonary vasoconstriction, and increased glucose demand. Infants with the greatest risk for hypothermia include those that are preterm, SGA, sick, requiring a prolonged resuscitation, or those with defects requiring surgery such as gastroschisis or omphalocele.[27]

Compared with the adult, the neonate has a limited ability to increase oxygen consumption, to produce heat by shivering, or to dissipate excess heat through sweating. The neonate maintains body temperature through basal metabolism, muscular activity, and chemical thermogenesis. The infant's primary mechanism of heat production in response to cold stress is chemical thermogenesis by metabolizing brown fat stores. This process requires increased oxygen consumption and increased glucose utilization. Preterm or hypoxic neonates are at increased risk for cold stress because of decreased stores of brown fat and/or their inability to metabolize it for the generation of heat production.[27]

The optimal temperature ranges for the newborn include the following:
- Skin: 36.2°C to 37.2°C
- Axillary: 36.5°C to 37.3°C
- Rectal: 36.5°C to 37.5°C[31,32]

Temperature must be frequently monitored during transport via skin temperature probes in transport incubators. Rectal temperatures are not recommended because of the high risk of perforation of the rectum.

Heat losses occur through convection, conduction, evaporation, and radiation.
- Radiation: Simple heat transfer from the body to the surrounding atmosphere
- Convection: Heat transfer from the body as air flows past (e.g., air currents, breezes)
- Evaporation: Heat transfer to water as it changes from liquid to gas (e.g., a wet infant)
- Conduction: Heat transfer between the body and objects in contact (e.g., a scale)

The neutral thermal environment is the range of environmental temperatures at which the neonate maintains a normal body temperature with minimal metabolic activity and oxygen consumption. During transport, the baby must be in a double-walled isolette set at a temperature that creates a neutral thermal environment (Table 29.5).[33]

When managing a baby in the hospital, the baby should be on a radiant warmer. Chemical mattresses and plastic wrap can also be beneficial in preparing the neonate for transport and should be considered for babies less than 32 weeks' gestation or those at high risk for developing hypothermia.[5] Carefully follow manufacturer guidelines with any commercial heat-generating products to prevent overheating or burns. Clear plastic wrap or commercial products can be applied directly (e.g., wrapping the infant) to minimize further heat loss, but avoid the head and airway to prevent suffocation. When transporting a neonate in severe cold conditions, thermal covers may be used over double-walled transport incubators to further maintain a neutral thermal environment for the neonate.

Rewarming neonates that are unintentionally hypothermic is generally done slowly, at rates under 0.5°C/h, to decrease complications such as apnea, hypotension from vasodilation, and arrhythmias.[27]

The neonate must also not become hyperthermia, which is associated with perinatal respiratory depression.

Respiratory Management: General Considerations

Many ill neonates have some degree of respiratory compromise. The transport team must perform careful and continuous assessment of respiratory status to provide adequate respiratory support before moving the patient to the transport incubator. This minimizes the likelihood of having to remove the baby from the transport incubator to perform interventions in a less controlled environment with fluctuating temperatures.

A normal neonatal respiratory rate is 30 to 60 breaths/min. Tachypnea can occur in neonates with pulmonary processes that impair gas exchange or from nonpulmonary processes that result in a metabolic acidosis. In either case, the respiratory center will respond by increasing the minute volume in an attempt to compensate for the developing acidosis. It is important to evaluate the baby's respiratory rate, work of breathing, gas exchange, presence of cyanosis, and oxygen saturations in the context of current oxygen supplementation. It can also be helpful to review chest x-rays and blood gas results because these can help guide ventilator and other treatment strategies.

Gas exchange is best evaluated by looking for regular, symmetric chest rise and fall and by listening to lung fields bilaterally for air flow.

Increased work of breathing is evidenced by nasal flaring, grunting, and retractions. Nasal flaring decreases airway resistance to improve airflow. Grunting represents an attempt to increase end-expiratory pulmonary pressures and improve the driving pressure of oxygen across the alveolar–capillary interface. Retractions occur when a neonate with poor lung compliance attempts to increase tidal volumes by using accessory respiratory muscles. This effort increases inspiratory force and draws the chest inward during inspiration, but retractions can also decrease the usable lung capacity and ventilation.

Hemoglobin desaturation can be evaluated by looking at the tongue and mucous membranes and through pulse oximetry. On examination, acrocyanosis is a self-limiting condition in which the neonate's hands and feet remain cyanotic for up to 48 hours after birth. It is generally not a pathologic finding. Central cyanosis (cyanosis in the tongue and mucous membranes) is a more significant finding. Pulse oximetry monitoring greatly enhances the ability to titrate oxygen delivery based on patient response and need. The oxygen saturation probe should be placed on a preductal on the right hand

TABLE 29-5	Neutral Thermal Environmental Temperatures				

Age and Weight	Starting Temperature (°C)	Range of Temperature (°C)	Age and Weight	Starting Temperature (°C)	Range of Temperature (°C)
0-6 hr			1501-2500 g	32.3	31.2-33.4
Under 1200 g	35.0	34.0-35.4	Over 2500 g (and >36 wk)	31.7	30.1-33.2
1200-1500 g	34.1	33.9-34.4	>72-96 hr		
1501-2500 g	33.4	32.8-33.8	Under 1200 g	34.0	34.0-35.0
Over 2500 g	33.9	32.0-33.8	1200-1500 g	33.5	33.0-34.0
(and >36 wk)			1501-2500 g	32.2	31.1-33.2
>6-12 hr			Over 2500 g	31.3	29.8-32.8
Under 1200 g	35.0	34.0-35.4	(and >36 wk)		
1200-1500 g	34.0	33.5-34.4	>4-12 days		
1501-2500 g	33.1	32.2-33.8	Under 1500 g	33.5	33.0-34.0
Over 2500 g	32.8	31.4-33.8	1501-2500 g	32.1	31.0-33.2
(and >36 wk)			Over 2500 g		
>12-24 hr			(and >36 wk)		
Under 1200 g	34.0	34.0-35.4	4-5 days	31.0	29.5-32.6
1200-1500 g	33.8	33.3-34.3	5-6 days	30.9	29.4-32.3
1501-2500 g	32.8	31.8-33.8	6-8 days	30.6	29.0-32.2
Over 2500 g	32.4	31.0-33.7	8-10 days	30.3	29.0-31.8
(and >36 wk)			10-12 days	30.1	29.0-31.4
>24-36 hr			>12-14 days		
Under 1200 g	34.0	34.0-35.0	Under 1500 g	33.5	32.6-34.0
1200-1500 g	33.6	33.1-34.2	1501-2500 g	32.1	31.0-33.2
1501-2500 g	32.6	31.6-33.6	>2-3 wk		
Over 2500 g	32.1	30.7-33.5	Under 1500 g	33.1	32.2-34.0
(and >36 wk)			1501-2500 g	31.7	30.5-33.0
>36-48 hr			>3-4 wk		
Under 1200 g	34.0	34.0-35.0	Under 1500 g	32.6	31.6-33.6
1200-1500 g	33.5	33.0-34.1	1501-2500 g	31.4	30.0-32.7
1501-2500 g	32.5	31.4-33.5	>4-5 wk		
Over 2500 g	31.9	30.5-33.3	Under 1500 g	32.0	31.2-33.0
(and >36 wk)			1501-2500 g	30.9	29.5-32.2
>48-72 hr			>5-6 wk		
Under 1200 g	34.0	34.0-35.0	Under 1500 g	31.4	30.6-32.3
1200-1500 g	33.5	33.0-34.0	1501-2500 g	30.4	29.0-31.8

Adapted from American Academy of Pediatrics: Committee on Fetus and Newborn: *Guidelines for perinatal case,* ed 2, Elk Grove Village, IL: 1988; American Academy of Pediatrics and American College of Obstetricians an Gynecologists.

Generally the smaller infants in each weight group require a temperature in the higher portion of the temperature range. Within each time range, the younger the infant, the higher the temperature required.

or wrist. This site evaluates oxygenation to the brain and heart, as it evaluates blood that is before the ductus arteriosus, so it is not affected by a ductal-level shunt, if one exists.[5,34] It may take up to 10 minutes for a baby to achieve an oxygen saturation of 95% after birth (see Table 29-2). Immediate care after delivery should be targeted to an age-appropriate saturation. After the first 10 minutes, preductal target oxygen saturations should be maintained between 91% and 95% unless there are conditions present that require adjustment, such as cardiac disease or pulmonary hypertension.[27,35]

Fetal hemoglobin and, accordingly, the fetal oxyhemoglobin dissociation curve, are different than those of adult patients. Fetal hemoglobin (hemoglobin-N) has a higher affinity for oxygen than adult hemoglobin, meaning that it binds oxygen at a lower oxygen tension but is reluctant to release the oxygen molecules. This is beneficial in utero to facilitate placental oxygen uptake. For the neonate, this means that the PaO_2 can be high with little change in oxygen saturation. This relationship is represented by a leftward shift of the oxyhemoglobin dissociation curve.[27,36] Remember that other factors causing a leftward shift are alkalosis and hypothermia, whereas acidosis and hyperthermia shift the curve to the right. With a right shift, it is more difficult to saturate the hemoglobin molecule, but it is easier to release the oxygen to the tissues (Fig. 29.3).

Blood gases supplement pulse oximetry in determining oxygenation along with assessing ventilation and pH.

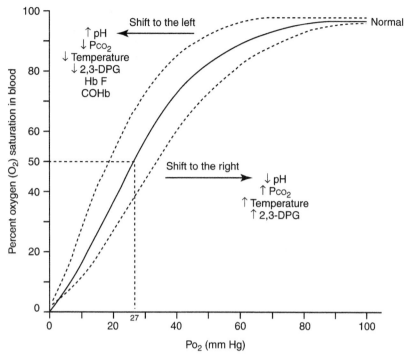

• **Fig. 29.3** Oxyhemoglobin dissociation curves: Normal and shifted. (From Schick L, Windle P. *PeriAnesthesia Nursing Core Curriculum: Preprocedure, Phase I and Phase II PACU Nursing,* ed 3, St. Louis, MO: Saunders; 2016.)

Newly born infants tend to have a mild metabolic acidosis, but usually have more normal blood gases within 48 hours. It is important to know the site from which the sample was drawn because normal values vary among arterial, venous, and capillary blood gas samples. Normal values are included in Table 29.6. The blood gas sample should also be interpreted in the context of the respiratory support being provided at the time the sample was obtained.

Respiratory Support

The first component of respiratory management is ensuring correct opening, positioning, and clearing of the airway. Following that, supplemental oxygen is often administered. Oxygen is a drug with associated risks and side effects, particularly lung injury and retinopathy of prematurity.[35] It is administered by a number of methods.

Blow-by or free-flow oxygen near the baby's face can be used on a short-term basis, but has two main drawbacks. First, accurate measurement of the exact amount of supplementation is impossible. Second, the flow of cold oxygen into the neonate's face may result in increased inappropriate heat-generating responses and vagal stimulation.

A low-flow nasal cannula delivers flow rates of 1 L/min or less.[37] Although commonly used, it is difficult to ascertain the inspired oxygen concentration because the baby entrains room air through the mouth and nose in addition to the supplied oxygen.

Nasal continuous positive airway pressure (nCPAP) is beneficial for infants with adequate respiratory effort but who exhibit increased work of breathing and/or increased oxygen requirements. It can be delivered via mask or nasal prongs, and mask CPAP can be given while the nCPAP is being set up. The early use of CPAP can reduce the need for intubation,

TABLE 29-6	**Normal Neonatal Blood Gas Values**			
Site	pH	PCO$_2$	PO$_2$	HCO$_3^-$
Arterial	7.35–7.45	35–45 mm Hg	50–90 mm Hg (term) 50–80 mm Hg (preterm)	22–26 mEq/L (term) 20–24 mEq/L (preterm)
Capillary	0.02–0.05 lower than arterial	8–14 mm Hg higher than arterial	30–41 mm Hg lower than arterial	2–3 mEq/L higher than arterial
Venous	0.01–0.03 lower than arterial	3–7 mm Hg higher than arterial	23–32 mm Hg lower than arterial	0.5–1.5 mEq/L higher than arterial

Data from Yapicioglu H, Ozlu F, Ozcan K, et al. Comparison of arterial, venous and capillary blood gas measurements in premature babies in newborn intensive care unit. *Cukurova Med J.* 2014; 39(1):117-124.

mechanical ventilation, and surfactant administration in newborns.[11,38,39] An AAP policy statement described it as the preferred initial approach to prevent neonatal respiratory distress syndrome (RDS). Neonates with an oxygen requirement that exceeds 60% to 70% should be evaluated for intubation.

High-flow nasal cannula (HFNC), with flow rates typically between 2 and 8 L/min, is increasingly being used instead of nCPAP devices.[38-41] The nasal prongs are smaller than prongs used with nCPAP and HFNC does not require a seal, which may cause less nasal trauma. It may also be easier to apply, and some believe that it improves carbon dioxide elimination.[37] The role of HFNC is still being evaluated; it appears to be at least not inferior to nCPAP.[42] A small device that heats and humidifies HFNC air is available for transport.

Noninvasive mechanical ventilation is used when the clinician is attempting to avoid endotracheal intubation. Nasal intermittent positive pressure ventilation augments nCPAP by delivering intermittent positive pressure breaths via nasal prongs. It is mainly used for infants requiring early support because of apnea or for postextubation. Although there is no current data to support the use of nasal intermittent positive pressure ventilation over nCPAP, early studies suggest nasal intermittent positive pressure ventilation reduces the frequency and severity of apnea and is better at reducing extubation failures in neonates.[43,44]

Invasive ventilation requires the placement of an ETT, with inherent risks for complications. Mechanical ventilation decreases work of breathing, improves overall gas exchange, and can recruit lung units. ETT and mechanical ventilation should be considered in infants with warning signs of respiratory failure, such as grunting with retractions, inability to maintain O_2 saturations, or respiratory insufficiency, that are not responsive to a trial of CPAP. Patients with inadequate respiratory effort require early intubation, as do babies with pathology that precludes positive pressure by other means, such as a CDH.

Traditionally, neonatal transport ventilators have provided time-cycled, pressure-limited ventilation. With this method of conventional mechanical ventilation, tidal volumes can have considerable fluctuation caused by lung compliance changes, ETT leaks, and the baby's spontaneous breathing.[45] Ventilation can also be delivered in a volume-targeted mode, which may be associated with decreased risk for barotrauma and associated chronic lung disease, less risk for pneumothorax, and decreased days of ventilation.[45-47] The goal with either mode is a returned tidal volume between 4 and 7 cc/kg. After ventilation is begun with empiric settings, subsequent adjustments are based on physical examination, chest x-rays, blood gases, and response to treatment.

High-frequency ventilation (HFV) delivers fast rates and small tidal volumes, via high-frequency oscillation ventilation (HFOV), high-frequency jet ventilation (HFJV), and high-frequency flow interruption (HFFI). The use of HFOV and HFJV in transport has historically been limited because of size, weight, battery life, and electromagnetic interference with aircraft avionics. Small, lightweight, pneumatically driven HFV devices are available for the transport environment.

> **• BOX 29.1 Mnemonic for Deterioration in Ventilation**
>
> - **D:** Dislodged endotracheal tube.
> - **O:** Obstructed endotracheal tube.
> - **P:** Pneumothorax in intubated or nonintubated patients.
> - **E:** Equipment, including the ventilator and gas sources.

There are differences in the mechanism of how gas exchange occurs with each device, and there are also similarities. For all devices, oxygenation is achieved by titrating FiO_2 and adjusting mean airway pressure. HFOV has active exhalation, whereas HFJVs and HFFIs have passive exhalation. Amplitude, which creates chest movement, is adjusted similarly on the HFO and HFFI, whereas HFJV requires conventional breaths to help recruit the lung.

With HFV, mean airway pressure is used to recruit the lung and improve oxygenation. Small changes in tidal volume (amplitude) have a big effect on carbon dioxide removal because alveolar ventilation during HFV is equal to tidal volume squared times frequency. Frequency is set to achieve optimal gas exchange based on the pathophysiology of the lung. Studies suggest that HFV with inhaled nitric oxide (iNO) is more successful in treating patients with severe lung disease and meconium aspiration syndrome than conventional mechanical ventilation, and suggest a benefit to using HFV for infants with CDH.[48-50]

Any infant treated with positive pressure is at increased risk for complications. Abdominal distention can also interfere with adequate ventilation, so patients with invasive or noninvasive ventilation should have a gastric tube in place venting air. Any sudden deterioration in an infant receiving PPV should prompt immediate evaluation, including patients receiving noninvasive PPV. The DOPE mnemonic is a reminder of potential causes (Box 29-1).[51]

Blood Pressure and Perfusion

Assessment of circulatory status should begin with an evaluation of the maternal history along with any delivery room complications. A history suggestive of hypovolemia as a basis for poor perfusion may include compression of the cord or a history of blood loss during the pregnancy, labor, or delivery. A history of maternal fever or infection may result in an infant with distributive or septic shock. Infants with a history of asphyxia may have myocardial dysfunction.

The physical assessment should include the evaluation of serial blood pressures (BPs) and pulses in upper and lower extremities, central capillary refill time (in the context of body temperature), and preductal and postductal oxygen saturations. For a normal BP, many clinicians use the criterion that the mean arterial BP in millimeters should be maintained at or greater than the baby's gestational age in weeks. Interestingly, this has not been empirically evaluated.[52,53] It is also important to pay attention to the pulse pressure, determined by subtracting the diastolic pressure from the systolic pressure. Normal pulse pressure for a term infant is 25 to 30 and for a preterm infant it is 15 to 25. A narrow pulse pressure can suggest heart failure, peripheral vasoconstriction, compression on the heart, or severe aortic valve stenosis. A wide pulse pressure can be suggestive of a patent ductus arteriosis (PDA), other cardiac abnormalities, and/or sepsis from warm shock.[27]

Shock is a major cause of neonatal morbidity and mortality, and sepsis is the most common source of shock in neonates.[54] Shock is characterized by inadequate tissue and organ perfusion that results in cellular dysfunction and, if not corrected, cellular damage can cause end organ failure and potential death. Adequate tissue perfusion is dependent on cardiac output, vascular integrity, and the ability of the blood to deliver oxygen and metabolic substrates and remove wastes.[55] It is important to differentiate simple hypotension from hypotension associated with uncompensated shock. Hypotension and poor perfusion in the absence of other shock symptoms are common problems in the neonate, especially in infants less than 1500 g.[27]

Shock can be classified in three categories: hypovolemic, cardiogenic, and distributive. These etiologies are not necessarily exclusive. In compensated shock, perfusion to vital organs (i.e., brain, heart, liver, kidneys) is maintained with absent or minimal changes noted in vital signs caused by compensatory mechanisms that maintain BP and blood flow. The transport team may observe an increase in capillary refill time; decreased pulse quality; tachycardia; pallor and/or cool peripheral skin; or neurologic changes such as hypotonia, lethargy, and irritability.[56] If the shock is not reversed, the neonate will be unable to maintain compensatory mechanisms, resulting in hypotension. Treatment of shock should begin before the development of hypotension and further cellular dysfunction.[52,56]

Treatment is aimed at the restoring adequate perfusion. An initial bolus of 10 mL/kg of normal saline solution infused over 15 to 30 minutes is a reasonable initial step in babies without evidence of pulmonary edema. If there is acute blood loss, packed red blood cells, including uncrossmatched type O negative cells, can be given. Each volume bolus should be followed by an assessment of pulmonary status before continuing to additional volume restoration. If cardiogenic shock is suspected initially or on subsequent examination, an inotropic agent is indicated. Patients with refractory hypotension may benefit from the addition of vasopressors such as dopamine, epinephrine, or norepinephrine. The administration of hydrocortisone can increase BP and reduce catecholamine requirement without serious adverse reactions.[53,57] The management of infection and septic shock is discussed in greater detail elsewhere in this chapter.

Pathologic Conditions of the Neonate

Respiratory Disorders
Surfactant Deficiency

The most common cause of respiratory distress in the preterm infant is RDS, formerly known as hyaline membrane disease (HMD). RDS is primarily caused by a deficiency of surfactant, but can also occur in the presence of extreme stress such as severe hypoxia.

The primary function of lung surfactant is to lower surface tension at the air–water interface of the alveoli, preventing atelectasis and improving compliance. Surfactant decreases surface tension in the alveolus during expiration, which allows the alveolus to maintain a functional residual capacity. The absence of surfactant results in poor lung compliance and atelectasis. Infants with surfactant deficiency have progressive respiratory distress symptoms such as increased work of breathing, accessory muscle use, retractions, nasal flaring and grunting, and increased oxygen support as a result of poor lung compliance. Characteristic radiographic findings include reticular granular pattern in the lungs and hypoexpansion. Infants may require minimal respiratory support to maximal mechanical ventilation. As discussed earlier, early use of nCPAP is recommended for babies with RDS.

Exogenous surfactant was approved for use by the Food and Drug Administration in 1990. Ten years of extensive clinical studies showed that exogenous surfactant treatment substantially reduces mortality, incidence of air leak, pulmonary interstitial emphysema, and other complications such as bronchopulmonary dysplasia.[58,59] Both natural surfactant extracts and synthetic preparations are available. Administration of exogenous surfactant may result in rapid improvement in lung volumes and compliance with subsequent overventilation and air leaks. The team should monitor the baby and the measured ventilator values carefully in the half hour after surfactant delivery. There is not a clear, proven best method to deliver surfactant.[60] Repeated doses at specific intervals may be indicated.[60]

Pneumonia

Pneumonia is typically of bacterial origin and can have early or late onset. Early-onset pneumonia is generally acquired from the mother and is seen within the first 3 days of life. It is often associated with rupture of membranes for more than 12 hours before delivery. However, a respiratory infection can occur in the fetus even in the presence of intact membranes. Symptoms of amnionitis and fetal infection include maternal fever or elevated white count, purulent or foul-smelling amniotic fluid, fetal tachycardia, loss of beat-to-beat variability, and premature labor. Late-onset pneumonia is associated with mechanical ventilation and prolonged hospitalization. See also the discussion of sepsis and septic shock elsewhere in this chapter.

Aspiration Pneumonia

Although aspiration of meconium is the most severe form of aspiration pneumonia, the neonate may also aspirate amniotic fluid or blood at the time of delivery. Typically, meconium aspiration occurs in term or postterm infants when meconium is passed and aspirated causing pulmonary disease, which leads to hypoxemia and acidosis. It is a leading cause of morbidity and mortality in term infants.[61] The presence of meconium in the amniotic fluid should alert the medical team to the possibility of acute or chronic in utero asphyxia, as well as the risk for meconium aspiration pneumonia.

Common symptoms of neonates with meconium or other substance aspiration include respiratory distress soon after birth, the appearance of a barrel chest caused by over-inflation, and tachypnea. Radiographic findings may reveal patchy bilateral densities. The presence of meconium in the bronchial tree causes obstruction to airflow and pneumonitis. Complications of meconium aspiration syndrome include pulmonary air leaks and persistent pulmonary hypertension (PPHN).

The transport goals for managing the neonate with aspiration pneumonia are maintaining oxygenation and ventilation and, if mechanically ventilated, minimizing barotrauma. To achieve optimal gas exchange, deep sedation and the use of neuromuscular blockade may be necessary. Agitation can contribute to an increased pulmonary vascular resistance (PVR), right-to-left shunting, and hypoxemia. Careful attention must be paid to maintaining adequate perfusion and BP, and to avoid acidosis. Antibiotic therapy is frequently started in these infants until sepsis has been ruled out as the case of in utero meconium release.

Pulmonary Air Leaks

Air leaks occur most commonly in neonates with underlying lung disease and are frequently seen with the use of positive airway pressure treatments.[62,63] The most common air leaks are pneumothorax and pneumomediastinum. Uncommonly, pneumoperitoneum and pneumopericardium could also occur. The infant with an air leak may appear nearly asymptomatic, with only muffled heart tones or absent/diminished breath sounds, or the infant's condition may deteriorate rapidly, necessitating immediate intervention. Assessment includes evaluation of breath sounds, shift in the location of point of maximum impulse (PMI), transillumination of the chest, and radiographic confirmation. To transilluminate the chest, place a cold light source on the chest. A normal chest will have a small and symmetric halo around the light source. A large and asymmetric light distribution suggests a pneumothorax. It can be very helpful to compare the light distribution bilaterally.

Neonates with a pneumothorax and minimal symptoms may only need a one-time needle thoracentesis and oxygen, or no treatment other than close monitoring. Infants with severe distress or with clinical indication of a tension pneumothorax need emergent needle decompression without delay for radiographic diagnosis (Figs. 29.4 and 29.5). For babies with an air leak of any type who are mechanically ventilated, minimizing the mean airway pressure will help to prevent the accumulation or reaccumulation of air. In the transport setting, transport medical personnel must consider the impacts of altitude changes on an air leak or air collection. Boyle's law describes that entrapped gas volume expands by about 3% for every 1000-foot increase in elevation.

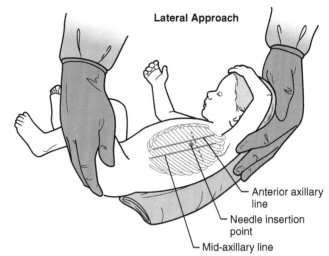

Lateral Approach

- Anterior axillary line
- Needle insertion point
- Mid-axillary line

• **Fig. 29.4** Needle insertion point.

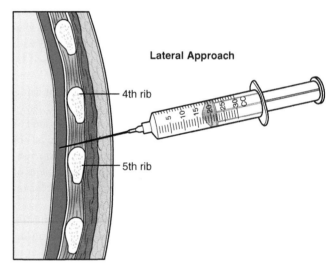

Lateral Approach

- 4th rib
- 5th rib

• **Fig. 29.5** Needle insertion.

Persistent Pulmonary Hypertension in the Newborn

PPHN of the newborn is a syndrome characterized by persistent elevated PVR that results in right-to-left (systemic-to-pulmonary) shunting at the ductus arteriosus or the foramen ovale and leads to hypoxemia in the presence of a structurally normal heart. This disease process is commonly seen in near-term infants with severe asphyxia, meconium aspiration syndrome, CDH, or sepsis. PPHN can also rise from idiopathic vascular abnormalities or arrested vascular development from CDH or other space-occupying chest lesions.

The clinical differentiation between cyanotic heart disease and PPHN can be difficult to make. A preductal and postductal oxygen saturation differential of over 10 mm Hg in the presence of profound hypoxemia suggests, but is not exclusive for, PPHN. The shunt can also occur centrally, across the foramen ovale. The hyperoxia test will also help distinguish PPHN from parenchymal disease. In this test, the patient is placed on 100% FiO_2 by hood or ETT for 10 minutes, and then a preducted arterial blood gas is drawn from the right radial artery. A significant increase in the PaO_2 to over 100 mm Hg during the test suggests parenchymal disease, whereas the absence of an increase favors PPHN or cardiac disease. Patients with PPHN may also demonstrate an improvement with hyperventilation to the high end of the normal respiratory rate range while on 100% oxygen, and those with heart disease will not.[64]

Treatment for PPHN is aimed at maintaining adequate oxygenation until the PVR begins to drop, which normally occurs in the first several days. Oxygen is a potent pulmonary vasodilator that is as effective as iNO when either is administered alone, so patients should receive 100% oxygen initially.[65-67] Maintaining a systemic BP higher than pulmonary pressure discourages right-to-left shunting. Typically, these infants are managed at the upper limits of normal through ensuring adequate circulating volume and cardiac output. Accepted parameters include a mean arterial pressure of 45 to 55 mm Hg or systolic BP of 50 to 70 mm Hg.

Infants unable to maintain adequate oxygenation with 100% oxygen and BP support may be considered for iNO therapy. Nitric oxide is a selective pulmonary vasodilator that targets the vascular smooth muscle cells surrounding the resistance arteries and creates an additive decrease in pulmonary vascular pressures beyond that of oxygen alone.[67] The iNO reduces the need for extracorporeal membrane oxygenation (ECMO) in term and late preterm infants with severe PPHN, but does not reduce non-ECMO mortality, length of stay, or adverse neurodevelopmental development. Up to 40% of babies with PPHN will not respond to, or sustain a response to, iNO.[68]

Once it diffuses into the bloodstream, nitric oxide binds to hemoglobin and is inactivated. This allows for pulmonary bed relaxation with minimal systemic side effects. The ultrashort half-life, under a second, does mean that interruptions of delivery to an NO-dependent patient must be avoided. A usual starting dose of iNO is 20 to 40 parts per million. If there is not a response within about 20 minutes of initiation, improvement is not usually seen with higher doses.[68-70] There is a trend toward increased off-label use of iNO in preterm infants (less than 34 weeks) that is not supported by evidence.[71]

Patients transported on iNO may benefit from deep sedation with neuromuscular blockade paralytics to minimize oxygen consumption and increases in PVR because of endogenous catecholamine release. Surfactant therapy decreases the need for ECMO in patients with PPHN that is secondary to mild parenchymal lung disease, but not for babies without concomitant parenchymal lung disease. Use varies among centers.[72,73]

Infants with severe PPHN who remain hypoxic even with maximum respiratory support and initiation of iNO may be considered for cardiopulmonary support from ECMO. ECMO is also used to treat neonates with RDS, PPHN, meconium aspiration syndrome, sepsis, and CDH. Indicators of severity of illness are standardized and require the use of calculations of the oxygen index (OI), as shown in the following oxygenation index formula[74]:

Oxygenation Index =
$$(FiO_2 * \text{Mean Airway Pressure} * 100) / PaO_2$$

Extracorporeal Life Support Organization severity indications include:
- OI greater than 40 for greater than 4 hours
- OI greater than 20 with lack of improvement despite prolonged (over 24 hours) maximal medical therapy or persistent episodes of decompensation
- Severe hypoxic respiratory failure with acute decompensation (PaO_2 greater than 40) unresponsive to intervention
- Progressive respiratory failure and/or pulmonary hypertension with evidence of right ventricular dysfunction or continued high inotropic requirement.[75]

When the severity of illness criteria has been met, specific criteria are also used for patient selection. Variability exists among ECMO centers on this specific selection criteria; however, examples include the following:
- Birth weight greater than 2000 g
- Gestational age over 34 weeks
- No uncontrolled bleeding
- No major intracranial hemorrhage
- Mechanical ventilation longer than 10 to 14 days
- No uncorrectable CHD
- No lethal congenital anomalies
- No irreversible brain damage[74-76]

The goal of ECMO is to support the lungs and heart until there is a reversal of the pulmonary and cardiac dysfunction. ECMO cannulation can be venous-venous (VV) or venous-arterial (VA). With VV ECMO, blood is removed from and then returned to the venous circulation. VV ECMO provides only pulmonary support by improving oxygenation and carbon dioxide removal. With VA ECMO, blood is removed from the venous circulation and returned to the arterial circulation. VA ECMO provides support for both the heart and lungs by decreasing cardiac work and oxygen consumption, improving cardiac output, and providing oxygenation and carbon dioxide removal.

Risks associated with ECMO include bleeding, blood clot formation, infection, and transfusion problems along with mechanical failure of the pump. The most common clinical complication is bleeding caused by the anticoagulation therapy required for the implementation of ECMO.[76] Potential hemorrhage sites include but are not limited to insertion sites of cannulas; chest tubes; peripheral IV lines; and intracranial, intrathoracic and abdominal areas.[76] Intracranial hemorrhages are the most serious complication associated with poor neurologic prognosis.[75,77]

Congenital Diaphragmatic Hernia

CDH occurs within the first few weeks of gestation. The cause has not been well defined; however, it is believed that CDH occurs because of failure of the pleuroperitoneal folds to close normally. Abdominal contents migrate into the thoracic cavity, compressing the developing lungs and blood vessels causing pulmonary hypoplasia and pulmonary hypertension. Generally CDH is an isolated event, although it can be associated with additional abnormalities. Left-sided defects account for 80% to 85% of all CDH and occur more often in males. Right-sided defects are associated with higher morbidity and mortality.[78]

Early detection of this defect is essential to quickly initiate appropriate therapy and surgical intervention, because bowel distention further compromises respiratory function beyond the structural defect. For babies with a prenatal diagnosis of CDH, a large-bore (10-Fr) orogastric tube should be inserted right away with the initiation of low intermittent suction. It is important to manage the airway early because these infants are at high risk for hypoxemia and acidosis, which will increase the risk of pulmonary hypertension. Avoid PPV with a facemask. When ventilation is necessary, immediate endotracheal intubation should be performed. Ventilatory management is aimed at maximizing ventilation while minimizing barotrauma, if possible, with lower inspiratory pressures and, as needed, higher respiratory rates. Preserving spontaneous respiration in these patients, if possible in the transport setting, can be beneficial.

Up to one-third of CDHs are diagnosed in the postnatal period, even in countries with robust ultrasound programs.[79] The typical presentation with postpartum diagnosis of CDH includes the early onset of respiratory distress, unequal or absent breath sounds, a shift in the PMI, and potentially scaphoid abdomen. Although scaphoid abdomen is listed as a classic sign, it is frequently not evident in the delivery room. Bowel sounds may be auscultated in the chest, and abdominal structures will be visible in the chest on a radiograph. The placement of a gastric tube before imaging will help illuminate gastrointestinal (GI) structures.

CDH used to be considered a surgical emergency. Recent studies have supported delayed surgery to permit physiologic stabilization. PPHN and shock frequently complicate the management of these infants. For babies with CDH and PPHN, evidenced by a wide prepostductal saturation difference, preserving ductal patency, supporting the right ventricle, and pulmonary vasodilation can be helpful. Published protocols recommend the use of iNO to treat pulmonary hypertension in newborns with CDH and may provide short-term oxygenation improvement before ECMO cannulation. The safety and efficacy of prolonged INO therapy in these patients has not been well established.[68,80-82]

Neonatal Heart Disease

Congenital heart disease (CHD) is the most common birth defect, and is estimated to occur once in every 110 births in the United States. Maternal factors that would suggest a high risk for cardiac disease are a family history of CHD, congenital infection, prepregnancy diabetes, and exposure to alcohol and drugs.[83,84]

The early signs of congestive heart failure are tachypnea and tachycardia, which makes distinguishing pulmonary inefficiencies from cardiac disease difficult. A detailed history of the onset of symptoms can be helpful. The immediate onset of respiratory symptoms at birth is more likely to indicate the presence of pulmonary disease, because few babies are born in active heart failure. Babies with cardiac disease are often "quietly tachypneic" initially, without other indications of respiratory distress. A chest x-ray should be obtained and evaluated in concert with clinical findings. An abnormal heart size with increased or decreased vascular markings may be suggestive of a heart defect.[84]

On assessment, tachypnea with low $PaCO_2$ is more indicative of nonpulmonary causes of respiratory distress such as cardiac anomalies or metabolic or neurologic disorders, whereas tachypnea accompanied by increased PCO_2 suggests pulmonary conditions. Cardiovascular findings suggestive of cardiac disease include pathologic murmurs (e.g., diastolic murmurs, systolic regurgitant murmurs, continuous murmurs associated with an abnormal examination), other abnormal heart sounds, hyperactive precordium, discrepant BPs or pulses between upper and lower extremities, and hepatomegaly. A baby with no murmur may still have significant heart disease.[84]

Preductal and postductal oxygen saturation monitoring can be used as a supportive diagnostic tool. Preductal oxygen saturation is measured on the right hand, and postductal oxygen saturation is measured on either foot. Preductal oxygen saturations more than 10 mm Hg higher than lower extremity saturations indicate right-to-left shunting from the pulmonary artery across the ductus arteriosus to the aorta. Preductal oxygen saturations less than lower extremity saturations may indicate transposition of great vessels. Remember that intracardiac shunting at the atrial or ventricular level will produce a decreased systemic oxygen saturation but not differential saturation between preductal and postductal sites.

Once the determination has been made that cyanosis in the newborn is caused by a fixed right-to-left shunt, the transport team should attempt to differentiate between shunting caused by PPHN and anatomic heart disease. Typically, infants with CHD present with a low $PaCO_2$ and a compensated or partially compensated metabolic acidosis. As described earlier, the infant who is hypoxic in room air but has a PaO_2 greater than 150 with 100% supplemental oxygen is more likely to have pulmonary disease than cyanotic heart disease or PPHN with a fixed right-to-left shunt. Patients with PPHN may also demonstrate an improvement with hyperventilation to the high end of the normal respiratory rate range while on 100% oxygen, whereas those with heart disease will not.[64]

If other causes of cyanosis have been ruled out and oxygen saturations do not increase greater than 75% even with

100% FiO_2, adequate ventilation, and fluids, a presumptive diagnosis of heart disease should be considered and the patient managed accordingly.

Neonatal cardiology and congenital heart defects represent a complex spectrum of conditions. Understanding normal neonatal anatomy, then considering the circulation effects of the defect and the effects of shunting across the duct (if present), can help conceptualize the patient's presentation and management (see Fig. 29.1). A simplified rubric, which may help make the defects and management more understandable, groups defects into four categories:

- Left outflow tract defects, ductal dependent for systemic blood flow
- Cyanotic defects, not ductal dependent
- Cyanotic defects, ductal dependent for pulmonary blood flow
- All other defects[84]

Approximately 20% of congenital heart defects are those with an anatomic obstruction to systemic blood flow, caused by coarctation or interruption of the aorta, critical aortic valve stenosis, or a hypoplastic left heart. In these patients, closure of the ductus arteriosus dramatically reduces systemic blood flow, causing pulmonary edema and shock. On examination, patients with aortic arch interruption or aortic coarctation classically have a BP gradient between higher upper extremity pressures and lower pressures in the legs. Patients with an obstruction to systemic blood flow benefit from preserved ductal patency with by continuous prostaglandin infusion.

Prostaglandin E1 is a continuous infusion medication that dilates the smooth muscle in the ductus arteriosus. It is indicated in patients who are known to have CHD that is ductal dependent for either systemic or pulmonary flow, and is also a reasonable intervention in patients who are persistently cyanotic and in whom the diagnosis of CHD cannot be clearly ruled in or out. This is often the case in the initial stabilization and transport settings.[85] Common side effects include apnea, fever, and hypotension. In consideration of the short half-life and critical nature of the drug, it is best to infuse prostaglandins through a separate IV site and to ensure that a second working IV is always available. Clinicians should consider the possibility of hypotension and apnea when starting prostaglandins on a neonatal patient, particularly at higher doses. There is some evidence that lower doses of the agent may be as effective as currently recommended doses, particularly in patients requiring ductal patency for pulmonary rather than systemic flow, and that lower doses reduce the incidence of side effects.[86,87]

In the patient with a left ventricular outflow tract that is ductal dependent for systemic flow, BP and cardiac output can be managed with volume resuscitation and inotropic medications. Hyperoxia and hypocarbia decrease PVR, increase left-to-right shunting across the ductus, and can worsen systemic perfusion and pulmonary edema. Accordingly, these patients are best managed with target preductal oxygen saturations between 75% and 85% and ventilation to a PCO_2 that is normal or in the higher end of the normal range, Continuous, simultaneous monitoring of the preductal and postductal oxygen saturations can demonstrate changes in the magnitude of the shunt across the ductus.

A number of heart lesions will create cyanosis as a result of the mixing of oxygenated and deoxygenated blood at the atrial or ventricular level but have preserved blood flow through the pulmonary artery and are generally not ductal dependent for pulmonary flow. These cases represent about 15% of CHD patients and include the tetralogy of Fallot, truncus arteriosus, total anomalous pulmonary venous return, and Ebstein's anomaly. Oxygen will improve pulmonary blood flow in these patients. The central mixing and need to balance systemic and pulmonary blood flow make the target preductal oxygen saturation 75% to 85% in these patients. Prostaglandin infusions are generally not required, unless there is severe disease represented by a persistent preductal saturation under 75% on supplemental oxygen.

A smaller number, about 9% of patients with CHD, have a defect creating cyanosis from reduced pulmonary blood flow. These patients, therefore, are dependent on an open ductus arteriosus for pulmonary blood flow. These defects include transposition of the great arteries, tricuspid atresia, pulmonary atresia, and the severe forms of tetralogy of Fallot and Ebstein's anomaly. In patients with an obstruction to pulmonary blood flow, higher inspired oxygen concentrations will reduce PVR and improve blood flow, so preserving ductal patency with a prostaglandin infusion is required to preserve pulmonary circulation. As with other patients who have cyanotic CHD, the target preductal oxygen saturation is between 75% and 85%. High levels of oxygen are also a stimulus for the PDA to close, which could worsen ductal-dependent lesions. Preductal and postductal saturations should be monitored continuously to evaluate both vital organ perfusion and a change in shunt magnitude.

Gastrointestinal Disorders

The transport team deals primarily with GI disorders related to obstruction, either functional or anatomic; infection; or externalized abdominal contents. Obstructions of the GI tract can occur anywhere from the esophagus through the anus. The management of all of these disorders primarily centers on decompression of the bowel, fluid management, antibiotic therapy, and respiratory support.

Esophageal Atresia/Tracheoesophageal Fistula

Esophageal atresia (EA) is a congenital defect that results in an interruption of the esophagus causing a loss of connection to the lower esophagus and stomach. The upper esophagus can end in a blind pouch or be associated with an abnormal connection to the trachea called a tracheoesophageal fistula (TEF). The incidence of EA/TEF is about 1 in every 4000 live births in the United States. Of these,

84% have an associated TEF. Interestingly, an "H-type" TEF without EA occurs approximately 4% of the time.[88,89]

These conditions may be difficult to diagnose. An obstetric history of polyhydramnios should increase the suspicion of upper GI obstruction. Patient findings suggesting EA include the inability to pass a gastric tube to the stomach, excessive oral secretions, and choking or coughing during feedings. Diagnosis can be confirmed with radiographs, particularly those showing a radiopaque catheter curled in the upper esophageal pouch or supplemented with contrast medium. Careful evaluation of the rest of the GI tract, the cardiovascular system, and the genitourinary system should be completed because of frequently associated anomalies.[88,89]

It is estimated that up to 60% of infants with EA/TEF have additional anomalies, including the VACTERL association. VACTERL is not specific to a genetic diagnosis but includes vertebral, anal, cardiac, TEF, renal, and limb defects.[88,90]

The majority of fistulas occur between the lower esophageal pouch and the trachea.[88] These fistulas allow air to pass from the respiratory tree into the stomach and gastric acid to reflux into the bronchial tree. These infants are at high risk for aspiration either from the oropharynx refluxing from the upper esophageal pouch or aspiration of gastric contents from the lower TEF. PPV should be avoided if possible, because it distends the stomach via the fistula and may interfere with ventilation or result in gastric perforation. A transport team caring for an infant with EA should place the patient semiprone position to minimize aspiration.[91] A gastric tube should be placed in the upper esophageal pouch and placed to suction. If a TEF is suspected, elevate the bed 30 degrees to reduce the risk of gastroesophageal reflux and aspiration.

Intestinal Obstructions

Common initial symptoms of intestinal obstruction include bilious vomiting, abdominal distention, feeding intolerance, large quantities of gastric contents at delivery, absence of an anal opening, and lack of stooling in the first 24 hours. An obstetric history of polyhydramnios suggests a GI obstruction. Although the presence of bilious vomiting in a newborn may be related to other causes, intestinal obstruction should be presumed until ruled out. Abdominal distention may be present depending on the level of the obstruction. The presence of tenderness, metabolic acidosis, or decreasing platelets may indicate a bowel necrosis or peritonitis and should be treated as an urgent problem.

Urgent cases include malrotations with volvulus and those with associated peritonitis, perforation, or suspected bowel necrosis.

Management includes decompression of the bowel with intermittent large-bore gastric suction, IV fluids, antibiotic therapy as indicated, and respiratory support. These infants may have large fluid requirements because of large interstitial fluid losses. Severe abdominal distention may compromise respiratory status. Evaluation of these neonates should include assessment of oxygen needs and ventilatory capacity with appropriate measures taken to correct deficits. In severe cases of peritonitis, sepsis and shock may also be present and should be treated appropriately.

Necrotizing Enterocolitis

Necrotizing enterocolitis (NEC) is an acquired disease characterized by intestinal damage ranging from mucosal injury to necrosis and perforation. It occurs in up to 10% of VLBW babies, with a mortality rate of up to 50%, but may also affect older, larger, and even term babies. For preterm infants, presentation is usually in the second or third week of life, with earlier onset as birth gestational age declines. For term infants, onset is usually in the first few days after birth, but NEC can present as late as 1 month. The genesis of NEC is poorly understood, with contributing factors believed to include hypoxia, feeding, sepsis, abnormal colonization of the bowel, GI ischemic-reperfusion injury, and the release of inflammatory mediators.[92]

Early recognition of risk factors and symptoms allows for early treatment. Systemic nonspecific signs include apnea, lethargy, poor feeding, and temperature instability. Abdominal symptoms include feeding intolerance with increased gastric aspirates, bile-stained gastric aspirates, increasing abdominal girth, and guaiac-positive stools. Progression of the disease results in increasing abdominal distention to the point of tautness, grossly bloody stools, abdominal wall erythema, and abdominal tenderness. Radiographic findings include dilated bowel loops, thickening of the bowel wall, and the classic sign of air in the bowel wall (pneumatosis intestinalis). Portal gas is a poor prognostic sign, and pneumatosis intestinalis is pathognomonic. The absence of radiographic findings does not rule out the diagnosis of NEC.[92]

The initial course of treatment includes cessation of enteral feedings and gastric decompression. Patients will require IV fluids and parenteral nutrition. They are usually started on broad-spectrum antibiotics such as ampicillin, gentamicin, and clindamycin or metronidazole. Surgery is always a consideration. It is mandatory for perforation or for necrotic intestine, both of which are suggested by pneumoperitoneum.[92]

Omphalocele/Gastroschisis

Although omphalocele and gastroschisis are two separate entities, their treatment during transport is essentially the same. An omphalocele occurs when the abdominal contents that protrude into the extra embryonic coelom at the base of the umbilical cord during embryonic development fail to return to the abdominal cavity in the 12th week of development. The defect is covered by an amniotic-peritoneal membrane in which the umbilical cord inserts. The membrane may be broken during delivery. The size of the defect may vary from a small hernia to inclusion of a large percentage of the abdominal contents. An omphalocele is often associated with other abnormalities and syndromes.[93] Gastroschisis, on the other hand, is a defect that occurs because of a disruption of the abdominal wall formation in the embryonic period. The defect is usually to the right of the umbilical cord and allows for evisceration of abdominal contents. Because the defect is normally very close to the umbilicus, it is frequently mistaken for an omphalocele. This defect, however, is not covered by a membrane. The defect occurs early in gestation, so the intestines may appear edematous with adhesions because they have been floating in the amniotic fluid for some time. Generally gastroschisis is categorized as simple, meaning it is not associated with other GI or chromosomal abnormalities.[94]

Both groups of infants are at risk for infection, large fluid losses, hypoglycemia, impaired bowel perfusion, and hypothermia. Treatment includes immediate wrapping of the defect with moist saline gauze and plastic wrap or, alternatively, placement of the neonate in a bowel bag to prevent fluid losses. The infant must have nothing by mouth and gastric suction applied to maintain bowel decompression. If the abdominal opening is extremely small, the patient may be at a high risk for bowel ischemia as a result of the constriction of blood flow. Caring for the child on his or her side may help reduce tension on the bowel and improve circulation. Careful monitoring and maintenance of temperature in normal range are essential in the management of these children with a skin defect. This increased need for thermogenesis also places them at risk for hypoglycemia and hypovolemia.

Neonatal Infections

Neonates are at risk for infections because of their immature immune system. Infections are acquired in utero, in the birth canal, or from external sources after birth. The most common neonatal infections are viral and bacterial pneumonia; sepsis; and infrequently, meningitis. Pneumonia has been addressed in the subsections on respiratory illnesses. Other neonatal infections include congenital cytomegalovirus, rubella syphilis, toxoplasmosis, neonatal hepatitis B, and herpes simplex virus.

Sepsis is categorized as either early-onset (EOS) or late-onset (LOS), differentiated by the appearance before or after 72 hours of life.[95,96] Infants with EOS often present during their hospitalization, whereas infants with LOS are often seen initially in outpatient settings such as emergency departments. Risk factors for EOS include maternal chorioamnionitis, rupture of membranes greater than 18 hours before delivery, premature labor, maternal illness, infection or fever, and maternal GBS colonization. LOS is thought to be caused by environmental organisms.

The infant with sepsis may have mild and subtle onset of symptoms or a fulminating course that results in rapid progression to shock. Common signs and symptoms include temperature instability, "does not look well," respiratory distress, tachycardia, apnea and bradycardia, lethargy, irritability, poor tone, and poor feeding. Poor perfusion and hypotension are considered late findings. An infant with any of these symptoms must be evaluated for potential sepsis. If the infant has meningitis, seizures must be added to the list of common presenting signs.

Evaluation of these infants includes a complete blood cell count with differential. A low absolute neutrophil count and an elevated ratio of immature-to-total neutrophils (I/T ratio), although not required for a diagnosis of sepsis, increases the level of suspicion for bacterial sepsis. The ANC is calculated with the equation (white blood cell count) × (segmented neutrophil percentage + band neutrophil percentage + metamyelocyte percentage). Normal ranges vary by postnatal age, and the Schmutz or Manroe chart describes normal values. The I/T ratio is a more rapidly calculated and interpreted guide. The ratio is calculated with the equation (percentage of band neutrophils + percent of metamyelocytes)/(percentage of segmented neutrophils + percentage of band neutrophils + percentage of metamyelocytes). An I/T ratio over 0.2 suggests infection, and an I/T ratio over 0.8 is associated with a higher risk of death from sepsis.[27]

Although the definitive diagnosis of septicemia requires positive blood culture results, infants with highly suspicious signs should be started on an appropriate empiric antibiotic regimen until culture results are available. Classic empiric antibiotic approaches include ampicillin, gentamycin, third-generation or fourth-generation cephalosporins, and antiviral agents. In the case of meningitis with seizures, examination of the cerebrospinal fluid (CSF) is indicated but should not delay antibiotic therapy and should probably also not delay transport. For these patients empiric ceftriaxone is usually added to the sepsis regimen.

Patients with severe sepsis or shock will require hemodynamic support with isotonic IV fluids and, as indicated, vasopressors and hydrocortisone.

Neurologic Disorders
Hypoxic-Ischemic Encephalopathy

Brain injuries that are caused by hypoxic-ischemia can cause neonatal encephalopathy, which carries risks for significant mortality and long-term morbidity. The mechanism of hypoxic injury can be maternal impaired oxygenation, insufficient placental perfusion, or intrapartum events that impair fetal oxygenation such as cord prolapse, uterine rupture, difficult extraction, or nuchal cord.

Targeted temperature management (TTM) with induced hypothermia is an effective therapy that improves neurologic outcomes in late preterm and term babies (≥36 weeks) with moderate to severe hypoxic-ischemic encephalopathy (HIE). The TTM involves lowering the infant's body temperature to slow biological processes, decreasing disease progression. A meta-analysis of six large published clinical trials showed a number needed to treat (NNT) six babies with moderate HIE to prevent one death or disability, and seven babies with severe HIE to prevent one death or disability.[97-99] In comparison, the NNT for the benefit of aspirin for patients with ST-elevation myocardial infarction is 42 patients.[100]

Current inclusion criteria require a highly specific age, an indicator of birth hypoxia, and an indicator of neurologic effect:

1. Chronologic
   * Gestational age of 36 weeks or more
   AND
   * 6 or fewer hours of life
2. Perinatal depression
   * Indicator of birth hypoxia: Apgar score of less than 5 at 10 minutes of age
   OR
   * pH less than 7.0, or base deficit greater than or equal to 16 mmol/L in an umbilical cord blood sample or any blood sample within the first hour of birth
   OR
   * Need for PPV at 10 minutes of life
3. Abnormal neurologic examination
   * Seizures
   OR
   * Abnormality in three of these categories
     o Spontaneous activity
     o Posture
     o Autonomic nervous system
     o Tone
     o Primitive reflexes
     o Level of consciousness
   OR
   * Moderate (Sarnat stage II) to severe (Sarnat stage III) encephalopathy[97,98]

The majority of large clinical trials have administered cooling by two methods: whole-body cooling and selective head cooling. There is limited research comparing the two methods, and no clarity demonstrating that either is safer or more effective.[101,102] Similarly, the optimal target temperature for cooling has not been determined. Most study protocols have maintained a temperature between 33.0°C and 35.0°C for 3 days.[98] It is clear that longer and deeper cooling do not improve outcomes.[103]

In the transport setting, both active and passive cooling can be used effectively. Active cooling in transport may increase the risk that babies will arrive with nontherapeutic hypothermia. Servo-controlled devices improve the effectiveness and safety of active cooling in transport.[104-107] Care must also be taken to prevent hyperthermia, which is associated with an increased risk of death and disability.[108] Monitor BP, HR, and capillary refill, and provide appropriate support of vital signs. As the metabolic rate decreases, so does the HR, so hypothermia does often cause a relative bradycardia that is well tolerated.

Neural Tube Defects

Neural tube defects (NTDs) are birth defects of the brain, spine, or spinal cord and are the most common congenital central nervous system (CNS) structural anomaly.[109] Failure of development of the neural tube early in gestation may result in a number of defects including anencephaly, encephalocele, meningocele, and myelomeningocele.

Open defects are more common and have exposed neural tissue with associated leakage of CSF. Myelomeningocele is the most common NTD. Patients with myelomeningoceles are at high risk for the subsequent development of a latex allergy, so all medical supplies used in caring for these patients should be latex free.[110] Assess the location, size and whether the defect is leaking CSF. An initial evaluation of spontaneous activity, muscle weakness or paralysis, and anal wink should be noted. The infant should be positioned off the defect during transport. Infection is a significant concern, so the defect should be covered by a sterile saline soaked dressing and then covered with plastic wrap to prevent heat loss. Consider antibiotic prophylaxis.

Closed defects are usually on the spine, and neural tissue is not exposed. It is not uncommon to be able to see the abnormality along the spine, which can present as a fluid-filled mass, a tuft of hair at the base of the spinal cord, an area of skin discoloration, or a lesion covered by skin without visible neural tissue. As noted with open lesions, an evaluation of spontaneous activity, muscle weakness, paralysis, and anal wink should be noted on assessment before transport.

Seizures

Seizures commonly occur in ill newborns and are often the first sign of a CNS disorder. There are many etiologies of neonatal seizures. The most frequently occurring are neonatal encephalopathy, intracranial hemorrhage, infection, metabolic disturbances, congenital abnormalities of the brain, and drug withdrawal.[111] Because of the immature nervous system of the newborn, infants rarely exhibit the generalized tonic-clinic seizures seen in adults and older children. Seizures in the newborn can be divided into four categories:

1. *Subtle:* These are frequently overlooked by caretakers. This type may consist of repetitive mouth or tongue movement, bicycling movements, eye deviation, repetitive blinking, staring, or apnea.
2. *Clonic (multifocal or focal):* These are typically characterized by slow, repetitive, rhythmic contractions of the limbs, face or trunk.
3. *Tonic (generalized or focal):* These may resemble posturing seen in older infants and children and may be accompanied by disturbed respiratory patterns. This type may also include tonic extension of limbs or tonic flexion of upper limbs and extension of lower limbs.
4. *Myoclonic:* These are characterized by multiple jerking motions of the upper (common) or lower (rare) extremities.

Seizure activity is frequently confused with jitteriness in the newborn. Jitteriness may be distinguished from seizures in the following ways:

* Sensitive to stimulus, whereas seizures are not.
* Characterized by tremors rather than the slow and fast phases of seizure activity.

- Can normally be stopped with flexing of the limb, as opposed to seizures, which do not respond to this maneuver.

In treatment of neonatal seizures, identification of the cause is important because it may prevent further injury. The obstetric and neonatal history may reveal risk factors for seizure disorders. Physical examination should be performed, along with laboratory studies including glucose; calcium; magnesium; sodium; blood gas; and in suspected infection, blood cultures. There is no consensus regarding an optimal treatment strategy, and there is limited helpful literature. Phenobarbital is the most commonly used initial antiepileptic agent in neonates, followed by either repeat doses of phenobarbital or second-line agents such as phenytoin, fosphenytoin, levetiracetam, or a benzodiazepine.[112,113] Serious side effects of these drugs may include respiratory or cardiovascular depression.

Developmental Care

It is important to incorporate developmental care interventions while transporting these small patients to decrease the risk of neurodevelopmental complications. Transport teams can consider the use of a gel-filled mattress to decrease the effects of vibration on infants, and nesting the infant with rolls or gel donuts serves to reduce stress by providing containment, positioning, and comfort.[25,114] Infants are exposed to excessive noise in the transport environment, which can create negative physiologic responses such as increased heart and respiratory rates and decreased oxygen saturation. Transport teams should consider interventions that decrease the noise levels. The use of earmuffs is associated with a reduction in noise level and adverse neonatal outcomes.[115,116]

Equipment

The transport of the neonate requires a skilled team and proper equipment. Medical equipment used in air medical operations should be electromagnetic interference-approved for flight.[117,118] If a team engages in multiple simultaneous transports, a full set of functioning equipment and appropriate caregiver skill mix is necessary for each neonate that is transported. The transport team should use safety and best industry practice for securing neonatal patients and also for securing themselves and their equipment.

Summary

Medical transport providers caring for neonates in any out-of-hospital environment must have training in the stabilization and care of the types of infants they may transport.[119] Attention to appropriate team composition and the availability of specialized equipment and medications is necessary to ensure safe transport of these patients. Competency in neonatal care, protocols, and procedures is essential to neonatal transport care.

References

1. Kugelman A, Colin AA. Late preterm infants: near term but still in a critical developmental time period. *Pediatrics*. 2013;132(4): 741-751.
2. Orr RA, et al. Pediatric specialized transport teams are associated with improved outcomes. *Pediatrics*. 2009;124(1):40-48.
3. *Tenth Edition Accreditation Standards of the Commission on Accreditation of Medical Transport Systems, in General Standards.* Sandy Spring, SC: CAMTS; 2015.
4. American Academy of Pediatrics. *Guidelines for air and ground transport of neonatal and pediatric patients.* 4th ed. Elk Grove Village, IL: American Academy of Pediatrics; 2015.
5. Weiner GM, Zaichkin JG. *Textbook of Neonatal Resuscitation.* Elk Grove Village, IL: American Academy of Pediatrics; 2016:xiii, 313.
6. Apgar V, Holaday DA, James LS, et al. Evaluation of the newborn infant; second report. *J Am Med Assoc.* 1958;168(15): 1985-1988.
7. Apgar V. A proposal for a new method of evaluation of the newborn infant. *Curr Res Anest Anal.* 1953;32(4):260-267.
8. Mullany LC. Neonatal hypothermia in low-resource settings. *Semin Perinatol.* 2010;34(6):426-433.
9. Wyckoff MH, et al. Part 13: Neonatal Resuscitation: 2015 American Heart Association guidelines update for cardiopulmonary resuscitation and emergency cardiovascular care. *Circulation.* 2015;132(18 suppl 2):S543-S560.
10. Al Takroni AM, et al. Selective tracheal suctioning to prevent meconium aspiration syndrome. *Int J Gynaecol Obstet.* 1998;63(3): 259-263.
11. Morley CJ, et al. Nasal CPAP or intubation at birth for very preterm infants. *N Engl J Med.* 2008;358(7):700-708.
12. SUPPORT Study Group of the Eunice Kennedy Shriver NICHD Neonatal Research Network, et al. Early CPAP versus surfactant in extremely preterm infants. *N Engl J Med.* 2010;362(21):1970-1979.
13. Dawes GS. *Foetal and Neonatal Physiology; A Comparative Study of the Changes at Birth.* Chicago, IL: Year Book Medical Publishers; 1968.
14. Peterson J, et al. Accuracy of the 7-8-9 Rule for endotracheal tube placement in the neonate. *J Perinatol.* 2006;26(6):333-336.
15. Garey DM, et al. Tidal volume threshold for colorimetric carbon dioxide detectors available for use in neonates. *Pediatrics.* 2008; 121(6):e1524-e1527.
16. Finn D, et al. Enhanced monitoring of the preterm infant during stabilization in the delivery room. *Front Pediatr.* 2016; 4:73.
17. Whitelaw CC, Slywka B, Goldsmith LJ. Comparison of a two-finger versus two-thumb method for chest compressions by healthcare providers in an infant mechanical model. *Resuscitation.* 2000; 43(3):213-216.
18. Wyllie J, et al. Part 11: Neonatal resuscitation. *Resuscitation.* 2011;81(1):e260-e287.
19. Iliodromiti S, et al. Apgar score and the risk of cause-specific infant mortality: a population-based cohort study. *Lancet.* 2014; 384(9956):1749-1755.
20. Freeman JM, Nelson KB. Intrapartum asphyxia and cerebral palsy. *Pediatrics.* 1988;82(2):240-249.
21. Watterberg KL, et al. The Apgar Score. *Pediatrics.* 2015;136 (4):819-822.
22. Executive summary: Neonatal encephalopathy and neurologic outcome, second edition. Report of the American College of Obstetricians and Gynecologists' Task Force on Neonatal Encephalopathy. *Obstet Gynecol.* 2014;123(4):896-901.

23. Mohamed MA, Aly H. Transport of premature infants is associated with increased risk for intraventricular haemorrhage. *Arch Dis Child Fetal Neonatal Ed.* 2010;95(6):F403-F407.

24. Schmid MB, et al. Prospective risk factor monitoring reduces intracranial hemorrhage rates in preterm infants. *Dtsch Arztebl Int.* 2013;110(29-30):489-496.

25. Malusky S, Donze A. Neutral head positioning in premature infants for intraventricular hemorrhage prevention: an evidence-based review. *Neonatal Netw.* 2011;30(6):381-396.

26. Rysavy MA, et al. Between-hospital variation in treatment and outcomes in extremely preterm infants. *N Engl J Med.* 2015;372 (19):1801-1811.

27. Karlsen K. *The S.T.A.B.L.E. Program Post-Resuscitation /Pre-Transport Stabilization Care of Sick Infants Guidelines for Neonatal Healthcare Providers.* 6th ed. Learner Manual. Stable: Park City, UT; 2013.

28. Committee on Fetus and Newborn, Adamkin DH. Postnatal glucose homeostasis in late-preterm and term infants. *Pediatrics.* 2011;127(3):575-579.

29. Brownell E, Howard CR, Lawrence RA, Dozier AM. Delayed onset lactogenesis II predicts the cessation of any or exclusive breastfeeding. *J Pediatr.* 2012;161(4):608-614.

30. Mathur NB, Krishnamurthy S, Mishra TK. Evaluation of WHO classification of hypothermia in sick extramural neonates as predictor of fatality. *J Trop Pediatr.* 2005;51(6):341-345.

31. Rutter N. Temperature control and its disorders. In: Rennie JM, ed. *Robersons Textbook of Neonatology.* London: Churchill Livingstone; 2005:267-279.

32. Knobel RB. Thermal stability of the premature infant in neonatal intensive care. *Newborn Infant Nurs Rev.* 2014;14(2):72-76.

33. Gardner SL, et al. *Merenstein & Gardner's Handbook of Neonatal Intensive Care.* Philadelphia, PA: Elsevier Health Sciences; 2015.

34. Mariani G, et al. Pre-ductal and post-ductal O_2 saturation in healthy term neonates after birth. *J Pediatr.* 2007;150(4):418-421.

35. Manja V, Lakshminrusimha S, Cook DJ. Oxygen saturation target range for extremely preterm infants: a systematic review and meta-analysis. *JAMA Pediatr.* 2015;169(4):332-340.

36. Castillo A, et al. Pulse oxygen saturation levels and arterial oxygen tension values in newborns receiving oxygen therapy in the neonatal intensive care unit: is 85% to 93% an acceptable range? *Pediatrics.* 2008;121(5):882-889.

37. Wilkinson D, et al. High flow nasal cannula for respiratory support in preterm infants. *Cochrane Database Syst Rev.* 2016;2: CD006405.

38. Papile L-A, et al. Respiratory support in preterm infants at birth. *Pediatrics.* 2014;133(1):171-174.

39. Dunn MS, et al. Randomized trial comparing 3 approaches to the initial respiratory management of preterm neonates. *Pediatrics.* 2011;128(5):e1069-e1076.

40. Shoemaker MT, et al. High flow nasal cannula versus nasal CPAP for neonatal respiratory disease: a retrospective study. *J Perinatol.* 2007;27(2):85-91.

41. Sakonidou S, Dhaliwal J. The management of neonatal respiratory distress syndrome in preterm infants (European Consensus Guidelines–2013 update). *Arch Dis Child Educ Pract Ed.* 2015; 100(5):257-259.

42. Lavizzari A, et al. Heated, humidified high-flow nasal cannula vs nasal continuous positive airway pressure for respiratory distress syndrome of prematurity: a randomized clinical noninferiority trial. *JAMA Pediatr.* 2016:1243 [Epub ahead of print].

43. Lemyre B, et al. Nasal intermittent positive pressure ventilation (NIPPV) versus nasal continuous positive airway pressure (NCPAP)

for preterm neonates after extubation. *Cochrane Database Syst Rev.* 2014;(9):CD003212.

44. Cummings JJ, et al. Noninvasive respiratory support. *Pediatrics.* 2016;137(1):e20153758.

45. Klingenberg C, et al. A practical guide to neonatal volume guarantee ventilation. *J Perinatol.* 2011;31(9):575-585.

46. Al Ethawi Y. Volume-targeted versus pressure-limited ventilation for preterm infants: a systematic review and meta-analysis. *J Clin Neonatol.* 2012;1(1):18-20.

47. Wheeler K, et al. Volume-targeted versus pressure-limited ventilation in the neonate. *Cochrane Database Syst Rev.* 2010;(11): CD003666.

48. Kinsella JP, et al. Randomized, multicenter trial of inhaled nitric oxide and high-frequency oscillatory ventilation in severe, persistent pulmonary hypertension of the newborn. *J Pediatr.* 1997; 131(1 Pt 1):55-62.

49. Datin-Dorriere V, et al. Experience in the management of eighty-two newborns with congenital diaphragmatic hernia treated with high-frequency oscillatory ventilation and delayed surgery without the use of extracorporeal membrane oxygenation. *J Intensive Care Med.* 2008;23(2):128-135.

50. Honey G, et al. Use of the Duotron transporter high frequency ventilator during neonatal transport. *Neonatal Netw.* 2007;26 (3):167-174.

51. Kleinman ME, et al. Part 14: pediatric advanced life support: 2010 American Heart Association Guidelines for Cardiopulmonary Resuscitation and Emergency Cardiovascular Care. *Circulation.* 2010;122(18 suppl 3):S876-S908.

52. Dempsey EM, Barrington KJ. Evaluation and treatment of hypotension in the preterm infant. *Clin Perinatol.* 2009;36(1):75-85.

53. Ng PC, et al. A double-blind, randomized, controlled study of a "stress dose" of hydrocortisone for rescue treatment of refractory hypotension in preterm infants. *Pediatrics.* 2006;117(2): 367-375.

54. Caresta E, et al. What's new in the treatment of neonatal shock. *J Matern Fetal Neonatal Med.* 2011;(24 suppl 1):17-19.

55. Schmaltz C. Hypotension and shock in the preterm neonate. *Adv Neonatal Care.* 2009;9(4):156-162.

56. Seri I, Markovitz B. Cardiovascular compromise in the newborn infant. In: Gleason CA, Devaskar SU, eds. *Avery's Diseases of the Newborn.* Philadelphia: Elsevier Saunders; 2012:714-731.

57. Ruoss JL, McPherson C, DiNardo J. Inotrope and vasopressor support in neonates. *NeoReviews.* 2015;16(6):e351-e361.

58. Bahadue FL, Soll R. Early versus delayed selective surfactant treatment for neonatal respiratory distress syndrome. *Cochrane Database Syst Rev.* 2012;11:CD001456.

59. Engle WA, American Academy of Pediatrics Committee on Fetus and Newborn. Surfactant-replacement therapy for respiratory distress in the preterm and term neonate. *Pediatrics.* 2008;121 (2):419-432.

60. Committee on Fetus and Newborn, American Academy of Pediatrics. Respiratory support in preterm infants at birth. *Pediatrics.* 2014;133(1):171-174.

61. Lee J, et al. Meconium aspiration syndrome: a role for fetal systemic inflammation. *Am J Obstet Gynecol.* 2016;214(3):366. e1-e9.

62. Jeng M-J, et al. Neonatal air leak syndrome and the role of high-frequency ventilation in its prevention. *J Chin Med Assoc.* 2012; 75(11):551-559.

63. Ho JJ, Subramaniam P, Davis PG. Continuous distending pressure for respiratory distress in preterm infants. *Cochrane Database Syst Rev.* 2015;(7):CD002271.

64. Warren JB, Anderson JM. Newborn respiratory disorders. *Pediatr Rev.* 2010;31(12):487-496.

65. Steinhorn RH. Neonatal pulmonary hypertension. *Pediatr Crit Care Med.* 2010;11(suppl 2):S79-S84.

66. Stark AR, Eichenwald ED. *Persistent pulmonary hypertension of the newborn.* Waltham, MA: UpToDate; 2016.

67. Atz AM, et al. Combined effects of nitric oxide and oxygen during acute pulmonary vasodilator testing. *J Am Coll Cardiol.* 1999;33(3):813-819.

68. Finer NN, Barrington KJ. Nitric oxide for respiratory failure in infants born at or near term. *Cochrane Database Syst Rev.* 2006;(4):CD000399.

69. Ichinose F, Roberts Jr JD, Zapol WM. Inhaled nitric oxide: a selective pulmonary vasodilator: current uses and therapeutic potential. *Circulation.* 2004;109(25):3106-3111.

70. Peliowski A, Canadian Paediatric Society, Fetus and Newborn Committee. Inhaled nitric oxide use in newborns. *Paediatr Child Health.* 2012;17(2):95-100.

71. Kumar P, et al. Use of inhaled nitric oxide in preterm infants. *Pediatrics.* 2014;133(1):164-170.

72. Nair J, Lakshminrusimha S. Update on PPHN: mechanisms and treatment. *Semin Perinatol.* 2014;38(2):78-91.

73. Lotze A, Mitchell BR, Bulas DI, Zola EM, et al. Multicenter study of surfactant (beractant) use in the treatment of term infants with severe respiratory failure. Survanta in Term Infants Study Group. *The J Pediatr.* 1998;132(1):40-47.

74. Chapman RL, et al. Patient selection for neonatal extracorporeal membrane oxygenation: beyond severity of illness. *J Perinatol.* 2009;29(9):606-611.

75. Extracorporeal Life Support Organization. *Guidelines for Neonatal Respiratory Failure: Supplement to the ELSO General Guidelines. Extracorporeal Life Support Organization.* Ann Arbor, MI: Extracorporeal Life Support Organization; 2013.

76. Carriedo H, Deming D. Therapeutic techniques: neonatal ECMO. *NeoReviews.* 2003;4(8):e212-e214.

77. Stocker CF, Horton SB. Anticoagulation strategies and difficulties in neonatal and paediatric extracorporeal membrane oxygenation (ECMO). *Perfusion.* 2016;31(2):95-102.

78. DeKoninck P, et al. Right-sided congenital diaphragmatic hernia in a decade of fetal surgery. *BJOG.* 2015;122(7):940-946.

79. Done E, et al. Prenatal diagnosis, prediction of outcome and in utero therapy of isolated congenital diaphragmatic hernia. *Prenat Diagn.* 2008;28(7):581-591.

80. Campbell BT, et al. Inhaled nitric oxide use in neonates with congenital diaphragmatic hernia. *Pediatrics.* 2014;134(2):e420-e426.

81. Puligandla PS, et al. Management of congenital diaphragmatic hernia: A systematic review from the APSA outcomes and evidence based practice committee. *J Pediatr Surg.* 2015;50(11):1958-1970.

82. Mohseni-Bod H, Bohn D. Pulmonary hypertension in congenital diaphragmatic hernia. *Semin Pediatr Surg.* 2007;16(2):126-133.

83. Mai CT, Riehle-Colarusso T, O'Halloran A, et al. Selected birth defects data from population-based birth defects surveillance programs in the United States, 2005–2009: featuring critical congenital heart defects targeted for pulse oximetry screening. *Birth Defects Res A Clin Mol Teratol.* 2012;94(12):970-983.

84. Karlsen KA, Tani LY. *S.T.A.B.L.E cardiac module: recognition and stabilization of neonates with severe CHD.* Salt Lake City, UT: S.T.A.B.L.E, Inc; 2003.

85. Donofrio MT, et al. Diagnosis and treatment of fetal cardiac disease: a scientific statement from the American Heart Association. *Circulation.* 2014;129(21):2183-2242.

86. Huang F-K, et al. Reappraisal of the prostaglandin E1 dose for early newborns with patent ductus arteriosus-dependent pulmonary circulation. *Pediatr Neonatol.* 2012;54(2):102-106.

87. Yucel IK, et al. Efficacy of very low-dose prostaglandin E1 in duct-dependent congenital heart disease. *Cardiol Young.* 2015;25(1):56-62.

88. Scott DA, et al. Esophageal atresia/tracheoesophageal fistula overview. In: Pagon RA, eds.: GeneReviews. Seattle, WA: University of Washington, Seattle; 2014.

89. Achildi O, Grewal H. Congenital anomalies of the esophagus. *Otolaryngol Clin North Am.* 2007;40(1):219-244.

90. Shaw-Smith C. Oesophageal atresia, tracheo-oesophageal fistula, and the VACTERL association: review of genetics and epidemiology. *J Med Genet.* 2006;43(7):545-554.

91. Pinheiro PF, Simoes e Silva AC, Pereira RM. Current knowledge on esophageal atresia. *World J Gastroenterol.* 2012;18(28):3662-3672.

92. Gephart SM, et al. Necrotizing enterocolitis risk: state of the science. *Adv Neonatal Care.* 2012;12(2):77-89.

93. Henrich K, et al. Gastroschisis and omphalocele: treatments and long-term outcomes. *Pediatr Surg Int.* 2008;24(2):167-173.

94. Arnold MA, et al. Risk stratification of 4344 patients with gastroschisis into simple and complex categories. *J Pediatr Surg.* 2007;42(9):1520-1525.

95. Sass L. Group B Streptococcal infections. *Pediatr Rev.* 2012;33(5):219-225.

96. Cohen-Wolkowiez M, et al. Early and late onset sepsis in late preterm infants. *Pediatr Infect Dis J.* 2009;28(12):1052-1056.

97. Committee on Fetus and Newborn, Papile LA, Baley JE, et al. Hypothermia and neonatal encephalopathy. *Pediatrics.* 2014;133(6):1146-1150.

98. Tagin MA, et al. Hypothermia for neonatal hypoxic ischemic encephalopathy: an updated systematic review and meta-analysis. *Arch Pediatr Adolesc Med.* 2012;166(6):558-566.

99. Jacobs SE, et al. Cooling for newborns with hypoxic ischaemic encephalopathy. *Cochrane Database Syst Rev.* 2013;(1):CD003311.

100. Randomised trial of intravenous streptokinase, oral aspirin, both, or neither among 17,187 cases of suspected acute myocardial infarction: ISIS-2. ISIS-2 (Second International Study of Infarct Survival) Collaborative Group. *Lancet.* 1988;2(8607):349-360.

101. Allen KA. Moderate Hypothermia: Is selective head cooling or whole body cooling better? *Adv Neonatal Care.* 2014;14(2):113-118.

102. Atici A, et al. Comparison of selective head cooling therapy and whole body cooling therapy in newborns with hypoxic ischemic encephalopathy: short term results. *Turk Arch Pediatr.* 2015;50(1):27-36.

103. Shankaran S, et al. Effect of depth and duration of cooling on deaths in the NICU among neonates with hypoxic ischemic encephalopathy: A randomized clinical trial. *JAMA.* 2014;312(24):2629-2639.

104. Fairchild K, et al. Therapeutic hypothermia on neonatal transport: 4-year experience in a single NICU. *J Perinatol.* 2010;30(5):324-329.

105. Sharma A. Provision of therapeutic hypothermia in neonatal transport: a longitudinal study and review of literature. *Cureus.* 2015;7(5):e270.

106. Chaudhary R, et al. Active versus passive cooling during neonatal transport. *Pediatrics.* 2013;132(5):841-846.

107. Akula VP, et al. A randomized clinical trial of therapeutic hypothermia mode during transport for neonatal encephalopathy. *J Pediatr.* 2015;166(4):856-861.e1-e2.

108. Laptook A, et al. Elevated temperature after hypoxic-ischemic encephalopathy: risk factor for adverse outcomes. *Pediatrics*. 2008;122(3):491-499.

109. Parker SE, et al. Updated National Birth Prevalence estimates for selected birth defects in the United States, 2004-2006. *Birth Defects Res A Clin Mol Teratol*. 2010;88(12):1008-1016.

110. Rendeli C, et al. Latex sensitisation and allergy in children with myelomeningocele. *Childs Nerv Syst*. 2006;22(1):28-32.

111. Silverstein FS, Jensen FE. Neonatal seizures. *Ann Neurol*. 2007;62(2):112-120.

112. Slaughter LA, Patel AD, Slaughter JL. Pharmacological treatment of neonatal seizures: a systematic review. *J Child Neurol*. 2013;28(3):351-364.

113. Hellstrom-Westas L, Boylan G, Agren J. Systematic review of neonatal seizure management strategies provides guidance on anti-epileptic treatment. *Acta Paediatr*. 2015;104(2):123-129.

114. Prehn J, et al. Decreasing sound and vibration during ground transport of infants with very low birth weight. *J Perinatol*. 2015;35(2):110-114.

115. Zahr LK, de Traversay J. Premature infant responses to noise reduction by earmuffs: effects on behavioral and physiologic measures. *J Perinatol*. 1995;15(6):448-455.

116. Duran R, et al. The effects of noise reduction by earmuffs on the physiologic and behavioral responses in very low birth weight preterm infants. *Int J Pediatr Otorhinolaryngol*. 2012;76(10): 1490-1493.

117. Bruckart JE, Licina JR, Quattlebaum M. Laboratory and flight tests of medical equipment for use in U.S. Army Medevac helicopters. *Air Med J*. 1993;1(3):51-56.

118. Nish WA, et al. Effect of electromagnetic interference by neonatal transport equipment on aircraft operation. *Aviat Space Environ Med*. 1989;60(6):599-600.

119. Cross B, Wilson D. High-fidelity simulation for transport team training and competency evaluation. *Newborn Infant Nurs Rev*. 2009;9(4):200-206.

30

The Pediatric Patient

LESLIE S. LEWIS

COMPETENCIES

1. Identify the differences between the pediatric and adult patient.
2. Perform a primary and secondary assessment of the pediatric patient in preparation for transport.
3. Provide an overview of selected pediatric illnesses and injuries.
4. Identify the equipment necessary to perform a competent pediatric transport.

We have all heard it before and it remains true to this day that a child is not a smaller version of an adult when it comes to providing medical care. To be successful in caring for the pediatric patient, the transport provider must be able to assess a child from across the room before the child's anxiety kicks in and alters his or her presentation. The pediatric provider must become skilled in the anatomic, physiologic, and developmental differences in children compared with adults. The pediatric provider must know how to differentiate age and developmental stage assessment findings along with their anatomic and physiologic differences to ensure that the correct, safe, and effective pediatric-specific intervention or treatment is implemented.

A Developmental Approach to Pediatric Assessment

The transport provider's challenge in caring for ill or injured children is impacted by the child's stage of development and growth patterns. Understanding the pediatric stages of growth and development helps the provider assess and treat the current condition of the patient appropriately. Children with special health care needs (CSHCNs) may be developmentally delayed compared with their chronologic age and present more of a challenge to the transport provider. The pediatric patient can present a variety of challenges to the transport provider, such as level of verbal communication, responses to invasive procedures, or the capacity to be separated from a family member, which may result in becoming a risk factor when traumatic injuries are involved. To be effective and to establish a safe, secure, and confident environment for both the child and the parent, it is essential for all pediatric transport providers to communicate with children of all ages and developmental stages. Doing so may require the provider to communicate at the child's level, or talk to the child even when they are nonverbal, and put into practice developmental skills to obtain an accurate assessment and treatment plan for each patient.[1-3]

When caring for the ill or injured child, the transport provider is also caring for the parents and possibly extended family members. Table 30.1 contains examples of developmental stages and approach strategies for pediatric patients. Injuries in children tend to follow an age and developmental-specific pattern. See Table 30.2 for examples of age-specific development and injury patterns.[1-3]

Pediatric Resuscitation

Resuscitation of the pediatric patient requires that transport team members have the knowledge and skills to care for this population. A number of transport programs located throughout the United States use specialized pediatric transport teams to support an infant or child during transport. Programs that use nonspecialized teams to transport pediatric patients require members to acquire additional training and education to support pediatric patients. According to the Commission on Accreditation of Medical Transport Systems, a specialty care pediatric transport is one that has a specialized team with the ability to support an infant or child with a life-threatening illness or injury. Specialized pediatric critical care transport teams are experienced, trained, and equipped to deliver definitive care away from the tertiary care center. These specialized teams provide an age-appropriate assessment and stabilization of the critically ill pediatric patient and are able to care for the parents of the child. When a specialized pediatric transport team is available, they should be considered for transport of critically ill or complex pediatric patients. Recent publications have shown improved care and better outcomes for neonatal and pediatric patients when the transport was provided by a specialized team.[3-5]

TABLE 30.1 Developmental Stages and Approach Strategies for Pediatric Patients

Stage of Development	Major Fears	Characteristics of Thinking	Approach Strategies
• Infants	• Separation and strangers	—	• Provide consistent caretakers • Reduce parent anxiety because it is transmitted to the infant • Minimize separation from parents
• Toddlers	• Separation and loss of control	• Primitive • Unable to recognize views of others • Little concept of body integrity	• Keep explanations simple • Choose words carefully • Let toddler play with equipment (stethoscope) • Minimize separation from parents
• Preschoolers	• Bodily injury and mutilation • Loss of control • The unknown and the dark • Being left alone	• Highly literal interpretation of words • Unable to abstract • Primitive ideas about the body (e.g., fear that all blood will "leak out:" if a bandage is removed)	• Keep explanations simple and concise • Choose words carefully • Emphasize that a procedure helps the child be healthier • Be honest
• School-age children	• Loss of control • Bodily injury and mutilation • Failure to live up to expectations of others • Death	• Vague or false ideas about physical illness and body structure and function • Able to listen attentively without always comprehending • Reluctant to ask questions about something they think they are expected to know • Increased awareness of significant illness, possible hazards of treatments, lifelong consequences of injury, and the meaning of death	• Ask children to explain what they understand • Provide as many choices as possible to increase the child's sense of control • Reassure the child that he or she has done nothing wrong and that necessary procedures are not punishment • Anticipate and answer questions about long-term consequences (e.g., what the scar will look like, how long activities may be curtailed)
• Adolescents	• Loss of control • Altered body image • Separation from peer group	• Able to think abstractly • Tendency toward hyperresponsiveness to pain (reactions not always in proportion to event) • Little understanding of the structure and workings of the body	• When appropriate, allow adolescents to be a part of decision making about their case • Give information sensitively • Express how important their compliance and cooperation are to their treatment • Be honest about consequences • Use or teach coping mechanisms such as relaxation, deep breathing, and self-comforting

From Sanders MJ. *Mosby's Paramedic Textbook*. 2nd ed. St. Louis: Mosby; 2000.

TABLE 30.2 Age-Specific Development and Injury Patterns

Age	Development	At-Risk Injuries
Infant 0–4 months	Feeding, holding, bonding, and dependence on caregivers	Aspiration, sudden infant death syndrome, bathing injuries (burns, near-drowning), environmental exposures (heat and cold), abuse, neglect, homicide, sexual assault, MVCs without proper restraint
Infant 4–8 months	Introduction of solid foods, teething, rolling side to side, sitting up, crawling	Falls, electrocution from cords and outlets, foreign body aspiration, toxic ingestions, MVC without proper restraint, burns, near-drowning, abuse, neglect, homicide, sexual assault, lacerations, fractures, head and spine injuries

	TABLE 30.2 Age-Specific Development and Injury Patterns—cont'd	
Age	**Development**	**At-Risk Injuries**
Infant 8–12 months	Crawling, walking, increased motor coordination (opening doors, latches, etc.)	Falls, aspiration, foreign body ingestion, toxic ingestion, pedestrian versus vehicle injuries, near-drowning, electrocution, motor vehicle collision without proper restraint, burns, suffocation, abuse, neglect, homicide, lacerations, fractures, head and spine injuries
Child 15 months to 3 years	Walking well and running, increased climbing skills, increased use of riding toys, use of utensils and cup, advanced motor skills (latches, doorways, match/lighter use) Emotionally, have increased desire for autonomy but have stranger anxiety Beginning to speak simple sentences	Falls, strike by vehicle as pedestrian or bike rider, burns, suffocation, near-drowning, toxic ingestions, foreign body aspiration, electrocution, MVC without proper restraint, abuse, neglect, homicide, lacerations, fractures, head and spine injuries
Child 4–9 years	Bike riding; swimming skills; entry into school systems; use of tools, firearms, and weapons; Increased exposures to nonfamily members, involvement in team sports; Use of seatbelts; Emotionally continue to increase autonomy with heightened body awareness and sensitivity to invasive examinations/procedures Rapidly increasing verbal skills	Toxic ingestions, foreign body aspiration, electrocution, MVC without proper restraint, abuse, neglect, homicide, sexual assault, lacerations, fractures, head and spine injuries
Child 10–12 years	Rapid physical growth; learning complex social skills; beginning of alcohol, tobacco, and drug experimentation; increased sexual experimentation; and involvement in largely physical team sports Use of motorized vehicles; Emotionally, have heightened awareness in gender differences, intense need for privacy, sense of responsibility, and need to be involved in decision making May experience clinical depression	Falls, strikes by vehicle as pedestrian or vehicle rider, burns, near-drowning, toxic ingestions, drug or alcohol overdose, foreign body aspiration, electrocution, MVC without proper restraint, abuse, neglect, homicide, sexual assault, suicide, complications of pregnancy or contraception, lacerations, fractures, head and spine injuries
Child 12–16 years	Increased incidence of risk-taking behaviors; increased autonomy in decisions of daily living; begin driving car; begin part-time jobs; increased sexual behavior; increased drug, alcohol, and tobacco use Emotionally, have increased body image disturbances, increased need for independence/decision making May suffer from clinical depression.	MVC, falls, occupational injuries, strikes by vehicle as pedestrian or bike rider, burns, near-drowning, toxic ingestions, drug or alcohol overdose, foreign body aspiration, electrocution, abuse, neglect, homicide, suicide, sexual assault, complications of pregnancy or contraception, lacerations, fractures, head and spine injuries

MVC, Motor vehicle collision.
From Holleran RS, ed. *ASTNA Patient Transport: Principles and Practice.* 4th ed. St. Louis: Mosby Elsevier; 2010.

Pediatric Airway Management/Respiratory Distress

Approximately 200,000 neonates and children are transported to a higher level of care in the United States annually. Airway management is a critical component of resuscitation. Almost half of the neonatal or pediatric critical care transports require respiratory intervention before transporting.[4] Pediatric respiratory emergencies are the most common cause of transports, hospital admissions, and a substantial number of deaths in children. An estimated 20% of all deaths in children are contributed to an acute respiratory infection in children 5 years of age and younger.[6-8]

Acute respiratory failure or arrest is the main cause of morbidity and mortality in critically injured or ill children. Airway management is one of the first steps initiated in stabilizing a pediatric patient for transport. It is essential in neonates, infants, and young children for the transport provider to be able to anticipate, rapidly recognize, and initiate appropriate interventions and treatment to prevent respiratory failure, cardiopulmonary arrest, or death. Respiratory failure is a result of the inability to provide oxygen and remove carbon dioxide to meet the metabolic demand of the child. Respiratory distress is divided into three categories mild, moderate, or severe.[6-12]

A child presenting with mild respiratory distress usually has no color changes, absent or mild retractions are present, air entry is mildly decreased, and the level of consciousness (LOC) is normal or the child may be restless with stimulation. A child presenting in moderate respiratory distress usually has no changes in color, with moderate retractions present. Air entry is moderately decreased, and the patient starts to become anxious and is restless with stimulation. Severe respiratory distress is when the child presents pale, dusky, or cyanotic; retractions are severe with the use of accessory muscles; air entry is significantly decreased; and the child's LOC is decreasing or becoming lethargic. Severe respiratory distress will lead to impending failure or arrest without intervention and treatment in infants and children. The trained transport provider should be able to recognize the severity of dyspnea, increasing tachypnea, decreased or poor air entry, tachycardia, cyanosis, impending fatigue, and changes in LOC before the child goes into failure or arrest, and prepares for immediate intubation of the child. See Table 30.3 for the most common causes of respiratory failure in children. See Table 30.4 for anatomic or physiologic causes for increased risk of respiratory failure in infants and children compared with adults.[6-13]

The goal of airway management is to secure the airway and achieve adequate tissue oxygenation and ventilation. Airway management in the prehospital setting may be difficult to achieve because of various injury patterns or conditions such as

TABLE 30.4 **Anatomic or Physiologic Causes for Increased Risk of Respiratory Failure in Infants and Children Compared With Adults[7,14,15,18]**

Causes	Anatomic or Physiologic
• High metabolic rate • Rapid desaturation	• Increases oxygen consumption to more than double adults • Lower functional residual capacity
• Increased risk of apnea • Increased risk of bradycardia • Increased resistance to breathing • Increased upper airway resistance	• Prematurity resulting in immature control of breathing • Incomplete maturation of sympathetic nervous system • Obligate nose breathers (usually up to 6 months of age) • Large tongues relative to the size of oral cavity • Epiglottis is large, floppy (impacts visualization of airway structures during direct laryngoscopy) • Smaller airway size, narrower at subglottic level (cricoid ring) • Airway softer, more pliable increasing chance of compression, collapse, or obstruction (e.g., agitation, illness, or pressure applied) • Larynx, trachea, and bronchi more compliant
• Increased resistance to breathing • Increased lower airway resistance	• Smaller airway size • Airway softer, more pliable increasing chance of compression, collapse, or obstruction (e.g., agitation or illness) • Increased airway chest compliance • Decreased elastic recoil
• Smaller lung volumes • Reduced surface area for gas exchange	• Significantly smaller number of alveoli (incomplete development) • Limited collateral pathways of ventilation (given that obstructed airways prevent alveoli to be ventilated by these alternative means predisposes those <3 yr of age to atelectasis, hypoxia, and hypercapnia)
• Decrease efficiency of respiratory muscles	• Decreased efficiency of diaphragm (poorly prepared to sustain increased workload of breathing) • Highly compliant ribs (horizontal ribs) • Poorly developed intercostal muscles
• Decreased endurance of respiratory muscles • Proportionately larger head particularly the occiput in infants and children	• Increased respiratory rate • Increases anatomic airway obstruction in supine position without a roll under shoulders for neck flexion • Inadequate positioning obstructs visualization of glottic opening during direct laryngoscopy

TABLE 30.3 **Common Causes of Respiratory Distress or Failure in Children**

Upper airway obstruction	• Croup • Epiglottitis • Foreign body aspiration
Lower airway obstruction	• Bronchiolitis • Status asthmaticus • Bronchopulmonary dysplasia
Lung disease	• Pneumonia • Acute respiratory distress syndrome • Pulmonary edema • Near-drowning
Causes affecting ventilation	• Neuromuscular disorders or myopathies • Infant botulism • Guillain-Barré syndrome • Chest wall trauma or malformations • Severe congenital scoliosis • Pleural effusion or pneumothorax
CNS issues affecting ventilation	• Status epilepticus • CNS infection • Trauma • Apnea of prematurity
Inability to meet oxygen demands of the body	• Hypovolemia • Septic shock • Cardiac insufficiency • Metabolic disorders

CNS, Central nervous system.
Adapted from Hammer, J. Acute respiratory failure in children. *Pediatr Respir Rev.* 2013;14(3): 2-13.

facial trauma, pharyngeal injury, or limited access to the patient or his or her airway. Congenital airway anomalies may be present and affect airway management in children. One of the most common congenital upper airway anomalies is choanal atresia or stenosis. There is an increased association of additional congenital anomalies associated with choanal atresia: CHARGE association, Trisomy 18 and 21, Apert syndrome, Crouzon syndrome, and Treacher Collins syndrome are a few of the most common. If bilateral choanal atresia is present the child will be in respiratory distress at birth and require emergency treatment with the placement of an oral airway. Pierre Robin sequence is another congenital anomaly with possible airway obstruction requiring airway management. Pierre Robin sequence is a triad of symptoms of micrognathia, glossoptosis, and laryngomalacia or tracheomalacia. Prone positioning may be effective in less severe presentations and if necessary a nasal airway may suffice for transport.[6-13]

Congenital craniofacial anomalies such as Crouzon, Apert, Pfeiffer, Treacher Collins, craniofacial macrosomia, or Goldenhar syndromes are syndromes with upper airway obstruction concerns for the transport provider. There are a large number of craniofacial anomalies associated with laryngotracheal malformations such as laryngeal atresia, laryngeal hypoplasia, laryngomalacia, vocal cord paralysis, laryngeal stenosis, webbing, and clefts. In addition to tracheobronchial anomalies, such as tracheal stenosis, tracheomalacia, and bronchomalacia, are also associated with craniofacial anomalies and increase airway obstruction in these children.[6-13]

Acquired upper airway obstructions the transport provider might encounter may be infectious or noninfectious. These include severe tonsillitis with adenoid enlargement such as with infectious mononucleosis, retropharyngeal and peritonsillar abscess, epiglottitis, croup, bacterial tracheitis, foreign body aspiration (FBA), anaphylaxis and angioedema, thermal injury from burns, caustic ingestion, or damage from referral endotracheal intubation (ETI) or tracheostomy.[6-13] These topics will be discussed in more detail later in the chapter.

In addition, referral facilities may not be competent or may be fearful of pediatric intubation. Failed or prolonged intubation attempts may be associated with negative consequences in children. A number of airway devices are available for neonatal and pediatric patient use with ETI the preferred method of choice to protect the child's airway, provide adequate oxygenation and ventilation, and prevent aspiration. Pediatric ETI requires the provider to have a high level of personal skills, experience, and recurrent training to maintain these skills.[6-13]

Pediatric Airway Anatomy

The anatomy of the pediatric airway is different from adult airway anatomy. The differences between the pediatric and the adult airway that may affect advanced airway management include the following[3,14-18]:

- Infants and younger children have larger occiputs in relation to their body size affecting optimal position of neck flexion in the supine position and may cause airway obstruction or interfere with visualization of the glottis opening. Improve airway positioning with a towel under child's shoulders.
- Small children have larger tongues in relation to the size of their mouth. The tongue is a common cause of airway obstruction when the child is in the supine position or has an altered mental status.
- Children have large and more vascular tonsils and adenoids compared with adults. Airway procedures or manipulation may cause bleeding and lead to partial airway obstruction with altered LOC.
- The larynx is anterior or more cephalad in infants and children compared with adults. The larynx is located opposite the C3 to C4 vertebrae in infants and children and may be as high as C2 to C3 in some infants. The larynx will drop to C4 to C5, possibly even C6, by late adolescence and in adults. This is a normal growth pattern in children that affects ETI. Because of the higher and more anterior airway configuration in infants and children, difficulty increases for some providers.
- The epiglottis is large and floppy in children younger than 3 years of age. In other children, the epiglottis is long, narrow, and floppy. In all children the epiglottis is angled away from the trachea. Using a straight blade, such as the Miller blade, is often required and effective in lifting the epiglottis out of the visual field for direct laryngoscopy.
- An omega-shaped epiglottis may be present, and is seen in children with laryngomalacia. An omega-shaped epiglottis may lead to positional inspiratory stridor in some children.
- The trachea is shorter (only 5 cm) in neonates and grows to 12 cm in adults. The trachea is narrow in younger children compared with adults. The short trachea tends to increase right mainstem intubations and self-extubations.
- In children younger than 10 years, the narrowest portion of the trachea has been identified as the cricoid process or ring. Newer studies suggest the anesthetized child has the greatest narrowing at the vocal cords. The subglottic region remains functionally the narrowest portion in the spontaneously breathing child. Pediatric cuffed and uncuffed endotracheal tubes (ETTs) are available. Pediatric advanced life support (PALS) recommends using cuffed ETTs for patients suspected of having high airway pressures, such as asthma or acute respiratory distress syndrome.
- The pediatric trachea may experience flexibility or collapse during episodes of agitation or partial airway obstruction as seen in children with croup. These children may require positive pressure ventilation (PPV) with bag-valve-mask ventilation (BVM) to stent open a partially occluded upper airway and may be considered an initial rescue for these children.
- The narrow tracheal lumen, the space between the tracheal rings, and the small size of the cricothyroid

membrane, creates a challenge when placing a needle or surgical cricothyroidotomy in the infant or child. In children younger than 10 years of age, a surgical cricothyroidotomy is not recommended as a rescue method; instead, a needle cricothyroidotomy should be attempted in these children. Based on animal studies, this method allows for oxygenation for an estimated 30 minutes while a definitive method of airway control is obtained.

The clinical implications affected by the pediatric airway compared with the adult airway include the following[3,14-18]:

- Infants are believed to be obligate nose breathers. The nares account for almost half the total airway resistance in these infants. Any secretions, edema, or obstruction can increase work of breathing and lead to respiratory distress in these children.
- Because of the small diameter of the nasal passages, even a small amount of edema or obstruction can markedly decrease air exchange, such as those seen in children with croup or respiratory syncytial virus (RSV).
- Posterior displacement of the tongue may cause airway obstruction. This increases in the supine position or with altered LOC.
- Control of the tongue with the laryngoscope blade may be difficult.
- The angle between the base of the tongue and the glottis opening is more acute, which makes straight blades more effective in visualizing the glottis in children.
- Control of the epiglottis with the laryngoscope blade may be more difficult.
- Because of the shape of the epiglottis, the Miller or straight blade is more popular compared with the curved Macintosh blade. The straight blade is placed under the epiglottis to elevate for visualization of the vocal cords.

The curved blade is placed in the vallecula and indirectly elevates the epiglottis from the glottic opening.

- A blind ETT placement may become caught at the anterior commissure of the vocal cords.
- Properly sized ETTs have a minimal air leak with ventilation. Cuffed ETTs are acceptable and recommended for anticipated higher airway pressure needs by PALS.
- Infants and young children tend to have a higher metabolic rate and consume oxygen twice that of adults. They also have a lower functional residual capacity resulting in lower intrapulmonary oxygen stores to use during periods of apnea or hypoventilation.
- The higher metabolic rate and lower functional residual capacity leads to a more rapid and abrupt desaturation in infants and children even with appropriate preoxygenation for airway interventions compared with adults.
- Infants and young children have small tidal volumes (6–8 mL/kg). Higher volumes or more aggressive PPV increases risk of iatrogenic barotrauma in these children.
- The nervous system of infants is affected more by the parasympathetic system because of the immature sympathetic nervous system increasing potential for bradycardia in response to hypoxia and further decreasing oxygen delivery.
- Vagal response is more prominent in infants and young children to airway suctioning or laryngoscope blade use.
- When children begin to experience airway difficulty without any intervention, they will decompensate more rapidly than adults.
- Airway adjuncts for respiratory distress are listed in Table 30.5.
- Noninvasive ventilation is used for pediatric respiratory distress, and the most common modalities are listed in Table 30.6.

TABLE 30.5 Airway Adjuncts for Respiratory Distress in the Pediatric Patient[3,19,22-24]

Nasal cannula (NC)	• Low-flow use only • 24%–44% FiO_2 with flows 1–6 L/min. • Should try to use humidity for all pediatric patients; best used with bubble humidifier • During transport may not be humidified
Simple oxygen mask	• 35%–60% FiO_2 with flows 6–10 L/min. • Higher concentrations of oxygen compared with an NC • May be used for transport
High-flow nasal cannula or Vapotherm	• Provides relative humidity of nearly 100% FiO_2 when warmed to 34°C–37°C. • Reduces work of breathing by washing out carbon dioxide from upper airway, humidification helps clear mucus from airways • Flow rates >2 L/min up to 30 L/min • Recent studies showing increased use in ED and during prehospital or interhospital transports
Nonrebreather mask with reservoir	• FiO_2 95% with flows 10–15 L/min • Reliably supplies the highest concentration of oxygen to a spontaneously breathing patient • Tight mask fit required to deliver higher concentrations of oxygen • If bag deflates patient may breathe in large amounts of exhaled carbon dioxide
Face tent	• Clear, plastic shell surrounds the child's head and upper body • 40%–50% FiO_2 using high-flow oxygen up to 15 L/min • Not sufficient if oxygen requirement >30% because of mixing of room air when tent is opened
Oxygen hood	• Oxygen hoods are clear, plastic cylinders that encompass the infant's head • 80%–90% FiO_2 with flow rates of >10–15 L/min. • Usually not large enough for children over 1 year of age

TABLE 30.5	**Airway Adjuncts for Respiratory Distress in the Pediatric Patient—cont'd**
Oropharyngeal airway (sizes 00 mm for neonates up to 110 mm for the extra-large adult patient)	• A plastic flange that displaces the tongue from the posterior pharynx and provides an oral opening for ventilation and suction • Placed with a tongue depressor and direct visualization in the unconscious child in those whose airway maneuvers (jaw thrust and chin lift) were unsuccessful at opening the airway • Contact with tongue and supraglottic structures may stimulate vomiting • Size determined with external measurement, with the flange at the level of the mouth, the tip should reach the angle of the jaw
Nasopharyngeal airway	• A flexible rubber tube that provides a conduit for air or oxygen from the nares to the posterior pharynx and provides ability to suction from the posterior pharynx • Tolerated in responsive or awake patients • Sizes determined with external measurement, with the airway approximated to equal the length from the tip of the nose to the tragus of the ear • Used in children with soft tissue upper airway obstruction • Lubricate well and gently insert into nares to avoid bleeding or injury
Self-inflating ventilation bag	• FiO_2 95%–100% with reservoir • Used to provide assisted ventilation and oxygen • Unable to provide blow-by oxygen • Does not require an oxygen source to function
Flow-inflating ventilation bag	• FiO_2 100% • Used to provide assisted ventilation and oxygenation • Able to provide blow-by oxygen • Must have an oxygen source to function • May require experience with use to be reliable

TABLE 30.6	**Noninvasive Ventilation Used in Pediatric Patients in Respiratory Distress[14,16-22]**
NIV	• The delivery of assisted ventilation without use of an advanced airway • NIV improves alveolar ventilation, oxygenation, and work of breathing • NIV avoids risks associated with advanced airways such as laryngeal injury and ventilator-induced lung injury
CPAP	• CPAP provides constant flow to maintain a set pressure to the lower airways • CPAP starts at 4–5 cm H_2O; adjust pressures to effect based on physiologic response up to 8–10 cm H_2O • CPAP increases functional residual capacity, which increases oxygenation, reduces airway resistance, and decreases work of breathing • Several positive pressure methods available to deliver CPAP such as nasal prongs, face mask, nasal mask
NPV	• Respiratory assistance in which subatmospheric pressure is applied intermittently using a cuirass or tank device externally that encompasses the chest • Expiration occurs as the pressure around the chest wall is returned to atmospheric levels • NPV it improves elimination of carbon dioxide without advanced airway[a]
BiPAP	• BiPAP provides two levels of positive airway pressure • Higher IPAP ranging from 2–25 cm H_2O • Lower EPAP ranging from 2–20 cm H_2O • Initial settings of IPAP of 8–10 cm H_2O and EPAP of 4–5 cm H_2O
Heated, humidified, high-flow nasal cannula	• Heated, humidified oxygen delivered by nasal cannula at high flow rates to decrease entrainment of room air • Comfortable and tolerated better than facemask or nasal masks • Improves oxygenation and ventilation, decreases work of breathing, reduces need for intubation, and allows earlier extubation • Mechanism of action of this mode is washout of nasopharyngeal dead space, which improves alveolar ventilation, decreases airway resistance, and improves pulmonary compliance, leading to lung recruitment • Positive pressure varies depending on flow rate and leakage around nares • Flow rates >2 to 30 L/min • Recent studies demonstrating increased use in emergency departments and during prehospital or interhospital transports

BiPAP, Bilevel positive airway pressure; *CPAP,* continuous positive airway pressure; *EPAP,* end-expiratory positive airway pressure; *IPAP,* inspiratory positive airway pressure; *NIV,* noninvasive ventilation; *NPV,* negative pressure ventilation.

Initial Management of Respiratory Distress/Arrest in the Pediatric Patient

- Perform a rapid assessment of the child because respiratory distress in children can quickly lead to cardiac arrest without intervention.
- Open the airway with either a jaw thrust or chin lift maneuver.
- Suction and position the patient.
- Provide oxygen, support breathing with bag-mask ventilation or any of the preceding airway adjuncts in Tables 30.5 and 30.6.
- Prepare for intubation.

Advanced Management of Respiratory Distress in the Pediatric Patient

Patients who present with or progress to respiratory distress may need more aggressive support than opening the airway and providing oxygen via an airway adjunct. These patients may need support from BVM ventilation (Box 30.1) with or without ETI. The provider should remember the best airway in a child is one you can oxygenate and ventilate. Research has demonstrated there is not a clear neurologic or survivable advantage between

ETI and BVM in pediatric patients 12 years of age or younger in the prehospital setting. According to the 2015 American Heart Association (AHA) guidelines, BVM ventilation may be effective and safer than ETI for short transport times or short out-of-hospital resuscitation. ETI for longer transport times is recommended given that it is difficult to maintain effective BVM ventilations for long periods of time and even harder in a moving vehicle.[3,6-9,16,17,19]

Pediatric resuscitation bags are shown in Fig. 30.1.

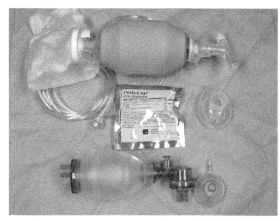

• **Fig. 30.1** Pediatric self-inflating resuscitation bags.

Endotracheal Intubation

ETI is considered one of the most effective and reliable methods of airway management in the pediatric patient for an array of reasons, which include the following[3,6-16]:

- Pediatric airway can be isolated ensuring adequate oxygenation and ventilation.
- Aspiration risk is decreased.
- Ventilations with chest compressions can be more efficient and coordinated.
- Improved control of inspiratory times and pressures.
- Positive end-expiratory pressure (PEEP) can be delivered.
- Endotracheal medications may be given during resuscitation measures when access cannot be obtained.
- Pulmonary toilet can be performed.

Indications for ETT in the pediatric patient[3,6-16] include:

- Anatomic or functional airway obstruction.
- Loss of airway protective reflexes in the unresponsive patient or in those at risk for aspiration of blood or vomit.
- Inadequate oxygenation from low oxygen saturations, pneumonia, or congestive heart failure.
- Inadequate ventilation form high end-tidal carbon dioxide ($EtCO_2$) or asthma.
- Respiratory distress leading to respiratory insufficiency, respiratory failure, or respiratory arrest.
- The need for high inspiratory pressures or PEEP.
- The need for mechanical ventilatory support.
- If patient transport is anticipated and patient is experiencing any of the previously mentioned issues.
- Intubation to protect the pediatric patient's airway during long transport times.
- Route for resuscitation medications before obtaining intravenous (IV) access.

Airway management is an initial step in stabilizing the pediatric patient. The reason for achieving airway control is to adequately oxygenate and ventilate the pediatric patient while decreasing potential for aspiration. Pediatric patients are at risk for rapid deterioration during intubation with increasing risk of bradycardia with desaturation with prolonged attempts. In addition, airway management in pediatric patients requires specialized equipment because of the differences in anatomy based on patient's size and age.[2,3,6-12]

ETI in the pediatric patient requires initial training, unique skill sets, clinical judgment, ongoing training, and experience to reliably perform in an effective, timely, and safe method. ETI requires specialized training to attain and maintain competency for the wide range of pediatric patient regarding age and size. Clinical experiences are becoming more limited because of the increased use of noninvasive ventilation devices available. Simulation offers the transport provider opportunities to develop, practice, and improve ETI skills without injury to a child using a number of different types of simulations from low fidelity to high fidelity. The high-fidelity–enhanced simulation is effective for the individual provider, team training, and system optimization and is a suitable tool for the assessment of the competency of the provider and team interaction during intubation of the pediatric patient.[2,3,6-12,20]

Pediatric providers must be able to assess, anticipate, and intervene in children with respiratory distress. It is crucial for providers to determine which patients will need aggressive airway management. The narrowest portion of the pediatric airway is subglottic at the cricoid ring in children less than 8 to 10 years of age. The shape of the pediatric trachea has led to uncuffed ETT use for intubation in these children. Recent literature has demonstrated that the pediatric airway is not as narrow as previously thought.[6] The 2015 AHA's PALS guidelines recommend the use of either cuffed or uncuffed ETTs for use during emergency intubations in children. Research has proven that cuffed ETTs are equally safe to use compared with uncuffed ETTs. The PALS guidelines suggest using cuffed ETTs for children when high airway pressures will be needed or suspected, such as those with asthma or acute respiratory distress. Cuffed ETTs have been shown to decrease the need for multiple intubations secondary to air leaking around an uncuffed ETT and does not increase adverse results such as damage to airway mucosa or subglottic area from overinflation in children of all ages. Pediatric cuffed ETTs are designed to use safely by managing cuff pressures with either a cuff manometer or by auscultating the air leak around the tube, which decreases the possibility of damage to the subglottic area. If the transport provider chooses to use a cuffed ETT, select an ETT that is one-half size smaller than the uncuffed ETT estimated to use by standard calculation. The team must be able to select the correct tube size, tube position, and cuff inflation pressure. The cuff inflation pressure should be less than 20 cm H_2O of water.[2,3,6-17]

There are several methods the provider may use to select the correct ETT size in pediatric patients including:

- Matching the outside diameter of the ETT to the child's little finger or nares.
- Use of the length-based resuscitation tapes, such as Broselow tape, which is recommended by advanced trauma life support (ATLS) and is fairly reliable to approximately 36 kg. Inaccuracies begin to appear if patient is tall or obese for age.
- For children older than 2 years, the formulas:

$$\text{Endotracheal tube size} = \frac{16 + \text{age in years}}{4}$$

Or

$$\text{Uncuffed endotracheal tube size (mm ID)} = \left(\frac{\text{age in years}}{4}\right) + 4$$

Or

$$\text{Cuffed endotracheal tube size (mm ID)} = \left(\frac{\text{age in years}}{4}\right) + 3$$

The depth of the ETT placement can be approximated by multiplying the internal diameter by 3 (e.g., 3.5 mm ETT × 3 is inserted to 10.5 cm). Gastric decompression is necessary in pediatric patients and selecting the correct size nasogastric or orogastric tube can be estimated by multiplying 2 by the size of the ETT.[3,6-17,21]

Preparing for ETI is a crucial step that is often not given enough respect. The pediatric provider who is prepared for complications that may occur can often prevent life-threatening events during this procedure. The necessary equipment is listed in Box 30.2.

The pediatric provider should have a backup plan in place in the event the provider is unable to ventilate or oxygenate the pediatric patient. Consider using oral or nasal airway adjuncts and attempt intubation. If unable to intubate the pediatric patient, consider using supraglottic rescue devices. If these devices are unsuccessful, consider needle or surgical airway procedures.[3,6,19-27]

Rapid sequence intubation is considered to be the universal method used for obtaining definitive airway management in the emergency setting. It is the combined efforts of pre-oxygenation, sedation, and a neuromuscular blockade used in rapid succession to optimize ETI in critically ill or injured patients. Rapid sequence intubation is the appropriate method used in pediatric patients to facilitate intubation. It is imperative for the provider to be adequately prepared for rapid sequence intubation in pediatric patients, which includes the readiness for unexpected situations or complications.[28-29] Rapid sequence intubation sedatives commonly used in pediatric patients are listed in Table 30.7. Common neuromuscular blockade medications used for pediatric rapid sequence intubation are listed in Table 30.8. Atropine sulfate is used to block the vagal responses in infants and children during ETI.[28-29]

Proper ETT placement is verified immediately after intubation by several methods[29]:
- Symmetric chest rise visualized.
- Auscultation of bilateral breath sounds begins high in the axillae.
- Absence of breath sounds or gurgling sounds in the stomach.
- Positive end-tidal CO_2 ($EtCO_2$) indicator via colormetric detector or capnography.

BOX 30.2   Equipment Necessary for Intubation[3,24-25,28-31]

- Oxygen delivery system (e.g., blow-by, nasal cannula, simple mask, nonrebreather, hood, tent, self-inflating bag, and flow-inflating bag)
- Bag-valve-resuscitation bag without pop-off valve
- Resuscitation masks of all pediatric sizes
- Oral and nasopharyngeal airways of all pediatric sizes
- Suction devices with pediatric sized catheters
- Pulse oximeter with pediatric probes
- Cardiac monitor
- If sedation and paralytics are used, rescue/reversal medications (e.g., naloxone) should be available
- Pediatric endotracheal tubes, sizes to include both uncuffed and cuffed 2.5, 3.0, 3.5, 4.0, 4.5, 5.0, 5.5 mm and 6.0-, 6.5-, 7.0-, and 8.0-mm cuffed (Fig. 30.2)
- Pediatric laryngoscope blade sizes 00 to 4 straight (e.g., Miller) and 1 to 4 curved (e.g., MacIntosh).
- Pediatric stylettes for endotracheal tubes sizes 2.5–8.0 mm
- Magill forceps both pediatric and adult
- End-tidal CO_2 detectors (disposable or in line) both pediatric and adult
- Rescue airway devices such as supraglottic airways
- Securing tape or device
- Weight-based measuring tape

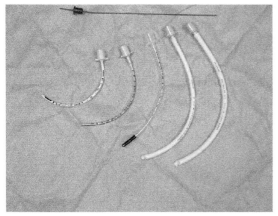

• **Fig. 30.2** Pediatric cuffed and uncuffed endotracheal tubes.

TABLE 30.7   Sedatives Commonly Used in Pediatric Rapid Sequence Intubation (RSI)

Sedative	Advantages	Disadvantages
Etomidate	• Hypotension rare • Effects observed quickly • Efficient	• Possible adrenal suppression seen with septic shock • Long acting neuromuscular blockades (NMBs) affect efficacy
Ketamine	• Potential for hypertension for patients exhibiting shock • Potentially may prevent post-RSI hypotension • Efficient	• Slower rate of administration compared to NMB med • Increased systemic vascular resistance may cause harm to patients in cardiogenic shock
Fentanyl	• Hypotension is rare • Efficient	• Possible rigid chest with rapid administration
Propofol	• Effects observed quickly • Efficient	• Potential hypotensive issues

NMB, Neuromuscular blockade; *RSI,* rapid sequence intubation.
Data from Mittiga MR, Rinderknecht AS, Kerrey BT. A modern and practical review of rapid-sequence intubation in pediatric emergencies. *Clin Pediatr Emerg Med.* 2015;16(3):172-185.

TABLE 30.8	Neuromuscular Blockade Commonly Used in Pediatric Rapid Sequence Intubation		
Neuromuscular Blockade	**Benefits**	**Risks**	
Succinylcholine	• Effects observed quickly • Short acting • Efficient	• Short acting and may need additional dosing • Hyperkalemia may occur • Additional dosing may cause bradycardia	
Rocuronium	• Safe to use with renal clearance (hyperkalemia) • Effects observed quickly (more efficient than vecuronium)	• Long acting, which may cause an issue if unable to intubate patient • Shorter duration compared with Vecuronium	
Vecuronium	• Safe to use with renal clearance (hyperkalemia)	• Long acting (longer compared with Rocuronium)	

Adapted from Mittiga MR, Rinderknecht AS, Kerrey BT. A modern and practical review of rapid-sequence intubation in pediatric emergencies. *Clin Pediatr Emerg Med.* 2015;16(3):172-185.

• Chest radiograph results, when clinically possible, should verify proper tube placement.

'Evidence and controversy in pediatric prehospital airway management exists and options include BMV, ETI, and supraglottic devices. Supraglottic airways have increased in popularity and use in the prehospital and emergency room settings because these devices are so easy to use, training is relatively simple, and they are dependable and quick to insert. Supraglottic devices do not offer a definitive airway in the prehospital setting. However, newer more advanced devices are offering greater seal pressures and the capacity to decompress gastric secretions to decrease potential aspiration. Supraglottic devices are usually used as rescue devices. Supraglottic airways have revealed a decrease in hands-on time during resuscitation, yet it is ambiguous as to whether any advanced airway offers a neurologic survival advantage compared with simple BVM in the prehospital setting. Supraglottic airways are considered to be first- or second-generation devices because the airway has gastric access. The first-generation supraglottic airways are simple airways attached to a mask resting over the glottic opening. The second-generation supraglottic airways have a gastric access channel for placement of gastric tube or venting of gastric contents. The second-generation devices offer a better second seal and as a result are able to support higher pressures compared with the first-generation devices. The second-generation supraglottic devices offer several advantages compared with the first-generation devices such as improved airway seal with the ability to reduce the risk of gastric insufflations, which ultimately allows for improved PPV and some protection against aspiration.[3,26,27,29,30]

Children who are designated as having a difficult airway or are unable to intubate by direct laryngoscopy may benefit by using supraglottic airways because they are potential conduits for ETI. The pros of using a supraglottic airway as an adjunct for intubation include the ability to be able to provide oxygen during intubation and relief of any upper airway obstruction in children designated with a difficult airway. Supraglottic airways are available in pediatric sizes and include the laryngeal mask airway (LMA), LMA Unique, LMA Supreme, and LMA ProSeal. The King LT-D and King LTS-D are available in pediatric >12 kg to adult sizes. The I-gel is available in neonatal 2 kg to adult >90 kg sizes. Air-Q and Air-Q SP are available in pediatric <7 kg to adult and pediatric <4 kg to adult sizes. Research comparing specific supraglottic airway devices, BVM, and ETT and associated neurologic outcomes has not been performed. Esophageal obturator airways such as the Combitube and oxygen-powered breathing devices are both not recommended in the pediatric population because of limited patient-appropriate sizes.[3,26,27,29,30]

No matter which advanced airway modality is used it is crucial for the provider to confirm proper placement, to provide adequate ventilation and oxygenation, and to promptly recognize displacement of the airway to improve pediatric advanced airway management during the prehospital or interfacility transports. Pulse oximetry, which is a noninvasive measurement of arterial blood oxygenation, has become a standard method of monitoring respiratory status for pediatric patients in prehospital or interfacility transports. Pulse oximetry is affected by movement, hypothermia, vasoconstriction, and poor perfusion, which are all common in the pediatric patient requiring transport.[6,17,31]

Exhaled carbon dioxide ($EtCO_2$) measurement is used to confirm correct placement of the airway and effectiveness of assisted ventilations. Colorimetric $EtCO_2$ is used to detect initial placement of ETTs in pediatric patients. Research has shown capnography improves time to detection of a dislodged ETT and the corrective actions necessary in pediatric patients. Freeman et al.[31] demonstrated that continuous capnograph waveforms may be useful for the assessment of pediatric ventilation regardless of airway (ETT, BVM, or supraglottic). Current literature and the 2015 AHA guidelines support BVM over ETI in the prehospital setting and using continuous capnograph may be an essential tool to ensure adequate ventilation in pediatric patients. Providing an adequate mask seal, with effective chest rise and breath sounds, is difficult to maintain and assess as providers are confronted with multiple tasks, environmental factors, limited space, and continuous movement from the mode of transport in the prehospital or interfacility setting. A useful tool for assessing adequate ventilations via ETT, BVM, or supraglottic device appears to be continuous capnography.[6,17,31]

Intubated pediatric patients are at high risk of extubation when loading and unloading the child in an aircraft or ground ambulance. If a change in the child's status occurs, consider the mnemonic DOPE to help identify the problem[6,31]:

D: Displacement of the ETT
O: Obstruction of the ETT
P: Pneumothorax
E: Equipment failure

Needle Cricothyroidotomy

Surgical airway in a child is rarely performed, but when it is it is potentially a lifesaving intervention. The pediatric provider must be able to recognize and manage the difficult airway in a child. Failing to recognize and respond in an appropriate manner can cause significant morbidity and mortality of that child. The inability to secure and control the child's airway via BVM, ETI, a supraglottic device, or because of facial injuries or an airway obstruction is an emergent situation requiring the pediatric provider to consider a surgical airway. An invasive airway in the pediatric patient is rare. A needle cricothyroidotomy is used for children 5 years of age or less. The Seldinger cricothyroidotomy is used on children older than 5 years of age. A surgical airway can be placed through the cricothyroid membrane on children older than 10 years of age (Fig. 30.3).[3,28-29,32]

Indications for needle cricothyroidotomy include the following:
• Complete airway obstruction
• Severe orofacial injuries
• Laryngeal tear or transaction
• Inability to secure the airway with the less invasive methods

The procedure for a needle cricothyroidotomy is shown in Box 30.3.

Complications of a needle cricothyroidotomy include the following:
• Inadequate ventilation that leads to hypoxia and death
• Aspiration of blood
• Esophageal laceration
• Hematoma
• Posterior tracheal wall perforation
• Subcutaneous or mediastinal emphysema
• Thyroid perforation

Passive aspiration may occur when using the needle cricothyroidotomy method. The size of this airway is small

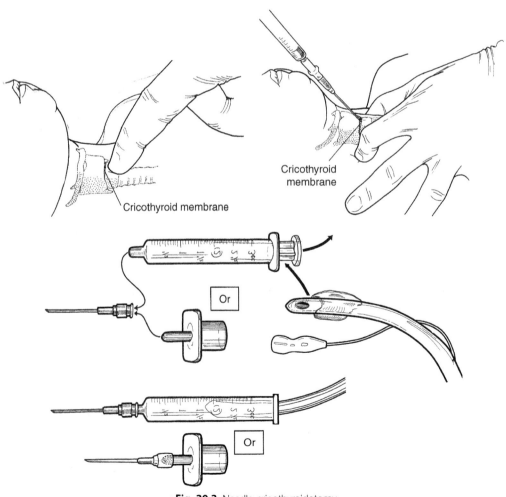

• **Fig. 30.3** Needle cricothyroidotomy.

• BOX 30.3 Needle Cricothyroidotomy

1. Place the patient in a supine position.
2. Assemble a 14-gauge, 8.5-cm, over-the-needle catheter to a 10-mL syringe.
3. Surgically prepare the neck with antiseptic swabs.
4. Palpate the cricothyroid membrane between the thyroid and cricoid cartilage.
5. Stabilize the trachea with the thumb and forefinger to prevent lateral movement.
6. Puncture the skin in the midline over the cricothyroid membrane with the 14-gauge needle attached to the syringe. A small incision with a #11 blade may facilitate passage of the needle.
7. Direct the needle at a 45-degree angle caudally.
8. Carefully insert the needle into the lower half of the cricothyroid membrane, aspirating as the needle is advanced.
9. Aspiration of air signifies entry into the tracheal lumen.
10. Remove the syringe and stylette while gently advancing the catheter downward into position, taking care not to perforate the posterior trachea.
11. Oxygen can then be delivered in a variety of ways. Commercial jet insufflators are available for this purpose. Oxygen can also be supplied by attaching the adapter from a #3.0 endotracheal tube to the catheter and ventilate with a resuscitation bag. Finally, oxygen tubing can be cut with a hole toward the end of the tubing, which is then attached to the catheter hub. Once attached to an oxygen source of 50 psi or greater, oxygen can be delivered by occluding the hole with the thumb. Regardless of the oxygen delivery source, inspiration should be provided for 1 second while passive exhalation is provided for 4 seconds.

From Holleran RS, ed. *ASTNA Patient Transport: Principles and Practice.* 4th ed. St. Louis: Mosby Elsevier; 2010.

and limited because of the lumen size, and it is more effective in oxygenation than ventilation. The child can only be oxygenated for about 30 to 45 minutes using this technique. Needle cricothyroidotomy is a temporary method to control a child's airway until ETT can be placed or the airway obstruction is removed.[3,28-29,32]

Selected Diagnoses With Respiratory Distress in the Pediatric Population

Asthma

Asthma prevalence in children is progressively increasing annually with an estimate of 6.8 million children currently diagnosed with asthma, or 9.3% of all children under the age of 18 years in the United States.[31,33] Asthma is not curable, nor can it be prevented, but it can be controlled. Asthma has a higher prevalence in children compared with adults. In children less than 18 years of age, males have a higher prevalence compared with females. Racial and socioeconomic differences exist with higher prevalence in Hispanic and African American children. In addition, children living below the federal poverty level also have a higher prevalence of asthma.[33,34]

Asthma is one of the most common chronic childhood diseases and is characterized by chronic airway inflammation, airway hyperresponsiveness, and intermittent and reversible bronchial constriction or obstruction. Pediatric asthma exacerbation (AE) is an acute episode that does not respond to standard therapy leading to a medical emergency. AEs are a common occurrence and a leading cause of acute hospital emergency department (ED) visits and hospital admissions. Asthma is also the leading cause of missed school days and work absences.[33,34]

Several studies have shown an increase in asthma prevalence and severity in children with asthma in association with low levels of vitamin D, acetaminophen use prenatally and in infancy, maternal diet during pregnancy including fast food and artificial sweetened soft drinks, increasing pollution levels, and obesity. Other factors impacting asthma development or exacerbation include environmental factors, allergens, and respiratory viruses.[33-38]

Approximately 80% of AEs are caused by viral respiratory infections. Rhinovirus (RV), RSV, coronaviruses (CVs), influenza A and B, parainfluenza viruses (PIVs), adenovirus (AV), human metapneumovirus (HMPV), human bocavirus, and enteroviruses are all related to AEs. RV is the most common pathogen causing AE in older children, and RSV is the most common in younger children.[38]

Clinical Presentation

A hallmark finding in patients experiencing an AE is expiratory wheezing. Asthma is the most common cause of chronic cough in children. Acute exacerbation signs and symptoms include coughing, dyspnea, chest tightness, and wheezing. Younger children reveal shortness of breath as decreased activity or verbalization. In children 5 years of age and younger, wheezing is the most common symptom associated with asthma. The child may present with nonspecific signs of respiratory distress including retractions, nasal flaring, cyanosis, accessory muscle use, and altered mental status. Coughing triggered by asthma may be recurrent or persistent and is usually associated with wheezing. Recurrent shortness of breath or during exercise increases the chance of an asthma diagnosis. If a child presents with hypoxia or saturations less than 92% he or she may require aggressive treatment. Severe AEs in children may cause tachypnea, tachycardia, and occasionally pulsus paradoxus. Accessory muscle use may indicate a severe AE. In severe AE, poor air exchange and movement without wheezing known as a silent chest is a sign of impending respiratory failure. Agitation or decreased mental status are signs of impending respiratory failure in children. Predictors of severe AE remain multifactorial.[32-40]

A detailed medical history is an important tool for the transport provider in the assessment of a child with wheezing. It is essential in determining causes other than asthma in a first-time wheezing patient. Questions to ask include age of patient, onset of symptoms, associated symptoms, history of asthma, history of ED visits, intensive care unit admission including if the child was on a ventilator within the past year, use of a short-acting β-agonist (SABA), compliance with controller medications, number and frequency of home treatments, and history of greater than or equal to 3 days of oral steroids in the last 3 months. A significant indicator of AE in a child is a recent ED visit for asthma.[32-43]

There are three reliable asthma scoring tools available for the provider to use to assist with the severity of the AE (Table 30.9).

Treatment

The primary goal of asthma treatment is the reversal of hypoxemia and control of contributing inflammatory responses. First-line therapy consists of supplementation of oxygen, the repeated administration of inhaled short-acting bronchodilators and anticholinergics, and early administration of corticosteroids either orally or intravenously. The most common bronchodilators and anticholinergics are albuterol and ipratropium bromide nebulized aerosols. A distinguishing characteristic of asthma is the response to bronchodilator or corticosteroids when symptomatic. In children, asthma is a clinical diagnosis.[33-43]

SABAs are the most effective treatment to relieve bronchospasm and reverse airway obstruction. SABAs use their sympathomimetic effects to exert bronchodilating effects by relaxing airway smooth muscle to relieve bronchospasm.

They also have secondary effects that enhance water output from bronchial mucous glands and improve mucociliary clearance. Albuterol and levalbuterol are the two available SABAs used in children. Airway inflammation occurs with AE, and corticosteroids are the most common treatment by suppressing cytokine production, granulocyte-macrophage colony-stimulating factor, and nitric oxide synthase activation and decreasing airway mucous production.[33-43]

Most guidelines suggest use of steroids in AE when the child does not respond to one inhaled SABA treatment. Prednisone, prednisolone, or dexamethasone are the most common corticosteroids administered for AE in children. Ipratropium bromide is an anticholinergic medication used in AE in children promoting bronchodilation without inhibiting mucociliary clearance. Children presenting with severe AE are often dehydrated because of poor oral intake and increased insensible losses from increased minute ventilation. The transport provider needs to consider a 20-mL/kg fluid bolus during transport and reassess. IV or subcutaneous terbutaline is a selective β_2-agonist and may be used in the management of acute severe AE in children. Magnesium sulfate is a bronchodilator used in the treatment of severe asthma by blocking calcium channels in respiratory smooth muscle. Magnesium also depresses muscle fiber excitability by inhibiting acetylcholine release and promoting bronchodilation. An additional treatment that may be used in children with AE is leukotriene receptor antagonists, such as montelukast, which blocks production of natural mediators involved in bronchoconstriction. Heliox is a gas blend of 20% oxygen and 80% helium that may be used for AE in children. Heliox is able to reduce turbulent flow and increase laminar gas flow, which ultimately improves airflow resistance in small airways. Heliox improves particle dispersion of aerosol treatments in the distal lungs, which helps remove carbon dioxide and decrease work of breathing in the child. If hypoxemia is present this therapy is not recommended. An additional method used in severe AE is noninvasive PPV (NiPPV) as an option to avoid intubation in children and improve their outcomes. ETT is indicated for children who are apneic or unresponsive and should be considered for those presenting with intractable hypoxemia, unresponsive respiratory acidosis, unresponsive to first-line asthma therapy medications, or worsening LOC.[33-43]

Early interventions are recommended for the treatment of AE in pediatrics by using the first-line treatment of oxygen, β-agonists, ipratropium bromide, and corticosteroids. For AE in children unresponsive to the first line of treatment, terbutaline, magnesium, Heliox and NiPPV are available and may be used before ETT.[32-33]

Croup

Croup is a common childhood upper airway viral infection called laryngotracheitis. It usually occurs in children ages 6 months to 3 years of age and in the fall and winter months. Sporadic cases may occur any time of year in older children.[3,13,44]

TABLE 30.9	**Pediatric Asthma Scores** *Tools Used to Assist the Provider in Classifying the Severity of Exacerbation*	
Preschool Respiratory Assessment Measure (PRAM)	**Pediatric Asthma Severity Score (PASS)**	**Pediatric Asthma Score (PAS)**
• A reliable, valid, and responsive tool to measure severity of airway obstruction in children 2–17 years of age	• A valid, reliable tool that determines pediatric asthma severity based on the physical exam findings in children 1–18 years of age	• A measurement tool with excellent face validity and good interobserver agreement for children >2 years of age
• Measures suprasternal retractions, air entry, wheezing, respiratory rate, and oxygen saturations	• Is limited because it only measures three clinical measures: wheezing, prolonged expiration, and work of breathing	• Measures respiratory rate, oxygen saturation, auscultatory findings, retractions, and dyspnea

Data from Kline-Krammes S, Robinson S. Childhood asthma: a guide for pediatric emergency medicine providers. *Emerg Med Clin North Am.* 2013;31(3):705-732.

Clinical Presentation

Croup symptoms mimic other respiratory diseases requiring the pediatric provider to make the appropriate differential diagnosis to ensure proper and effective interventions. Croup resulting from a viral infection is most frequently caused by PIV type 1 and occasionally type 3. Diagnosis is usually determined from the history and physical examination. In most cases of viral croup the symptoms are self-limiting and resolve on their own. Patients generally present with an upper respiratory tract infection, low-grade fever, and coryza. As the symptoms progress, inspiratory stridor may be present characterized by a barking cough with mild to moderate respiratory distress including nasal flaring, respiratory retractions, and stridor. Croup may also present with a sudden barking cough, hoarseness, and stridor. The most reliable symptoms to establish the severity of the disease is stridor and severity of retractions indicating narrowing of the subglottic area. A chest x-ray (CXR) will exhibit the "steeple" sign. If the inflammation extends to the bronchi, rhonchi and wheezing will be present. The provider must rule out epiglottis and retropharyngeal abscess because croup presentation is so similar. When assessing the child with suspected croup, it is essential to keep the child calm by allowing the parent to continue to hold the patient to prevent exacerbation of respiratory distress symptom and excessive narrowing of the child's airway.[3,13,44]

Treatment

The recommended treatment of choice for croup is a single dose of systemic corticosteroid. The current evidence supports using dexamethasone as the preferred steroid based on its longer half-life. Nebulized budesonide is indicated for mild to moderate or moderate to severe croup if the child is vomiting or unable to take oral steroids. Current evidence recommends nebulized epinephrine for children with moderate to severe croup. The provider must remember nebulized epinephrine has a 2-hour or less duration and the child may rebound. On rare occasions, severe croup may exhibit upper airway edema or obstruction requiring ETI for oxygenation and ventilation of the child.[3,13,44]

Epiglottitis

Epiglottitis is a rare bacterial infection of the supraglottic larynx, which is the area of the larynx superior to the vocal folds. If not recognized and treated properly it becomes a potentially life-threatening condition. Epiglottitis primarily affects children ages 2 to 6 years of age before the introduction of the conjugated *Haemophilus influenzae* type b (Hib) vaccine. There has been a decline in pediatric cases of epiglottitis since the introduction of the Hib vaccine. Epiglottis may be seen in older children and adults presenting with atypical symptoms. Epiglottitis risk factors include lack of immunity for Hib and immunodeficiency.[3,13,45]

Clinical Presentation

A child presenting with epiglottitis has a toxic appearance with a history of rapid onset of symptoms of high fever, noisy breathing, sore throat, and inability to tolerate secretions. Epiglottitis is second only to croup as a cause for infectious stridor and muffled voice. Presenting symptoms include fever, drooling, or spitting up of secretions caused by supraglottic edema and suprasternal and subcostal retractions. The child presents anxious and in the classic tripod positioning by leaning forward with arms extended for support, and jaw thrust forward or in the sniffing position with head up, neck forward, with mouth open to maintain airway. These positions help increase air entry. Altered mental status, mottled skin, and cyanosis are impending signs of airway obstruction and circulatory collapse. The provider must be able to recognize these signs because of the potential for life-threatening airway obstruction.[3,13,45]

Treatment

Assessing a patient with suspected epiglottitis is rapid with the patient remaining in a position of comfort usually in the parents' lap and should never be forced to change positions or be agitated. Obtain a history from the parents on time of onset of symptoms, any sick contacts, immunization status, medications, and their last meal. The provider must be prepared to secure the airway if necessary. The most qualified practitioner available to secure the airway in the event of an acute obstruction should be called to the bedside. Noninvasive monitoring can usually be applied without upsetting the patient. The presence of hypoxia may represent impending airway obstruction. The toxic-appearing patient must have his or her airway secured by an anesthesiologist or the ear, nose, and throat physician before any other intervention should be completed such as laboratory work or obtaining IV access. A lateral neck x-ray may help rule out other causes of stridor and respiratory distress. An edematous epiglottis will have a "thumb print" appearance on a lateral neck x-ray if epiglottitis is present. The aryepiglottic folds may also appear enlarged. Airway management, if possible, should be performed in the operating room. Because of the high risk of this procedure, the plan for securing the airway is discussed with the most experienced physician providers available and they are the only ones allowed to intervene. Securing the airway is a critical procedure requiring equipment for ETI, cricothyroidotomy, and tracheostomy and must be ready and in the patient's room. If the airway cannot be secured by ETI and the patient begins to deteriorate, the provider must consider a tracheostomy. Once the airway is secured, obtain cultures and begin third-generation cephalosporins; ceftriaxone or cefotaxime are the treatment of choice because they are able to eliminate Hib infection.[3,13,45]

Foreign Body Aspiration (FBA)

FBA is a common pediatric emergency and a significant cause of morbidity and mortality in children. In fact, FBA is the sixth most common cause of accidental deaths in children. FBA occurs when a foreign object becomes accidently lodged anywhere within a child's respiratory tract. Seventy percent of FBA occurs in children 3 years of age and younger with the peak incidence at 2 years of age. Factors increasing the risk for aspiration include immature dentition, poor chewing ability and swallowing coordination, the epiglottis positioned higher, the ease with which toddlers and infants are distracted, talking or crying while eating, and oral exploration. Organic foreign bodies such as nuts and seeds are the most common types of items aspirated by children. Other organic items include food, food-related items, fruits, and bones. The most common inorganic foreign objects aspirated are coins, pins, beads, small toy parts, small batteries, and pen caps. Organic foreign objects produce an inflammatory response and may make the obstruction worse and shorten the asymptomatic period. The inorganic foreign objects may remain asymptomatic for longer periods of time.[46-51]

Button batteries are smooth and shiny and appealing to young children, and the incidence of battery foreign body ingestion has increased 80% over the last 10 years in young children. An ingested battery can pass the esophagus and remain uneventful through the gastrointestinal (GI) system. However, the complications can be devastating if the battery becomes lodged in the esophagus or nasal cavity. Once the battery is impacted in either the esophagus or nasal cavity it generates an external electrolytic current and releases a toxic alkaline solution causing significant liquefactive necrosis in the surrounding tissues within 4 to 6 hours. Button battery aspiration or ingestions should be considered a medical emergency.[46-54]

Clinical Presentation

Foreign objects are aspirated into the right mainstem bronchus more often followed by the left mainstem bronchus; the trachea; the larynx; and finally, both bronchi. Upper airway aspiration or ingestion may cause a mechanical obstruction of the airway with asphyxiation if it becomes lodged in the larynx. There is a 45% mortality rate if the larynx is completely obstructed. Balloons are the most common cause of mortality in children. It is crucial for providers to consider FBA or ingestion as a differential diagnosis when a child presents without any symptoms or presents with acute onset of respiratory symptoms regardless of the initial lack of evidence to support it when the physical examination and CXR are normal. The most sensitive predictor of a true FBA in a child is a positive history or witnessed event from the parents. Choking or coughing has a high sensitivity associated with a proven FBA or ingestion. Physical examination of a child with suspected FBA is not as sensitive as a positive history. Only 40% of children will actually present with the classic triad of symptoms such as choking, coughing, and unilateral wheezing or decreased air entry.[46-54]

Most children who present with FBA or ingestion are often not witnessed. The classic triad of symptoms such as choking, coughing, and unilateral wheezing or decreased air entry usually indicates the foreign object is in the bronchial

tree. The clinical presentation of children suspected of FBA will depend on the location of the foreign object. Tracheal FBA may present with various levels of respiratory distress, stridor, or an acute life-threatening obstruction. The most common symptom is paroxysmal cough, which is a natural defense response to remove the foreign body from the airway. Other clinical symptoms include stridor, cyanosis, unilateral decreased air entry, fever, wheezing, and dyspnea.[46-54]

Children may present with an *upper airway obstruction* from an FBA with stridor, hoarseness, drooling, and some degree of respiratory distress depending on the location of the aspirated foreign object. *Lower airway obstruction* in children may present with wheezing and unilateral decreased breath sounds on the affected side in children with FBA. Persistent coughing can present in both upper and lower airway obstructions as well.[46-54]

FBA or ingestion necessitates prompt diagnosis and management. Delaying the diagnosis greater than 24 hours is associated with a 2.5 times increased risk of serious acute complications. The delayed diagnosis of a foreign body may result in an unrelenting cough, recurrent pneumonia, atelectasis, emphysema, laryngeal edema, laryngeal trauma, and hypoxic encephalopathy. Additional complications include pneumothorax, hydropneumothorax, pneumomediastinum, subcutaneous emphysema, pleural thickening, bronchiectasis, bronchial stenosis, or pulmonary abscess.[46-54]

The most common signs and symptoms of button battery aspiration or ingestion include vomiting, difficulty feeding, mild abdominal pain, cough, and bloody nasal discharge. Button battery ingestion and impaction is misdiagnosed as an upper respiratory tract infection in the absence of a history of battery ingestion. A magnet is another object increasingly being ingested by young children. Most magnets are smooth and will pass through the GI tract without complications; however, multiple magnets attract each other and will attract through different loops of the bowel causing the movement to stop and potentially cause mural pressure necrosis leading to bowel perforation, fistula formation, volvulus, obstruction, abdominal sepsis, and ultimately death.[46-54]

Treatment

If a child presents with complete obstruction, emergent airway procedures must be initiated. This may include the Heimlich maneuver, jaw thrust chin lift maneuver, and opening nasal or oral airways. If these procedures do not improve the child's respiratory distress, direct laryngoscopy may be required to either remove the foreign body with Magill forceps or to place an ETT past the obstruction. If all of these interventions are unsuccessful, an emergent cricothyrotomy or tracheostomy is essential to prevent morbidity or mortality in the child. Partial airway obstructions in a child with FBA are more common than the complete obstruction of the child's airway. These children should be treated as if they are heading for an emergency. Allow these children to remain with their parents and in a position of comfort while preparing for an emergent intervention should the foreign body become completely obstructed. Preparation includes preparing intubation equipment for airway management such as the bag and mask, ETTs, stylette, Magill forceps for foreign body removal, and set up for an emergent needle or surgical cricothyroidotomy.[46-54]

The emergent treatment of FBA is based on the child's presentation with or without symptoms. It is imperative to obtain a history of possible FBA in a child, physical examination, and CXR. If there is a lack of clinical symptoms additional diagnostic testing is required to confirm FBA in children. If an object is radiopaque it will be easily seen on CXR, but not all foreign objects are radiotransparent. The indirect findings on CXR if the object is not radiopaque will be overinflation, atelectasis, lung infiltrates, or consolidation. Normal CXRs have been found in 30% of children presenting with FBA. A multidetector computed tomography (MDCT) with virtual bronchoscopy is a noninvasive diagnostic tool that may be used. The disadvantage is the radiation exposure the child will endure from the CT. The rigid bronchoscopy was the procedure of choice in the past for retrieval of the foreign object in children and was considered the gold standard treatment for children. The disadvantage of this modality is that the child requires general anesthesia and the inability to reach the peripheral airways. The most popular modality currently used is the flexible bronchoscopy to remove foreign objects in children and as a diagnostic indicator. This treatment is relatively easy and safer than a rigid bronchoscopy and only requires local anesthesia. The flexible bronchoscopy is able to reach the distal airways to remove the foreign object, remove mucous or blood plugs, and allow bronchoalveolar lavage and vacuum aspiration if necessary. The only limitation of the flexible bronchoscopy is if the foreign object is too large to pass through the scope or the forceps are unable to grasp the object.[46-54]

Bronchiolitis

Bronchiolitis is the most common lower respiratory tract infection affecting infants and toddlers. It is an acute infection with an inflammatory component resulting in obstruction of the small airways. Bronchiolitis occurs in children between the ages of 0 to 24 months of age with peak incidence occurring at 3 to 6 months of age. It is diagnosed clinically with the primary symptoms of difficulty breathing, coryza, poor feeding, coughing, rhinorrhea, wheezing, and crepitus on auscultation. Bronchiolitis is associated with viral infections with the most common being RSV, which aligns seasonally beginning in the winter through to the spring typically. Additional viruses associated with bronchiolitis include RV, PIV, AV, metapneumovirus, and *Mycoplasma*. Bronchiolitis caused by RV infects the lower respiratory tract and triggers AEs in children. This viral pathogen is associated with a higher morbidity.[55-57]

Clinical Presentation

The incubation period for bronchiolitis caused by RSV is between 2 and 8 days; children will shed this virus for 3 to 8 days and infants have been found to shed RSV for up to 4 weeks. Bronchiolitis presents with a 1- to 3-day history with signs and symptoms of upper respiratory tract infection including nasal congestion or discharge, cough, and lowgrade fever; after the third day of wheezing, signs of respiratory distress with increased work of breathing and retractions are seen. Bronchiolitis patients have a higher fever with causative agent AV compared with RSV in children. Presenting signs and symptoms typically include tachypnea, mild intercostal and subcostal retractions, expiratory wheezing, prolonged expiratory phase with coarse or fine crackles on auscultation, and hypoxemia, which is present with oxygen saturations less than 93%. The child's clinical course may be mild in severity or severe with signs of apnea and deteriorating respiratory status requiring hospitalization. Severity of bronchiolitis is determined after assessment of the child's fluid status, tachypnea, nasal flaring, retractions, grunting, cyanosis, change in LOC, and apnea.[55-57]

Treatment

Bronchiolitis diagnosis is determined based on patient history, physical findings, and the season. Treatment of bronchiolitis is based on the infant or toddler's signs and symptoms and is supportive. The goal of therapy is to maintain adequate oxygenation and hydration. Infants having difficulty eating will need to have IV fluids for hydration or nasogastric tube for feeds. An infection of the airway in infants and young children increases the risk of respiratory failure because infants are obligate nasal breathers. The infants exhibiting respiratory distress may require supplemental oxygen to maintain oxygen saturations higher than 90%. Evidence supports nasal suctioning of children with bronchiolitis but not deep suctioning of the pharynx or larynx to provide temporary relief. Bronchodilator use with bronchiolitis is controversial, and the evidence demonstrates inconsistent improvement when using bronchodilator therapy. Nebulized epinephrine is an adrenergic agent with improved clinical significance in the treatment of bronchiolitis in the transport, emergency room, and hospital setting, but not in the home. It is thought that the additional vasoconstrictor properties reduce microvascular leakage and mucosal edema in children with bronchiolitis. Steroids may be given to potentially assist with reducing airway inflammation and edema. Additional treatments for bronchiolitis include nebulized 3% saline and high-flow nasal cannula (HFNC) with the delivery of heated and humidified oxygen from 8 to 40 L/min. The clinical course is usually self-limiting, usually lasting 7 to 10 days in healthy children, and requires longer (up to 28 days) recovery time for those children with preexisting conditions or premature infants. An increased risk for severe bronchiolitis occurs in premature infants, those less than 36 weeks' gestation, infants less than 12 weeks of age, and children with preexisting illnesses such as congenital heart disease (CHD) or chronic lung disease. Children in severe distress who are unresponsive to treatment may need ETI and mechanical ventilation.[55-57]

Pneumonia

Community-acquired pneumonia (CAP) is a major cause of mortality and the leading cause of hospitalization in children 5 years of age or younger. The majority of pathogens detected are viral and include RSV, RV, AV, PIV, and CV. RSV was the most common cause of pneumonia in children 2 years of age or younger. RV was the next most common cause of pneumonia in children. AV, PIV, and CV are the next most common. Bacterial pathogens are also a source of pneumonia in children. The most common bacterial pathogens causing pneumonia in children less than 2 years of age include *Streptococcus pneumoniae*, group B streptococci, gram-negative bacilli, *Staphylococcus aureus* and *Chlamydia trachomatis*. The bacterial pathogens causing pneumonia in children 2 to 5 years of age include *S. pneumoniae* and *S. aureus*. The most common bacterial pathogens causing pneumonia in children older than 5 years of age include *S. pneumoniae* and *Mycoplasma pneumoniae*. The best prevention of pneumonia in children is vaccination.[58-60]

Clinical Presentation

The World Health Organization (WHO) considers a diagnosis of CAP when a previously healthy child presents with signs of lung disease caused by an infection acquired outside of the hospital. Clinical signs of pediatric pneumonia are nonspecific in mild to moderate pneumonia in young children, making it difficult to diagnose, which leads to unnecessary antibiotic therapy. See Table 30.10 for risk factors and signs and symptoms of community acquired pneumonia.[58-61]

CXRs are not effective in differentiating viral and bacterial CAP or mild to moderate infection. Pneumonia, bronchiolitis, and reactive airway disease in children have similarities in clinical presentation and CXRs in children less than 5 years of age.[58-61]

Treatment

There has been a significant diversity in the use of diagnostic tests and antibiotic selection and use for CAP in children. The Pediatric Infectious Diseases Society and the Infectious Diseases Society of America developed guidelines in 2011 for the clinical management of CAP in the pediatric population, and these have been accepted by the American Academy of Pediatrics (AAP) and American College of Emergency Physicians (ACEP). These guidelines were established to promote appropriate diagnostic testing and a reduction in excessive use of broad-spectrum antibiotics in pediatric patients with CAP. The pediatric CAP guidelines recommend not obtaining diagnostic laboratory work or radiographic imaging as well as reducing or preventing excessive use of broad-spectrum antibiotics in children presenting with mild to moderate CAP in the ambulatory care setting. This includes not routinely obtaining blood cultures in children who are fully immunized and are nontoxic

appearing. A strong recommendation is that CXRs are not necessary for suspected CAP unless presenting with respiratory distress with hypoxemia, or for children who failed to improve after initial antibiotic treatment. These guidelines do recommend diagnostic testing including complete blood count; C-reactive protein (CRP); procalcitonin; influenza and viral polymerase chain reaction (PCR) testing, which screens for influenza A and B; PIV 1, 2, and 3; AV; RSV; and HMPV. Also recommended are a blood culture as well as a CXR along with the initiation of narrow-spectrum antibiotics for children presenting with moderate to severe CAP.[58-65]

Treatment for pediatric pneumonia is primarily supportive. If the child is presenting with mild respiratory distress and oxygen saturations less than 92%, then initiate oxygen therapy via nasal cannula. A moderate increase in work of breathing may require more than the nasal cannula. These children may begin exhibiting atelectasis, restrictive or obstructive lung disease, and oxygen saturations 90% or less on room air or nasal cannula and may require more assistance such as HFNC or Vapotherm if in the hospital setting. In the transport environment a nonrebreather, continuous positive airway pressure (CPAP), or other noninvasive mode of ventilation may be needed. If the patient deteriorates and advances to severe respiratory distress or failure with tachypnea, apnea, hypoxia, fatigue, he or she may require noninvasive ventilation or advance airway management with an ETT and mechanical ventilation. Children with CAP may need fluid resuscitation or hydration and need IV access because of their inability to take fluids by mouth caused by their respiratory status or insensible fluid losses. It is necessary to obtain blood cultures if initiating antibiotics in these patients. Patients who present with moderate to severe respiratory distress, worsening respiratory status, are toxic appearing, have changes in LOC, fail to respond to antibiotics, dehydration, and are less than 6 months of age should be admitted to the hospital.[58-65]

Pertussis

Pertussis or whooping cough is an endemic vaccine-preventable highly contagious disease. It is caused by the *Bordetella pertussis,* which is a gram-negative coccobacillus that is a highly contagious acute infection of the human respiratory tract responsible for a significant increase in morbidity and mortality, especially in infants younger than 6 months of age. Pertussis usually spreads to susceptible individuals through respiratory droplets aerosolized through paroxysms of coughing or sneezing by those infected who are in close contact. Most infants are infected by their parents or siblings. If pertussis is suspected, an important question for the transport team to ask would be if the parent's immunizations are up to date. Pertussis is commonly referred to as whooping cough or the 100-day cough. The incidence of pertussis is highest among infants, children 7 to 10 years of age, and adolescents in the United States. Despite widespread vaccination the incidence of pertussis has increased dramatically over the past 25 years with identified contributing factors

TABLE 30.10	**Community Acquired Pneumonia (CAP) in Children**[58-65]
Factors Associated With Incidence and Severity	• Prematurity • Congenital heart disease • Gastroesophageal reflux disease • Reactive airway disease • Smoke exposure • Neuromuscular disease • Immunosuppressed • Malnutrition • Underweight • Low socioeconomic status • Childcare attendance

Common Physical Findings	• Initial physical findings (key in clinical diagnosis of CAP)
	  • Fever
	  • Tachypnea (most significant clinical sign in children)
	  • Increased work of breathing
	  • Breath sounds: crackles, rhonchi, wheezing
	  • Coughing
	• Indicators for hospitalization
	  • Oxygen sats <92%
	  • Delayed capillary refill
	  • Lethargy
	  • Decrease LOC

Diagnostic Testing	• Chest x-ray (CXR)
	  • Often used to diagnose CAP
	• CXR or ultrasound rule out effusions
	  • Pleural effusions are most significant predictor of bacterial pneumonia
	  • Alveolar infiltrate suggests bacterial over viral
	  • Interstitial infiltrates may be viral or bacterial
	• Lab work
	  • C-reactive protein (CRP), CBC/D, Procalcitonin, erythrocyte sedimentation rate (ESR) (limited use in bacterial diagnosis of CAP)
	  • Nasopharyngeal swab: PCR assay (tests for 8 respiratory viruses)
	  • Tracheal aspirate (limited use in diagnosis)
	  • Blood cultures (studies indicate cultures do not change management)

Antibiotic Treatment	• Amoxicillin
	  • First choice for children 60 days of age to 5 years of age
	• Azithromycin (Zithromax)
	  • For patients allergic to penicillin or beta-lactam antibiotics
	  • Children 5 years to 16 years
	• Clarithromycin (Biaxin)
	• Erythromycin

Supportive Care	• Acetaminophen (Tylenol) or Ibuprofen (Motrin) used to treat additional symptoms accompanying CAP in children
	  • Fever
	  • Localized and referred pain in chest and/or abdomen
	  • Headache
	  • Arthralgia

From Koppolu, R, Simone S. *Medical and surgical management of pediatric pneumonia.* <https://www.napnap.org/sites/default/files/userfiles/education/2015SpeakerHO/213-%20Koppolu%20%26%20Simone.pdf>; 2016.

being parental refusal of immunizations and potential waning immunity after acellular pertussis vaccinations.[66-68]

Clinical Presentation

The most common clinical signs of pertussis infections are prolonged and paroxysmal coughing and inspiratory stridor, which makes the classic whooping cough sound. A pertussis diagnosis is difficult in young children and may go unrecognized when coinfections are present, such as RSV and AV. The classic presentation of pertussis includes paroxysms of coughing, an inspiratory whoop, and posttussive emesis. These classic symptoms occur as a primary infection in unvaccinated children younger than 10 years of age. It may also occur in vaccinated children and adults, but the symptoms are usually not as severe. Pertussis, the cough of 100 days, is divided into three stages. The catarrhal stage presents with symptoms similar to an upper viral respiratory infection with a cough and coryza, and fever is uncommon or low grade. Infants develop severe complications including failure to thrive

(FTT), apnea, respiratory failure, seizure, and death. The cough in this stage gradually increases in severity instead of improving, and the coryza remains the same. This stage usually lasts 1 to 2 weeks. The risk of transmission is greatest during the catarrhal stage. In the second, or paroxysmal stage, the coughing spells increase in severity. The paroxysmal cough is distinctive with a long series of coughs with little or no inspiratory effort. The child may gag, become cyanotic, or appear to be struggling to breathe. The whoop noise is forced inspiratory effort following a coughing spell and is not always present. Posttussive emesis is common, especially in children younger than 1 year of age. The paroxysmal stage usually lasts 2 to 8 weeks with the coughing episodes increasing in frequency during the first couple of weeks. It remains the same for 2 to 3 weeks, and then the coughing will gradually decrease. The convalescent stage is when the cough subsides and lasts over several weeks to months.[66-70]

Treatment

When a case of pertussis is identified, all exposed individuals should be notified and offered preventative treatment if necessary. This preventative treatment should include the team that transported the patient. Supportive care is the primary management for pertussis. Antibiotic therapy is imperative, or the child will remain contagious throughout the majority of the illness. Treatment with antibiotics is important for infants younger than 6 months of age because they have an increased risk for severe complications. Pertussis is identified by either a pertussis culture or positive PCR within 6 weeks of cough onset in children less than 1 year, or 3 weeks of cough onset in children older than 1 year. The initiation of antibiotic therapy should be started based on clinical suspicion and not waiting on laboratory confirmation since it may take up to a week for the result. The most common antibiotic used to treat pertussis is azithromycin. Consider admitting children less than 6 months of age to

the hospital because they have an increased risk of severe or fatal pertussis.[66-70]

Anaphylaxis

Anaphylaxis is a serious and potentially life-threatening systemic reaction in children occurring after contact with an allergy triggering substance. The systems affected include cutaneous, mucosal (80%–90%), respiratory (70%), cardiovascular (45%), GI (45%), and central nervous systems (CNSs; 15%). The incidence of allergic or anaphylactic reactions in the pediatric population is increasing annually. It is imperative for prehospital providers to rapidly assess, diagnose, and treat anaphylaxis appropriately to decrease mortality and morbidities in the pediatric population.[71-72]

Clinical Presentation

Anaphylaxis is a clinical diagnosis. A complete blood count and a comprehensive metabolic panel have been long established as unreliable and not practical in identifying anaphylaxis in children. The three most common allergens causing anaphylaxis in children are food (e.g., tree nuts, peanuts, fish, shellfish, eggs, fruits, dairy products), medications (e.g., penicillin), and insect stings and bites (e.g., honeybees, bumblebees, yellow jackets, hornets, wasps). See Table 30.11 for signs and symptoms of pediatric anaphylaxis.[71-73]

Treatment

Initial treatment of the pediatric patient experiencing anaphylaxis begins with a quick, thorough assessment of the child's airway, breathing, and circulation and rapid administration of intramuscular (IM) epinephrine, which is the treatment for controlling symptoms and decreasing morbidities and mortalities. Epinephrine is the drug of choice

TABLE 30.11	Signs and Symptoms of Pediatric Anaphylaxis[72-73]		
Cutaneous/Mucosa	**Upper Respiratory**	**Cardiovascular**	**Treatment Options**
• Urticaria (hives)	• Stridor	• Chest pain	1st Line Therapy
• Angioedema	• Dysphonia	• Tachycardia	• Epinephrine IM
• Flushing	• Hoarseness	• Bradycardia	(anterolateral thigh)
• Pruritus	• Swollen lips, tongue, or palate	• Hypotension	
• Periorbital	• Sneezing	• Dysrhythmias	
• Lips, tongue, palate	• Rhinorrhea	• Cardiac arrest	
• Throat, uvula	• Bronchospasm		
	• Upper airway obstruction		
Gastrointestinal	**Central Nervous System**		
• Abdominal pain	• Sense of impending doom	**2nd Line Therapy**	
• Nausea, vomiting	• Fussy, irritable	• Antihistamines	
• Diarrhea	• Drowsy, Decreased LOC	• Corticosteroids	
	• Dizziness	• Aggressive fluid resuscitation	
	• Confusion		
	• Headache		
	• Anxiety		

for treating pediatric anaphylaxis and should be given as soon as diagnosis is suspected. The initial recommended dose of epinephrine is 0.01 mg/kg of a 1:1000 solution intramuscularly such as in the child's thigh. This dose may be repeated every 5 to 15 minutes. Even though most patients experiencing anaphylaxis respond to one or two doses of epinephrine, the prehospital provider must be prepared for advanced airway management in a child experiencing anaphylactic reaction because deterioration in respiratory status may occur quickly. If the child does not respond to epinephrine and upper airway edema occurs, rapid sequence intubation medications are not recommended, and if unable to place an ETT, the child may require a needle cricothyroidotomy. Capnography use during transport assists in detecting early ventilatory changes in children with anaphylaxis, because hypoxemia may be a late sign of impending airway compromise in children.[71-74]

Metabolic Acidosis

Metabolic acidosis is a common finding in pediatric patients. The anion gap (AG) is used to classify pediatric causes of metabolic acidosis. The AG is usually calculated as the difference between sodium (Na^+), a major cation, and the major measured anions chloride (CL^-) and bicarbonate (HCO_3^-) using the following formula: $AG (mEq/L) = (Na^+) - (Cl^- + HCO_3^-)$. An elevated AG is caused by an increase in unmeasured anions such as lactate or β-hydroxybutyrate in the blood. AG can also be elevated with hypokalemia, hypocalcemia, or hypomagnesium. In newborns, an elevated AG is greater than 16 mEq/L and in children it is greater than 14 mEq/L.[3,75]

There are no clinical features of pediatric metabolic acidosis; instead infants and children present with symptoms of their underlying condition. An example of this is lactic acidosis, which presents with signs and symptoms of sepsis or shock with poor tissue perfusion, cool extremities, and hypotension. The most obvious clinical finding in acute metabolic acidosis caused by respiratory compensation is tachypnea. In metabolic acidosis, respiratory compensation results in a lower PCO_2 and will raise the pH in the direction of normal. Inadequate compensatory response may be an indication of unrecognized respiratory insufficiency, disease, or impending failure. Metabolic acidosis is diagnosed by obtaining a blood gas with pH less than 7.36, a decrease in blood HCO_3 levels, and a decrease in PCO_2 with respiratory compensation. A 1-mm Hg decrease in PCO_2 usually results in a 1 mmol/L decrease in HCO_3 levels. Identifying the cause of metabolic acidosis is essential in guiding treatment options. Initial evaluation includes a detailed history, physical examination, and basic laboratory testing, and with the initial diagnostic tests an AG is needed. Identification and management of the underlying cause of metabolic acidosis is essential and needs to occur quickly. Pediatric causes of metabolic acidosis are listed in Table 30.12.[3,75]

TABLE 30.12	Pediatric Causes of Metabolic Acidosis		
	Large anion gap (MUDPILES)	**Normal anion gap**	**Small anion gap**
	M = methanol	Renal tubular acidosis	Hypoalbuminemia
	U = uremia or chronic renal failure	Vomiting	Nephrotic syndrome
	D = diabetic ketoacidosis	Diarrhea	
	P = propylene glycol	Addison's disease	
	I = infection, inborn errors or metabolism	Acetazolamide	
	L = lactic acidosis	Enteric fistulas	
	E = ethanol		
	S = salicylates		

Data from Kher K, Sharron M. *Approach to the child with metabolic acidosis.* https://www.uptodate.com/contents/approach-to-the-child-with-metabolic-acidosis#H628739007; 2016.

Endocrine and Metabolic Emergencies

Children presenting with a suspected endocrine or metabolic disorder imparts a challenge for providers if there is no underlying condition, because the signs and symptoms of these disorders are nonspecific and similar to those seen in children experiencing other emergencies. These nonspecific symptoms may lead to a delayed or missed diagnosis resulting in serious morbidities and mortalities such as cerebral dysfunction leading to coma or death, which may be seen in diabetic ketoacidosis (DKA), hypoglycemia, or adrenal insufficiency. See Table 30.13 for signs and symptoms common to these emergencies.[76,77]

Hypoglycemia

Hypoglycemia is when the blood glucose concentration is 60 mg/dL with alterations in LOC occurring with 50 mg/dL in plasma and 44 mg/dL in whole blood. If hypoglycemia

TABLE 30.13	Signs and Symptoms of Pediatric Endocrine and Metabolic Emergencies[77,196]	
CNS Impairment:	**Cardiovascular:**	**Metabolic Acidosis:**
Lethargy		Kussmaul's respirations
Irritability	Tachycardia	Nausea
Tremors	Hypotension	Vomiting
Seizures	Shock	Poor feeding
Altered LOC		Weight loss
Coma		Failure to thrive
Hypotonia		
Cheyne–Stokes respirations		

continues beyond 48 hours it requires an evaluation of the underlying cause. The causes of hypoglycemia are age dependent. Hypoglycemia in children from birth to 6 months of age is the result of an increase in glucose utilization as seen with hyperinsulinism, small-for-gestation age infants, asphyxiated neonates, infants born to diabetic mothers, Beckwith–Wiedemann syndrome, defects in ketone production, carnitine deficiency, inadequate fat stores, infection, or fever. Decreased hepatic glucose are enzyme deficiencies or inadequate glycogen stores, or liver failure. Children 6 months to adolescence experience hypoglycemia either from increased glucose utilization or decreased hepatic glucose production.[76,77]

Treatment

Initial labs are bedside glucose, serum glucose, liver function tests, electrolytes, and urinalysis including ketones. Hypoglycemia treatment is initially nonspecific until the underlying cause is identified. The goal is to restore normal glucose concentrations to support CNS and renal metabolic needs of the child. Emergent treatment is usually 2 to 3 mL/kg of dextrose 10% and ongoing dextrose infusion 5% to 20% to maintain euglycemia. Reassess glucose levels after interventions. More intensive laboratory work is required to diagnose the underlying cause if continues beyond the first 48 hours of life.[76,77]

Adrenal Insufficiency

Adrenal insufficiency causes are either central, which are abnormalities in the hypothalamus or pituitary gland, or primary to the adrenal glands. If a child is receiving steroids to treat asthma, leukemia, organ transplantation, an autoimmune disorder, or replacement steroids for central or primary hypoadrenalism, they are at risk of an adrenal insufficiency crises during an acute, febrile illness. Adrenal insufficiency from any cause results in the inability of the child to maintain electrolyte balance, plasma volume, blood pressure, and glucose levels when experiencing stress, and may have a fatal outcome without glucocorticoid replacement.[76,77]

Treatment

Children with adrenal insufficiency may exhibit weakness, anorexia, vomiting, weight loss, salt craving, and hyperpigmentation. The child with adrenal insufficiency will present with tachycardia; hypotension; and signs of shock including pale color, poor perfusion, cool clammy skin, alterations in LOC, or coma. The comprehensive metabolic panel will demonstrate adrenal insufficiency with hyponatremia, decreased bicarbonate, increased chloride level, a normal AG, metabolic acidosis, and a low glucose level. The initial treatment for children with adrenal insufficiency crisis is to restore tissue perfusion with a 20-mL/kg bolus of normal saline to treat hypotension or dehydration. Hypoglycemia is treated with a glucose bolus of 2 to 3 mL/kg of 10% dextrose and a stress dose of a glucocorticoid such as hydrocortisone 2 to 3 mg/kg.[76,77]

Hyponatremia

Hyponatremia is noted when serum Na^+ is less than 135 mEq/L. Causes of hyponatremia are considered to be disorders of sodium homeostasis when the movement of free water into the extracellular space surpasses its loss. Fundamental causes of hyponatremia include hypovolemic from renal losses caused by diuretics, mineralocorticoid deficiency, renal tubular dysfunction, cerebral salt wasting, vomiting, diarrhea, and burns. Other causes include nephritic syndrome, acute or chronic renal failure, or water intoxication.[76,77]

Treatment

Initial signs and symptoms of hyponatremia are CNS changes from cerebral edema with anorexia, lethargy, or apathy, which may progress to the child being disoriented and agitated and experiencing seizures, Cheyne-Stokes respirations, hyporeflexia, and coma. Neuromuscular weakness and vomiting may be present. The comprehensive metabolic panel is the initial laboratory test. Hyponatremia treatment is usually initiated when the sodium level is below 125 with a hypertonic 3% saline solution of 1-mL/kg per hour IV infusion, which will correct the sodium level by 1 mEq/L per hour and monitor serum sodium levels during infusion.[76,77]

Hypernatremia

Hypernatremia is a disorder of water metabolism. The loss of free water from the kidneys or GI tract exceeding the loss of sodium will lead to hypernatremia. Osmotic dieresis, diabetes insipidus, and gastroenteritis or excessive sodium intake either by mouth or intravenously will lead to hypernatremia. Patients with a normal thirst mechanism rarely experience hypernatremia.[76,77]

Treatment

The signs and symptoms of hypernatremia result from intracellular CNS dehydration. Rapid correction of hypernatremia may result in cerebral edema. It is recommended to correct the serum sodium level slowly by less than 0.5 mEq/L hour to decrease any unwanted side effects. In hypovolemic children, isotonic 0.9% saline is used initially to correct fluid deficits over a 36- to 48-hour period of time and then transition over to 0.45% saline solution for maintenance. If the child is experiencing diabetes insipidus, then the drug of choice is DDVAP. If the child is in a hypervolumic state such as those with Cushing's syndrome, then he or she will require diuretic therapy using hydrochlorothiazide.[76-77]

Diabetic Ketoacidosis

Diabetes mellitus is one of the most common pediatric and adolescent diseases worldwide. A major complication of diabetes is DKA, which is the leading cause of overall morbidity and mortality in children and adolescents with type

1 diabetes. Cerebral edema is the cause of morbidity and mortality in children with DKA. It is estimated that cerebral edema results in less than 1% of all DKA presentations, and 50% to 60% of those children will not survive. DKA is characterized by the metabolic triad of hyperglycemia, AG metabolic acidosis, and ketonemia resulting from an absolute or relative insulin deficiency and an excess of counterregulatory hormone. DKA presents with hyperglycemia leading to osmotic urinary dieresis with subsequent dehydration. The body responds to the dehydration by stimulating a stress response with counterregulatory hormone production, leading to greater insulin resistance, which results in a vicious cycle of hyperglycemia and continued fluid losses. Ultimately DKA causes severe dehydration and electrolyte abnormalities in these children.[78-81]

Clinical Presentation

DKA typically presents with the classic triad of symptoms of polyuria, polydipsia, and weight loss with or without polyphagia. Abdominal pain and nausea and vomiting are also common presenting symptoms. Late signs and symptoms result in changes in mental status; Kussmaul respirations; and fruity, sweet-smelling breath. DKA is diagnosed if a child presents with hyperglycemia with a blood glucose level greater than 200 mg/dL, venous pH less than 7.3 or bicarbonate (HCO_3) concentration less than 15 mmol/L, ketonuria, and ketonemia. DKA severity has three different presenting categories: mild DKA presents with a venous pH less than 7.3 and HCO_3 less than 15 mmol/L, moderate DKA presents with venous pH less than 7.2 and HCO_3 less than 10 mmol/L, and severe DKA presentation is a venous pH less than 7.1 and HCO_3 less than 5 mmol/L.[78-81]

The goal of therapy for DKA is reversal of the ketoacidosis and not the return of glucose levels to normal. Important initial labs are a venous blood gas, complete blood count, comprehensive metabolic panel, and β-hydroxybutyrate or urine ketones. Current practice guidelines recommend pediatric resuscitation if necessary in these patients, obtain IV access, monitor hourly vital signs, neurologic checks, monitor blood glucose, and accurate fluid intake and output. Children with new-onset DKA younger than 5 years of age or with significant acidosis, hypocapnia, or azotemia are at a higher risk of developing cerebral edema. DKA management is fluid resuscitation to rehydrate and improve tissue perfusion and glomerular filtration rate, corrections of ketoacidosis and hyperglycemia through the inhibition of lipolysis and ketogenesis with insulin infusion, restoration of electrolyte balances, and the prevention of complications such as cerebral edema.[78-81]

Treatment

Initial fluid resuscitation in pediatric patient is a 10- to 20-mL/kg fluid bolus over 1 to 2 hours. This dose can be repeated if the patient is hemodynamically unstable. To prevent the risk of cerebral edema and herniation, fluid resuscitation must not go beyond 40 to 50 mL/kg in the first 4 hours of treatment. The total replacement fluids include both maintenance and deficit replacement fluids and should not exceed two times the maintenance rate.[78-81]

Initial replacement fluids are normal saline in pediatric DKA patients. Initially no dextrose is in the replacement fluids, but as the hyperglycemia improves from the insulin infusion, a dextrose infusion is started and titrated to control the drop in the blood glucose levels while maintaining the insulin infusion. If the child's blood glucose is higher than 250 mg/dL, then replacement fluids are only normal saline. Once the blood glucose level falls below 250 mg/dL, replacement fluids should change to a two-bag system with one being normal saline and the other 5% dextrose to slow the decline of the patient's blood glucose levels. If the patient's blood glucose falls below 150 mg/dL, then the dextrose should be changed to 10% solution.[78-81]

Rehydration alone can slowly drop the blood glucose levels in pediatric DKA patients, but an insulin infusion is essential to suppress the lipolysis and ketogenesis that controls DKA. Insulin infusion treatment is started after volume resuscitation has started and initial labs are obtained to know the patient's potassium level. Low-dose insulin infusion at 0.1 units/kg per hour is started and continues at this rate until the ketoacidosis has resolved. The patient's high glucose levels usually will improve or be close to normal before the acidemia resolves. Because of this, the insulin infusion must continue until the ketoacidosis is resolved with a pH greater than 7.3, HCO_3 greater than 15 mmol/L, β-hydroxybutyrate less than 1 mmol/L, and closure of the AG. During fluid replacement for DKA patients, the dextrose fluids are titrated to prevent hypoglycemia from occurring while maintaining the insulin infusion. It is imperative to monitor frequent blood glucose levels and the neurologic status of these children.[78-81]

Congenital Heart Disease

CHD or defects are those present at birth. These defects change the blood flow through the heart and may involve the interior walls of the heart, valves in the heart, or the arteries or veins that carry blood to or away from the heart. CHD may present as a simple heart defect without any presenting symptoms to complex heart defects presenting with life-threatening symptoms. CHD is now the most common type of birth defect. It is estimated that there are close to one million adolescents and young adults worldwide living with CHD.[82-85]

A universal screening tool for newborns for critical CHD is endorsed by the AAP, AHA, and the American College of Cardiology. The Centers for Disease Control and Prevention (CDC) reported in 2015 that almost all states have established legislation, regulation, or hospital guidelines supporting newborn screening for CHD. This tool was designed to screen newborns before discharge using pulse oximetry. Screening should be performed after 24 hours of life or as late as possible before discharging the patient home. Screening performed before 24 hours is not as reliable as later screening because the child may still be in transition from intrauterine to extrauterine conditions. A positive screen indicates the patient needs further evaluation to identify the cause and may require the child be transferred to a designated center capable of treating CHD.[85]

Clinical Presentation

Acyanotic heart defects are defects in which oxygenated blood is shunted from the left (systemic) side of the heart to the right (pulmonary) side. Cyanotic heart defects are defects in which blood from the right (pulmonary) side of the heart mixes with oxygenated blood from the left (systemic) side and enters the systemic circulation. This defect will present itself within minutes of delivery to the first few weeks of life when the patent ductus arteriosus (PDA) closes. The PDA may provide the only means of pulmonary blood flow requiring prostaglandin E1 (PGE) to be started. These defects may require a shunt in the newborn period. The mixing blood flow heart defects may require emergent surgical palliation or surgery to survive. Patients with mixing blood flow heart defects may present extremely ill with severe acidosis and in a shock state, for example, if the child is born with transposition of the great arteries (TGA) and has a patent septum and no septal defect is present. Total anomalous pulmonary venous return (TAPVR) defects are a surgical emergency if the veins are obstructed below the diaphragm and do not allow blood to return to the heart. The child born with left ventricular outflow tract resulting in an obstruction to blood flow out of the heart will be critically ill if the ductus arteriosus has closed. It is imperative that transport providers remember that any neonate presenting in shock that is not responding to airway control, fluid resuscitation, and vasopressors has left ventricular outflow tract obstruction until proven otherwise, and PGE must be started immediately. See Table 30.14 for signs and symptoms of CHD.[82-85]

Acquired Heart Disease

Acquired heart disease occurs after birth and is a result of damage to the heart from an inflammatory process affecting the endocardium, myocardium, pericardium, conduction system, or coronary arteries from a viral or bacterial infection.[82-84]

TABLE 30.14	Congenital Heart Defects, Presenting Signs and Symptoms[82-84]			
Classification	Acyanotic Heart Defects	Cyanotic Heart Defects	Mixed Blood Flow Defects	Obstructive Blood Flow Defects
PBF	Increased PBF	Decreased PBF	Mixed PBF	Left-sided obstructive blood flow
Shunt	Left to right shunting	Right to left shunting	Shunting direction depends on size and pressure in the lungs	Obstructed blood flow
Early signs	Tachypnea caused by excessive PBF	Cyanosis, may present at birth or in first few weeks of life when PDA closes PDA may be only source of PBF	May be a surgical emergency at birth if TGA does not have an ASD or large patent foramen ovale for mixing of blood It is also a surgical emergency in TAPVR if veins are obstructed	Must start PGE immediately or will quickly develop metabolic acidosis and shock if PDA closes
Congenital heart disease	PDA, ASD, VSD, atrioventricular canal defect (atrioventricular canal)	Tricuspid atresia, pulmonary atresia, tetralogy of Fallot, pulmonary stenosis, Ebstein's anomaly	TGA, TAPVR, truncus arteriosus	Coarctation of the aorta, aortic stenosis, interrupted aortic arch, hypoplastic left heart syndrome
Presenting signs and symptoms	Respiratory distress, diaphoresis with feeds or activity, poor weight gain, FTT, enlarged heart, pulmonary edema, CHF	Murmur, tachypnea, shortness of breath, irritable, diaphoresis, difficulty feeding, poor weight gain, FTT, fatigues easily, may need to start PGE to reopen or maintain PDA, CHF, cardiomegaly, arrhythmias	Cyanosis, CHF, murmur may or may not be present, tachypnea, emergent atrial septostomy may be needed to stabilize TGA, may require PGE infusion to open or maintain PDA TGA on chest x-ray may appear as an egg on a string TAPVR may appear as a snowman on chest x-ray	Tachycardia, tachypnea, decreased perfusion, pallor, cyanosis, murmur may or may not be present, CHF, decreased pulses, cardiomegaly on chest x-ray Without PGE to open PDA will quickly deteriorate to metabolic acidosis and shock

ASD, Atrial septal defect; *CHF,* cardiac heart failure; *FTT,* failure to thrive; *PBF,* pulmonary blood flow; *PDA,* patent ductus arteriosus; *PGE,* prostaglandin; *TAPVR,* total anomalous pulmonary venous return; *TGA,* transposition of the great arteries; *VSD,* ventricular septal defect.

Kawasaki Disease

Kawasaki disease (KD) is the leading cause of acquired heart disease in children. There is no definitive test to diagnose KD. The hallmark of KD is fever of at least 5 days, and the presence of four of these symptoms: conjunctivitis; erythema of the lips and oral mucosa; rash; unilateral cervical adenopathy; and erythema to the palms and soles, with induration and desquamation to the fingers. The goal of initial management is to reduce the inflammation and reduce the risk of coronary artery damage or aneurysms. Treatment in the acute phase includes aspirin and IV immunoglobulin.[82-84]

Myocarditis

Myocarditis is an inflammation of the cardiac muscle and the leading cause of dilated cardiomyopathy in children. Congestive heart failure (CHF) is the hallmark sign of myocarditis, and myocarditis is the most common cause of acute CHF. The child has a viral illness 10 to 14 days before onset of symptoms. Treatment is inotropes, afterload reducers, diuretics, antibiotics, and support therapy.[82-84]

Pericarditis

The hallmark of pericarditis is inflammation of the pericardium. The most common cause in infancy is a virus such as coxsackie, AV, or influenza. Acute pericarditis may be secondary to *S. pneumoniae* or *S. aureus*. Postpericardiotomy syndrome occurs following cardiac surgery. Symptoms of acute pericarditis include precordial chest pain made worse by breathing, coughing, or movement; pericardial friction rub; and fever. Treatment requires blood cultures and nonsteroidal antiinflammatory medications to treat discomfort. If an infectious cause is suspected, pericardiocentesis may be required.[82-84]

Endocarditis

Endocarditis is inflammation of the endocardium affecting a valve. Infective endocarditis (IE) is an uncommon but life-threatening infection in children. CHD is a significant risk factor for IE. A fever and murmur are always present. The child usually presents with fulminant disease with a septic appearance. If the patient presents with sepsis, then severe valvular dysfunction, conduction disturbances, or embolic events may occur and empirical antibiotic treatment must be initiated until the specific organism is able to be isolated for appropriate antibiotic treatment.[82-84]

Cardiomyopathy

Cardiomyopathy is disease of the myocardium. The heart muscle becomes abnormally thick, stiff, or enlarged, affecting the heart's ability to pump and maintain its rhythm. Dilated cardiomyopathy is the most common type. The heart becomes enlarged and weakened and has many causes but may be familial. Hypertrophic cardiomyopathy occurs when one or more of the ventricles become thickened, and usually affects adolescents. It is associated with abnormal heart rhythms, and can lead to sudden death. Hypertrophic cardiomyopathy runs in families. Restrictive cardiomyopathy is the rarest form affecting children. The chambers of the heart become stiff, are unable to fill adequately with blood, and have associated abnormal heart rhythms. Symptoms in infants include difficulty breathing, diaphoresis, poor weight gain, and irritability, and older children may have a heart murmur, fatigue, heart palpitations, dizziness, fainting, and difficulty exercising. Treatments include diuretics, fluid restriction, inotropes, antiarrhythmic medications, pacemaker, or a heart transplant.[82-84]

Arrhythmias

Cardiac arrhythmias in children are often caused by an underlying CHD, especially following open heart surgery. Certain CHDs are associated with a higher incidence of cardiac arrhythmias including tetralogy of Fallot, corrected TGA, TAPVR, large atrial and ventricular septal defects, atrioventricular canals, aortic and subaortic stenosis, and congenital mitral stenosis. The most common postoperative arrhythmias include supraventricular tachycardia, ventricular tachycardia, sick sinus syndrome, and complete heart block. Other causes of arrhythmias in children include congenital complete heart block, Wolff-Parkinson-White syndrome and long QT syndrome. Acquired heart diseases associated with arrhythmias include viral myocarditis, KD, and cardiomyopathies.[82-84]

Congestive Heart Failure

CHF occurs when the cardiovascular system is unable to deliver oxygen and nutrients to the tissues at a rate that meets the metabolic demands, or the supply is inadequate for demand. CHF affects preload, afterload, contractility, and heart rate. CHD is the most common cause of CHF in children. Symptoms of CHF include poor feeding, which is a red flag to the provider; the patient is diaphoretic and tachypneic with feeds; slow weight gain or FTT; and small for age. Symptoms include tachypnea, retractions, nasal flaring, cardiomegaly, hepatomegaly, tachycardia with weak pulses, diaphoresis, cool extremities, a gallop, pulmonary effusions, and decreased urine output. Treatment of CHF includes decreasing oxygen consumption with bed rest, sedations, nutrition, antipyretics, and if necessary mechanical ventilation to improve oxygen delivery to the body. Medical management includes medications to increase contractility of the heart such as digoxin, decreasing workload, diuretics, and milrinone. If these are ineffective, surgical intervention may be required.[82-84]

Advanced Trauma Life Support: ABCDEs of Trauma Care

American College of Surgeons (ACS) established the systematic approach for the rapid assessment of traumatic injuries and implementation of lifesaving interventions of the patient's identified injuries, vital signs, and mechanism of injury (MOI). The systematic approach involves a rapid primary survey to identify life-threatening injuries, resuscitation, secondary survey, and the initiation of definitive care. This process is considered to be the ABCDEs of trauma care, and it helps the provider to identify life-threatening injuries by using the following sequence:

A: Airway maintenance with cervical spine protection
B: Breathing and ventilation
C: Circulation with hemorrhage control
D: Disability–neurologic status
E: Exposure/environmental control

This process was initially developed for the adult trauma patient, but the principles of the ABCDEs of initial assessment are the same for children.[3,86]

Pediatric Trauma

Pediatric trauma is the leading cause of morbidity and mortality in children over 1 year of age. Head injuries are the most common injury reported. Motor vehicle collisions (MVCs) are the leading cause of severe pediatric trauma and deaths. Research, education, and injury prevention programs designed to decrease pediatric-related trauma injuries including MVCs and related injuries are a priority for trauma centers, regulatory governmental agencies, trauma support groups and societies, and the automotive industry.[87-89]

Physiologic and Psychological Considerations

Almost all medical transport providers have heard about how children are not smaller versions of adults but rather unique and continually evolving. A child's anatomic, physiologic, and psychological differences separate them considerably from the adult. The unique anatomic and physiologic differences in children as well as the severity of injuries support the need for children to be transported to facilities that are experienced; that have pediatric-appropriate equipment; and that are capable of recognizing, diagnosing, and treating pediatric traumatic injuries and embrace family presence. Research studies have demonstrated an increase in survival rates and decreases in mortality and morbidities when pediatric patients are treated at pediatric trauma centers (PTCs) or adult trauma centers with pediatric capabilities.[87-89]

Size and Body Surface Area

A significant physical characteristic of children is their smaller size, which exposes their vulnerability. The intense energy transferred from falls, car bumpers, or any form of blunt force trauma results in a greater force applied per unit of body area in children. This is because children have smaller total body mass, lesser amounts of elastic connective tissue, a pliable skeleton, and a compact location of internal organs. These features have been shown to increase the incidence of multiple organ injuries in children. Children have thinner skin, less subcutaneous tissue, and a higher body surface area to mass ratio compared with adults. These factors result in an increased thermal energy loss and reduces the child's ability to autoregulate his or her temperature or maintain normothermic. Brief exposure can quickly lead to hypothermia, which can prolong coagulation, alter CNS function, and increase the risk of mortality in pediatric trauma.[87-90]

Skeletal Structure

Children have pliable incomplete calcification of their skeletons and many active growth plates. The pliability of the pediatric patients' skeletal structures may result in their internal organs being injured without damage to the overlying bony structures. An example would be the pediatric patient presenting with a pulmonary contusion from blunt force trauma in the absence of any rib fractures. Pediatric patients have many active growth centers or plates, which if injured, require a pediatric orthopedic surgeon consult to prevent any long-term morbidities. A child should be suspected of having significant trauma to underlying organs and structures if skeletal thoracic fractures are identified because it takes a massive amount of energy to inflect these fractures.[87-89]

Psychological Status

Interacting with pediatric patients requires the provider to understand age-appropriate developmental levels and key milestones. It is crucial for providers to interact with injured children according to their developmental level. An ill or injured child may regress to an earlier developmental stage. Interactions with children should be based on the developmental level depicted. Medical transport providers should become familiar with normal developmental milestones in children so they will know when the child is age appropriate or regressing developmentally from the stressful event (see Table 30.1 and Table 30.2).[3,89-91]

Evidence has demonstrated that family presence during resuscitation and invasive procedures is beneficial to patients and their families. Family presence at a child's bedside meets the psychological needs of the patient in a time of crisis and helps the parents to understand the severity of their child's condition and witness all the efforts by the medical team to help their child. Family presence has been shown to improve medical decision making, patient care, communication with the health care team, and patient and family satisfaction.[92-93]

Approximately 200,000 specialty neonatal and pediatric critical care transports occur each year, making family-centered care a relevant issue. A majority of pediatric critical care transport teams support parents going along with their child on ground transports, but because of aircraft performance issues with weight and balance, configuration, or individual program policy constraints, a smaller number of transport programs allow parents on air medical transports. Parental accompaniment has now become a measure of quality on pediatric critical care transports.[92,93]

Long-Term Effects of Traumatic Injury

Long-term quality of life in children following traumatic injuries, and the subsequent effects on their growth and development, is a significant concern. Pediatric patients have to recuperate from a traumatic injury as well as continue the process of normal growth and development. The physiologic and psychological effects of traumatic injuries may impact the child's long-term quality of life, especially if the injury affects physical characteristics by altering functionality and growth, leaving physical scars, or causing traumatic brain injury (TBI) type changes cognitively and behaviorally. Evidence has shown children may have alterations in cognition and behavioral changes up to a year following an injury. Social, affective, and learning disabilities are present in a large number of seriously injured children. Data have shown that up to 25% of children in an MVC experience posttraumatic stress disorder. Most children and their parents will experience resolution of mild trauma symptoms without the need for psychological or psychiatric treatment. However, traumatic experiences can impact children and their families long after the actual event. Some children and their families may benefit from psychosocial support or interventions. Pediatric injuries and hospitalizations also create a considerable burden on parents and siblings including financial burdens, time away from work, and separation from their other children. All medical facilities should have a multidisciplinary team of social workers, child life specialists, psychiatrists, psychologists, and chaplains to help patients and their families deal with the long-term after effects of traumatic experience.[3,86,89,94-95]

Primary Survey

The goal of the primary survey is to rapidly survey the injured child to identify underlying injuries and reverse potential life-threatening conditions. During the primary survey, the assessment and management are the same for adults and children. The differences include the amount of blood, fluids, and medications; size of the child; degree and swiftness of heat loss; and injury patterns. The ABCDE algorithm identifies life-threatening injuries by following the sequence in order of airway maintenance with cervical spine protection, breathing and ventilation, circulation with hemorrhage control, disability and neurologic status, and exposure/environmental control including complete removal of clothes to expose the patient and prevent hypothermia. The primary survey includes frequent reassessments following interventions to confirm or exclude injuries requiring immediate intervention. Remember to consider the pediatric patient's unique physiologic and anatomic differences because they are essential for proper assessment and treatment.[3,86,89]

Airway and Cervical Spine Protection

Airway patency is critical to prevent severe morbidities and mortalities in the pediatric patient. Airway management is an initial step in stabilizing the pediatric trauma patient. Achieving adequate airway control is necessary to adequately oxygenate and ventilate the pediatric patient while decreasing potential for aspiration. Failure to provide early and aggressive airway management in children leads to hypoxia, respiratory failure, and arrest.[3,7,86,89,96]

An open airway is the number one priority in the initial assessment. The pediatric airway is anatomically different from the adult airway. The child's larger tongue and the position of the larynx being anterior and more cephalic in the neck increases the level of difficulty during laryngoscopy compared with adults. Children have a disproportion between the size of the head and midface. The child's large occiput forces passive flexion of the cervical spine while the child is lying supine, and the airway is more likely to be compromised and obstructed. In the absence of trauma, the pediatric patients' airways are best protected by placing them in the "sniffing" position, which is a slightly superior and anterior position of the midface. In the presence of trauma, the "neutral" position best protects both the cervical spine and ensures adequate airway opening. Placing a towel or blanket of approximately 2- to 3-cm thickness under the shoulders and posterior thorax will help the child achieve a more anatomically neutral position (Fig. 30.4). In the pediatric trauma patient, the neck should be kept immobilized to prevent hyperextension at the C1-C2 and prevent hyperflexion at C5-C6. With traumatic injuries, manual stabilization of the cervical spine should be maintained during airway management and until the child is immobilized. (Immobilization of the cervical spine is addressed later in the chapter.)[3,7,86,89,96]

The airway in the unresponsive child should be opened using the jaw thrust without head tilt maneuver to open the airway while a team member maintains manual stabilization to protect the cervical spine. If the child is unconscious, an oropharyngeal airway will give support to keep

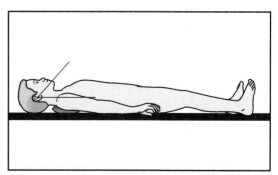

• **Fig. 30.4** Neutral positioning of a child on a backboard for proper alignment.

the tongue out of the hypopharynx but may cause vomiting if the child has an intact gag reflex. An oral airway should be placed with direct visualization with a tongue blade to prevent oral trauma and bleeding.[3,7,30,86,89,96]

Once the airway is opened and suctioned for debris or secretions, supplemental oxygen should be provided. Patients with inadequate respiratory rates, impaired ventilation, or an inability to protect the airway from secretions or emesis should have the airway protected with ETI. BVM ventilation with 100% oxygen is the best method to use initially to provide assist ventilations in the unresponsive child while preparing for ETI. The transport provider should remember the best airway in a child is one you can oxygenate and ventilate. Research has demonstrated there is no clear neurologic or survivable advantage between ETI and BVM in pediatric patients 12 years of age or younger in the prehospital setting. According to the 2015 AHA guidelines, BVM ventilation may be effective and safer than ETI for short transport times or short out-of-hospital resuscitation.[3,6-9,16-17,19,28,29,31,86]

Nonelective nasal intubations should not be performed on children younger than 12 years of age because of the acute angle to the glottis. This makes this procedure extremely difficult for maintaining a neutral cervical spine position. Needle (<5 years of age or Seldinger technique >5 years of age) or surgical (children older than 10 years of age) cricothyroidotomy may be necessary to control the child's airway if intubation is unsuccessful or facial trauma prevents ETI.[3,28,29,32]

Rapid sequence induction standardized medication protocols exist for the majority of transport programs to simplify rapid sequence intubation and allow efficient airway management of the critically injured child. Pediatric patients are at risk of rapid deterioration during intubation with an increased risk of bradycardia with desaturation for prolonged attempts. These standardized protocols outline the use of IV medications to facilitate ETI while avoiding potential complications associated with induction, such as bradycardia and desaturations.[3,28,29,86,96]

Currently the National Association of EMS Physicians (NAEMSP), ACEP, and ACS Committee on Trauma (COT) support the use of drug-assisted intubation in the prehospital environment. Differences continue to exist between transport programs concerning which rapid sequence intubation medications are the best or preferred for children who have suffered traumatic injuries.[3,26,28,29,86,95-96]

It is necessary to have an accurate patient weight to provide proper medication dosages during the rapid sequence intubation procedure. Infants and children have a pronounced vagal response to ETI, and many rapid sequence intubation protocols use atropine sulfate at the initial medication to block the vagal response to laryngoscopy.[3,26,28,29,86,95-96]

Hypoxia is a major cause of bradycardia in the pediatric patient, which is another reason preoxygenation is performed in children. Bradycardia should be treated rapidly during any airway procedure using the BVM for assisted ventilation with supplemental oxygen and atropine, if not already administered. Atropine is followed by a short-acting sedative and a short-acting neuromuscular blocking agent. Several rapid sequence intubation medications fulfill these requirements and can be safely used in children. The medications used in rapid sequence intubation and management of the pediatric airway were discussed in more detail earlier in this chapter.[3,26,28,29,86,95-96]

Rescue airways such as the esophageal obturator or the Combitube are not usually recommended in the pediatric population because of limited patient-appropriate sizes. Supraglottic airways have increased in popularity and use in the prehospital setting because of ease of use, relatively simple training, dependability, and quick insert. Supraglottic devices do not offer a definitive airway in the prehospital setting; however, newer more advanced second-generation devices are offering greater seal pressures and the capacity to decompress gastric secretions, which decreases potential aspiration. Supraglottic devices are usually not used as rescue devices in the prehospital setting. Supraglottic devices were discussed in more detail earlier in the chapter.[3,26-28,30,86]

ETI is the most reliable method of establishing a secure airway and oxygenating and ventilating a pediatric trauma patient. ETI indications, procedure, and new AHA and PALS recommendations for cuffed or uncuffed ETT use with pediatric trauma patients was discussed in detail earlier in this chapter.[9,17]

Breathing

After control of the airway and cervical spine immobilization has been achieved, attention is then turned to oxygenation and ventilation of the pediatric trauma patient. All trauma patients need supplemental oxygen. Evaluation of the child's respiratory status and the ability to recognize early signs of distress are essential in the management of the pediatric trauma patient because subtle findings of respiratory distress are often missed. The patient's respiratory rate is the first assessment step when evaluating respiratory status. Children have varying normal rates of respiration that decrease with age. It is important to know what the normal respiratory rates are for the different pediatric ages. For example, a healthy infant breathes 40 to 60 times per minute, whereas an older child will have normal respiratory rates of 20 breaths/min. Tachypnea is an early but nonspecific sign of respiratory distress. Bradypnea is a late sign of distress and often signifies impending cardiopulmonary arrest. Hypoxia is the most common cause of respiratory arrest in children.

When viewed with other physical findings, the assessment of a child's respiratory rate provides a much more accurate assessment of the overall respiratory status.[3,86,89]

A child's work of breathing increases with respiratory distress. Increased work of breathing in children may present with any of the following clinical signs and symptoms:

- Nasal flaring
- Retractions: intercostals, subcostal, substernal, clavicular, supraclavicular
- Head bobbing

- Grunting
- Tripod positioning
- Stridor
- Snoring
- Altered respiratory rate: tachypnea, bradypnea, or apnea
- Adventitious breath sounds: wheezing, rales, or rhonchi
- Paradoxical respirations: seesaw respirations
- Pallor
- Decreased gag reflex
- Decreased or absent breath sounds
- Cyanosis, which is a late sign of distress

Any of these changes calls for supplemental oxygen support and, depending on the severity of the child's respiratory distress, may necessitate BVM ventilations or advanced airway control with ETT.[3,86,89]

Selected Traumatic Injuries Contributing to Respiratory Distress

Chest trauma accounts for approximately 10% of all trauma affecting children. However, it is quite significant because of the considerable mortality associated with it. Chest trauma is either nonpenetrating or blunt (does not involve opening the chest) and usually involves a high-energy impact to multiple areas of the body or penetrating trauma (causes an open wound). More than 80% of pediatric thoracic trauma results from blunt injury.[3,86,97]

Injuries as a result of blunt force chest trauma can be classified into the four types:

1. Chest wall injuries causing rib fractures, sternal fractures, or a flail chest
2. Pulmonary injuries causing pulmonary contusion, pneumothorax, hemothorax, tracheobronchial disruption, or diaphragmatic injury
3. Cardiovascular injuries resulting in myocardial contusion, cardiac tamponade or rupture, aortic disruption, or pulmonary vascular injury
4. Esophageal injuries including an esophageal rupture

Chest trauma is second only to head injuries as a cause of accidental death in children. The physiologic differences in pediatric patients change the patterns of injury. Chest or thoracic trauma is a common cause of respiratory distress in children. The compliant nature of the pediatric thoracic cage allows for significant blunt force trauma that apparently compresses the ribs and sternum without any fractures, which allows the transfer of high-energy trauma to a child's internal structures and organs. The most common pattern of pediatric chest trauma is a high-energy blow that may involve other regions of the body. Over half of children with chest trauma also have head, abdominal, and limb injuries. The elastic consistency of the ribs protects children from sustaining rib fractures or mediastinal injury or it may decrease rib fractures from occurring; thus, rib and mediastinal fractures are uncommon in children. The provider should be concerned about the underlying organs if rib fractures are present. The thinness of the chest wall may cause the respiratory assessment to be more difficult because breath sounds may be referred from one area of the chest to another, making diagnosis more difficult. The mobility of the mediastinal structures increases the susceptibility of pediatric patients to develop a tension pneumothorax. Pneumomediastinum is rare and relatively benign in the majority of pediatric cases.[3,86,97]

Tension Pneumothorax

A tension pneumothorax occurs when air enters into the pleural space on inspiration and is unable to escape on expiration. The air leaks into the thorax and pressures rise rapidly affecting ventilation on that side, which relocates the mediastinum toward the contralateral side and the pressure then interferes with venous return. Tension pneumothorax presents with distension of the hemithorax, dyspnea, hypotension, absence of breath sounds, and hyperresonance together on the affected side, with increased jugular venous pressure, cyanosis, and tracheal deviation (which is a late sign). Subcutaneous emphysema may be noted with tactile examination of the chest. Intubation with mechanical ventilation may increase risk of a tension pneumothorax because PPV increases intrathoracic pressure. Tension pneumothoraces are diagnosed clinically indicating emergent intervention without the delay of CXR confirmation.[3,86,97-98]

Treatment for Tension Pneumothorax

Adequate treatment can be a needle decompression followed by a chest tube or insertion of the chest tube. The most common initial treatment is a needle decompression with a large-bore IV catheter placed into the intrapleural space at the second intercostal space midclavicular line of the affected side of the chest. The placement of an age-appropriate size chest tube at the fifth intercostal space at the anterior midaxillary line on the affected side is the definitive treatment. Chest tubes should have a one-way flutter valve attached or be placed to water seal drainage to prevent reaccumulation of air. Tension pneumothoraces should always be treated before transport.[3,86,97-98]

Simple Pneumothorax

A simple pneumothorax may be caused by either blunt or penetrating trauma. In pediatric patients, a simple pneumothorax occurs in the absence of rib fractures from blunt trauma occurring during inspiration when the glottis is closed causing an abrupt increase in the intrathoracic alveolar pressure and subsequent alveolar rupture. The lung will collapse when air enters the potential space between the visceral and parietal pleura. As the lung tissue collapses, a ventilation and perfusion are affected because blood perfusing the collapsed area is no longer oxygenated. Signs and symptoms of a simple pneumothorax are dyspnea, decreased or absent breath sounds on the affected side, hyperresonance on the affected side, and chest pain that radiates to the shoulder area. Respiratory distress may be present or develop over time or with ascent in a fixed-wing aircraft. Subcutaneous emphysema may be present with tactile examination of the chest.[3,97-98]

Treatment for Simple Pneumothorax

Treatment of a simple pneumothorax consists of the placement of an age- and size-appropriate chest tube in the fifth intercostal space at the anterior midaxillary line on the affected side. Chest tubes should be attached to one-way flutter valves or water seal drainage to prevent reaccumulation of air. A suspected simple pneumothorax without signs of severe respiratory or cardiovascular compromise should be evaluated by CXR secondary to other conditions (e.g., traumatic diaphragmatic hernia) and may have similar clinical findings. All pneumothoraces greater than 20% or any pneumothoraces present in patients who are intubated and on mechanical ventilation or will need PPV should be treated with a chest tube before transport or ascending in an air medical transport vehicle.[3,97-98]

Open Pneumothorax

An open pneumothorax occurs when a penetrating injury allows free movement of air in and out of the pleural space causing collapse of the lung with impaired ventilation. An open pneumothorax is characterized by the presence of a penetrating chest wound, dyspnea, chest pain, and hyperresonance and decreased breath sounds over the affected side of the chest. An audible "sucking" sound may be heard during inspiration and expiration.[3,97-98]

Treatment for Open Pneumothorax

Treatment for an open pneumothorax requires treatment for both the lung collapse and the penetrating chest wound. A sterile occlusive dressing, taped on three sides, should be immediately placed over the wound. The dressing is taped on three sides to allow for venting of the pleural space by lifting the dressing should reaccumulation of air in the pleural air occur. If untreated, reaccumulation of pleural air can lead to a tension pneumothorax. After the wound is treated, a chest tube should be inserted as discussed previously to treat lung collapse and prevent a tension pneumothorax during transport. A chest tube should be placed remotely from the penetrating wound to decrease the risk of intrathoracic infection and initiate antimicrobial treatment.[3,97-98]

Hemothorax

Hemothorax occurs when blood collects in the pleural space from either blunt or penetrating trauma. The most common causes are lung laceration or laceration of an intercostal vessel producing a potential severe or massive hemothorax, which would require immediate drainage and a possible blood transfusion in pediatric patients. Massive hemothorax of this type is rare in children. Hemorrhage exceeding 20% to 25% of the child's blood volume not only will cause hypovolemic shock but also restricts the intrathoracic space, necessitating an intervention. Blood losses of 4% per hour require surgical intervention, but this rarely occurs in pediatric patients. Signs and symptoms of a hemothorax present with dyspnea, chest pain, decreased or absent breath sounds over the affected side, and dullness to percussion on the affected side of the chest. Tachycardia; tachypnea; cool, pale, diaphoretic skin; and hypotension (signs of shock) may also be present.[3,86,97-98]

Treatment for Hemothorax

Management of hemothorax should begin with resuscitative efforts with oxygenation, ventilation, control of external bleeding, and fluid resuscitation if needed. Aggressive fluid resuscitation can dilute the remaining blood and clotting factors, which interferes with the body's ability to form clots, control bleeding, and hemostasis. Once a hemothorax exceeds 20% to 25% of the child's blood volume mark, signs of hypovolemic shock will be present. Initial treatment may be intubation and mechanical ventilation, and the placement of age- and size-appropriate chest tube placed in the fifth intercostal space of the anterior midaxillary line. The chest tube then needs to be placed to water seal drainage with suction. These interventions will allow time for transport to a surgical center or for the decision for an emergent thoracotomy. This rarely occurs in pediatric patients. A venous hemorrhage may stop with an increase in intrathoracic pressures, which will allow the patient to stabilize without surgical intervention. Remember that clamping the chest tube is a temporary measure until an emergent open thoracotomy can be performed. Fluid resuscitation for blood loss may be needed.[3,86,97-99]

Flail Chest

The elasticity of children's ribs protects against fractures, even in the presence of significant energy transfer or blunt force trauma. A significant blunt force causing multiple adjacent rib fractures in several places along the chest wall allowing a segment of the chest to move separating from one another is a rare incident in pediatric trauma but may be the most common severe pediatric injury providers treat. Multiple and extensive rib fractures damage the rigidity of the rib case and produce a flail chest. A flail chest leads to paradoxical respiratory effort in which the thoracic wall collapses during inspiration and compromises gas exchange. It may be rare in pediatric patients but usually has underlying lung involvement or damage when it does occur. A flail chest may occur more often in older adolescents. In addition to the paradoxical chest wall movement on the affected segment during inspiration and expiration, chest pain, dyspnea, hypoxia, and cyanosis are present.[3,97-100]

Treatment for Flail Chest

A flail chest in pediatric patients is often diagnosed by CXR. CT of the chest may be indicated to assess the extent of underlying injuries. Most rib fractures do not require specific interventions except for pain control and supportive interventions. However, when the rib cage is unstable in children presenting with multiple fractures in multiple places, it may be helpful to use adhesive bandages or other methods in an attempt to make the chest wall more rigid and prevent the paradoxical movements. If this method is ineffective, and a flail chest cannot be stabilized, the child will require intubation and mechanical ventilation, which is the only intervention to preserve adequate gas exchange. Management focuses on supportive measures to control pain and prevent atelectasis and pneumonia. The underlying pulmonary contusion associated with flail chest is a major concern in pediatric patients. These injuries can be difficult to manage because the contusion to the lungs are sensitive to being over and under resuscitated.[3,97-100]

Pulmonary Contusion

Pulmonary contusion and lacerations are the most common pediatric thoracic injuries. Pulmonary contusion can occur in the absence of overlying rib fractures and is an injury resulting from direct compression of the parenchyma by a significant blunt force high-energy trauma or the violent displacement of the lung, which can lead to more severe life-threatening injuries. A pulmonary contusion can occur even in the absence of rib fractures. Pulmonary contusion occurs when kinetic energy from some form of blunt force is transferred to a child's chest wall damaging the lung parenchyma. This results in damage to the alveolar spaces, hemorrhage, and edema, and the contusion may interfere with gas exchange affecting the respiratory status of the child. Damage to the child's lung includes alveolar collapse from extravasation of fluid into the interstitium and inactivation of surfactant as well as ventilation-perfusion mismatch, which causes hypoxia. If left untreated, respiratory arrest may occur. Presenting symptoms of a pulmonary contusion in children includes dyspnea, tachypnea, bloody sputum, and possibly obvious chest wall injuries. Clinical appreciation of pulmonary contusions on examination may be difficult; however, the provider should maintain a high index of suspicion for pediatric patients with thoracic injuries or those involved in rapid deceleration injuries. Radiographic changes may not appear until 24 hours after injury. Pulmonary contusions can be reabsorbed and the lung repaired after several days, but this can cause substantial damage, which may increase the risk of an infection. If the child also has a lung laceration with the contusion, it is usually associated with air leaks, pneumothorax, and eventually a hemothorax.[3,97-100]

Treatment for Pulmonary Contusion

Pulmonary contusion treatment management in children centers around the oxygenation, ventilation, cardiovascular support, and the immediate management of life-threatening injuries. Initially, pulmonary contusions in children may be associated with significant MOIs and multiorgan involvement, and the initial assessment may require life-threatening

complications to be addressed. Pulmonary contusions may not be symptomatic and present with a normal CXR that is not indicative of a contusion. When the child presents asymptomatic, this phase deteriorates within 24 to 72 hours from the initial traumatic event and diagnosis is made by CXR and the child exhibiting signs of respiratory distress.[3,97-100]

Complications associated with pulmonary contusion are pneumonia or acute respiratory distress syndrome. Diagnosis may be made if the provider is highly suspicious for a significant MOI to the chest, or the child is complaining of chest pain and tenderness, or if external contusions are noted. These symptoms and injuries are associated with additional internal injuries such as a pneumothorax or hemothorax. Most pulmonary contusions are scarcely symptomatic by themselves. In these rare situations, the affected area is large and will limit gas exchange surface area resulting in hypoxia, hypercarbia, and acidosis.[3,97-100]

Definitive treatment of pulmonary contusion in children is supportive with rigorous monitoring for respiratory deterioration, supplemental oxygen, assisted ventilations, and other supportive interventions such as pain control, inhaled nitric oxide, and positioning. There is limited evidence demonstrating any benefits of broad-spectrum antibiotic administration to prevent an infection from damaged lung tissue, but it is widely accepted and ordered. Extracorporeal membrane oxygenation (ECMO) is regarded as a supportive therapy for pulmonary contusions in those pediatric patients unable to oxygenate and ventilate to prevent further lung damage from barotraumas.[3,97-101]

Diaphragmatic Rupture

Traumatic diaphragmatic rupture (TDR) usually results from blunt or penetrating injuries to the upper abdomen or lower thorax resulting in rupture or herniation of the diaphragm. It is a relatively uncommon injury in pediatric patients but should be considered in cases of thoracoabdominal injury. TDR commonly affects the left side more frequently because the internal structures on the left side are weaker and the liver offers extra protection and support to the right hemidiaphragm. On rare occasions a penetrating instrument may tear the diaphragm directly, but more often TDR is a result of high-energy blunt force trauma to thoracoabdominal structures. Blunt force trauma severe enough to tear the diaphragm usually has spleen or liver involvement. Diagnosis of TDR is often difficult because the signs may not stand out on CXRs, the presenting symptoms may resemble other conditions or injuries, or the severity of the other injuries distracts the provider from detecting diaphragmatic injuries. Rapid diagnosis and identification of TDR injuries and any other associated injuries are essential to prevent life-threatening herniation from the abdominal organs being pushed into the thorax causing lung compression, shifting of mediastinal structures, obstruction, ischemia, sepsis, and death. TDR is characterized by dyspnea, dysphagia, chest pain, sharp shoulder pain, auscultation of bowel sounds over the lower thorax, and decreased breath sounds over the affected side of the chest.[3,97,99-100,102]

Treatment for Diaphragmatic Rupture

Pediatric traumatic rupture of the diaphragm is a rare event that occurs more often on the left side and always requires surgical treatment. CXR and multidetector CT (MDCT) are the most commonly used modalities used to diagnose TDR. The definitive treatment for diaphragmatic rupture is surgical repair. Clinical support with intubation, mechanical ventilation, and gastric decompression are necessary before transport or surgical intervention. Adequate gastric decompression must be provided to these patients during air medical transports. The definitive treatment for TDR is surgical repair.[3,97,99-100,102]

Tracheobronchial Injuries

Tracheobronchial ruptures (TBRs) caused by blunt chest trauma are rare but potentially fatal in pediatric patients. TBRs are life-threatening ruptures of the trachea or bronchi usually located between the cricoid cartilage and the carina or division of the bronchi. The majority of these injuries are a result of blunt force trauma, usually from MVCs. The elasticity of the thoracic cage of young children protects them from sustaining injuries to the external chest wall. However, in the presence of severe blunt force trauma, the child's intrathoracic structures may be compressed without any external evidence of injury. High-energy blunt force trauma or crush syndrome can cause a rapid increase in tracheobronchial pressure and may account for the blowout perforation of the trachea without the presence of rib or sternal fractures. The majority of tracheal injuries occur close to the carina with the right mainstem bronchus affected more frequently than the left. Major tracheobronchial injuries are life-threatening, resulting in severe respiratory distress and hemodynamic instability requiring rapid interventions. Any damage to the tracheobronchial wall permits air leaks, which potentially can present as a tension pneumothorax, pneumomediastinum, and subcutaneous emphysema. Presenting signs and symptoms of tracheobronchial injury may include dyspnea; hemoptysis; coughing; palpable subcutaneous emphysema of the neck, face, and thoracic areas; respiratory distress; absent breath sounds on the affected side of the chest; a persistent air leak from a pneumothorax that reaccumulates after insertion of chest tube. Hamman's sign, a crunching or rasping sound auscultated over the precordium synchronized with the patient's heartbeat, may also be appreciated with mediastinal emphysema. The transport provider should suspect tracheobronchial injury in a child if, after successful chest tube placement, a pneumothorax reaccumulates after chest tube insertion while continuing to water seal drainage and suction.[3,97-99,101,103]

Treatment for Tracheobronchial Injuries

Pediatric patients with major tracheobronchial trauma usually die from associated injurie before reaching the hospital.

This injury's initial clinical presentation may be inconsistent and vague making management extremely difficult or the child presents in severe cardiopulmonary distress. Prompt recognition, diagnosis, and surgical treatment are essential prognostic indicators for survival in these rare injuries with high mortality rates. Manage the patient's airway with intubation and mechanical ventilation, and begin resuscitation for hemodynamic instabilities. Perform needle decompression for tension pneumothoraces, and chest tube placement for drainage is indicated. A persistent, large-volume air leak in spite of adequate chest drainage is a significant indicator for a large tracheobronchial tear or injury. A large tracheobronchial tear could develop a massive pneumothorax and become a life-threatening event. In these cases, air under tension accumulates not only in the pleural space, but also in the mediastinum and neck and even in the subcutaneous tissue. A CXR is the most informative diagnostic tool for this injury. Any disturbance of the tracheobronchial air column, massive atelectasis, deep cervical emphysema, and pneumomediastinum, in association with the pneumothorax, are highly suggestive of a severe TBR. The fallen lung sign is pathognomonic of a total rupture of one of the main pulmonary bronchi. A critical diagnostic tool for diagnosing TBR is bronchoscopy. It should be performed by experienced thoracic surgeons or pulmonologists and remains the gold standard for establishing this diagnosis. All of these patients must be closely monitored for reaccumulation of air that may result in a tension pneumothorax during transport. If after chest tube and ventilation management fails to reestablish patient stability, ECMO heart and lung supportive therapy may be used for ventilatory support in the absence of severe bleeding or intracranial hemorrhage. Surgical intervention for repair of TBR injuries is necessary.[3,97-99,101,103]

Sternal Fractures and Rib Fractures

The elasticity and flexibility of the thoracic cage protects children from being subjected to chest wall injuries such as a rib fractures, flail chest, or sternal fractures. Rib and sternal fractures are rather rare in children but are seen in adolescent patients. Infants presenting with rib fractures should raise a red flag for the provider to consider child abuse. Infants presenting with rib fractures from suspected child abuse are a result of an anteroposterior compression of the chest seen in the shaken and squeezed child. A single or isolated rib fracture is not a common occurrence in children and should be investigated further by the provider for associated or underlying injuries because of the significant blunt energy transfer needed to accomplish this injury.[3,97,99-100,104-105]

Blunt force trauma or compression of the chest causes rib fractures in children. Rib fractures in children are associated with an increased risk of severe injuries, and the transport provider should be prepared to manage the potential for severe internal injuries. Rib fractures from blunt force trauma may puncture the pleural cavity, resulting in a pneumothorax, or lacerate the intercostal artery, an internal mammary gland, or the lung parenchyma, which may result in a hemothorax. Rib fractures from blunt trauma cause more internal injuries in children compared with compression injuries. Chest wall compression resulting in rib fractures presents with lateral segments of the ribs fracturing outward. Fractures of the sternum are rarely seen or occur in children. It takes a substantial blunt force to the chest of a child for this injury to occur. The transport provider should be cognizant of damage to underlying internal structures of children presenting with rib and or sternal injuries or fractures. Cardiac contusions, pulmonary contusions, and aortic injuries may be detected with sternal and/or rib fractures. Rib fractures in children are a common source of pain and discomfort, affecting the depth and quality of the child's respiratory effort, and splinting of respirations, dyspnea, ecchymosis, and possibly crepitus may be seen. Sooner or later, untreated rib fractures will damage underlying structures.[3,97,99-100,104-105]

Treatment Sternal Fractures and Rib Fractures

It is essential to control the pain of children presenting with rib or sternal fractures. These children may require ventilatory support, and will need a physical examination and diagnostic testing to evaluate underlying structure damage. A CXR is usually an adequate diagnostic tool to identify rib fractures. The oblique views may help identify nonaccidental injury and should be considered if child abuse is suspected. CT of the chest should be considered to rule out intrathoracic injuries if the child has first rib fractures, sternal fractures, and posterior sternoclavicular fracture dislocations.[3,97,99-100,104-105]

Laryngotracheal Injuries

Pediatric laryngotracheal injuries result from blunt neck trauma and are extremely rare in children. Presenting symptoms in children may be nonspecific and without the provider suspecting this diagnosis early it is easily overlooked, especially in those presenting with multisystem injury involvement. Laryngotracheal injuries are potentially fatal in children if the provider fails to recognize it early and initiate appropriate interventions. The incidence of pediatric neck trauma with motor vehicle accidents is increasing in the pediatric population from rapid deceleration. Other MOIs for pediatric laryngotracheal trauma include clothesline injuries to the neck while riding motorcycles, all-terrain vehicles, and snowmobiles when the child strikes a stationary object. Also, high-impact sports and martial arts can cause a clothesline injury. Other MOIs include direct trauma to the neck form fists, feet, or blunt weapons, or strangulation from hanging, ligature suffocation, or manual choking, and falls.[106-107]

Treatment of Laryngotracheal Injuries

The signs and symptoms of laryngotracheal injuries include hoarseness, dysphonia, aphonia, odynophagia, dysphagia, cervical tenderness, cervical crepitus, hemoptysis, stridor, and respiratory distress. It is important to determine when managing a suspected laryngotracheal trauma whether the child is stable or unstable. An injury classification exists for laryngotracheal injuries from group one, which includes minor hematoma without fracture, to group five, which includes a complete laryngotracheal separation. Children who are unstable with laryngotracheal trauma or suspected trauma may be in respiratory distress and require interventions. The provider should use supplemental oxygen, a jaw thrust or chin lift to open the child's airway, and begin gentle mask ventilation. It is important to avoid aggressive BVM to prevent or decrease worsening of cervical emphysema, which will affect adequate ventilation. Intubation is high risk with laryngotracheal trauma because of the potential to lose the airway. If the child is unstable, a tracheostomy is considered the standard method for securing the airway for a suspected laryngotracheal injury in the field. Laryngotracheal injuries are associated with additional injuries to the cervical spine, esophagus, and vascular structures of the neck. Chest and neck x-rays are required to evaluate cervical spine fractures, subcutaneous emphysema, pneumothorax, or pneumomediastinum. A CT scan will provide information about the child's airway anatomy, cartilage fractures, cervical spine fractures, or vascular injuries. Airway management is controversial because of the extremely high risk of losing the airway with this injury.[106-107]

Diagnostic Adjuncts for Thoracic Trauma

Thoracic trauma is second only to accidents and unintentional injuries as the leading causes of morbidity and mortality in pediatric patients. In children, more than 80% of all thoracic injuries are the result of blunt trauma. Pediatric trauma patients frequently present first to an outside hospital (OH) before being transported to a level I PTC for specialized and definitive care. Frequently, the OHs have already performed a CT scan before transfer. This imaging is often unnecessary, according to ATLS recommendations, which stress that CT scans should not be performed at the OH when transferring the child out for treatment, or if they are not clinically indicated. OHs obtaining CT scans on pediatric trauma patients before transfer to a PTC results in a delay of care, exposes the child to excessive radiation, and increases health care costs. CT imaging has dramatically increased over the last few years, and with this escalation comes considerable risk to the pediatric patient. Children are still experiencing growth and development and concern is growing that exposure to ionizing radiation may predispose children to radiation-induced malignancies. Taking into account the risks of radiation-induced cancer from CT scans, PTCs have adopted a variety of dose-reduction techniques and reconstructive models that substantially decrease radiation exposure without decreasing the diagnostic quality of the images produced.

ATLS guidelines recommend using CXRs as the initial diagnostic tool for the assessment of thoracic injuries after physical examination. CXRs are quick, portable, and can promptly diagnose common thoracic complications such as a pneumothorax, hemothorax, and mediastinal irregularities.

There are no established guidelines for using chest CTs instead of CXRs for pediatric blunt trauma patients. The lack of regulation or guidelines contributes to the remarkable increase in the use of chest CT and the resultant decrease in CXRs for initial diagnostic imaging for pediatric blunt chest traumas. Many studies evaluated the MOI, rib fractures, contusions, and pneumothorax in pediatric blunt thoracic injuries and demonstrated that CTs were not necessary in the majority of trauma cases because the added information obtained frequently did not change the plan of care for these patients. This information suggests the importance of developing a strict imaging guideline for pediatric blunt trauma patients to limit excessive exposure to CT radiation while not compromising the quality of useful diagnostic information. Chest CT offers enhanced imaging of intrathoracic structures and increases the diagnosis of pediatric intrathoracic injuries; however, this added information does not frequently change the overall care of the pediatric trauma patient. CXR is a valuable screening tool for pediatric blunt trauma patients, and the provider should manage this patient without a routine chest CT being performed. After obtaining the initial CXR on these trauma patients, those presenting with an abnormal mediastinal silhouette on CXR should proceed with a chest CT to evaluate the child for vascular injuries. Also, a chest CT should be done on pediatric patients with suspected thoracic spine injuries and fractures because the thoracic spine is the most commonly injured section of the pediatric patient.[3,108-109]

Circulation

In the initial trauma assessment, circulation is the third step of the primary survey to determine the circulatory status of the patient. In trauma, the assessment of circulatory status focuses on the estimation and treatment of fluid and blood loss associated with traumatic injuries. The physiologic differences in pediatric patients make this assessment more difficult than in adults, especially if the provider is not aware of these differences. The provider should also know the pediatric patient's normal vital sign parameters. Together with the knowledge of the physiologic difference in pediatric patients, this will help the provider establish an accurate diagnosis. In pediatric trauma patients, the evaluation and management of the circulation status includes recognition of circulatory compromise, an accurate estimation of the pediatric patient's weight and circulatory volume, fluid resuscitation, blood replacement, venous access, assessments of the adequacy of resuscitation with urine output, and thermoregulation status.[3,86,89,95]

Physical Examination

Pediatric patients with traumatic injuries resulting in fluid and blood loss may present with the following clinical signs and symptoms[3,86,89]:

- An altered LOC. Preverbal children may be unable to recognize parents or caregivers.

- A decreased response to stimuli or the environment. This is often recognized when the child exhibits a decreased response to painful procedures such as IV starts or a reduction of fractures.
- Restlessness or anxiety.
- Confusion or irritability.
- Dry mucous membranes or absence of tears.
- Tachypnea.
- Tachycardia. In the early stages of shock, tachycardia may be the only indicator of blood loss or shock.
- A change in the child's skin color. Pediatric patients may appear ashen, pale, mottled, or cyanotic.
- Capillary refill greater than 3 seconds, which may be a sensitive indicator of circulatory status in children. It is important to monitor the child's thermoregulation because hypothermia will also increase the capillary refill time.
- Peripheral pulses change and become weak and thready with severe shock in children.
- Skin is cool mostly in the extremities and diaphoretic.
- Difficulty in obtaining a blood pressure in pediatric patients is caused by vasoconstriction from catecholamine release and decreased cardiac output (CO).
- Children have unique compensatory mechanisms in moderate to severe shock states to maintain normotensive blood pressure because of sustained catecholamine response.
- Blood pressure is a late indicator of circulatory status in children. Other clinical indicators as listed earlier are often more sensitive indicators. Hypotension and bradycardia after traumatic injuries in children are ominous late clinical findings and need to be treated aggressively.
- Decreased or absent breath sounds.
- Decreased urine output.
- Placing a urinary catheter early in the care of traumatically injured children is essential for assessment of circulatory status and effectiveness of resuscitation.
- End organ perfusion (i.e., kidneys) decreases with fluid or blood loss and is reflected with oliguria or anuria.
- Maintenance of 1 to 2 mL/kg per hour of urine output is the goal of circulatory support in the pediatric patient.
- Circulatory compromise in children can often be subtle and must be found with a careful physical examination. Waiting for major changes in vital signs or laboratory studies increases patient morbidity and often makes resuscitation more difficult.
- Monitoring of the patient is necessary during the assessment and resuscitation of children with traumatic injuries. Cardiac monitoring and pulse oximetry monitoring can aid in initial assessment and monitoring of ongoing patient status.
- A normal pulse oximetry reading does not accurately reflect tissue oxygenation, which is an indicator that trauma patients should receive supplemental oxygenation.

Laboratory studies helpful in the assessment of the pediatric trauma patient's circulatory status include the following:

- A complete blood cell count, especially hematocrit levels.
- Serum, finger or heel stick glucose measurement.
- Electrolytes.
- Arterial and venous blood gases. A decrease in the pH indicates acidosis is developing from oxygen debt and anaerobic metabolism. Elevated $PaCO_2$ indicates respiratory acidosis and impaired ventilation. A decreased PaO_2 is indicative of hypoxia in the child. A decreased HCO_3 is indicative of the buffering of acidosis. Blood gases are helpful in the initial assessment of ventilation and fluid status in the injured child.
- Lactate level.
- Urinalysis for measurement of specific gravity.

Diagnostic studies that may be helpful in assessment of circulatory status of trauma patients include:

- Chest radiography for evaluation for hemothorax, aortic injury, or pulmonary contusion.
- Head and cervical spine CT scan for evaluation of intracranial bleeding and spinal cord injury (SCI).
- Abdominal and pelvic CT scan.
- Pelvis radiography for evaluation for pelvic fractures.
- Long-bone radiography, especially of the femurs, which can account for considerable blood loss in children.

Once the circulatory status is revealed, concentrated efforts are aimed at the prevention of further fluid loss by controlling external bleeding and replacement of fluid or blood loss. Fluid resuscitation is discussed at length later in this chapter.[3,86,89]

Selected Traumatic Injuries Can Lead to Fluid or Blood Loss or Circulatory Compromise

Any injury causing bleeding or fluid loss potentiates hemodynamic instability without treatment. The following injuries are high risk for major blood or fluid loss in the pediatric trauma patient.[3,86]

Head Injuries and Scalp Lacerations

The head is the most frequently injured area in a child and the most common causes of TBI in the pediatric population. Causes of TBI in children vary by age. Falls are the most common cause of TBI in younger children. Motor vehicle accidents, other accidents, and sports injuries are the most common in older children and teenagers. MVCs are reported to be the major cause of TBI-related deaths in children. Nonaccidental trauma (NAT) is a significant cause of TBI in infants and any child with an unexplainable head injury.[3,86,89]

Pediatric patients have an estimated circulating volume of 80 mL/kg. Infants have a proportionately larger head to body ratio, and an associated larger blood volume in their head leads to hypovolemia in the presence of intracranial hemorrhage. Infants with open fontanelles and open cranial sutures may have increased bleeding and intracranial pressure (ICP). Epidural, subdural, subarachnoid, and intraventricular hemorrhages are four types of internal bleeding on the brain in a child; they can cause significant to lethal amounts of blood loss in pediatric patients. Scalp and head lacerations are vascular in nature, and bleeding may be profuse with the potential for substantial blood loss to occur in children and may require aggressive fluid resuscitation and direct pressure. Support of the child's circulatory status with fluid resuscitation may take precedence over the treatment of increased ICP with TBI. (Head injuries are discussed in depth later in the chapter).[3,86,89,108]

Facial and Mandibular Injuries

Facial fractures are relatively uncommon in pediatric patients with mandibular fractures being the most common of all facial fractures of childhood. MVCs, fall from a height, bicycle injury, sports-related injury, violence or assault, and NAT are the most common MOIs. Concomitant injuries with pediatric maxillofacial injuries include concussion, intracranial hemorrhage, cervical spine injury (CSI), and skull fractures. Concomitant intracranial, chest, abdominal, and extremity injuries emphasize the high-energy impact required to induce mandibular fractures in children. The bony structures of the skull are incredibly vascular, and like facial injuries they can bleed copiously when injured. Patients with Le Fort fractures or open mandibular fractures may need aggressive resuscitation. The majority of profuse bleeding associated with pediatric facial trauma may be from lacerations and soft tissue injuries. The vascularity of the face makes clinical findings often obvious with frank external bleeding noted. After airway control is achieved, some patients may need oral and retropharyngeal packing to control bleeding. Marked facial swelling and ecchymosis may also be present with these injuries. Monitor for cerebrospinal fluid leakage in children with maxillofacial injuries.[3,95,109-111]

Treatment of Facial and Mandibular Injuries

Evaluating pediatric facial injuries involves following the principles of trauma management with the initial or primary survey started of the child's airway to clear and secure the airway, breathing, and bleeding control while maintaining immobilization of the cervical spine because of concomitant injuries. Hypovolemic shock may result in children from excessive blood loss from injuries to the extremely vascular face. Bleeding may require resuscitation because of the amount of blood loss, especially with open Le Fort fractures. Consider that the patient may have a TBI and maintain adequate systolic blood pressure to ensure adequate cerebral perfusion pressure (CPP) when resuscitation measures are needed. Depending on the child's response to crystalloid support during resuscitation, blood products may be needed until bleeding is under control. After the child is stabilized, move on to the secondary survey for a more detailed examination of the child's head, face, and neck to identify any additional injuries.[3,95,109-111]

Massive Hemothorax

Massive hemothorax is discussed in the previous section.

Cardiac Injury

Blunt cardiac injury (BCI) is uncommon in children. It is usually associated with high-energy mechanisms such as MVCs. Diagnosis of BCI is difficult in children because presenting signs and symptoms and external signs are limited or absent. The child presenting with any of the following symptoms—ecchymosis, abrasions, or deformity to the chest wall; focal rib tenderness; muffled heart tones; new-onset murmur; abnormal upper and lower extremity pulses; rib fractures; and pulmonary contusion in the presence of blunt force trauma—should be considered at risk for BCI.[3,104,112-113]

The chest wall of a child is more susceptible to underlying injuries such as BCI because of the elastic, compliant rib cage, which transmits more kinetic energy to a child's intrathoracic internal structures without fractures in blunt force trauma. Most BCI's may not be diagnosed and will resolve without interventions, and those that are diagnosed usually have additional presenting symptoms on CXR, abnormal electrocardiogram (ECG), or physical examination.[3,97,104,112-113]

Treatment for Cardiac Injuries

BCI occurs most often from MVCs, falls, and crush injuries. Direct impact to the precordium from a projectile is less common but increasing in frequency. Rapid deceleration is the most common MOI resulting in BCI. BCI in children is associated with pulmonary contusion and rib fractures. Prehospital management of BCI is difficult in the field. Follow the principles of ATLS with rapid transport to the closest trauma center. Children with blunt chest trauma may present with respiratory or cardiac compromise or immediate life-threatening injuries, and an initial rapid assessment is necessary to initiate control of airway, breathing, and circulation. Immediate interventions are implemented to treat life-threatening injuries such as cardiac tamponade, commotio cordis, or injury to the great vessels.[3,97,104,112-114]

Commotio Cordis

Commotio cordis is a type of BCI that occurs in athletes and is increasing in frequency because of sports-related injuries. Commotio cordis results from a projectile, such as a baseball, striking the child's chest during a susceptible time in the cardiac cycle resulting in ventricular fibrillation and sudden cardiac death in the child.[3,104,112-115]

Treatment for Commotio Cordis

Perform the primary survey, which is the initial rapid assessment and stabilization of the child; identify life-threatening injuries; and initiate immediate treatment for any BCI in children. If commotio cordis is suspected or witnessed, immediately begin cardiopulmonary resuscitation (CPR). Survival for this BCI requires immediate CPR and early automated external defibrillator use for survival; without these two interventions survival is poor in children.[3,104,112-115]

Cardiac Tamponade

Cardiac ventricular rupture is rare in children but is the most common cause of death from blunt trauma. The right ventricle is the chamber most frequently injured because the location is anterior to the chest and under the sternum. Because of the increased pliability of the pediatric rib cage, rib fractures may be absent in the child with a cardiac injury. Pericardial tamponade most frequently occurs with injury to the heart or great vessels. It can be caused by either blunt or penetrating trauma to the chest. Children with blunt thoracic injuries commonly have few signs and symptoms to suggest a cardiac injury is present. The classic triad of jugular venous distension, muffled heart sounds, and hypotension (referred to as Beck's triad) is difficult to detect in pediatric patients. Another classic sign of cardiac tamponade is pulsus paradoxus, which is when the child's blood pressure falls more than 10 mm Hg during inspiration. Data indicate this occurs in less than 50% of pediatric patients with pericardial tamponade, so it is not reliable for the diagnosis of pericardial tamponade. Jugular venous distension, and an elevated central venous pressure, can be missed in smaller children because of smaller necks and increased subcutaneous tissue and cannot be a reliable sign. Remember that other clinical conditions may occur, such as hypovolemia, or environmental concerns, such as noise, can make this diagnosis difficult. It only takes a small amount of blood to interfere with cardiac activity because of the child's small pericardial sac. Fortunately, removal of this small amount of blood will drastically improve cardiac function.[3,104,112-116]

Cardiac tamponade should be considered in all patients with blunt or penetrating thoracic injuries. Pulseless electrical activity in the absence of tension pneumothorax and hypovolemia is highly suggestive of cardiac tamponade. Another sign of cardiac tamponade is pulsus paradoxus, which is described earlier, and is not reliable for the diagnosis of pericardial tamponade. Kussmaul's sign, which is a rise in venous pressure with inspiration when breathing spontaneously, is a true paradoxical venous pressure abnormally associated with cardiac tamponade. Both of these are extremely difficult to assess in the transport setting but can be indicative of cardiac tamponade.[3,104,112-116]

Treatment of Cardiac Tamponade

The treatment of cardiac tamponade includes immediate supportive treatment with IV crystalloid to transiently increase filling pressure and improve CO, but definitive treatment includes pericardiocentesis to evacuate fluid. The most optimal method would be under ultrasound guidance, but this is not part of the transport provider's normal arsenal of equipment.

Pericardiocentesis

Treatment of this injury is rapid pericardiocentesis to decompress the pericardium. A subxiphoid approach with a spinal needle or an over-the-needle catheter attached to a 30-mL syringe with a three-way stopcock is the preferred method of aspiration of blood from the pericardial sac. The needle is directed to the pericardium at a 45-degree angle during aspiration. Cardiac monitoring to assess for ventricular arrhythmias or irritability is essential. Aspiration of a small amount of pericardial nonclotting blood may be all that is needed to temporarily relieve symptoms and see an improvement in hemodynamic status caused by the injured myocardium's ability to self-seal. Pericardiocentesis may not be diagnostic or therapeutic when the blood in the pericardial sac has clotted. Transport to an appropriate facility for definitive cardiac care is always necessary.[3,86,104,112-116]

Myocardial Contusion

Myocardial contusion occurs when blunt force is delivered to the myocardium causing injury. Cardiac contusion is the most common cardiac injury after blunt trauma. With relatively smaller amounts of subcutaneous fat and cartilaginous ribs, children are at great risk for this injury. Only mild symptoms, such as palpitations or precordial or chest pain, may be present following injury. Additional symptoms such as arrhythmias and decreased CO may occur but are not common in the immediate postinjury period. The absence of obvious chest wall trauma does not rule out the diagnosis of cardiac injury. Pediatric patients with blunt thoracic trauma serious enough to cause pulmonary contusion or rib fractures are at high risk for myocardial contusion. Because of the potential for complications and the difficulty in making a definitive diagnosis, a high index of suspicion for myocardial contusion should be held in patients with blunt chest trauma. Monitor patient for complications of myocardial contusion, which include hypotension, conduction abnormalities, or wall motion abnormalities on echocardiography. Common arrhythmias include premature ventricular contractions, unexplained sinus tachycardia, atrial fibrillation, and bundle branch blocks (primarily on the right); ECG may show ST segment abnormalities indicating myocardial infarction.[3,86,104,112-116]

Treatment of Myocardial Contusion

Treatment of myocardial contusion is supportive. Patients need at least 24 hours of cardiac monitoring. The risk for sudden arrhythmia decreases greatly after 24 hours. Significant arrhythmias should be treated with advanced cardiac life support (ACLS) and PALS protocols, and cardiology consultation may be indicated.[3,86]

Traumatic Aortic Disruption

Traumatic aortic disruption or blunt aortic injury (BAI) resulting from blunt chest trauma is a rare injury in children and most die at the scene of the traumatic injury. The chance of survival is increased with rapid detection and surgical intervention. Rapid deceleration is the most common MOI resulting in BAI from MVCs or falls from great heights. Children who survive may present with hypotension, unequal upper and lower pulses or decreased blood pressures in the lower extremities compared with upper extremities, and paraplegia. Occasionally, children may present with minimal or no evidence of chest wall trauma. If the child has rib fractures or suspected pulmonary contusion, suspect BAI. If CXRs are available, a widened superior mediastinum, an abnormal contour of the aortic knob, and a left hemothorax or pleural effusion may be seen. Patients with aortic rupture who have a chance of survival are those with a partial laceration at the level of the ligamentum arteriosum and survive because of a contained hematoma at the site. Unexplained persistent hypotension is usually not related to this injury, and other bleeding sources should be sought. A transected aorta that bleeds freely into the left chest can cause profound hypotension but is quickly fatal (in minutes) without operative intervention. Clinical signs and symptoms of this injury are often absent, and a high index of suspicion must be maintained for patients with MOIs that involve rapid deceleration. CXR findings that may be indicative of major vessel injury are listed in Box 30.4. False-positive and negative x-ray findings are possible, so any patient with suspected aortic injury should receive more testing. Angiography continues to be the gold standard for diagnosis, but CT scan of the chest and transesophageal echocardiography may also show aortic injury.[3,86,112-116]

• BOX 30.4   Chest X-Ray Findings That May Indicate Major Vessel Injury

- A widened mediastinum
- Obliteration of the aortic knob
- Deviation of the trachea to the right
- Obliteration of the space between the pulmonary artery and the aorta
- Depression of the left mainstem bronchus
- Deviation of the esophagus or the gastric tube to the right
- Widened paratracheal stripe
- Widened paraspinal interfaces
- Presence of a pleural or apical cap
- Left hemothorax
- Fractures of the first or second rib or scapula

From Holleran RS, ed. *ASTNA Patient Transport: Principles and Practice.* 4th ed. St. Louis: Mosby Elsevier; 2010.

Treatment of Traumatic Aortic Disruption

Transport patient to a center capable of caring for a child with a cardiothoracic injury. Treatment of this injury is operative repair either with resection and grafting or primary repair. Hemothoraces should be treated as described previously, and fluid resuscitation should be provided based on the patient's hemodynamic status.[3,86,115-116]

Penetrating Cardiac Trauma

Research is limited regarding pediatric penetrating cardiac trauma. Penetrating cardiac trauma may be associated with a hemopericardium and tamponade. Penetrating trauma resulting from gunshot wounds tends to cause larger injuries to the chest and presents with blood loss and hypovolemia. Small penetrating injuries to the pericardium can heal spontaneously over time. The right ventricle is injured more often in penetrating trauma because of its anterior location. Penetrating injury to multiple chambers of the heart has a significant mortality attached. Rapid resuscitation and early transfer to the operating room at a definitive facility will significantly decrease mortality.[3,86,115-116]

Abdominal Injuries

Abdominal trauma is the most common cause of unrecognized fatal injury in children. Blunt abdominal trauma is the third most common cause of trauma-related deaths in children. Approximately 90% of abdominal trauma is blunt force and 10% is penetrating. Intraabdominal injuries are more common in patients with the seatbelt sign than those children without. The presence of the seatbelt abrasion sign should trigger the provider to suspect significant intraabdominal injuries that may require acute interventions. The anatomic differences in children predispose them to abdominal injuries. Children have larger solid organs in relation to their size, less subcutaneous fat, and less developed musculature of the abdomen resulting in less protection from injury. They also have a protruding abdomen placing vital organs closer to impacting forces and a small thorax with elastic compliant ribs that decreases protection, especially to the liver and spleen. The spleen and liver are the most frequently injured organs, followed by the kidneys, small bowel, and pancreas.[3,86,89,117-121]

The most common MOIs for blunt abdominal trauma in children are MVCs, auto versus pedestrian injury, bike versus car, and falls. Bicycle handlebar injuries, sports, incidents involving all-terrain vehicles, and NAT are additional MOIs causing internal abdominal injuries in children. The mortality rate in children after blunt abdominal trauma is rare but increases as more abdominal structures are identified as injured. It is difficult to perform examinations of abdominal injuries of pediatric patients because of their fear of being examined or the pain from other injuries that are distracting the child and interfering with the assessment. Preverbal children are unable to describe or relate pain.

Abdominal findings can be subtle and are often missed on initial examination. The transport provider should maintain a high index of suspicion or awareness for potentially serious underlying injuries in children presenting with multiple traumatic injuries.[3,86,89,117-121]

Treatment of Abdominal Injuries

The initial management of children with suspected intraabdominal injury (IAI) should be to follow the ATLS guidelines for diagnosis and treatment of immediately life-threatening injuries. During stabilization, children with signs of IAI and hemodynamic instability that do not respond to fluid resuscitation and blood transfusion calls for an emergent laparotomy. Following the primary survey, the provider should begin the secondary survey of hemodynamically stable children who are suspected of blunt IAI to identify any missed injuries. The secondary survey helps identify other indicators for observation, or laboratory evaluation. Imaging with a focused assessment with sonography for trauma (FAST) is a useful tool in the initial and secondary evaluation, or an emergent laparotomy may be needed in unstable patients.[3,86,89,117-121]

Penetrating abdominal trauma in children from gunshot or stab wounds accounts for approximately 10% of all abdominal injuries. Bullets may cause extensive damage from the high kinetic energy of the projectile, and the blast effect can change the route of the bullet after it enters the body, increasing damage along the bullet's path. The small intestine is injured more often than the large bowel, which is injured more than the liver in penetrating abdominal trauma. Penetrating trauma is usually easily identified in the primary survey through inspection.

The risk of complications may be expected by the presentation of clinical shock, number of organs injured, amount of blood transfusions the child required, and other associated thoracic injuries. Exploratory laparotomy is currently the gold standard for managing penetrating abdominal injuries in children.[3,86,89,117-121]

New data are immerging indicating that selective nonoperative management may be a safe treatment option for children who are hemodynamically stable after clinical examination and radiographic evaluations are performed. The use of a minimally invasive laparoscopic surgery may be used for those hemodynamically stable. The Pediatric Emergency Care Applied Research Network (PECARN) conducted a study and established a prediction rule encompassing seven patient history and physical examination variables, without labs or ultrasonographic information, that were able to identify children with blunt torso trauma at very low risk for IAI, which successfully limited CT scans and invasive treatment methods.[3,86,89,117-122]

Blunt abdominal trauma must be suspected and discovered from historical information, MOI, and physical examination. During the secondary survey, the provider monitors closely for subtle signs of hemorrhagic shock such as compensation for hypovolemia with tachycardia that progresses to a narrowed pulse pressure (20 mm Hg or less); delayed capillary refill time; pallor; mottling; cool, clammy skin; decreased urine output; or altered mental status in children. Although not definitive, these findings may indicate ongoing intraabdominal hemorrhage. Remember, children can lose up to 30% of their blood volume before systolic blood pressure begins to trend down, which allows a significant intraabdominal hemorrhage to occur. Physical signs indicating increased suspicion for IAI in children include ecchymosis, especially in the umbilical or flank areas; abrasions; tire track marks; seatbelt sign in restrained passengers; abdominal tenderness; abdominal distension; peritoneal irritation indicated with abdominal wall rigidity; or pain in the left shoulder induced by palpation of the left upper quadrant (Kehr's sign); or absent bowel sounds indicating a prolonged ileus. Signs of abdominal injury are variable and may evolve over time, which necessitates serial examinations. The stomach and bladder (unless contraindicated because of injury) need to be decompressed and the child examined for abrasions and contusions. If the child remains awake and alert, gentle palpation may demonstrate significant pain and tenderness, but the accuracy of the provider's assessment may be affected if distracting injuries are present.[3,86,89,117-121]

Seatbelt Sign (Syndrome) and Injuries

Seatbelt use in an MVC is the single most effective process to decrease morbidity and mortality in children. The use of lap and shoulder seatbelt restraints reduces the risk of fatal injuries to children 5 years of age and older. It is important to ensure the child is using the seatbelts correctly and has the lap belt positioned correctly low across the thighs and not across the abdomen, which will reduce intraabdominal injuries in children. Seatbelt sign or syndrome presents with erythema, ecchymosis, or abrasions across the abdominal wall, intraabdominal injuries to both hollow (more common) and solid (less common) organs, and spinal fractures of the lumbar spine (Chance fracture, which is most often from L2 to L4 in children). Additional signs and symptoms may include abdominal pain or tenderness indicating an increased risk of internal injuries.[3,86,89,123-125]

The MOI related to the seatbelt sign is a rapid deceleration resulting in compression of the lower abdomen and sudden hyperflexion of the upper torso around the seatbelt, leading to crushing of the abdominal content against the spine. The MOI related to the seatbelt sign is a significant force being transmitted to the abdomen and spine necessitating a thorough examination by the provider. Children who present with seatbelt sign are considerably more likely to sustain intraabdominal injuries involving the mesentery, bowel, and pancreas, compared with those without seatbelt signs. There is not a reported association of solid organ (liver or spleen) injuries involved with this presenting sign. Intraabdominal injuries are more common in patients presenting with the seatbelt sign than without. The transport provider should be cognizant and prepared to provide rapid interventions for the child with seatbelt sign. In addition, a SCI presents in half of the children with seatbelt sign.[3,86,89,118,123-125]

Treatment for Seatbelt Sign

The initial management of children with suspected IAI resulting from the seatbelt sign or syndrome is to follow the ATLS guidelines for diagnosis and treatment of immediately life-threatening injuries. The provider needs to maintain a high level of suspicion for internal injuries in these patients and perform serial clinical examination and appropriate diagnostic tests in patients not proceeding immediately to laparotomy. Treatment may include observation, IV fluids, blood transfusion, labs, emergent laparotomy (unstable) and potential CT (stable).[3,86,89,118,123-125]

Diagnostic Adjuncts for Abdominal Trauma

The FAST is a quick noninvasive method for evaluating for free intraperitoneal fluid suggestive of abdominal injuries, but CT remains the gold standard for diagnosing abdominal injuries. Treatment is trending toward serial monitoring of hematocrit, bed rest, and additional imaging studies, and less toward surgery. CTs are associated with significant radiation exposure, and now there are data suggesting children exposed to CT will develop cancer (such as thyroid cancer), later in life. The diagnostic peritoneal lavage (DPL) can be used to quickly diagnose or exclude the presence of internal bleeding. The DPL is a diagnostic tool used less often because of increased uses of CTs and FAST modalities. DPL is used more often in unstable children or those presenting with inconsistent examination.[3,86,89,117-118]

Nonaccidental Abdominal Trauma

Abdominal injury in NAT is a documented reason why children are hospitalized. Abdominal injuries in children from NAT are frequently significant with an escalating need for surgical interventions. If a child presents with an abdominal injury and NAT is known or suspected, CT of the abdomen and pelvis with contrast should be performed for both diagnostic testing and forensic evidence. NAT injuries of the bowel have a high rate of occurrence, but the liver, spleen, and pancreas are injured more often in children. The abdominal injuries present in a child suspected of NAT are frequently quite severe and may require surgery. Abdominal trauma is the second most common cause of fatal child abuse after head injuries. Children with abdominal injuries from NAT will usually also present with coexisting injuries including head injuries, thoracic trauma including rib and clavicle fractures, and pulmonary contusions. Identifying NAT in the setting of known abdominal trauma is important to protect the child from future abuse and also guide diagnostic investigation. Recognition of abdominal injuries in the presence of NAT or suspected abuse is challenging as a result of the unclear clinical histories, delayed presentations, and vague or nonspecific patient complaints. Delays in diagnosing abdominal injuries from NAT may contribute to poor outcomes in these children. A large number of children with abdominal injuries from NAT may not have any physical signs such as bruising or their x-ray does not demonstrate changes indicative of NAT. Physical signs may include hypoactive bowel sounds or abdominal bruising. Labs are not always clear-cut and helpful in diagnosing NAT. Findings of anemia and leukocytosis are not reliable indicators of abdominal trauma and may occur without significant injuries. Patients with aspartate aminotransferase (AST) or alanine aminotransferase (ALT) greater than 80 IU/L should trigger the transport provider to suspect abdominal trauma. Additional labs to consider are lipase, amylase, and urinalysis. The transport provider should maintain a high level of suspicion for NAT in patients who have both hollow viscous injuries and solid organ injuries in children.[3,86,89,117-119]

Spleen and Liver Injuries

The liver and spleen are the most common, potentially life-threatening organs injured in children. The majority of all injuries to the liver and spleen are from blunt force trauma in children. The prognosis for both types of injury depends mainly on the presence or absence of associated injuries, especially TBI and chest trauma. Solid organ injuries are common in pediatric patients who suffer major or multisystem trauma. With isolated or single-system trauma, the spleen is the most commonly injured abdominal organ. The ribs of children only partially protect the liver and spleen, and the remainder of these organs extends below the rib cage. The pliability of a child's rib cage, the large segments of the spleen and liver extending below the ribs, less subcutaneous fat, and weak musculature of the abdomen all increase the risk of internal injuries to the liver and spleen when the MOI is from a blunt force.[3,86,117-121]

The MOI may be a direct force to the epigastric area, tearing away the blood supply as a result of rapid deceleration, penetrating injury from fractured rib, or crushing injury against the spinal column. The liver and spleen are incredibly vascular, and disruption of the vascular supply to these organs can result in massive hemorrhage. Clinical signs may be subtle but may include point and rebound tenderness, radiation of pain to the left shoulder from injuries to the spleen, ecchymosis or an abrasion to the upper abdominal quadrants, lower rib fractures, and abdominal distention. Signs of shock may be present when there is significant injury to these organs.[3,86,117-121]

Treatment of Spleen and Liver Injuries

Initial assessment of an injured child should follow the ATLS guidelines to identify life-threatening injuries that have a negative effect on the airway, breathing, and circulation. Identification of abdominal injuries occurs with the secondary survey after the pediatric patient is stabilized through interventions performed in the primary survey.[86]

Clinical signs of injury to the spleen or liver will include signs and symptoms of hypovolemia shock with tachycardia, delayed capillary refill, pallor, altered mental status, decreased urine output, hypotension, abdominal contusions with signs of ecchymosis, abrasions as a result of seatbelt or bicycle handle bars injuries, or abdominal distension. Other clinical signs are tenderness over the abdominal areas, right upper quadrant tenderness that may indicate an injury to the liver, or left upper quadrant tenderness that may indicate an injury to the spleen. Orogastric tube insertion facilitates the abdominal examination by reducing aspiration of gastric contents and decreases distention from swallowed air. Patients presenting with signs and symptoms of hypovolemia require fluid resuscitation with crystalloid solutions and possibly blood transfusions to reverse the hypovolemic shock until definitive treatment is received to control bleeding of the liver or spleen. Unstable children with blunt trauma to the abdomen who do not improve with fluid resuscitation of 40 to 60 mL/kg of normal saline or lactated Ringer's solution IV, followed by packed red blood cells of 10 mL/kg IV, require emergent exploratory laparotomy. Transport pediatric trauma patients to a definitive center capable of performing serial observations or damage control surgery to stop the hemorrhage.[3,86,117-121,126]

Nonoperative management of the hemodynamically stable pediatric trauma patient with spleen or liver (solid organs) injuries is a treatment option with low rates of failure; nonoperative failure is when the child requires surgical intervention. Obtaining a CT following blunt abdominal trauma has provided the recognition of active bleeding of the spleen or liver by identifying the IV contrast or blush, which is a reliable indicator of significant organ injury. Nonoperative management of blunt abdominal trauma with suspected liver or spleen injury is the standard of care for the stable pediatric trauma patient. Unstable pediatric patients may require surgical intervention with a splenectomy. Research has shown that pediatric patients presenting with contrast blush on CT were successfully treated with the nonoperative method following serial examinations, labs (especially hematocrit), treatment with blood products, and if necessary angiography. This method demonstrated far less blood product requirement for children than surgical intervention of a splenectomy, which sets up the child for postsplenectomy sepsis.[3,86,117-122,126]

Nonaccidental Solid Organ Injuries

The liver and pancreas are the most frequently injured solid organs from NAT. The left lobe of the liver is the most frequently injured in NAT and most likely from central assault, which is the opposite injury sustained in accidental traumas. In NAT, liver lacerations may be present without signs or symptoms. Liver lacerations can be identified by checking for abnormal levels of transaminase. Transaminase assists in detection of occult liver injuries and these levels may help determine the age of the hepatic injury. The determination of the age of the hepatic injury may not only help identify the individual responsible for inflicting the blunt force injuries to the child but may help the provider to recognize a fabricated history of how the child was injured. In children with NAT liver injury, the ALT may be higher than the AST, indicating that the liver injury is older than 12 hours. Hepatic and splenic injuries from NAT present with MOIs similar to accidental traumas and include lacerations, fractures, hematomas, and rupture and hepatic lacerations, which are the most common. Linear lacerations through the liver, known as bear claw lacerations, are the most common in children and are identified at imaging, and are a result of compression applied to the hepatic parenchyma. The majority of blunt NATs affecting the liver or spleen are treated nonoperatively.[86,117-119,126]

Pancreatic Injuries

The pancreas is the fourth most common solid organ injury in children following injuries to the spleen, liver, and kidneys. The pancreas is not as vascular as the liver and spleen, and major blood loss is very rare. Blunt trauma injury to the pancreas is difficult to diagnose immediately after the injury because of the retroperitoneal location of the trauma, the lack of reliable signs and symptoms, and the limited sensitivity on common imaging modalities. The most common complications are the formation of pancreatic fistulae, pancreatitis, and the development of pancreatic pseudocysts, which usually present weeks after injury. The nonoperative management of minor pancreatic injury is well accepted with grade I and II injuries. The treatment of grade III and higher are more serious pancreatic injuries with capsular, ductal, or parenchymal disruption in pediatric patients, and the treatment is controversial. Pancreatic injury is determined on an elevated serum amylase, lipase levels, and CRP, CT, ultrasonography or endoscopic retrograde cholangiopancreatography (ERCP).[3,86,117-118,120-121]

The most common MOIs are pedestrian versus automobile, NAT, injuries received in an MVC, or handlebars of a bicycle. The actual MOI usually involves compression of the pancreas against the rigid spinal column or direct blunt force. Severe pancreatic intraabdominal injuries may require immediate surgical intervention, and other less severe injuries may be treated with nonoperative management. An isolated pancreatic injury may have a delay of hours or days before the onset of abdominal symptoms. The symptoms following injury include abdominal pain, nausea, and vomiting and fever and may be nonspecific but should increase the level of suspicion for pancreatic injury following blunt abdominal trauma. An example would be a bicycle handlebar injury. Serum amylase levels are obtained for all children with blunt abdominal trauma, but they do not correlate to the severity of injury and should not be used as a diagnostic measure in patients. A CRP level greater than 150 mg/dL at 48 hours helps differentiate between mild or severe pancreatitis. The serum lipase level may be used only to exclude salivary amylase in cases of head and neck injuries.[3,86,117-118,120-121]

CT imaging obtained on admission is a valuable tool when positive for pancreatic injury because it identifies the location of the trauma and grading of injuries is usually accurate. CT should not be used as a study of exclusion. The failure of the CT scan to detect pancreatic injuries on admission does not suggest diagnostic inaccuracy, but rather the evolving nature of pancreatic injuries. Class III injuries missed on initial CT scans are typically later diagnosed on ERCP. Such injuries are allowed to progress to pseudocysts. Ultrasound scans are used to document and follow-up in children in whom pseudocysts develop during hospitalization. Management of pancreatic injuries is determined by the severity and location of the injury and the presence or absence of associated abdominal injuries. Pancreatic injury is an unusual complication of blunt abdominal trauma, usually is minor (grade I or II), with pancreatic ductal disruption occurring in a minority of cases (grade III or higher). Children with pancreatic injuries without ductal disruption do not appear to suffer increased morbidity following conservative management, and children presenting with ductal disruption may require operative intervention.[3,86,117-118,120-121]

Nonaccidental Pancreatic Injuries

The average age of a child with NAT pancreatitis is less than 3 years of age and is younger than children with pancreatitis from other MOIs. The majority of traumatic pancreatitis is secondary to NAT. In the absence of a plausible history, such as an MVC or bicycle handlebar injury, the provider should suspect that the traumatic pancreatitis is from NAT. Imaging to detect pancreatic injury in children may be limited. If the CT is obtained immediately after the trauma it may not detect a majority of injuries to the pancreas. The most common CT finding following a NAT pancreatic injury in children is fluid in the lesser sac. Any finding of any peripancreatic fluid without other abdominal injuries is indicative of pancreatic injury.[126]

Hollow Viscous Injuries

Blunt abdominal trauma is common in pediatric patients but rarely results in significant hollow visceral injuries. For children to have damage to hollow visceral organs requires powerful blunt force mechanisms that cause associated injuries to the solid visceral organs resulting in a delayed diagnosis and treatment of the hollow viscous organs. The most common hollow visceral injury is a jejunal perforation, followed by injury to the duodenum, colon, and finally the stomach. Most of these injuries result from a direct force such as an MVC, seatbelt injury, bicycle handlebar injury, or falls. The MOI is usually rapid acceleration or deceleration of the intestinal structures near a fixed anatomic point, such as the ligament of Treitz, or the trapping of bowel between the seatbelt and the spine. Definitive management of children evaluated for hollow viscous injury as a result of blunt abdominal trauma is dependent on the child's clinical findings. Most of these injuries will require surgical intervention.[3,86,117,121,127]

Nonaccidental Hollow Viscous Injuries

Hollow viscous injuries account for just over 10% of all intraabdominal injuries in NAT that require hospitalization. Bowel injury resulting from NAT is significantly higher than accidental bowel injuries. The duodenum and proximal jejunum are the most commonly injured hollow viscous organs in NAT. Other associated NAT injuries are to the gastric area, bladder, and colon. The duodenum and proximal jejunum are high-risk injuries in NAT secondary to their location at the ligament of Treitz and the concentration of force from a punch or kick to the epigastric area. Bowel injuries from NAT can range from localized hematoma to bowel perforation, or an intramural hematoma, which is the most common bowel injury associated with NAT. Bowel injuries may also have mesenteric tears or contusions. A disruption of the mesentery from NAT may cause bowel ischemia. Children presenting with bowel perforation and peritonitis frequently go directly to surgery without any imaging. Free air on CXR is indicative of intraperitoneal free air and that the bowel has perforated. The provider must remember that NAT injuries often involve both the peritoneal and the retroperitoneal duodenum, and a plain x-ray may not be sufficient to identify and diagnose all NAT injuries. Bowel perforation from blunt trauma secondary to NAT may not be identified on a CT scan, making it a difficult diagnosis. Findings of pneumoperitoneum or leakage of oral contrast material are diagnostic of intestinal perforation but are insensitive and are seen most frequently in patients with clinical peritonitis who would proceed to surgery regardless of the CT results. The most common finding in bowel or mesenteric injury is unexplained intraperitoneal fluid. However, this finding is not predictive of injury, and patients with isolated intraabdominal free fluid at CT can follow a nonoperative approach that includes serial abdominal examinations.[126,127]

Stomach Injuries

Stomach injuries rarely occur as a result of blunt abdominal trauma but may occur as a result of a lap belt, air bag, or handlebar injuries. Abdominal pain occurring after blunt abdominal trauma should have the provider suspecting hollow visceral organ injury. Perforation is the most common gastric injury. Pediatric trauma patients develop gastric dilation from crying or assisted ventilation and may lead to circulatory and respiratory compromise if untreated. All pediatric patients with multisystem injury or those who need assisted ventilation should have their stomachs decompressed with a gastric tube to prevent these complications. Gastric tubes can be used if the patient does not have known or suspected facial or head injuries. Orogastric tubes are safer than nasal tubes until facial and head trauma are eliminated. Initial management of children with suspected blunt hollow viscous injuries requires adherence to ATLS guidelines related to immediate life-threatening injuries for diagnosis, treatment, and appropriate resuscitation. Peritonitis is more common in patients with perforations of the stomach.[3,86,117,121]

Duodenal Injuries

The most common hollow viscous injury is the jejunal perforation. This injury is suggestive of NAT if there is no other history of abdominal trauma in children. High-energy blunt forces, direct blows to fixed points such as the ligament of Treitz or the ileocecal valve, or sudden deceleration causing a shearing force at the mesenteric attachment may cause injuries to the jejunum. A mesenteric injury may affect the blood supply to the small intestine and may lead to delayed perforation from ischemic necrosis. This injury presents with pain and tenderness to palpation 12 to 24 hours after the injury. Peritoneal signs are vague because the jejunal contents are not as acidic as those of the stomach. The small intestine contents are less acidic than stomach contents and have limited or no signs of peritoneal irritation. The bacterial count is low but still has the potential to cause sepsis, abdominal abscess, or infection. Treatment is supportive and requires surgical intervention. MVCs are the most common cause of duodenal injuries in children followed by NAT.[3,86,117,121]

Nonaccidental Duodenal Injuries

Duodenal injuries require special consideration given their high association with NAT in young children. In children 3 years of age and younger the majority of duodenal injuries are caused by NAT. A duodenal hematoma may be the first recognizable sign indicating NAT. Clinical presentation in cases of NAT is often delayed, and delay in presentation with duodenal injuries carries a higher rate of complications, with increased rates of abscess formation and sepsis.[126]

Genitourinary Injuries

Traumatic injuries to the genitourinary system are rarely fatal in children, but they may be associated with hemorrhage and hypovolemic shock. In pediatric blunt abdominal trauma, the most injured solid organ is the kidney. Children are at a greater risk of kidney injury because of the pliable elastic rib cage permitting compression during rapid deceleration. The kidneys are anatomically large for the child's abdomen and pelvis size, and the lack of perirenal fat contributes to increased risks of renal injury in children exposed to blunt abdominal trauma. The management goals of pediatric renal trauma are to protect the renal parenchyma and minimize patient morbidity by treating life-threatening injuries. Life-threatening emergencies are rapidly recognized and evaluated by using ATLS rapid primary assessment with the objective to decrease or limit unnecessary surgical interventions. Clinical findings may be subtle, and hematuria is not considered a sensitive indicator of injury. Treatment of these injuries is supportive and may require surgical evaluation. Most blunt pediatric renal injuries are low, grade I to III, and are seen more in male children usually older than 6 years of age. Management is evolving toward a conservative approach with a high rate of success in grade IV renal injuries in which no life-threatening bleeding is present. The most frequent causes of renal trauma in children include all-terrain vehicles, dirt bikes, falls, MVCs, bicycles, and sporting activities. The majority of pediatric abdominal renal trauma is handled without surgical intervention. The anatomic position of the pediatric bladder offers protection from pelvic fractures. Bladder rupture is more common in children than adults and occurs as a result of the child's shallow pelvis. The genitourinary system in children can be injured by vehicle restraints in deceleration injuries or by falls with direct blunt trauma. As with many abdominal injuries, a high index of suspicion must be maintained for patients with MOIs likely to cause trauma to the genitourinary system.[3,86,117,121-123,128]

Nonaccidental Kidney Injuries

Isolated hematuria or renal injury may occur in 25% of cases of IAI secondary to NAT. NAT resulting in renal injuries is common in children hospitalized with intraabdominal trauma. Reported NAT injuries include hematomas, contusions, and renal vascular injuries. Renal injuries should be graded using the American Association for the Surgery of Trauma Organ Injury Scale. Renal lacerations are graded by the involvement of the renal collecting system. CT imaging requires testing during the excretory phase to detect urinary bleeding. NAT resulting in low-grade lesions, such as ill-defined hypoattenuating parenchymal contusions and small subscapular hematomas, will usually resolve without long-term sequelae. A shattered kidney (multiple lacerations and fragmentation) and complete renal devascularization are the most severe (grade V) renal injury. Treatment of NAT renal injuries is aimed at renal preservation, with the first choice being nonoperative management.[126]

Pelvic Injuries

Pediatric pelvic fractures are rare injuries and are associated with a higher morbidity and mortality than any other orthopedic injuries. Pelvic fractures are rare in children and caused by a high-energy mechanism. The pediatric pelvis contains more cartilage, is more elastic, and can absorb a greater amount of force without having fractures occurring. One of the most disturbing complications related to pelvic fractures is the extensive bladder and/or urethral injuries (BUIs). Patients with these injuries often require multiple urologic extensive procedures and experience long-term sexual and psychological dysfunction. Bladder injuries are uncommon regardless of the sex, and urethral injuries are seen more often in males. The diagnosis of a pelvic fracture with associated BUI is often difficult to make in the field or the ED, particularly in female children. The reason for this is likely multifactorial, such as BUIs are often sustained after major trauma involving multiple organ systems; the provider may be treating life-threatening injuries during the trauma resuscitation; younger children may not be able to adequately communicate and localize their pain; increasing the risk for an unrecognized injury; and last, the classic signs and symptoms associated with urethral injuries, such as blood at the meatus or perineal hematoma, are often absent. When pediatric pelvic fractures occur they are associated with a higher likelihood of morbidity and

mortality. One major cause of this morbidity is BUI. When BUI is missed, the outcome is often poor. Up to 23% of BUIs may be missed on the initial examination on males and up to 40% on females. On average, these missed injuries may not be detected until almost 3 days later. If the diagnosis of BUI is delayed, patients may develop a wide variety of complications including septic shock, pelvic abscess, peritonitis, myonecrosis of the thigh, and bladder entrapment.

The key to a good outcome without complications lies in the early detection of BUI. The majority of children with pelvic fractures, however, are severely injured and do not have BUI.

Children have more pliable bones with thicker periosteum in their pelvic bones. In pediatric patients, avulsion fractures of the pelvis and isolated pelvic ring fractures are more common. Significant force is required for the child to sustain a complete pelvic ring disruption involving the posterior elements. Pelvic fractures are rare in young children but can be common traumatic injuries in late adolescence. Mechanisms of injuries include motor vehicle crashes and falls with direct blunt trauma. Fatal hemorrhage in the retroperitoneal area is associated with these fractures and requires prompt immobilization and aggressive fluid resuscitation. Clinical findings include obvious visual asymmetry, instability and pain to palpation, pain with adduction of the legs, and ecchymosis. These findings may also present with profound hypotension and shock.[3,86,128-133]

Treatment of Pelvic Injuries

Debate continues on the most appropriate method to use for stabilizing pediatric pelvic fractures for transport. Each transport program should have pediatric protocols related to pelvic support during transport. Stabilization with sheet strapping and external immobilizers are splinting options, dependent on the fracture patterns and orthopedic surgeon availability. Pelvic fractures without hemodynamic instability may only need close observation during transport. Fatal hemorrhage seen with adults is rare in pediatric pelvic fractures. The bleeding that occurs with pediatric pelvic fractures is usually associated with solid organ injuries. Identification and treatment of the life-threatening injuries should be the primary focus of the initial acute management in children presenting with pelvic fractures. More aggressive immobilization should be used for pediatric patients with clinical signs of hemorrhage or hypovolemic shock. Fluid resuscitation with crystalloids (normal saline or lactated Ringer's solution) and blood products may be necessary. Plain x-rays have limited sensitivity for detecting pediatric pelvic fractures. CT scan is the gold standard for pelvic fracture diagnosis and assessment in children, but the advantages of CT should be considered against any long-term risks or effects of excessive radiation exposure.[3,86,128-133]

Femur Fractures

Femur fractures in children can cause a significant amount of blood loss. Femur fractures are rare but are the most common cause of hospitalization for pediatric orthopedic injuries. The treatment for femur fractures is based on age and injury with a tendency toward operative stabilization. The femur is the largest bone in the body. In pediatric trauma, a child with a suspected femur fracture may also have associated injuries or life-threatening injuries when linked to high-impact trauma such as an MVC. In infants and toddlers, NAT and falls are the most common causes of femur fractures. In toddlers to older children, falls are the most common cause of femur fractures. Motor vehicle versus pedestrian collisions, MVCs, and sports-related injuries are the most common causes of femur fractures in older children and teenagers. A pediatric injury pattern involving children who are hit by a motor vehicle and sustain a femur fracture, severe head injury, and chest and abdominal injury is commonly called Waddell's triad. Femur fractures are associated with significant trauma in children, and one should suspect multiple injuries in any child who is involved in any trauma with significant blunt force.[3,86,134-135]

Treatment of Femur Fractures

Most femur fractures in children may be diagnosed based on clinical presentation. Common presenting symptoms include localized tenderness, swelling, obvious deformity, shortening, and/or crepitus on palpation. Monitor for indications and associated proximal femur fracture, such as pain in the hip joint and other signs such as an externally rotated leg position. The skin needs to be carefully inspected for signs of an open fracture. Initiate antibiotics as soon as possible with any open fracture. All fractures should include a careful neurovascular examination distal to the fracture site before and after splitting to make sure the fracture has not damaged arteries or nerves. Pediatric femur fractures are considered to be a significant injury with the potential to lose a large amount of blood, which mandates early and urgent interventions. Pediatric patients with femur fractures who have been involved in a high-speed MVC should undergo ATLS standard trauma evaluation to establish an airway and cervical spine immobilization as well as evaluation for breathing and circulation compromise requiring vascular access for fluid resuscitation caused by blood loss in the femur.[3,86,134-135]

After assessment of neurovascular function and administration of appropriate analgesics, fractured femurs should be aligned and immobilized. Traction splints, air splints, or a variety of commercial splints can be used for immobilization. Monitor air splints for pressure increase or decrease with altitude changes. After alignment and immobilization of the child's femur, a neurovascular assessment should always be repeated. Fluid resuscitation with crystalloid and blood products may be necessary. For those children with isolated femur fractures, immobilization and pain management are the goals of treatment.[3,86,134-135]

Vascular and Venous Injuries

Trauma is one of the leading causes of morbidity and mortality in children. Vascular injuries in children are relatively uncommon. In children, vascular trauma creates challenges because of the child's small arteries, vasospasm of these small arteries, decreased intravascular volume, the vessel growth potential, and significance of long-term durability. Early identification and rapid interventions for vascular injuries are essential to prevent significant morbidity and mortality from massive blood loss in these children. It is challenging in pediatric vascular trauma patients to pinpoint a diagnosis because the signs and symptoms of an internal vascular injury may be cloaked by the child's physiologic ability to compensate hemodynamically for an extended period of time. Providers must maintain a high index of suspicion for associated injuries. Knowledge of the potential patterns of injury and management options are essential to limit long-term disability. Vascular injuries in children resulting from blunt trauma most often occur via the sharp edge of fractured bones. Vascular injury in pediatric trauma may be associated with significant morbidity and mortality from acute or delayed ischemia secondary to acute blood loss, arterial dissection, hematoma, aneurysm, or thrombosis.[136-137]

Treatment of Vascular and Venous Injuries

Clinical imaging techniques such as ultrasound, CT, CT angiography, traditional angiography, and DPL may be used as diagnostic aids, and the use of newer imaging modalities such as MDCT scanning may be the preferred method for assessing pediatric vascular trauma. Nonoperative management of traumatic venous injuries is rarely supported because a delay in definitive management may be detrimental to survival. Consideration for operative intervention is the preferred management of venous injuries, especially if coexisting arterial injury is suspected. Surgical repair of venous injury in children requires specialist surgical technique, instruments, and perioperative support. To allow for growth later in life, interrupted sutures may be used for primary repair of venous injuries in children. Synthetic grafts are usually not effective for venous repair in younger children.[136-137]

Poor prognostic indicators increasing mortality risk in pediatric trauma patients are poor surgical access, blunt MOI with a shearing mechanism, delayed diagnosis, and the presence of additional traumatic injuries such as a head injury. Mortality in pediatric traumatic venous injuries increased if the inferior vena cava or hepatic veins were injured. Pediatric vascular injuries are primarily caused by blunt force mechanisms and affect the upper and lower extremities. Blunt force trauma causing vascular injuries in children is usually associated with sharp edges of fractured bones. Definitive management for pediatric vascular injuries is operative management. Repair techniques are graft or patch angioplasty, end-to-end anastomosis, and interposition grafts. Pediatric vascular injuries have an increase in morbidity as a result of the small size of the damaged arteries, need for blood vessel growth along with child, and long-term patency of the vascular repairs. Children presenting with vascular or venous injuries, or both, should be transferred to a designated PTC for surgical intervention to decrease morbidity and mortality and optimize long-term patient outcomes.[136-137]

Disability

The fourth step in the primary survey is the neurologic assessment of an injured child, which is the disability component of the primary survey. Traumatic head or brain and spinal cord injuries are the most common causes of disability in the pediatric trauma patient. Head injuries continue to be the leading cause of death in children injured from traumatic events. Children have anatomic differences that predispose them to head injuries, such as their relatively large head size compared with their body surface area; open fontanelles; cranial sutures, which can allow for a significant increase in intracranial swelling; and poorly developed neck and upper extremity musculature offering less protection to the head and neck.[3,86,89]

The neurologic assessment of the primary survey includes a quick assessment of the child's neurologic function by evaluating pupillary responses and calculating the child's Glasgow Coma Scale (GCS) or the Alert, Verbal, Pain, Unresponsive (AVPU) Pediatric Response Scale. This should be done at the end of the primary survey or before administration of sedatives, narcotics, or paralytics. Assessment of the child's neurologic status should be repeated for any improvement or deterioration. The more extensive neurologic evaluation should be deferred until the secondary survey to evade interruption or slowing down of the primary survey. It is important to establish a baseline GCS in children with a TBI to evaluate an evolving intracranial injury and the associated neurologic status changes. A rapid neurologic assessment evaluates a child's LOC, pupil size and reaction, and motor response, which help assess the level of a SCI. The GCS should be calculated using age-specific criteria. The three main components of the GCS are eye opening, verbal responses, and motor response; the motor response score has been found to be the best predictor of outcome after TBI. Pupillary assessment includes an evaluation of pupil size and response to light and can easily and rapidly be assessed. Causes of a decreased LOC in an injured child include TBI, hypoxemia, poor cerebral perfusion, or hypovolemic shock.[3,86,89,136-141]

Level of Consciousness

The rapid and reliable assessment of LOC is essential to identify the neurologic status of an acutely ill or injured child and to recognize early signs of deterioration. Neurologic status is obtained quickly with the assessment of pupil response to light and use of one of the standard scoring tools used in pediatrics such as the AVPU Pediatric Response and the GCS. The causes of a decreased

LOC in children can be numerous and include respiratory distress or failure with hypoxia or hypercarbia, hypoglycemia, seizures, infection, shock, brain injury, or trauma. Determining LOC is a crucial step in the management of the critically ill or injured child. The GCS is the most commonly used standard scoring tool and provides reliable, objective assessment of neurologic status by measuring eye opening, verbal response, and extremity movements. This scoring tool is validated in the assessment of children with head injuries and universally accepted for assessment of LOC in all other neurologic injury or illnesses. The GCS score is the most commonly used and reliable indicator of severity of TBI in all patients. The GCS is a validated standard scoring tool but requires skill for the provider to use consistently between patients. The use of the AVPU mnemonic (A is awake and alert, V is only responsive to verbal stimuli, P is only responsive to painful stimuli, and U is completely unresponsive) is a simplified version of the GCS. The AVPU scale is a commonly used assessment tool to rapidly measure the child's LOC and is accepted by the AHA PALS course. The AVPU responsiveness scale appears to provide a rapid, simple method to assess the critically ill child's LOC, and is an easier LOC scoring tool for prehospital personnel to use with children. Transport teams that are dedicated neonatal or pediatric carriers will tend to use the more common GCS for children. The AVPU is far easier to use and remember for the prehospital provider who is not a pediatric specialist.[3,86,89,138-139,142]

Pediatric Traumatic Brain Injury

Pediatric TBI is a leading cause of morbidity and mortality in the United States. For the most part, TBIs in children occur secondary to falls, being struck by an object or struck against a stationary object, MVCs, sports, bicycles, and NAT. The GCS is a clinical classification tool used to quantify the severity of TBI using the patient's best pupil, verbal, and motor responses. A mild TBI is considered to have a GCS range of 13 to 15, a moderate TBI score between 9 and 12, and a score of 8 or less is deemed to be a severe TBI. Long-term quality of life in children who have sustained a TBI can range from mild to severe deficits in academic, neurocognitive, neurobehavioral, and psychosocial skills.[139,142-143]

Etiology of Pediatric TBI

Causes of pediatric TBI can vary by age in children. In young children, falls are the most common cause of TBI. Younger children have large heads compared with body size and while they are developing coordination skills they frequently fall. In older children and adolescents, MVCs, other accidents involving a bicycle or motorcycle, and sports injuries are the most common causes of TBI. The older child age group starts to exhibit risk-taking behaviors, which increases the opportunity for brain injuries to occur. The majority of deaths related to TBI in children older than 1 year of age are the result of MVCs. In infants less than 1 year of age, NAT is the most common cause of TBI and is considered a significant problem. Any child who presents with an unexplainable head injury should be considered NAT until ruled out. A clinical sign used to predict an intracranial injury along with a head injury is the presence of a scalp hematoma. A scalp hematoma in the temporal/parietal or occipital areas of the child's skull increases the risk of an associated linear skull fracture being present. Any time the child presents with a scalp hematoma, the transport provider needs to suspect a linear skull fracture until proven otherwise. The infant who has an open anterior fontanel may allow a large amount of blood loss into this space before the child will decompensate.[139,143-145]

Table 30.15 lists the low-risk predictors established by the PECARN predictive rule for identification of a significant brain injury in children without advanced imaging or interventions. A child presenting without any of these symptoms usually does not require CT scans or invasive interventions; instead, observation of these children is performed. Table 30.16 lists the moderate and high risks associated with clinically significant TBI signs and symptoms in children and the recommendations for either neurologic observation or the need for neuroimaging with CT scan or MRI.[139,143-146]

TABLE 30.16	Signs/Symptoms Observed in Children Considered a Moderate and High Risk for a TBI[144,145,147]
Moderate Risk	**High Risk**
Treatment Indicates Observation or Probable Neuroimaging by CT Scan or MRI	*Treatment Crucial for Emergent Neuroimaging by Either CT Scan or MRI*
• Vomiting that resolves without intervention • Brief or unknown LOC • Headache • History of lethargy or irritability with infants may be resolved • Parents report infant not acting right • Severe mechanism of injury (e.g., motor vehicle crash, fall > 3 feet) • Scalp hematoma (e.g., temporal, parietal, or occipital) • Skull fracture > 24 hours • Unwitnessed traumatic injury • Any traumatic injury in infant < 3 months	• Suspicion of NAT in infants or children • Persistent vomiting • New onset seizure activity following injury • Altered mental status • Prolonged LOC • Bulging fontanelles in infants • Focal neurologic findings • Basilar or depressed skull fracture

LOC, Level of consciousness; *NAT,* nonaccidental trauma.

TABLE 30.15	Pediatric Emergency Care Applied Research Network (PECARN) Rule: A Validated Prediction Tool Used to Identify Children with Low Risk of a Significant TBI

Age in Years	Clinical Criteria*
<2	GCS < 15 Parental reports of child not acting normal Altered mental status reported > 5 second loss of consciousness Mechanism of injury severe (e.g., motor vehicle crash, fall > 3 feet) Temporal, parietal, or occipital scalp hematoma Palpable skull fracture is detected
≧2–18	GCS < 15 Altered mental status reported Documented loss of consciousness Mechanism of injury severe (e.g., motor vehicle crash, fall > 3 feet) Vomiting Severe headaches Signs of a basilar skull fracture detected

GCS, Glascow Coma Scale.

*Children presenting without any of the following established predictors are considered low risk for a significant TBI and a CT is not recommended.

Pediatric Primary Brain Injuries

Brain injuries are classified as either primary or secondary. Primary brain injury is the result of a mechanical force or damage incurred by the initial injury to the brain. The most common mechanisms causing a primary brain injury are when an object strikes a child's head, when the brain strikes the inside of the skull, or an acceleration-deceleration type of accident. Primary brain injuries are classified as focal or diffuse and may occur simultaneously. Focal injuries are scalp injuries, skull fractures, soft tissue injuries, or extraaxial hemorrhages such as an epidural, subdural, subarachnoid, or intraventricular hemorrhage. Diffuse injuries are intracranial lesions such as diffuse axonal injuries, cortical contusions, intraparenchymal hemorrhages, or vascular injuries. These injuries are usually a result of acceleration-deceleration forces.[139,143-145]

Pediatric Secondary Brain Injuries

Secondary brain injuries are not mechanically induced; instead, they are the result of events occurring after the initial brain injury and are a result of hypotension, hypoxemia, hypercapnia, hypoglycemia, and intracranial hypertension. Secondary brain injuries may develop rapidly within minutes of the initial insult to the brain and continue to evolve over hours to days. The most common causes of pediatric secondary brain injury are hypotension and hypoxemia and are associated with increased morbidities and mortalities in children. Research shows that correcting hypoxemia in a child with a TBI prior or during transport is associated with a significant increase in survival and a decrease in morbidities. This makes secondary brain injury prevention a critical intervention and primary goal of prehospital patient transport, EDs, and pediatric intensive care management.[139,143-146]

Standard Trauma Guidelines

Recommendations are for patients with a primary TBI to receive cardiopulmonary and hemodynamic support resuscitation to decrease or reduce secondary brain injuries caused by hypoxia, hypotension, and increased ICP. If the ICP is uncontrollable with positioning and medical management with sedation, then narcotics, paralytics, and osmotic diuretics may be needed. The two most common scoring tools are the AVPU Pediatric Response Scale and the GCS, which were discussed in more detail in a previous section.[138,140,147]

Pupillary Response

The pupils should be assessed for size, equality, and light response. Pupils that are fixed, dilated, unequal, sluggish, poorly reactive, or nonreactive to light and accommodation may be indicative of intracranial hypertension, increased ICP, or brainstem involvement. Direct trauma to the eye may also cause pupillary dysfunction; therefore, ocular findings should be correlated with the rest of the neurologic assessment. The transport provider needs to assess the child's pupils before administration of medications for intubation, seizure control, or paralytics.[3,88,93,139,142]

Motor Responses

Children with increased ICP have decreased or abnormal responses to pain. Decorticate and decerebrate posturing may be present. Flaccidity with severe head injury and paralysis from spinal cord injuries may be found on initial examination. The GCS has three areas assessed: are eye opening, verbal responses, and motor response to stimulation with the motor response score being the best predictor of long-term outcome in children after TBI. The motor response is regarded as a good indicator of the ability of the child's CNS to function properly to stimulation. The best way to elicit motor responses in the child with altered LOC is to apply pressure to one of the child's fingertips, to pinch the trapezius muscle at the base of the child's neck and upper shoulder area, and to apply pressure to the supraorbital notch. The child will respond with normal or abnormal flexion motor responses or no response using these three methods. Normal flexion will occur rapidly after stimulation and the arm will move away from the child's body. Abnormal flexion will respond slowly to the applied stimulation, the arm will move toward the body and across the chest with the forearm rotating and thumb clenched, and the child's legs will extend to the stimulation. Factors affecting motor responses in children include spinal cord injuries, peripheral nerve injuries, extremity injuries affecting movement, pain, or the inability to understand the provider or developmental delays.[3,86,89,139,142]

Pediatric TBI: Airway Control, Initial Stabilization, and Cervical Spine Immobilization

For children with TBI, prehospital providers should provide an initial rapid assessment of the patient's airway, breathing, circulatory status, and GCS for any other indicators of disability. The goals of initial stabilization and resuscitation include providing adequate oxygen delivery and ventilation, fluid resuscitation, and prevention of secondary damage to the child's brain. Cervical spine (C-spine) immobilization is recommended for all patients with possible cervical spine or SCI and is included in the initial stabilization of a child with TBI. Children with head injuries may have associated spinal injuries and should be C-spine immobilized and secured on a pediatric-designed immobilization device for transport until a SCI can be ruled out. Cervical spine injuries are closely associated to TBIs in children. The MOI causing the head injury is closely associated and increases the risk of cervical injuries in children. Maintaining manual C-spine immobilization is essential during airway control and stabilization of these children to prevent any cervical damage to these children.

Airway control and stabilization of the child with a TBI begins with the provider securing a stable airway with ETI. In children who are hemodynamically unstable or have low GCS scores, medications to intubate and secure an airway may not be used to potentially prevent hypotension causing a secondary brain injury. Rapid sequence intubation uses analgesia, sedatives, and paralytics to create optimal conditions to perform an emergent intubation. Caution must be observed during the use of rapid sequence intubation medications to prevent hypotension from occurring after administration. Rapid sequence intubation sedative medications midazolam and propofol may cause hypotension in these children and subsequent secondary brain injury while controlling the airway. Paralytics such as vecuronium prevent neurologic examination for an extended period of time and should be avoided. Most commonly used paralytics for rapid sequence intubation include succinylcholine and rocuronium and are the most frequently used in pediatric patients with TBI. Evidence supports the use of etomidate for intubation with a decrease in ICP. Fentanyl is another popular rapid sequence intubation medication for children. There is conflicting research on the usefulness of lidocaine with intubations in children. It is an optional medication that may have the ability to lessen the effects of ICP. Most Emergency Medical Service (EMS) programs and specialty transport teams have established protocols concerning which medications are appropriate for intubating children with TBIs.[3,86,89,139,143,147-148]

Adequate Ventilation

Pediatric patients requiring assisted ventilation via bag and mask or ETI benefit from $EtCO_2$ monitoring to ensure hyperventilation and hypoventilation do not occur. Hyperventilation occurs when the PCO_2 is less than 35 mm Hg and decreases cerebral blood flow, which may contribute to cerebral ischemia and secondary brain injury. Transient hyperventilation with an $EtCO_2$ goal of 30 to 35 mm Hg can be performed on the pediatric patient with signs of increased ICP and herniation, and in the patient with increased ICP refractory to osmotic agents. It is essential to maintain control of the child's airway and maintain adequate ventilation with an $EtCO_2$ of 35 to 40 mm Hg. This will significantly decrease any long-term morbidities in these children. The pediatric TBI guidelines recommend avoiding mild hyperventilation with a $PaCO_2$ less than 35 mm Hg and severe hyperventilation with a $PaCO_2$ less than 30 mm Hg to decrease risk of secondary brain injury. Pediatric TBI research has shown that avoiding hypercapnia and hypocapnia for the first 48 to 72 hours after the initial head injury is associated with the child's survival. Guidelines for prehospital transport of pediatric patients with a TBI recommend that after gaining control of the child's airway it is essential to maintain adequate ventilation management and the use of $EtCO_2$ monitoring. This is the most effective method used to monitor the child's ventilatory efforts during transport.[139,143,147-149]

Circulation

Fluid resuscitation in children begins with isotonic fluid boluses of 20 mL/kg with consideration given to the need for blood products in a pediatric patient who sustained a significant blood loss. Hypotension in the pediatric patient with TBI is a predictor of poor outcome. Evidenced-based TBI guidelines support CPP thresholds, and new research has shown that CPP targets should be age specific. These thresholds for CPP goals are above 50 mm Hg or 60 mm Hg in adults, above 50 mm Hg in 6 to 17 year olds, and above 40 mm Hg in 0 to 5 year olds and seem to be appropriate targets for preventing cerebral ischemia and secondary brain injury. Recent studies demonstrated that systemic hypotension had an inconsistent relationship to events of low CPP, but an elevated ICP was significantly related to all low CPP events across all the age groups. This data stressed the importance of controlling the child's ICP at all times and treating systolic blood pressure at specific moments. Hypotension after severe TBI increases the risk of secondary brain injury resulting in reduced perfusion to the child's brain. After initial resuscitation, it is important for the provider to maintain the child's circulatory status with an effective blood pressure. This is crucial to the child with TBI to ensure that autoregulation of the CPP is not impaired. Children are able to preserve their blood pressure and may initially only exhibit signs of hypovolemia as tachycardia. Tachycardia in the child with suspected TBI requires immediate evaluation. The preservation of a stable mean arterial blood pressure is important to provide adequate cerebral perfusion and oxygenation and decrease secondary brain injury.[139,143,150]

Intracranial Hypertension and Treatment Options

Primary and secondary injuries may lead to increased ICP in children with TBI. When the ICP is high, the direct brain tissue damage impairs the cerebral blood flow and metabolic regulation. In children with a TBI, a GCS of less than or equal to 8 indicates severe TBI with an increased risk of intracranial hypertension. Elevated ICP is one of the causes of secondary brain injury in these children and is associated with poor outcomes. Low GCS scores on the motor response section of the GCS may indicate intracranial hypertension. Increased ICP occurs frequently in children with severe TBI who do not demonstrate spontaneous motor function with the GCS evaluation. When the provider is able to successfully decrease ICP in children with TBIs, evidence shows a significant improvement in clinical outcomes with decreased morbidities. There are several methods available to help reduce ICP and secondary brain injuries: positioning the patient with head elevated and midline, the use of sedation, hyperosmolar medications such as mannitol and 3% hypertonic saline, and paralytic medications. Hyperosmolar therapy decreases elevated ICP through an osmotic effect, which is accomplished with either mannitol at 1 g/kg or 3% hypertonic saline at 5 to 10 mL/kg in children. Both mannitol and 3% sodium have a low penetration across the blood-brain barrier, creating an osmotic gradient effect in the patient's circulating blood, but this osmotic effect requires an intact blood-brain barrier for it to be effective. Recent studies have shown that 3% hypertonic saline given as a bolus was more effective than mannitol in lowering the cumulative and daily ICP spikes after a severe TBI in children. Additional studies have shown these two hyperosmolar medications are equally effective in treating increased ICP in pediatric TBI patients. Successfully controlling the child's ICP improves clinical outcomes in children by preventing secondary brain injuries.[139,143,150-152]

Seizures after Traumatic Brain Injury or Antiseizure Prophylaxis

Posttraumatic seizures may occur following TBI in children. The percentage of occurrence is directly related to the severity of the brain injury. Seizures are more common in children less than 3 years of age with severe head injuries, depressed skull fractures, cerebral edema, or intraparenchymal hemorrhages. Seizures increase the child's metabolic demands of the brain resulting in increased ICP leading to secondary brain injury. Antiseizure prophylaxis decreases the incidence of posttraumatic seizures in children with TBI. Common medications used for antiseizure prophylaxis are fosphenytoin, phenytoin, and levetiracetam. Common medications for posttraumatic seizures include lorazepam and diazepam, which both can be given rectally, and midazolam, which may be given nasally or rectally. Other medications include fosphenytoin, phenytoin, or phenobarbital. Monitor patient's vital signs closely with administration of these medications to prevent hypotension and secondary brain injury from a decrease in CPP.[3,139,143]

Positioning

Maintaining the patients head up at 30 degrees while secured on a pediatric immobilization device while maintaining the patient's head midline with commercial devices or towel rolls unless prohibited by other injuries will assist to decrease ICP in the child by promoting venous drainage and consequently improving CPP.[3,139,143]

Environmental Issues

Control of noise, especially in the transport setting, is important in controlling acute elevations in ICPs. Unless prohibited by patient injury, earplugs or earmuffs can decrease noise stress on patients. Adequate sedation and pain management can help decrease ICP.[3]

Reevaluation

Continuous monitoring and reevaluation of the patient is performed during primary and secondary surveys, especially with children experiencing a neurologic impairment. It is necessary during transport to assess for deterioration of patient status, increases in ICP, and effectiveness of medical interventions.[139]

Mild to Moderate Traumatic Brain Injury: Imaging

The goal of caring for children with mild to moderate TBI is to identify significant intracranial injury while limiting unneeded imaging and unnecessary radiation exposure. Most children with mild TBI are at low risk for long-term neurologic complications or deficits. The prevalence of intracranial hemorrhage in children with mild TBI is relatively low and increases if the child has an underlying neurologic disorder such as ventriculoperitoneal shunt, scalp laceration, visible skull fracture, and neurologic findings. PECARN developed the childhood head injury predictive rule, which identifies children at high risk for necessitating neurosurgical intervention and at medium risk for having a brain injury on imaging.[139,146]

Spinal Cord Injuries

Spinal cord injuries (SCIs) in children are rare and increases in prevalence in adolescents. SCIs occurring in children are rarely observed as an isolated injury but more often combined with additional injury patterns. Because of their anatomic differences, children are predisposed to cervical spinal injuries (CSIs). Pediatric CSIs are rare but devastating resulting in the

child's death or life-changing neurologic damage. Pediatric CSIs are rare because the level of injury is different and they carry a much higher morbidity and mortality compared with adults. It is important to understand pediatric CSI patterns in relation to MOI, treatment, and neurologic outcomes in children. An accurate, rapid diagnosis and management are necessary to avoid potentially devastating injuries to children. The size of the head in a child is proportionally larger compared with their body, resulting in acceleration and deceleration at high-impact speeds, which causes more stress to the upper cervical spine. The fulcrum sits at the C2-C3 level in a child, and as the child ages it tends to move lower to the C5-C6 level. The incomplete ossification of the vertebral bodies, underdeveloped spinal processes, and ligamentous laxity are the reason children have a decreased incidence of CSIs. The anatomic and developmental differences, cervical spine stability, and the injury pattern in the pediatric patient is significantly different from the adult. After 10 years of age the injury pattern begins to be similar to that of an adult. The most common types of pediatric CSIs are fractures of the vertebral body, followed by subluxation. Table 30.17 lists the CSI MOI and injury classification based on the age of the child.[153-156]

TABLE 30.17		
Age of Child	**Mechanism of Injury for CSI**	**Injury Classification of CSIs**
<2 years of age	• Motor vehicle crash (MVC) • falls	• Axial area affected • Most common area is atlanto-occipital dislocation,* which affects the occiput through C2 • Uncommon for young children to experience SCIWORA
2–7 years of age	• MVC • Falls • Child versus motor vehicle	• Axial area affected • Atlanto-axial rotator subluxation** • Atlanto-occipital dislocation most common (occiput through C2)
8–15 years of age	• Sports injuries • MVC • Falls • Diving accidents	• Subaxial injuries occur with subaxial vertebral body fractures, which affects C3-C7 more frequently (are common and often miss diagnosed) • SCIWORA is more common in this age group

*Atlanto-occipital dislocation—highly unstable, potentially devastating ligamentous neurological injury.
** Atlanto-axial rotator sublaxation—injury to C1-C2 causing impairment in rotation of the neck.
CSI, Cervical spine injury; *SCIWORA,* spinal cord injury without any radiographic abnormality.
Adapted from Leonard JR, Jaffe DM, Kuppermann N, Olsen CS, Leonard JC. Cervical spine injury patterns in children. *Pediatrics.* 2014;133(5): e1179-e1188.

SCI without any radiographic abnormality (SCIWORA) affects older children more often. All three of these types of CSIs are commonly associated with comorbid head injuries. SCIWORA is the diagnosis given to children experiencing neurologic deficits associated with the cervical spinal cord in the absence of abnormalities on radiographs or CTs. Magnetic resonance imaging (MRI) has become a common imaging modality in spinal trauma because of its enhanced ability to identify soft tissue lesions such as discoligamentous injuries, cord hematomas, cord edema, cord transections, and neurocompressive injuries, which are not seen on radiographs or CT scans. MVCs, falls, and NAT are more common MOIs for children younger than 8 years of age diagnosed with SCIWORA. Sports-related injuries such as gymnastics, diving, horseback riding, football, and wrestling are more common MOIs in older children.[153-156]

Imaging to Detect Traumatic Injuries of the Cervical Spine in Children

CSI may be rare in children but the potential consequences are devastating. The most sensitive and specific methods of clearing cervical spines in children are not known. Over the last decade, cervical spine CT for pediatric patients has increased considerably making it the standard modality used to detect CSIs in children. A cervical spine CT scan is not only costly, but the long-term risk of radiation exposure to children is an increasing concern because the use of CT imaging has become more popular in evaluating patients. Cervical radiation exposure increases the risk of developing thyroid cancer in children. Ionizing radiation doses delivered by CT scans are 100 to 500 times higher than conventional x-rays.

There has been a growing interest in creating guidelines for the clearance of the pediatric cervical spine to reduce significant exposure of CT scan radiation and yet be effective to clear CSIs. Two commonly validated clinical decision guidelines established to clear adult cervical spine are the National Emergency X-Radiography Utilization Study (NEXUS) criteria and the Canadian C-Spine Rule (CCR). The NEXUS criteria and the CCR do not specifically address clearance of the pediatric cervical spine. One guideline in the literature was the NEXUS criteria adapted to minimize radiation exposure while clearing the pediatric cervical spine. Protocols have been developed to facilitate safe clearance of pediatric cervical spines clinically or through the use of modalities exposing children to less extreme forms of radiation. Based on concerns for ionizing radiation exposure, the University of Iowa Trauma Service developed a Pediatric Cervical Spine Clearance Protocol for children younger than 10 years of age. The guidelines are moving away from CT scan as the primary modality; initial imaging is plain x-rays and then decide if additional imaging with MRI or CT is warranted.[156-159]

Plain Radiography

Anteroposterior and lateral plain x-rays are commonly used as initial screening x-rays. They can identify the majority of cervical spine fractures, but may need to be repeated for a more adequate visualization. The lateral plain radiograph should be the first test to screen for pediatric CSI. The sensitivity of the lateral neck x-ray is relatively high and increases with children older than 8 years. Anteroposterior views usually do not increase sensitivity. In the cooperative child who is over 5 years of age and able to follow commands, the odontoid open mouth x-ray is an additional view that is used to detect dens or burst fractures of C1. An oblique view provides enhanced views of the posterior elements of the neck and subluxation. The odontoid and oblique views are not recommended for initial examination but can be considered when initial views are indeterminate or the clinical scenario suggests a specific bony injury is present. Flexion-extension x-rays are additional views of the cervical spine. These may be considered in the stable trauma patient who has persistent neck pain regardless of normal lateral and anteroposterior x-rays.[158-159]

Magnetic Resonance Imaging

An MRI does not have the ionizing radiation risks associated with CT. Compared with CT, MRI has higher sensitivity for spinal cord and soft tissue injuries but is less sensitive than CT in detecting bony injuries. The MRI is more difficult to obtain compared with the CT scan in an acutely injured child because of limited availability, and the length of time required to obtain adequate MR images frequently requires sedation in children. The role of MRI in CSI is in the detection of significant CSIs in obtunded patients who cannot be examined clinically. An obtunded patient with a normal MRI finding can have his or her cervical spine safely cleared and can reduce the length of time in a cervical collar. MRI imaging may be cost-efficient if used appropriately. An MRI protocol for obtunded children has saved each patient a significant amount of money likely related to a shorter immobilization time and hospital stay.[158-159]

Computed Tomography

CT scans are superior in sensitivity for detecting acute CSIs compared with plain x-rays. However, current evidence does not support the use of CT scans as a standard screening tool for children with a potential traumatic CSI. In children, most injuries found on cervical spine CT are also noted on plain radiography. CT scans in children are associated with a longer ED length of stay, higher resource use of ED staff, and a significant exposure of ionizing radiation to the child. Children are more sensitive to the carcinogenic effects of ionizing radiation. Among the plain x-rays, MRI, and CT imaging technologies, CT scans are of the greatest concern regarding children because of the high levels of ionizing radiation associated with this technology and the estimated increase in the child's lifetime cancer risk associated with the scans. Long-term radiation risks associated with CT scans in children is the rationale for why the industry is adopting other modalities to evaluate CSIs in children.

CT scans expose patients to significantly more radiation than plain x-rays. As an example, one head CT scan before the age of 10 years results in one excess brain tumor per 10,000 patients. An approach to reducing radiation exposure for pediatric patients in which a cervical spine CT is indicated is a focused CT. The CT focuses a beam directly to a specific level of concern. A focused CT from occiput to C3 increases sensitivity for diagnosing CSI while limiting radiation exposure.[158-159]

Spinal Protection

A review of the literature was unable to determine whether the effect of full spinal immobilization in pediatric trauma patients was helpful or harmful to the child's mortality, neurologic injury, spinal stability, or adverse effects. There are two goals for spinal protection in children: to limit current damage and prevent a secondary injury. Full spinal immobilization is considered the standard of care for all children meeting the injury criteria for transport to a trauma center with the conviction that maintaining the child's spine in a neutral position and minimizing spine motion during transport will limit neurologic injury. Children who sustain blunt trauma are frequently placed in full spinal immobilization in an effort to protect the cervical spine from further injury. However, given the rare association of CSIs in children, the potential harmful effects, if they present themselves, may prevail over any potential benefit of immobilization for most children.[160-165]

The ACEP states that spinal motion restriction should be the preferred practice because true spinal immobilization is impossible. Without sufficient data, there is only guidance from experts in the field of pediatric trauma, which recommends full spinal immobilization of pediatric trauma patients to protect a child's cervical spine. There is insufficient data in children to support standards of treatment; instead, there are recommendations from the Congress of Neurologic Surgeons, the ACS-COT, and the NAEMSP for spinal immobilization of all patients in the presence of either suspicion of a CSI or an MOI with the potential to cause CSI in a child. The recommendations suggest fully immobilizing the child using a cervical collar and an appropriately sized backboard for transporting children to minimize risk of CSI after trauma. If at all possible, try to use a pediatric-designed backboard. Adult backboards are unable to immobilize and restrict a child correctly, and they promote neck flexion in a child. Use of either a blanket or padding to elevate the shoulders and upper thoracic area or have a backboard with an occipital recess to bring the pediatric spine into better neutral alignment is recommended. The padding or blanket should extend continuously from the shoulders through the thoracic and lumbar spine to the pelvis to maintain a neutral alignment of the child's entire spine. Padding under the shoulders only flexes the thoracic and lumbar spine of a child. Additionally, if you are using an adult backboard or an oversized backboard on a child, consider adding padding between the edges of the board and the child. This will pad the open areas between the sides of the backboard and the child under the straps and fill the open triangle area preventing lateral movement of the child on the backboard.[160-165]

Devices for younger children include the Pedi-Pac, Pedi-Boards, Pedi-Air, MedKids Baby Board, pediatric vacuum mattresses, Papoose board, and Kendrick Extrication Device (KED), which have demonstrated safe and effective immobilization tools for providers. The KED can be used for both extrication and immobilization but still requires a blanket or padding to maintain a neutral position.[160-165]

Application of Proper Spinal Immobilization

The most important intervention in the transport of children with known or suspected SCI is proper spinal protection. Before application of cervical collars and a backboard, jewelry and necklaces should be removed to prevent interference with radiologic examinations and possible pressure injuries. Care should also be taken to remove sharp debris, such as glass, from the patient to prevent further injury. One provider will maintain manual stabilization of the child's cervical spine while the other places an appropriately sized firm cervical collar. An improperly sized collar can interfere with respirations or cause inappropriate extension of the child's cervical spine. An appropriately fitting cervical collar has the child's chin rests in the chin piece with the collar below the child's ears, and resting on the clavicles. Cervical collars are designed and available to fit newborns up to adults. Infants may be too small for a properly fitted cervical collar or the transport provider may not have the appropriately sized collars available. In these circumstances, a towel roll may be used to immobilize the cervical spine. A towel roll must prevent flexion and extension and align the cervical spine in a neutral position. If a towel roll cannot achieve these goals, manual control may need to be continued until child is transported to a definitive center.[160-165]

Once a cervical collar has been applied, the child is then logrolled and placed on a backboard. One person should provide manual control of the collared cervical spine, with another person at the child's shoulders and hips and another at the child's hips and legs. Opposite the patient, one person should be in place to position the backboard. The person controlling the cervical spine may then lead the command to turn the patient as a unit onto his or her side. This is the time for the provider not involved in the logrolling of the patient to inspect and palpate the patient's back and spine, assessing for step-offs, injuries, or pain. Inspection and palpation of the head, neck, and spine should be performed to assess for lacerations, hematoma, cerebrospinal fluid (CSF) or bloody drainage from the ears or nose, depressed skull fractures, or step-off in the spinal column. All inspection and palpation should be performed on children while maintaining manual cervical spine control and logrolling with spinal precautions in place.[160-165]

Although evaluation of the spine and back are not technically part of the primary survey, these assessments are best performed with the patient placed on a backboard, which is necessary for transport protection of the cervical spine. Children younger than 8 years of age have disproportionately large heads, so padding under the shoulders on the board is necessary to keep the cervical spine in a neutral position. As mentioned earlier, the entire spine of the child needs to be in a neutral position so the blanket or padding should continue to the child's pelvis. The backboard can be positioned at a 30- to 45-degree angle and the child then rolled onto it. Once the patient is centered on the board, lateral stabilization of the cervical spine with blanket rolls or blocks and securing the head with straps or tape should be performed. The final step in spinal immobilization is securing the body to the board with straps (securing the chest, hips, and knees). Straps should be secure enough to allow turning the board from side to side without movement of the patient's body. This turning may be necessary in the unintubated patient who has periods of emesis during transport. Suction should be readily available for any patient secured to a backboard. A neurologic examination should precede and follow all spinal immobilization procedures.[160-165]

Even with expert guidance, the diligence of consistent spinal immobilization with appropriately sized equipment for children is highly variable or not done at all. Children younger than 2 years of age are more vulnerable and at a higher risk for severe high-level cervical injuries and are unable to communicate effectively any signs or symptoms of the injury, yet these are the ones who are not fully immobilized with a cervical collar and pediatric sized backboard. A study found a correlation between eight factors and CSIs in children suggesting the need to provide full spine immobilization. They include altered mental status; focal neurologic findings; neck pain; torticollis; substantial torso injury; and medical conditions predisposing the child to CSI such as Down syndrome, diving injury, or high-risk MVC.[160-165]

Removal of a Child From a Child Safety Seat With Maintenance of Spinal Immobilization

Infants and young children up to about 8 years of age may still require car seats or booster seats when riding in a car. Those secured correctly may never need spinal immobilization. The literature reports controversy over whether to remove a child from their car seat or to transport them in their car seat. Any child with an unstable airway, respiratory, or circulatory status must be removed from their car seat. If the child remains in their car seat, it is impossible for the transport provider to perform a full primary and secondary survey of the child and potential injuries may be missed. Children with an ejected car seat, damage to the car seat, or a car seat with a high back should always be removed from their car seat. Without doing so the transport provider would be unable to provide emergent interventions including intubation, aspiration prevention, or venous access.[3,86,163]

Removing a child from a car seat requires the initiation of manual cervical spine immobilization by one provider. The other provider will remove or cut the shoulder harness,

and move the safety bar out of the way. Position the child safety seat at the foot of the backboard. Tip the child safety seat back, and lay it down on the backboard. One person then slides his or her hands along each side of the patient's head until they are behind the patient's shoulders. The head and neck are now supported laterally by that person's arms. A second person should then take control of the patient's body. On the instruction of the person holding the head, slide the child out of the safety seat onto the backboard and immobilize as described previously.[3,86,163]

Adverse Effects of Spinal Immobilization

Full spinal immobilization is common in children who are victims of blunt trauma to protect the child's cervical spine from further injury. Because children infrequently suffer cervical injury the potential harmful effects of full spine immobilization may outweigh any potential benefit for the majority of children. Studies have documented children who are immobilized following a traumatic incident report more pain; increased pain on arrival to the ED; and are at a higher risk of undergoing radiographic imaging of the cervical spine and a higher hospital admission rate compared with those children who are not immobilized in the field, regardless of the injury severity reported. Pain caused by spinal immobilization may be confused with the actual traumatic injury, which may lead to unnecessary diagnostic evaluations and exposure to ionizing radiation from CT scan of the cervical spine. Additional adverse effects include increased risk of aspiration and skin breakdown if left on a hard backboard for an extended period of time.[3,161,163-165]

Exposure and Environment

The final segment of the primary survey is exposure of the traumatically injured child. The child's clothing is removed to allow a visual inspection of the body for rapid identification and to decrease the chance of missing any obvious injuries and initiate treatment of multiple injuries if warranted. This step requires a team effort to maintain manual cervical spine stabilization and logroll the child. This allows the provider to assess and inspect the child's back and spine for step-offs or other deformities, tenderness, or other external injury. If warranted, a rectal examination may be done at this time. Even though this is not officially part of the primary survey, it falls into place naturally because very little additional time is needed to complete it and the child must be logrolled anyway to be place on a backboard for transport. Remember to place a pad or blanket under the shoulders down to the pelvis to maintain a neutral spinal alignment, especially for children younger than 8 years of age. Immediately cover the child with warm blankets after exposing the child for examination to minimize heat loss. It is important to be more vigilant with infants and young children because they are more vulnerable to heat loss secondary to their large surface area (head) in relation to their body volume. The patient's temperature should be obtained in this step and reassessed during transport. Additional methods used to help prevent heat loss include increasing the room if in an ED or the ambulance for transport and Bair hugger or overhead heat lamp if available.[3,86,89,143,166]

Hypothermia

Hypothermia is a decrease in the body's core temperature caused by inadequate body temperature regulation or excessive environmental cold stress. Hypothermia can be accidental, such as an environmental exposure, or intentional, such as with therapeutic hypothermia. Hypothermia can occur rapidly with submersion injuries or gradually as a result of exposure to ambient temperatures. Hypothermia is a core temperature below 35°C (95°F). The stage of hypothermia has a major impact on both recognition and treatment. Hypothermia is considered mild with a core temperature of 32°C to 35°C (90°F–95°F), moderate with a core temperature of 28°C to 32°C (82°F–90°F), or severe with a core temperature below 28°C (82°F). Infants and children are at a higher risk of hypothermia because of their larger ratio of surface area to body mass, limited glycogen stores to support heat production, a young infant's inability to increase heat production through shivering, and a decreased ability to recognize and avoid hypothermic exposure. Heat is lost from the body by radiation, conduction, convection, evaporation, and respiration. The clinical features of hypothermia depend on the stage of hypothermia. See Box 30.5 for the stages and clinical features of hypothermia.[3,86,166]

Management of Hypothermia

Successful management of the hypothermic child depends on the stage of hypothermia and rapid assessment of the patient following the ABDCDEs of the primary survey along with the treatment of the injury or other medical conditions including effective rewarming interventions. In the prehospital environment, suspicion of hypothermia is vital and should be considered with not only the children exposed to the environment but those who may have an altered mental status. Accurate core temperature in children with hypothermia is essential to proper treatment and interventions. Prehospital providers must avoid exertion and excessive handling of the hypothermic patient during rescue or securing on the stretcher. Patients with hypothermia because of these actions may mobilize cold and acidic blood to the heart increasing the potential for cardiac arrhythmias or arrest. Many patients arrive at the hospital colder than at the scene. Patient rescue, transport, and treatment of hypothermic patients involves risks of iatrogenic cooling. During transport, the prehospital provider provides passive rewarming strategies by doing everything possible to prevent further heat loss by removing wet clothing, gently covering the patient with blankets, increasing the ambient temperature in the mode of transport, warming IV fluids if possible, and giving heated humidified oxygen. External rewarming of children with moderate to severe hypothermia in transport is usually avoided because it requires active external rewarming, which is difficult in the transport environment.[3,88,166-167]

Active external rewarming techniques include applying heat externally to the child using a forced air rewarming device, radiant heat, and applying heat packs. Active external rewarming has the potential to promote further cooling, hypotension from rewarming shock, ventricular fibrillation, or asystole in patients. It is important to warm the trunk before the extremities.

Active internal rewarming techniques are invasive ways to rewarm a child. These include continued efforts from the passive and active external rewarming with heated humidified oxygen and warmed IV fluids. Invasive techniques of rewarming used for severe hypothermia include heated saline lavage of the pleura, bladder, stomach, or peritoneum. Another method of active internal rewarming is ECMO and is used for severe hypothermia in children who are unresponsive to the other methods or have absent circulation.[3,88,166,167]

Treatment of Mild Hypothermia

Patients with environmental exposure and mild hypothermia respond well to passive rewarming by removal of wet clothing and drying the skin, active external rewarming with forced air heating blanket and radiant heat lamp, and administering warmed IV normal saline. Continual monitoring of core temperature and continuous monitoring of cardiac rhythm and circulatory status is essential to demonstrate that the child is responding to the appropriate methods of rewarming.[3,88,166-167]

• BOX 30.5   Stages and Clinical Signs of Hypothermia[166,167]

Mild Stage: Core temperature 32-35°C or 90-95°F
   Signs: Conscious, mild tachycardia, shivering, piloerection, cyanosis, pallor, acrocyanosis, vasoconstriction, delayed capillary refill time, increased metabolism, possible hypertension
Moderate Stage: Core temperature 28-32°C or 82-90°F
   Signs: Loss of compensatory shivering, altered mental status, lethargy, clumsiness, confusion or delirium, irrational behaviors such as paradoxical undressing, slurred speech, decreased heat production, circulatory insufficiency and instability, vasodilation starts, hypovolemia, decreased metabolism, decreasing cerebral blood flow, diuresis, extravasation of fluids, decreasing blood

pressure and heart rate, decreasing respiratory depression and ventilation
Severe Stage: Core temperature less than 28°C or 82°F
   Signs: Unconscious – suspended cerebral activity, no shivering, loss of thermoregulation, vasodilation, decreased heart rate and cardiac output, decreased stroke volume, decreased cardiac conduction, increased cardiac irritability, slowed nerve conduction, vital signs may or may not be present, erythema and edema, muscle rigidity, stupor or coma, bradycardia progressing to absent pulses, fixed and dilated pupils, ventricular fibrillation, asystole

Determine the underlying cause of the child's mild hypothermia if an environmental exposure is not the cause. The most common causes of mild hypothermia in children are sepsis, hypoglycemia, hyponatremia, hypothyroidism, adrenal insufficiency, and burns. Hypothermia is most frequently associated with sepsis in infants and in children with gram-negative sepsis. Drugs affecting the child's CNS or endocrine or metabolic diseases may be the underlying cause of mild hypothermia in children. Diagnostic testing and appropriate treatment should be initiated to correct the hypothermia.[3,88,166-167]

Treatment of Moderate or Severe Hypothermia

Children with moderate to severe hypothermia require intensive support of the airway, breathing, and circulation in addition to rewarming. Hypoventilation may be a physiologic finding in moderate or severe hypothermia. Gentle respiratory support is safe and should be provided as needed by providing warmed humidified 100% oxygen via nonrebreather mask for all patients. If status is deteriorating, initiate BVM ventilation and prepare for intubation. ETI is performed if the child continues to deteriorate and respiratory failure occurs along with uncompensated shock or cardiac arrest. ETI should not be delayed in the hypothermic child if the child's status indicates it is needed. Monitor closely for cardiac arrhythmias during intubation. Children with severe hypothermia intubation may be more difficult because of muscle rigidity. In children with severe hypothermia, the heart rate and respiratory effort may be slow and difficult to detect. Research shows to initiate CPR immediately if no signs of life are found in a child with severe hypothermia. Hypothermia induces vasoconstriction making vascular access difficult in children. Vascular access is imperative for the child to improve because aggressive infusion of warmed IV fluids for volume expansion is one of the primary treatments for moderate to severe hypothermia. It requires the placement of two large-bore peripheral IVs or, if this is not possible, placement of an intraosseous (IO) needle or a central line in the femoral vein and begin normal saline 20 mL/kg of volume using high-capacity warmers and tubing and rapidly infuse warm saline. The child may require another 20-mL/kg fluid bolus because aggressive and ongoing volume expansion is usually required while treating hypothermia. Hypoglycemia is a common finding with hypothermia and requires treatment. Rhythms associated with moderate to severe hypothermia include perfusing bradycardic rhythms such as sinus bradycardia, first degree heart block, and atrial fibrillation. In moderate to severe hypothermia, these rhythms are considered adequate for maintaining sufficient oxygen delivery. Atropine and epinephrine are usually not given because rewarming usually corrects these rhythms to a more normal rhythm. The nonperfusing cardiac rhythms include ventricular fibrillation, ventricular tachycardia without a pulse, and pulseless electrical activity or asystole and are commonly seen with moderate to severe hypothermia.[3,88,166-167]

Aggressive active internal rewarming or extracorporeal rewarming with ECMO are usually the primary treatments for these children. If a perfusing rhythm does not return with rewarming, immediately begin CPR and continue aggressive rewarming measures. The efficacy of epinephrine is decreased with severe hypothermia. There is limited data to support administration of epinephrine during rewarming strategies. To promote the return of spontaneous circulation (ROSC), follow the 2015 pediatric cardiac arrest algorithm along with aggressive rewarming techniques, but avoid excessive doses of epinephrine. Attempts at rewarming the child should not delay transport to a critical care facility that has the ability to provide all the necessary treatments to reverse the severe hypothermia including extracorporeal capabilities with ECMO.[3,88,166-167]

Heatstroke

Hyperthermia is a life-threatening condition with a core temperature of greater than or equal to 40°C (104°F) with CNS dysfunction in patients with environmental exposure to heat. Classic heatstroke occurs from environmental exposure to heat and is common in younger children who are unable to escape from a hot environment, such as those left in a car or those with underlying chronic medical conditions that impair thermoregulation such as cystic fibrosis and CHD. Exertional heatstroke occurs in young healthy children who are engaging in heavy exercise during times of high ambient temperature and humidity, such as teenage athletes. Heat-related illness is the third major cause of death in adolescents behind traumatic and cardiac causes of death. The highest rate of nonfatal heat illnesses are high school athletes, especially football players.[3,168]

Children receive serious heat-related injuries when the critical thermal maximum (CTM) is exceeded, which is the degree of elevated body temperature and the duration of heat exposure before cell damage occurs. Evaporation is the primary mechanism of heat loss in a hot environment. The diagnostic criteria for children with heatstroke are elevated core temperature greater than or equal to 40°C (104°F) and CNS abnormalities following environmental heat exposure. Temperature elevation increases oxygen consumption and metabolic rate, causing hyperpnea and tachycardia. CNS symptoms may be subtle or cause impaired judgment or inappropriate behavior, seizures, delirium, hallucinations, ataxia, dysarthria, or coma. Additional clinical signs associated with heatstroke include tachycardia, tachypnea, flushed and warm or diaphoretic skin, and vomiting and diarrhea. Patients with heatstroke may present with coagulopathy, with purpura, hemoptysis, hematemesis, melena, or hematochezia. Above 42°C (108°F) patients are at risk for multiorgan failure.[3,168]

Treatment of Heatstroke

Any child with an LOC with exertion in warm weather or found in a heated car should be treated as a child with a heatstroke. The diagnosis of heat-related illness is challenging in the prehospital setting. Core temperature may not be obtained and by arrival of EMS some cooling measures have usually already been performed. The prehospital provider's best method of cooling pediatric patients is removal from the source of heat stress, and rapid initiation of cooling is the treatment initiated. The risk of morbidity and mortality in children with heat-related illness is associated with duration of hyperthermia exposure. One method is ice water immersion, if the equipment and trained personnel are available, or an evaporative external cooling in the field. Prehospital cooling should start before or at the same time EMS is activated. Evaporative cooling methods in the field or in the ambulance are done by spraying the patient with water or saline. Additionally, decrease ambient temperature in the ambulance with air conditioners on high speed and manually fanning the patient. Apply ice packs to the child's axilla, groin, and neck, along with the administration of room temperature IV fluids.[3,168]

Initial stabilization may include the need for basic or advanced control of airway and breathing if CNS effects are causing respiratory depression from coma or seizure activity. All patients with heatstroke require venous access either with two large-bore IVs, IOs, or central access. Fluid resuscitation is dependent on the type of heatstroke. The provider can administer IV fluids at room temperature, but monitor closely to prevent fluid overload. Children with classic nonexertional heatstroke are only mildly to moderately hypovolemic, but with exertional heatstroke they are more moderately to severely hypovolemic and may require 20 to 40 mL/kg of normal saline or more. Altered mental status may resolve after oxygenation and adequate tissue perfusion, and normothermia is achieved. If seizures develop, treat with benzodiazepines as needed. All children with heatstroke after stabilization and rapid cooling should be admitted to a pediatric critical care unit because the child remains at high risk for end organ failure and metabolic and coagulation abnormalities. The child with heatstroke is at risk and should be evaluated for rhabdomyolysis with hyperkalemia, hypocalcemia, hyperphosphatemia, disseminated intravascular coagulation, acute kidney injury, hyponatremic dehydration, cardiogenic shock with low systemic vascular resistance (SVR), cerebral edema, and liver failure.[3,168]

Near-Drowning

Drowning and submersion injuries are the leading causes of accidental death and morbidities in children. Over 500,000 deaths globally each year are attributed to drowning. The CDC reported in 2010 that drowning was the leading cause of accidents and death in children ages 1 to 4 years, the second leading cause of death in children ages 5 to 9 years, and the third leading cause of death in children ages 10 to 14 years. Drownings can be broken down by the type of water (i.e., freshwater or saltwater) and temperature. Warm water drownings occur in temperatures greater than or equal to 20°C (68°F), and cold water drownings occur in temperatures less than or equal to 20°C (68°F). The most common locations of drowning in children occur in freshwater, including lakes, rivers, and other natural bodies of water; followed by swimming pools; then bathtubs or buckets; and then saltwater, which is the smallest percentage. Infant drownings are highest in swimming pools at home.[3,169]

Risk factors identified for children are epilepsy, congenital long QT syndrome, catecholaminergic polymorphic ventricular tachycardia, hyperventilation before swimming, hypoglycemia, and hypothermia. In older children alcohol and illicit drugs are contributors to drowning. The drowning process usually begins with voluntary breath holding then small amounts of water are aspirated into the airway, triggering a coughing reflex and laryngospasm. The child cannot breathe because of the laryngospasm so exchange of gas stops, leading to hypoxia, hypercarbia, and acidosis. As arterial oxygen tension decreases, laryngospasm is relieved and additional water is aspirated by the child, leading to cerebral hypoxemia, which causes the child to lose consciousness and become apneic followed quickly by cardiac arrest. The entire drowning process usually takes place within seconds to minutes. Intrapulmonary shunting of blood through poorly ventilated lungs is the primary pathophysiologic process of drowning. Contributing to this process of intrapulmonary shunting includes bronchospasm, impaired alveolar–capillary gas exchange from aspirated fluid within the alveolar space, surfactant inactivation and washout, decreased surfactant production because of alveolar damage, and atelectasis causing pulmonary edema and a ventilation/perfusion mismatch. After 24 hours an infectious or chemical pneumonitis may occur from aspiration of gastric contents or type of water from near nonfatal drowning. Hypoxia, acidosis, and hypothermia contribute to cardiovascular dysfunction or dysrhythmias. Permanent neurologic damage is common in the survivors of near-drowning. The amount of damage is determined by the duration and severity of the initial hypoxic-ischemic injury.[3,169]

Management of Near-Drowning

Pediatric survivors of near-drowning almost universally have two things in common: limited submersion times and excellent initial resuscitative care. The first priority in managing a child who has a near-drowning event is to reverse hypoxemia by restoring adequate oxygenation and ventilation. Initial efforts focus on airway, breathing, and circulation. Oxygen, with or without mechanical ventilation support, is the first line of therapy. The child breathing spontaneously and able to maintain an oxygen saturation greater than 90% or a partial pressure of oxygen greater than 90 mm Hg with a fraction of inspired oxygen of 0.5 may be able to remain on the nonrebreather mask with oxygen therapy alone. Children who are apneic or exhibiting respiratory depression require ETI using a rapid sequence induction technique. Intubation not only secures an airway but also protects against aspiration of gastric contents and allows for suctioning of the airway and effective oxygenation and ventilation if copious pulmonary edema develops. Mechanical ventilation with PEEP should be used. In the event of suspected CSIs, the provider needs to avoid hyperextension of the neck during resuscitation. Immobilization of the cervical spine is based solely on the history of submersion by witnesses. The most frequent complication of children who drown is regurgitation and aspiration of stomach contents, which causes more damage to the lungs and affects oxygenation. All victims of drowning with evidence of shock need IV fluid resuscitation with normal saline with the initial fluid boluses starting at 20 mL/kg. If IV access cannot be obtained in a timely manner because of ongoing CPR or extreme vasoconstriction, IO access should be performed. Decreased CO with high systemic and pulmonary vascular resistance occurs secondary to hypoxia associated with near-drowning. This injury may persist even after adequate oxygenation, ventilation, and perfusion have been established requiring the initiation of inotropic agents to improve CO and reestablish adequate tissue perfusion. Reverse the child's hypothermia slowly.[3,169]

Secondary Survey

The secondary survey begins after the primary survey (ABCDEs) is completed and resuscitative efforts are initiated. A complete head-to-toe evaluation of the trauma patient should be completed to assess for non–life-threatening injuries including a complete history, physical examination, and reassessment of vital signs and interventions. This evaluation requires each region of the body to be examined completely by inspection; palpation; and, where appropriate, auscultation and percussion. Ideally, this survey should take place during transport rather than at the scene of injury. The potential for missing an injury or facility to realize the impact of an injury is significant, especially in the unresponsive or unstable patient. Assessment for lacerations, fractures, abrasions, ecchymosis, ocular and dental injuries, and areas of swelling or edema are included in the secondary survey. Any part of the body not fully assessed during the primary survey should now be evaluated for injury. A full set of vital signs should also be completed. A complete neurologic examination is performed including repeating the GCS score. If time permits, dressing of wounds and immobilization of fractures can now take place. Frequent reassessment of the patient's primary survey and effectiveness of medical interventions should be ongoing during transport. Neurovascular assessments before and after immobilization of fractures are necessary. Obtain the child's weight either by caregiver history or by use of a length-based resuscitation tape. Cardiac monitors and pulse oximeters (if not already in place) should be applied. A radio report to receiving facilities should also be completed at this time and before arrival to the receiving facility.[3,86,89]

Nonaccidental Trauma or Neglect

According to the CDC abusive head trauma is an injury to the skull or intracranial contents of a baby or child younger than 5 years of age caused by intentional abrupt impact and violent shaking. NAT is a leading cause of childhood traumatic injury and death in the United States. Physical and sexual abuse of children is a frequent, disturbing, and significant problem. When a child is harmed, those who provide emergency care, such as prehospital providers, may be the first to respond to the child's injury or situation. The ability to detect NAT, maltreatment, and neglect is a necessary skill for any person involved in the care of children. Adequate education and training is imperative for prehospital providers. They should know how to assess, suspect, report, and document concerns of NAT. This will not only help the child but also improve the overall quality of prehospital care of these children. Careful consideration of patient findings and caregiver history is crucial in identification of children in need of intervention.[3,88,170]

Abuse may be physical, emotional, or sexual. Acts that deprive children of their basic needs such as food and clothing are more appropriately called neglect. Children born premature or with multiple medical conditions are a higher risk of experiencing NAT. Shaken baby syndrome is a common form of NAT identified in these children and described by a triad of symptoms, which includes subdural hematoma, retinal hemorrhage, and encephalopathy suggesting MOI with tearing of the bridging veins secondary to shaking the child. All states have statutes that require reporting of suspected maltreatment or neglect. It is important to be aware of the local statutes and community support options available in your area. Physicians, nurses, police officers, social workers, prehospital personnel, and other adults who interact with children should all be aware of historical and physical findings that are indicators for abuse or neglect. These findings are listed in Box 30.6. Keep in mind that some of these injuries can occur in the absence of abuse. A careful history of mechanisms and supervision is critical in children with these clinical findings. It is a requirement of

---

> • **BOX 30.6** **Historical Indicators of Child Abuse, Neglect, or Maltreatment**
>
> Caregiver history incongruent with the mechanism of injury and actual injuries
> Caregiver history incongruent with child's developmental abilities
> Delay in seeking medical treatment
> Patterned or unusual marks on the child's body
> Injuries of various age or injuries of multiple types
> A caregiver who denies knowledge of how an injury occurred
> A caregiver whose response to the child's injury is not appropriate
> A caregiver who expresses over or under concern for the seriousness of the child's injury
> A recent change in caregivers
> No preexisting medical condition that describes the child's injury
> Inconsistencies or changes in the history provided
> Emphasis of unimportant details or unrelated minor problems by the caregiver
> Previous treatment for suspicious or unexplained injuries
> Caregivers who seek medical attention for the child's injuries in other area hospitals
> Bypassing a closer emergency department to seek care at a department further away
> Tension or hostility between caregivers or tension or hostility directed at the child or staff
> An uncooperative caregiver
> Injuries that could have been prevented with closer supervision
>
> From Holleran RS, ed. *ASTNA Patient Transport: Principles and Practice.* 4th ed. St. Louis: Mosby Elsevier; 2010.

• BOX 30.7   Clinical Signs and Symptoms of Child Abuse, Neglect, or Maltreatment

- Behavioral
- Inappropriate reactions to procedures
- Frightened of caregiver
- Goes easily to strangers; uncharacteristic for child's age
- Extreme apprehension with other children's crying
- Bruises–Potentially inflicted bruises include the following:
  - Bruises to the face, neck, chest, abdomen, back, flank, thighs, or genitalia
  - Bruises in various stages of healing
  - Bruises suggestive of being struck by an object
  - Pinch marks; pairs of crescent-shaped bruises
  - Fingerprint or thumb patterns
  - Bruises suggestive of being kicked
  - Bruises to the mouth, gums, or buccal mucosa
  - Multiple or symmetric bruises or marks
- Burns–Characteristics of intentionally inflicted burns include the following:
  - Immersion burn; circumferential and often symmetric "stocking" pattern burns to the feet, "glovelike" pattern
  - Burns to hands, doughnut pattern burn to buttocks
  - Burns with sharply demarcated edges without splash burns
  - Ligature or rope burns to wrists, ankles, torso, or neck
  - Cigarette or cigar burns, especially on typically concealed areas
  - Contact burns: dry uniform print may be in the configuration of an object used to cause the burn (e.g., grill)
  - Symmetric burns
  - Splash patterns in unusual sites (e.g., genitals) or splash patterns with separated areas
  - Burn to the dorsum of the hand
- Delays in seeking treatment

- Bites and other marks–Characteristics of potentially inflicted marks include the following:
  - Down-turned lesions at the corners of the mouth, caused by being gagged
  - Human bites; crescent-shaped bruises with circular lesions; individual tooth marks may be present; a distance greater than 3 cm between the third tooth and canine on each side indicates a bite caused by an adult or child older than 8 years of age
- Head injuries suggestive of abuse include the following:
  - Skull fractures; multiple complex or bilateral skull fractures in an infant
  - Cerebral edema with retinal hemorrhages (common in shaken baby syndrome)
  - Subdural hematoma or subarachnoid hemorrhage
  - Traction alopecia and scalp swelling from hair pulling
- Skeletal fractures suggestive of abuse include the following:
  - Multiple fractures in different stages of healing or untreated healing fractures
  - Unusual fractures: ribs, scapula, sternum, vertebrae, distal clavicle
  - Metaphyseal injuries that have the appearance of tufts, chips, or "bucket handles" causing arcs of bone
  - Spiral fractures of long bones
  - Transverse fractures
  - Repeated fractures at the same site, multiple bilateral or symmetric fractures

From Holleran RS, ed. *ASTNA Patient Transport: Principles and Practice.* 4th ed. St. Louis: Mosby Elsevier; 2010.

---

emergency care providers to report abuse and to make sure to document the case number in the charting. Box 30.7 lists signs and symptoms of child abuse, neglect, or maltreatment.[3,88,170]

Federal legislation provides the foundation for state laws on child injury by identifying a minimum set of injuries and behaviors that classify abuse and neglect of children. The Federal Child Abuse Prevention and Treatment Act (CAPTA) and the CAPTA Reauthorization Act of 2010 outline the minimum standards of child abuse and neglect for states to follow with their own classifications.

Sexual Abuse

Children who suffer sexual abuse may present with vague somatic symptoms or behavioral changes. Sexual abuse should always be considered in patients with equivocal clinical findings. Other children may present for care after revealing abuse to a caregiver. Sexual abuse of children occurs primarily in the preadolescent years. Females are more likely to be sexually abused than males in the preadolescent group, with males less likely to report sexual abuse. See Table 30.18 for signs and symptoms of sexual abuse in children. Care in the transport setting should include treatment of medical issues with psychological support of the patient.[3,171]

Shock and Shock Management

Shock in pediatric patients is one of the leading causes of morbidity and mortality because of the failure to supply enough oxygen to meet the tissue oxygen demand. This causes tissue hypoxia and increases anaerobic metabolism. Elevated serum lactate levels reflect the anaerobic metabolism related to cellular hypoxia and are considered to be an important indicator of impaired tissue perfusion in patients.[3,172-173]

Shock can develop from an array of conditions resulting in insufficient circulating blood volume (preload), changes in vascular resistance (afterload), heart failure (contractility), and obstruction to flow. Early recognition of shock and prompt treatment is essential for reversing the effects and improving patient outcomes.[3,172-173]

The current American College of Critical Care Medicine recommendations that the diagnosis of shock include early fluid resuscitation with crystalloids such as normal saline or Ringer's lactate, followed by initiation of vasoactive medications such as dopamine or epinephrine as a first line, epinephrine for cold shock and norepinephrine for warm shock, and hydrocortisone for those with potential risk of adrenal insufficiency.[3,172-173]

There are several etiologies of shock, and the underlying pathology is inadequate tissue oxygenation. The goal of shock management is the support of oxygen delivery and CO.

TABLE 30.18	**Sign and Symptoms of Sexual Abuse in Children**
Genital-Rectal	• Clinical signs may be absent
	• Bruising, lacerations, or abrasions to the genital or rectal area
	• Bleeding or itching from the urethral, anal, or genital areas
	• Pain or burning in the genital or anal area
	• Vaginal or penile infection or discharge
	• Foreign body revealed in the vaginal, urethral, or rectal areas
	• Inflammation or irritation of the vagina and/or vulva
	• Anal inflammation or irritation
	• Sexually transmitted disease beyond the newborn period
	• Pregnancy of young adolescent child
	• Dysuria with urination
	• Frequent urinary tract infections
Medical	• Anorexia causing weight loss
	• Unexplained abdominal pain
	• Chronic daily headaches
	• Enuresis and/or encopresis in school-aged children
	• Chronic constipation
	• Painful urination or defecation
	• Bruises to the soft or hard palate
Behavior Changes	• Clinging behaviors
	• Uncontrollable, hyperactive temper tantrums, aggression, or self-injury
	• Accident-prone, self-destructive with intentional self injuries
	• Sleep disturbances, nightmares, or night terrors
	• Loss of appetite
	• Excessive fears, phobias
	• Depression, withdrawal from family and friends, and low self-esteem
	• Social interatctions with peers
	• Failing in school
	• Self-medication and substance abuse
	• Suicidal ideation or attempts
	• Specific inappropriate details of sexual contact or behaviors
	• Promiscuity, prostitution, sexual abuse or violence on others
	• Hypersexuality
	• Compulsive masturbation

Adapted from Bechtel K, Bennett BL. Evaluation of sexual abuse in children and adolescents. In: UpToDate, August 2016. Wiley JF (ed.), UpToDate, Waltham, MA. (Accessed on June 07, 2017.) Retrieved from https://www.uptodate.com/contents/evaluation-of-sexual-abuse-in-children-and-adolescents.

Etiologies of Shock

There are several etiologies of shock:

- *Hypovolemic shock* is the most common type of shock experienced by children. It develops when intravascular volume is insufficient to maintain tissue perfusion. The decrease in intravascular volume results in a decreased preload, which decreases CO leading to an increase in SVR and increased capillary refill. Sources of volume loss include vomiting; diarrhea; osmotic dieresis; capillary leak from sepsis; and intraabdominal processes with third space losses such as pancreatitis, intussusception, appendicitis, burn injuries, hemorrhage, inadequate fluid intake, or insensible losses.[3,172-174]
- *Distributive shock,* also called vasodilatory shock, results from a decrease in system vascular resistance, with abnormal distribution of blood flow resulting in inadequate tissue perfusion. Causes of distributive shock include sepsis, anaphylaxis reaction, and acute injury to the spinal cord or brain (neurogenic shock). Sepsis is the most common etiology seen in children. Anaphylaxis is another cause and manifests as an immediate, potentially life-threatening systemic reaction to an external source, which is usually an allergic IgE-mediated immediate hypersensitivity reaction. Neurogenic shock is a relatively rare occurrence following an acute injury to the spinal cord or CNS resulting in a loss of sympathetic venous tone.[3,172-174]

- *Cardiogenic shock* results from pump failure because of intrinsic cardiac disease resulting in the inability of the heart to provide adequate CO. This decreased cardiac contractility is a result of CHD, myocarditis, myocardial contusion, myocardial ischemia, cardiomyopathy, or cardiac arrhythmia. Physiologic signs of cardiogenic shock include tachycardia, increased SVR, and decreased CO.[3,172-174]
- *Obstructive shock* is caused by an acquired obstruction of systemic blood flow from the heart, which causes abrupt impairment of CO resulting in blood flow physically obstructed with an increased vascular resistance. Obstructive shock is caused by cardiac tamponade, tension pneumothorax, massive pulmonary embolism, CHD with ductal-dependent lesions such as hypoplastic left heart syndrome or critical aortic stenosis. It may also present when the ductus arteriosus closes during the first few weeks of life.[3,172-174]

Assessment and Diagnosis

Children can compensate for circulatory dysfunction by increasing heart rate, SVR, and venous tone while maintaining normal blood pressures with poor tissue perfusion present. The challenge for providers is to recognize children in shock before hypotension develops, which is a late sign. The cause of shock is not always known before treatment must be initiated. A systematic approach is needed to assess and diagnose children presenting with poor perfusion. This is done by the provider identifying features of the child's history, physical examination, and ancillary studies that may suggest the underlying condition. The goals of initial evaluation of shock in children require immediate identification of life-threatening conditions, rapid recognition of circulatory collapse, and early classification of the type and cause of the shock.[3,174,175]

Historical data to help the provider identify the condition causing shock include the following[3,174]:

- A history of fluid loss caused by vomiting, diarrhea from gastroenteritis, DKA, or GI bleeding.
- Hypovolemic shock caused from hemorrhage caused by a solid organ injury from blunt abdominal trauma, obstructive shock with a tension pneumothorax or cardiac tamponade, or neurogenic shock with an SCI.
- Fever or immunocompromise caused by chemotherapy, sickle cell disease, or inherited immunodeficiencies may indicate septic shock.
- A history of exposure to an allergen such as a bee sting or food causing anaphylactic shock.
- Septic shock may develop as a result of exposure to toxins such as β-blockers, calcium channel blockers, or cardiac glycosides.
- Cardiogenic shock may present in patients with chronic heart disease such as cardiomyopathy or complex CHD.
- Adrenal crisis must be considered in a patient at risk for adrenal insufficiency, such as children receiving chronic steroid therapy, hypopituitarism, or neonates with sepsis.

Signs and Symptoms

The clinical presentation of shock in children is variable with several common signs and symptoms including tachycardia and signs of poor perfusion.

Common clinical signs and symptoms of shock include the following[3,176]:

- Tachycardia is a common and important indicator. It is also a nonspecific finding and seen with other common childhood conditions such as fever, pain, and anxiety, which can cause tachycardia without poor perfusion.
- Skin changes are present in most shock states because of the child's regulatory processes compensating for decreased or poor effective tissue perfusion. Vasoconstrictive mechanisms redistribute blood from the peripheral, splanchnic, and renal vessels to maintain coronary and cerebral perfusion resulting in the child's skin being cool, clammy, pale, mottled, or diaphoretic. Conversely, in early distributive shock the child has peripheral vasodilation and the skin may be flushed and hyperemic. This is also seen when there is a failure of the child's regulatory mechanisms to maintain peripheral vascular resistance and is a sign of irreversible shock.
- Impaired LOC in children is a sign of impaired cerebral perfusion. The child may initially be listless, restless, anxious, confused, irritable, show decreased levels of responsiveness to the environment, be agitated, or not interact with parents. The child's mental status will continue to deteriorate and become obtunded, and coma results as shock worsens.
- Tachypnea is present.
- Decreased or absent urine output occurs with a decreased glomerular filtration rate secondary to shunting of renal blood flow to other organs.
- Lactic acidosis develops resulting in progressive tissue hypoperfusion, which is caused from inadequate delivery of oxygen to the tissues and decreased clearance of lactate by the kidneys, liver, and skeletal muscle.
- Decreased or absent bowel sounds.
- Changes in pulse quality may occur with pulses being weak, thready, or absent.
- May have difficulty obtaining a blood pressure.
- Hypotension is a late and ominous sign in children. The compensatory vasoconstriction that is very effective early in the shock state with systemic blood pressure maintained in the normal range along with poor perfusion present begins to fail. Bradycardia and hypotension should be recognized as ominous signs and should be aggressively treated in children.

According to the AHA PALS guidelines, shock can be primarily separated into stages: compensated, decompensated, and irreversible. See Table 30.19 for a description of each stage.[3,173-174]

Many of the preceding clinical signs and symptoms are not specific to shock and need to be considered in relation to history and patient presentation. Measures of end organ perfusion such as LOC, urinary output, heart rate, and pulse quality may be the most helpful assessment factors in patients with suspected shock.

Diagnostic aids for children in shock include the following[3,174]:

- Cardiopulmonary monitor.
- Pulse oximeter. If the child is exhibiting poor perfusion this may prevent an accurate reading, but a normal reading does not rule out the child's need for supplemental oxygen.
- CXR to rule out cardiomegaly, pulmonary infection, pneumothorax or hemothorax.
- Laboratory studies to obtain include a complete blood count, glucose, and electrolytes with a lactate level.
- Arterial or capillary blood gases are helpful in monitoring the child's acidosis caused by oxygen debt and anaerobic metabolism, but also monitor the child's oxygenation and ventilation status. Obtaining serial blood gases can be useful to monitor effectiveness of interventions.
- For suspected septic shock, cultures of blood, body fluids, sputum, CSF, wounds, and indwelling devices may be obtained to determine whether there is a source of potential infection.

TABLE 30.19	Stages of Shock and Physiologic Response	
Compensated	**Decompensated**	**Irreversible**
• Homeostatic mechanisms rapidly compensate for diminished perfusion and systolic blood pressure maintained within normal range • Heart rate initially increased • Signs of peripheral vasoconstriction with cool skin, decreased peripheral pulses, and oliguria can be found as perfusion becomes more compromised	• Compensatory mechanism become overwhelmed • Heart rate markedly elevated and hypotension develops • Sign and symptoms of organ dysfunction such as alerted mental status result of poor brain perfusion appear • Systolic blood pressure is maintained in normal limits in children until they have lost 30%–35% of their circulating volume • Once hypotension develops, the child deteriorates rapidly to cardiovascular collapse and cardiac arrest	• Progressive end organ dysfunction leads to irreversible organ damage and death • Tachycardia may be replaced by bradycardia and blood pressure becomes very low • Process is often irreversible regardless of resuscitative efforts

From Waltzman ML. Pediatric shock. *J Emerg Nurs.* 2015;41(2):113-118.

- A urinary catheter should be placed for accurate measurement of the child's urine output.
- Urinalysis to assess for the presence of blood, ketones, bacteria, glucose, and specific gravity measurement.

Treatment of Shock

Successful management of children with shock requires the rapid initiation of aggressive treatment. The provider should implement a goal-directed or systematic approach for most patients presenting with shock because the cause is not always known. During initial stabilization, assessment, and observation, indications that help determine the etiology of the shock should be sought. This will provide the most optimal therapy and quickly identify children who may be harmed by the therapy or who are not responding to the initial approach.[3,172-173,175]

- Rapid assessment to quickly determine the presence and suspected type of shock.
- Initial management of hypovolemic, distributive, and cardiogenic shock should focus on fluid resuscitation with isotonic crystalloid solution appropriate to the type of shock and specific pharmacologic therapies, as indicated, once the etiology of shock is identified.
- Interventions must be administered in a rapid sequence, with evaluation of physiologic indicators before and after each intervention.
- Physiologic indicators include blood pressure, central and peripheral pulses, mental status, and urine output.
- Several physiologic indicators can be monitored noninvasively during the initial management of shock such as mean arterial pressure. Clinical experience suggests that quality of central and peripheral pulses, skin perfusion, mental status, and urine output are useful signs for assessing response to therapy interventions.
- Heart rate is an important physiologic indicator of circulatory status. For children with shock, tachycardia is a compensatory response to poor tissue perfusion. A

positive response to treatment would be a decrease in the child's heart rate with fluid therapy.
- Continue monitoring and provide supportive treatment for the child after showing signs of improvement in perfusion.
- Achieving a normal blood pressure is essential for the patient who has hypotensive shock.
- If obstructive shock is present, it requires emergent recognition and treatment of the cause (e.g., tension pneumothorax or hemothorax, cardiac tamponade, CHD with closure of the ductus arteriosus, or pulmonary embolism). If shock is caused by a cardiac arrhythmia, such as supraventricular tachycardia, then treatments to restore normal sinus rhythm are essential initial steps.

Venous Access in Children

Before fluid resuscitation can begin on children with suspected shock, venous access must be obtained. Sites for venous access in children include the following[3]:
- Percutaneous peripheral attempts (limited to two attempts).
- IO needle placement.
- Saphenous vein cutdown.
- Percutaneous placement in the femoral vein.
- Percutaneous placement in the subclavian vein.
- Percutaneous placement in the external jugular vein. This site should not be used if a cervical collar is in place.
- Percutaneous placement in the internal jugular vein.

Hypovolemic Shock

Intravascular fluid losses from hemorrhage, vomiting, diarrhea, osmotic diuresis, or capillary leak are the principal elements of hypovolemic shock. The management of hypovolemic shock focuses on fluid replacement and preventing ongoing fluid loss. Vasoactive medications will not improve the child's perfusion status; the tank must be filled first. Administer 20 mL/kg normal saline or lactated Ringer's solution for hypovolemic shock for most children and repeat as needed. Each bolus should be infused over 5 to 10 minutes. Rapid infusion of fluids should be performed with caution in children with severe malnutrition.[3,172-173,175]

For children who have not improved after receiving a total of 60 mL/kg over 30 to 60 minutes consider the following[3,172-173,175]:

- The amount of fluid lost may be underestimated as with burn injuries or there may be significant ongoing fluid loss from hemorrhage secondary to blunt abdominal trauma or capillary leak syndrome associated with bowel obstruction.
- Other conditions may be causing or contributing to shock (i.e., a child with multiple trauma who has an SCI).
- It is not a first-line treatment but colloids are an option for patients with hypoalbuminemia (albumin <3 g/dL) or hyperchloremic metabolic acidosis who have not improved after initial therapy with at least 60 mL/kg of crystalloid solutions.
- Patients with hemorrhagic shock who have not improved should receive blood and require definitive treatment for the cause of hemorrhage. Delaying fluid resuscitation for traumatic hemorrhagic in children is not recommended.
- Hypovolemic shock is uncommon in children with DKA. Patients in DKA whose perfusion does not improve with 10 mL/kg of isotonic fluid should be evaluated for other causes of shock.

Cardiogenic Shock

A history of heart disease, an abnormal cardiac examination, and worsening clinical status with fluid resuscitation are suggestive of cardiogenic shock. Additional findings suggestive of cardiogenic shock include a gallop rhythm, pulmonary rales, jugular venous distention, hepatomegaly, tachycardia out of proportion to fever or respiratory distress, cyanosis unresponsive to oxygen, and absent femoral pulses. If these signs are present, a smaller isotonic crystalloid fluid bolus of 5 to 10 mL/kg infused over 10 to 20 minutes will decrease the chances of exacerbating heart failure. If needed, an additional 5- to 10-mL/kg aliquots may be given if needed for improvement in physiologic indicators. Cardiogenic shock is less common than other forms of shock in children, and early consultation with a pediatric cardiologist is recommended.[3,172-173,175]

Cardiogenic shock management issues include the following[3,172-173,175]:

- Cardiogenic shock should be considered for any child without an easily identifiable cause for shock whose condition worsens with fluid therapy.
- Some children with poor cardiac function may also be volume depleted. Fluid should be administered slowly and in boluses of 5 to 10 mL/kg and reassess.

- Treatment with dobutamine or phosphodiesterase enzyme inhibitors such as milrinone can improve myocardial contractility and reduce SVR (afterload).
- Cardiac arrhythmias (e.g., supraventricular or ventricular tachycardia) should be addressed before fluid resuscitation.

Distributive Shock

Distributive shock is characteristic of a marked decrease in SVR. This form of shock does well with both fluid resuscitation and vasopressor infusions depending on the underlying etiology, septic shock, anaphylactic shock, or neurogenic shock. Septic shock management is recommended by the American Critical Care Medicine guidelines for neonates and children with septic shock and includes the following[3,172-173,175-179]:

- Treatment with 20-mL/kg crystalloid bolus over 5 to 10 minutes and repeat until perfusion improves or until the child develops rales or hepatomegaly.
- Correct hypoglycemia and hypocalcemia.
- Begin antibiotics after cultures obtained.
- Septic shock may be classified as cold or warm shock based on clinical findings. Children in cold septic shock exhibits cool extremities, delayed capillary refill, and poor pulses. They also have low CO and elevated SVR in an attempt to maintain perfusion pressure. Warm shock presents with vasodilation, low SVR, increased CO, clinical quick capillary refill, warm extremities, and bounding pulses. Traditionally, it was thought that septic shock was a cold shock, but recent data suggest community-acquired septic shock usually does not present as cold shock. Hospital-acquired or central line-associated septic shock frequently presents as warm shock.
- Fluid refractory shock will need inotropic support. To reverse cold shock start dopamine and titrate infusion; if resistant, initiate epinephrine infusion and titrate. To reverse warm shock, initiate and titrate a norepinephrine infusion.
- Catecholamine-resistant shock will need hydrocortisone started if patient is at risk for adrenal insufficiency.
- Cold shock with normal blood pressure is managed by titrating fluids and epinephrine infusion; consider starting milrinone.
- Cold shock with low blood pressure requires titration of fluids and epinephrine; consider adding norepinephrine.
- Warm shock with low blood pressure is managed by titrating fluids and norepinephrine; consider adding vasopressin.
- Refractory septic shock not responding to fluid resuscitation and inotropes may need ECMO therapy.

When the child has a history of allergies and/or the presence of stridor, wheezing, urticaria, or facial edema, anaphylactic shock is suggested. Children with possible anaphylaxis should receive IM epinephrine, IV or IM diphenhydramine, and steroids, in addition to rapid infusions of normal saline. Wheezing should be treated with nebulized albuterol. Patients with cardiovascular collapse or those that respond poorly to IM epinephrine may require epinephrine intravenously.[3,172-174,177-179]

Neurogenic shock refers to hypotension, usually associated with bradycardia, as a result of an interruption of the autonomic pathways in the spinal cord causing decreased vascular resistance. Patients with traumatic SCI may also suffer from hemodynamic shock related to blood loss and other complications. An adequate blood pressure is believed to be critical in maintaining adequate perfusion to the injured spinal cord, limiting secondary ischemic injury. Appropriate mean arterial pressure for age should be maintained using IV fluids, transfusion, and pharmacologic vasopressors as needed. Bradycardia caused by cervical spinal cord or high thoracic spinal cord disruption may require external pacing or administration of atropine.[3,172-174,177-179]

Obstructive shock causes include tension pneumothorax, cardiac tamponade, hemothorax, pulmonary embolism, or ductal-dependent congenital heart defects and require specific interventions to relieve the obstruction to blood flow.[3,172-174,177-179]

Damage Control Resuscitation

Trauma is the leading cause of death in children. Hemorrhage continues to be the leading cause of preventable traumatic deaths in children. Damage control resuscitation (DCR) is intended to improve patient outcomes through alleviation of the lethal triad of acidosis, hypothermia, and coagulopathy. The ACS adopted both DCR and permissive hypotension in adults in the ATLS curriculum. DCR is designed to use on patients with severe uncontrollable hemorrhage and requires large amounts of blood products. DCR is not intended for those who respond to initial fluids without further interventions. Children have physiologic differences compared with adults when presenting with hypovolemic shock, such as the ability to compensate for approximately 45% circulating blood loss before shock is reflected in the child's blood pressure. This physiologic response suggests that permissive hypotension may not be a good choice in children, especially if they have a head injury and adequate CPP is indicated. The goal of initial resuscitation in children is hemodynamic stability and restoration of adequate tissue perfusion with an end point of urine output greater than 1 mL/kg per hour. It is important to remember to prevent hypothermia during fluid resuscitation because hypothermia may result in vasoconstriction, acidosis, and consumptive coagulopathy. Along with preventative hypothermic measures, the prehospital provider should initiate fluid resuscitation starting with 20 mL/kg fluid bolus of Ringer's lactate or isotonic sodium chloride solution. This may be given up to two times, and then the provider should consider blood components. In the prehospital environment, excessive volume replacement (overresuscitation) with crystalloids in injured children increases the tendency for higher rates of multiorgan failure and mortality.[180-181]

Children with evidence of hemorrhagic shock who fail to respond to fluid resuscitation should begin receiving blood and blood products. Guidelines are not well established in pediatric trauma patients describing the best time to switch from crystalloid fluids to blood and blood products. Current data suggest early identification of coagulopathy and the need to treat patients with red blood cells, fresh frozen plasma, and platelets in a 1:1:1 unit ratio, limiting the use of crystalloid administration. This may improve survival in pediatric patients with severe traumatic injury and life-threatening bleeding.[180-181]

American Heart Association 2015 Updates

The 2015 AHA guidelines update for CPR and emergency cardiovascular care were released in November 2015. The summary of 2015 pediatric basic life support and quality of CPR recommendations include the following[3,17,182]:

- Continue the sequence from 2010 guidelines by initiating CPR with C-A-B over the original A-B-C.
- New algorithms for one-rescuer and multiple rescuer health care provider (HCP) pediatric CPR have been separated into two separate algorithms. They have added the use of cell phones with speakers to activate an emergency response and continue conversation with dispatcher to assist the lay rescuer with CPR.
- Provide chest compressions that depress the chest at least one-third of the anteroposterior diameter of the chest in pediatric patients. This is approximately 1.5 inches in infants and 2 inches in children. In adolescents (children who have reached puberty) use the recommended adult depth compression of at least 2 inches but no greater than 2.4 inches.
- For simplicity and absence of sufficient pediatric evidence, the 2015 guidelines recommend using the adult compression rate of 100 to 120 per minute for infants and children.
- Conventional CPR (rescue breaths and chest compressions) should be provided for infants and children because most pediatric arrests have a primary respiratory component, which necessitates ventilation as part of effective CPR. However, because compression-only CPR can be effective in patients with a primary cardiac arrest, if rescuers are unwilling or unable to deliver breaths, then rescuers can perform compression-only CPR for infants and children in cardiac arrest.
- Early, rapid IV administration of isotonic fluids is accepted as a cornerstone of therapy for septic shock. For children in shock, an initial fluid bolus of 20 mL/kg with frequent reassessment is used.
- A large study of fluid resuscitation conducted in children with severe febrile illnesses in a resource-limited setting found worse outcomes to be associated with IV fluid boluses. Recommendations are for the administration of IV fluid boluses to be conducted with extreme caution because they may be harmful in children with febrile illness in settings with limited access to critical care resources such as mechanical ventilation and inotropic support.
- There is no evidence to support the routine use of atropine as a premedication to prevent bradycardia in

emergency pediatric intubations. It may be considered in situations in which there is an increased risk of bradycardia.

- If invasive hemodynamic monitoring is in place at the time of a cardiac arrest in a child, it may be reasonable to use it to guide CPR quality.
- Recommend HCPs monitor physiologic parameters during resuscitation, and $EtCO_2$ is the only recommended parameter that can easily monitored in the field.
- Amiodarone or lidocaine are equally acceptable treatment for shock-refractory ventricular fibrillation or pulseless ventricular tachycardia in children.
- Vasopressor use in resuscitation recommends giving epinephrine during cardiac arrest.
- Extracorporeal CPR may be considered for children with underlying cardiac conditions who have an in-hospital cardiac arrest (IHCA).
- Temperature should be monitored continuously and fever should be treated aggressively in comatose children in the first few days after IHCA or OHCA.
- For comatose children resuscitated from OHCA, maintain either 5 days of normothermia at 36°C to 37.5°C or 2 days of initial continuous hypothermia of 32°C to 34°C followed by 3 days of normothermia.
- For children remaining comatose after IHCA, there are insufficient data to recommend hypothermia over normothermia.
- After ROSC, fluids, inotropes, and vasopressors should be used to maintain a systolic blood pressure above the fifth percentile for age. Intraarterial pressure monitoring should be used continuously to monitor blood pressure and identify and treat hypotension.
- After ROSC in children, titrate oxygen to achieve normoxemia with oxygen saturations greater than 94%. Oxygen should be weaned to target saturations in the range of 94% to 99%. The goal should be to strictly avoid hypoxemia while maintaining normoxemia.
- Post-ROSC ventilation strategies should focus on a $PaCO_2$, which avoids extremes of hypercapnia and hypocapnia.
- Neonatal resuscitation suggests a delayed cord clamping for 30 seconds for both term and preterm infants who do not require resuscitation at birth.
- It is no longer recommended to intubate the nonvigorous meconium-stained amniotic fluid infant who presents with poor muscle tone and inadequate breathing efforts. PPV should be initiated if the infant is not breathing or the heart rate is less than 100 beats/min.
- During resuscitation of term and preterm newborns, the use of a three-lead ECG for the rapid and accurate measurement of the newborn's heart rate is recommended.
- Resuscitation of preterm newborns of less than 35 weeks' gestation should be initiated with low oxygen (21%–30%), and the oxygen concentration should be titrated to achieve a preductal oxygen saturation approximating the interquartile range measured in healthy term infants after vaginal birth at sea level. Initiating resuscitation of preterm newborns with high oxygen (65% or greater) is not recommended.

Additional Pediatric Medical and Trauma Conditions

Seizures

Status epilepticus (SE) is one of the most common pediatric neurologic emergencies. The mortality in children is up to 3%. Morbidities include cognitive and neurodevelopmental impairments, epilepsy, and recurrent SE. SE refractory to the initial antiepileptic medications is associated with poor outcome. SE is defined as any continuous convulsive seizure activity or intermittent convulsive seizure activity lasting more than 30 minutes without regaining consciousness between the seizures. SE in children is the most common life-threatening neurologic emergency. Classification of SE falls into four categories. Acute symptomatic SE occurs because of a neurologic insult such as trauma, CNS infection, or metabolic disorders. Remote symptomatic SE includes patients with neurologic disorders, such as chronic encephalopathies, which predispose these children to seizures. Idiopathic seizures are those that occur in known epileptic patients who abruptly stop taking anticonvulsant medications. The febrile SE includes epileptic seizures associated with fever lasting more than 30 minutes without CNS infection.[183-185]

Children begin to suffer neurologic damage when seizures last 30 minutes or longer and can be complicated by focal neurologic deficits, cognitive impairment, behavior problems, airway compromise, or other adverse events. Seizures account for the second most common condition requiring EMS pediatric transport. Several studies in the pediatric prehospital literature compared administration routes of benzodiazepines for seizure patients and found similar results between the IV route and the IM, intranasal (IN), buccal, and rectal routes. The literature suggests alternative routes of administration (specifically IM, IN, and buccal) are equally effective and comparable as IV, with the same side effect profiles; therefore, they should be considered preferentially for children in the prehospital setting. EMS providers can administer benzodiazepine to a seizing child as quickly as possible and repeat if seizure persists longer than 5 to 10 minutes. Avoid giving more than two doses of benzodiazepines because of an increased risk of respiratory depression. The most commonly seen adverse effect of benzodiazepines is respiratory depression. Hypoglycemia is an infrequent but important cause of pediatric seizures, and can be easily and quickly identified via the use of a point-of-care glucometer.[183-185]

Concussive Head Injuries in Children

Concussions in children and adolescents account for 90% of all TBIs. It is estimated that one in five children will experience a concussion by the age of 10 years. Falls and sports-related activities are the most common causes of concussions. Concussion is a form of mild TBI that occurs as a result of a direct impact to the child's head or impact to the body that transmits forces to the head. Common early symptoms include headaches, dizziness, vertigo or imbalance, lack of awareness of surroundings, brief loss of consciousness, and nausea and vomiting. Confusion is a hallmark sign of concussions and may include amnesia usually of the traumatic event and occasionally the preceding event.[186-187]

There is emerging evidence that repetitive concussions may cause persistent neurocognitive changes. Repetitive concussions have been a contributing factor to neurodegenerative conditions including chronic traumatic encephalopathy, posttraumatic stress disorder, substance abuse, anxiety, and depression.[186-187]

The prehospital provider will be transporting more concussive children because of the rising numbers of children actively engaging in sports-related activities. Another factor increasing concussions numbers is the media bringing concussions to the forefront and discussing professional athletes who are beginning to experience long-term deficits from concussions experienced years before.[186-187]

Pediatric Dog Bites and Attacks

Dog bites are common in the United States and can result in significant morbidity in pediatric patients. The injuries may range from superficial wounds to life-threatening head and neck injuries, and fatalities. It is estimated that 4.5 million ED visits are for animal bites each year, with 85% to 90% being dog bites, and 40% accounting for significant pediatric trauma involving prehospital emergency transport, with 10 to 20 animal-related pediatric fatalities every year. There is no single dog breed responsible for all animal bites. However, the Pit bull and Rottweiler breeds are responsible for the majority of human fatalities over the last 20 years. The majority of dog bite victims are children and they involve the head, neck, and face. Adolescents receive the majority of dog bites to their extremities. Psychological trauma may result and manifest itself in fear and nightmares and is documented to have an adverse effect on quality of life for both the child and parents. Dog bite injuries frequently affect the head, neck, and facial areas of children and are the most common reason for emergency transport. These injury areas are vascular, tissue damage could be extensive, and the child's airway may be affected. It is essential to clean these wounds effectively, and treatment is usually primary closure by a plastic surgeon to limit scarring morbidities and secondary infections in children. These children will require antibiotics, tetanus, and possibly rabies prophylaxis.[188-190]

Prehospital Pain Management in Children

Pain is commonly seen in prehospital care. The under recognized and inadequate treatment of pain is associated with adverse physiologic and emotional effects such as slower healing, emotional trauma, and alterations in pain processing. Children whose pain is untreated can have lasting effects into adulthood including fear of medical encounters, posttraumatic stress disorder, and misuse of medical care. Pain is an important part of the body's response to tissue injury, and the intensity is related to the extent, severity, and location of injury. Untreated pain can lead to shock from pain making pain management one of the most important therapies needed in the patient after trauma, especially for children. Pain management in the child with an injury should include nonpharmacologic and pharmacologic interventions. Nonpharmacologic interventions include ice packs and immobilization of fractures. If these measures are ineffective in relieving pain, then pharmacologic methods are needed. Correctly providing pain management in the injured child after injury significantly affects the disease prognosis. The prehospital care provider needs to ensure that each child transported has their pain level assessed and documented in the chart and appropriate interventions should be provided.[191-192]

Children With Special Needs

It is estimated that there are more than 12 million CSHCNs in the United States. CSHCNs are one of the fastest growing populations that use a significant proportion of health care resources within their communities. As medical technology and understanding of chronic conditions improve and surgical interventions such as repair of congenital heart defects, gastroschisis, omphalocele, and myelomeningocele continue to improve, these children are living longer and more fulfilling lives at home with their families. These children present daily challenges for their families, but they especially present a unique set of challenges for the prehospital provider. The prehospital provider is frequently unfamiliar with their medical issues and the medical technology that they need to sustain themselves at home.

CSHCNs are those who require additional long-term needs greater than 6 months that are more significant than the general population, and they are technology dependent (i.e., ventilator dependent) or have significant behavioral or developmental disorders (i.e., autism). The need for emergency services in this population is not uncommon, and EMS prehospital providers are frequently responding to medical and traumatic emergencies involving children with severe cardiac, pulmonary, or neurologic conditions, or more advanced technologies such as mechanical ventilation, tracheostomies, gastrostomy or jejunostomy tubes, central venous lines, and ventriculoperitoneal CSF shunts.

In 1997, the EMS for Children program assembled a special task force designed to explore the growing emergency care needs for this population and to focus on ways to improve the quality of prehospital care delivered to children with complex medical health issues. The task force and local hospitals are working to help identify these patients in the community to help the prehospital provider be more prepared to care for the children in their area.

Prehospital providers may require additional education to be able to provide the appropriate care and transport needs of these patients. The prehospital provider should remember to use the patient's family members or caregivers as a valuable resource of knowledge regarding the child's routine care because they manage most issues that occur with the child and have been trained in the maintenance and operation of the child's medical devices and technology. There is new information available with the addition of the emergency information form (EIF) to help provide additional information for the prehospital provider. Because of concerns that the family member may not be as knowledgeable regarding the child's care or a language barrier, both the American AAP and the ACEP recommends a copy of the EIF for the CSHCN be placed a in the freezer of the child's home, so that it can be located quickly and easily in the event of a medical emergency. The emergency transport of CSHCN for definitive medical care requires that the prehospital provider has adequate information in caring for the patient to be able to provide the highest level of care during transport. CSHCN children would be better cared for if the prehospital provider was able to transport to a pediatric facility. Because this may not always be an option, once the child is stabilized, the interfacility transport of the child to a pediatric center may be done by a specialized pediatric transport team. Research has shown specialized pediatric transport teams improve overall care and outcomes in these children.[191-192]

Behavioral and Mental Health Issues

Prehospital EMS transports for nonemergent pediatric health issues are considerable and drastically rising. Transporting a pediatric psychiatric patient can be challenging, with a child acting out or it is unclear if the child is reacting normally to stress in the environment, or if there is an imminent risk of harm to self or others, and parents who are either anxious or apprehensive. It is estimated that one in five children ages 13 to 18, or over 21%, will experience a severe mental disorder at some point during their life, and for children ages 8 to 15 the estimate is 13%.[193-195]

The etiology of pediatric psychiatric diagnoses is extensive and influenced by a multitude of variables that may be internal or external to the patient. Many of these variables are not modifiable, such as genetic predisposition and personality, or a response to environmental factors, such as family dynamics. Factors that may affect a psychiatric illness in a child include intelligence; social abilities; and having some kind of talent, such as an athletic ability, which can minimize the negative effects of the illness. The patients who are substance abusers almost always seem to exacerbate the course of the psychiatric illness. A large number of pediatric psychiatric patients begin to show symptoms during early childhood and early recognition, intervention, and treatment may modify the effects or control the illness and hopefully prevent severe dysfunction as the child goes into young adulthood. See Table 30.20

TABLE 30.20	Pediatric Psychiatric Diagnoses With Age of Onset 5 to 12 Years		
	Intermittent Explosive Disorder (IED)	Reactive Attachment Disorder (RAD)	Pervasive Developmental Disorder (PDD)
	Periods of aggression or violence followed by remorse, guilt, or anxiety	History of severe abuse, neglect, abandonment in infancy There is a persistent, prolonged disregard for the physical and emotional well-being of the child by caregivers	This disorder includes autism and Asperger's syndrome Symptoms may be noticed by parents in infancy but typically around 3 years, these children have impairments in social interaction and communications skills, many have difficulty with spoken language, and do not grasp social cues (i.e., humor, facial expressions or body language)
	Precipitating event such as a restriction or limit set by others, but child reacts out of proportion to situation Unmanageable aggression or violence is reason for transport to emergency department	Child has difficulty with trust, empathy, establishing healthy relationships At younger ages exhibiting disturbing behaviors such as cruelty to animals and other children, lying, stealing, sexually acting out is common Impulsiveness, aggression, agitation, and unmanageable behaviors are reason they are transported	These children are hypersensitive to noise and lights, have ritualistic behaviors and a rigid adherence to routines These children have exaggerated emotional reactions Uncontrollable behavior is one of the reasons for transport or they truly have a medical illness
	Key strategy for dealing with IED is to establish rapport with child to reduce anxiety and provide reassurance	Children with RAD develop other disorders during adolescence such as conduct disorder, oppositional defiance disorder, or borderline personality disorder	May need to ask parents for advice about the best methods to interact with the child

Data from Gilbert SB. Beyond acting out: Managing pediatric psychiatric emergencies in the emergency department. *Adv Emerg Nurs J.* 2012;34(2):147-163.

TABLE 30.21	Adolescent Psychiatric Disorders With Age Onset of 13 to 17 Years		
Major Depressive Disorder	**Oppositional Defiant Disorder**	**Conduct Disorder**	**Borderline Personality Disorder**
Adolescents are at high risk for depression and multiple stressors from home, school, and relationships	Disorder unique to children and adolescents characterized by behavioral problems at home and school	Teenagers tend to have more severe behavioral problems than those with ODD	History of early childhood abuse, neglect, and abandonment, growing up without a sense of being protected or nurtured and developing poor coping skills
They overwhelm the teenager's normal coping mechanisms	Open defiance of rules, arguing with adults and peers, difficulty taking responsibility	Behaviors are more aggressive, threatening, and without concern for others	BPD traits emerge in adolescence and continues into adulthood
Parental conflict, relationship breakups, and educational difficulties are the most common precipitating factors	In school children with ODD have trouble making and keeping friends; they are difficult to redirect; and need to be in control and have the last word whether it is with parents, peers, or other adults	History of cruelty to animals or younger children, sexual deviancy with use of force, tendency to provoke physical fights	These are characterized by dramatic attention-seeking behaviors, self-harming, suicidal gestures, anger, defensive, resistant to interventions from others, and blames parents rather than take responsibility for their behaviors
Others include being the victim of bullying, which increases depression and suicidal ideation	Etiology is unclear but has associations with history of neglect, family dysfunction, and abuse or chaotic home situation	Lack of respect for authority, complete disregard for rules	Teens are often hypersensitive to criticism from adults, even under normal circumstances
Adolescents do not have perspective or understand the inevitable changes that occur over time, and many choose to end or attempt to end their lives	They present with anger and are resentful and uncooperative , which is most common reason for transport	Manipulative behaviors include lying and blaming others	Quick to anger if directly confronted or challenged about their behaviors
Depression leads to a loss of rational, objective thinking	They may easily be frustrated or irritated but typically they are not violent or aggressive unless provoked	Truancy, running away, and substance abuse are common	During transport they become more anxious and agitated if they sense disapproval
Teenagers feel excessively guilty, isolated, and embarrassed	Teenagers with ODD are more likely to engage in risky behaviors, experiment with substances, and have minor legal issues	Ring leaders and encouraging others to break the rules or laws; lack of empathy, compassion, and concern for others, which allows them to engage in cruel acts without regret	Anxiety may be expressed as argumentativeness, resistance, or hostility
They may be overly sensitive to criticism		Treatment options are minimal but some behavioral modifications may result from early intensive interventions such as therapeutic residential treatment	Manipulative behaviors are a tactic to get their needs met or gain control of the situation
These parents of these children have no idea anything is wrong until they attempt an overdose and require emergent transport		Long-term outcomes tend to be poor, and many of these adolescents develop antisocial and sociopathic personality disorders as adults	

BPD, Borderline personality disorder; *ODD,* oppositional defiant disorder.
Data from Gilbert SB. Beytond acting out: Managing pediatric psychiatric emergencies in the emergency department. *Adv Emerg Nurs J,* 2012;34(2):147-163.

for pediatric psychiatric disorders affecting children 5 to 12 years of age. See Table 30.21 for adolescent psychiatric disorders. The pediatric EMS prehospital provider will be transporting a great deal more of these children because of the significant rise in the number of pediatric and adolescent mental health psychiatric disorders and substance use being diagnosed. The prehospital EMS provider will be transporting either from an out of control behavioral outburst in the home or at school, or a child who has inflicted injury to themselves such as cutting, or a teenager who has overdosed on a medication or attempted to hang or shoot his or herself in an attempt to commit suicide. The knowledge of these disorders may help the provider with a safe transport.[193-195]

References

1. Chiocca EM. *Advanced Pediatric Assessment.* 2nd ed. New York: Springer Publishing; 2015.
2. Fuchs S, Pante MD, eds. *Pediatric Education for Prehospital Professionals.* 3rd ed. Burlington, MA: Jones and Bartlett; 2014.
3. Holleran RS, ed. *ASTNA Patient Transport: Principles and Practice.* 4th ed. St. Louis, MO: Mosby Elsevier; 2010.
4. Stroud MH, et al. Pediatric and neonatal interfacility transport: Results from a national consensus conference. *Pediatric.* 2013; 132(2):359-366.
5. Commission on Accreditation of Medical Transport Systems, ed. *Tenth Edition Accreditation Standards of The Commission on Accreditation of Medical Transport Systems.* 10th ed. Sandy Springs, SC: CAMTS; 2015.

6. Anders J, Brown K, Simpson J, Gausche-Hill M. Evidence and controversies in pediatric prehospital airway management. *Clin Pediatr Emerg Med.* 2014;15(1):28-37.

7. Hammer J. Acute respiratory failure in children. *Paediatr Respir Rev.* 2013;14(2):64-69.

8. Smith KA, et al. Risk factors for failed tracheal intubation in pediatric and neonatal critical care specialty transport. *Prehosp Emerg Care.* 2015;19(1):17-22.

9. Hansen M, et al. Out-of-hospital pediatric airway management in the United States. *Resuscitation.* 2015;90:104-110.

10. Piegeler T, et al. Advanced airway management in the anaesthesiologist-staffed helicopter emergency medical service (HEMS): A retrospective analysis of 1047 out-of-hospital intubations. *Resuscitation.* 2016;105:66-69.

11. Nadler I, McLanders M, Sanderson P, Liley H. Time without ventilation during intubation in neonates as a patient-centered measure of performance. *Resuscitation.* 2016;105:41-44.

12. Eber E. Respiratory emergencies in children. *Paediatr Respir Rev.* 2013;14(2):62-63.

13. Pfleger A, Eber E. Management of acute severe upper airway obstruction in children. *Paediatr Respir Rev.* 2013;14(2):70-77.

14. Nagler J. *Emergency Airway Management in Children: Unique Pediatric Considerations.* In: UpToDate, June 2016. Wiley JF (ed.), UpToDate, Waltham, MA. Accessed on June 07, 2017. Retrieved from https://www.uptodate.com/contents/emergency-airway-management-in-children-unique-pediatric-considerations.

15. Mick NW. Airway management in patients with abnormal anatomy or challenging physiology. *Clin Pediatr Emerg Med.* 2015;16(3):186-194.

16. Wing R, Armsby CC. Noninvasive ventilation in pediatric acute respiratory illness. *Clin Pediatr Emerg Med.* 2015;16(3):154-161.

17. de Caen AR, et al. Part 12: Pediatric advanced life support: 2015 American heart association guidelines update for cardiopulmonary resuscitation and emergency cardiovascular care. *Circulation.* 2015;132(18 suppl 2):S526-S542.

18. Belanger J, Kossick M. Methods of identifying and managing the difficult airway in the pediatric population. *Am Assoc Nurse Anesth.* 2015;83(1):35-41.

19. Bailey P. *Continuous Oxygen Delivery Systems for Infants, Children, and Adults.* In: UpToDate, August 2016. Wiley JF (ed.), UpToDate, Waltham, MA. Accessed on June 07, 2017. Retrieved from http://www.uptodate.com/contents/continuous-oxygen-delivery-systems-for-infants-children-and-adults.

20. Emerson B, Shepherd M, Auerbach M. Technology-enhanced simulation training for pediatric intubation. *Clin Pediatr Emerg Med.* 2015;16(3):203-212.

21. Heyming T, et al. Accuracy of paramedic Broselow tape use in the prehospital setting. *Prehosp Emerg Care.* 2012;16(3):374-380.

22. Milesi C, et al. High-flow nasal cannula: Recommendations for daily practice in pediatrics. *Ann Intensive Care.* 2014;4:1-7.

23. Long E, Babl FE, Duke T. Is there a role for humidified heated high-flow nasal cannula therapy if paediatric emergency departments? *Emerg Med J.* 2016;33(6):386-389.

24. Fan G, Diao B, Zhang Y. Application of modified oropharyngeal airway in emergency care of patients with traumatic brain injury. *Int Med J.* 2014;21(2):163-165.

25. American Academy of Pediatrics, et al. Equipment for ground ambulances. *Prehosp Emerg Care.* 2014;18(1):92-97.

26. Ostermayer DC, Gausche-Hill M. Supraglottic airways: the history and current state of prehospital airway adjuncts. *Prehosp Emerg Care.* 2014;18(1):106-115.

27. Huang A, Jagannathan N. The role of supraglottic airways in pediatric emergency medicine. *Clin Pediatr Emerg Med.* 2015;16(3):162-171.

28. Mittiga MR, Rinderknecht AS, Kerrey BT. A modern and practical review of rapid-sequence intubation in pediatric emergencies. *Clin Pediatr Emerg Med.* 2015;16(3):172-185.

29. Walls R, Murphy M, eds. *Manual of Emergency Airway Management.* 4th ed. Philadelphia, PA: Lippincott Williams & Wilkins; 2012.

30. Jagannathan N, Ramsey MA, White MC, Sohn L. An update on newer pediatric supraglottic airways with recommendations for clinical use. *Pediatr Anesth.* 2015;25(4):334-345.

31. Freeman JF, Ciarallo C, Rappaport L, Mandt M, Bajaj L. Use of capnographs to assess quality of pediatric ventilation with 3 different airway modalities. *Am J Emerg Med.* 2016;34(1):69-74.

32. Peters J, et al. Indications and results of emergency surgical airways performed by a physician-staffed helicopter emergency service. *Injury.* 2015;46(5):787-790.

33. World Allergy Organization. *Treatment of Asthma in Children 5 Years and under, Based on Different Global Guidelines.* http://www.worldallergy.org/professional/allergic_diseases_center/treatment_of_asthma_in_children/; 2015.

34. Kline-Krammes S, Robinson S. Childhood asthma: A guide for pediatric emergency medicine providers. *Emerg Med Clin North Am.* 2013;31(3):705-732.

35. Koninckx M, Buysse C, de Hoog M. Management of status asthmaticus in children. *Paediatr Respir Rev.* 2013;14(2):78-85.

36. Sordillo JE, et al. Prenatal and infant exposure to acetaminophen and ibuprofen and the risk for wheeze and asthma in children. *J Allergy Clin Immunol.* 2015;135(2):441-448.

37. Hollenbach JP, Cloutier MM. Childhood asthma management and environmental triggers. *Pediatr Clin North Am.* 2015;62(5):1199-1214.

38. Akturk H, et al. Impact of respiratory viruses on pediatric asthma exacerbations. *J Pediatr Infect.* 2016;10(1):14-21.

39. Bush A, Fleming L. Diagnosis and management of asthma in children. *Br Med J.* 2015;350:h996.

40. Misra SM. The current evidence of integrative approaches to pediatric asthma. *Curr Probl Pediatr Adolesc Health Care.* 2016;46(6):190-194.

41. Doymaz S, Schneider J, Sagy M. Early administration of terbutaline in severe pediatric asthma may reduce incidence of acute respiratory failure. *Ann Allergy Asthma Immunol.* 2014;112(3):207-210.

42. Schwarz ES, Cohn BG. Is dexamethasone as effective as prednisone or prednisolone in the management of pediatric asthma exacerbations? *Ann Emerg Med.* 2015;65(1):81-82.

43. Ohn M. Jacobe S. Magnesium should be given to all children presenting to hospital with acute severe asthma. *Paediatr Respir Rev.* 2014;16(4):319-321.

44. Nierengarten MB. Diagnosis and management of croup in children. *Contemp Pediatr.* 2015;32(3):31-33.

45. Adil EA, Adil A, Shah RK. Epiglottitis. *Clin Pediatr Emerg Med.* 2015;16(3):149-153.

46. Lowe DA, Vasquez R, Maniaci V. Foreign body aspiration in children. *Clin Pediatr Emerg Med.* 2015;16(3):140-148.

47. Cevik M, et al. The characteristics and outcomes of foreign body ingestion and aspiration in children due to lodged foreign body in the aerodigestive tract. *Pediatr Emerg Care.* 2013;29(1):53-57.

48. Chapman T, Sandstrom CK, Parnell SE. Pediatric emergencies of the upper and lower airway. *Appl Radiol.* 2012;41(4):10-17.

49. Adramerina A, et al. How parents' lack of awareness could be associated with foreign body aspiration in children. *Pediatr Emerg Care.* 2016;32(2):98-100.

50. Hegde SV, Hui PKT, Lee EY. Tracheobronchial foreign bodies in children: Imaging assessment. *Semin Ultrasound CT MRI.* 2015; 36(1):8-20.

51. Singh H, Parakh A. Tracheobronchial foreign body aspiration in children. *Clin Pediatr.* 2014;53(5):415-419.

52. Ettyreddy AR, et al. Button battery injuries in the pediatric aerodigestive tract. *Ear Nose Throat J.* 2015;94(12):486-493.

53. Liao W, Wen G, Zhang X. Button battery intake as foreign body in Chinese children. *Pediatr Emerg Care.* 2015;31(6):412-415.

54. Strickland M, Rosenfield D, Fecteau A. Magnetic foreign body injuries: A large pediatric hospital experience. *J Pediatr.* 2014; 165(2):332-335.

55. Teshome G, Gattu R, Brown R. Acute bronchiolitis. *Pediatr Clin North Am.* 2013;60(5):1019-1034.

56. Aziz N, Yousuf R, Gattoo I, Latief M. Clinical predictors of hospital admission in children aged 0-24 months with acute bronchiolitis. *Int J Pediatr.* 2015;3(2.1):75-79.

57. Casey G. Bronchiolitis: A virus of infancy. *Nurs N Z.* 2015; 21(7):20-24.

58. Jain S, et al. Community-acquired pneumonia requiring hospitalization among U.S. children. *N Engl J Med.* 2015;372(22):2166-2168.

59. Elemraid MA, et al. Changing clinical practice: Management of paediatric community-acquired pneumonia. *J Eval Clin Pract.* 2014;20(1):94-99.

60. Esposito S, Principi N. Unsolved problems in the approach to pediatric community-acquired pneumonia. *Curr Opin.* 2012;25(3): 286-290.

61. Koppolu R, Simone S. *Medical and Surgical Management of Pediatric Pneumonia.* Retrieved from https://www.napnap.org/sites/ default/files/userfiles/education/2015SpeakerHO/213-% 20Koppolu%20%26%20Simone.pdf; 2016.

62. Tam PI, Hanisch BR, O'Connell M. The impact of adherence to pediatric community-acquired pneumonia guidelines on clinical outcomes. *Clin Pediatr.* 2015;54(10):1006-1008.

63. Hoshina T, et al. The utility of biomarkers in differentiating bacterial from non-bacterial lower respiratory tract infection in hospitalized children: Difference of the diagnostic performance between acute pneumonia and bronchitis. *J Infect Chemother.* 2014;20(10):616-620.

64. Esposito S, et al. Measurement of lipocalin-2 and syndecan-4 levels to differentiate bacterial from viral infection in children with community-acquired pneumonia. *BMC Pulm Med.* 2016; 16(1):1-8.

65. Neuman MI, et al. Emergency department management of childhood pneumonia in the United States prior to publication of national guidelines. *Acad Emerg Med.* 2013;20(3):240-246.

66. Staudt A, Mangla AT, Alamgir, H. Investigation of pertussis cases in a Texas county, 2008-2012. *South Med J.* 2015;108(7): 452-457.

67. Pavic-Espinoza I, et al. High prevalence of Bordetella pertussis in children under 5 years old hospitalized with acute respiratory infections in Lima, Peru. *BMC Infect Dis.* 2015;15(1):1-7.

68. Cornia P, Lipsky BA. *Pertussis Infection: Epidemiology, Microbiology, and Pathogenesis.* In: UpToDate, October 2015. Baron EL (ed.), UpToDate, Waltham, MA. Accessed on June 07, 2017. Retrieved from https://www.uptodate.com/contents/pertussis-infection-epidemiology-microbiology-and-pathogenesis.

69. Yeh S, Mink CM. *Pertussis Infection in Infants and Children: Clinical Features and Diagnosis.* In: UpToDate, Jan 2017. Torchia MM (ed.), UpToDate, Waltham, MA. Accessed on June 07, 2017. Retrieved from https://www.uptodate.com/contents/pertussis-infection-in-infants-and-children-clinical-features-and-diagnosis.

70. Cornia P, Lipsky BA. *Pertussis Infection in Adolescents and Adults: Treatment and Prevention.* In: UpToDate, April 2017. Baron EL (ed.), UpToDate, Waltham, MA. Accessed on June 07, 2017. Retrieved from https://www.uptodate.com/contents/pertussis-infection-in-adolescents-and-adults-treatment-and-prevention.

71. Sidhu N, et al. Evaluation of anaphylaxis management in a pediatric emergency department. *Pediatr Emerg Care.* 2016;32(8):508-512.

72. Tiyyagura GK, Arnold L, Cone DC, Langhan M. Pediatric anaphylaxis management in the prehospital setting. *Prehosp Emerg Care.* 2014;18(1):46-51.

73. Zilberstein J, McCurdy MT, Winters ME. Anaphylaxis. *J Emerg Med.* 2014;47(2):182-187.

74. Carrillo E, Hern HG, Barger J. Prehospital administration of epinephrine in pediatric anaphylaxis. *Prehosp Emerg Care.* 2016;20(2):239-244.

75. Kher K, Sharron M. *Approach to the Child with Metabolic Acidosis.* In: UpToDate, July 2016. Kim MS (ed.), UpToDate, Waltham, MA. Accessed on June 07, 2017. https://www.uptodate.com/contents/approach-to-the-child-with-metabolic-acidosis.

76. Park E, Pearson NM, Pillow MT, Toledo A. Neonatal endocrine emergencies. *Emerg Med Clin North Am.* 2014;32(2):421-435.

77. Barker JM, Bajaj L. Hypo and hyper: Common pediatric endocrine and metabolic emergencies. *Adv Pediatr.* 2015;62(1):257-282.

78. Hsia DS, Alimi A, Coss-Bu JA. Fluid management in pediatric patients with DKA and rates of suspected clinical cerebral edema. *Pediatr Diabetes.* 2015;16(5):338-344.

79. Bakes K, et al. Effect of volume of fluid resuscitation on metabolic normalization in children presenting in diabetic ketoacidosis: A randomized controlled trial. *J Emerg Med.* 2016;50(4):551-559.

80. Brink SJ. Paediatric and adolescent diabetic ketoacidosis. *Pract Diabetes.* 2014;31(8):342-347.

81. Olivieri L, Chasm R. Diabetic ketoacidosis in the pediatric emergency department. *Emerg Med Clin North Am.* 2013;31(3):755-773.

82. Barata IA. Cardiac emergencies. *Emerg Med Clin North Am.* 2013;31(3):677-704.

83. Yates MC, Rao PS. Pediatric cardiac emergencies. *Emerg Med Open Access.* 2013;3(6):1-7.

84. Altman CA. *Identifying Newborns with Critical Congenital Heart Disease.* In: UpToDate, June 2016. Armsby C (ed.), UpToDate, Waltham, MA. Accessed on June 07, 2017. Retrieved from https://www.uptodate.com/contents/identifying-newborns-with-critical-congenital-heart-disease.

85. Oster M. *Newborn Screening for Critical Congenital Heart Disease Using Pulse Oximetry.* In: UpToDate, Mar 2017. Armsby C (ed.), UpToDate, Waltham, MA. Accessed on June 07, 2017. Retrieved from https://www.uptodate.com/contents/newborn-screening-for-critical-congenital-heart-disease-using-pulse-oximetry.

86. American College of Surgeons. *Advanced Trauma Life Support for Doctors: ATLS Student Course Manual.* 9th ed. Chicago, IL: American College of Surgeons; 2013.

87. Stewart TC, et al. A comparison of injuries, crashes, and outcomes for pediatric rear occupants in traffic motor vehicle collisions. *J Trauma Acute Care Surg.* 2013;74(2):628-633.

88. Centers for Disease Control and Prevention. *CDC Childhood Injury Report.* Retrieved from http://www.cdc.gov/safechild/child_injury_data.html; 2015.

89. McFadyen JG, Ramaiah R, Bhananker SM. Initial assessment and management of pediatric trauma patients. *Int J Crit Illn Inj Sci.* 2012;2(3):121-127.

90. Kelleher DC, et al. Factors associated with patient exposure and environmental control during pediatric trauma resuscitation. *J Trauma Acute Care Surg.* 2013;74(2):622-626.

91. Bullock JA, Haddow GD, Coppola DP. *Managing Children in Disasters: Planning for their Unique Needs.* Boca Raton, FL: Taylor and Francis Group; 2010.

92. Guzzetta C. Family presence during resuscitation and invasive procedures. *Crit Care Nurse.* 2016;36(1):e11-e14.

93. Joyce CN, Libertin R, Bigham MT. Family-centered care in pediatric critical care transport. *Air Med J.* 2015;34(1):32-36.

94. Forgey M, Bursch B. Assessment and management of pediatric iatrogenic medical trauma. *Curr Psychiatry Rep.* 2013;15(2):340.

95. Seid T, Ramaiah R, Grabinsky A. Pre-hospital care of pediatric patients with trauma. *Int J Crit Illn Inj Sci.* 2012;2(3):114-120.

96. Ballow SL, Kaups KL, Anderson S, Chang M. A standardized rapid sequence intubation protocol facilitates airway management in critically injured patients. *J Trauma Acute Care Surg.* 2012;73(6):1401-1405.

97. Tovar JA, Vasquez JJ. Management of chest trauma in children. *Paediatr Respir Rev.* 2013;14(2):86-91.

98. Air & Surface Transport Nurses Association. *Transport Professional Advanced Trauma Course.* 6th ed. Aurora, CO: Air & Surface Transport Nurses Association; 2015.

99. Snyder SR, Kivlehan SM, Collopy KT. Thoracic trauma: What you need to know. *EMS World.* 2012;41(7):60-66.

100. Lima M, ed. *Pediatric Thoracic Surgery.* Milan, Italy: Springer-Verlag Italia; 2013.

101. Ballouhey Q, Fesseau R, Benouaich V, Leobon B. Benefits of extracorporeal membrane oxygenation for the major blunt tracheobronchial trauma in the paediatric age group. *Eur J Cardio-Thoracic Surg.* 2013;43(4):864-865.

102. Okur MH, et al. Traumatic diaphragmatic rupture in children. *J Pediatr Surg.* 2014;49(3):420-423.

103. Ballouhey Q, et al. Management of blunt tracheobronchial trauma in the pediatric age group. *Eur J Trauma Emerg Surg.* 2013;39(2):167-171.

104. Kadish H. *Chest Wall Injuries in Children.* In: UpToDate, Mar 2016. Wiley JF (ed.), UpToDate, Waltham, MA. Accessed on June 07, 2017. Retrieved from https://www.uptodate.com/contents/chest-wall-injuries-in-children.

105. Flaherty EG, Perez-Rossello J, Levine MA, Hennrikus WL. Evaluating children with fractures for child physical abuse. *Pediatrics.* 2014;133(2):e477-e489.

106. Hernandez DJ, Jatana KR, Hoff SR, Rastatter JC. Emergency airway management for pediatric blunt neck trauma. *Clin Pediatr Emerg Med.* 2014;15(3):261-268.

107. Chatterjee D, et al. Airway management in laryngotracheal injuries from blunt neck trauma in children. *Pediatr Anesth.* 2016;26(2):132-138.

108. Golden J, et al. Limiting chest computed tomography in the evaluation of pediatric thoracic trauma. *J Trauma Acute Care Surg.* 2016;81(2):271-277.

109. Puckett Y, et al. Imaging before transfer to designated pediatric trauma centers exposes children to excess radiation. *J Trauma Acute Care Surg.* 2016;81(2):229-235.

110. Swanson EW, et al. Application of the mandible injury severity score to pediatric mandibular fractures. *J Oral Maxillofac Surg.* 2015;73(7):1341-1349.

111. Al Shetawi AH, et al. Pediatric maxillofacial trauma: A review of 156 patients. *J Oral Maxillofac Surg.* 2016;74(7):1420.e1-1420.e4.

112. Flint PW, et al. *Cummings Otolaryngology-Head and Neck Surgery.* 6th ed. Philadelphia, PA: Elsevier Saunders; 2015.

113. Mendez DR. *Overview of Intrathoracic Injuries in Children.* In: UpToDate, Feb 2016. Armsby C (ed.), UpToDate, Waltham, MA. Accessed on June 07, 2017. Retrieved from http://www.uptodate.com.libproxy.usouthal.edu/contents/overview-of-intrathoracic-injuries-in-children.

114. Legome E, Kadish H. *Cardiac Injury from Blunt Trauma.* In: UpToDate, Jan 2016. Grayzel J (ed.), UpToDate, Waltham, MA. Accessed on June 07, 2017. Retrieved from https://www.uptodate.com/contents/cardiac-injury-from-blunt-trauma.

115. Mendez DR. *Initial Evaluation and Stabilization of Children with Thoracic Trauma.* In: UpToDate, May 2017. Wiley JF (ed.), UpToDate, Waltham, MA. Accessed on June 07, 2017. Retrieved from https://www.uptodate.com/contents/initial-evaluation-and-stabilization-of-children-with-thoracic-trauma.

116. Kamdar G, Santucci K, Emerson BL. Management of pediatric cardiac trauma in the ED. *Clin Pediatr Emerg Med.* 2011; 12(4):323-332.

117. Maeda K, Ono S, Baba, K, Kawahara I. Management of blunt pancreatic trauma in children. *Pediatr Surg Int.* 2013;29(10): 1019-1022.

118. Mendez DR. *Overview of Blunt Abdominal Trauma in Children.* In: UpToDate, April 2017. Wiley JF (ed.), UpToDate, Waltham, MA. Accessed on June 07, 2017. Retrieved from http://www.uptodate.com.libproxy.usouthal.edu/contents/overview-of-blunt-abdominal-trauma-in-children.

119. Holmes JF, et al. Identifying children at very low risk of clinically important blunt abdominal injuries. *Ann Emerg Med.* 2013;62(2):107-116.

120. Guyther JE. Advances in pediatric abdominal trauma: What's new in assessment and management. *Trauma Rep.* 2016;17(5):1-15.

121. Wesson DE. *Liver, Spleen, and Pancreas Injury in Children with Blunt Abdominal Trauma.* In: UpToDate, Oct 2016. Wiley JF (ed.), UpToDate, Waltham, MA. Accessed on June 07, 2017. Retrieved from http://www.uptodate.com.libproxy.usouthal.edu/contents/liver-spleen-and-pancreas-injury-in-children-with-blunt-abdominal-trauma.

122. Tran S, Kabre R. Selective nonoperative management of pediatric penetrating abdominal trauma. *Pediatr Emerg Med.* 2014; 15(3):219-222.

123. Paris C, Brindamour M, Ouimet A, St-Vil D. Predictive indicators for bowel injury in pediatric patients who present with a positive seat belt sign after motor vehicle collision. *J Pediatr Surg.* 2010;45(5):921-924.

124. Biswas S, Adileh M, Almogy G, Bala M. Abdominal injury patterns in patients with seatbelt signs requiring laparotomy. *J Emerg Trauma Shock.* 2014;7(4):295-300.

125. Borgialli DA, et al. Association between the seat belt sign and intra-abdominal injuries in children with blunt torso trauma in motor vehicle collisions. *Acad Emerg med.* 2014;21(11):1240-1248.

126. Sheybani EF, et al. Pediatric nonaccidental abdominal trauma: What the radiologist should know. *Radiographs.* 2014;34(1): 139-153.

127. Guzzo H, Middlesworth W. *Hollow Viscus Blunt Abdominal Trauma in Children.* In: UpToDate, Oct 2016. Wiley JF (ed.), UpToDate, Waltham, MA. Accessed on June 07, 2017. Retrieved from http://www.uptodate.com.libproxy.usouthal.edu/contents/hollow-viscus-blunt-abdominal-trauma-in-children.

128. Dangle PP, et al. Evolving mechanisms of injury and management of pediatric blunt renal trauma-20 years of experience. *Urology.* 2016;90:159-163.

129. Lee JN, et al. Predictive factors for conservative treatment failure in grade IV pediatric blunt renal failure. *J Pediatr Urol.* 2016;12(2):93.e1-e7.

130. Fiechtl J. *Pelvic Trauma: Initial Evaluation and Management.* In: UpToDate, Jan 2017. Wiley JF (ed.), UpToDate, Waltham, MA. Accessed on June 07, 2017. Retrieved from http://www.uptodate.com/contents/pelvic-trauma-initial-evaluation-and-management.

131. Delaney KM, et al. Risk factors associated with bladder and urethral injuries in female children with pelvic fractures: An analysis of the National Trauma Data Bank. *J Trauma Acute Care Surg.* 2016;80(2):472-476.

132. Shaath MK, et al. Associated injuries in skeletally immature children with pelvic fractures. *J Emerg Med.* 2016;51(3):246-251.

133. Ortega HW, et al. Patterns of injury and management of children with pelvic fractures at a non-trauma center. *J Emerg Med.* 2014;47(2):140-146.

134. Stone KP, White K. *Femoral Shaft Fractures in Children.* In: UpToDate, Mar 2017. Wiley JF (ed.), UpToDate, Waltham, MA. Accessed on June 07, 2017. Retrieved from http://www.uptodate.com/contents/femoral-shaft-fractures-in-children.

135. Kliegman RM, et al. eds. *Nelson Textbooks of Pediatrics.* 19th ed. Philadelphia, PA: Elsevier Saunders; 2011.

136. Rowland SP, et al. Venous injuries in pediatric trauma: Systematic review of injuries and management. *J Trauma Acute Care Surg.* 2014;77(2):356-363.

137. Wahlgren CM, Kragsterman B. Management and outcome of pediatric vascular injuries. *J Trauma Acute Care Surg.* 2015;79(4):563-567.

138. Hoffmann F, et al. Comparison of the AVPU scale and the pediatric GCS in prehospital setting. *Prehosp Emerg Care.* 2016;20(4):493-498.

139. Lumba-Brown A, Pineda J. Evidence-based assessment of severe pediatric traumatic brain injury and emergent neurocritical care. *Semin Pediatr Neurol.* 2014;21(4):275-283.

140. Youngblut JM, Caicedo C, Brooten D. Preschool children with head injury: Comparing injury severity measures and clinical care. *Pediatr Nurs.* 2013;39(6):290-298.

141. Fuhrman BP, Zimmerman J, eds. *Pediatric critical care.* 4th ed. Philadelphia, PA: Elsevier Mosby; 2011.

142. Glasgow Coma Scale. *The Glasgow Structured Approach to Assessment of the Glasgow Coma Scale.* Retrieved from http://www.glasgowcomascale.org/; 2015.

143. Ducharme-Crevier L, Wainwright M. Acute management of children with traumatic brain injury. *Clin Pediatr Emerg Med.* 2015;16(1):48-54.

144. Burns ECM, et al. Scalp hematoma characteristics associated with intracranial injury in pediatric head injury. *Acad Emerg Med.* 2016;23(5):576-582.

145. Medscape. *Classification and Complications of Traumatic Brain Injury.* Retrieved from http://emedicine.medscape.com/article/326643-overview#a1; 2016.

146. Schutzman S. *Minor Head Trauma in Infants and Children: Evaluation.* In: UpToDate, April 2017. Wiley JF (ed.), UpToDate, Waltham, MA. Accessed on June 07, 2017. Retrieved from http://www.uptodate.com/contents/minor-head-trauma-in-infants-and-children-evaluation.

147. Pitfield AF, Carroll AB, Kissoon N. Emergency management of increased intracranial pressure. *Pediatr Emerg Care.* 2012;28(2):200-204.

148. Agrawal D. *Rapid Sequence Intubation (RSI) in Children.* In: UpToDate, May 2017. Wiley JF (ed.), UpToDate, Waltham, MA. Accessed on June 07, 2017. Retrieved from http://www.uptodate.com/contents/rapid-sequence-intubation-rsi-in-children.

149. Hansen G, Vallance JK. Ventilation monitoring for severe pediatric TBI during interfacility transport. *Int J Emerg Med.* 2015;8:41.

150. Allen BB, et al. Age-specific cerebral perfusion pressure thresholds and survival in children and adolescents with severe traumatic brain injury. *Pediatr Crit Care Med.* 2014;15(1):62-70.

151. Mangat HS, et al. Hypertonic saline reduces cumulative and daily intracranial pressure burdens after severe traumatic brain injury. *J Neurosurg.* 2015;122(1):202-210.

152. Taha AA, Westlake C, Badr L, Mathur M. Mannitol versus 3% NaCl for management of severe pediatric traumatic brain injury. *J Nurse Pract.* 2015;11(5):505-510.

153. Leonard JR, et al. Cervical spine injury patterns in children. *Pediatrics.* 2014;133(5):e1179-e1188.

154. Huisman TAGM, et al. Pediatric spinal trauma. *J Neuroimaging.* 2015;25(3):337-353.

155. Sun R, et al. A pediatric cervical spine clearance protocol to reduce radiation exposure in children. *J Surg Res.* 2013;183(1):341-346.

156. Mahajan P, et al. Spinal cord injury without radiologic abnormality in children imaged with magnetic resonance imaging. *J Trauma Acute Care Surg.* 2013;75(5):843-847.

157. Rosati SF, et al. Implementation of pediatric cervical spine clearance guidelines at a combined trauma center: Twelve-month impact. *J Trauma Acute Care Surg.* 2015;78(6):1117-1121.

158. Tat ST, Mejia MJ, Freishtat RJ. Imaging, clearance, and controversies in pediatric cervical spine trauma. *Pediatr Emerg Care.* 2014;30(12):911-918.

159. McMahon PM, et al. Protocol to clear cervical spine injuries in pediatric trauma patients. *Radiol Manage.* 2015;37(5):42-48.

160. Leonard JC, et al. Factors associated with cervical spine injury in children after blunt trauma. *Ann Emerg Med.* 2011;58(2):145-155.

161. Leonard JC, Mao J, Jaffe DM. Potential adverse effects of spinal immobilization in children. *Prehosp Emerg Care.* 2012;16(4):513-518.

162. Clemency BM, et al. Patients immobilized with a long spine board rarely have unstable thoracolumbar injuries. *Prehosp Emerg Care.* 2016;20(2):266-272.

163. Collopy KT, Kivlehan SM, Snyder SR. *Pediatric Spinal Cord Injuries.* Retrieved from http://www.emsworld.com/article/10736962/pediatric-spinal-cord-injuries; 2012.

164. Kim EG, et al. Variability of prehospital spinal immobilization in children at risk for cervical spine injury. *Pediatr Emerg Care.* 2013;29(4):413-418.

165. White IV CC, Domeier RM, Millin MG. EMS spinal precautions and the use of the long backboard– resource document to the position statement of the National Association of EMS Physicians and the American College of Surgeons committee on trauma. *Prehosp Emerg Care.* 2014;18(2):306-314.

166. Corneli HM. *Hypothermia in Children: Clinical Manifestations and Diagnosis.* In: *UpToDate,* August 2016. Wiley JF (ed.), UpToDate, Waltham, MA. Accessed on June 07, 2017. Retrieved from https://www.uptodate.com/contents/hypothermia-in-children-clinical-manifestations-and-diagnosis.

167. Corneli JM. *Hypothermia in Children: Management.* In: UpToDate, Dec 2016. Wiley JF (ed.), UpToDate, Waltham, MA. Accessed on June 07, 2017. Retrieved from https://www.uptodate.com/contents/hypothermia-in-children-management.

168. Ishimine P. *Heat Stroke in Children.* In: UpToDate, Oct 2016. Wiley JF (ed.), UpToDate, Waltham, MA. Accessed on June 07, 2017. Retrieved from https://www.uptodate.com/contents/heat-stroke-in-children.

169. Semple-Hess J, Campwala R. *Pediatric Submersion Injuries: Emergency Care and Resuscitation*. Retrieved from http://cdn7.slremeducation.org/wp-content/uploads/2015/02/Peds0614-Submersion-Injuries.pdf; 2014.

170. Paul AR, Adamo MA. Non-accidental trauma in pediatric patients: a review of epidemiology, pathophysiology, diagnosis and treatment. *Transl Pediatr*. 2014;3(3):195-207.

171. Bechtel K, Bennett BL. Evaluation of sexual abuse in children and adolescents. In: UpToDate, March 2017. Wiley JF (ed.), UpToDate, Waltham, MA. Accessed on June 07, 2017. Retrieved from https://www.uptodate.com/contents/evaluation-of-sexual-abuse-in-children-and-adolescents.

172. Friedman ML, Bone MF. Management of pediatric septic shock in the emergency department. *Clin Pediatr Emerg Med*. 2014;15(2):131-139.

173. Waltzman ML. Pediatric shock. *J Emerg Nurs*. 2015;41(2):113-118.

174. Waltzman M. *Initial Evaluation of Shock in Children*. In: UpToDate, Feb 2017. Wiley JF (ed.), UpToDate, Waltham, MA. Accessed on June 07, 2017. Retrieved from https://www.uptodate.com/contents/initial-evaluation-of-shock-in-children.

175. Waltzman M. *Initial Management of Shock in Children*. In: UpToDate, August 2016. Wiley JF (ed.), UpToDate, Waltham, MA. Accessed on June 07, 2017. Retrieved from https://www.uptodate.com/contents/initial-management-of-shock-in-children.

176. Waltzman M. *Physiology and Classification of Shock in Children*. In: UpToDate, Feb 2017. Wiley JF (ed.), UpToDate, Waltham, MA. Accessed on June 07, 2017. Retrieved from https://www.uptodate.com/contents/initial-evaluation-of-shock-in-children.

177. Thompson GC, Macias CG. Recognition and management of sepsis in children: Practice patterns in the emergency department. *J Emerg Med*. 2015;49(4):391-395.

178. Kim YA, Ha EJ, Jhang WK, Park SJ. Early blood lactate area as prognostic marker. *Intensive Care Med*. 2013;39(10):1818-1823.

179. Weiss SL, Pomerantz WJ. *Septic Shock: Rapid Recognition and Initial Resuscitation in Children*. In: UpToDate, May 2017. Wiley JF (ed.), UpToDate, Waltham, MA. Accessed on June 07, 2017. Retrieved from https://www.uptodate.com/contents/septic-shock-rapid-recognition-and-initial-resuscitation-in-children.

180. Marjanovic V, Budic I. Fluid resuscitation and massive transfusion protocol in pediatric trauma. *Acta Fac Med Naiss*. 2016;33(2):91-99.

181. Hughes NT, Burd RS, Teach ST. Damage control resuscitation: Permissive hypotension and massive transfusion protocols. *Pediatr Emerg Care*. 2014;30(9):651-656.

182. American Heart Association. *Highlights of the 2015 American Heart Association: Guidelines Update for CPR and ECC*. Retrieved from https://eccguidelines.heart.org/wp-content/uploads/2015/10/2015-AHA-Guidelines-Highlights-English.pdf; 2015.

183. Carey JM, Shah MI. Pediatric prehospital seizure management. *Clin Pediatr Emerg Med*. 2014;15(1):59-66.

184. Fernandez IS, et al. Time from convulsive status epilepticus onset to anticonvulsant administration in children. *Neurology*. 2015;84(23):2304-2311.

185. Barzegar M, Mahdavi M, Behbehani AG, Tabrizi A. Refractory convulsive status epilepticus in children: etiology, associated risk factors and outcome. *Iran J Child Neurol*. 2015;9(4):24-31.

186. Browne GJ, Dimou S. Concussive head injury in children and adolescents. *Aust Fam Physician*. 2016;45(7):470-476.

187. Semple BD, et al. Repetitive concussions in adolescent athletes–translating clinical and experimental research into perspectives on rehabilitation strategies. *Front Neurol*. 2015;6:1-16.

188. Ellis R, Ellis C. Dog and cat bites. *Am Fam Physician*. 2014;90(4):239-243.

189. O'Brien DC, et al. Dog bites of the head and neck: An evaluation of a common pediatric trauma and associated treatment. *Am J Otolaryngol*. 2015;36(1):32-38.

190. Garvey EM, Twitchell DK, Ragar R, Egan JC, Jamshidi R. Morbidity of pediatric dog bites: A case series at a level one pediatric trauma center. *J Pediatr Surg*. 2015;50(2):343-346.

191. Rutkowska A, Skotnicka-Klonowicz G. Prehospital pain management in children with traumatic injuries. *Pediatr Emerg Care*. 2015;31(5):317-320.

192. Browne LR, et al. Prehospital opioid administration in the emergency care of injured children. *Prehosp Emerg Care*. 2016;20(1):59-65.

193. Gilbert SB. Beyond acting out: Managing pediatric psychiatric emergencies in the emergency department. *Adv Emerg Nurs J*. 2012;34(2):147-163.

194. Knowlton AR, et al. Pediatric use of emergency medical services: the role of chronic illnesses and behavioral health problems. *Prehosp Emerg Care*. 2015;20(3):362-368.

195. National Alliance on Mental Illness. *Mental Health by the Numbers*. Retrieved from http://www.nami.org/Learn-More/Mental-Health-By-the-Numbers; 2016.

31

Military Patient Transport

CHRISTOPHER T. PAIGE, TIMOTHY L. HUDSON, AND KATHLEEN FLARITY

COMPETENCIES

1. Describe the military en route care patient transport system used in humanitarian and combat action.
2. Describe military roles (Roles 1–4) of care within the military en route care patient transport system.
3. Identify different military medical service (Air Force, Army, and Navy) capabilities.
4. Identify military patient transport platforms (air, sea, and ground).
5. Identify the military medical training needed for transport personnel.
6. Recognize special military patient transport situations.

This chapter describes the US military en route care patient transport system deployed during combat and humanitarian operations. Not unlike the US medical system, the deployed military health care system is an integrated system that accomplishes triage and emergency treatment and then transports the patient to the appropriate level of care or returns the member to duty. Essentially the military built a state-of-the-art trauma system in some of the most austere and dangerous locations for humanitarian and military operations other than war or wartime contingencies.[1] At the point of injury (POI), first aid is initiated. The patient is then rapidly transported through multiple medical support roles to include emergency medical response (Fig. 31.1), advanced trauma surgery (Fig. 31.2), and patient transport (Figs. 31.3 and 31.4) toward hospital definitive care. (Note: The views expressed in this chapter are taken from published articles and Department of Defense [DoD] doctrine. It is not to be taken as an official policy or position of the DoD or the US Government.)

Within the DoD, the Air Force, Army, and Navy each have their own independent service surgeons general and doctrines. In the past, by design, the different medical services generally "took care of their own," with each service caring for its members (i.e., Army soldiers seeing Army providers) and the Navy, in addition to their own service, charged with Marine medical care. This was a logical system, with each of the military services charged with service-specific

tasks. The Navy and Marines primarily are tasked with the oceans and coastal areas, the Army with land security, and the Air Force with aerospace. However, today's military operations are vastly more complicated, with the Navy, Marines, Army, and Air Force frequently sharing missions in and around the battle space in what are called joint operations. In addition, coalition partners and host nation military resources are frequently embedded together in operations. Joint Operations present a unique challenge to the military patient transport system. The interdependent Air Force, Army, and Navy medical transport capabilities must be interoperable and interchangeable.[2] This chapter references the Joint Publication (JP-02) Health Services Support dated July 26, 2012, as well as specific service medical doctrine to describe the Military Health System patient movement, its requirements, and its capabilities.[3]

Roles of Care

To best understand US military en route care patient transport, one must first understand the different roles of patient care. After being introduced to the military medical roles of care, one can more easily understand the different transportation platforms, capabilities, capacities, and resources found in the combat arena.

Military *roles* refer to the capability of care and are in sequential order of a patient's movement through the military medical system.[4] This can be somewhat confusing at first because the role numbers are opposite to the civilian system of the American College of Surgeons trauma levels. In the military system, the lower the role, the less capability of providing the patient with a full complement of medical and surgical services. The purpose of creating graduating roles is for service members to be evaluated, treated, and released to duty at the lowest role possible.[4] If medical care needed by the service member cannot be administered at a certain role of care, then they are transported to a higher role. Of note, in the urban environment, like Afghanistan and Iraq, where there is no "frontline," it is not uncommon for the transportation of a patient to go directly from Role 1 to Role 3.[5] In recent conflicts surgical intervention has been moved closer to combat, which has increased the ability to receive more immediate Role 2 care.[5]

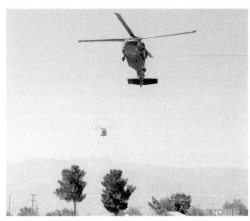

• **Fig. 31.1** Two Army UH-60 Black Hawks arriving on scene to evacuate injured soldiers.

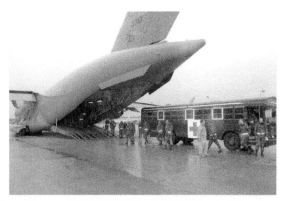

• **Fig. 31.4** Loading patients for intertheater patient transportation on an Air Force C-17.

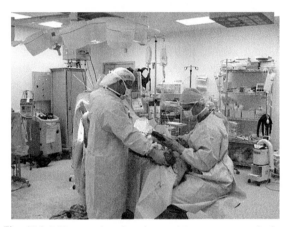

• **Fig. 31.2** Military patient in advanced trauma surgery in forward location.

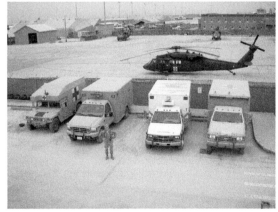

• **Fig. 31.3** Some military ground and air intratheater transport capabilities.

Role 1

Role 1 is described by Joint Publication JP-02 as "The first medical care military personnel receive (also referred to as unit-level medical care), p. xii."[3] Role 1 begins at the *POI.*[7] *POI care* begins with patient assessment and triage, and is conducted immediately to identify whether life-saving measures must be taken. These measures encompass actions such as maintenance of airway, hemorrhage control, and prevention of shock. POI care is accomplished by the individual first on scene, which can be a nonmedical provider trained as a combat lifesaver or self-aid/buddy care (SABC).[8] The *nonmedical provider* (soldier, sailor, airman, or marine) is trained to perform first-aid procedures to begin early lifesaving treatment such as basic airway control with nasopharyngeal airway, controlling bleeding including hemostatic agent dressing, or combat application tourniquet (CAT). The primary focus is stabilization of the patient condition and transport to a higher role of care.

This is not the only care available to the warrior. Frequently a Navy *corpsman* or Army or Air Force *medic* (a trained emergency medical technician) is embedded within the combat team and is on scene to provide trauma care. In addition to emergency care, many are trained in public health, disease prevention, and evaluation of diseases and injuries that are not related to battle. This training is often provided by medical briefings dependent on the geographic area of operations and based on current epidemiologic trends.

Role 2

For support of the many medical needs of a security force, small medical teams are placed far forward near combat operations. They are commonly referred to as *battalion aid stations* (BASs). The team includes a physician, physician assistant, and medics. Traditionally, surgical intervention is minimal at the BAS. However, in an effort to bring more surgical capability closer to the POI, mobile trauma teams are attached to the BAS. The Marines (staffed by Navy medical providers) have a forward resuscitative surgical system (FRSS) attached to the BAS, and the Army has their forward surgical team (FST). This shift to trauma teams being more capable and more forward occurred from lessons learned in combat in Iraq in 2003.[9] Role 2, therefore, ". . . provides advanced trauma management and emergency medical treatment including continuation of resuscitation started in Role 1."[7]

This capability (Fig. 31.5) does not have inpatient bed capability but may have increased access to primary care,

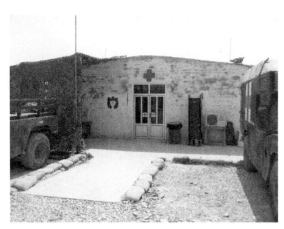

• **Fig. 31.5** Emergency entrance to a Role 2 facility.

laboratory, emergency dental, combat stress/mental health, optometry, and basic radiography, and can be augmented with surgical assets. Each service has a similar but slightly modified capability at Role 2. The patient is triaged to determine transport priority based on current medical assets and the patient's condition. At times, patients can be treated and returned to duty. If needed, emergent care, including resuscitation, is provided and more complete medical and surgical measures are taken. Because the Role 2 facility is close to combat operations, the relative safety of the tactical situation at times dictates what extent of medical

care can be administered. Data from combat experience suggest minimal intervention at Role 2 (2 hours or less) provides a better outcome.[10-12]

The Air Force Role 2 capabilities include the mobile field surgical team (frequently called "M-Fast") and the small portable expeditionary aeromedical rapid response (SPE-ARR) Team. Both are used similar to the FRSS of the Navy and FST of the Army to augment surgical capabilities in a combat or humanitarian theater. Additionally, expeditionary medical support (EMEDS) Basic and EMEDS + 10 are available to expand Role 2 medical services. These incorporate a 25-person SPEARR team and include multiple operating rooms (ORs) and 6 and 10 beds, respectively. These components are integral to the remainder of the Air Force Theatre Hospital System.

The Navy can place an amphibious ready group (ARG) offshore during a humanitarian crisis or war. The ARG consists of up to six ships with assault helicopters on deck. These helicopters are used for assault but can double as both amphibious assault and patient transport platforms. One ship in the ARG is called a casualty receiving and treatment ship. It has up to 45 beds, four ORs, and 17 intensive care beds (see Box 31.1 for more information on Role 2 capabilities among the services).

After stabilization, the patient is packaged for en route care transport to the next role of care, an Army combat support hospital (CSH; pronounced "cash"), an Air Force EMEDS, or a Navy fleet hospital.

• BOX 31.1 Role 2 Capabilities

US Army

Treatment Platoon
Basic/emergency treatment is continued.
Packed red blood cells (type O, Rh positive and negative), limited radiography, laboratory, and dental.
20 to 40 cots with 72-hour holding.
No surgical capability.

Forward Surgical Team
Continuous operations for up to 72 hours.
Life-saving resuscitative surgery, including general, orthopedic, and limited neurosurgical procedures.
Twenty-person team with one orthopedic and three general surgeons, two nurse anesthetists, critical care nurses, and technicians.
Operational within 1 hour of arrival at the supported company.
May be transported by ground, fixed-wing, or helicopter; some are airborne deployable.
Two operating tables for a maximum of 10 cases per day and for a total of 30 operations within 72 hours.

Postoperative Intensive Care for up to 8 Patients for up to 6 Hours. US Air Force

Mobile Field Surgical Team
Five-person team (general surgeon, orthopedist, anesthetist, emergency medicine physician, and OR nurse/technician).
Ten life-saving/limb-saving procedures in 24 to 48 hours from three backpacks.
Designed to augment an aid station or flight line clinic.

Small Portable Expeditionary Air Medical Rapid Response Team
Ten-person team: five-person M-FST, three-person critical care transport/two-person preventive medicine team (flight surgeon, public health officer).
Stand-alone capable: 7 days, 10 life-saving/limb-saving procedures in 24 to 48 hours. Designed to provide surgical support, basic primary care, postoperative critical care, and preventive medicine for early phase of deployment.
Highly mobile unit, with all equipment fitting into one pallet-sized trailer.

Expeditionary Medical Support Basic
Medical and surgical support for an airbase, sick call, resuscitative surgery, dental care, limited laboratory, and radiography capability.
Twenty-five staff includes SPEARR.
Four holding beds/one OR table.
Ten life-saving/limb-saving procedures in 24 to 48 hours.

Can Augment: 10 Beds/56-Person Staff (EMEDS + 10). US Navy

Forward Resuscitative Surgical System
Rapid assembly, highly mobile.
Resuscitative surgery for 18 patients within 48 hours without resupply.
One OR, two surgeons (general/orthopedic).
No holding capability.
No intrinsic evacuation capability.

• BOX 31.1 Role 2 Capabilities—cont'd

Typically augmented with an en route care team to allow for evacuation capability.

Also requires host unit for logistics and security.

Surgical Company

Provides surgical care for a marine expeditionary force. Basis of allocation is one per infantry regiment.

Three ORs, 60-bed capability.

Patient holding time up to 72 hours.

Stabilizing surgical procedures.

Casualty Receiving and Treatment Ships

Provides medical care for an amphibious ready group.

Helicopter assets with casualty receiving capability.

Laboratory, radiography.

Fleet surgical team: three to four physicians, one surgeon, one certified registered nurse anesthetist, and support staff.

Augment: two orthopedic, two general surgeons, and oral maxillofacial surgeon with dental unit.

Excellent casualty flow capability because of large helicopter flight deck. Forty-seven to 48 beds, four to six ORs, 17 intensive care beds.

EMEDS; Expeditionary medical support; *M-FST,* mobile field surgical team; *OR,* operating room; *SPEARR,* small portable expeditionary aeromedical rapid response.

Role 3

Role 3 medical assets are the highest level of medical care available within the combat theater and allow for inpatient hospital beds within the theater.[5] These Role 3 facilities are similar in trauma/surgical capability to a US civilian Level 1 or 2 trauma center. Most are modular (Fig. 31.6), with the exception of the fleet hospital. Modular build allows medical planners to tailor medical personnel and the size of facility to actual or predicted requirements. The fleet hospital provides up to 500 beds and is comparable with the Army Role 3 hospital. It is equipped to provide resuscitation, initial wound surgery, and postoperative treatment. Patients at a Role 3 hospital are stabilized for continued transport through the en route care system or returned to duty. Role 3 capability is similar between the services and has proven to be interoperable, interchangeable, and interdependent with deployment rotations.[5] The Army CSH Role 3 facilities can have up to 248 beds, which are usually divided into 48 intensive care unit beds and 200 intermediate care beds (medical/surgical). The surgical capability can provide up to six ORs. Surgical services include general, orthopedic, urologic, dental, and oral maxillofacial. Units include a robust blood bank, laboratory, radiology to

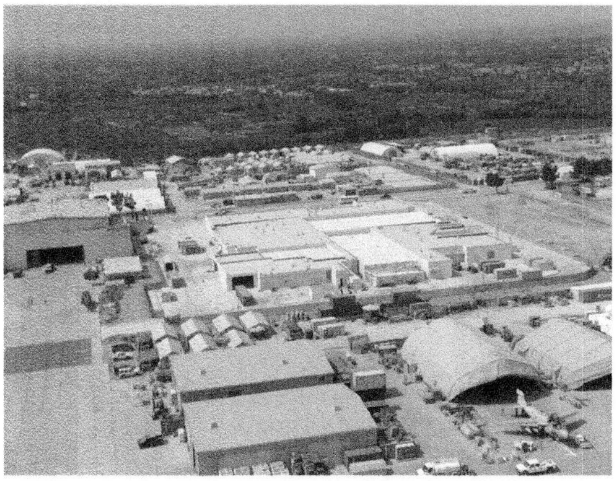

• **Fig. 31.6** Role 3 facility. Note proximity to airport for intertheater movement.

include computed tomographic scan and magnetic resonance imagery, nutrition, and physical therapy. It also provides preventative medical surveillance capability to monitor disease and nonbattle injury. This clinic also provides outpatient psychiatry and inpatient neuropsychiatric consultation services.

In the CSH the early-entry hospitalization element and the hospital augmentation element combine for a total of 84 beds (44 and 40, respectively). The hospital company provides hospitalization for up to 164 patients, consisting of two wards that provide critical care nursing for up to 24 patients and seven wards that provide intermediate nursing care for up to 140 patients.

An Air Force Role 3, traditionally the EMEDS + 25, is a 25-bed facility. It includes 84 personnel and two OR tables that can accomplish 20 operations within 48 hours. The Air Force EMEDS + 25 capability can be increased by the addition of specialty teams such as vascular/cardiothoracic; neurosurgery; obstetrics/gynecology; ear, nose, and throat; and ophthalmology.[4]

Traditionally, Role 3 medical care was provided by field hospitals within theater but outside combat operations. Iraq and Afghanistan operations have used the en route care patient transport system directly from combat Role 2 facilities to a fixed facility like Landstuhl Regional Medical Center in Germany (Fig. 31.7). Humanitarian operations (a natural disaster, such as tsunami, hurricane, or earthquake) have the option to deploy the naval ship Mercy or Comfort as a Role 3 platform (Fig. 31.8). The Role 3 facility is designed for treatment and evaluation of patients with the goal to return the warrior to duty. If patients are unable to return to combat duty, they are transported to their home unit or to one of the Role 4 hospitals in the United States.

Role 4

Role 4 hospitals, located in the United States and other safe havens, provide complete medical care and maintain all general and specialty capabilities. These include DoD hospitals such as Walter Reed National Military Medical Center and

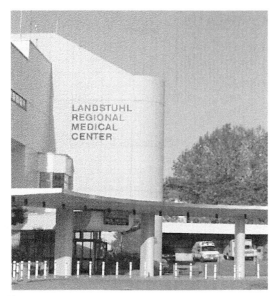

Fig. 31.7 Landstuhl Regional Medical Center, a Role 3 facility.

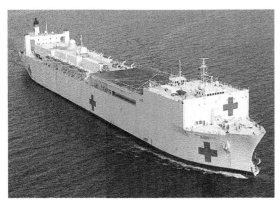

Fig. 31.8 Role 3 hospital ship, T-AH Mercy.

San Antonio Military Medical Center. The focus in these facilities is on medical, surgical, rehabilitative, mental health, and convalescent care.

En Route Care: Military Patient Transportation System

Within the military medical system, during combat operations, en route patient transportation involves moving patients intratheater and intertheater.[7] This movement takes a collaborative effort of the military medical system. For example, it is not unusual for a wounded Marine to be treated initially by another Marine, followed by a Navy corpsman, an Army surgeon, and an Air Force flight nurse (FN), all during transport through Roles 1 to 4. Common means of military patient transport are summarized in Table 31.1 and discussed in the following sections.

Intratheater: Roles 1 to 3
Point of Injury Care Providers

En route care is a continuation of care during transport, from POI to rehabilitation.[13] En route care builds with critical care capability as the patient moves through the system. Rapid, appropriate care and transport help return individuals to their units or out of theater to a facility that provides the needed definitive care.[14] To provide rapid care, medical and surgical assets have been moved closer to combat operations. Each soldier is trained in first aid, "self-aid and buddy care (SABC), or combat casualty care.[8] Ideally, help comes from an embedded medical specialist: the team "doc," which is a Navy corpsman or Army combat medic with specific training for resuscitation, triage, and packaging for transport. They are trained in combat arms as well

TABLE 31.1	**Common Means of Military Patient Transport**	
Capability	**Employment**	**Litter Spaces/Seats Available**
Fireman's carry	Intratheater: CASEVAC or MEDEVAC	One example of carries from POI
NATO litter	Intratheater and Intertheater: MEDEVAC and aeromedical evacuation	All transport platforms are designed to NATO litter specifications
M997 four-litter HMMWV	Intratheater: CASEVAC or MEDEVAC	4 litter (max) 8 ambulatory (max) Combination of litter/ambulatory 2/4
Black Hawk UH-60A	Intratheater: CASEVAC or MEDEVAC	6 litter (max) 7 ambulatory (max) Combination of litter/ambulatory 3/4 (max)
Sea Knight CH-46	Intratheater: CASEVAC or MEDEVAC	15 litter (max) 25 ambulatory (max) Combination of litter/ambulatory 6/15 (max)
Ambus	Intratheater: MEDEVAC	20 litter (max) 44 ambulatory (max)

TABLE 31.1	Common Means of Military Patient Transport—cont'd	
Capability	**Employment**	**Litter Spaces/Seats Available**
Hercules C-130	Intratheater: aeromedical evacuation	74 litter (max) 92 ambulatory (max) Combination of litter/ambulatory 50/27
Globemaster C-17	Intertheater: aeromedical evacuation	36 litter (max) 102 ambulatory (max) Combination of litter/ambulatory 36/54
KC-135 Stratotanker	Intertheater: aeromedical evacuation	15 litter (max) 50 ambulatory (max) Combination of litter/ambulatory 15/24
Osprey CV-22	Air Force: special operations	9 litter 24 ambulatory
MRAP ambulance or RG33 HAGA	Intratheater	4 Litter 8 Ambulatory
Mercy T-AH	Intertheater Intratheater: Role 3 capability	1000 hospital beds (max) Combination of services 21 operating rooms/20 recovery 80 intensive care beds 900 medical/surgical

HAGA, Heavy armored ground ambulance; *HMMWV,* high mobility multipurpose wheeled vehicle; *MRAP,* mine-resistant ambush protected; *NATO;* North Atlantic Treaty Organization; *POI,* point of injury.

as emergency medical treatment. These professionals are trained in spinal stabilization and extrication, advanced airway support (e.g., intubation and cricothyrotomy), and emergency surgical procedures, such as chest decompression, use of CAT, and emergency laceration repair and combat gauze to control hemorrhage.

Notable differences between the Army and Navy are found regarding how they support en route casualty evacuation. The US Army uses a dedicated medical evacuation platform (air or ground ambulance) that is staffed with trained flight medics or nurses (medical evacuation or MEDEVAC). The Navy often uses transport vehicles designed for multiple use (air or ground). This use of vehicle of opportunity (not necessarily fitted for a medical specific mission) is called casualty evacuation (or CASEVAC).

Casualty Evacuation

Once POI care is provided and the decision to transport has been made, a number of options are exercised. Usually, the most rapid option is referred to as casualty evacuation or *CASEVAC.* These patients are moved from the POI to medical treatment with a military vehicle of opportunity. With minimal defense systems and when the scene is unsafe, a medical transport platform is not typically brought into active combat zones.[15] CASEVAC transport to a Role 1 to 3 facility may or may not be coordinated or announced. CASEVAC is frequently used in military operations in urban terrain because of the limited number of landing zones for rotor-wing medical evacuation

platforms. At times, application of first aid/buddy aid and rapid transport to the nearest treatment facility in a vehicle of opportunity is faster and safer. Basically, the military on scene are prepared to "load-and-go" to the nearest medical facility.

Ground Transportation

The US Army has the largest intratheater medical ground evacuation capability for collecting, regulating, and caring for US military personnel. Numerous medical *ground transport* platforms exist. These platforms are largely dedicated field ambulance vehicles that are operated by two basic emergency medical technicians with typical basic life support medical supplies and equipment similar to that found in a civilian ambulance.

Traditionally, casualties are first taken to a BAS or medical platoon. From the POI, the casualty can be taken to one of these areas directly on a military stretcher called a North Atlantic Treaty Organization (NATO) litter (see Table 31.1) or more frequently by tactical vehicles such as the armored high mobility multipurpose wheeled vehicle (HMMWV; pronounced HUMVEE), Stryker, or mine-resistant ambush protected (MRAP) vehicle (RG33 heavy armored ground ambulance [HAGA]).

If available, a HAGA (Figs. 31.9 and 31.10) is used in a high-risk environment. Soft-skinned ambulances such as the M996 or M997 (see Table 31.1) are not used forward of a BAS because of limited protection against small-arms fire.

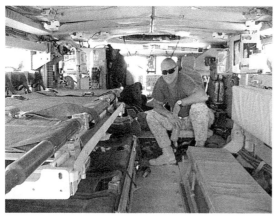

• **Fig. 31.9** Ramp used to load patient into a heavy armored ground ambulance.

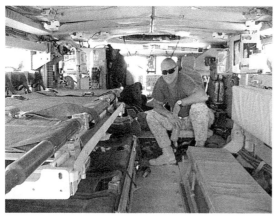

• **Fig. 31.10** Litter mounted on top and bottom left in a heavy armored ground ambulance (patient litter system).

Based on the combat situation, a casualty could be transferred from a BAS to a Role 2 or Role 3 facility with an M996 or M997 ambulance. However, this transfer is occurring less because of the urban environment of current conflicts. The risk from improvised explosive devices and ambush attacks has made it necessary to use armored transport vehicles for casualty transport to a protected forward operating base.

The wheeled ambulance is designed for field use; it can operate on paved and secondary roads, trails, and cross-country terrain and can operate in all weather conditions. Electrical power access is provided to operate the onboard

medical equipment. Before evacuation of casualties, the medical personnel must configure an evacuation platform to accommodate the types and number of patients. After configuring the platform, they prioritize, load, and appropriately secure the casualties to ensure safe transport and patient access during evacuation. Casualties are normally loaded head first in the field ambulance. However, if the casualty requires access to a specific injured side, the patient can be loaded feet first. A M996 ambulance can accommodate two litter patients and one ambulatory patient. The M997 and the M113 tracked ambulance can accommodate four litter patients and one ambulatory or a total of eight ambulatory patients.[16]

Medical Evacuation

MEDEVAC involves the rapid movement of a patient with a medically staffed and equipped vehicle. A classic example of this is the UH-60 Black Hawk, the MEDEVAC workhorse of the Army (Fig. 31.11). This rotary medical capability is taught at a tri-service Joint En Route Care Course (JECC).

The transport can be from a battlefield (on scene) to a medical treatment facility or movement between medical treatment facilities. In 2012 the flight medic program expanded to include the critical care flight paramedic. A nurse does not generally accompany a MEDEVAC to the POI location. Care is provided by flight paramedics between roles of care unless the patient being transported is in critical condition. In a critical care transport, a critical care nurse and a flight paramedic accompany the patient. Critical care patients from Role 1 or Role 2 FST or FRSS frequently have abdomens left open, with paralytics, sedatives, narcotics and are ventilated.[17] The transport route is frequently unsafe, and control of the combat area of operations (air and surface) is a challenge.[6] Enemy attacks during transport are possible. This risk requires the provider to wear combat gear (weapon, ammunition, Kevlar helmet, and body armor) and fly or drive with rapid evasive moves, which makes care an exponential challenge.[18] In 2007, the US Army conducted more than 12,000 helicopter patient transports in Afghanistan and Iraq in support of combat operations.[18]

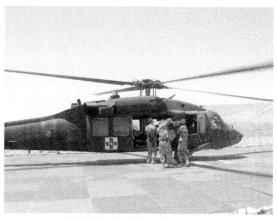

• **Fig. 31.11** UH-60 Black Hawk helicopter.

Most of these transports (>75%) were casualties who required surgery. These transports included Role 2 to 3 transports.[18]

Aeromedical Evacuation

Aeromedical evacuation (AE) is an Air Force–specific mission that uses fixed-wing resources to evacuate the ill and wounded under the care of qualified AE crew members both intratheater and intertheater. AE uses an integrated multiplatform capability. The crews are universally qualified on multiple aircraft and provide care on any of the following: C-130 or C-17, for intratheater; C-17 or KC-135, for intertheater (see Table 31.1); and some on C-21s, which are Learjet 35s converted for military usage. Other opportune fixed wing aircraft can also be used. More than 186,000 AE patient movements have been successfully completed since the onset of operations Iraqi Freedom, New Dawn, and Enduring Freedom, with a 98% survival rate.[19]

AE crews, FNs, and AE technicians (AETs) provide en route medical support necessary to reduce the loss of life, limb, and eyesight (Fig. 31.12). The specific number of crew members depends on the length of the flight, patient acuity, and number of patients. Typically, an urgent or priority intratheater mission is shorter in flight time and will be called to evacuate and care for only a few patients. This may only require one FN and two AETs. A standard crew for other missions that may be carrying larger patient loads for longer flight times is two FNs and three AETs. For an extended crew duty day (24 hours) the standard crew will be augmented with another FN and AET. The team may be larger based on other circumstances and directed by the chief nurse/commander. The AE environment is dynamic, and each crew member is required to maintain clinical expertise, accountability, knowledge, and skill to manage patients in flight. The team leader, one of the FNs known as the medical crew director (MCD), is also responsible for operational medical mission management.

For transport of critical patients, the AE crew may be augmented by one of various specialty teams. One example

is the critical care air transport team (CCATT) and Royal Air Force (RAF) Critical Care Air Support Teams (CCASTs) providing the AE system's core critical care capability by delivering care to severely ill or injured patients during air transport.[22] This team consists of one physician, one critical care nurse, and a cardiopulmonary technician. An augmentation to the AE team, the specialty team works with and receives mission operational direction from the MCD.

The Air Force works jointly with other US military services to improve emergency care for service members critically injured in combat by using tactical critical care evacuation teams (TCCETs). The three-person teams are comprised of an emergency medicine or critical care physician, a certified nurse anesthetist, and an emergency department nurse or intensive care/critical care nurse and fly mostly on rotary-wing aircraft.[19] The TCCET-E is an enhanced five-person team who specialize in emergency trauma care with an in-flight surgical capability to transport and treat patients with acute, life-threatening injuries. These crews often fly on a fixed-wing aircraft to give the emergent medical and surgical capability and capacity a wider range.[20] The five-person TCCET-E crew also flies with the standard AE crew.

Augmenting specialty teams to the AE system has resulted in rapid critical patient treatment and transport. Moving an injured patient from a Role 1 to a Role 4 facility in the continental United States was a process that sometimes took more than a month during the Vietnam War. Today it is not unusual to take as few as 36 hours. The speed of the process, combined with improvements in body armor and surgical care, has made a life-saving difference in survival rate among wounded soldiers. Some of the success is from the location of AE crews close to Roles 1 to 3, CCATT development, and the effective and efficient use of airframes.[6]

Other specialty teams that may augment AE include the US Army flight burn team from San Antonio Medical Center, Texas; the lung team from Landstuhl Regional Medical Center in Germany; and the neonatal unit teams located throughout the military medical system. The United Kingdom's four-person medical emergency response team is comprised of an emergency medicine physician, a critical care nurse, and two paramedics and is another example of a specialty team. This team's designated aircraft platform is a CH-47.

How Patient Transport Is Initiated

Intratheater

A "911" call is not used in a combat zone, but the ability to get MEDEVAC capabilities on scene is just a call away. All combat movements are monitored on a communication channel by an operations center. If casualties are sustained or reinforcements are needed, the operations center is notified and reinforcements are dispatched. If a helicopter evacuation is necessary, the operations center establishes a

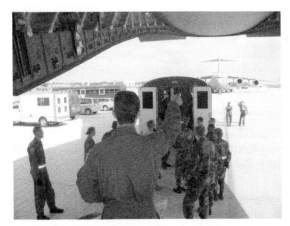

• **Fig. 31.12** Medical crew director directing a patient on load (on ramp of C-17).

location, and the medical requirements are relayed through a MEDEVAC request. This method is most common from POI to Role 2 or 3 care but can include interfacility transfers as well between equally rated facilities. This may be done because a fixed-wing transport is needed and the other facility is located near an airfield. For the longer transports, the Air Force is notified for fixed-wing assets.

Air Force patient movement begins when a patient movement request (PMR) is made from the attending physician to the validating flight surgeon. The flight surgeon is located in the Patient Movement Requirements Center (PMRC), with an FN, administrative technician, and medical service officer. The PMRC assists the referring physician creating the PMR and patient preparation for flight. The PMRC then contacts the Air Operations Center, specifically the AE control team (AECT). The AECT is staffed by AETs and nurses who work with the C-130, KC-135, and C-17 pilot and crew representatives. The process can have an aircraft and AE crew on the way in 1 hour.[21]

Intertheater

Intertheater AE is accomplished the same way as intratheater AE. The facility contacts the PMRC. A PMR is submitted. The AECT finds an aircraft. The patient is then moved out of the combat theater and to a Role 3 or Role 4 facility for definitive care.

Training

Point of Injury Care Providers

Moving medical treatment closer to each service member is best accomplished by requiring each service to train for trauma. Training starts with basic first aid. The focus is on teaching each member of the service (soldier, sailor, marine, and airman) how to care for themselves or their buddy if they are injured. The Air Force calls it SABC, the Army calls it self aid/buddy aid, the Navy calls it first aid, and the Marines call it basic life-saving first aid.[8] The Combat Life Savers Course is provided to all combat Marines. The military's combat medical training has as its foundation material based on a course called Tactical Combat Casualty Care. Although the training varies slightly, each course focuses on basic airway management, hemorrhage control, and communicating for help and transport. For the medical specialist in each service, further trauma training is provided.

The Army sends combat medics through a course called Health Care Specialist for nearly 5 months. A medic assigned to a MEDEVAC unit is trained at the JECC where the focus is enhancement of trauma life support skills from the POI to initial treatment locations.[18] In addition to the trauma training, special training is provided for chemical, biologic, and radiation exposure.

Maintenance of currency is accomplished through military and civilian continuing education programs, online training, and different symposiums and conventions. In addition, the

Air Force, Army, and Navy have contracted with civilian trauma centers around the United States to exercise trauma skills before deployment to combat zones.

Ground Transport

Currently, although the Air Force trains and tests to the National Registry for Emergency Medical Technicians, no formal ground transport courses are sponsored by any of the services. Most medics and nurses are trained on the job.

Rotor-Wing Transport

Initially, limited training was provided for the hospital-based critical care nurse in transporting patients in rotor-wing aircraft. In 2004 the US Army initiated the JECC to give a more formal orientation to transport nursing. This course is now a tri-service course coordinated by the Army Medical Department Center and School Program of Instruction at Fort Rucker, Alabama. The JECC provides trauma transport training to Joint Service, Coalition Forces, DoD, and other federal government organizations. It teaches patient transport specifics for rotary-wing aircraft. This course includes 80 hours of distance learning including 2 weeks' on-site education including operationalization of medical skills using complex simulations and extensive aircraft training. The course includes didactic and practical applications of flight transport trauma management concepts, effective communication, crew resource management, and roles of the transport provider.[18] In addition to flight patient care, flight physiology, water survival, combat survival, emergency egress, and communications are covered.

Fixed-Wing Transport

The fixed-wing military transport training is an Air Force responsibility. Originally developed in the 1940s, the FN/AET course covers communications, logistics, safety, air operations, patient considerations, the stresses of flight, altitude physiology, a systems review of altitude-related illnesses, and the effects of altitude on other diagnoses. Included is a review of the AE system, communication of patient needs, and the roles of supporting agencies. In addition, there is a focus on the equipment used in the AE system and the logistics of patient movement items (monitors, suction machines, etc.) and how they are maintained in such a large system. The course is combined with a 2-week survival course that covers combat survival, evasion, and water survival. The FN and AETs then attend a formal training unit (FTU) for their AE initial qualification (AEIQ) for 3 weeks. The FTU provides standardized ground and in-flight training on multiple airframes in a simulated environment at Wright-Patterson Air Force Base, Ohio. The training encompasses communications, logistics, safety, air operations, aircraft systems, and simulated patient care in flight. Students in the AEIQ course undergo 5 days of classroom training, 2 days of off-site ground training, 6 days in a C-130 simulator, and 2 days for testing and equipment evaluation followed by 3 days of in-flight evaluations at the end of the program. When the students graduate, they are qualified aircrew members.

The airframes focused on during training include the C-130, C-17, and KC-135. This course is open to all services and frequently has Army, Navy, Department of Homeland Security (DHS), and allied nation health providers in attendance.

Special Operations

Each of the services has special operations capabilities: Army Special Forces, Navy SEALs, and Air Force Para Rescue Jumpers. Each is trained in nonconventional assisted recovery. These teams may be tasked to recover a prisoner of war or someone who has been shot down behind enemy lines. The Army calls this personnel recovery, the Navy terms it tactical recovery of aircraft and personnel, and the Air Force refers to it as combat search and rescue.[2] Each rescue team has a member that is trained to the paramedic level. These specialists work on platforms that combine combat tactics with medical capabilities. Common search and rescue vehicles are the HH-60G Pave Hawk (Army), the CV-22 Osprey (Air Force), and the MH-46 Sea Knight (Navy; see Table 31.1).

Department of Homeland Security

US Coast Guard

Similar to combat search and rescue, the US Coast guard has the capability to move patients from an austere environment (out at sea) to a hospital. With search and rescue being an almost daily operation, these professionals are trained to the paramedic level. The common transport vehicles are the HH-65 Dolphin, the HH-60 Jayhawk, and the C-130.

US Immigrations and Customs Enforcement

The DHS has found itself in need of transporting undocumented and arrested foreigners that are sometimes ill or injured. The DHS sends nurses to the Air Force Flight Nurse Course for training. They commonly use fixed-wing aircraft and use nurses with transport backgrounds as Immigrations and Customs Enforcement employees.

Department of Health and Human Services

US Public Health Service

The US Public Health Service (USPHS) Commissioned Corps is made up of more than 6500 full-time, well-trained, highly qualified public health professionals. USPHS falls under the leadership of the Assistant Secretary of Health and the Surgeon General within the Department of Health and Human Services (HHS). In the spring of 2014, when the World Health Organization declared a public health emergency caused by the Ebola outbreak in Sierra Leon, Liberia, and Guinea, the United States leveraged the "whole of government" when the State Department asked the DoD and the HHS to coordinate a humanitarian response that would address the current outbreak. Military medicine deployed an Air Force EMEDS + 25 with a USPHS medical staff group (Centers for Disease Control Ebola Response Team) to Liberia. Additionally, the US Air Force developed a transport isolation system (TIS) capable of transporting up to four patients in a C-17 cargo aircraft. The units are capable of negative airflow, which keeps contaminants inside the TIS and an air-filtration system circulates clean air up to 24 times an hour. Portable chemical toilets are set up inside for patients. This combined government effort was the first of its kind and proved to be both innovative and effective.

Peacetime Operations

Military Operations Other Than War

In times of natural disaster or humanitarian relief, either in the United States or abroad, the US military medical system can be mobilized. Requests from individual state governments or other nations for medical assistance are frequent to the US military. Support may include search, recovery, care, and transport from special operations assets or any of the available medical platforms mobilized in war.

Local Agreements

When not at war, the military frequently uses civilian services for patient transport. Many communities have agreements for sharing resources. These agreements allow the military (a federal agency) to respond to emergencies outside the "gate" of a military reservation or to transport patients from the military treatment facility to a local hospital with a higher level of care. In addition, these agreements set lines of communication and define the support that can be provided if a local community is overwhelmed in a mass casualty situation. These agreements also increase the capabilities for the local community in a disaster response. In addition, they allow the military transport system to bring patients needing further treatment to a higher level of care at a civilian organization. Frequently, unit deployments account for varied reliability in this relationship. A civilian ambulance company that responds to emergencies on military installations is not unusual, even if it has an organic well-trained, robust medical transport capability.

Summary

Military medical systems are utilized for a wide spectrum of operations, including humanitarian relief, disaster response, homeland security, small-scale contingencies, and major theater war. The military medical system is planned, deployed, and constructed from the ground up to support military action or humanitarian relief. The medical system must be able to support this action anytime and anywhere in the world. Within the military medical system, the Air Force, Army, and Navy work to combine different military medical transport platforms that move patients rapidly from the POI to definitive care. Soldiers, marines, airmen, and sailors know if they are ever injured, even in the most remote location, they will be rapidly triaged, treated, and transported to the highest level of medical care necessary. The interdependence of the Air Force, Army, and Navy patient transport system is supported by highly skilled and trained transport medical personnel. By providing joint interoperable and interchangeable platforms, military en route care and patient transport saves lives. Many of the lessons learned in military medicine during combat operations have been applied to and now benefit medicine in the civilian sector.

References

1. Eastridge BJ, Jenkins D, Flaherty S, et al. Trauma system development in a theater of war: experiences from Operation Iraqi Freedom and Operation Enduring Freedom. *Mil Med.* 2006;61(6):1366-1373.

2. Joint Publication (JP 3-50) Personnel Recovery dated 4 December, 2014. https://doctrine.af.mil/download.jsp?filename=3-50-Annex-Personnel-Recovery.pdf. Accessed 06.13.17.

3. Joint Publication (JP-02) Health Services Support dated July 26, 2012. http://dtic.mil/doctrine/new_pubs/jp4_02.pdf. Accessed 07.05.17.

4. Borden Institute, Emergency War Surgery. *Chapter 2, Roles of Medical Care (United States).* 2013. http://www.cs.amedd.army.mil/borden/FileDownloadpublic.aspx?docid=80035d1a-f208-473d-993b-6debfb17db91. Accessed 09.05.17.

5. Butler Jr FK. Tactical medicine training for SEAL mission commanders. *Mil Med.* 2001;166(7):625-631.

6. Gawande A. Casualties of war: military care for the wounded from Iraq and Afghanistan. *N Engl J Med.* 2004;351(24):2471-2475.

7. Joint Publication (JP 4-02) Doctrine for Health Service Support in Joint Operations dated 26 July 2012. http://www.dtic.mil/doctrine/new_pubs/jp4_02.pdf. Accessed 06.13.17.

8. Air Force Instruction 36-2644. Self-aid and buddy care training. US Air Force; 19 August 2014.

9. Peck M. Golden hour surgical units prove worth. *Mil Med Technol.* 2003;7(5).

10. Holcomb JB, Stansbury LG, Champion HR, et al. Understanding combat casualty care statistics. *J Trauma.* 2006;60(2):397-401.

11. Kotwal RS, Montgomery HR, Kotwal BM, et al. Eliminating preventable death on the battlefield. *Arch Surg.* 2011;146(12):1350-1358.

12. Langan NR, Eckert M, Martin MJ. Changing patterns of in-hospital deaths following implementation of damage control resuscitation practices in US forward military treatment facilities. *JAMA Surg.* 2014;149(9):904-912.

13. Marbry RL. Impact of critical care trained flight paramedics on casualty survival during helicopter evacuation in the current war in Afghanistan. *J Trauma Acute Care Surg.* 2011;73(suppl 1):S32-S37.

14. *US Department of the Army March 2008 TRADOC Pamphlet 525-66, Military Operations Force Operating Capabilities.* Washington, DC. Available at www.tradoc.army.mil/tpubs/pams/p525-66.pdf. Accessed 00.11.16.

15. Butler FK Jr, Holcomb JB, Giebner SD, et al. Tactical combat casualty care 2007: evolving concepts and battlefield experience. *Mil Med.* 2007;172(11 suppl):1-19.

16. *US Department of the Army 1992 Field Manual 8-10-6: Medical Evacuation in a Theater of Operations; Tactics, Techniques, and Procedures.* Washington, DC: US Department of the Army.

17. Riha GM, Kiraly LN, Diggs BS, et al. Management of the open abdomen during the global war on terror. *JAMA Surg.* 2013;148(1):59-64.

18. Hudson TL, Morton RT. Critical care transport in a combat environment: building tactical trauma transport teams predeployment and intra-theater. (unpublished).

19. Ricks M. *New Tactical Care Teams Aim to Save More Lives.* http://www.shadowspear.com/vb/threads/new-af-tccet-teams-and-mission-creep-defined.14387/; 2012 Accessed 09.05.17.

20. Savan J. *New Air Force Concept for Aeromedical Evacuation to Meet Challenges in Africa.* http://www.stripes.com/news/new-air-force-concept-for-aeromedical-evacuation-to-meet-challenges-in-africa-1.259333; 2013.

21. Ingalls N, Zonies D, Bailey JA, et al. A review of the first 10 years of critical care aeromedical transport during operation Iraqi Freedom and Operation Enduring Freedom. The importance of evacuation timing. *JAMA Surg.* 2014;149(8):807-813.

22. Tipping RD, Macdermott SM, Davis C, Carter TE. *Air Transport of the Critical Care Patient in Combat Anesthesia: The First 24 Hours.* http://www.cs.amedd.army.mil/FileDownloadpublic.aspx?docid=57ab806b-df57-42d7-85b4-5f96907faf92; Accessed 9 May 7, 2017.

32

Professional Issues

RENEÉ SEMONIN HOLLERAN, PATRICIA CORBETT, AND CHERYL ERLER

COMPETENCIES

1. Integrate the concepts related to professional practice, including legal, ethical, and family care, into the transport environment.
2. Promote the use of research and evidence-based practice in the transport environment.
3. Implement the use of quality management and Just Culture in the transport environment.

There are multiple professional issues that are a part of patient transport. Many involve patient care. Most require being familiar with complicated concepts and staying aware of the ever-changing knowledge related to these issues.

Many of these issues require decisions to be made that affect both the patient and the transport team before, during, and after transport. Clinical decision making is an important skill for all transport personnel and is a necessary part of the professional issues experienced in the transport process.

This chapter addresses some of the common professional issues faced by transport teams including legal concerns; ethical decision making; competent, safe, and quality patient care; a culture of fairness; family concerns; research; and evidence-based practice (EBP).

Legal Issues

Knowledge of legal principles is necessary for members of the transport team. Registered nurses and other members of the transport team practice in a unique setting in which they must become familiar with a myriad of regulations, legal principles, and laws. Examples include the scope of practice of transport team members; Federal Aviation Administration, and Federal Communications Commission regulations; and state and local regulations that direct ground transport vehicles. The education and training of the transport team must include information on the various laws and regulations pertinent to transport practice. Specific laws such as the Consolidated Omnibus Reconciliation Act (COBRA) and the Emergency Medical Treatment and Labor Act (EMTALA) provide guidelines and regulations of which the transport team must be aware to provide safe and competent patient care.[1-12]

An Overview of the Law

Law comprises all of the rules and regulations by which a society is governed. Statutes are laws made by governmental bodies, and they vary from state to state. Statutes must comply with applicable federal law. The various acts applicable to nursing practice (e.g., the state nurse practice acts) are examples of statutory law. Statutes frequently require written rules and regulations for enforcement. Administrative agencies write administrative law and the rules and regulations that enforce the statute. The State Boards of Nursing are administrative agencies that promulgate administrative law. Case law, or judicial law, varies from state to state. Legal issues brought before the courts are interpreted based on the facts of a particular case.[1-20]

Criminal law permits legal action to be filed by the state for behavior that is offensive or harmful to society. Transport nurses may be charged with a criminal offense for a violation of either the State Nurse Practice Act or safe nursing practices (e.g., a charge of assault for treating a patient who explicitly refused or withdrew consent, or a charge of criminal negligence when a serious medical error caused a patient's death). *Civil law,* in contrast to criminal law, permits an action to be filed by an individual for monetary compensation. *Tort law* is used most commonly in civil cases related to medical and nursing care. Compensation is requested for the person wrongfully injured by the actions of another.[1-12]

Negligence and malpractice are often incorrectly used as interchangeable terms. *Negligence* is a deviation from accepted standards of performance. *Malpractice* is based on a professional standard of care and the professional statutes of the caregiver. The same types of acts form the basis for negligence and malpractice.[1-12]

Standards of care are another important concept of which transport teams must be aware. Standards of care are created in multiple ways, including by law, regulation, or case law. Numerous standards of care are applied to patient transport. Many come from professional associations such as the Air & Surface Transport Nurses Association (ASTNA) and the Commission on Accreditation of Medical Transport Systems (CAMTS). These standards are used to determine whether the care provided in the transport process is the generally accepted or expected care that should occur in similar circumstances. These standards are routinely used by legal experts and presented to juries in determination of whether malpractice has occurred.[1-12]

Elements of Malpractice

The elements of malpractice that must be present are shown in order of priority in Box 32.1. First, a *duty* must be present. The duty may be a contract, statute, or voluntary assumption of care of a patient by a transport nurse. It is created by the development of a nurse–patient relationship and not merely employment status.[1-12]

Once a duty is established to exist, the second element is a *breach of duty.* Breach of duty may occur as a result of malfeasance (act of commission) or nonfeasance (act of omission).[1-12] Administration of the wrong medication is malfeasance, whereas failure to follow a procedure is nonfeasance.[1-12]

The third element is *foreseeability.* Foreseeability involves whether one could reasonably expect certain events to cause specific results.[1-12]

The fourth element in malpractice is *causation.* A reasonable cause-and-effect relationship must be shown between the breach of duty and the injury.[1-12] The two types of causation are (1) in fact and (2) proximate. *Proximate cause* occurs when the result is directly related to the act. *Cause in fact* occurs when the breach of duty owed causes the injury.[1-12]

The fifth element is *injury.* The patient must be harmed physically, financially, or emotionally in a discernible way.[1-12]

The sixth element is *damages.* Damages are compensatory in nature and may be of different types. *General damages* are inherent to the injury itself. *Special damages* are losses and expenses incurred as a result of stress and emotional pain produced by the injury. *Punitive damages* are requested for an alleged malicious intent or willful or wanton misconduct.[1-12]

• BOX 32.1   Elements of a Malpractice Case

Presence of duty
Breach of duty
Foreseeability
Causation
Injury
Damages

In certain circumstances, the doctrine of *res ipsa loquitor,* "let the thing speak for itself," is used. The elements that must be proved are causation, injury, and damages. Commonly, *res ipsa loquitor* is used in situations in which the patient was unconscious or in surgery at the time the injury occurred.[1-12]

Statute of Limitations

Filing a lawsuit is under a *statute of time limitations.* Generally, if malpractice is alleged after a traumatic injury, the statute of limitations is 2 years; in cases of disease, it is at the time discovered. The exception is in pediatric cases. The statute of limitations is extended until the minor is emancipated or reaches the age of majority (established by state law).[1-12]

Types of Liability

Intentional Torts or Criminal Acts

Assault or battery, or both, may be either *criminal* or *tort* (civil). *Assault* is placing an individual who has not given consent into a situation in which he or she fears immediate bodily harm. *Battery* is the touching of a person without his or her consent. Battery can also occur with the touching of anything connected with a person (clothing, purse, and jewelry) without consent. Damages for battery may be punitive or nominal as well as compensatory.[1-20]

Other types of intentional torts are, briefly, false imprisonment, which is the unjustifiable detention of a person without his or her consent, and invasion of privacy, which is a key concept in issues related to confidentiality. The patient has the right to privacy of medical information. Photographs may not be taken and information may not be released without consent. Some situations are newsworthy, and the public's right to know can exceed the patient's right to privacy. Knowledge of statutes and knowledge of relevant laws related to consent is vital. Defenses often used against intentional torts are consent (discussed later in this chapter), self-defense, defense of others, and necessity.[1-20]

Quasiintentional Torts

A *quasiintentional tort* protects an individual's interest in a person's reputation, privacy, and freedom from legal action that is unfounded. It is a legal action that arises from damages inflicted on a person's reputation or privacy. Examples of such a tort include defamation of character, libel, and breach of confidentiality. Tort law does not actually protect a person; it just provides an avenue through the courts to seek compensation for damages done.[1-20]

Vicarious Liability

Vicarious liability is defined as one party being responsible for the actions of another. The doctrine of *respondeat superior,* "let the master respond," has been used frequently when nurses are accused of malpractice. As a result of this doctrine, the employer has an obligation to ensure that employees perform duties in a competent safe manner. Two elements must be shown: (1) the injured party must prove that the employer had control over the employee; and (2) the negligent act occurred in the scope and course of the employment. Vicarious liability can be found with either malfeasance or nonfeasance of the employee.[1-20]

Courts have attached judgments directly against institutions for corporate negligence. Hospitals have found themselves accountable as an entity when the duty is owed directly to the patient and not through employees. Types of corporate duties attached directly to the institution are outlined in Box 32.2.[1-20]

Product Liability

An increase has been seen in *product liability* cases, which are mixtures of tort and contract law. The sale of a product places the manufacturer, processor, or nonmanufacturing seller at risk for a product liability case should injury to a person or person's property occurs. Delivery of a service without the sale of the product is generally not substantial enough for a successful product liability suit. However, court decisions have been inconsistent in separating the sale of product from delivery of a service. *Collective liability* may occur when several manufacturers have participated in a cooperative activity. *Alternative liability* occurs when two or more manufacturers commit separate acts.[1-20]

Abandonment

The principles related to abandonment are important to transport nurse practice. *Abandonment* occurs with unilateral termination of the nurse–patient relationship without consent from the patient. Abandonment can also occur if the care of the patient is transferred to someone less qualified. Questions may arise regarding abandonment any time there is a demonstration of disregard for the patient's welfare, unreasonable practices, or both. The various types of transports should be reviewed by each program and evaluated to ensure that potential abandonment issues are addressed. George[5] suggested that the act of dispatching an ambulance was presumptive of voluntary assumption of a

---

• BOX 32.2 Examples of Corporate Duties Owed Directly to the Patient

Duty of reasonable care in maintenance and use of equipment
Availability of equipment and services
Duty of reasonable care in selecting and retaining employees
Adoption and assurance of compliance with rules related to administrative responsibility for patient care
Selection and retention of medical staff

---

duty to a patient. This assumption should be considered in development of communication center protocols.[14,17]

Consent Issues

Many medical tort claims are related to *consent issues. Informed consent* requires more than a patient's signature on a consent form. The suggested treatment must be presented to the patient with a discussion of all material risks, consequences, and available alternatives. If the patient refuses the first treatment option, other treatment options should be explained. Informed consent requires understanding on the part of the patient.[1-20]

Consent can be written or oral. Nurses are frequently asked to obtain signatures on consent forms. Before the patient signs, the nurse should determine that the patient understands the purpose of the consent. *Expressed consent* occurs with written or oral acknowledgment. *Implied consent* occurs when a patient is compliant with a request (extending arm for phlebotomy, allowing placement of nasal prongs, etc.). Implied consent is frequently operational in emergency situations. Most consent statutes allow for treatment of life-threatening emergencies if the patient is unable to consent because it is the reasonable thing to do. One should be cautious, however, not to exceed the limits of implied consent. If the patient is physically or mentally incapable of consenting, implied consent is operative in the case of a true emergency. In the absence of a true emergency, consent should be obtained before treatment from a person who is authorized to consent.[1-20]

Consent for treatment of minors is reserved for a parent or legal guardian. Implied consent is used for minors with life-threatening emergency conditions. The parents or legal guardian should be contacted as soon as possible for notification and consent. Most states have laws related to emancipated minors who can consent before the age of majority. In addition, minors may be allowed to consent for treatment of certain conditions such as sexually transmitted diseases, pregnancy, and substance abuse.[1-20]

Refusal to consent or *withdrawal of consent* is sometimes a murky question. A common issue is the refusal of a blood transfusion because of religious beliefs. If the treating physician believes that a blood transfusion is necessary and the patient refuses, an attempt can be made to obtain a court order. However, in the field, the competent patient's wishes must be respected. The court uses a balancing test to weigh one right against the other. The court tends to support the right of the patient to make a knowing choice in refusing consent. The exception is in the case of minors. If the court is convinced a child needs life-saving measures, compelling state's interest in the child usually overrides the parent's interest.[1-20]

Documentation

The purpose of documentation is to document care and treatments given, validate continuity of care between health professionals, establish a record of patient care so that it can be reviewed for continuity and continuing education and research, provide data for reimbursement and cost analysis, and legally protect the caregiver. Transport team members may receive subpoenas for a deposition many years after the actual transport. The documentation of the transport will help provide important information for the deposition if that documentation is written well.[1-3,13-15,21-32]

The medical record of a patient belongs to the hospital or transport service, although the patient has a right to the information contained therein. The *medical record* is the documentation of the patient's course of treatment. It serves as a means of communication between various providers of service. It protects the legal interests of the patient, the hospital, and the health care practitioner. The patient's privacy must be protected in these situations. The Health Insurance Portability and Accountability Act (HIPAA) and transport are briefly discussed later in this chapter. The contents of the medical record should be factual and based on objective data.[16,17,23,25,33]

The medical record should be:

- Brief, concise, accurate, and thorough
- Include all interventions performed and response to interventions
- Clearly written and legible
- Without judgmental terms
- Timely

Abbreviations are strongly discouraged today. The Joint Commission offers guidelines on the use of abbreviations. Only approved abbreviations should be used. The entries should be readable, concise, and complete. The patient description should be objective and include the patient's appearance, signs and symptoms, and interventions and responses. Documentation should occur in a timely fashion. If an untoward incident occurs, an event report should be completed and appropriate personnel notified. Today, several computer-based transport records are available; however, these programs must provide the components of patient documentation pertinent to the transport service using the program. Several advantages to computer-based documentation include the ability to read the documentation, time stamping of procedures and medication administration, recordkeeping of transport team interventions, and retrieval of data for research and continuous quality improvement (CQI). The transport record should "tell the story" of the transport process. An important piece of the story is the history of present illness, including a time line of events before the transport. Many critical decisions are made based on the time line of events. However, it is important to remember that the transport team may not know the exact time line of events until after completion of a transport. Documentation of any deviations from protocols and orders obtained from medical control is also important.[1-20]

Only designated personnel should review charts, and such a review must comply with relevant privacy legislation. Records are an important component of the CQI process and a way to document transport team competencies.[16,17,23,25,33]

Health Insurance Portability and Accountability Act

HIPAA became effective in 1996. It is a federal law intended to protect patient health information and simplify the means by which health care providers electronically file and transmit health care claims. These safeguards currently apply to all protected health information, including electronic, written, and photographic forms. The HIPAA law has three different rules with specific compliance guidelines. The *Transaction and Code Set Rule* is primarily related to billing and requires that the transport team ensure that the appropriate information is documented to enhance this process. The *Privacy Rule* designates that private health information (PHI) about the patient be safeguarded and restricted. Finally, the *Security Rule* outlines how PHI should be protected, including encryption of transmitted data and physical security of a facility in which PHI is stored. HIPAA has presented a challenge to transport teams who must be careful and consistent in how information about the patient is provided and used. Implications to transport teams include the following:

- Transport team members must undergo mandatory HIPAA training.
- Oral and written information about the patient must be protected. Information about the patient should be appropriately stored.
- Patients should receive a Notice of Privacy Practices. This notice is not given during the transport process but should be provided after the emergency has passed.
- Transport teams may share PHI about the patient with providers at a scene and at a referring hospital without a patient's consent, contact a base station and provide radio reports, provide follow-up on the patient for quality improvement purposes, and provide selected information with involved law enforcement.[16,17,23,25,33]

Information may also be shared without the patient's consent when information is needed related to the monitoring and controlling of communicable disease, injury, or disability; disclosure for compiling statistics, such as for births and deaths; reporting of adverse events to the Food and Drug Administration and disclosure to government oversight committees; disclosure to evaluate work place injuries; and organ donation programs and certain law enforcement personnel. Examples of information that may be shared with law enforcement personnel include child maltreatment, PHI sought through the court system, and disclosure of limited information in the process of identifying a suspect. Transport team members must become aware of the implications of HIPAA to the patients that they transport and their practice.[16,17,23,25,33]

Consolidated Omnibus Budget Reconciliation Act/Emergency Medical Treatment and Active Labor Act[16]

The COBRA law was passed in 1986 and it contained the EMTALA law.[16] It is sometimes referred to as the antidumping statute. The essential components of the EMTALA include the following:

1. All patients who present to an emergency department (ED) should receive a nondiscriminatory medical screening to determine whether a medical emergency is present.
2. A patient with a medical emergency must be stabilized within the capabilities of the transferring hospital and within reasonable probability that no material deterioration in the patient's clinical condition will occur.
3. If the patient must be transferred for further care, a receiving hospital must have accepted the patient and have the appropriate equipment and staff available to care for the patient.
4. The referring hospital must send all copies of medical records, diagnostic studies, and informed consent documents, and the patient must be transported with the appropriate vehicle and personnel.

If the patient's condition is unstable, the transfer certification must address the following[16]:

- Patient's condition
- Benefits of transfer
- Risk of transfer
- Specific information about the receiving facility, including that patient report was called to the receiving facility
- Description of the mode of transportation
- Patient or designate must sign a consent and certify how the transfer was initiated (patient request, physician request, or other)
- The form should be witnessed, and the patient or designate must sign that he or she understands the risks and benefits of transfer

In 1990, the COBRA law underwent further revisions that broadened the scope of who is subject to the law. The law now includes all participating physicians and any other physician responsible for the examination, treatment, or the transfer of the patient at the participating hospital.[16] Further clarifications of EMTALA were released by the Department of Health and Human Services, Centers for Medicare and Medicaid Services in September 2003. The document was titled "Clarifying Policies Related to the Responsibilities of Medicare-Participating Hospitals in Treating Individuals with Emergency Medical Condition (Final Regulation).[1-3,13-15,21-32] Violations of COBRA/EMTALA legislation include financial penalties and potential loss of government funding.

The transport team needs to be aware of potential violations (e.g., a transfer that may be based on financial reasons instead of patient need) and notify the appropriate authorities when a violation has occurred.[1,16,21,25,32]

Clarification of Hospital Helipads

In 2004, site review guidelines from EMTALA helped to clarify the use of hospital helipads by Emergency Medical Services (EMS) personnel.[1,17] An ambulance may meet a helicopter team on the helipad of Hospital A for transfer to Hospital B without triggering any EMTALA obligation unless the ambulance crew requests medical assistance from Hospital A.[32] If medical assistance is requested, Hospital A becomes responsible for EMTALA compliance.

If Hospital A owns the ambulance that requests the assistance of the helicopter on Hospital A's helipad, Hospital A has an EMTALA obligation if the patient is transported from the scene of an emergency response, subject to the exceptions under the "ambulance rule."[1,16,17]

Diversion

In the past 15 years, ED and hospital patient *diversion* has become a major issue in the United States. Initially, it was seen in larger cities, but it has now become an issue across the entire country and even the world.[15,22,25,27] Causes of diversion include use of the ED by nonurgent cases; inadequate staffing; decrease in the number of EDs available in given areas of the country; use of ancillary services, such as computed tomographic or magnetic resonance imaging scans; and hospital bed shortages. No matter the cause, diversion does have an impact on transport programs.[1,2,4,12,16,17,30,34] According to EMTALA, hospitals with specialized services such as trauma and burn centers do not have a "right" to divert; however, they can use diversion to help manage patient flow. Hopefully, this assists with keeping patients safe and improving quality of care.[15]

Transport teams must be aware of diversion policies in the communities in which they serve and be a part of how these policies are developed. This awareness also includes the role of the transport program in the event of a disaster.

Mission diversion, as explained by Williams,[9] is not specifically involved with EMTALA regulations. However, similar to the resource issues identified in ED overcrowding and diversion, there are many times a transport program may have to direct limited resources to meet multiple responses. Transport programs should have written policies and procedures about how and when missions are diverted, what priorities are used to determine which missions are diverted, who makes the decision to divert or redirect the patient, how transport teams are notified, and what type of documentation is required when a diversion occurs.

Medical Direction During Interfacility Patient Transfers

Responsibility for the patient during transport is an important legal concept that must be understood by transport team members. Transfer of patients from one institution to another has become a fundamental part of patient care today. The chapter on patient preparation for transport identified some of the multiple reasons a patient may need transfer and transport. The section in this chapter describes the federal regulations related to patient transfer and transport as pointed out by EMTALA. According to COBRA/EMTALA, unless otherwise specified, patient care during transport is the responsibility of the transferring physician and hospital. The transferring physician is responsible for the following[1,11,12,16,17,28]:

- Identifying the appropriate receiving facility
- Writing transfer orders
- Identifying the appropriate transport team, equipment, and treatment that are needed during the transport process

The authority that governs patient care during transport varies from state to state and is based on the type of transport team that is with the patient. Medical responsibility for the patient should be arranged before the transport process is initiated. For example, a transport team may be composed of a nurse and a physician. Because a physician is present, medical direction could come from that person. Other options for medical direction during transport include the following:

- Transferring physician assumes medical direction.
- Receiving physician assumes medical direction.
- Medical director of the transport service assumes medical direction.
- Responsibility may be shared and predefined with a transfer of medical direction en route because of long distances (e.g., on international transports).

Transport teams should have policies, procedures, and protocols in place to address medical direction during transport, and education for clinicians should be provided on these policies and procedures. The transport service and its medical director are responsible for providing safe competent care during the process.

Scope of Practice

Statutes, rules, or a combination of the two defines the *scope of practice*. Some of the statutes that govern members of the transport team include the scope of practice as stated in State Nurse Practice Acts or EMS statutes. The Nurse Practice Acts establishes licensure requirements for nurses. Most states require mandatory licensure before either the title or actions are permitted. Exceptions are generally related to students, new graduates, and transport through a state's jurisdiction.[3,9] Box 32.3 illustrates the common elements of nurse practice acts as an example of a scope of practice.

Chapter 2 described the roles of specific members of the transport team. Most of these members practice in an expanded role. Before practicing in an expanded role,

---

• BOX 32.3 Elements of Nurse Practice Acts

Definition of professional nursing
Requirements for licensure
Exemptions
Licensure across jurisdictions
Disciplinary action and due process requirements
Creation of Board of Nursing
Penalties for practicing without a license

---

transport team members should review the pertinent nurse, EMS, medical, and pharmacy practice acts; attorney general's opinions; and recent judicial decisions that govern their practice. The institution's policies and procedures should be investigated and followed to ensure that the scope of practice for the transport team is clearly defined. This is also done with the transport services medical director. The CAMTS outlines in its standards the role of the medical director.[3,9]

In addition to scope of practice, the standards of care that govern the professional practice of the transport team members must be reviewed. *Internal standards* are set by the role of the team member, job descriptions, and policies and procedures. *External standards* are established by state boards of nursing, professional and specialty organizations, and federal guidelines.[3,9,11,12] In cases of purported deviation from the standard of care, the external standards may be submitted as evidence, expert witnesses used, or both. Professional publications may be submitted to assist the jury in understanding the expected standard of care.[3,9,11,12]

ASTNA developed standards and guidelines that include rotor-wing transport, fixed-wing transport, ground transport, and commercial escort.[20] This document is available on the ASTNA website (http://astna.org/) as well as position statements related to patient transport. Other members of the transport team including the International Association of Flight Paramedics and the Association of Air Medical Physicians provide additional examples of external standards that guide the practice of patient transport.

Ethical Issues

Today, transport team members are faced with many ethical dilemmas, including who to transport and by what method; when not to transport, especially if patient resuscitation is futile; and being asked or forced to transport patients in unsafe environments, for example, when the weather is less than optimal. Some transport teams are forced to make decisions about whether to transport a patient with equipment or problems that they have inadequate experience handling because of competition or fear of revenue loss.[4,26,27,29,35-42]

Ethical Decision Making in the Transport Environment

Ethical decisions are generally made based on a set of specific values, which include the following[27,35]:

- *Patient autonomy:* Allowing patients to make decisions about their health care.
- *Beneficence* versus *malfeasance:* The benefit of the transport outweighs the potential harm the transport could cause.
- *Veracity:* Honesty, telling the truth, open patient care and health care provider relationships; veracity should also extend to statement of purpose for the transport program.

- *Justice:* Fairness for the patient and, at times, the community that the transport program serves.

Unfortunately, multiple demands may influence the transport decision, including competition, lack of experience, and concern about employment.

The availability of equipment, advanced life support skills, and personnel has contributed to the development of a *technologic imperative*.[4,27,29,35-42] In other words, because it exists, it must be used. Patients, families, and communities have come to expect access to the newest and best technologies and that everything should be available for everyone.

In 1995, Iserson and colleagues[37,38] developed a model that is still pertinent to making ethical decisions in the transport environment. This model includes the following:
- Problem perception: Is there a problem?
- List alternatives: Identify solutions and barriers.
- Choose an alternative.
- List the consequences of the actions chosen.
- Consider one's own personal beliefs when making the decision.
- Evaluate the decision.

Ethical decision making is a dynamic process. The transport team cannot ignore previous experience or the personal beliefs of the team members and those with whom the team is working. These things are never easy, but they cannot be overlooked.

To Transport or Not to Transport

As health care costs continue to increase, the cost of patient transport and appropriate use of services have become important issues that many transport programs must address. Deciding when to transport a patient who has sustained cardiac arrest, whether as a result of trauma or a medical problem, continues to be one of the most difficult dilemmas faced by many transport programs. Research has shown that survival rates of patients who have out-of-hospital cardiac arrests range from 1.0% to 11.4%. There are multiple factors that influence survival and many cannot be controlled by the transport team. Many survivors sustain severe neurologic injury, and the quality of their life is impaired.[4,27,29,35-42]

Whether to transport a patient who may be dead in the field remains a difficult decision and has profound ethical implications. The public also has come to expect both EMS and transport programs to come to the rescue of all who need medical assistance, which attaches additional pressure to the decisions that must be made related to the transport of a patient who is in full arrest.

The transport team must always be critical when making an ethical decision related to the transport of patients who have sustained cardiac arrest. *Critical* means thoughtful and reflective of the means, goals, and implications of this practice.[4,27,29,35-42] The transport team must consider the feelings of those who have been caring for the patient; the wishes of the patient's family, if present; and whether everything has truly been done for the patient.

Education, critical examination of the facts, and evaluation of one's personal values related to death and dying should assist the transport team in developing guidelines for when not to transport and with difficult transport decisions. Case presentations, literature reviews, and the use of clinical guidelines are some methods that may be used to make moral practice decisions. As pointed out by Mattox in 1993,[43] "both society and trauma resuscitators [must] accept that the patient who has a fatal injury [should] die with dignity, not being subject to extensive and expensive resurrection techniques."

Ethical decision making can be challenging in the transport environment. It must encompass care values, compassion, accountability, and commitment to the people served by the transport service. Transport teams should discuss troubling patient transports. Decision-making protocols should include all members of the transport team, the patients, and the communities that they serve.

As health care technology progresses and presents new challenges, health care personnel must never lose sight of the rights of their patients. In addition, they must never lose sight of their duties to provide care in a safe, supportive professional transport environment.

The Family in Transport

Patient care during transport is generally focused on meeting the physiologic needs of an acutely ill or injured patient. However, the patient is generally a part of a family, although the definition of the term may vary. A family may be described in legal, cultural, religious, or personal terms. The families of today are as diverse as the people who live in them.[22,31,32,34,44-46]

Although transport team members are accustomed to the transport environment and process, they should not forget that this experience is new and often frightening for the family members of a seriously ill or injured person. The transport team must consider care of the family to be an extension of patient care and not an additional task that needs to be accomplished. The support that health care professionals provide to a patient's family during the initial stages of the patient's crisis can be invaluable. Contact with a transport team or ED employees may be the family's first interaction with health care personnel in this emergency. The family's perception of the response of these health care providers can be the impetus to either healthy or ineffective coping. Ideally, early interventions aimed at decreasing the family's stress should be performed to prevent the breakdown of the family structure.[10,24,31,32,44,45]

Unfortunately, death is an inherent part of the transport process. Some patients die before transport, and the role the family may play in this dying process can make patient care particularly arduous for the transport team. Whether the family is allowed to be present during resuscitation attempts is an issue that has been gaining attention from both health care professionals and the public. Families will demand to be a part of the resuscitation so that they can at least say goodbye to their loved ones no matter where the resuscitation takes place.[10,24,31,32,44,45]

Family Issues Relating to Transport of the Patient

Family members of critically ill or injured patients are already under stress,[22,31,32,34,44-46] and the need to transport the patient on a fixed-wing aircraft, helicopter, or ground vehicle adds to that level of stress.[22,31,32,34,44-46] Decisions concerning care must be made quickly, and the patient's family members often feel uninformed and unsure, especially if they have limited medical knowledge. Because time is a factor, the family has no opportunity to elicit medical information and request second opinions.

Family members may feel uncomfortable relaying concerns about the transport to the health care providers and transport team. Some concerns are related to the medical treatment rendered or even the safety of transport. Other concerns may include the following[10,24,31,32,44,45]:

- Separation from their loved one for the duration or distance of the transport
- Uncertainty about the events that necessitated transfer and transport of the patient
- Lack of understanding of the medical diagnosis
- The referring physicians, nurses, and transport team members are unfamiliar to the family and patient

Because most patients who need critical care transport have injuries or illnesses that are sudden and unplanned, family members usually do not have time to prepare for the emergency. If they have never been exposed to this type of crisis, they may not have the coping skills needed to effectively manage the stress entailed.[10,24,31,32,44,45]

Referring Facility

The transport team should make every effort to speak with the patient's family before leaving the referring facility. This interaction may be as simple as an introduction, such as "Hi, my name is Jane Doe, and I am the transport nurse who will be with your family member during the transport." During this interaction, the team can assess the family. The team can then alert personnel at the receiving hospital's social or pastoral service department if it appears that the family may need their assistance. The transport team can also take this opportunity to determine the family's plans for traveling to the receiving hospital and get an estimate of their time en route. Family members should be notified of the transport vehicle's intended destination, and they should be told where to report once they arrive at the receiving facility. If necessary, directions to the receiving hospital can be given to the family. Many transport programs provide individual maps for this purpose. When possible, the family should be provided with a specific individual name or place they may ask for when arriving at the receiving facility. The transport team can offer to contact the family via cell phone at the conclusion of the transport. This practice is particularly useful with pediatric patients to help alleviate parental anxiety.[22,31,32,34,44-46]

• **BOX 32.4** **Family Needs of Patients Transported via Helicopter**

Family members of patients who need helicopter transport perceived that they lacked the following:
1. The opportunity to see the patient before he or she was put in the helicopter
2. Information about who would take care of the patient in transport
3. Information about the safety of air transport
4. Directions to the receiving hospital
5. Knowledge about how the patient fared during the transport

---

The transport team may pause before leaving the institution to allow family members to say goodbye to the patient. This is especially important if the patient's injuries are life-threatening; in this case, the family may not have another opportunity to speak to the patient before he or she dies. In this author's experience, the opportunity to say goodbye to the patient is greatly appreciated by the family. In most cases, depending on the severity of the patient's injuries, the transport can be delayed for a few minutes without negative effects on the patient's outcome. These simple interactions between the family and the transport team are invaluable in helping to alleviate the family's stress.[22,31,32,34,44-46]

Fultz and colleagues[45] conducted a study to identify the information needs of family members regarding air medical transport. The information needs rated as very important by family members included what was wrong with the patient, why the patient had to be flown to another facility, and where the patient could be found at the receiving hospital. Box 32.4 lists the important needs that most family members perceived as being unmet.[45] The results of this research are important no matter how the patient is transported. Transport programs should use this information as a guide when providing care to the family to better care for the needs of the patient's family.

Joyce et al.[46] found that a family member was four times more likely to accompany a pediatric patient if the vehicle for transport was an ambulance. Reasons that may have influenced this included safety restrictions related to weight and balance; a family member's "fear of flying"; or a preference to have a personal vehicle available at the receiving destination. The authors also noted that in pediatric critical care transport, parental accompaniment has become a measure of quality as well as predictor of family satisfaction related to the transport.

Receiving Facility

Information concerning the patient's family members should be communicated to the receiving hospital to facilitate continuity of care. The social services department of the receiving hospital can be alerted to cases in which their services may be especially needed. Personnel at receiving hospitals want to know whether the family plans to travel to their hospital. Because large distances must sometimes be covered by ground, an estimated time of arrival is useful. Knowledge of the family's plans can be helpful in case the patient's condition deteriorates and consent to perform particular procedures is needed. The hospital may need to know the family's wishes for treatment if the patient's condition is life-threatening. Organ procurement issues can be considered if the staff knows when and if the family intends to arrive. These issues are particularly important if the patient is a minor.

Family members frequently leave the referring facility as soon as the decision is made to transfer the patient, and they may arrive at the receiving hospital ahead of the patient. In this case the referring nurse can notify the receiving hospital of the family's departure for their facility. If the receiving hospital is aware of the family's intended time of arrival, they can direct the family to the appropriate area in the hospital.

Transporting Family Members

Family members frequently ask whether they can travel to the receiving facility with the patient. In this era, patients and families are more assertive in making their requests known to the medical community. Research continues to show that patients, families, and health care providers can benefit from family presence.[44]

The decision to transport a family member is based on multiple factors, some more important than others. The personal feelings of a team member should not interfere with a decision on what is best for the patient and family. The entire transport team should provide input, but safety should always be the overriding principle. In air transport, the pilot has the final word. It is always as clear in the ground transport environment because issues that drive this decision such as weight and balance are not as clearly defined in the ground transport environment. Safety for the entire team is the primary factor on which to base this decision when concern exists about the possibility of family interference.

Other factors the team may take into consideration when deciding whether to transport members of the patient's family are the patient's age, the seriousness of the patient's condition, other transportation available to the family, and the length of the transport time. Box 32.5 provides examples of inclusion and exclusion criteria for transport of family members.

Some transport vehicles, particularly air medical, are not capable of carrying an additional passenger because of performance factors or space limitations. Although the aircraft may have the capability of carrying extra passengers, some limitations, including engine power, effects of weather on equipment performance, and the amount of weight the aircraft can safely carry, determine whether an additional passenger can be brought aboard.

Parents often ask whether they can accompany their child on the transport. Determination of whether the presence of

---

• BOX 32.5 Examples of Inclusion/Exclusion Criteria for Determination of Whether Family Members Should Accompany a Patient During Air Medical Transport

Inclusion of family members during air medical transport may be desirable in the following cases:
The referring facility is far from the receiving facility, and the family has no other means of transportation.
The patient is near death, and the family wishes to be with the patient during his or her last moments.
The patient is a child and would benefit from being accompanied by a parent.
The family and the patient both strongly want the family to accompany the patient.
Exclusion of family members during air medical transport may be desirable in the following cases:
Inclusion of the family member will interfere with patient care.
The family member's weight exceeds permissible parameters.
The family member is overly anxious and poses a danger to the safety of the transport.
The landing zone is walled in on three sides, and the pilot must do a vertical takeoff.
A crew member has a concern about a family member.
Weather conditions are marginal.
The family member has a fear of flying.
The family member gets motion sickness.
The distance between the two facilities is short.
The patient's condition is unstable and requires extensive care.

---

the family member will pose a problem during transport is important because of an inappropriate level of anxiety. All family members exhibit some anxiety; thus anxiety should not rule out the possibility of the person going on the transport. The determination must be made on the basis of whether inclusion of the family members will interrupt the transport team's duties if they sit in the front or interfere with care to the patient if they sit in the back. It cannot be stressed enough that if transporting the family member in any way jeopardizes safety or care, the family member should not be transported.[22,31,32,34,44-46]

The transport team may want to exclude the family from the transport when the weather is marginal. This factor can apply to either a ground or an air vehicle. Diversions or precautionary landings require extra concentration on the part of the pilot; thus interference with flying can occur if the pilot has to explain what is happening or calm a worried passenger. Ground vehicle drivers need to be able to address their full concentration on roads that may be ice covered or if visibility is impaired by fog.

Once the determination to transport family members is made, they need a safety briefing by the pilot in an air medical vehicle or the driver in a ground vehicle. The family member should be directed to the transport vehicle for the briefing while the patient is being prepared for the transport; this gives the pilot or driver an appropriate amount of time to conduct the safety briefing. The extra passenger can be belted in the seat and be ready for departure. If this is done before the patient reaches the vehicle, the transport is not delayed.

Many times the transport team must make a split-second decision as to whether the family can be transported with the patient. Experience helps to make this decision process easier. No specific rules exist for including or excluding the family. Each situation must be assessed separately. In many instances, family members are not allowed to accompany the transport team. The possibility of transporting family members should not be automatically ruled out by the transport team because at times it is appropriate and would be beneficial if the team made an effort to include the family.

If family members accompany the transport team, the risk of increased emotional difficulty always exists for the transport team. However, the benefits to the patient and family when emotional support is provided far outweigh the emotional risks to the transport team. One must always look at each situation for what provides the best care for both patient and family.[22,31,32,34,44-46]

Family Presence During Resuscitation

The presence of family members during attempts to resuscitate a patient is an emotionally charged topic that is gaining the attention of health care practitioners and the public. Whether families should be allowed to view resuscitation is a topic of controversy among the medical community. Providing emotional support for family members can be difficult. Before health care providers determine the stance they will take on this issue, they should familiarize themselves with the literature, discuss the issue with others who have participated in a resuscitation attempt with family members present, and ask themselves the following question: If my child or family member needed to be resuscitated, would I want to be there? Box 32.6 lists other questions that practitioners should consider when dealing with this issue. A major point to keep in mind is that in most situations, the risks to the health care provider in emotionally supporting the family do not outweigh the benefits that are provided for the family.

Family Presence Program

Foote Hospital in Michigan[31] is a pioneer in the family presence program. The Foote Hospital program was initiated because of two instances in which family members refused to leave the patient during a resuscitation attempt. After these two instances occurred, a survey was sent to the families of patients who had been resuscitated in the Foote Hospital ED. The survey asked whether they would have wanted to be present during the resuscitation attempt of their family member if they had been given the opportunity. Seventy-two percent of the respondents indicated that they would have liked to have been present. These results showed the staff at Foote Hospital the need for a formalized family presence program.[31] Foote Hospital approached the issue by developing a formalized program. Initially, a chaplain or social worker provides the family with information about the condition of the patient and determines whether the family would like to view the resuscitation attempt. During the time that the chaplain or social worker is with the family, the medical personnel perform any necessary invasive procedures. After the invasive procedures have been completed, the chaplain or social worker accompanies the family into the resuscitation room and stays with them to provide support and information. Because the medical staff has very little responsibility for providing support to the family, they can then keep their attention focused on the resuscitation. If further invasive procedures are needed, family members are asked to step out of the room.[31]

The nurses at Foote Hospital, who were informally surveyed before the program was initiated, had two main concerns: (1) that the family would interrupt patient care and (2) that outward expressions of grief by family members would make it difficult for nurses to perform their job. They also had a fear that they would be observed doing or saying something that would upset the family. Box 32.7 lists reasons that health care providers give for not wanting family members to be present during resuscitation attempts. Stress for the family is another concern cited by nurses.

The literature confirms that family members have a desire to be present during resuscitation attempts and that this process helps them in their grief work.[31] After Foote Hospital's program was established, a survey revealed that three of

---

> **• BOX 32.6** **Questions to Be Considered by Health Care Providers in Evaluation of Whether Family Members Should Be Present During Resuscitation Attempts**

1. How do you feel about allowing family members to participate in a resuscitation attempt?
2. Have you ever facilitated family participation in a resuscitation attempt?
3. Have you ever experienced a situation in which family members participated in a resuscitation attempt?
4. What, if anything, makes you feel uncomfortable about participation of family members in a resuscitation attempt?
5. What, if anything, would make you feel more comfortable about participation of family members in a resuscitation attempt?

> **• BOX 32.7** **Reasons Given by Health Care Providers for Excluding Family Members During Resuscitation Attempts**

The family may disrupt or interfere with patient care.
Outward expressions of grief by family members might make control of their own emotions difficult or impossible for staff members.
The experience may be too traumatic for the family.

four staff members supported the program. They believed that the program benefited the family even if it was emotionally harder for the staff. Follow-up research with family members who were present during resuscitation attempts showed that the program was successful and that it helped in the grief process. Many family members commented that they were glad to see that everything possible was done for their loved one. One family member commented that he was glad to be able to say goodbye before the patient died.[31]

Time and societal influences have changed views about health care and health care management. Most family members like to be involved in every aspect of the patient's life, except when it comes to hospitalization. It has been the way that "modern" health care has been delivered that has marginalized the role of both the patient and family in the care.[32]

Multiple nursing associations including ASTNA, the Emergency Nurses Association, and the American Association of Critical Nurses have influenced and helped develop a role for the family during resuscitation. Nursing's persistence and vision have influenced other organizations such as the American Heart Association (AHA) and the American College of Surgeons. In the new AHA guidelines, the role of the family is expanded, and family presence is an important consideration to the delivery of care.[32]

When family members are encouraged to become involved in the situation, they feel supported and useful and have a sense of some control, which enhances the health care provider–family relationship. Family members who are frustrated and angry because they do not know what is happening to the patient are actually harder to manage and take more time than those who are kept informed. Health care providers must keep in mind that family members may not feel comfortable expressing their feelings, especially if they think these feelings are contradictory to the nurse's feelings. Asking family members what is best for them helps the transport team attain the goal of being a family advocate.[10,24,31,32,44,45]

Implications for Patient Transport

Transport team members and emergency personnel are exposed to situations in which family members may be in close proximity during the resuscitation process. Nurses have a wealth of information on this topic that comes from personal experience, and they should relate these experiences to other health care providers. Nurses should be on the forefront of supporting family presence; this support can play an important role in changing health care practices.[10,24,31,32,44,45]

When transport teams resuscitate a patient outside the hospital in the presence of prehospital care providers or referring hospital personnel, the code should always be conducted in a professional manner. Because transport team members are never on their "own turf," the care they provide is open for scrutiny by all bystanders. Less noise and chaos are generally present during a resuscitation attempt by a transport team than in a hospital simply because fewer people are present. Transport nurses can attest to the fact

that a code can be successfully run with fewer people than are used in a hospital. Speaking in normal calm tones during a code seems to have a calming effect on those present; thus simply decreasing the noise level during a resuscitation attempt lessens the degree of chaos.[10,24,31,32,44,45]

One factor the transport team must consider when giving emotional care to the family outside the hospital is the lack of ancillary support services, such as social services or pastoral care. The transport team must adjust to this lack of support services and find other innovative ways to provide care to the family without jeopardizing patient care.

Although not everyone is prepared to view resuscitation attempts, the literature supports the fact that many persons wish to be present when attempts are made to resuscitate a family member. The presence at resuscitation attempts is helpful for working through grief. Transport nurses and all transport team members should be patient advocates in the true sense of the word by asking the family what they want and by helping them to achieve their goals.

Bereavement After Sudden Death in the Field

When patients are pronounced dead in the field or are not transported from a referring facility, their families may not be able to benefit from support services available when patients are taken to the receiving facility. Family members often have many questions after the death of a loved one. If family members are at the scene, the transport team should make an attempt to interact with them. If at all possible, the family should be encouraged to view the patient's body at the scene.

The initial shock experienced by family members may prevent them from knowing what questions to ask. The team can talk to the family about the facts that led up to the incident and explain the possible injuries that caused the death. Family members often do not remember what was said to them as much as they remember the attitude of the person who was talking to them.

Common responses of family members to the death of a patient are anger and hostility. These feelings are the result of a lack of control, frustration, and helplessness over the events surrounding the illness and death. Expressed anger often disguises underlying fears and anxieties that need to be addressed. Angry persons often discourage health care professionals from helping them, thus leaving them feeling lonely and isolated.

Transport teams can help the family to understand that the advanced care that their team delivered was the best care possible. The public may not be aware that the transport team is capable of providing the same care that is delivered in an ED; they may be under the impression that the best care possible is that which is given in the hospital. They may believe that the role of the transport team is to provide rapid transport and that the gold standard of care is provided in the hospital.

The transport team is responsible for giving care to the victim and emotional care to the family. If at all possible, the transport team should assist the prehospital care providers in talking with the family. Because of the nature of transport operations, the team cannot always stay at the scene and assist the family. If the team cannot stay, the team's assessment of the family may be an impetus for initiating a referral for follow-up. If the base station is associated with a hospital, the social services department may be able to assist with the follow-up. The team may be involved with this follow-up at a later date by calling the family and repeating some of the medical information that the family either did not understand or were not capable of comprehending at the time of the patient's death.

Emotional care of the family is an important part of patient transport. The transport team may need additional education and increased awareness of their potential impact in this area. Understanding the diversity of patients and families may aid in providing care to the patient before, during, and after the transport. The development of policies and procedures that address the needs of families related to transport must be a part of every transport program. Family care is an integral part of transport practice.[10,24,31,32,44,45,47]

Research

Research is systematic inquiry that uses disciplined methods to answer questions or solve problems with an ultimate goal of developing, refining, and expanding a body of knowledge.[48] The goal of health care research is the validation of existing knowledge or discovery of new knowledge that provides the evidence or direction necessary to guide quality clinical practice. Nurses are responsible for using knowledge gained through research to define and refine critical care transport practices. The field of critical care transport is a relatively new area of research compared with other medical and nursing specialties. It offers a wide spectrum of potential research questions based on method of transport and patient populations transported. Clinical practice can serve as a rich source of research ideas that include clinical observations, validation of treatment guidelines, testing of new procedures, replication of previous studies, and identification of gaps in existing medical or nursing literature. Additional areas for research in critical care transport include, but are not limited to, staff education, program administration, patient safety, economic concerns, development of a safety culture, health care delivery systems, and quality evaluation.

The research process is consistent across all disciplines. However, research studies are often accorded greater credibility when the research team is multidisciplinary. Approaches to research may be qualitative or quantitative. *Quantitative research* includes systematic collection of numeric information, whereas *qualitative research* involves systematic collection of subjective data. The selection of one or the other or both methodologies typically depends on the question of interest. Research may also be grossly classified as basic or applied. *Basic research* is conducted to expand a body of knowledge, whereas *applied research* is performed to find answers or solutions to existing problems. Applied research tends to be of greater immediate utility for defining best practices.[48]

Before initiation of the research process, a fundamental understanding of common terms is essential. Box 32.8

• BOX 32.8 Definition of Terms

Cluster sampling: A process in which the sample is selected by randomly choosing smaller and smaller subgroups from the main population.

Convenience sampling: A process in which a sample is drawn from conveniently available subjects.

Internal validity: The degree to which the changes or differences in the dependent variable (the outcome) can be attributed to the independent variable (intervention or group differences). This is related to the degree to which extraneous variables are controlled.

Judgmental sampling: Another name for purposive sample.

Population: All subjects of interest to the researcher for the study.

Purposive sampling: A process in which subjects are selected by investigators to meet a specific purpose.

Quota sampling: A process in which the subjects are selected by convenience until the specified number of subjects for a specific subgroup is reached. At this point, subjects are no longer selected for that subgroup, but recruitment continues for subgroups that have not yet reached their quota of subjects.

Sample: A small portion of the population selected for participation in the study.

Sampling: A process used for selecting a sample from the population.

Simple random sampling: A process in which a sample is selected randomly from the population, with each subject having a known and calculable probability of being chosen.

Snowball sampling: A process in which the first subjects are drawn by convenience; these subjects then recruit people they know to participate, and they recruit people they know, and so forth.

Stratified random sampling: A process in which a population is divided into subgroups and a predetermined portion of the sample is randomly drawn from each subgroup.

Systematic random sample: A process in which a sample is drawn by systematically selecting every nth subject from a list of all subjects in the population. The starting point in the population must be selected randomly.

Threats to Validity

Assignment of subjects: Changes in the dependent variable are a result of preexisting differences in the subjects before implementation of the intervention.

Biophysiologic measures: Measures of biologic function obtained through use of technology, such as electrocardiographic or hemodynamic monitoring.

Blocking: Assignment of subjects to control and experimental groups based on extraneous variables. Blocking helps to ensure that one group does not get the preponderance of subjects with a specific value on a variable of interest.

Concurrent validity: Criterion-related validity in which the measures are obtained at the same time.

• BOX 32.8 Definition of Terms—cont'd

Construct validity: A form of validity in which the researcher is not as concerned with the values obtained by the instrument but with the abstract match between the true value and the obtained value.

Content validity: Concern with whether the questions asked, or observations made, actually address all of the variables of interest.

Criterion-related validity: The results from the tool of interest are compared with those of another criterion that relates to the variable to be measured.

Determination of stability: Only appropriate when the value for the variable of interest is expected to remain the same over the time period examined.

External validity: The degree to which the results can be applied to others outside the sample used for the study.

Face validity: The instrument looks like it is measuring what it should be measuring.

Hawthorne effect: Subjects respond in a different manner just because they are involved in a study.

History: Natural changes in the outcome variable are the result of another event inside or outside the experimental setting but are attributed to the intervention instead.

Instrumentation: Changes in the dependent variable are the result of the measurement plan rather than the intervention.

Internal consistency: The degree to which items on a questionnaire or psychological scale are consistent with each other.

Interrater reliability: The degree to which two or more evaluators agree on the measurement obtained.

Loss of subjects: Changes in the dependent variable are a result of differential loss of subjects from the intervention or control groups.

Maturation: Changes in the dependent variable are a result of normal changes over time.

Observation: The activity of interest is observed, described, and possibly recorded via audiotape or videotape.

Predictive validity: Criterion-related validity in which measurement with one instrument is used to predict the value from another instrument at a future point in time.

Psychological scale: Usually a number of self-report items combined in a questionnaire designed to evaluate the subject on a particular psychological trait, such as self-esteem.

Reliability: The degree of consistency with which an instrument measures the variable it is designed to measure.

Self-report: The variables of interest are measured by asking the subject to report on the perception of the value for the variable.

Stability: Determination of the degree of change in a measure across time.

Validity: How well the tool measures what it is supposed to measure.

---

contains definitions of useful research terms. The initial step in the research process is identification of the question of interest. The question should be clear and specific. For example, what is the incidence rate of hypothermia in patients transported via air? Another research question might focus on identification of the relationship between an independent variable (the intervention variable) and one or more dependent variables (the outcomes measured). Such a question might read: What is the relationship between hypovolemia and hypothermia? An example of a qualitative study questions is how do family members of patients transported via air perceive the level of care provided? Once a specific question has been selected, a literature review can be conducted to identify existing studies and determine their levels of evidence. Pertinent studies then need to be critiqued for research strength and may be evaluated with established critique guidelines that focus on each step of the research process. Some questions to consider include the following:

1. How many subjects are in the study, and how was sample size determined?
2. Was the research design appropriate to answer the research question?
3. What are the results of the study? Are the results valid? Can they be generalized to the transport (or other specific) setting?
4. Will the results of the study impact clinical care or project design?

The research design forms the general structure of the study, and multiple designs may be used. A common mistake made by novice researchers is failure to fit the research question into the appropriate study design. An example is use of a quantitative design (seeking to make statistical predictions) when a qualitative design (an in-depth exploration of subjective information) would better answer the research question. Box 32.9 lists several common research designs. Experimental study design elements include manipulation, randomization, and control. According to Thompson and Panacek,[49] *manipulation* is the ability of the researcher to interact with study subjects to effectively direct the independent variable. Manipulation is evidenced in interventional studies in which one group receives an intervention, whereas a control group does not. *Randomization* ensures that all subjects have an equal chance of assignment to either the control or the experimental group. *Control* refers to the researcher's ability to limit the influence of confounding or extraneous variables. Studies with a true experimental design contain all three of these elements. However, most clinical studies are not true experiments and are therefore classified as quasiexperimental studies, because one or more of these three key elements is missing.

• BOX 32.9 Classifications of Research Designs

1. True experimental
2. Quasiexperimental
   Cohort
   Group sequential
   Cross sectional
3. Nonexperimental
   Case control
   Historical
   Surveys, questionnaires
   Case series
   Case reports

Once a research project involving human subjects has been designed, an *institutional review board* (IRB) must review and approve the study. The function of an IRB is to ensure that subject rights are protected. Some IRBs also evaluate the validity and methodology of the research proposal. Whenever human subjects are involved in research, informed consent or a consent waiver must be obtained from the IRB. One of the roles of an IRB is to ensure that researchers have honored the tenets of informed consent, which include verifying that the patient has shown decision-making ability, that the patient was not coerced, and that the study has been thoroughly explained. Subjects must be free to refuse participation without jeopardizing access to treatment. All subjects need to be assured of anonymity and their right to withdraw from the study at any time. Research in the prehospital environment can make obtaining timely informed consent difficult.[18] Exceptions have been made for life-threatening situations. In 1996 a Waiver of Informed Consent Guidelines for emergency research was established under federal rule (21CFR 50.24). It was revised in 2011 and updated in April 2013.[40] The federal guidelines, referred to as the Final Rule, outline qualifying criteria for subjects (Box 32.10). Researchers must ensure that the criteria for these exceptions have been included in the research proposal.

After a research design has been selected, the sample identified, and data collected, the data need to be analyzed and the results interpreted. The specific research design dictates the techniques used to for data analysis. *Descriptive statistics* summarizes quantitative data and allow the researcher to describe what occurred in the sample. *Inferential statistics tests* are used to determine differences between two or more samples. Qualitative data require nonstatistical analysis procedures. A major problem for clinical researchers is interpreting research findings because numbers can be used to say many things. Also, some findings of statistical significance may have little or no clinical significance. Any conclusions drawn from the data must actually be supported by the data.[48,50]

The final components of clinical research are presentation and dissemination of the data. Professional associations and journals afford many opportunities to share results and link study conclusions to the work of other researchers.

• BOX 32.10   Emergency Exception to Informed Consent

- Subject is in life-threatening situation.
- Subject is unable to consent because of condition.
- No time to contact legally authorized representative for subject.
- Available treatments are untested or deemed unsatisfactory.
- Possibility must exist that subject will benefit from treatment.
- Prior community consultation and public disclosure of study protocol.

Research in the transport environment can present some unique challenges including coordination of study protocols with other departments, institutions, and agencies; inability to control the study environment; the simultaneous need for urgent care delivery; and complications associated with obtaining and ensuring informed consent. The dissemination of findings contributes to the weight of evidence necessary for practice.

Research in the transport environment can present some unique challenges including coordination of study protocols with other departments and institutions, an uncontrolled environment, the need for urgent acute care delivery, and the complications of obtaining and ensuring informed consent. Communication and collaboration are the keys to assembling a research team and identifying issues to facilitate a smooth research process.

Evidence-Based Practice

Worldwide attention has been focused on the need for health care providers to be accountable for delivery of safe quality care based on scientific information and knowledge of "best practices." *Evidence-based medicine* (EBM) is a term that originated in the 1980s at McMaster Medical School, Hamilton, Ontario. Canada, Australia, and Great Britain are credited with the early EBM movement to promote health care best practice decisions. EBM, as defined by Sackett and colleagues,[50] is the conscientious, explicit, and judicious use of current best practice information for making decisions about the care of patients. EBP includes integration of individual clinical expertise with the best available clinical evidence from systematic research.[51] EBP is a problem-solving approach to the delivery of health care that combines the best evidence from well-designed studies with a clinician's expertise and a patient's preferences and values.[52] A number of EBP models for nursing care are found in the literature, two of which are the Advancing Research and Clinical Practice Through Close Collaboration model, developed by Melnyk and Fineout-Overholt, and the Iowa model, developed by Titler and colleagues.[50,51]

The EBM process involves categorization of clinical practices according to the strength of the evidence. The general categories include systematic reviews, clinical evidence, and clinical practice guidelines. Levels of evidence (Box 32.11) are also referred to as the hierarchy of evidence. Systematic reviews and meta-analyses of randomized clinical trials (RCTs) are considered the strongest level of evidence (level I), and opinions and reports of expert committees are considered the weakest (level VII).[18,48-53]

EBP guidelines provide direction for dealing with many common clinical situations. A number of electronic resources provide access to systematic reviews and EPB guidelines. Transport team members should become familiar with databases that impact their practice. The *Agency for Health Care Research Quality* is a good example.[21] Although systematic reviews are considered the highest level of evidence,

Level I

Systematic reviews
Meta-analyses of RCTs
Evidence-based clinical practice guidelines based on systematic reviews of RCTs

Level II

Well-designed RCTs (one or more)
Single nonrandomized trials

Level III

Noncontrolled trials without randomization
Systematic reviews of correlational/observational studies

Level IV

Well-designed case-control and cohort studies
Single correlational/observational studies

Level V

Systematic reviews of descriptive and qualitative studies

Level VI

Single descriptive or qualitative studies

Level VII

Opinions of authorities or reports of expert committees

RCT, randomized controlled trials.
Adapted from Ackley BJ, Swan BA, Ladwig G, Tucker S. *Evidence-Based Nursing Care Guidelines: Medical-Surgical Interventions*. St. Louis, MO: Mosby-Elsevier; 2008.

some have design flaws. The practitioner needs to ask the following questions when evaluating any study:

- Is the study of high scientific merit, and does it have an appropriate research design?
- Are results consistent from study to study?
- Are all clinical outcomes, including benefits and potential harm, addressed?
- Does my patient population of interest correspond to patients described in the studies?[21]

For identification of best practice information, the clinician needs to formulate an appropriate clinical question that narrows the scope of the literature search. PICO, a model developed by faculty at McMaster University, Ontario, is a strategy used for framing the clinical question. PICO is an acronym in which P stands for patient or population of interest, including diagnosis, age, and gender; I is for intervention, such as a medication or treatment; C is for comparison (not every question has a comparison component); and O is for outcome, which may include a primary and secondary outcome (Box 32.12).[54] A sample clinical question might be Do patients with traumatic brain injury who are intubated during prehospital transport have fewer metabolic acid-base disturbances than patients who are not intubated? This question involves a comparison group, but not all questions do. In a search of the literature, limiting electronic searches to articles with the terms "evidenced-based" or "systematic reviews" can help narrow your search.[54]

Quality Management

Patient transport has become a crucial part of modern health care. As the health care system faces dwindling financial resources, ongoing financial justification and proof of improved patient outcomes is necessary to justify the high cost of transport services. For many transport programs, *quality management* (QM) is often viewed as a time-consuming activity with little measurable impact on actual patient outcomes. This section provides an overview of the QM process for transport programs and suggests several practical methods for evaluation of patient transport and improvement of systems of care.

Definition of Terms: Quality Assurance versus Continuous Quality Improvement

A veritable alphabet soup of quality terms has glutted health care. For the sake of clarity, it is important to define the terminology. *Quality assurance* (QA) implies a traditional approach to outcome evaluation. It includes such activities as monitoring specific indicators and comparing results with predetermined thresholds or standards. Unfortunately, health care providers sometimes perceive traditional QA in a negative light because it is associated with the perception that individuals are doing a poor job or are not complying with certain standards. As an alternative to traditional QA,

Components of the Clinical Question	Patient	Intervention	Comparison (Optional)	Outcome
Question	Description of the patient or population of interest	Intervention or therapy of interest (e.g., medication, treatment) or prognostic factor	Alternative medication, treatment, etc., for comparison	The clinical outcome, including a time frame if appropriate
Example	In patients with anxiety	Does music therapy	Or support groups	Reduced hospital visits

CQI, *total quality management* (TQM), and many derivations of these concepts have been used in the health care arena over the last few decades. These terms are often used interchangeably, but they embrace essentially the same concepts. The CQI approach is radically different from traditional QA, but not all individuals who use the terms appreciate the differences.

CQI and QA practices differ radically in approaches to motivation, leadership, methodology, and organization. Traditionally, health care providers have been motivated to perform QA activities primarily to meet externally mandated regulatory requirements (e.g., The Joint Commission). Conversely, the focus of CQI activities is to please customers. Patients are informed consumers with discriminating tastes in health care services. Although few choices may be available in emergency transport situations, patients and families have certain expectations of health care providers, regardless of the setting.

General components of a QM program include the following[3,55,56]:

- Program mission statement
- Program vision statement
- Program value statement
- Goals and objectives
- Delineated critical success factors
- Definition of the scope of practice of the transport program
- Decision on an approach to QM
- Chosen methodology
- Established reporting procedures
- Development of recommendations for action
- Establishment of evaluation intervals

The role of a leader in a CQI program differs dramatically from that of a leader in a QA program. In a QA program, quality initiatives are typically the responsibility of a middle manager or a QA coordinator. The entire responsibility for ensuring quality is relegated to this individual. In a CQI program, accountability for quality rests with the organization's leaders, who must be committed to the CQI initiative in both word and deed.

Perhaps the greatest difference between the CQI and QA approaches is the methodology used. The QA approach has typically focused on retrospective audits, quality indicator monitoring, and less than rigorous studies. With this approach, decisions can be made based on weak data and personal opinions. CQI methodology relies on statistics and facts, not feelings and assumptions. In addition, CQI methodology stresses a standardized problem-solving approach designed to yield predictable evidence-based results.

Finally, the organizational culture in a program committed to CQI is fundamentally different; all processes and plans are centered on the customer (patients and families). Quality customer service is a core value in CQI organizations. Employees are empowered to meet the needs of the customer by implementing changes and making decisions without being unduly encumbered by bureaucratic rules and regulations.

Just Culture: Quality Care Without Blame

QA, CQI, or TQM should always occur within a no-blame culture. Transport team members may be reluctant to acknowledge breeches in protocols, incidents, or events if the sense that someone will be punished. However, accountability should never be underplayed. Mistakes may occur, but intentional high-risk behaviors should not be tolerated.

The transport environment is stressful. Decisions need to be made rapidly and, depending on the condition of the patient, an incorrect decision may yield serious consequences. Adverse events can result from normal transport care such as medication administration, equipment failure, or challenging interventions such as intubations in the transport vehicle.

Admitting and evaluating a near-miss, adverse event, or an error in the transport environment is ethical and provides an opportunity to improve the quality of patient care and promote patient safety.[39] However, many transport team members may feel unsupported, or fearful of repercussions if they admit or report an error. Factors identified that hinder transport teams "speaking up" include authority gradients (social status, educational level, professional status, and perceived expertise) and challenging someone with more authority (Medical Direction versus the transport team).[40,57]

In 1999, the Institute of Medicine published a book titled *To Err is Human,* which challenged health care providers to identify, admit (tell the patient or family), and develop ways to learn from "our mistakes." This set the foundation for a "Just Culture."[57]

According to Frazer and Smith[57] Just Culture "defines and differentiates behaviors and provides guidelines on how to deal with each type of behavior, to manage risk and prevent adverse outcomes, such as incidents and accidents" (p. 83). The transport QM program should encourage a "culture" that allows for transport team members to safely "disclose" errors. These disclosures should result in plans of care, changes in practice, and ways to notify and involve both the patient and family in how the error will be addressed including financial costs when indicated.[39,56,57] Lu et al.[39] provided an example of an "Error disclosure conversations to patients" (p. 219). These are summarized in Box 32.13.[39]

Quality Management Model for Air Medical Transport

Both CAMTS and ASTNA provide a framework for the development of a QM program for a medical transport program. A summary of these components, including quality indicators, are contained in Box 32.14.[3,20]

Despite some inherent limitations, traditional QA activities have merit in the medical transport environment. Transport programs might be inclined to discard QA methods completely to adopt an exclusive CQI approach; however, a combination of the two methods may be the

BOX 32.13 Family Support Related to Errors

- Focus goals and outcomes around the needs of the patient/ family
- Present information in language the patient/family can understand
- Convey the facts surrounding the error
- Explain how medical ramifications will be managed
- Describe the steps that have been or will be taken to prevent reoccurrence of the error
- Reassure patient/family that they will not have any additional financial costs because of the error
- Apologize and express regret for the error

From Lu D, Guenther E, Wesley A, Gallagher T. Disclosure of harmful medical errors in out-of-hospital care. *Ann Emerg Med.* 2013;61(2)215-221.

BOX 32.14 Components of Quality Assurance Program and Suggested Quality Indicators From the Commission on Accreditation of Air Medical Transport Systems Quality Management Flow Chart

- QM program linked to risk management
- QM integrated with other components of the transport program, for example, Communications and Safety Management System
- Written QM plan
- Regularly scheduled QM meetings
- Monitoring and evaluation process driven by aspects of care
- Indicators and thresholds or other criteria:
  - Patient safety
  - Interfacility patients not transported bedside to bedside
  - Out-of-range cabin temperatures without risk mitigation
  - Arrest during transport (i.e., CPR)
  - Two-patient transports
  - Single-medical-provider transports
  - Fatigue-risk management (such as use of time-outs, utilization of fatigue-risk management tools)
  - Communications
    - ETA accuracy
    - Accuracy of coordinates (RW)
    - Weather at time of request and during transport if changes occur
    - Request times from acceptance to lift-off or departure times
  - Clinical indicators
    - Based on scope of care
  - Levels of care
- Evidence of action plans
- Evidence of the reporting of QA activities
- Evidence of outcome studies
- Evidence of annual goal establishment

CPR, Cardiopulmonary resuscitation; *ETA,* estimated time of arrival; *QA,* quality assurance; *QM,* quality management; *RW,* rotor wing.

most effective way to evaluate and improve care. Both QA and CQI methodologies can be integrated into a program's overall QM strategy. QA activities can serve as a stimulus for multidisciplinary CQI teams because the transport process encompasses multiple phases and persons. The remainder of this chapter uses the term quality management

to imply a blending of the best aspects of traditional QA and CQI.

Assignment of Accountability: The Staff-Based Approach to Quality Management

Medical transport services managers are ultimately accountable for their program's quality activities. However, involvement of all transport team members in the QM program (from inception through monitoring, data collection, change, and evaluation) is the only way to achieve commitment at all levels. Managers can delegate many activities to committees or individuals, such as a QM coordinator, but top-down support and involvement are essential components of an effective QM program. Executive level involvement is demonstrated by financial support for individuals assigned QM responsibilities. These individuals must receive adequate training and be allowed paid time away from routine duties to complete QM activities and projects. Some medical transport services hire QM coordinators who are assigned the bulk of the QM workload. Whether the QM coordinator is a full-time staff member or an individual who works part time, one individual must be accountable for overseeing the process. Failure to assign accountability results in disorganization and lack of QM program direction.

The success or failure of a medical QM program is also related to the degree to which team members are involved in its development, implementation, and ongoing maintenance. If a QM program is conceived and implemented with little or no involvement on the part of those who deliver care, it is likely to be perceived negatively. If, on the other hand, all team members are given an opportunity to contribute to QM program development, personal investment on the part of the staff improves the chances of program success.

Quality Management Committee

Development of a QM committee is one way to promote staff involvement in the QM process. The QM committee approach promotes "ownership" of the QM program on the part of the transport team. The participation of transport team members may be used as part of the program's clinical advancement system. Committee membership may be determined by application, appointment, or election. Whatever the approach, members must be committed to the goals of the committee. Bylaws that address QM committee structure, reporting mechanisms, voting privileges, attendance requirements, and so on can serve to heighten members' sense of commitment to the aims of the committee.

Quality Management Program Organizational Strategies

The most effective QM programs are well organized and multifaceted. Programs that rely too heavily on one monitoring method risk missed opportunities for improvement. However, management of multiple or simultaneous studies and indicators can be overwhelming. A written QM plan is an effective organizational tool. The plan provides the infrastructure for quality initiatives and facilitates a systematic and organized monitoring and evaluation process. The development of such a plan is straightforward; however, certain essential components must be included.

First, the content of the QM plan must be based on the transport program's scope of service, which describes the types of patients transported and how they are transported. For instance, a transport program that transports 80% of its patients from the scene of injury has a different scope of care or service than a neonatal transport program. A statement that clearly summarizes the essence of the services provided by the particular program and by its crew members could read: "Our program provides rapid assessment, diagnosis, and treatment of critically ill or injured patients of all ages from the scene of injury and between care facilities." With this statement as a framework, QM personnel can begin to develop standards, identify high-risk high-volume aspects of care, and target appropriate strategies to monitor them.

Identification of Important Aspects

Important aspects of care to evaluate include areas that are high risk, problem prone, or low volume. Events with these characteristics have the greatest impact on patient outcome, costs, and program functioning. Care interventions, such as physical assessment, documentation, medication administration, invasive procedures, and response to requests for service, are examples of important aspects of medical transport care.

Indicator Development

Indicators are well-delineated objective measures of compliance with a particular standard. Potential indicators of physical assessment after endotracheal intubation include the following:
1. Bilateral breath sounds are documented on all patients after intubation.
2. Esophageal intubations are recognized and corrected.

Thresholds and Benchmarks

The final step in development of a written QM plan is establishment of the level at which lack of compliance with a given standard or quality indicator is considered unacceptable and necessitates intervention. This level, usually expressed as a percentage, is known as the *threshold*. Some experts prefer the use of the term *benchmark* when implying an externally determined performance level. National professional associations have sometimes published suggested thresholds, but little research has supported their validity. Whether this will change in the future remains to be seen.

However, lack of current data does not preclude a transport program from identifying its own thresholds and benchmarks.

When no national data are available with which to validate a certain level of performance, how does one realistically assign thresholds? First, thresholds must be attainable and practical. Thresholds that are so high they cannot be met are unrealistic. Conversely, there are high-risk indicators for which failure to meet the standard 100% of the time could result in deleterious patient outcomes. For example, the threshold for the indicator "esophageal intubations are recognized and corrected" should be 100%.

Establishment of Priorities for Monitoring and Evaluation[3,56]

A written QM plan outlines all general categories of care monitored in a given time period, how often these aspects of care are monitored, and the methods used. Actual implementation of these activities can be daunting. A prioritization tool is needed to determine which activities should be undertaken first. A *decision matrix* is a simple but valuable way to prioritize QM efforts. It is usually most effective when completed by a group, such as the QM committee, or a similar planning structure. The following example describes the use of a decision matrix.

The XYZ Transport Program QM committee meets the first week of January to establish quality initiatives for the coming year. During this meeting, group members brainstorm to identify clinical and operational nursing, paramedic, respiratory therapy, administration, aviation, medical, mechanical, and communications issues. As a result of their brainstorming, the QM committee targets 10 important opportunities for improvement. Areas of concern include interfacility bedside times, intubation success rates, medical control contact documentation, maternal transport team composition, chest pain management documentation, fetal monitor interpretation, refueling turnaround times, compliance with transport guidelines, referral hospital satisfaction, and pediatric fluid management. To decide which of these issues will be addressed first during the coming year, the QM committee consults a decision matrix and identifies their five highest priority issues to determine where they need to focus the greatest efforts.

Utilization Appropriateness

A comprehensive transport program QM plan monitors appropriate indicators and uses findings from monitoring activities as a stimulus for the inclusion of all who are involved in the transport process. Another component of a comprehensive QM program is the evaluation of transport appropriateness. Utilization evaluation is an essential piece of the greater quality picture, yet this important element is often overlooked by many transport services.[1,3,56]

The criteria for a medically appropriate transport are controversial and remain to be validated. Several professional organizations have proposed utilization appropriateness criteria. Each program must develop a mechanism to screen for transport appropriateness, both prospectively and retrospectively. In development of criteria, several general considerations should be kept in mind. First, does the patient's condition dictate the need to minimize scene or interhospital transport time? Second, what distances, local geography, or traffic conditions might justify various transportation alternatives? Third, what is the availability of appropriate vehicles and personnel? Fourth, what are the prevailing weather conditions that might interfere with air or ground transport? Finally, what are the costs of various transportation alternatives? With these considerations as a framework, the transport program can develop criteria for appropriate use of medical transport resources.

Legal Considerations for Quality Management

One of the most under acknowledged considerations in the development of a QM program involves the legal issues that surround the quality evaluation process.[9-12,14,25,56,57] Laws that protect QM activities and personnel involved in data collection from the threat of subpoena and liability vary significantly from state to state. In fact, in some states, the confidentially of QM documentation has been challenged. This section examines the importance of state discoverability, immunity, and admissibility laws to the QM process and the legal protection of individuals involved in QM activities.

For an understanding of the ramifications of state legislation on the QM process, a few legal terms must be defined. *Discovery* is a term used to describe the acquisition of information and evidence before a trial, via oral or written deposition or other means. Laws governing rules of procedure and evidence vary significantly by state. *Admissible evidence* is anything that is allowed as evidence by a court. Information not typically considered discoverable is not automatically precluded from admissibility if it comes to light by means other than the formal discovery process. For example, if a plaintiff's attorney stumbles on undiscoverable QM data stored in sloppy personnel files or carelessly placed in patient records, certain states allow this information to be admitted as evidence.

A *subpoena* is a directive from the court requiring a witness to appear before the court. A subpoena can also force a witness to produce any written evidence that may be pertinent to the case. The difference between subpoena and discoverability becomes problematic because they are two separate legal processes. State laws that prevent discoverability may not necessarily prevent subpoenas. These issues are further confused by the often unclear and ambiguous language used in these laws, which leaves interpretation up to individual courts.

State laws defining the protection of QM data and QM activities from discoverability, subpoena, and admissibility should have considerable impact on the planning, design, and implementation of a transport service's QM plan.

These laws have implications regarding the protection of both the health care providers monitored and the data derived from QM activities. Without protective legislation, persons who initiate QM activities place themselves and their colleagues at risk. In addition, transport programs that implement QM plans with inadequate knowledge of peer-review statutes in their state place the transport service at risk. Each transport program should consult with an attorney to determine the rules within their service area.

Once a transport program has adequate knowledge of applicable discoverability and peer-review statutes, several additional precautions need to be taken to ensure protection under the law. Examples of activities include the following:

1. Written memoranda regarding adverse patient outcomes, medication errors, and reasons for transport delay (whether valid or otherwise) should not be circulated through the transport program for review.
2. Written documentation of such incidents should never be kept in employee personnel files, which may be discoverable and admissible in court.
3. Data derived from QM studies should be contained within the QM system. A helpful method is to title all QM data, reports, and summaries with "XYZ Transport Service's Quality Management Program: Confidential."
4. If the actual number of the state's peer-review protective statute and its wording are known, the transport program can affix this wording to all documents relating to QM.
5. Explicit discussion of sensitive patient care information should not occur in the open forum of the transport service's weekly or monthly chart review. This practice, although it has educational merit, places all crew members who hear about the incident at risk for subpoena.
6. Any memoranda or other written materials, such as incident reports, should not make references to the source of the data.[10,24,31,32,44,45,58]

Laws that affect QM activities are diverse and often ambiguous. Statutes in many states have gone unchallenged. Because of complexities in law, program administrators must obtain legal assistance when tackling these issues.

Summary

Multiple professional issues are involved in patient transport. This chapter examined some of the topics that are commonly experienced before, during, and after transport. What is important is that these are professional, multidisciplinary, collaborative issues that must include all the members of the transport team and at times the patient and the family.

Knowledge of the law and legal doctrine is a necessary component of the transport process. Transport team members must be familiar with both the internal and professional standards that describe their scope of practice and profession. Ignorance of the law harms not only the health care provider but also the patients that they serve.

Care of the family is an important part of patient transport. The transport team may need additional education and increased awareness of their potential impact in this area. Transport team members must develop an understanding of the diversity of patients and their families to provide holistic care during the transport process. The development of policies and procedures that address the needs of families related to transport must be a part of every transport program. The care of a patient's family is as important as the care of the patient.

Research is important because it identifies, describes, and communicates EBP related to the care of patients during critical care transport. It provides a systematic approach for review and analysis of data to develop optimal clinical practice guidelines. Critical care transport research can be particularly difficult because of the environment in which it is conducted and the challenges faced when studying critically ill and injured patients.

QM in the transport environment remains among the greatest challenges a program must face. A framework for a QM process has to be practical and comprehensive. The transport team must feel able to practice in a just and safe environment.

As health care and patient transport continues to move into the 21st century, these issues and more will continue to be a challenge. Patients, families, and those who use transport teams and programs expect safe and competent patient care based on a knowledge of applicable law, research, EBP, and CQI.

References

1. American College of Emergency Physicians (ACEP). Appropriate interfacility patient transfer. *Ann Emerg Med.* 2016;67(5):690.
2. Burt CW, McCaig LF, Valverde R. Analysis of ambulance transports and diversions among US emergency departments. *Ann Emerg Med.* 2006;47(4):317-326.
3. Commission on Accreditation of Air Medical Transport Systems (CAMTS). *Accreditation Standards.* 10th ed. Andersonville, TN: CAMTS; 2015.
4. Geiderman J, Marco CA, Moskop J, et al. Ethics of ambulance diversion. *Am J Emerg Med.* 2015;33(6):822-827.
5. George JE. *Law and emergency care.* St. Louis, MO: Mosby; 1980.
6. Hoot NR, Aronsky D. Systemic review of emergency department crowding: causes, effects and solutions. *Ann Emerg Med.* 2008;52(2):126-136.
7. Kelen G, Peterson S, Pronovost P. In the name of patient safety, let's burden the emergency department more. *Ann Emerg Med.* 2016;67(5):737-740.
8. Magauran BG. Risk management for the emergency physician: competency and decision-making capacity, informed consent, and refusal of care against medical advice. *Emerg Med Clin North Am.* 2009;27(4):605-614, viii.
9. Williams A. Legal issues in air and ground transport. In: Blumen I, (Editor in Chief). *Principles and Directions of Air Medical Transport.* Salt Lake City, UT: Air Medical Physicians Association; 2015: 170-194.
10. William J. Family presence during resuscitation: To see or not to see. *Nurs Clin North Am.* 2002;37(1):211-220.
11. York-Clark D, Stocking J, Johnson J, eds. *Flight and Ground Transport Nursing Core Curriculum.* Denver, CO: Air & Surface Transport Nurses Association; 2006.
12. York-Clark D, Johnson J, Stocking J, Treadwell D, Corbett P, eds. *Critical Care Transport Core Curriculum.* Aurora, CO: Air & Surface Transport Nurses Association; 2017.
13. American Academy of Pediatrics. *Air and Ground Transport of Neonatal and Pediatric Patients.* 3rd ed. Elk Grove Village, IL: AAP; 2007.
14. Beahan S. Legal issues in medical records/health information management. In *Practical Guide to Clinical Computing Systems.* 2nd ed. 2015:167-178.
15. Cushing M. *Nursing Jurisprudence.* East Norwalk, CT: Appleton & Lange; 1988.
16. Emergency Medical Treatment and Active Labor Act, as established under the Consolidated Omnibus Budget Reconciliation Act (COBRA) of 1985 (42 USC 1395 dd) and 42 CFR 489.24; 42 CFR 489.20 (EMTALA regulations).
17. Fanaroff J. Legal issues in pediatric transport. *Clin Pediatr Emerg Med.* 2013;14(3):180-187.
18. Requarth JA. Informed consent challenges in frail delirious, demented, and do-not-resuscitate adult patients. *J Vasc Radiol.* 2015; 26(11):1647-1651.
19. Thibeault SM, ed. *Transport Professional Advanced Trauma Course.* 6th ed. Aurora, CO: Air & Surface Transport Nurses Association; 2015.
20. Treadwell D, James S, Arndt K, Werth R. *Standards for Critical Care and Specialty Transport.* Aurora, CO: Air & Surface Transport Nurses Association; 2015.
21. Agency for Healthcare Research Quality. http://www.ahrq.gov/; 2016 Accessed 19.06.16.
22. American Heart Association. *Family Support.* https://eccguidelines.heart.org/index.php/circulation/cpr-ecc-guidelines-2/part-3-ethical-issues/?strue=1&id=5-1; 2015 Accessed 18.06.16.
23. Baker EF, Moskop JC, Geiderman JM, et al. Law enforcement and emergency medicine: An ethical analysis. *Ann Emerg Med.* 2016;68(5):599-607.
24. Beachley M. Evolution of the trauma cycle. In: McQuillan KA, Makic MB, Whalen E, eds. *Trauma Nursing: From Resuscitation to Rehabilitation.* 4th ed. St. Louis, MO: Saunders; 2009:1-18.
25. Ben-Assuli O. Electronic health records adoption, quality of care, legal and privacy issues and their implementation in emergency departments. *Health Policy.* 2015;119(3):287-297.
26. Boehringer BK, Tilney P. An elderly man in cardiac arrest on a ski slope. *Air Med J.* 2015;34(2):62-63.
27. Campbell TW. Do death attitudes of nurses and physicians differ? *Omega.* 1983;14(1):43-49.
28. Carruba C. Role of medical director in air medical transport. In: Blumen I, (Editor in Chief). *Principles and Directions of Air Medical Transport.* Salt Lake City: Air Medical Physicians Association; 2015:89-96.
29. Chester A, Harris T, Hodgetts T, Keefe N. Survival to discharge after cardia arrest attended by a doctor-paramedic helicopter emergency medical service: An Utstein-style multiservice review of 1085 activations. *J Emerg Med.* 2015;49(4):439-447.
30. Clark J. That transport was appropriate, wasn't it? *Air Med J.* 2015;35(1):16-18.
31. Doyle CJ. Family participation during resuscitation: An option. *Ann Emerg Med.* 1987;16(6):673-675.
32. Dwyer T. Predictors of public support for family presence during cardiopulmonary resuscitation: A population based study. *Int J Nurs Stud.* 2015;52(6):1064-1070.

33. Lazar RA. *EMS Law: A Guide for EMS Professionals*. Rockville, MD: Aspen; 1989.

34. Emergency Nurses Association. *Trauma Nursing Core Course*. 7th ed. Emergency Nurses Association: Des Plaines, IL; 2014.

35. Erler CJ, Thompson CB. Ethics, human rights and clinical research. *Air Med J*. 2008;27(3):110-113.

36. Guyette F, Reynolds J, Frisch A, Post Cardiac Arrest Service. Cardiac arrest resuscitation. *Emerg Med Clin North Am*. 2015;33 (3):669-690.

37. Iserson K, Sanders A, Mathieu D. *Ethics in Emergency Medicine*. Tucson, AZ: Galen Press; 1995.

38. Kraus C, Marco C. Shared decision making in the ED: Ethical consideration. *Am J Emerg Med*. 2016;34(8):1668-1672.

39. Lu D, Guenther E, Wesley A, Gallagher T. Disclosure of harmful medical errors in out-of-hospital care. *Ann Emerg Med*. 2013;61 (2):215-221.

40. U.S. Department of Health and Human Services Food and Drug Administration Office of Good Clinical Practice Center for Drug Evaluation and Research Center for Biologics Evaluation and Research Center for Devices and Radiological Health. *Guidance for Institutional Review Boards, Clinical Investigators, and Sponsors. Exception from Informed Consent Requirements for Emergency Research*. http://www.fda.gov/downloads/RegulatoryInformation/ Guidances/UCM249673.pdf; March 2011 Updated April 2013 Accessed 19.06.16.

41. Venkat A, Huckstein JV, Dhindson HS. Ethical issues in air medical transport. In: Blumen I, (Editor in Chief). *Principles and Directions of Air Medical Transport*. Salt Lake City, UT: Air Medical Physicians Association; 2015:32-38.

42. Von Vopelius-Feldt J, Coulter A, Benger J. The impact of prehospital critical care team on survival from out-of-hospital cardiac arrest. *Resuscitation*. 2015;96:290-295.

43. Mattox K. "Ideal" posttraumatic parameters. *J Trauma*. 1993;34 (5):734.

44. Flanders SA, Strasen JH. Review of evidence about family presence during resuscitation. *Crit Care Clin North Am*. 2014;26(4):533-550.

45. Fultz JH. Air medical transport: What the family wants to know. *J Air Med Transp*. 1993;12(11-12):431-435.

46. Joyce C, Libertin R, Bigham M. Family centered care in pediatric critical care transport. *Air Med J*. 2015;34(1):32-36.

47. Hansen M, Hansen E. Left behind: Caring for children in families experiencing patient transport. *Air Med J*. 2014;33(2): 69-70.

48. Polit DF, Beck CT. *Nursing Research: Generating and Assessing Evidence for Nursing Practice*. 9th ed. Philadelphia, PA: Wolters, Kluwer/Lippincott Williams & Wilkins; 2011.

49. Thompson CB, Panacek EA. Research study designs: experimental and quasi-experimental. *Air Med J*. 2006;25(6):242-246.

50. Sackett DL, Rosenberg WM, Gray JA, et al. Evidence based medicine: what it is and what it is not. *BMJ*. 1996;312(7023): 71-72.

51. *The Well-Built Clinical Question: The EBM Process*. http://hsl.lib. unc.edu/services/evidence-based-practice-resources; 2015 Accessed 19.06.16.

52. Messer SB. Evidence-based practice. *Encyclopedia of Mental Health*. 2nd ed. Amsterdam: Elsevier; 2016:161-189.

53. Melnyk BM. Integrating levels of evidence into clinical decision making. *Pediatr Nurs*. 2004;30(4):323-325.

54. Ham-Baloji W, Jordan P. Systemic review as a research method in post graduate nursing education. *Health SA Gesonheid*. 2016;21(1): 120-128.

55. Eppich W. "Speaking up" for patient safety in the pediatric emergency department. *Clin Pediatr Med*. 2015;16(2):83-89.

56. Hutchison T, Rorie D, Hinze N. Quality management, process improvement and patient safety. In: Bumen I, ed. *Principles and Direction of Air Medical Transport*. Salt Lake City, UT: Air Medical Physicians Association; 2015:130-151.

57. Frazer E, Smith D. In search of excellence. In: Bumen I, ed. *Principles and Direction of Air Medical Transport*. Salt Lake City, UT: Air Medical Physicians Association; 2015:83-89.

58. Institute of Medicine. *To Err Is Human*. http://www.nap.edu/ read/9728/chapter/1; November 1999 Accessed 19.06.16.

33

Accreditation for Air and Ground Medical Transport

EILEEN FRAZER

Accreditation means to give authority or reputation; to trust; to accept as valid or credible. Most medical professionals are familiar with the term accreditation because of the organization that accredits hospitals, the Joint Commission. The history of accreditation for hospitals is an interesting one that laid the foundation for other accrediting agencies to follow.

History of the Joint Commission

In 1915, the American College of Surgeons (ACS), recognizing the need to standardize patient care in hospitals, allocated $500.00 to establish standards to promote quality patient care.[1] Hospitals in 1915 were not necessarily places patients went to be cured; instead they were places patients went to die. Medical knowledge was minuscule compared with today's world. Penicillin had not yet been discovered, and although aseptic technique was used in surgery, no effective medications were available to manage postoperative infections.[2]

By 1917, the ACS developed a one-page list of requirements they called Minimum Standards for Hospitals. An on-site inspection was developed by the ACS in 1918 to determine whether hospitals with more than 100 beds could meet compliance with the Minimum Standards for Hospitals. More than 700 hospitals throughout the United States were evaluated in the first year, and only 89 (13%) met the requirements of the minimum standards requirements. Although these results were dismal, the inspection raised the awareness of the medical community, who were ready to accept the need for standardization and a verification process to improve quality.

More than 3000 hospitals were voluntarily surveyed by 1951. With the growth and overwhelming success of voluntary accreditation for hospitals, the ACS organization became overwhelmed and invited other organizations to participate. The Joint Commission on Accreditation of Hospitals (JCAH) was chartered in 1951 with the ACS and the following participating organizations: The American College of Physicians, the American Medical Association, the Canadian Medical Association, and the American Hospital Association.[3]

Later in the 1950s, the Canadian Medical Association withdrew to form its own national organization, and JCAH expanded to include health care outside the hospital environment, such as home health, mental health, and ambulatory health care. This expansion eventually resulted in a name change to the Joint Commission on Accreditation of Healthcare Organizations or JCAHO, known as *the Joint Commission* today.[2]

The White Paper Calls for Improved Emergency Medical Services

The Joint Commission was well established before standards even existed for medical transport. In fact, problems in transport were not even identified until 1966 when the white paper titled "Accidental Death and Disability: The Neglected Disease of Modern Society"[4] was published by the National Academy of Science. At that time, helicopter transport for the civilian population was unheard of, and standardization did not exist for ground transport vehicles or for the medical attendants who accompanied patients. Untrained personnel in the back of a mortician's vehicle did 50% of the ground transports, whereas fire, police, or volunteer groups performed the other 50%.[1]

The white paper triggered legislation that specifically addressed Emergency Medical Services and even suggested the use of helicopters.[1]

The Maryland State Police Aviation Division developed the earliest known public service helicopter system in 1969. A few hospital-based helicopter programs were seen by the mid-1970s, but the growth of these types of services did not really peak until the mid-1980s. At this time, hospitals were regionalizing, with specific hospitals recognized as centers of excellence in one or more specialty areas. Trauma center designation often included a helicopter program or access to a helicopter program, which was an added impetus to the growth in the number of helicopter services.

Also, the Vietnam experience proved a sharp decrease in mortality rates because of the rapid response of helicopters in transporting the injured from the field to definitive care. From a civilian perspective, the Golden Hour theory by Dr. R. Adams Cowley of the Shock Trauma Unit of Baltimore proposed that a critically injured patient had a precious 60 minutes to obtain definitive surgical treatment after an injury to survive.[5] The Golden Hour theory and the Vietnam experience[1] were frequently touted as reasons for a hospital, especially a trauma center, to start a helicopter service.

In 1980, a new organization, the Association of Hospital Based Emergency Air Medical Services (ASHBEAMS; the name was later changed to the Association of Air Medical Services [AAMS]), was formed. This organization started as a forum for administrators and personnel to get together and network with other hospital-based helicopter programs. No standards were available at this time, so those assigned to start up a hospital-based helicopter program usually had no air transport experience, no pattern to follow, and no awareness of the potential hazards and managers who understood the risks even less. The aviation component (aircraft, pilots, and maintenance) was contracted from an aviation vendor. Pilots were usually Vietnam veterans who were still operating under the oath they practiced in the military—complete the mission. Care providers were thrust into the unfamiliar aviation environment without standardized transport training and with the ingrained attitude that the patient, not safety, always comes first. Clearly all were well intentioned, but as more and more accidents began to occur, it was recognized that the profession needed standardization, not unlike the ACS recognized the need for standards in hospitals in the early 1900s.[4,6]

In 1985, 16 air medical accidents with 12 fatalities occurred.[3] The Federal Aviation Administration (FAA) was concerned, and the press began to alert the public. At the time, ASHBEAMS had minimal guidelines addressing patient care issues, but when the press started to focus on the number of air medical accidents, ASHBEAMS began to meet with other national groups, such as the Helicopter Association International (HAI), the National Flight Nurses Association (NFNA), National Flight Paramedics Association (NFPA), and the National EMS Pilots Association (NEMSPA), to develop consensus standards on safety and operational practices.

In 1986, the ASHBEAMS Safety Committee started a peer review safety audit called Priority One, with use of the safety guidelines that had been developed through the consensus process of the organizations listed previously. Priority One was beta-tested at Duke University in Durham, North Carolina and at the Staff for Life Program in Columbia, Missouri. As a result of these visits, the Safety Committee found that patient care standards specific to the transport environment were needed as well as safety guidelines to make the process complete. Therefore a feasibility study was performed to determine the need and viability of an accreditation program specifically for air medial transport.

Part of the feasibility study involved dialog with the Joint Commission and other accrediting bodies. Many organizational leaders felt that the Joint Commission should incorporate transport standards into its accreditation process and then layer in the air medical profession, which would negate the expense and effort needed to create another accrediting agency. However, the Joint Commission was not interested in responsibility for standards addressing the aviation environment, and stated that it was completely out of their field of expertise. Also, in the late 1980s, helicopter services were starting to be outsourced or privately owned and no longer sponsored or based at hospitals. Typically, fixed-wing medical transport services were privately owned and operated by an aviation company with no connections to hospitals. Both types of services were completely outside the realm of the Joint Commission.

Accreditation Organization Founded for Air Medical Transport

In 1989, with the feasibility study completed and presented, ASHBEAMS members voted to fund start-up costs for an air medical accreditation agency. Conceptually, this organization would be separate and independent of ASHBEAMS and would be made up of member organizations so that each member organization had equal representation on the Board of Directors.

The following seven organizations met on July 13, 1990, in Kansas City, Missouri, to form the Commission on Accreditation of Air Medical Services (CAAMS): the American College of Emergency Physicians, the AAMS, the National Association of Air Medical Communication Specialists, the National Association of EMS Physicians, the NEMSPA, the NFNA (now called Air & Surface Transport Nurses Association [ASTNA]), and the NFPA (now called the International Association of Flight and Critical Care Paramedics [IAFCCP]).

CAAMS was formally incorporated in Pennsylvania as a nonprofit organization. The mission of CAAMS was and is to improve the quality of patient care and safety of the transport environment. Along with the tools for the new organization's foundation, such as the articles of incorporation, policies, and bylaws, the most important task for the new board was to develop the accreditation standards.

All accrediting organizations have a similar process of site visits that usually occur every 3 years to verify compliance with standards. However, the standards are what define the site survey process. Medical transport services that apply for accreditation are awarded or are withheld from accreditation based on compliance with the accreditation standards. Therefore the standards must be attainable, measurable, and consistent with current practice.

Accreditation Standards

To gain acceptance of the accreditation standards, CAAMS used guidelines and standards from many of the organizations mentioned previously (ASHBEAMS, HAI, NFNA, NEMSPA, and NFPA) to begin the process. In an attempt to create a document that would address both safety and patient care issues, the CAAMS board studied the National Transportation Safety Board's accident reports to determine whether a standardized practice, policy, or procedure could have prevented an accident. The CAAMS board also worked with officials from the FAA who were specifically assigned to be a liaison with the air medical profession.

In some cases, the accreditation standards exceeded FAA regulations, and in some cases, the regulation was copied into a standard to provide needed emphasis on a particular issue. For example, an FAA regulation is that personnel and passengers must be seat-belted for all takeoffs and landings.[6] However, during site visits, medical personnel would often tell site surveyors that if they were busy with the patient on liftoff or landing, they did not bother with the seatbelts. Indeed, in some of the survivable air medical accidents, several medical attendants received serious back and spinal injuries because they were not secured in their seatbelts on liftoff.

Before the first edition of *Accreditation Standards* was published in 1991, numerous drafts were mailed to organizations and individuals affiliated with the air medical transport profession. CAAMS also held a public hearing at the air medical transport conference in September 1990 in Nashville, Tennessee, to gather opinions and suggestions for the draft of standards that were distributed.

Accreditation standards are revised every 3 years to keep abreast of current practice. The following broad topics included in the Accreditation Standards are each supported by specific criteria (Box 33.1).

Site Surveyors

Several accrediting agencies in related health care fields were willing to share copies of their policies and qualifications for site surveyors when CAAMS was developing its new accrediting agency. One of those organizations, the Commission on Accreditation of Rehabilitation Facilities (CARF), was very generous and allowed the Executive Director of CAAMS to participate in its site surveyor training course. Subsequently, the course developed by the CAAMS Site Surveyor Selection Committee was based on the principles of CARF's program. Originally, in 1991, there were 35 applicants for the 12 site surveyor positions. Applicants were chosen based on the requirements and on their level of experience. Applicants were required to have a minimum of 4 years' experience and a background in two of the four following categories: aviation, communications, medical, and management, with a heavy emphasis on management experience. The first site surveyor training class was held in 1991, with classes repeated every 2 to 3 years to keep up with attrition and site-visit demands.

> **• BOX 33.1   Commission on Accreditation of Medical Transport Systems Accreditation Standards**

General Standards*

Medical Section
Medical Direction and Clinical Supervisor
　　Medical Personnel
　　Staffing
　　Training
Commercial Escorts

Aircraft/Ambulance Section
Medical Configuration
Operational Issues
Aircraft/Ambulance equipment
Communications

Management and Administration Section
Management/Policies
Utilization Review
Quality Management
Infection Control

Rotor-Wing Standards

Certificate of the Aircraft Operator
Weather and Weather Minimums
Pilot Staffing and Training
Maintenance
Helipad and Refueling
Community Outreach

Fixed-Wing Standards

Certificate of the Aircraft Operator
Aircraft

Weather and Weather Minimums

Pilot Staffing and Training
Maintenance
Community Outreach

Ground Interfacility Standards

Vehicles
Driver Qualifications
Maintenance and Sanitation
Mechanic
Policies

*Apply to all modes of transport.

Past and Future Challenges

In 1997, CAAMS changed its name to the Commission on Accreditation of Medical Transport Systems (CAMTS) to capture a wider range of potential applicants and to accommodate the need for standards and accreditation for critical care ground services. Many of these ground mobile intensive care unit (MICU) services consisted of pediatric and neonatal specialty teams, and many were part of an already existing air service. The services needed to be able to have their entire transport program accredited. Although the Commission on Accreditation of Ambulance Services exists for ground emergency services, it does not have standards that specifically address critical care. Therefore CAMTS developed the ground standards (critical care standards were already in place) and began to fill this void in 1997 when it offered accreditation for ground critical care services as well as air medical services. In 2000 CAMTS also included basic life support (BLS) and advanced life support (ALS) ground standards to accommodate the transport services that either provided air or critical care ground services and also provided BLS and ALS ground transport.[2,5]

As mentioned previously, most medical professionals understand accreditation because of exposure to the hospital accrediting agency (the Joint Commission). However, in developing an air medical accreditation process, aviation professionals had to be educated on the purpose and goals of accreditation. Although the aviation component was accustomed to regulations, the aviation professionals were not familiar with accreditation and did not understand the need for yet another process when most believed they were already overregulated by the FAA. The fixed-wing community was particularly baffled. Most fixed-wing transport services were owned and managed by private aviation operators who were totally unfamiliar with the term accreditation. CAAMS worked through the NEMSPA, as one of its member organizations, to try to gain wider acceptance and also developed a formal Aviation Advisory Committee to involve the fixed-wing community, managers from the major EMS Aviation Operators, and the FAA. The purpose of the Aviation and Safety Advisory Committee, which meets annually, is to provide updated information and to provide a forum for gathering input from the aviation professionals.

Another challenge facing the accreditation of air medical programs through CAMTS was the volatile health care market of the 1990s. Hospitals were closing, merging, or buying up other hospitals, and if transport was part of hospital's system, it suddenly needed to show a positive financial outlook or cease to exist, which was quite a turnaround from the 1980s when hospitals did not worry about what the helicopter cost as long as it brought patients into the hospital and was available as a visible marketing tool. Therefore when the focus shifted to the bottom line of the budget, many hospital-based helicopter programs were fighting for survival and had difficulty justifying the cost of accreditation.

Since the year 2000, CAMTS has been meeting the demands of a rapidly changing air medical and ground transport community. A simple one-helicopter program based at one specific hospital is no longer the norm. With private business and aviation companies hiring their own medical teams and outsourcing communication centers, scheduling a site visit has become much more complicated. In many cases, a team of three or more site surveyors is necessary to visit all the satellite bases, maintenance centers, and communication centers that may be a part of a single program.

An increase in the number of applicants for accreditation has also been experienced as state and local EMS agencies move toward requiring CAMTS accreditation. In 2008 nine states (Colorado, Massachusetts, Maryland, Michigan, New Hampshire, New Mexico, Rhode Island, Utah, and Washington) and several county agencies in California and Nevada had regulations that required air medical services to achieve CAMTS accreditation. CAMTS is placed in a potentially litigious position, especially if a medical transport service does not meet the standards and does not receive accreditation. The CAMTS Board of Directors prefers that states provide "deemed status" to CAMTS accredited services for accredited programs that have met or exceeded higher standards than the minimal standards usually required by government agencies. In addition, there are legal challenges to states that require CAMTS accreditation based on the 1978 Airline Deregulation Act.[7] The primary focus was on the competitive market environment for air carriers. To ensure that states would not undo federal deregulation with regulation of their own, Congress included a preemption provision as follows: "A State, political subdivision of a state, or political authority of at least 2 states, may not enact or enforce a law, regulation, or other provision having the force or effect of law related to *price, route, or service* of an air carrier that may provide air transport." Because some of the CAMTS Accreditation Standards exceed Federal Aviation Regulations regarding pilot training and certain operating criteria, such as higher weather minimums, states that require CAMTS accreditation are being challenged in federal court. For this reason, states that previously required CAMTS accreditation are moving away from this requirement in their regulations.

Many services apply for accreditation and reaccreditation not because they are required to do so by state regulations or by contracts but for the obvious benefits of accreditation such as outside auditing, accreditation as a marketing tool, competitive edge, and reimbursement advantages as well as discounted insurance premiums for liability and medical malpractice policies.[8,9]

Many medical transport services also find a number of intangible benefits as a result of going through the accreditation process, such as more cohesive working relationships, team building, a revitalized pride, and professionalism among personnel. Along with these benefits, the program receives a listing of the contingencies or areas that do not meet the intent of the accreditation standards or are not in compliance with the accreditation standards. This list of concerns and deficiencies is used for performance improvement that is reported back to CAMTS in follow-up reports (see Boxes 33.1 and 33-2).

Today, 21 member organizations are involved, with each sending one representative to serve on the board of directors. Board members make all of the accreditation decisions, create and update policies, and revise the Accreditation Standards. In addition to the founding organizations listed earlier, CAMTS is proud to include the following member organizations:

Aerospace Medical Association (AsMA)
Air Medical Operators Association (AMOA)
Air Medical Physicians Association (AMPA)

Air & Surface Transport Nurses Association (ASTNA)

American Academy of Pediatrics (AAP)

American Association of Critical Care Nurses (AACN)

American Association of Respiratory Care (AARC)

American College of Emergency Physicians (ACEP)

American College of Surgeons (ACS)

Association of Air Medical Services (AAMS)

Association of Critical Care Transport (ACCT)

Emergency Nurses Association (ENA)

European HEMS @ Air Ambulance Committee (EHAC)

International Association of Flight & Critical Care Paramedics (IAFCCP)

International Association of Medical Transport Communications Specialist (IAMTCS)

National Air Transportation Association (NATA)

National Association of EMS Physicians (NAEMSP)

National Association of Neonatal Nurses (NANN)

National Association of State EMS Officials (NASEMSO)

National EMS Pilots Associations (NEMSPA)

United States Transportation Command (USTRANSCOM)

In the fall of 2015, CAMTS published its 10th edition of *Accreditation Standards* that reflect changes in current health care and transport practices. This edition also address international medical transport services as appropriate to the country of residence and the specific regulator of that country as referenced by the term "Authority Having Jurisdiction". These standards were in development for 3 years, and various drafts and town hall meetings were held to discuss the changes and suggestions from constituents. Types of care are specifically defined by the qualifications of the medical team along with equipment, medications, interventions, and quality metrics in the 10th edition. Although the Patient Care section of the standards is more specific, the scope of this edition has been broadened to address other modes of medical transport. The term "surface vehicle" used throughout the document refers to vehicles such as ground ambulance, boat, snowmobile, all-terrain vehicle, and so forth being used for patient care and transport. CAMTS also added a category titled "Special Operations." These are services that provide medical care and/or potential medical transport that do not necessarily fit within the previous sections of these standards. Some examples include medical coverage at sporting, concert, or special events; special public safety operations (such as tactical rescue or "SWAT" callouts); and citizen recovery from potentially unstable environments.[9]

In November 2015, CAMTS registered CAMTS EU in Europe and Switzerland. CAMTS EU is a stand-alone nonprofit organization that is based in Switzerland with the same mission, vision, and values as CAMTS. This new organization will provide availability and focus on international policies and practices. CAMTS EU was created to serve constituents outside of North America recognizing not only cultural differences but government restrictions and laws of other countries while maintaining the integrity of the process in the United States and Canada.

Internationally, there is more interest and applications for accreditation and a heightened interest with the CAMTS EU presence. There are three CAMTS-accredited services in the United Kingdom, one in South Africa, and three in Thailand. In addition, CAMTS conducted consults in Europe, Brazil, Saudi Arabia, and the Far East.

CAMTS has trained four European site surveyors and will be adding more international medical transport professionals to the pool of 65 U.S. and Canadian site surveyors. Site surveyors represent all disciplines involved in medical transport so that a site visit is planned with surveyors who have the appropriate experience and background. None of the current site surveyors has less than 10 years' experience in medical transport.

It is the diversity and wealth of experience of the site surveyors and board members that provide CAMTS with the strength and integrity to offer accreditation to medical transport services in North America and abroad and to continually improve medical transport services for patients now and in the future.

Other Accreditation Bodies

CAMTS serves as the primary accreditation body for medical transport systems. However, several other agencies have come into the transport market over the years. These accreditation bodies provide accreditation processes for air or ground or both. Table 33.1 contains examples of some of these other bodies.

TABLE 33.1 Examples of Other Accrediting Bodies for Medical Transport

Association	Accreditation Offered
National Accreditation Alliance Medical Transport Applications	Air and ground transport
Commission on Accreditation on Ambulance Services	Ground transport
European Airmedical Institute (EURAMI)	Air Ambulance accreditation

Summary

Accreditation provides a framework for program evaluation and improvement. It also demonstrates to the public and the patients that a transport program complies with specific standards to ensure safe and competent patient transport.

References

1. Helicopter Association International. *Helicopters 1948–1998: a Contemporary History HAI.* Alexandria, VA: Helicopter Association International; 1998.
2. Duffy M, Joint Commission on Accreditation of Healthcare Organizations. *An Introduction to the Joint Commission: its Survey and Accreditation Processes, Standards, and Services.* Chicago, IL: Joint Commission on Accreditation of Healthcare Organizations; 1988.
3. R Frazer. Air medical accidents: 20-year search for information. *Air Med.* 1999;5(5):34.
4. Samuels D, Bock H, et al. *Air Medical Crew National Standard Curriculum.* Pasadena, CA: ASHBEAMS; 1988.
5. Rhodes M, Perline R, Aronson J, Rappe A. Field triage for on-scene helicopter transport. *J Trauma.* 1986;26(11):963-969.
6. AIM/FAR: *§91,105 Flight Crewmembers at Stations.* Washington, DC: Federal Aviation Administration; 2017.
7. Richardson JG. *Health and Longevity.* Philadelphia, PA: Home Health Society; 1914.
8. Commission on Accreditation of Air Medical Systems. *Accreditation Standards of the Commission on Accreditation of Medical Transport Systems.* 7th ed. Anderson, SC: CAAMS; 2006.
9. Commission on Accreditation of Medical Transport Systems. *2015 Accreditation Standards of the Commission on Accreditation of Medical Transport Systems.* 10th ed. Anderson, SC: CAMTS; 2015.

34

Wellness

JAN L. EICHEL AND RENEÉ SEMONIN HOLLERAN

COMPETENCIES

1. Identify the components of a healthy lifestyle.
2. Describe how to integrate the components of a healthy lifestyle into the transport environment.
3. Identify causes of critical incident stress in the transport environment.
4. Discuss methods to manage critical incident stress in the transport environment.

Introduction

Transport professionals who care for the critically ill may need reminders to care for themselves. This is part of the elusive "work/life balance" for which we strive. As medical professionals, the benefit of a healthy lifestyle is obvious to us. The more difficult task is identifying healthy individual actions and making them a regular habit. It has been said that all who work in emergency medical services (EMS) and medical transport are dealing with sleep deprivation, fatigue, and stress.[1]

Some obstacles to a work/life balance include erratic schedules, availability of healthy foods, poor sleeping conditions while at work, and stressors (both home and work). Lack of preparation may lead to overall poor choices. Considering the attention transport professionals give to clinical preparation, it would seem ironic to have a lack of preparation for self-care. Just as they prepare and check their tools for airway management, they would be well advised to prepare their food, schedules, and other tools to maintain a healthy lifestyle.

Components of a Healthy Lifestyle

A healthy lifestyle is known to mitigate stress. When individuals develop healthy methods of managing stress, these effects can be managed with less detrimental long-term effects. Without balance, stressors become overwhelming and the exhaustion phase may become the norm rather than the anomaly.[2]

Diet

A balanced diet is important to help counteract the effects of stress and to help maintain a healthy body.[3] Caffeine appears to be a favorite among transport professionals; however, caffeine is a strong stimulant that is known to produce a stress reaction on the body. The avoidance of caffeine helps individuals feel more relaxed and helps sleep patterns.[4] Caffeine is found in coffee, tea, soda, and chocolate. If used, it is best consumed before lunch and with a balanced meal. Alternatives to caffeine, such as green or herbal teas, are acceptable and often healthier.[3]

Individuals often use alcohol as a relaxation tool. Alcohol stimulates the secretion of adrenaline and results in nervous tension, irritability, and insomnia, thus increasing stress.[5] Limiting alcohol to a single glass of wine with dinner is a healthier alternative.

Fried foods and high-fat foods depress the immune system. Because stress depresses the immune system, transport professionals should restrict intake of fatty fried foods. A supply of healthy alternatives that can be made readily available, such as granola or high-protein bars, is helpful to avoid unhealthy fast food options.[3]

Whole grains promote the production of serotonin in the body, which increases a sense of well-being. Yellow, green, and leafy vegetables are rich in vitamins and minerals, help boost the production of serotonin, and help boost the immune system, helping to counteract the effects of stress on the body.

Meal regularity, which may favor weight management and metabolic health, is another important aspect of the balanced diet. The meal pattern of three regular meals and two healthy snacks has been shown to stabilize glucose and favor metabolic health.[6] This is an obstacle for the busy transport provider, but with adequate planning and preparation small meals every 4 hours can be achieved.

Caffeine and candy are not the best options when your energy is low and your schedule is busy. The ideal food that will provide lasting drive is one rich in protein, fiber, and complex carbohydrates. Some of the best options for snacks or smart choices for a lunchtime meal that will keep your energy up are shown in Box 34.1.

<table>
<tr><td colspan="2">• BOX 34.1 Foods That Boost Energy</td></tr>
</table>

• BOX 34.1 **Foods That Boost Energy**

One ounce of almonds
Air-popped popcorn
Two tablespoons of peanut butter
Salmon
Bananas
Kale
Oatmeal
Pistachios
Hummus
Six ounces low-fat Greek yogurt

Exercise

Exercise mitigates stress in several ways. Exercising releases endorphins that chemically make an individual feel better. Exercise also stops the production of the chemicals that are produced during the fight-or-flight phase of stress.[5]

Exercise does not have to be extremely strenuous or take a long period of time. Any movement that engages the cardiovascular and musculoskeletal system produces positive effects.[7] Team sports or activities with a partner also add to the benefits of exercise. Walking during a break or using the stairs can accomplish exercise. There are many ways to monitor progress and track goals or create a competitive game out of it. Associated weight loss can also prove beneficial as well as strength-building exercises that improve work performance and reduce the risk of on-the-job injuries.

Laughter

Laughter has been found to be an effective stress management tool.[8] Laughter allows for the release of endorphins that produce feelings of euphoria and relaxation. Laughter has been proven to benefit both neuroendocrine and cardiac systems and has shown improved clinical courses for chronically and acutely ill individuals.[9] Watching a funny movie, visiting a comedy club, or joking with friends can help relieve stress through humor.

Verbalization of Feelings

Individuals often keep feelings of stress internalized for fear of showing weakness or loss of control.[10] When sharing feelings that involve stress, individuals should not minimize their feelings or the feelings of others. Transport professionals should share their concerns with others but must also be willing to seek professional help if these feelings begin to jeopardize their sense of well-being.

Sleep

Although inadequate sleep periods may not solely produce stress among transport professionals, sleep deprivation is associated with increased risk for accident and injury.[11-14]

Disruption in circadian rhythm and shortened sleep cycles have been found to increase stress and increase the risk for injury and accident in transport professionals.

Transport professionals can minimize the effects of shift work by minimizing secondary jobs, maintaining a consistent sleep pattern when not on duty, and avoiding activities that can disrupt sleep patterns (such as alcohol, caffeine, and exposure to electronic screens before sleep).

Preventative Care

Preventative care includes health services like screenings and check-ups. They are used to prevent illnesses, disease, and other health problems, or to detect illness at an early stage when treatment is likely to work best. Transport providers should be offered a medical screening as included in an annual wellness program by the employer. It may include tuberculosis testing, vaccinations, hearing evaluations, screening for depression, and counseling on lifestyle choices such as smoking cessation. If incorporated into the work environment, it becomes part of the culture and may increase compliance.

Immunizations

Included in the risk assessment for the transport provider is the increased exposure to pathogens. Each year the Advisory Committee on Immunization Practices approves immunization schedules recommended for persons living in the United States. It is approved by the American College of Physicians, the American Academy of Family Physicians, the American College of Obstetricians and Gynecologists, and the American College of Nurse-Midwives.[15]

Keeping in mind that recommendations may change, a transport provider may use this guideline for deciding which immunizations would be beneficial, based on risk factors associated with the type of patients they care for and areas of travel, local versus international. For example, in the US 4100 cases of bacterial meningitis occurred each year between 2003 to 2007.[16] Although not as contagious as the common cold, it can be transmitted through saliva and occasionally through close, prolonged general contact with an infected person (i.e., the transport environment). There are currently vaccines available for three types of bacteria that can cause meningitis[16]:

- *Neisseria meningitidis*
- *Streptococcus pneumoniae*
- *Haemophilus influenzae* type b (Hib)

Evaluation of your scope of service and risk of exposure should be part of your risk assessment for all vaccinations.

Stress in Transport Medicine

The transport environment and the nature of the industry expose transport professionals to frequent stress in both their professional and personal lives. The challenges of transport expose these individuals to stress not commonly addressed by other professions. Continual changes in health care and clinical services provide a tumultuous arena for the provision of care.

In addition to outside stressors, there are many directly encountered during the physical transport. Stressors of transport include hypoxia, barometric pressure changes, thermal changes, decreased humidity, vibration, noise, fatigue, and gravitational forces. These physiologic stresses are discussed in depth in Chapter 4.

Rules and laws govern transport programs and undoubtedly add to the transport provider's stress as well. It is a challenge to balance the desire for safety and the patient's need for rapid transport.

Sometimes stress in the transport environment can be good. For instance, it can help one develop skills needed to manage potentially threatening situations. However, stress can be harmful when it is severe enough to become overwhelming and may lead to a loss of control.

Strong emotions like fear, sadness, or other symptoms of depression are normal, as long as they are temporary and do not interfere with daily activities. If these emotions last too long or cause other problems, then it is a different story.

Physical or emotional tension are very often signs of stress. They may be the reaction to a situation that causes anxiety or feelings of being threatened. Stress can be positive and lead to learning new skills as a team or negative such as when dealing with the effects of a natural disaster. Symptoms of stress are included in Box 34.2.

It is difficult to summarize how to mitigate stress in a few paragraphs. Much research has been done and professional help is available in many forms including Employee Assistance Programs, Community Mental Health Centers, or practitioners in private practice. Feeling emotional, nervous, or having trouble sleeping can be a normal reaction to stress. Having a healthy lifestyle and getting the right support can put experiences and problems in perspective. Stressful feelings should lessen in a few days or weeks. Some

---

> **• BOX 34.2** **Symptoms of Stress**
>
> Common reactions to a stressful event include the following:
> - Disbelief and shock
> - Tension and irritability
> - Fear and anxiety about the future
> - Difficulty making decisions
> - Being numb to one's feelings
> - Loss of interest in normal activities
> - Loss of appetite
> - Nightmares and recurring thoughts about the event
> - Anger
> - Increased use of alcohol and drugs
> - Sadness and other symptoms of depression
> - Feeling powerless
> - Crying
> - Sleep problems
> - Headaches, back pains, and stomach problems
> - Trouble concentrating

> **• Box 34.3** **Tips to Feel Better**
>
> - Eat healthy, well-balanced meals.
> - Exercise on a regular basis.
> - Get plenty of sleep.
> - Give yourself a break if you feel stressed out.
> - Talk to others. Share your problems and how you are feeling and coping with a parent, friend, counselor, doctor, or pastor.
> - Avoid drugs and alcohol. Drugs and alcohol may seem to help with the stress. In the long run, they create additional problems and increase the stress you are already feeling.
> - Take a break. If your stress is caused by a national or local event, take breaks from listening to the news stories, which can increase your stress.
> - *Recognize when you need more help.* If problems continue or you are thinking about suicide, talk to a psychologist, social worker, or professional counselor.

---

tips for beginning to feel better are in Box 34.3.[9] *Recognize when you need more help.* If problems continue or you are thinking about suicide, talk to a psychologist, social worker, or professional counselor.

Critical Incident Stress

Critical incident stress (CIS) can occur with one specific incident or situation. Critical incidents usually involve a perceived threat to a person physically or the physical health of others. Critical incidents are determined by the effect on a person's sense of safety and security and "competency in the world."[5]

There is no shortage of CIS in EMS. The comradery that supports emergency personnel also makes them feel a loss that much more. Examples of personal CIS include line-of-duty deaths among EMS or law enforcement personnel, assaults, sexual abuse, child abuse, suicide, attempted suicide, or unexpected death of a loved one. Global critical incidents include acts of terrorism, natural disasters, mass casualty homicides, or responding to mass casualty events. It has been noted that the more media attention given to the event the greater the risk of CIS.[5,17]

The most common symptoms of CIS that occur among transport professionals include anxiety and fear for personal safety.

Critical Incident Stress Management

Critical incident stress management (CISM) is an interventional protocol designed to help deal with major traumatic events.[5] CISM is highly structured and requires specific standardized training for individuals involved in the processes after a major event. The seven components to CISM are preincident education, individual crisis or peer support, demobilization, defusing, debriefing, family support, and referral services. Grief and loss sessions are included when deaths are involved.

Grief and loss sessions are provided after the death of an individual involved in a critical incident. These sessions help those involved to work through the grief process and deal with the sense of loss involved in the critical incident.[5]

Crisis management briefings are used to keep participants informed "before, during and after crisis to present facts, facilitate a brief, controlled discussion" and provide information about the critical incident. These briefings may be adjusted as information about the critical incident changes.[5]

Resources are available for the management of the stress, which is an integral part of patient transport. Some of these resources are noted in Box 34-4.

Summary

Wellness may be the most elusive portion of your career. The transport provider is often the self-motivated, diligent, and perseverant type. They are accustomed to achieving a goal by overcoming ever-changing obstacles. While we care for our patients, it is important to care for ourselves as well. Small steps on a day-to-day basis, may help lead to a long, healthy life and rewarding career.

References

1. Overton JW, Shiparski L, Authier PD. Individual Provider Wellness and Self-care. In: Overton J, Frazer E, eds. *Safety and Quality in Medial Transport Systems: Creating an Effective Culture.* Burlington, VT: Ashgate Publishing Co; 2012:235-251.

2. Kaye B, Jordan-Evans S. *Love'em or Lose'em.* San Francisco, CA: Berrett-Koehler; 1999.

3. Blackwood A. Food + stress. body + soul. 2007;24(20):64.

4. Goudreau J, Edmondson G, Conlin M. Dispatches from the war on stress. *Bus Week.* 2007;4045:74.

5. Mitchell J. *Critical Incident Stress Debriefing* (CISD). http://www.info-trauma.org/flash/media-f/mitchellCriticalIncidentStressDebriefing.pdf. Accessed 29.04.17.

6. Alhussain M, Macdonald I, Taylor M. Irregular meal-pattern effects on energy expenditure, metabolism, and appetite regulation: a randomized controlled trial in healthy normal-weight women. *Am J Clin Nutr.* 104(1):21-32.

7. Johnson TD. Address your stress, for a healthier life. *Nations Health.* 2008;38(3):24.

8. Alessia K. Stop stressing and start relishing life. *Nat Health Vegetarian Life.* Autumn 2008;46.

9. Sahakian A, Frishman WH. Humor and the cardiovascular system. *Altern Ther Health Med.* 2007;13(4):56-58.

10. North C, Wraa C. *Stress: Taming Your Shadow 2000.* Critical Care Transport Medicine Conference; April 18, 2000.

11. Frakes MA, Kelly JG. Shift length and on-duty rest patterns in rotor-wing air medical programs. *Air Med J.* 2004;23(6):34-39.

12. Frakes MA, Kelly JG. Off-duty preparation for overnight work in rotor wing air medical programs. *Air Med J.* 2005;24(5):215-217.

13. Frakes MA, Kelly JG. Sleep debt and outside employment patterns in helicopter air medical staff working 24-hour shifts. *Air Med J.* 2007;26(1):45-49.

14. Thomas F, Hopkins RO, Handrahan DL, et al. Sleep and cognitive performance of flight nurses after 12-hour evening versus 18-hour shifts. *Air Med J.* 2006;25(5):216-225.

15. Advisory Committee on Immunization Practices, Centers for Disease Control and Prevention. Available at http://www.cdc.gov/vaccines/acip/index.html. Accessed 04.06.16.

16. Centers for Disease Control and Prevention. *Bacterial Meningitis.* Available at http://www.cdc.gov/meningitis/bacterial.html. Accessed 04.06.16.

17. Battles ED. An exploration of post-traumatic stress disorder in emergency nurses following Hurricane Katrina. *J Emerg Nurs.* 2007;33(4):314-318.

Appendix A

Post-Accident Resource Document

Introduction

Air medical transport services provide an essential life-saving function in the healthcare and aviation systems. These services are generally high profile in nature and attract positive attention from the media. Although air medical crashes are rare, when they occur, they instantly become an intensely emotional event.

This document describes the various phenomena experienced by members of an air medical program after an aircraft incident. Its intended purposes are to assist air medical program leaders in progressing through the necessary critical functions necessary after a crash and to address the short-term and long-term issues and decisions.

Phase I: The First Few Hours: Initial Shock and Reaction

When an air medical crash occurs, the timeliness and quality of information conveyed may vary depending on the circumstances. Notification of the crash may come to the communications center via scene witnesses (e.g., emergency medical services [EMS], police, fire, and bystanders) or from the media. Rotor-wing crashes, which likely occur during takeoff or landing, usually are a witnessed event, whereas a fixed-wing crash may occur in a rural area far from the program's base of operation. With the advent of scanners, alpha-numeric paging systems, and media access to crash information, flight team members may receive information directly before official notification from a program representative.

Post-Accident Incident Plan

The program's post-accident incident plan (PAIP) becomes the road map for the communications center staff to initiate the necessary critical steps that enhance crew survival and limit the program's liability. Priorities are:
- Verification of facts: crash location, other pertinent details.
- Dispatch of rescue crews: civil air patrol, air medical, or ambulance response to the crash site.
- Activation of notification list according to the PAIP.
- Notification of security for crowd control at the base of operation or hospital.

Role of Program Leadership

The air medical program administrator's role involves developing organization around the process, ensuring that the PAIP is followed, and ensuring that appropriate roles are assigned. Provision of medical care to the victims of the crash, both air medical crew members and others involved in the crash, should be a high priority. The program leader should also ensure that the appropriate notifications are made to administration, the public relations director, the Part 135 operator (aviation site manager or lead pilot), and regulatory agencies such as the National Transportation Safety Board (NTSB), Federal Aviation Administration (FAA), and state health department. Flight team members must be notified of the event and directed to come to the program site where resources are available and factual information can be shared.

Family Member Notification

As the person in charge, the program leader must ensure that family members of the onboard crew are notified. Ideally, this notification should occur in person. The program leader should send a responsible person to the location of the family members whenever feasible. Often, the media broadcast the information regarding the crash before notification of the family can occur. Minimally, this notification should occur via phone. A private area at the facility, but away from the flight team, should be identified for the family members to gather. An individual should be assigned to provide factual information and to meet the needs of the family members. The program leader should communicate facts only, not speculate.

In the first few hours, a critical incident stress-diffusing session needs to be organized. An agency of choice is identified to conduct this session, and as many crew members as possible should be present.

Dealing With the Media

An appropriate individual must be assigned to deal with the media. The media should have a place to convene away from the crash site or the flight team. A proactive approach to information sharing helps to limit speculation on the part of the media. When possible, one of the program leaders should be designated as a liaison for information sharing with the public relations official.

Decision to Remain in Service

A decision to remain in service may need to be addressed quickly if the program operates multiple aircraft. The program administrator needs to quickly assess whether continued service is appropriate depending on the flight team members' readiness to respond to a request for service. Such a decision should put safety first, keeping in mind that the profound effects on the air medical crew may minimize their effectiveness in providing patient care and in paying attention to safety principles for anywhere from hours to days after a crash. Flight team members need time to seek information and process the events and results of the crash.

During this period, the availability of other air medical transport programs in the area should be considered. If possible, their communications centers are notified of the program's situation and informed that flight requests may be referred to their programs.

The program leader should also identify the scene coordinator, someone from the aviation team (pilot or mechanic) who should be assigned to coordinate activities at the crash site. The role of this individual is to coordinate the efforts of the various investigating agencies and to provide information to these agencies and the program administrator. This individual also is the liaison to the Part 135 operator.

Critical Incident Stress Management

An air medical crash invokes a critical incident stress (CIS) response for many individuals both inside and outside of the program. Therefore, the program leadership must recognize that psychologic assistance in dealing with the stress response and grieving process should be a required step for all members of the air medical team. Details about the assistance (who provides it, how it is provided, and who participates) should be identified in the post-accident incident planning process. Because individuals may not be able to adequately assess their own level of stress response, mandatory participation in the critical incident stress management (CISM) session is beneficial.

The mental health professionals involved in the CIS response can provide crucial assistance in assessment of individual readiness for return to flight. This assessment of all team members, including the program leader, is a crucial component of any PAIP and provides the information needed to determine the right time to return the program to service.

Despite CISM interventions and readiness assessments, air medical team members may experience a wide variety of post-stress phenomenon, such as hypervigilance (e.g., obsession over the sighting of wires in and around the landing zone) or flashbacks (e.g., triggered by a nighttime flight with circumstances similar to the crash). Such phenomena may limit a team member's ability to perform his or her role. Strategies such as doubling up flight team members or adding flight team members on board as staffing and aircraft configurations allow can be helpful as individuals return to perform their role on the aircraft after any critical incident.

Anger is an emotion commonly experienced by flight team members as a normal reaction to catastrophic loss and post-traumatic stress. Although individuals need to work through their anger, if misdirected, this anger may be destructive to the rebuilding process. One-on-one counseling may be necessary to address individual stress reactions to an event.

After a crash, team members are likely to continue in their role as members of the air medical team. This involvement provides an opportunity to experience regular acknowledgment and support from coworkers who can directly relate to their feelings. Commonly, some staff resign 6 to 12 months after a crash. The number of staff resigning is based on numerous factors, such as support both in and outside of work and individual ability to cope with the work-related tragedy.

Phase II: The First 24 Hours: Initial Development of a Plan

The decision regarding the continuation of the air medical service is likely to occur in the first 24 hours and is often the ultimate test of the agency's support of the air medical program. If this decision is not addressed in the first few hours, this may become an essential decision to make and communicate to customers. The media can be a good source of distributing this information. Emergency medical services (EMS), public service groups, and communications centers should be notified of the return to service.

Management of the Media

Any positive relations developed with the media may pay off as the intense news coverage occurs. Regular news conferences and flight team interviews should be conducted as appropriate. The public needs to know that the flight team can go on and that the program will continue. Providing the human side of this situation to the media may cause a switch in focus from the negative aspects of the event. The local media (television and print) are likely to cover this topic daily for several days to weeks. Flight program staff need to expect this so that they are not overwhelmed by the amount of media coverage.

Interaction With Family Members

Interactions with family members of the crash victims should be planned. Program administration needs to contact family members to express concern and to determine whether their needs are being met.

Family members of the air medical team may want to participate in a debriefing. The CISM team may be appropriate for this activity and the staff debriefing. In addition, family members may benefit from meeting with one of the program's pilots and representatives from administration. Their need for information is heightened, especially with regard to program safety. Meeting the needs of team members' families goes a long way in gaining the individual support necessary for return to work in the flight program.

Keeping Leadership Informed

Daily briefings to the CEO, Board of Directors, and line managers should be provided. The program leadership may have difficulty with use of objective decision-making skills during the crisis. The objectiveness of second-order people can assist with this and validation of decision making.

Communication With the Air Medical Team

Updated information from administration, planned CISM interventions, interaction with media, and successes (e.g., positive encounters and support from peers or customers) should be provided. Regular staff meetings and ongoing CISM interventions, such as diffusing, debriefings, one-on-ones, and further individual counseling sessions, may be needed on a daily basis for the first week or two. This time is an opportunity to share information, common feelings, and experiences.

Neighboring air medical programs and the Concern Network should be contacted, if this has not already occurred. The industry recognition and support that results may be beneficial to the staff and program leadership.

Legal Issues

The legal consequences of a crash quickly become apparent. Attorneys, risk managers, and the insurance carrier should be notified as early as possible. Leadership should be prepared to share the PAIP and steps taken to mitigate the event.

Phase III: Days 2 to 5: Implementation and Modification

During this phase, many of the realities of the crash become evident. The agencies that surround the program need to get back to business, whereas the air medical team members and leadership may continue to experience difficulty in coping with daily encounters and tasks.

Care of the Injured Victims

In the case of crash survivors, care of the injured crew members may necessitate special attention to confidentiality issues, especially if the care takes place at the program's base hospital or trauma center. Flight team members commonly make regular visits to an injured flight team member. Their preoccupation with the injured team member's medical condition and concern for family members may delay the individual's return to flying.

Human Resources

The human resources department staff is essential in assisting with the processing of forms for injured and deceased employees. The staff may be able to contact the hospital chaplain to coordinate support for the rest of the hospital staff or agency employees.

Replacement of the Aircraft

Plans to replace the aircraft should be underway with a plan for return to service. It is helpful to the flight team to know the plan for going back into service. All equipment on board the aircraft needs to be replaced. Use of the equipment list should ease the process of identification of capital purchases required. When possible, an individual in the purchasing department should be designated to handle the process of timely equipment replacement. Equipment vendors may be able to provide loaner units to facilitate getting the aircraft back into service in a timely manner.

Identification of the tail number for the replacement aircraft may become a sensitive issue for flight team members. Retiring the tail number of the crash vehicle and starting again is often wise. Flight teams may have a useful role in tail number selection. Several tasks appropriate to delegate to the flight team are symbolic of the program moving forward, such as ordering and restocking the replacement aircraft. Opportunities to empower the staff with appropriate decisions may provide a mechanism to move beyond the immediate crisis.

Psychologic Support for Staff

Ongoing assessment of team readiness to return to work and available ongoing psychologic support are necessary to plan and communicate need. Staff must understand the necessity of ongoing psychologic care, especially if individuals are not coping effectively with the stress. Inappropriate group dynamics may become evident as a coping mechanism, necessitating an intervention for the entire group.

Funeral Planning

Death in the line of duty often translates to a public funeral, a ritual observed by firefighters, EMS personnel, and police officers. The EMS community is likely to communicate this expectation early. Often, the outpouring of expected involvement cannot be contained and may result in a public funeral. In many cases, the next of kin of the deceased may need to be convinced that a public funeral is in order. A trusted member of the EMS community who has experience in planning a public funeral (e.g., a member of a local fire department) should be identified. This person may be invaluable in planning with the family and program leadership an otherwise overwhelming event. Religious officials need to be involved in the planning along with the family so that the funeral plans are culturally sensitive to meet the needs of the family (e.g., Native American burial practices) and those of the community at large.

In addition, regular meetings with the designated individuals planning the public funeral are necessary to ensure that the air medical program and staff needs are met. Municipal and state police involvement may be necessary to ensure that a processional of rescue vehicles can occur.

The air medical service leadership should consider taking the flight teams out of service to allow attendance at the funerals because participation in this ritual is an essential part of the healing process. Once again, neighboring flight programs can be called to cover air medical transport requests. Several hours of down time after each funeral may be needed before team members can return to service.

Memorial Services

Memorial services may occur in addition to the public funeral. The CISM team and mental health workers can give advice regarding the appropriate timing for the memorial service. The service should provide an opportunity for team members to share personal remarks and eulogies. This service can provide a sense of closure for some team members and an opportunity to move forward in the recovery process.

Participation in the funeral and memorial service is essential for all flight program staff. The aircraft may be taken out of service for this time, and coverage by other air medical services may be requested. A neighboring air medical service can be asked to reposition aircraft to better cover the region, which reduces the chance of air medical team members missing the service and conveys to the community the program's commitment to provide service.

Request for Memorials

Individuals or groups in the community may find a need to memorialize the aircraft crash site and deceased crew members. These issues may raise sensitivities with family members and the flight team, especially if suggestions are not consistent with the wishes of the family or flight team. Decisions dealing with these requests can be distracting and time consuming. Keep in mind that these issues do not need to be dealt with right now. An urgent decision is rarely necessary. In many cases, delegating this responsibility to the public relations department may be appropriate.

Delayed Issues

Formal Investigation

As the formal investigation continues, announcements of findings should be shared with key personnel in a timely manner. The program leader may need to adopt a strategy to relay information to air medical teams before media reports. Ongoing regular meetings with the staff may be beneficial.

Evaluate Program Safety

A plan to evaluate the program's safety program should include a review of:
- Safety and operational policies and procedures.
- Safety education for staff.
- Quality and effectiveness of crew resource management (CRM) training.
- Community outreach safety education.
- Quality of the program's safety culture.

Review of these processes is a necessary step in providing reassurance for all members of the air medical team, administration, and risk management offices, with respect to the program's commitment to safety. A plan to evaluate safety helps to avoid the pitfall of reacting to requests based on stress and emotion rather than methodology. The flight team, operator, and administration should be involved. The effectiveness of the PAIP is evaluated and revised as necessary. An independent safety audit may be the choice to ensure objectivity. A timetable for implementation of recommendations should be developed.

Legal Issues

We exist in a litigious society, and the number and nature of suits filed may be surprising. The news of such suits may become a significant distraction to the air medical teams as they work to reenter the flight environment. Some issues to keep in mind are:
- Insurance subrogation, the legal doctrine of substituting one creditor for another, can lead to litigation involving customers, which could become an image problem for the program if the insurance provider sues the customer in the name of the operator or aircraft owner. Working closely with the legal department to support and reassure customers may be essential to preserve a positive working relationship.
- Filing deadlines and statutes of limitations should be anticipated so that the flight team and public relations director can be prepared to manage the media. Often, announcements of lawsuit filings appear in the press. Knowledge of lawsuits may generate a negative emotional response by air medical teams. Because safety policy, procedures, and communications logs are likely to be subpoenaed, such documents may be archived as manuals are updated.

Final Outcome of Lawsuits

Several years are often necessary to settle lawsuits that result from an air medical crash. This possibly may be reported in the media. A relationship should be developed with legal counsel regarding their commitment to communication with the program when legal activity is likely to attract the media's interest. Keeping flight teams informed is essential.

Emotional Support for Program Leadership

To perform in the midst of an overwhelmingly emotional event, the leader may deny his or her own feelings of fear, grief, and anger to move the program forward. Although this denial may be necessary initially, if this process goes on for too long, the program may move on and leave the program leadership emotionally destitute and dysfunctional. Program managers must set aside some time to go through a formal grieving process and recognition of the intense impact the event has on them. Professional counseling is needed for all individuals involved. Without this assistance, inappropriate methods of dealing with the stress may eventually impair the long-term effectiveness of the manager. The help of a professional counselor should be sought in a confidential setting, preferably away from the work environment. Time away from work with family and friends needs to be planned.

Anniversaries

The anniversary of a crash is a time of special recognition for the team and family members. The program leader should be prepared to deal with special requests for time off and recognize that the staff may need to be together. A meeting of the staff with an opportunity to talk about feelings may be beneficial and should be offered to the flight team. Mental health workers should be available if team members need to speak in confidence about their feelings around the anniversary.

Each anniversary is acknowledged in various ways by the staff. If the psychologic needs of the staff and program leadership are regarded as a high priority, it is easier to deal with each anniversary.

Bibliography

Dodd R. Factors related to occupant crash survival in emergency medical services helicopters. *Aviat Sci Technol.* 1992.

Hawkins M. Personal protective equipment in helicopter EMS. *Air Med J.* 1994;4(94):123-126.

Low R, Sousa J, Dufresne D, et al. *IFR Capability Lowers Accident Rates of Civilian Helicopter Ambulances: A Multifactorial Epidemiologic Study.* Greenville, NC: East Carolina University School of Medicine; 1997.

Mitchell J, Bray G. *Emergency Services Stress: Guidelines for Preserving the Health and Careers of Emergency Personnel.* Englewood Cliffs, NJ: Prentice-Hall; 1990.

Mitchell J, Everly G. *Critical Incident Stress Debriefing: An Operations Manual for the Prevention of Traumatic Stress Among Emergency Services and Disaster Workers.* 2nd ed. Ellicott City, MD: Chevron; 1996.

National Transportation Safety Board (NTSB). *Safety Study, Commercial Emergency Medical Service Helicopter Operations, Report Number NTSB/SS-88/01. NTSB.* Washington, DC: NTSB; 1988.

Schneider C. Dollars and sense. *Air Med.* 1997;21(4).

POST-CRASH ADMINISTRATIVE CHECK LIST

Action Steps	Completion Date/Time	Comments
I. First 2 Hours		
A. Activate PAIP.		
1. Emergency/medical response to crash site.		
2. Complete notification list.		
3. Decide whether to remain in service (multiple aircraft).		
4. Identify and activate:		
a. Scene coordinator.		
b. Base site coordinator.		
c. Accident investigation team.		
5. Identify a coordinator for the media.		
6. Convene flight team members.		
a. Provide updated information.		
b. Plan for initial CISM intervention.		
c. State expectation for ongoing CISM interventions.		
B. Notify family members, in person as applicable.		
C. Ensure that various coordinators have a checklist.		
II. First 24 Hours		
A. Liaison with public relations regarding managing the media.		
B. Interact with family members.		
C. Develop a plan to address flight team family member needs and CISM intervention.		
D. Inform leadership of plan.		
E. Schedule a meeting with air medical team for information sharing and CISM.		
F. Notify attorneys, risk managers, and insurance carrier.		
III. First 2 to 5 Days		
A. Notify Human Resources, employee benefits, employment status, agency support.		
B. Develop and communicate plan for aircraft replacement.		
C. Develop and implement a plan for ongoing psychologic support for staff.		
D. Designate an individual to plan a public funeral as indicated.		
E. Designate individual to plan memorial service.		
F. Identify a contact person to deal with requests for memorials.		
IV. Delayed Issues: 5 Days to 2 Weeks and Beyond		
A. Formal investigation: communicate initial findings.		
B. Evaluate program safety.		
C. Keep track of legal issues and communicate to staff:		
1. Insurance subrogation.		
2. Filing deadlines/statute of limitations.		
3. Final outcome of lawsuits.		
D. Provide emotional support for program leadership. If not already done, it is time to make a plan.		
E. Anniversaries: plan meetings with staff and honor requests for time off.		

Add items to checklist as necessary.

Index

Printed and bound by CPI Group (UK) Ltd, Croydon, CR0 4YY

08/05/2025

01864689-0001